HEAD AND NECK

Grabb's Encyclopedia of Flaps

THIRD EDITION

Volume I

HEAD AND NECK

Grabb's Encyclopedia of Flaps

THIRD EDITION

Editors

Berish Strauch, MD
Professor of Plastic Surgery
Albert Einstein College of Medicine
Bronx, New York

Luis O. Vasconez, MD
Professor of Surgery and Director
Division of Plastic Surgery
University of Alabama Medical Center, Birmingham
Chief Plastic Surgeon
University of Alabama Hospital
Birmingham, Alabama

Elizabeth J. Hall-Findlay, MD
Plastic Surgeon
Banff Mineral Springs Hospital
Banff, Alberta, Canada

Bernard T. Lee, MD
Instructor in Surgery
Harvard Medical School
Division of Plastic and Reconstructive Surgery
Beth Israel Deaconess Medical Center
Boston, Massachusetts

Wolters Kluwer | Lippincott Williams & Wilkins
Health
Philadelphia • Baltimore • New York • London
Buenos Aires • Hong Kong • Sydney • Tokyo

Acquisitions Editor: Brian Brown
Managing Editor: Michelle La Plante
Marketing Manager: Lisa Parry
Project Manager: Bridgett Dougherty
Senior Manufacturing Manager: Benjamin Rivera
Creative Director: Doug Smock
Production Service: Nesbitt Graphics, Inc.

© 2009 by LIPPINCOTT WILLIAMS & WILKINS, a WOLTERS KLUWER business
530 Walnut Street
Philadelphia, PA 19106 USA
LWW.com

Library of Congress Cataloging-in-Publication Data

Grabb's encyclopedia of flaps / editors, Berish Strauch ... [et al.]. -- 3rd ed.
    p. ; cm.
Includes bibliographical references and index.
ISBN 978-0-7817-6432-2
ISBN 978-0-7817-6600-5
1. Flaps (Surgery) I. Grabb, William C. II. Strauch, Berish, 1933- III.
Title: Encyclopedia of flaps.
[DNLM: 1. Surgical Flaps. 2. Reconstructive Surgical Procedures. WO 610G727 2009]
RD120.8.G78 2009
617.9'5--dc22

                                                    2008024234

Care has been taken to confirm the accuracy of the information presented and to describe generally accepted practices. However, the authors, editors, and publisher are not responsible for errors or omissions or for any consequences from application of the information in this book and make no warranty, expressed or implied, with respect to the currency, completeness, or accuracy of the contents of the publication. Application of the information in a particular situation remains the professional responsibility of the practitioner.

The authors, editors, and publisher have exerted every effort to ensure that drug selection and dosage set forth in this text are in accordance with current recommendations and practice at the time of publication. However, in view of ongoing research, changes in government regulations, and the constant flow of information relating to drug therapy and drug reactions, the reader is urged to check the package insert for each drug for any change in indications and dosage and for added warnings and precautions. This is particularly important when the recommended agent is a new or infrequently employed drug.

Some drugs and medical devices presented in the publication have Food and Drug Administration (FDA) clearance for limited use in restricted research settings. It is the responsibility of the health care provider to ascertain the FDA status of each drug or device planned for use in their clinical practice.

To purchase additional copies of this book, call our customer service department at (800) 638-3030 or fax orders to (301) 223-2320. International customers should call (301) 223-2300.

Visit Lippincott Williams & Wilkins on the Internet: at LWW.com. Lippincott Williams & Wilkins customer service representatives are available from 8:30 am to 6 pm, EST.

10 9 8 7 6 5 4 3 2 1

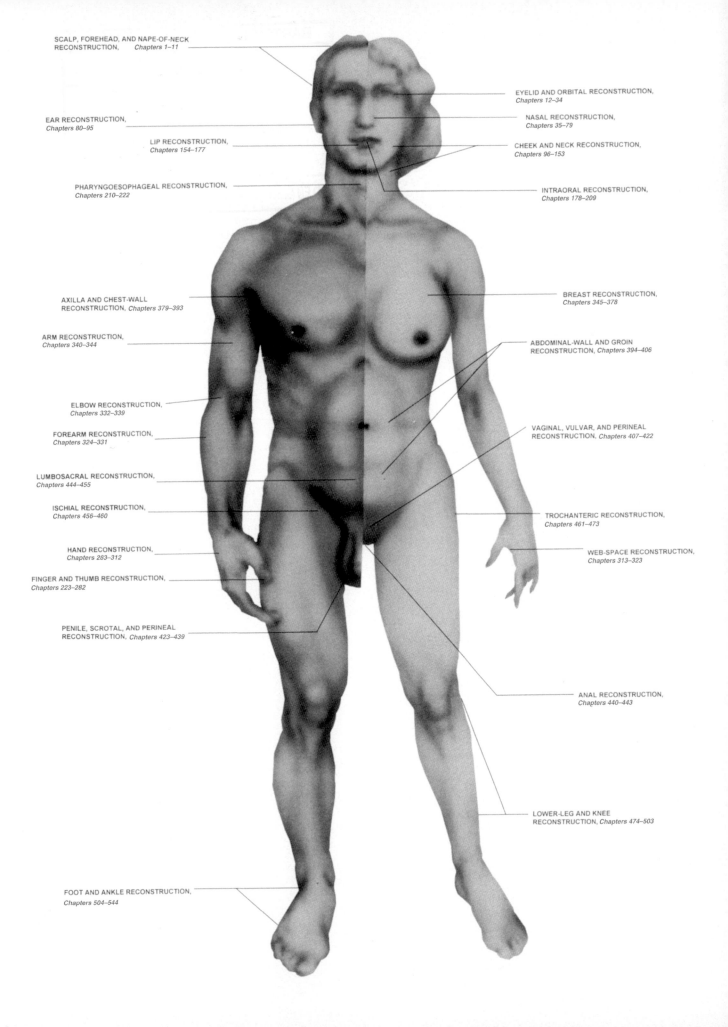

SCALP, FOREHEAD, AND NAPE-OF-NECK RECONSTRUCTION, *Chapters 1–11*

EYELID AND ORBITAL RECONSTRUCTION, *Chapters 12–34*

EAR RECONSTRUCTION, *Chapters 80–95*

NASAL RECONSTRUCTION, *Chapters 35–79*

LIP RECONSTRUCTION, *Chapters 154–177*

CHEEK AND NECK RECONSTRUCTION, *Chapters 96–153*

PHARYNGOESOPHAGEAL RECONSTRUCTION, *Chapters 210–222*

INTRAORAL RECONSTRUCTION, *Chapters 178–209*

AXILLA AND CHEST-WALL RECONSTRUCTION, *Chapters 379–393*

BREAST RECONSTRUCTION, *Chapters 345–378*

ARM RECONSTRUCTION, *Chapters 340–344*

ABDOMINAL-WALL AND GROIN RECONSTRUCTION, *Chapters 394–406*

ELBOW RECONSTRUCTION, *Chapters 332–339*

FOREARM RECONSTRUCTION, *Chapters 324–331*

VAGINAL, VULVAR, AND PERINEAL RECONSTRUCTION, *Chapters 407–422*

LUMBOSACRAL RECONSTRUCTION, *Chapters 444–455*

ISCHIAL RECONSTRUCTION, *Chapters 456–460*

TROCHANTERIC RECONSTRUCTION, *Chapters 461–473*

HAND RECONSTRUCTION, *Chapters 283–312*

WEB-SPACE RECONSTRUCTION, *Chapters 313–323*

FINGER AND THUMB RECONSTRUCTION, *Chapters 223–282*

PENILE, SCROTAL, AND PERINEAL RECONSTRUCTION, *Chapters 423–439*

ANAL RECONSTRUCTION, *Chapters 440–443*

LOWER-LEG AND KNEE RECONSTRUCTION, *Chapters 474–503*

FOOT AND ANKLE RECONSTRUCTION, *Chapters 504–544*

To my wife, and children, and especially to my grandchildren, David Michael,
Kimberly Ann, Carolyn Beth, Alexandra Rae, and Matthew Jost.

BERISH STRAUCH, MD

To my wife, Diane, my daughters, Cristina, Nessa and Rachel, and to
my grandchildren, Francesca and Elisa, for their continued support
and joy they have given me throughout the years.

LUIS VASCONEZ, MD

To my mother, Betty Hall, who has been an inspiration to all her children;
and to my own three children, Jamie, David and Elise,
who have become very enjoyable young adults.

ELIZABETH J. HALL-FINDLAY, MD

To my wife, Britt, for her unwavering love, support, and sacrifice.
I am truly fortunate to be married to such an amazing woman.
To my sons, Brodie and Teddy, for the never-ending joy they bring.
Finally, to my parents, who share a contagious thirst for knowledge.

BERNARD T. LEE, MD

D. L. Abramson, MD
42A East 74th Street,
New York, New York 10021

W. P. Adams, Jr., MD
Children's Medical Center
Parkland Memorial Hospital
Veteran's Administration Medical Center
Zale Lipshy University Hospital
Baylor Medical Center
5323 Harry Hines Boulevard
Dallas, Texas 75235-9132

J. E. Adamson, MD, FACS (Retired)
P. O. Box 695
Linville, North Carolina 28646

J. Aftimos, MD
Centre Hospitalier D'Agen
Rue des Héros de la Résistance
F-47000 Agen, France

Galip Agaoglu, MD
Department of Plastic Surgery
The Cleveland Clinic Foundation
Cleveland, Ohio

F. C. Akpuaka, MBBS (Ibadan), FRCS (Ed), FRCS (Glasgow), FWACS, FICS
Professor of Plastic Surgery, College of Medicine, Abia State
University, Uturu, Nigeria
Director of Plastic Surgery
Plastic Surgery Unit
St. Francis Hospital
2 Richard Street
Asata-Enugu, Nigeria

R. S. Ali, MD
Department of Plastic and Reconstructive Surgery
Castle Hill Hospital
Castle Road
Cottingham, United Kingdom

R. J. Allen, MD
Division of Plastic Surgery
Medical University of South Carolina
Charleston, South Carolina

E. C. Almaguer, MD
Chief of Plastic Surgery, Santa Rosa Medical Center,
San Antonio
Baptist Hospital System
343 West Houston, #211
San Antonio, Texas 78205

C. Angrigiani
Posadas 1528 PB
Buenos Aires
Argentina

P. Andrades, MD
Assistant Professor
Division of Plastic Surgery and
Division of Maxillofacial Surgery
University of Chile Clinical Hospital
Hospital del Trabajador
Santiago, Chile

N. H. Antia, FRCSEng, FACSHon (Deceased)

S. Arena, MD (Retired)
125 Greenwood Road
Fox Chapel
Pittsburgh, Pennsylvania 15238

R. V. Argamaso, MD, FACS (Deceased)

L. C. Argenta, MD
North Carolina Baptist Hospital
Bowman-Gray Plastic Surgery
Medical Center Boulevard
Winston-Salem, North Carolina 27157

S. Ariyan, FACS
Yale-New Haven Hospital
Connecticut Center for Plastic Surgery
60 Temple Street, Suite 7C
New Haven, Connecticut 06510

D. P. Armstrong, MD, FACS
Community Memorial Hospital of San Buenaventura
Clinical Faculty, UCLA, Division of Plastic Surgery
168 North Brent Street, Suite 403
Ventura, California 93003

C. Arrunátegui, MD
Department of Plastic Surgery
Hospital da Santa Casa de Misericordia
Belo Horizonte, Brazil

H. Asato, MD
Assistant Professor
Department of Plastic and Reconstructive Surgery
University of Tokyo Hospital
7–3-1 Hongo Bunkyo-ku
Tokyo 113, Japan

E. Atasoy, MD
University of Louisville
Christine M. Kleinert Institute for Hand and Microsurgery
225 Abraham Flexner Way, Suite 700
Louisville, Kentucky 40202–1817

C. Augustin, MD
Centre Hospitalier D'Agen
29, Bd. de la République
F-47000 Agen, France

J. M. Avelar, MD
Albert Einstein Hospital, São Paulo
Al Gabriel Monteiro
Da Silva 620
01442–000 São Paulo-SP, Brazil

K. Azari, MD
Assistant Professor
Division of Plastic Surgery
University of Pittsburgh Medical Center
Pittsburgh, Pennsylvania

H. A. Badran, MB, BCh, FRCS, FRCSEd
Head, Department of Plastic Surgery
Ain Shams University
98 Mohamed Farid Street
Cairo 11111, Egypt

G. J. Baibak, FACS
3634 West Bancroft Street
Toledo, Ohio 43606

B. N. Bailey, MD, FRCS
Oxford Regional Health Authority
Stoke Mandeville Hospital
Mandeville Road
Aylesbury, Buckinghamshire, HP21 8AL
United Kingdom

V. Y. Bakamjian, MD (Retired)
Roswell Park Cancer Institute
Department of Head and Neck Surgery
Elm and Carlton Streets
Buffalo, New York 14263

C. R. Balch, MD
Naples Community Hospital
201 Eight Street, South, Suite 102
Naples, Florida 34102

T. Barfred, MD, PhD
Assistant Professor of Surgery, Odense University
Head of Hand Surgery, Department of Orthopaedic Surgery,
Odense University Hospital, Odense, Sweden
Head of Hand Surgery
Section of Orthopaedic Surgery
Odense University Hospital
500 Odense, Denmark

Marguerite P. Barnett, FACS
530 South Nokomis Avenue, Suite 6
Venice, Florida 34285

R. L. Baroudi, MD
Rua Bahia 969
São Paulo, SP 01244–001
Brazil

J. N. Barron, MS, FRCSEd, FRCSEng (Deceased)

F. E. Barton, Jr., MD
Baylor University Medical Center
Parkland Hospital
Presbyterian Hospital
Mary Shiels Hospital
411 North Washington Avenue, #6000 LB 13
Dallas, Texas 75246–1774

R. M. Barton, FACS
Vanderbilt University Hospital
Nashville Virginia Hospital
Baptist Hospital
Vanderbilt University Hospital
Medical Center South, Room 230
Nashville, Tennessee 37232

J. Baudet, MD
Professor of Plastic and Reconstructive Surgery
University of Bordeaux
Chief of Department of Plastic and Reconstructive Surgery
C.H.U.-Hôpital du Tondu
Groupe Pellegrin-Tondu
Place Amélie Raba-Léon
F-33076 Bordeaux, France

C. Beard, MD (Retired)
University of California, San Francisco
400 Parnassus Avenue, Suite 750-A
San Francisco, California 94143

R. W. Beasly, MD
Professor at NYU Medical Center
Director of Hand Surgery at Bellevue Hospital Center
Hand Surgery Associates
310 East 30th Street
New York, New York 10016–8303

Col. D. W. Becker, Jr., MD
Wilford Hall USAF Medical Center, San Antonio, Texas
2200 Bergquist Drive, Suite 1
Lackland AFB, Texas 78236–5300

H. Becker, MD, FACS
Boca Raton Community Hospital
5458 Town Center Road
Boca Raton, Florida 33486–1009

Professeur T. Bégué, MD
Chirurgie Orthopédique-Traumatologique et Réparatrice de
l'Appareil Locomoteur
Hôpital Avicenne
125, route de Stalingrad
F-93009 Bobigny Cedex, France

F. C. Behan, FRACS, FRCS
91 Royal Parade
Parkville 3052
Melbourne, Victoria
Australia

M. S. G. Bell, MD
Suite 306
340 McLeod Street, South
Ottawa, Ontario, Canada, K2P 1A4

T. Benacquista, MD
Einstein Weiler Hospital
Department of Plastic and Reconstructive Surgery
Albert Einstein College of Medicine and
Montefiore Medical Center
3331 Bainbridge Avenue
Bronx, New York 10467

M. Ben-Bassat, MD
Deputy-Chief
Department of Plastic Surgery
Beilinson Hospital
Tel Aviv, Israel

S. P. Bhagia, MD
Baugh Farzana Plastic Surgery Centre, Agra, India
4/14 Baugh Farzana
Agra 282 002, India

S. K. Bhatnagar, MD
Professor in Plastic Surgery
Department of Plastic Surgery
King George's Medical College
Lucknow 226 003, India

S. Bhattacharya, MS, MCh, FICS
Awadh Hospital, Lucknow
Neera Hospital, Lucknow
Star Hospital, Gorahpur
Consultant Plastic Surgeon and Oncologist
C-907 Mahanagar
Lucknow 226 006, India

S. L. Biddulph, MD
Chief Hand Surgeon, Johannesburg Hospital
Houghton 2050, South Africa

E. Biemer, MD
Department of Plastic Surgery
Technical University of München
Ismaningerstrasse 22
D-81675 München, Germany

J. H. Binns, MD
Wayne State University
540 East Canfield
Detroit, Michigan 48201

R. J. Bloch, MD
R. Sampaio Viana 628
Paraiso-São Paulo 04004–002
Brazil

J. G. Boorman, MD
Queen Victoria Hospital
East Grinstead
West Sussex, RH19 3DZ United Kingdom

L.J. Borud, MD
Instructor in Surgery
Department of Surgery
Harvard Medical School
110 Francis Street, Suite 5A
Boston, Massachusetts 02215

J.-L. Bovet, MD
Unité de Chirurgie de la Main
Clinique Jean-Villar
F-33520 Burges, France

J. B. Boyd, MD, FRCS, FRCS(C), FACS
Cleveland Clinic Hospital, Ft. Lauderdale
Broward General Hospital, Ft. Lauderdale
Holy Cross Hospital, Ft. Lauderdale
Imperial Point Hospital, Ft. Lauderdale
North Ridge Hospital, Ft. Lauderdale
Department of Plastic and Reconstructive Surgery
Cleveland Clinic Florida
3000 West Cypress Creek Road
Ft. Lauderdale, Florida 33309

R. J. Brauer, MD
Greenwich Hospital, Connecticut
49 Lake Avenue
Greenwich, Connecticut 06830–4519

N. K. Breach, MB, FRCS, FDSRCS
Department of Surgery
Royal Marsden Hospital
Downs Road
Sutton SM2 5PT, United Kingdom

T. D. R. Briant, MD, FRCS(C), FACS
Honorary Consultant, St. Michael's Hospital
32 Dale Avenue
Toronto, Ontario, Canada, M4W 1K5

T. R. Broadbent, MD (Retired)
2635 St. Mary's Way
Salt Lake City, Utah 84108

M. Brones, MD, FACS
Grossman Burn Center at Sherman Oaks Hospital,
California
Suite 102
4849 Van Nuys Boulevard
Sherman Oaks, California 91403

M. D. Brough, MD
University College London Hospitals
Royal Free Hospital
The Consulting Suite
82 Portland Place
London W1N 3DH, United Kingdom

E. Z. Browne, Jr., MD, FACS
Cleveland Clinic
Department of Plastic and Reconstructive Surgery
Cleveland Clinic Foundation
9500 Euclid Avenue
Cleveland, Ohio 44195

C. D. Bucko, MD, FACS
Scripps Memorial Hospital, La Jolla, California
Panerodo Hospital
University of San Diego Medical Center
Sheerp Memorial Hospital
Mission Bay, Columbia
Suite B
9900 Genesee Avenue
La Jolla, California 92037

J. Bunkis, MD, FACS
4165 Blackhawk Plaza Circle, Suite 150
Danville, California 94506–4691

G. C. Burget, MD, FACS
Clinical Assistant Professor, Section of Plastic Surgery,
The University of Chicago Hospitals
2913 North Commonwealth Avenue, Suite 400
Chicago, Illinois 60657

J. A. Butler, MD, FACS
Wausau Hospital
Saint Michael's Hospital, Stevens Point, WI
North Central Wisconsin Plastic Surgery, SC
425 Pine Ridge Boulevard, Suite 202
Wausau, Wisconsin 54401

H. S. Byrd, MD, FACS
Baylor University Medical Center
Children's Medical Center
Zale Lipshy University Medical Center
Suite 6000 LB 13
411 North Washington Avenue
Dallas, Texas 75246

D. Calderón, MD
Hospital del Trabajador
Ramon Carnicer, 185-5 Piso
Providencia
Santiago, Chile

W. Calderón, MD
Professor of Surgery
University of Chile
Chief of Plastic Surgery
Service Hospital del Trabajador
Santiago, Chile

M. A. Callahan, MD, FACS
Eye Foundation Hospital
St. Vincent's Hospital
Medical Center East Outpatient Surgery
700 South 18th Street, Suite 511
Birmingham, Alabama 35233

R. R. Cameron, MD (Retired)
38330 Sweetwater Drive
Palm Desert, California 92211–7048

G. W. Carlson, MD
Wadley R. Glenn Professor of Surgery
Department of Surgery
Associate Program Director
Division of Plastic Surgery
Emory University School of Medicine
Atlanta, Georgia

C. E. Carriquiry, MD
Associate Professor, Plastic Surgery, School of Medicine,
Universidad de la República Montevideo-Uruguay
21 de Setiembre 2353 Ap. 201
Montevideo 11200, Uruguay

N. Carver, MS, FRCS, FRCS(Plast)
Department of Plastic and Reconstructive Surgery
Royal London Hospital
St. Bartholomew's Hospital
London, E1 1BB United Kingdom

V. M. Casoli, MD
Department of Plastic and Reconstructive Surgery
C.H.U.-Hôpital Du Tondu
Groupe Pellegrin-Tondu
Place Amélie Raba-Léon
F-33076 Bordeaux, France

P. C. Cavadas, MD, PhD
Head of the Reconstructive Surgery and Microsurgery Unit
Hospital Vírgen del Consuelo
Hand Transplant Surgery Unit
"La Fe" University Hospital
Valencia, Spain

A. Cerejo, MD
Consultant Neurosurgeon
Hospital S. Joao Medical School
Oporto, Portugal
Avenida Vasco Da Gama
Ed. Silva porto, BL.C, 9B
4490 Povoa de Varzim, Portugal

L. A. Chait, MD
Johannesburg Group of Teaching Hospitals
211 Parkland Clinic
Junction Avenue Park
Johannesburg, South Africa

R. Chandra, MS, MCh
Professor, Plastic Surgery
King George's Medical College
Lucknow 226 003, India

R. A. Chase, MD
Professor, Stanford University School of Medicine
Department of Surgery
Stanford, CA 94305

P. Chhajlani, MD
"Ganga Jamuna Apartments"
South Tukoganj, Near Nath Mandir
Indore 452 001, India

D. R. H. Christie, MBChB, FRACR
John Flynn Hopital, Tugun, Australia
Eastcoast Cancer Centre
Inland Drive
Tugun, QLD 4224, Australia

Y. K. Chung, MD
Yonsei University Wonju College of Medicine
Wonju Christian Hospital
Ilsandong
Wonju, Korea

M. E. Ciaravino, MD
Attending Plastic Surgeon
St. Joseph's Hospital
Houston, Texas
3805 West Alabama, #3105
Houston, Texas 77027

B. E. Cohen, MD, FACS
Academic Chief and Director, Plastic Surgery Residency
Program, Cohen and Cronin Clinic
Director, Microsurgical Research and Training Laboratory,
St. Joseph Hospital, Houston
Plastic and Reconstructive Surgery
Cohen and Cronin Clinic
1315 Calhoun, Suite 920
Houston, Texas 77002

C. C. Coleman, Jr., MD, FACS (Retired)
Consultant Plastic Surgeon, Clinical Professor of Surgery,
University of Virginia, Charlottesville, Virginia
Visiting Professor, University of Virginia
P. O. Box 558
Irvington, Virginia 22480–0558

J. J. Coleman III, MD, FACS
University Hospital
Riley Hospital
Wishad Hospital
VA Medical Center
Professor of Surgery
Director, Division of Plastic Surgery
Indiana University
Emerson Hall 235, 545 Barnhill Drive
Indianapolis, Indiana 46202

P. Colson, MD
Head Surgeon
Burn Unit
Saint Luke's Hospital
34, Place Bellecour
F-69002 Lyons, France

M. B. Constantian, MD, FACS
Adjunct Assistant Professor of Surgery, Dartmouth
Medical School
Active Staff, Department of Surgery (Plastic Surgery),
St. Joseph Hospital and Southern New Hampshire
Regional Medical Center
Nashua, New Hampshire
19 Tyler Street, Suite 302
Nashua, New Hampshire 03060

L. M. Cordero, MD (Deceased)

R. J. Corlett, MD
Royal Melbourne Hospital
Preston and North Gate Community Hospital
766 Elizabeth Street
Melbourne 3000, Australia

H. Monteiro Da Costa, MD
Professor and Consultant Plastic Surgeon,
Plastic and Reconstructive Unit, S. Joao Hospital,
Medical School, Oporto
Consultant Plastic Surgeon, Matosinhos and Vila Nova Eaia
Hospitals, Oporto
Professor in Plastic Surgery
Rua do Corvo, 323
Pr. da Granja
4405 Arcozelo VNG, Portugal

E. D. Cronin, MD, FACS
Chief of Plastic Surgery Section, St. Joseph Hospital
Plastic and Reconstructive Surgery
Cohen and Cronin Clinic
1315 Calhoun, Suite 920
Houston, Texas 77002

T. D. Cronin, MD (Deceased)

J. W. Curtin, MD
Rush-Presbyterian-St. Luke's Medical Center,
Chicago, Illinois
1180 Hill Road
Winnetka, Illinois 60093

R. K. Daniel, MD, FACS
Hoag Memorial Hospital/Presbyterian Hospital, California
1441 Avocado Avenue, Suite 308
Newport Beach, California 92660–7704

S. K. Das, MD, FACS, FRCS
St. Dominic's Hospital
River Oaks Hospital
River Oaks East Hospital
University of Mississippi Medical Center
Mississippi Methodist Medical Center
Parkview Hospital, Vicksburg
Division of Plastic Surgery
University of Mississippi Medical Center
2500 North State Street
Jackson, Mississippi 39211

J. E. Davis, MD
Matricula No. 7101
Vincente Lopez 2653, Argentina

R. De la Plaza, MD
Director, Plastic Surgery Department, La Luz Clinic,
Madrid
Clínica de Cirugía Plástica y Estética
Salou, 28
E-28034 Madrid, Spain

A. L. Dellon, MD, FACS
Professor, Plastic and Neurosurgery,
The Johns Hopkins University School of Medicine
2328 West Joppa Road, Suite 325
Lutherville, Maryland 21093

G. H. Derman, MD
Attending Staff, Rush-Presbyterian-St. Luke's
Medical Center
Attending Staff, Evanston Hospital
Assistant Professor, Rush Medical College, Chicago, Illinois
4709 Golf Road, Suite 806
Skokie, Illinois 60076–1258

B. Devauchelle, MD, PhD
Department of Maxillofacial Surgery
Centre Hospitalier Universitaire
Amiens, France

C. J. Devine, Jr., MD
400 West Brambleton Avenue, Suite 100
Norfolk, Virginia 23510–1115

I. K. Dhawan, MD
Department of Surgery
Al Mafraq Hospital
Abu Dhabi, India

Dr. A. D. Dias, MS
Professor Emeritus, L.T.M.G. Hospital, Sion, Mumbai
St. Thereza Hospital, Agashi, Virar
"Shanti Sadan"
157-B Perry Road
Bandra, Mumbai 400 050, India

R. O. Dingman, MD (Deceased)

T. A. Dinh, MD
Division of Plastic Surgery
Baylor College of Medicine
6560 Fannin, Suite 1034
Houston, Texas 77030

M. I. Dinner, MD, FACS
Meridia Hillcrest Hospital
Assistant Clinical Professor
Case Western Reserve Medical School
3755 Orange Plaza
Cleveland, Ohio 44122–4455

B. H. Dolich, MD
Albert Einstein College Hospital and Montefiore
Medical Center
New York Eye & Ear Hospital
1578 Williamsbridge Road
Bronx, New York 10461

R. V. Dowden, MD, FACS
Meridia Hillcrest, Mt. Sinai, University Hospital
6770 Mayfield Road, Suite 410
Mayfield Heights, Ohio 44124

G. A. Drabyn, MD, FACS
Riverside Methodist Hospital
3545 Olentangy River Road, Suite 130
Columbus, Ohio 43214

J. M. Drever, MD, FRCS
Etobicoke General Hospital
Cosmetic Surgery Hospital
135 Queens Plate Drive, Fifth Floor
Toronto, Ontario, Canada, M9W 6V1

J.-L. Ducours, MD
Centre Hospitalier D'Agen
Service de Chirurgie Maxillo-faciale
Centre Hospitalier
86 boulevard Sylvain Dumon
F-47000 Agen, France

G. M. Duncan, MChB, FRACS
Plastic Surgical Unit
Hutt Hospital
Private Bag
Lower Hutt, New Zealand

E. C. Duus, MD
Comanche County Memorial Hospital
Southwest Medical Center
5604 Southwest Lee Boulevard, Suite 310
Lawton, Oklahoma 73505–9663

W. Dzwierzynski, MD
Professor of Plastic Surgery
Medical College of Wisconsin
Milwaukee, Wisconsin

A. S. Earle, MD, FACS
Professor (Emeritus) of Plastic Surgery
Case Western University School of Medicine
1656 Emerald Green Court
Deltona, Florida 32725

D. S. Eastwood, MD (Retired)
St. Kames's University Hospital, Leeds, United Kingdom
Leeds University Hospital
11, North Park Road
Roundhay
Leeds LS8 1JD, United Kingdom

B. W. Edgerton, MD
Kaiser Permanente, West Los Angeles
Plastic Surgery Department
6041 Cadillac Avenue
Los Angeles, California 90034

M. T. Edgerton, MD
University of Virginia Health Sciences Center
Department of Plastic Surgery
Charlottesville, Virginia 22908

P. Egyedi, MD, DMD, PhD
Department of Oral and Maxillofacial Surgery
Utrecht University Hospital
P.O. Box 85500
NL-3508 GA Utrecht, The Netherlands

L. Eisenbaum, MD, PC
Colorado Medical Center of Aurora
Longmont United Hospital
Plastic and Reconstructive Surgery
Esthetic and Hand Surgery
Presbyterian Aurora Medical Center
750 Potomac Street, Suite 201
Aurora, Colorado 80011

M. M. El-Saadi, MD
Assistant Professor of Plastic Surgery
Zagazig University Hospital
Zagazig, Egypt

D. Elliot, MA
Woodlands
Woodham Walter
Essex
United Kingdom

R. A. Elliott, Jr., MD, FACS
P.O. Box 39
Slingerlands, New York 12159

L. F. Elliott, MD
Northside Hospital
St. Joseph's Hospital
Piedmont Hospital
Scottish-Rite Children's Hospital
975 Jonson Ferry, Suite 500
Atlanta, Georgia 30342

N. I. Elsahy, MD, PC, FRCS(C), FACS, FICS
Southern Regional Medical Center, Riverdale, Georgia
6524 Professional Place, Suite A
P.O. Box 1318
Riverdale, Georgia 30274

A. J. J. Emmett, MB, BS, FRCS, FRACS
Honorary Consultant, Princess Alexandra Hospital,
Brisbane, Australia
Woodgreen
128 Osborne Road
Bowral NSW 2576, Australia

D. N. F. Fairbanks, MD
Clinical Professor of Otolaryngology, George Washington
University School of Medicine, Washington, DC
Sibley Memorial Hospital, Washington, DC
3 Washington Circle, Northwest, Suite 305
Washington, DC 20037–2356

G. R. Fairbanks, MD
St. Mark's Hospital
Cottonwood Hospital, Primary Children's Medical Center
Bonneville Surgical Center
1151 East 3900 South, B110
Salt Lake City, Utah 84124

R. S. Feingold, MD
Assistant Clinical Professor in Plastic and Reconstructive
Surgery, Albert Einstein College of Medicine
Long Island Jewish Medical Center
Montefiore Medical Center
New York Hospital Medical Center of Queens
North Shore University Hospital
Winthrop-University Hospital
900 Northern Boulevard
Great Neck, New York 11021

M. Feldman, MD, FACS
Shore Memorial, Somers Point, New Jersey
Feldman Plastic Surgery, P. A.
222 New Road, Suite 6
Linwood, New Jersey 08221

A.-M. Feller, Prof. Dr. med.
Chairman, Department of Plastic Surgery
Behandlungszentrum Vogtareuth
Krankenhausstrasse 20
D-83569 Vogtareuth, Germany

R. J. Fix, MD, FACS
University of Alabama at Birmingham
The Children's Hospital of Alabama
Veterans Administration Medical Center
University of Alabama, Plastic Surgery MEB 524
1813 Sixth Avenue, South
Birmingham, Alabama 35294

A. E. Flatt, MD, FRCS
Baylor University Medical Center, Dallas, Texas
Clinical Professor, SW Medical School, Dallas, Texas
Consultant Emeritus in Hand Surgery,
U.S. Air Force
Director of Education
George Truett James Orthopaedic Institute
Baylor University Medical Center
3500 Gaston Avenue
Dallas, Texas 75246-9990

L. Fonseca Dos Santos, MD
Service d'Orthopedie
Hôpital Trousseau
26 Avenue de Dr. A Netter
F-75012 Paris, France

G. Foucher, MD
Head of SOS Main, Strasbourg
4 Bd. du President
F-67000 Strasbourg, France

M. Fox, MD, FACS
4001 Kresge Way, Suite 320
Louisville, Kentucky 40207-4640

J. D. Franklin, MD, FACS
Erlanger Health System, Memorial Hospital
Hutcheson Medical Center
Plaza Ambulatory Care Center
979 East Third Street, Suite 4002
Chattanooga, Tennessee 37403

A. Freiberg, MD, FRCS(C), FACS
Division of Plastic Surgery
Toronto Western Hospital
399 Bathurst Street
Edith Cavell Wing, 4-304
Toronto, Ontario MST 2S8, Canada

R. Fujimori, MD
Department of Plastic Surgery
Kyoto University
465 Kajii-cho Kawar
Kyoto 602, Japan

T. Fujino, MD, FACS, DrMedSci
Professor and Chairman
Department of Plastic Surgery
Keio University School of Medicine
35 Shinanomachi Shinjukuku
Tokyo 160, Japan

L. T. Furlow, Jr., MD, FACS
Clinical Professor, University of Florida College of Medicine,
Gainesville, Florida
3001 Northwest 28th Terrace
Gainesville, Florida 32605

D. W. Furnas, MD, FACS
University of California, Irvine Medical Center
St. Joseph Hospital, Orange
Childrens Hospital of Orange County
VA Hospital, Long Beach
University of California Irvine Medical Center
Division of Plastic Surgery
101 City Drive
Orange, California 92868–2901

F. N. Gahhos, MD
Venice Hospital
135 San Marco Drive
Venice, Florida 34285

A. Gardetto, MD
Professor of Plastic and Reconstructive Surgery
General Hospital of Brixen
Brixen, Italy

P. M. Gardner, MD
Assistant Professor, Department of Surgery,
Division of Plastic Surgery
University of Alabama at Birmingham
1600 7th Avenue South, ACC 322
Birmingham, Alabama 35233

N. W. Garrigues, MD
Scripps Memorial Hospital
Assistant Professor, University of California, San Diego
3405 Kenyon Street, Ste. 401
San Diego, California 92110–5007

J. S. Gaul, MD (Retired)
Charlotte, North Carolina

K. E. Georgeson, MD
University of Alabama Hospitals
The Children's Hospital of Alabama
1600 7th Avenue, South, ACC 300
Birmingham, Alabama 35233

G. S. Georgiade, MD
Duke University Medical Center—Surgery
P.O. Box 3960
Durham, North Carolina 27710

R. Ger, MD, FRCS
Albert Einstein College of Medicine
1300 Morris Park Avenue
Bronx, New York 10461

V. C. Giampapa, MD, FACS
89 Valley Road
Montclair, New Jersey 07042–2212

A. Gilbert, MD
15 rue Franklin
F-75016 Paris, France

D. A. Gilbert, MD, FRCS(C), FACS
Norfolk General Hospital
Children's Hospital of the King's Daughters
De Paul Hospital
Maryview Hospital
Plastic Surgery Associates, Inc.
400 West Brambleton Avenue, Suite 300
Norfolk, Virginia 23510

R. P. Gingrass, MD, SC
Elmbrook Hospital, Brokfield, Wisconsin
St. Joseph's Hospital, Milwaukee, Wisconsin
Plastic and Reconstructive Surgery
9800 West Bluemound
Milwaukee, Wisconsin 53226

F. Giraldo, MD, PhD
Plastic and Reconstructive Unit, University of Málaga
Regional Hospital "Harlos Haya," Málaga, Spain
Plastic and Reconstructive Unit
Regional Hospital "Carlos Haya"
E-29010 Málaga, Spain

D. W. Glasson, MD, FRACS
Wellington Hospital, Wellington, NZ
Hutt Hospital, Lower Hutt, NZ
Bowen Hospital, Wellington, NZ
Plastic Surgery Specialists
140 Ghuznee Street
Wellington 1, New Zealand

A. M. Godfrey, MB, BCh
Consultant Plastic Surgeon
Nuffield Acland Hospital and Nuffield Orthopaedic Centre, Oxford
The Paddocks Hospital, Bucks, and
The Ridgeway Hospital, Wilts
Felstead House
23 Banbury Road
Oxford OX2 6NX, United Kingdom

R. D. Goldstein, MD, FACS
Assistant Clinical Professor
Albert Einstein College of Medicine
Montefiore Medical Center
Bronx, New York 10461

R. M. Goldwyn, MD, FACS
Clinical Professor of Surgery, Harvard Medical School
Division of Plastic Surgery, Beth Israel Deaconess
Medical Center, Boston, MA
1101 Beacon Street
Brookline, Massachusetts 02146

D. J. Goodkind, MD
Yale-New Haven Hospital
Clinical Instructor of Surgery, Yale University
136 Sherman Avenue, South, Suite 205
New Haven, Connecticut 06511–5236

B. Gorowitz, MD
Department of Plastic and Reconstructive Surgery
C.H.U.-Hôpital Du Tondu
Groupe Pellegrin-Tondu
Place Amélie Raba-Léon
F-33076 Bordeaux, France

L. J. Gottlieb, MD, FACS
Professor of Clinical Surgery, Plastic and
Reconstructive Surgery
Department of Surgery
University of Chicago, Illinois
5841 South Maryland Avenue, MC 6035
Chicago, Illinois 60637

D. P. Green, MD
9150 Huebner Road, Suite 290
San Antonio, Texas 78229

B. M. Greenberg, MD, FACS
833 Northern Boulevard, Suite 115
Great Neck, New York 11021

J. M. Griffin, MD, FACS
Piedmont Hospital
Associate Clinical Professor, Department of Surgery
Emory University School of Medicine
Northside Hospital
Scottish Rite Children's Medical Center
Center for Plastic Surgery
365 East Paces Ferry Road
Atlanta, Georgia 30305–2351

B. H. Griffith, MD, FACS
Northwestern Memorial Hospital
Children's Memorial Hospital
Rehabilitation Institute of Chicago
Chief of Plastic Surgery, Shriners Hospital for Crippled
Children
Northwestern University Medical Center
251 East Chicago Avenue, Suite 1026
Chicago, Illinois 6061–2641

A. R. Grossman, MD, FACS
The Grossman Burn Center
Sherman Oaks Hospital, California
4910 Van Nuys Boulevard, Suite 306
Sherman Oaks, California 91403–1728

P. H. Grossman, MD
Grossman Burn Center
Sherman Oaks Hospital, California
4910 Van Nuys Boulevard, Suite 306
Sherman Oaks, California 91403

J. C. Grotting, MD, FACS
Children's Hospital of Alabama
Baptist Medical Center-Montclair
The Eye Foundation
Baptist Medical Center-Princeton
Health South Medical Center
Brookwood Medical Center
Outpatient CareCenter
McCollough, Grotting & Associates Plastic Surgery
Clinic P. C.
1600 20th Street, South
Birmingham, Alabama 35205

B. K. Grunert, PhD
Medical College of Wisconsin
Froedtert Memorial Lutheran Hospital
Children's Hospital of Wisconsin
9200 W. Wisconsin Avenue
Milwaukee, Wisconsin 53226

C. R. Gschwind, MD
The Centre for Bone and Joint Diseases
Royal North Shore Hospital, St. Leonards
Department of Hand Surgery
Hand and Microsurgery Unit
Royal North Shore Hospital
St. Leonards, NSW 2065, Australia

J. Guerrerosantos, MD
Chairman and Plastic Surgeon-In-Charge
Jalisco Institute for Reconstructive Surgery
Chairman and Professor, Division of Plastic and
Reconstructive Surgery, University of Guadalajara, Mexico
Garibaldi 1793
Col. L de Guevara
Guadalajara, Jalisco, 44680, Mexico

P. J. Gullane, MD
Otolaryngologist-in-Chief, Toronto Hospital, Toronto
Site Leader, Head and Neck Surgery, Princess Margaret
Hospital and Toronto Hospital
Staff Otolaryngologist, Mount Sinai Hospital, Toronto
Consultant Otolaryngologist
North York General Hospital, Toronto
200 Elizabeth Street, East
Toronto, Ontario, Canada, M5G 2C4

J. P. Gunter, MD, FACS
Presbyterian Hospital of Dallas
Parkland Memorial Hospital
Baylor University Medical Center
8315 Walnut Hill Lane, Suite 125
Dallas, Texas 75231–4211

B. Guyuron, MD, FACS
Medical Director of Zeeba Clinic
Clinical Professor of Plastic Surgery
Case Western Reserve University
29017 Cedar Road
Lyndhurst, Ohio 44124

K. F. Hagan, MD, FACS
Vanderbilt University Hospital, Baptist Hospital,
Columbia Centennial, The Atrium
Nashville Surgery Center
Vanderbilt University Medical Center
2100 Pierce Avenue
230, MCS
Nashville, Tennessee 37232–3631

E. J. Hall-Findlay, MD, FRCS
Plastic Surgeon
Banff Mineral Springs Hospital
Suite 340, Cascade Plaza
317 Banff Avenue
Banff, AT TOL 0C0, Canada

G. G. Hallock, MD, FACS
Consultant in Plastic Surgery, The Lehigh Valley and Sacred
Heart Hospitals, Allentown, Pennsylvania
St. Luke's Hospital, Bethlehem, Pennsylvania
1230 South Cedar Crest Boulevard, Suite 306
Allentown, Pennsylvania 18103

S. K. Han, MD, PhD
Professor of Plastic Surgery
Korea University College of Medicine
Seoul, Korea

R. Happle, MD
Department of Dermatology
University of Münster
Schlossplatz 2
D-4400 Münster, Germany

K. Harii, MD
Graduate School of Medicine, The University of Tokyo
Department of Plastic and Reconstructive Surgery
University of Tokyo Hospital
7–3-1 Hongo Bunkyo-ku
Tokyo 113, Japan

D. H. Harrison, MD
Regional Plastic Surgery Centre, Mount Vernon,
Northwood, UK
Flat 33, Harmont House
20 Harley Street
London WIN 1AA, United Kingdom

S. H. Harrison, MD, FCRS (Retired)
The Plastic Surgery
Mount Vernon Hospital
Rickmansworth Road
Northwood HA6 2RN, United Kingdom

C. R. Hartrampf, Jr., MD, FACS
St. Joseph's Hospital
Atlanta Plastic Surgery
Suite 500, 975 Johnson Ferry
Atlanta, Georgia 30342–1619

S. W. Hartwell, Jr., MD
Emeritus Staff, The Cleveland Clinic Foundation
9500 Euclid Avenue, E48
Cleveland, Ohio 44195–5257

A. Hayashi, MD
Assistant Professor, Department of Plastic and
Reconstructive Surgery, Toho University Hospital
Department of Plastic and Reconstructive Surgery
Toho University School of Medicine
6–11–1 Ohmorinishi, Ohta-ku
Tokyo 143, Japan

F. R. Heckler, MD, FACS
Director, Division of Plastic Surgery
Allegheny General Hospital, Pittsburgh, Pennsylvania
Clinical Associate Professor of Plastic Surgery, University of
Pittsburgh, School of Medicine, Allegheny General Hospital
320 East North Avenue
Pittsburgh, Pennsylvania 15212

T. R. Heinz, MD
University of Alabama Hospitals
The Children's Hospital of Alabama
Veteran's Administration Medical Center
University of Alabama at Birmingham
Plastic Surgery
1813 6th Avenue, South (MEB-524)
Birmingham, Alabama 35294–3295

C. Heitmann, MD, PhD
Department of Plastic, Reconstructive and Hand Surgery
Markuskrankenhaus
Frankfurt am Main
Germany

V. R. Hentz, MD
Stanford University Hospital
900 Welch Road, Suite 15
Palo Alto, California 94304

C. K. Herman, MD
Medical Director of Plastic Surgery
Pocono Health Systems
100 Plaza Court, Suite C
East Stroudsburg, PA 18301
Assistant Clinical Professor of Surgery (Plastic Surgery)
Albert Einstein College of Medicine, New York, NY 10467
Private practice, 988 Fifth Avenue, New York, NY 10021

H. L. Hill, Jr., MD
Tallahassee Memorial Medical Center, Florida
Tallahassee Single Day Surgical Hospital
Tallahassee Plastic Surgery
1704 Riggins Road
Tallahassee, Florida 32308

B. Hirshowitz, FRCS
Emeritus Professor of Plastic and Reconstructive Surgery
Faculty of Medicine
Technion-Israel Institute of Technology, Haifa
55 Margalit Street
Mount Carmel
Haifa 34464, Israel

J. G. Hoehn, MD, FACS
St. Peter's Hospital
Samuel Straton Veterans Administration
Albany Medical Center
The Child's Hospital
Albany Memorial Hospital
Albany Plastic and Reconstructive Surgery Center
Four Executive Park Drive
Albany, New York 12203

W. Y. Hoffman, MD, FACS
University of California, San Francisco Medical Center
Associate Professor of Plastic Surgery
University of California, San Francisco
350 Parnassus, Suite 509
San Francisco, California 94117–3608

J. Holle, MD
Institute of Anatomy
Medical University of Vienna
Department of Plastic and Reconstructive Surgery
Wilhelminen Hospital
Vienna, Austria
Krapfenwald G 9
Vienna, A1190, Austria

T. Honda, MD
Department of Plastic and Reconstructive Surgery
Tokyo Women's Medical University
8-1 Kawada-cho, Shinjuku-ku, 162-0054
Tokyo, Japan

C. E. Horton, MD
Sentara Norfolk General Hospital
Bon Secours DePaul Hospital
Children's Hospital of The King's Daughters
229 West Bute Street, Suite 900
Norfolk, Virginia 23510

A. S. Hoschander, MD
Resident
Department of Surgery
Long Island Jewish Medical Center/North Shore University Hospital
Manhasset, New York

W. Hu, MD
Centre Hopitalier Universitaire de Brest
Hôpital de la Cavale Blanche
F-29200 Brest, France

T. Huang, MD
Clinical Professor of Surgery
University of Texas Medical Branch
326 Market Street
Galveston, Texas 77550-5664

D. J. Hurwitz, MD
University of Pittsburgh Medical Center
Children's Hospital of Pittsburgh
Plastic and Reconstructive Surgery
Aesthetic and Craniofacial Surgery
University of Pittsburgh Medical Center
3471 Fifth Avenue
Pittsburgh, Pennsylvania 15213

J. J. Hurwitz, MD, FRCS(C)
Ophthalmological Executive Committee,
University of Toronto
Opthalmologist-in-Chief, Mount Sinai Hospital
Professor of Ophthalmology, University of Toronto
Director of Oculoplastics Programme
University of Toronto
600 University Avenue, Suite 408
Toronto, Ontario, Canada, M5G 1X5

Y. Ikuta, MD
Department of Orthopedic Surgery
Hiroshima School of Medicine
Kasumi 1–2-3
Hiroshima 734, Japan

O. Iribarren, MD
Department of Surgery
Surgery Service and Office of Nosocomial Infections Control
Saint Paul Hospital, School of Medicine
Universidad Catolica del Norte
Larrondo 1080
Videla s/n
Coquimbo. IV Region, Chile

F. Iselin, MD
Director of Hand Service
Department of Surgery, Centre de Chirugie de la
Main-Urgences Mains
Hôpital Nanterre
Paris, France

T. I. A. Ismail, MD
29 Nawal Street
Aguiza-Giza
Cairo, Egypt

Y. Itoh, MD, PhD
National Defense Medical College
Division of Plastic and Reconstructive Surgery
Department of Dermatology
3–2 Namiki
Tokorozawa, Saitama 359, Japan

Y. Iwahira, MD
Department of Plastic Surgery
Toho University Hospital
6–11–1 Ohmorinishi, Ohta-ku
Tokyo 143, Japan

H. Izawa, MD
Associate Professor
Department of Plastic and Reconstructive Surgery
St. Marianna University School of Medicine
2–16–1 Sugao
Myamae-ku, Kawasaki 216, Japan

Z. H. Jabourian, MD
Clinch Valley Medical Center, #2300
Richlands, Virginia 24641

I. T. Jackson, MD, DSc(Hon), FACS, FRCS, FRACS(Hon)
Institute for Craniofacial and Reconstructive
Surgery
Diplomate of the American Board of
Plastic Surgery
Institute for Craniofacial and Reconstructive
Surgery
3rd Floor, Fisher Center
16001 West 9 Mile Road
Southfield, Michigan 48075

R. V. Janevicius, MD, PC
Elmhurst Memorial Hospital, Elmhurst, Illinois
Plastic and Reconstructive Surgery
360 West Butterfield Road, Suite 230
Elmhurst, Illinois 60126

H. Janvier, MD
St. Luke's Hospital
34, Place Bellecour
69002 Lyons, France

V.T. Joseph, MBBS, FRCSEd, FRACS, MMED(Surgery), FAMS
Chairman, Division of Pediatric Surgery
KK Woman's & Children's Hospital
100 Bukit Timah Road
Singapore 229899

B. B. Joshi, MS
Mahatma Gandhi Hospital
Parel
Mumbai 400 012, India

J. Juri, MD
National University
Calle Viamonte 430
Buenos Aires, Argentina 1053

M. J. Jurkiewicz, MD, FACS, FRCS
Emory Affiliated Hospitals
25 Prescott Street, Northeast
Atlanta, Georgia 30308

J. B. Kahl, MD, FACS
Director of Plastic Surgery Residency & Department Head,
Christ Hospital
Head of Department of Plastic Surgery, Mercy Hospital
Active Staff, Bethesda Hospitals
Children's Hospital of Cincinnati
Jewish Hospital and
Deaconess Hospital
President, Montgomery North Plastic Surgery Center
Staffs of Providence, St. Luke, Good Samaritan
Clinical Instructor, University of Cincinnati
10545 Montgomery Rd., #100
Cincinnati, Ohio 45242

W. J. Kane, MD
Mayo Clinic
905 14th Avenue, Southwest
200 1st Street, Southwest
Rochester, Minnesota 55905

E. N. Kaplan, MD
1515 El Camino Real, Suite D
Palo Alto, California 94306

I. Kaplan, MB, ChB
Professor of Surgery and Incumbent of Chilewich Chair of
Plastic Surgery
University of Tel Aviv
Head, Department of Plastic Surgery
Belinson Medical Center
Petah-Tiqva 76 100, Israel

I. B. Kaplan, MD
Plastic Surgery Associates, Inc.
400 West Brambleton Avenue, Suite 300
Norfolk, Virginia 23510–1115

M. R. Karapandžić, MD
Belgrade University
Studenski Trg 1
1101 Belgrade 6, Yugoslavia

A. Karev, MD
Head, Department of Hand Surgery, Kaplan Hospital
Rehovot POBA 76100 Israel

R. B. Karp, MD
Courtesy Staff, Suburban Hospital, Bethesda, MD
11510 Old Georgetown Road
Rockville, Maryland 20852

R. G. Katz, MD
3500 Fifth Avenue
Pittsburgh, Pennsylvania 15213

J. C. Kelleher, MD, FACS
Microsurgery Fellow
Division of Plastic Surgery
Department of Surgery
University of Mississippi Medical Center
Jackson, Missouri

A. F. Kells, MD, PhD
Microsurgery Fellow
Division of Plastic Surgery
Department of Surgery
University of Mississippi Medical Center
Jackson, Mississippi

J. M. Kenkel, MD
University of Texas, Southwestern, Dallas, Texas
5323 Harry Hines Boulevard
Dallas, Texas 75235–9132

C. L. Kerrigan, MD, FRCS
Mary Hitchcock Memorial Medical Center
Lebanon, New Hampshire
Veteran Affairs Medical Center, White River Junction, VT
Dartmouth-Hitchcock Medical Center
One Medical Center Drive
Lebanon, New Hampshire 03756

M. Keyes-Ford, PAC (Deceased)

A. A. Khashaba, MD
Assistant Professor of Plastic Surgery
Zagazig University
4 Dr Ahmed Nada Street
Heliopolis, Cairo, Egypt

R. K. Khouri, MD, FACS
Baptist Hospital, Miami, FL
Doctors Hospital, Miami, FL
Cedars Hospital, Miami, FL
Dermatology and Plastic Surgery Center
328 Crandon Blvd., Suite 227
Key Biscayne, Florida 33149

Y. Kikuchi, MD
Department of Plastic and Reconstructive Surgery
Tokyo Women's Medical University
8-1 Kawada-cho, Shimjuku-ku, 162-0054
Tokyo, Japan

S. K. Kim, MD, PhD
Professor
Department of Plastic and Reconstructive Surgery
Dong-A University School of Medicine
Dong-A University Hospital
Seo-Gu
Busan, Korea

K. S. Kim, MD, PhD
Department of Plastic and Reconstructive Surgery
Chonnam National University Medical School
Dong-gu, Gwangju, Korea

Y. Kimata, MD
Professor
Department of Plastic and Reconstructive Surgery
Okayama University
Graduate School of Medicine, Dentistry and
Pharmaceutical Sciences
Shikata-cho, Okayama, Japan

B. Kirkby, MD
Associate Professor
The Royal Dental College
Copenhagen, Denmark

H. W. Klein, MD, FACS
Mercy Hospitals, Sacramento
Sutter Affiliated Hospitals
University of California, Davis
Suite 202
8120 Timberlake Way
Sacramento, California 95823–5412

S. Kobayashi, MD
Head and Professor of Department of Plastic and
Reconstructive Surgery, Iwate Medical University
19–1 Uchimaru Morioka-shi, Iwate 020
Japan

R. Kolachalam, MD
6848 Tiffany Circle
Canton, Michigan 48187

H. Koncilia, MD
Department of Plastic and Reconstructive Surgery
Wilhelminen Hospital, Vienna, Austria

I. Koshima, MD
Associate Professor of Plastic and Reconstructive Surgery
Plastic and Reconstructive Surgery
Kawasaki Medical School
577 Matsushima, Kurashiki City
Okayama 701–01, Japan

S. S. Kroll, MD, FACS (Deceased)

G. Kronen, MD
1115 Mallard Creek Road
Saint Matthews, Kentucky 40207-2489

J. E. Kutz, MD
Clinical Professor of Surgery (Hand)
University of Louisville School of Medicine
Christine M. Kleinert Institute for Hand and
Micro Surgery
225 Abraham Flexner Way, Suite 850
Louisville, Kentucky 40202

R. Kuzbari, MD
Associate Professor of Plastic Surgery
Wilhelminenspital
Montleartstrasse 37, A-1160
Vienna, Austria

S. Kwei, MD
North Shore Plastic Surgery
4 Centennial Drive, Suite 102
Peabody, Massachusetts 01960

H. P. Labandter, MD, FRCS
Herzlia Medical Center
7 Ramot Yam
Herzlia Pituach, Israel

L. Landín, MD
Assistant Surgeon
Reconstructive Surgery and Microsurgery Unit
Hand Transplant Surgery Unit
"La Fe" University Hospital
Valencia, Spain

V. C. Lanier, Jr., MD
300 Crutchfield Street
Durham, North Carolina 27704

N. Laud, MD
Lokmaya Tilak Municipal General Hospital
and Medical College
Saraswati Nilayam
Hindu Colony, Dadar
Mubai (Mumbai) 14, 400 014 India

S. A. Lauer, MD
Department of Ophthalmology
Albert Einstein College of Medicine and
Montefiore Medical Center
111 East 210th Steet
Bronx, New York 10467

D. Le Nen, MD
Centre Hopitalier Universitaire de Brest, France
Hôpital de la Cavale Blanche
F-29200 Brest, France

B. T. Lee, MD
Instructor in Surgery
Department of Surgery
Harvard Medical School;
Division of Plastic and Reconstructive Surgery
Beth Israel Deaconess Medical Center
Boston, Massachusetts

C. Lefevre, MD
Service d'Orthopedie, C.H.U.
Hôpital de la Cavale Blanche
F-29200 Brest, France

P. Leniz, MD
Burn and Plastic Surgery Unit
Hospital del Trabajador de Santiago
Santiago, Chile

A. G. Leonard, FRCS
Northern Ireland Plastic & Maxillofacial Service
The Upper Ulster Hospital
Dundonald, Belfast BT16 0RH
Northern Ireland, United Kingdom

M. A. Lesavoy, MD, FACS
UCLA Medical Center
Harbor-UCLA Medical Center
Santa Lionica-UCLA Medical Center
VA Medical Center-West Los Angeles
Division of Plastic and Reconstructive Surgery
UCLA School of Medicine
64–128 CHS, Box 951665
Los Angeles, California 90095–1665

M. Lester, MD
Assistant Professor
Department of Plastic and Reconstructive Surgery
University of Florida
Gainesville, Florida;
2 Council Street
Charleston, South Carolina 29401

L. A. Levine, MD
Lake Forest Hospital
Department of Urology
Rush-Presbyterian-St. Luke's Medical Center
1725 W. Harrison Street, Suite 917
Chicago, Illinois 60612

M. L. Lewin, MD (Deceased)

J. R. Lewis, Jr., MD, FACS (Deceased)

V. L. Lewis, Jr., MD
Professor of Clinical Surgery
Northwestern University Medical School
707 North Fairbanks Court
Suite 1210, Chicago, Illinois 60611

R. W. Liebling, MD
Associate Professor
Albert Einstein College of Medicine and
Montefiore Medical Center
Department of Plastic and Reconstructive Surgery
Jacobi Medical Center
1825 Eastchester Road
Bronx, New York 10461

B.-L. Lim, MD
Department of Hand Surgery
Singapore General Hospital
Outram Road
Singapore 0316

Chi-hung Lin, MD
Chang Gung Memorial Hospital
Kweishan
Taoyuan, Taiwan

W. C. Lineaweaver, MD
Professor and Chief, Division of Plastic Surgery
University of Mississippi Medical Center
Jackson, Mississippi

P. C. Linton, MD, FACS
Emeritus Professor of Plastic Surgery
University of Vermont College of Medicine
30 Main Street
Burlington, Vermont 05401

G. D. Lister, MD
Division of Plastic Surgery
University of Utah Medical Center
50 Medical Drive
Salt Lake City, Utah 84132

J. W. Little, III, MD, FACS
1145 19th Street, Northwest, Suite 802
Washington, DC 20036

J. W. Littler, MD (Deceased)

S. Llanos, MD
Burn and Plastic Surgery Unit
Hospital del Trabajador de Santiago
Centre for Health Research and Development
Universidad de los Andes
Chile

P. Lorea, MD
SOS MAIN Strasbourg
Strasbourg, France

M. M. LoTempio, MD
Fellow
Division of Plastic Surgery
Medical University of South Carolina

E. A. Luce, MD, FACS
Chief, Division of Plastic Surgery and Kiehn-DesPrez
Professor at University Hospitals of Cleveland/Case Western
Reserve University
Division of Plastic Surgery
11100 Euclid Avenue
Cleveland, Ohio 44106–5044

H. W. Lueders (Retired)
Community Hospital, Monterey, California
4007 Costado Road
Pebble Beach, California 93953

J. R. Lyons, MD
Yale-New Haven Hospital
Hospital St. Raphael
New Haven, Connecticut
330 Orchard Street
New Haven, Connecticut 06511–4417

S. E. MacKinnon, MD, FACS
Shoenberg Professor and Chief, Division of Plastic and
Reconstructive Surgery, Department of Surgery
Washington University School of Medicine
Division of Plastic Surgery and Reconstructive Surgery
One Barnes-Jewish Hospital Plaza, Suite #17424
St. Louis, Missouri 63110

W. B. Macomber, MD
Albany Medical College
1465 Western Avenue
Albany, New York 12203

N. C. Madan, MD
Associate Professor of Surgery
All India Institute of Medical Sciences
New Delhi, India

K. T. Mahan, DPM
Presbyterian Medical Center of University of Pennsylvania
St. Cigner Medical Center
Bethesda National Naval Medical Center
Pennsylvania College of Podiatric Medicine
The Foot and Ankle Institute
810 Race Street
Philadelphia, Pennsylvania 19107–2496

A. M. Majidian, MD
Grossman Burn Center at Sherman Oaks Hospital, California
2080 Century Park East, Ste 501
Los Angeles, California 90067

S. Malekzadeh, MD
Resident, University of Maryland Medical System,
Baltimore, MD
University of Maryland Medical System
22 S. Greene Street
Baltimore, Maryland 21201

R. T. Manktelow, MD
The Toronto Hospital
Mount Sinai Hospital
Hospital for Sick Children
Etobreske General Hospital
St. Michael's Hospital
The Toronto Hospital
Western Division
399 Bathurst Street 5WW835
Toronto, Ontario, Canada M5T 2S8

C. H. Manstein, MD
Chief, Division of Plastic Surgery, Jeans Hospital,
Philadelphia
Assistant Professor of Surgery, Temple University
School of Medicine, Philadelphia
Manstein Plastic Surgery Associates
7500 Central Avenue, Suite 210
Philadelphia, Pennsylvania 19111–2434

B. Maraud, MD
Centre Hospitalier D'Agen
17, Rue de Strasbourg
F-47000 Agen, France

D. Marchac, MD
Hôpital Necker Enfants Malades, Paris, France
130 rue de la Pompe
F-75116 Paris, France

J. M. Markley, MD, FACS
St. Joseph Mercy Hospital, Ann Arbor
University of Michigan Medical Center, Ann Arbor
Suite 5001–5008
5333 McAulery Drive
Ann Arbor, Michigan 48106

D. R. Marshall, FRACS
Monash University
Wellington Road
Melbourne
Victoria 3618, Australia

D. Martin, MD
Department of Plastic and Reconstructive Surgery
C.H.U.-Hôpital Du Tondu
Groupe Pellegrin-Tondu
Place Amélie Raba-Léon
F-33076 Bordeaux, France

Y. Maruyama, MD
Department of Plastic and Reconstructive Surgery
Toho University School of Medicine
6–11–1 Ohmorinishi, Ohta-ku
Tokyo 143, Japan

Professeur A. C. Masquelet
Chirurgie Orthopédique-Tramatologique et
Réparatrice de l'Appareil Locomoteur
Hôpital Avicenne
125, route de Stalingrad
F- 93009 Bobigny Cedex, France

J. K. Masson, MD
Mayo Clinic
102 Southwest Second Avenue
Rochester, Minnesota 55905–0008

A. Matarasso, MD, FACS, PC
Manhattan Eye, Ear, & Throat Hospital
Albert Einstein College of Medicine and Montefiore Medical
Center
Plastic and Reconstructive Surgery
1009 Park Avenue
New York, New York 10028

S. J. Mathes, MD
University of California, San Francisco Hospitals
and Clinics
Department of Surgery
San Francisco, California 94143–0932

H. S. Matloub, MD, FACS
Professor of Plastic Surgery and Director of Hand Fellowship
Program, Froedtert Hospital
Children's Hospital of Wisconsin
Veteran's Administration Hospital
Department of Plastic and Reconstructive Surgery
Medical College of Wisconsin
9200 West Wisconsin Avenue
Milwaukee, Wisconsin 53226

K. Matsuo, MD
Department of Plastic and Reconstructive Surgery
Shinshu University School of Medicine
3-1-1 Asahi, Matsumoto 390, Japan

J. W. May, Jr., MD, FACS
Chief of Division of Plastic Surgery
Massachusetts General Hospital
Massachusetts General Hospital, Rm. 353
Ambulatory Care Center, Ste. 453
15 Parkman Street
Boston, Massachusetts 02214–3139

J. G. McCarthy, MD, FACS
New York University Medical Center
Bellevue Hospital Center
Manhattan Eye, Ear & Throat Hospital
NYU Medical Center
550 First Avenue
New York, New York 10016

J. B. McCraw, MD, FACS
Professor of Plastic Surgery
University of Mississippi
2500 North State Street
Jackson, Mississippi 39216-3600

I. A. McGregor, MD
7 Ledcameroch Road
Bearsden,
Glasgow G61 4AB, Scotland
United Kingdom

S. Medgyesi, MD
Consultant Plastic Surgeon
Rigshospitalet
Copenhagen, Denmark

J. Medina, MD
Hand surgeon
Department of Orthopedics
Las Palmas
Gran Canaria
Spain

B. C. Mendelson, FRCSE, FRACS, FACS
The Avenue Hospital, Melbourne, Australia
109 Mathoura Road
Toorak, Victoria 3142
Australia

N. Menon, MD
Microsurgery Fellow
Stanford University Medical Center
Division of Plastic Surgery
Palo Alto, California

R. Meyer, MD
Postgraduate Professor ISAPS (IPRAS)
Centre de Chirurgie Plastique
4-Avenue Marc-Dufour
CH-1007 Lausanne, Switzerland

D. R. Millard, Jr., MD, FACS
Jackson Memorial Hospital
Miami Children's Hospital
1444 Northwest Fourteenth Avenue
Miami, Florida 33125

R. L. Mills, MD
751 South Bascom Avenue
San Jose, California 95128–2604

T. Miura, MD
Chukyo University
101 Tokodate, Kaizu-cho
Toyota, Aichi, 470–03, Japan

J. R. Moore, MD
Associate Professor of Orthopedic Surgery
The Johns Hopkins University School of Medicine
1400 Front Avenue, Suite 100
Lutherville, MD 21093–5355

S. C. Morgan, MD
Huntington Memorial Hospital
Arcadia Methodist Hospital
USC-LA County Medical Center
10 Congress Street, Suite 407
Pasadena, California 91105–3023

K. Morioka, MD
Department of Plastic and Reconstructive Surgery
Tokyo Women's Medical University
Tokyo, Japan

A. M. Morris, MD
Dundee University
Dundee, DD1 9SV, Scotland
United Kingdom

W. A. Morrison, MD
Plastic Surgeon and Deputy Director
Microsurgery Research Centre
St. Vincent's Hospital
Melbourne, Australia

H. Müller, MD, DMD (Deceased)

W. R. Mullin, MD, FACS
Jackson Memorial
Cedar Medical Center
Children's Medical Center
Plastic Surgery Centre
1444 Northwest 14th Avenue
Miami, Florida 33125

J. C. Mustardé, MD
90 Longhill Avenue
Ayr, Scotland, KA7 4DF, United Kingdom

F. Nahai, MD
Professor of Plastic Surgery, Emory University
Emory University Clinic
1365 Clifton Road, Northeast
Atlanta, Georgia 30322

J. E. Nappi, MD
Riverside Methodist Hospital
3400 Olentauey River Road
Columbus, Ohio 43214

M. Narayanan, MD
Medical Advisor
Ramalingam Medical Relief Centre
Madras, India

T. M. Nassif, MD
Hospital dos Servidores do Estado
Chief, Department of Reconstructive Microsurgery
Hospital dos Sevidores do Estado
22281 Rio de Janeiro RJ, Brazil

Vu Nguyen, MD
Assistant Professor
Division of Plastic Surgery
University of Pittsburgh Medical Center
Pittsburgh, Pennsylvania

J. M. Noe, MD
Harvard Medical School
25 Shattuck Street
Boston, Massachusetts 02115

K. Nohira, MD
Hokkaido University, Department of Plastic and
Reconstructive Surgery
Keiyukai Sapporo Hospital, Division of Plastic Surgery
Chief of Soshundo Plastic Surgery
Otemachi Building 2F
Minami-1, Nishi-4, Chuo-ku
Sapporo 060, Japan

J. D. Noonan, MD, FACS
Albany Medical Center
St. Peter's Hospital, Children's Hospital
1465 Western Avenue
Albany, New York 12203–3512

M. Nozaki, MD
Department of Plastic and Reconstructive Surgery
Tokyo Women's Medical University
8-1 Kawada-cho, Shimjuku-ku, 162-0054
Tokyo, Japan

K. Ohmori, MD
Department of Plastic and Restorative Surgery
Tokyo Metropolitan Police Hospital
2-10-41 Fujima Chiyoda-ku
Tokyo 102, Japan

S. Ohmori, MD (Deceased)

H. Ohtsuka, MD
Associate Professor
Ehime University Hospital
Surgical Division
Section of Plastic and Reconstructive Surgery
Shitsukawa, Shigenobu-cho,
Onsen-gun, Ehime 791–0295, Japan

C. Orreteguy, MD
Centre Hospitalier-Villeneuve Sur Lot
19, Bd. de la Marine
F-47300 Villeneuve Sur Lot, France

M. Orticochea, MD
Montevideo University School of Medicine
Montevideo, Uruguay

A. I. Pakiam, MD, FACS
Hospital of Saint John and St. Elizabeth
London, United Kingdom

C. E. Paletta, MD, FACS
Associate Professor, Division of Plastic and
Reconstructive Surgery, St. Louis University Hospital
Cardinal Glennon Children's Hospital
Veterans Administration–St. Louis
St. Mary's Health Center
St. Louis University
Associate Professor, Division of Plastic Surgery
3635 Vista at Grand
St. Louis, Missouri 63110–0250

F. X. Paletta, MD, FACS (Retired)
3635 Vista at Grand
St. Louis, Missouri 63110–0250

B. Panconi, MD
Department of Plastic and Reconstructive Surgery
of the Hand
Hôpital Pellegrin-Tondu
Place Amélie Raba-Léon
F-33076 Bordeaux, France

S. D. Pandey, MS, MCh
Professor, Hand Surgery
King George's Medical College
Lucknow 226 003, India

W. R. Panje, MD
Rush-Presbyterian-St. Luke's Medical Center, Chicago, Illinois
1725 Harrison Street, Suite 340
Chicago, Illinois 60612

G. S. Pap, MD, DDS, FACS (Retired)
Plastic and Reconstructive Maxillo-Facial Surgery
2403 Spring Creek Road
Rockford, Illinois 61107

C. Papp, MD
Head, Department of Plastic and Reconstructive Surgery
Hospital of Barmherzige Brüder
Salzburg, Austria

A. M. Pardue, MD, FACS
Los Robles Regional Medical Center
Thousand Oaks, California
1993 West Potrero Road
Thousand Oaks, California 91361

K.J. Park, MD, PhD
Assistant Professor
Department of Surgery
Dong-A University Medical Center
3 go 1, Dongdaesin-dong, Seo-Gu, Busan 602-716
South Korea

S. W. Parry, MD
Tulane Medical Center
Professor of Surgery, Tulane University
Tulane Medical Center Hospital and Clinic
1415 Tulane Avenue
New Orleans, Louisiana 70112–2605

A. Patel, MD
Resident
Department of Otolaryngology
The New York Eye & Ear Infirmary
New York, New York

R. M. Pearl, MD, FACS
Stanford University Hospital
Kaiser Hospital, Santa Clara
Physician-in-Chief
The Permanente Medical Group
900 Kiely Boulevard
Santa Clara, California 95051–5386

James M. Pearson, MD
Chief Resident
Department of Otolaryngology
The New York Eye & Ear Infirmary
New York, New York

I. J. Peled, MD
Chairman, Department of Plastic Surgery
Rambam Medical Center
Technion Institute of Technology, Medical School
Department of Plastic Surgery
Rambam Medical Center
Haifa, Israel

P. Pelissier, MD
Chef de Clinique
Service de Chirurgie Plastique et Reconstructrice
Hôpital du Tondu-Pellegrin
F-33076 Bordeaux, France

A. D. Pelly, MD
Plastic Surgery Unit
The Prince of Wales Hospital
195 Macquarie Street
Sydney 2000, Australia

Y. P. Peng, RWH Pho, FRCS
Consultant
Department of Hand and Reconstructive
Microsurgery
National University Hospital, Singapore;
Emeritus Professor of Orthopaedic Surgery
National University of Singapore

J. O. Penix, MD
Sentard Norfolk General Hospital
Surgical Director of Neurological Surgery
Children's Hospital of the King's Daughters
Neurosurgical Associates
607 Medical Tower
Norfolk, Virginia 23507

J. M. Peres, MD
Department of Plastic and Reconstructive Surgery
C.H.U.-Hôpital Du Tondu
Groupe Pellegrin-Tondu
Place Amélie Raba-Léon
F-33076 Bordeaux, France

M. Pers, DrMed
Head, Department of Plastic Surgery
University of Copenhagen
Rigshospitalet
Copenhagen, Denmark

J. Perssonelli, MD
St. Paul Hay Hospital
Av. Moema 170/111
04082-002 São Paulo SP, Brazil

V. Petrovici, MD
Department of Surgery, University of Cologne
Merheim Hospital
Bachemerstrasse 267
D-50935 Köln, Germany

R. W. H. Pho, MBBS, FRCS
Professor in Orthopaedic Surgery
National University of Singapore
Chief, Department of Hand and Reconstructive Microsurgery
National University Hospital
5 Lower Kent Ridge Road
Singapore 119074

K. L. Pickrell, MD (Deceased)

M. J. Pidala, MD
Western Reserve Medical Center
1930 State Route 59
Kent, Ohio 44240

J. L. Piñeros, MD
President of the Chilean Society of Burns
Burn and Plastic Surgery Unit
Hospital del Trabajador de Santiago
Santiago, Chile

P. Poizac, MD
Centre Hospitalier D'Agen
17, rue de Strasbourg
F-47000 Agen, France

B. Pontén, MD
Department of Plastic Surgery
University of Uppsala
750 14 Uppsala, Sweden

L. Pontes, MC
Plastic Surgery Unit
Department of Surgical Oncology
Portuguese Institute of Oncology
Porto, Portugal

J. A. Porter, MD
Clinical Professor of Surgery
Northeastern Ohio Universities College of Medicine
Summa Health Systems
55 Arch Street, Suite 3D
Akron, Ohio 44304

M. A. Posner, MD
Clinical Professor of Orthopaedics
New York University School of Medicine
Chief of Hand Services, Hospital for Joint Diseases
Chief of Hand Services, Lenox Hill Hospital
2 East 88th Street
New York, New York 10128

Z. Potparic, MD
University of Miami School of Medicine
Division of Plastic Surgery
Miami, Florida 33136

N. G. Poy, MD (Retired)
Scarborough General Hospital, Scarborough, Ont, Canada
4151 Sheppard Avenue, East
Scarborough, Ontario, Canada M1S 1T4

J. N. Pozner, MD
Assistant Clinical Professor of Plastic Surgery
The Johns Hopkins Hospital, Baltimore, MD
Plastic and Aesthetic Surgery
1212 York Road, Suite B101
Lutherville, Maryland 21093

G. Pradet, MD
Centre de Chirugie de la Main-Urgences Mains
Hôpital Nanterre
Paris, France

F. E. Pratt, MD (Retired)
P.O. Box 417880
Sacramento, California 95841

J. J. Pribaz, MD
Brigham & Women's Hospital, Boston
Children's Hospital, Boston
Associate Professor/Chief, Hand and Microsurgery
Department of Surgery/Division of Plastic Surgery
Brigham and Women's Hospital
75 Francis Street
Boston, Massachusetts 02115

J. M. Psillakis, MD
Professor of Plastic and Reconstructive Surgery
University of Sao Paulo, Brazil
Av. Cauaxi 222
Ed. San Martin 703
Barueri 06454-020, Brazil

C. L. Puckett, MD, FACS
University of Missouri Hospital and Clinics
Professor and Head
Division of Plastic and Reconstructive Surgery
University of Missouri
One Hospital Drive
Columbia, Michigan 65212

C. Radovan, MD (Deceased)

S. S. Ramasastry, MD
University of Illinois at Chicago Medical Center
Cook County Hospital, Chicago, Illinois
Mount Sinai Hospital, Chicago, Illinois
820 South Wood Street, (M/C 958) 515 CSN
Chicago, Illinois 60612

O. M. Ramirez, MD, FACS
Greater Baltimore Medical Center
Professor, The Johns Hopkins University
School of Medicine
Franklin Square Hospital, Baltimore
Plastic and Aesthetic Surgery
1212 York Road Suite, B-101
Lutherville-Timonium, Maryland 21093–6240

Y. Ramon, MD
Department of Plastic Surgery
Rambam Medical Center, Haifa
4A Mapu Avenue
Haifa, 34361 Israel

V. K. Rao, MD, MBA
University of Wisconsin Hospital and Clinic
University of Wisconsin Medical School
600 Highland Avenue
Madison, Wisconsin 53792

D. A. Campbell Reid, MD, FRCS
Consultant Plastic Surgeon
Plastic and Jaw Department
Fulwood Hospital
Fulwood
Sheffield, S10 3TD, United Kingdom

R. S. Reiffel, MD, PC, FACS
White Plains Hospital
St. Agnes Hospital
Westchester Medical Center
12 Greenridge Avenue, Suite 203
White Plains, New York 10605

J. F. Reinisch, MD, FACS
Head, Division of Plastic Surgery
Childrens Hospital Los Angeles
University Hospital
Associate Professor of Clinical Surgery, University of
Southern California School of Medicine
Division of Plastic Surgery
Childrens Hospital Los Angeles
4650 Sunset Boulevard, MS #96
Los Angeles, California 90027

A. J. Renard, MD, FACS
3845 Bee Ridge Road
Sarasota, Florida 34233–1160

J. E. Restrepo, MD
Clínica Soma
Medellin, Columbia

C. A. Rhee, MD
2879 Hempstead Turnpike, Suite 204
Levittown, New York 11756

M. Ribeiro, MD
Plastic Surgery Unit
Department of Surgical Oncology I
Portuguese Institute of Oncology
Porto, Portugal

D. Richard, MD
Centre Hospitalier D'Agen
Rue Lamennais
F-47000 Agen, France

R. A. Rieger, MBBS, FRCS, FRACS
327 S. Terrace
Adelaide 5001, Australia

R. Roa, MD
President of the Chilean Burn Association;
Assistant Professor
Medical School, Universidad de los Andes
Santiago, Chile

G. A. Robertson, MD
Victoria Hospital, Winnipeg, Manitoba
Manitoba Clinic
790 Sherbrook Street
Winnipeg R3A 1M3, Canada

J. F. R. Rocha, MD
Laboratoire d'Anatomie de l'UER
Biomedicale de Saint Peres
Hôpital Trousseau
Paris, France

C. Rodgers, MD, FACS
Rose Medical Center
Swedish Hospital
Porter Hospital
Littleton Hospital
4600 Hale Parkway, Suite 430
Denver, Colorado 80220

E. Roggendorf, Dr.sc.med. (Deceased)

M. C. Romaña, MD
Hôpital d'Enfants Armand-Trousseau, Paris
Consultant Surgeon
Department of Orthopaedic and Reconstructive Surgery
for Children
Hôpital Trousseau
26 Avenue A. Netter
F-75012 Paris, France

T. Romo III, MD
Director of Facial Plastic and Reconstructive Surgery
Department of Otolaryngology Head and Neck Surgery
Lenox Hill Hospital
The Manhattan Eye, Ear and Throat Hospital
New York, New York

E. H. Rose, MD
Assistant Clinical Professor (Plastic Surgery)
The Mount Sinai Medical School, New York, NY
Attending Staff, The Mount Sinai Medical Center and
Lenox Hill Hospital, New York, NY
Founder and Director, The Aesthetic Surgery Center,
New York, NY
The Aesthetic Surgery Center
895 Park Avenue
New York, New York 10021

M. Rousso, MD
Senior Lecturer of Surgery
Hadassah Hebrew University, Jerusalem
Head of Hand Surgery and Day Care Surgery
Misgav Ladach General Hospital
POB 90
Jerusalem 91000, Israel

R. T. Routledge, MD, FRCS (Retired)
Chief of Plastic Surgery Department
Frenchay Hospital
Bristol, United Kingdom

R. C. Russell, MD, FACS, FRCS
Memorial Hospital, Springfield, IL
St. John's Hospital, Springfield, IL
Illini Hospital, Pittsfield, IL
Southern Illinois University School of Medicine
Plastic Surgery 1511, P.O. Box 19230
Springfield, Illinois 62794

R. F. Ryan, MD, FACS (Retired)
Emeritus Professor of Surgery (Plastic Reconstructive),
Tulane Medical School, New Orleans, LA
Perido Bay Country Club
5068 Shoshone Drive
Pensacola, Florida 32507

F. J. Rybka, MD, FACS
Mercy Hospital
Sutter Hospital
Professor of Plastic Surgery, University of California, Davis
San Juan Medical Plaza, Suite 350
6660 Coyle Avenue
Carmichael, California 95608–6312

M. N. Saad, MD
Honorary Consultant Plastic Surgeon
Wexham Park Hospital, Slough
Consultant Plastic Surgeon
The Thames Valley Nuffield Hospital, Slough and
The Princess Margaret Hospital
Osborne Road, Windsor
Berks SL4 3SJ, United Kingdom

H. Saito, MD, PhD
Fukui Medical University
Matsuoka-cho, Yoshida-gun
Fukui, Japan

S. Sakai, MD
Associate Professor
Department of Plastic and Reconstructive Surgery
St. Marianna University School of Medicine
2-16-1 Sugao
Myamae-ku, Kawasaki 216, Japan

R. H. Samson, MD
Sarasota Memorial Hospital
Columbia Doctors Hospital
Vascular Associates of Sarasota
4044 Sawer Road
Sarasota, Florida 34233

J. R. Sanger, MD, FACS
Medical College of Wisconsin
9200 West Wisconsin Avenue
Milwaukee, Wisconsin 53226

J.R. Ramón Sanz, MD
Head of Department of Plastic and Reconstructive Surgery
"Marqués de Valdecilla" University Hospital
Santander, Spain

G. H. Sasaki, MD, FACS
St. Luke Medical Center
Huntington Memorial Hospital
Arcadia Methodist Hospital
Plastic and Reconstructive Surgery
800 South Fairmount Avenue, Suite 319
Pasadena, California 91105

K. Sasaki, MD
Chief Professor of Nihon University School of Medicine
Department of Plastic and Reconstructive Surgery
Nihon University School of Medicine, Oyaguchi
Itabashi-ku, Tokyo Japan

R. C. Savage, MD, FACS
Assistant Clinical Professor, Division of Plastic Surgery,
Harvard Medical School
Needham Medical Building
111 Lincoln Street, Suite 3
Needham, Massachusetts 02192

H. Schaupp, MD (Retired)
University ENT Hospital
Frankfurt-am-Main, Germany

L. R. Scheker, MD
Christine M. Kleinert Institute for Hand and Microsurgery
Assistant Clinical Professor of Plastic and
Reconstructive Surgery
University of Louisville
225 Abraham Flexner Way, Suite 700
Louisville, Kentucky 40202–3806

R. R. Schenck, MD, FACS
Associate Professor and Director
Section of Hand Surgery
Senior Attending, Departments of Plastic and
Orthopaedic Surgery
Rush-Presbyterian-St. Luke's Medical Center
1725 Harrison Street, Rm 263
Chicago, Illinois 60612–3828

J. D. Schlenker, MD
Christ
Little Co. of Mary
Palos Community
Holy Cross
Illinois Valley Community Hospital
6311 West 95th Street
Chicago, Illinois 60453

J. Schrudde, MD
University of Köln
Osterriethwed 17
D-50996 Köln, Germany

M. A. Schusterman, MD, FACS
Clinical Associate Professor of Plastic and
Reconstructive Surgery
Baylor College of Medicine, Houston, TX
7505 South Main Street, Suite 200
Houston, Texas 77030

S. P. Seidel, MD
Cullman Regional Medical Center
Woodland Community Hospital
Walker Baptist Medical Center
Seidel Plastic Surgery
2035 Alabama Highway #157
Cullman, Alabama 35055

D. Serafin, MD, FACS
Professor, Chief of Plastic Reconstructive
Maxillary Oral Surgery
Duke University Medical Center
P.O. Box 3372
Durham, North Carolina 27710–0001

R. E. Shanahan, MD, FACS
Emeritus Staff, The Toledo Hospital
Emeritus Clinical Associate Professor of Surgery
Medical College of Ohio at JOCTPC
5945 Barkwood Lane
Toledo, Ohio 43560

L. A. Sharzer, MD, FACS
Albert Einstein College of Medicine and
Montefiore Medical Center
Westchester Square Hospital, NY
Beth Israel Hospital, NY
212 East 69th Street
New York, New York 10021

W. W. Shaw, MD, FACS
Professor, Chief, Division of Plastic Surgery
UCLA School of Medicine
Room 64-140 CHS
10833 LeConte Avenue
Los Angeles, California 90095

R. W. Sheffield, MD, FACS
Cottage Hospital, Santa Barbara, CA
1110 Coast Village Circle
Santa Barbara, California 93108

A. Shektman, MD
332 Washington Street
Suite 355
Wellesley, Massachusetts 02181

S. M. Shenaq, MD, FACS
The Methodist Hospital, Texas Medical Center
St. Luke's Episcopal Hospital, Texas Medical Center
Texas Children's Hospital, Texas Medical Center
Ben Taub General Hospital, Texas Medical Center
Veteran's Administration Hospital, Texas Medical Center
Institute for Rehabilitation and Research, Texas
Medical Center
Diagnostic Center Hospital, Texas Medical Center
Poly Ryan Memorial, Richmond, Texas
Northeast Medical Center Hospital, Humble, Texas
Professor of Surgery, Division of Plastic Surgery
Baylor College of Medicine
6560 Fannin Street, Suite 800
Houston, Texas 77030

G. H. Shepard, MD
Riverside Regional Hospital Medical Center
Newport News, Virginia
Mary Immaculate Hospital
Newport News, Virginia
895 Middle Ground Boulevard, Suite 300
Newport News, Virginia 23606

M. M. Sherif, MD
Associate Professor
Department of Plastic and Reconstructive Surgery
Aim Shams University, Cairo, Egypt
2(A) Al Sayed Abou Shady Street, Flat 606
Heliopolis, Cairo 11361, Egypt

K. C. Shestak, MD
Division of Plastic Surgery
University of Pittsburgh
Pittsburgh, Pennsylvania

Y. J. Shin, MD
Department of Plastic Surgery
College of Medicine
Chungnam National University
640 Taesa-Dong, Jung-ku, Taejeon
301-040 Korea

Y. Shintomi, MD
Soshundo Plastic Surgery Hospital
Director of Soshundo Plastic Surgery
Otemachi Building
Minami-1, Nishi-4, Chuo-ku
Sapporo 060, Japan

G. F. Shubailat, MD, FRCS, FACS
Member of the Senate, Jordan Parliament
CEO and Chairman of the Board, Chief of Plastic Surgery,
Amman Surgical Hospital
P. O. Box 5180
Amman 11183, Jordan

M. Siemionow, MD, PhD, DSc
Professor of Surgery
Director of Plastic Surgery Research
Department of Plastic Surgery
Cleveland Clinic
Cleveland, Ohio

C. E. Silver, MD
Professor of Surgery
Albert Einstein College of Medicne
Chief of Head and Neck Surgery
Montefiore Medical Center
111 East 210th Street
Bronx, New York 10467–2401

R. P. Silverman, MD
Chief, Division of Plastic Surgery
University of Maryland Medical Center
Baltimore, Maryland

F. A. Slezak, MD
Professor of Surgery, Northeastern Ohio Universities
College of Medicine, Department of Surgery
Summa Health Systems, Akron, Ohio
55 Arch Street, Suite 3D
Akron, Ohio 44304

C. J. Smith, MD
Swedish Hospital
Providence Hospital
Northwest Hospital
1221 Madison Street, Suite 1102
Seattle, Washington 98104–1360

E. Durham Smith, MD, FRACS
Senior Associate, University of Melbourne
Melbourne, 3052
Victoria, Australia

R. J. Smith, MD (Deceased)

J. W. Snow, MD
St. Vincent's Hospital
1820 Barrs Street, Suite 701
Jacksonville, Florida 32204

B. C. Sommerland, FRCS
Great Ormond St. Hospital for Children, London
St. Andrew's Hospital, Billeriay, Essex
Consultant Plastic Surgery
The Old Vicarage
17 Lodge Road
Writtle
Chelmsford, CMI 3H4, United Kingdom

J. T. Soper, MD
Professor, Department of Gynecological Oncology
Duke University
Division of Gynecologic Oncology
Duke University Medical Center
Durham, North Carolina 27715–3079

M. Soussaline, MD
Institut Gustave Roussy Villefrief
Clinique Ste. Genevieve
Plastic and Cosmetic Surgery Department
American Hospital
46, Boulevard Saint-Jacques
F-75014 Paris, France

D. Soutar, MD
Clinical Director, Consultant Plastic Surgeon
Honorary Senior Lecturer, University of Glasgow
Plastic Surgery Unit
Canniesburn Hospital
Bearsden
Glasgow, G61 1QL, Scotland, United Kingdom

M. Spinner, MD
557 Central Avenue
Cedarhurst, New York 11516–2136

M. Spira, MD, FACS
Chief of Plastic Surgery, St. Luke's Episcopal Hospital,
Houston, Texas
Baylor College of Medicine
6560 Fannin, Suite 800
Houston, Texas 77030

R. K. Srivastava, MD
Athens Regional Medical Center, Athens, Georgia
180 St. George Place
Athens, Georgia 30606

D. A. Staffenberg, MD, DSc (Honoris Causa)
Chief, Plastic Surgery
Surgical Director, Center for Craniofacial Disorders
Montefiore Medical Center
The Children's Hospital at Montefiore
Associate Professor
Clinical Plastic Surgery, Neurological
Surgery, Pediatrics
Albert Einstein College of Medicine
Bronx, New York

W. R. Staggers, MD
Thomas Hospital, Fairhope, AZ
South Bladwin Hospital, Foley, AZ
188 Hospital Drive, Suite 203
Thomas Hospital Medical Office Center
Fairhope, Arizona 36532

R. S. Stahl, MD, MBA
Associate Chief, Department of Surgery, Yale-New Haven
Hospital
Clinical Professor of Surgery, Yale University School of
Medicine
Yale New Haven Hospital, CB228
20 York Street
New Haven, Connecticut 06504

R. B. Stark, MD, FACS (Retired)
35 East 75th Street, 12C
New York, New York 10021

D. N. Steffanoff, MD (Retired)
114 Via Valverde
Cathedral City, California 92234

H.-U. Steinau, MD
BG-Universitätsklinik Bergmannsheil
Department of Plastic Surgery, Burn Center
Bürkle de la Camp Platz 1
D-44789 Bochum, Germany

M. Steiner, MD
Burn and Plastic Surgery Unit
Hospital del Trabajador de Santiago
Santiago, Chile

H. R. Sterman, MD
Albert Einstein College of Medicine and
Montefiore Medical Center
Holy Name Hospital
870 Palisade Avenue, Suite 203
Teaneck, New Jersey 07666

T. R. Stevenson, MD
Professor and Chief
Division of Plastic Surgery
University of California Davis Medical Center
2315 Stockton Boulevard
Sacramento, California 95817

W. Stock, MD
Ltd. Arzt f. Plast. Chirugie
Chirurgische Klinik
Nussbaumstrasse 2
D-80336 München 2, Germany

M. F. Stranc, MD
Head of Plastic Surgery Section, Health Sciences Center,
Winnipeg, Manitoba
Victoria Hospital, Winnipeg, Manitoba
Manitoba Clinic
790 Sherbrook Street
Winnipeg, Canada, R3A 1M3

W. E. Stranc, MD
Victoria Hospital
Winnipeg, Manitoba, R3A 1M3, Canada

B. Strauch, MD, FACS
Professor
Albert Einstein College of Medicine
5 Flagler Drive Bainbridge Avenue
Rye, New York 10580

V. V. Strelzow, MD, FACS, FRCS(C)
16300 Sand Canyon Avenue, Suite 704
Irvine, California 92618–3707

J. H. Sullivan, MD
Clinical Professor, University of California
San Francisco, California
220 Meridian Avenue
San Jose, California 95126–2903

I. Suzuki, MD
Associate Professor
Department of Plastic and Reconstructive Surgery
St. Marianna University School of Medicine
2-16-1 Sugao
Myamae-ku, Kawasaki 216, Japan

W. M. Swartz, MD, FACS
University of Pittsburgh Medical Center
5750 Centre Avenue, Suite 180
Pittsburgh, Pennsylvania 15206

E.-P. Tan, FRCS(Ed), FRACS
2 St. John's Avenue
Gordon, New South Wales 2072, Australia

M. J. Tavis, MD, FACS (Deceased)

G. Allan Taylor, MD, FRCS(C)
Assistant Professor of Surgery
University of Ottawa Medical School
Chief, Division of Plastic Surgery
Ottawa Civic Hospital
737 Parkdale Avenue
Ottawa, Ontario, Canada K1Y 4E9

G. I. Taylor, MD
Royal Melbourne Hospital
766 Elizabeth Street
Melbourne 3000, Australia

H.O.B. Taylor, MD
Plastic Surgery Resident
Harvard Plastic Surgery Program
Boston, Massachusetts

B. Teimourian, MD, FACS
Attending Surgeon, Suburban Hospital, Bethesda, MD
5402 McKinley Street
Bethesda, Maryland 20817

S. Terkonda, MD
University of Alabama at Birmingham, University Hospital
Instructor, Division of Plastic Surgery
University of Alabama at Birmingham, MEB-524
1813 Sixth Avenue, South
Birmingham, Alabama 35294

J. K. Terzis, MD
Sentara Hospitals
International Institute of Microsurgical Research
Eastern Virginia Medical School
330 West Brambleton Avenue
Norfolk, Virginia 23510

M. R. Thatte, MS, MCh (Plastic)
Mumbai Hospital Institute of Medical Sciences
Shushrusha Citizen's Co-Operative Hospital
Consultant Plastic Surgeon
167-F, Dr. Ambedkar Road
Dadar, Mumbai 400 014, India

R. L. Thatte, MD
Consultant Plastic Surgeon, Bhatia Hospital, Mumbai, India
Apartment 46
Shirish Co-op Housing Society
187 Veer Savarkar Marg
Mumbai 400 016, India

H. G. Thomson, MD, FACS
555 University Avenue, Suite 180
Toronto, Ontario, Canada M5G 1X8

G. R. Tobin, MD, FACS
Professor and Director, Division of Plastic Surgery
University of Louisville Hospitals
Department of Surgery
University of Louisville
Louisville, Kentucky 40292

M. A. Tonkin, MD
Clinical Associate Professor and Head, Hand and Peripheral
Nerve Surgery, Royal North Shore Hospital of Sydney
Department of Hand Surgery
The Royal North Shore Hospital of Sydney
Block 4, Level 4
St. Leonards, New South Wales, 2065, Australia

B. A. Toth, MD
Pacific-Presbyterian Medical Center
Assistant Clinical Professor, University of California, San
Francisco
2100 Webster Street, Suite 424
San Francisco, California 94115–2380

H. Tramier, MD
Service d'Orthopedie - Traumatologie - Chirurgie Pediaturgie
Centre Hospitalier, Aubogne Cedex
41, rue Saint-Jacques
F-13006 Marseille, France

G. Trengove-Jones, MD
Sentara Norfolk General Hospital
Sentara Leigh Hospital
De Paul Hospital
Childrens Hospital of the King's Daughters
Department of Plastic Surgery
Eastern Virginia Medical School
Norfolk, Virginia 23501–2401

W. C. Trier, MD, FACS (Retired)
6321 Seaview Avenue, NW, #20
Seattle, Washington 98107–2671

T.-M. Tsai, MD
Jewish Hospital
Suburban Hospital
Alliant Hospitals
University Hospital
Clark County Hospital, Indiana
Shriners Hospital, Lexington, Kentucky
Audubon Hospital
Caritas Hospital
Christine M. Kleinert Institute for Hand and Micro Surgery
225 Abraham Flexner Way, Suite 850
Louisville, Kentucky 40202

M. Tschabitscher, MD
Department of Microsurgical and
Endoscopic Anatomy
Medical University of Vienna
Vienna, Austria

Y. Ullmann, MD
Deputy Head, Department of Plastic and
Reconstructive Surgery, Rambam Medical Center
Faculty of Medicine (Bruce), Hatechnion, Haifa
Department of Plastic Surgery
Rambam Medical Center
Haifa 31096, Israel

S. Unal, MD
Department of Plastic Surgery
The Cleveland Clinic Foundation
Cleveland, Ohio

J. Unanue, MD
Centre Hospitalier Ter de Villeneuve Sur Lot
19 Bd. de la Marine
F-47300 Villeneuve Sur Lot, France

J. Upton, MD, FACS
Beth Israel Deaconess Medical Center, Boston, MA
Children's Hospital, Boston, MA
830 Boylston Street, Suite 212
Chestnut Hill, Massachusetts 02167

M. L. Urken, MD, FACS
Professor and Chairman, Department of Otolaryngology
Mt. Sinai Medical Center
Box 1189, One Gustave L. Levy Place
New York, New York 10029–6574

E. J. Van Dorpe, MD
Plastic Surgery Department
Onze Lieve Vrouw
Kortrijk, Belgium

F. Van Genechten, MD
Saint Augustinus-Saint Camillus Hospital, Antwerp, Belgium
Virga Jesse Hospital, Masself, Belgium
Oude Maasstraat. 1
B-3500 Hasselt, Belgium

L. O. Vasconez, MD, FACS
Chief Plastic Surgeon
University of Alabama at Birmingham Medical Center
Professor of Surgery and Chief
Division of Plastic Surgery
University of Alabama, Birmingham
1813 6th Avenue, South (MEB-524)
Birmingham, Alabama 35294-3295

T. R. Vecchione, MD
Associate Clinical Professor of Surgery, Division of Plastic
Surgery USSD, San Diego, CA
Senior and Past Chief of Staff, Children's Hospital of San Diego
Senior and Past Chief of Plastic Surgery, Morcy Hospital,
San Diego, CA
Senior and Past Chief of Plastic Surgery, Sharp Memorial
Hospital, San Diego, CA
306 Walnut Avenue, Suite 212
San Diego, California 92103

Professor R. Venkataswami, MS, MCh, FAMS, FRCS (EDIN), DSC (Hon)
Emeritus Professor, Dr M.G.R. Medical University
Chennai, Tamilnadv India
99 Dr. Algappa Chettiar Road
Chennai 600 084, India

R. J. J. Versluis, MD
Department of Otorhinolaryngology and
Head and Neck Surgery
Kennemer Gasthuis Deo
Velserstraat 19
NL-2023 EA Haarlem, The Netherlands

L. Vidal, MD
Department of Plastic and Reconstructive Surgery
C.H.U.-Hôpital Du Tondu
Groupe Pellegrin-Tondu
Place Amélie Raba-Léon
F-33076 Bordeaux, France

C. Vlastou, MD
Director, Department of Plastic and Reconstructive Surgery,
Diagnostic and Therapeutic Center of Athens "HYGEIA"
105-7 Vas Sovias Avenue
Athens 11521, Greece

V. E. Voci, MD, FACS
Presbyterian Hospital, Charlotte, NC
McRoy Hospital, Charlotte, NC
Gaston Memorial Hospital, Gastonia, NC
Voci Center Cosmetic Plastic Surgery, P.A.
2027 Randolph Road
Charlotte, North Carolina 28207–1215

H. D. Vuyk, MD
Gooi-Nord Hospital, Department of Otolaryngology,
Head and Neck Surgery
Rijksstraatweg 1
NL-1261 AN Blaricum, The Netherlands

S. C. Vyas, MD
Oakwood Hospital, Dearborn, MI
22260 Garrison
Dearborn, Michigan 48124

M. Wada, MD
Higasishinagawa Clinic
Higasishinagawa 3-18-8
Shinagawaku, Tokyo, Japan

M. S. Wagh, MS, MCh
Lecturer in Plastic Surgery, LTMG Hospital
Sion, Mumbai 400 022, India
601-602, B-Wing
Shantiwar
Shantivan Housing Complex
Borivali Suite 212(E), Mumbai 400 066, India

R. L. Walton, MD, FACS
University of Chicago Hospitals
University of Chicago - MC 6035
Plastic Surgery
5841 South Maryland Avenue
Chicago, Illinois 60637

A. Wangermez, MD
Centre Hospitalier D'Agen
Rue Lamennais
F-47000 Agen, France

P. H. Warnke, MD
Department of Oral and Maxillofacial Surgery
University of Kiel
Kiel, Germany

H. Washio, MD, FACS
Attending Staff, Plastic Surgery, St. Luke's–Roosevelt
Hospital Center, New York, New York
580 Park Avenue
New York, New York 10021

J. T. K. Wee, MD (Deceased)

F-C. Wei, MD
Professor and Chairman
Department of Plastic and Reconstructive Surgery
Chang Gung Memorial Hospital
199 Tung Hwa North Road
Taipei 10591, Taiwan

A. J. Weiland, MD
The Hospital for Special Surgery, New York, New York
The Hospital for Special Surgery
535 East 70th Street
New York, New York 10021–4872

N. Weinzweig, MD, FACS
Associate Professor of Plastic Surgery and Orthopaedic
Surgery, University of Illinois
Cook County Hospital
Associate Professor of Plastic Surgery and Orthopaedic
Surgery
University of Illinois
Division of Plastic Surgery M/C 958
820 South Wood Street, 515 CSN
Chicago, Illinois 60612–7316

A. W. Weiss, Jr., MD
St. Luke's Hospital
Associate Professor of Surgery, Michigan State University
College of Human Medicine
800 Cooper Street, Suite 1
Saginow, Michigan 48602–5371

M. R. Wexler, MD
Head, Department of Plastic and Aesthetic Surgery, Hand
Surgery and the Burn Unit, and Professor of Plastic Surgery,
Hebron
University, Hadassah Medical Center
Department of Plastic and Aesthetic Surgery
Hadassah University Hospital
Jerusalem 91120, Israel

W. White, MD (Deceased)

J. S. P. Wilson, FRCS
The Cromwell Hospital
London, United Kingdom

C. Windhofer, MD
Department of Plastic and Reconstructive Surgery
Hospital of Barmherzige Brüder
Salzburg, Austria

M. S. Wong, MD
Assistant Professor
Division of Plastic Surgery
University of California, Davis
Sacramento, California

J. E. Woods, MD, PhD, FACS
Mayo Medical Center, Rochester, MN
Emeritus Staff
Division of Plastic and Reconstructive Surgery
Mayo Clinic
200 First Street, Southwest
Rochester, Minnesota 55905

A. P. Worseg, MD
Department of Plastic and Reconstructive Surgery
Wilhelminenhospital
Vienna, Austria

E. F. Worthen, MD (Retired)
3504 Forsythe Avenue
Monroe, Louisiana 71201

Y. Yamamoto, MD, PhD
Assistant Professor, Department of Plastic and
Reconstructive Surgery
Hokkaido University School of Medicine
Kita 15, Nishi 7, Kitaku
Sapporo 060, Japan

N.W. Yii, MD
Division of Plastic Surgery
Wexham Park Hospital
Slough, Berkshire SL2 4HL,
United Kingdom

M. Young, MD
Grossman Burn Center at Sherman Oaks Hospital,
California
4929 Van Nuys Boulevard
Sherman Oaks, California 91403

N. J. Yousif, MD
Froedtert and Memorial Lutheran Hospital
9200 West Wisconsin Avenue
Milwaukee, Wisconsin 53226

P. Yugueros, MD
Mayo Medical Center, Rochester, MN
Division of Plastic and Reconstructive Surgery
Mayo Clinic
200 First Street, Southwest
Rochester, Minnesota 55905

L. S. Zachary, MD, FACS
University of Chicago, Division of Plastic Surgery
5841 South Maryland Ave. P.O. Box MC 6035
Chicago, Illinois 60637–1463

S. Zenteno Alanis, MD
Chief of Service
Department of Plastic and Reconstructive Surgery
Hospital General de Mexico
Providence 400 Penthouse
Mexico 12, D.F.

F. Zhang, MD, PhD
Professor
Division of Plastic Surgery
University of Mississippi Medical Center
Jackson, Mississippi

E. G. Zook, MD, FACS
Memorial Medical Center and St. John's Hospital
Southern Illinois University School of Medicine
Institute for Plastic Surgery
PO Box 19230
747 North Rutlidge Street
Springfield, Illinois 62794–1511

R. M. Zuker, MD, FRCS(C), FACS
Head, Division of Plastic Surgery
The Hospital for Sick Children
Professor of Surgery, Department of Surgery
University of Toronto
Head, Division of Plastic Surgery
The Hospital for Sick Children
555 University Avenue, Suite 1524B
Toronto, Ontario, Canada M5G 1X8

Since our last edition of *Grabb's Encyclopedia of Flaps*, major evolutionary changes have occurred in the field of reconstructive plastic surgery. The explosion of perforator flap sites and the techniques of harvesting the pedicle without extensive sacrifice of the underlying muscles are well represented in this new edition.

In the last ten years, the field of transplantation has also been further advanced by plastic surgeons. Face and hand allotransplantation represents some of the most exciting advances in all of medicine, and we have tried to provide a glimpse of this emerging field with the inclusion of two articles on facial transplantation. What was once science fiction has now become reality and may one day even become commonplace.

The changes in the reconstructive ladder are evident in all arenas. With the widespread success of microsurgery, many defects are currently reconstructed with the most complex free tissue transfers as the primary option, jumping straight to the top of the ladder. On the other hand, negative pressure devices have revolutionized wound care management and, in many cases, has supplanted tissue coverage, moving many potential defects rapidly down the ladder.

More than 12,000 citations in the literature on flaps were reviewed, and 43 new chapters were added to this third edition. Many of the older chapters were revised or brought up to date. The new edition includes flaps, both pedicle and microvascular, for reconstruction of the face, orbits, lips, and nose. The latest techniques in nasal reconstruction, including local mucosal flaps as well as providing total reconstruction of the nasal support and lining with microvascular forearm flaps, have been added. Use of innervated muscle for tongue reconstruction is presented. In the hand volume, many new flaps have been added for reconstruction of the palm, the fingers, and the metacarpals. Breast surgery articles, including the use of medial and lateral pedicles, are new to this edition. A major inclusion has been the addition of the multiple perforator flaps used for breast reconstruction. Articles on reconstruction of the chest and abdomen have been chosen, as have the latest techniques for lower extremity reconstruction.

In adding all of these new choices, the editors were faced with a dilemma. How do we keep the concept of an encyclopedic atlas, while still staying within the confines of hard copy pages and costs of printing? The decision was made to keep all of the previous articles but to list some of the lesser used flaps by chapter title and author only in the printed text so that the reader is aware of these choices. In the online edition, all of the articles, new and old, are presented with full text and illustrations. Of course, editorial opinions at the beginning of the chapters have been maintained to help the reader make prudent reconstructive decisions. To access these complete articles, go to www.encyclopediaofflaps.com.

The third edition of this encyclopedia would not have been possible without the dedication provided by Dr. R.D. (Lee) Landres. In addition, we would like to thank the editorial staff at Lippincott Williams & Wilkins. To all the authors who contributed new chapters or provided revisions of their original chapters in a timely fashion, we extend our thanks, as we are deeply indebted to them.

Berish Strauch, MD
Luis O. Vasconez, MD
Elizabeth J. Hall-Findlay, MD
Bernard T. Lee, MD

In the last ten years, evolutionary changes in the use of flaps in reconstructive plastic surgery have resulted in increased flap reliability, as well as in more definitive reconstruction of particular defects. Currently, there is much less dependence on the use of flap delays and on random skin flaps. The reconstructive surgeon is now provided with a choice not only of skin flaps, but also of composite flaps which may contain skin and muscle, muscle alone or, in cases where bony defects are also involved, associated bone flaps. There is no longer a requirement for empirical questions about whether or not a particular flap will have an adequate blood supply. We presently think in terms of reliable flaps with a known blood supply and a determinate reliability. Where this is not yet possible, the reconstructive surgeon is likely to consider a free microvascular flap.

Another important change is our independence from the so-called reconstructive ladder, according to which surgeons followed the precept of using the simplest method and then advancing to a more complex one. Nowadays, the objective should always be to utilize the best method first, the one that will fulfill the requirements of the reconstruction, even though it may be the most complex, for example, a microvascular composite flap.

It was impossible for the authors to have included every flap that has been described since the first edition. In fact, considerable care has been taken in choosing proven and reliable flaps. Over 10,000 citations in the literature on flaps were reviewed and 120 new and revised chapters were added to the second edition. A considerable number of chapters describing procedures that have not been proven clinically reliable have been deleted. The editors have also added appropriate editorial comments that should be helpful to the reader wherever these seemed indicated.

Undertaking publication of the second edition of the encyclopedia would not have been possible, had it not been for the dedication and immense help provided by the editorial assistance of Dr. R. D. (Lee) Landres. We would also like to thank the editorial staff at Little, Brown and Company, whose work on this second edition has been taken over by Lippincott-Raven Publishers. Additionally, our sincere thanks to all the authors who contributed new chapters or revision of the original chapters in a timely fashion. We are indebted to them.

B. S.
L. O. V.
E. J. H.-F.

An important and very broad area of plastic surgery entails the coverage of defects throughout the body. These defects are usually covered by flaps, of which we now have a great variety. For approximately 50 years, from the introduction of the tubed flap until the middle 1960s, most flaps were tubed. Although we realized that blood supply was important for survival of the tubed flap, it was not until the end of the 1960s that we began to pay attention to the distinct arterial and venous supplies of different flaps. Axial flaps, musculocutaneous flaps, fasciocutaneous flaps, and microvascular free flaps were introduced in the decade of the 1970s. These were rapidly used in great numbers, with clinical applications throughout the body. The concept of "delay" of flaps has just about been abandoned. It is extremely advantageous that we now have a multitude of flaps that can be applied for the coverage of particular defects.

A flap can be designed and made with an adequate dimension with the knowledge of its exact blood supply; one needs only proper execution to be assured of a consistent, satisfactory, and acceptable result. This great number and variety of the flaps that differ not only in their design, but also in their type, as far as the blood supply is concerned, is "wonderful" for the experienced surgeon, but it also may present a quandary for the student plastic surgeon. The young surgeon may not have the clinical experience of having performed many and different flaps for a similar defect. There is usually no problem with execution of the procedure, but the clinical judgment that some learn by previous clinical errors may be supported by consideration and proper description of available options.

This *Encyclopedia* attempts to provide choices for the closure of particular defects throughout the body. Recognized experts described how to execute a particular flap, and each flap is presented in a uniform format, emphasizing the indications and anatomy, including the blood supply, surgical technique, complications, and safeguards. Selected editorial comments are included as a guide to the reader.

The multiauthored format has been chosen to give each author, often the originator of the flap, an opportunity to explain the procedure, and in each chapter the editors have rewritten only to maintain the uniform format, always attempting to keep the authors' information unchanged.

This *Encyclopedia* is intended to serve as a stimulus to experienced surgeons to refresh their memories about a multitude of options for particular defects so that they may choose what, in their judgment, will give a safe, predictable, and acceptable result. This work also will show the student of plastic surgery the numerous options and will teach him or her to choose the most appropriate one and to consider a great many factors that can play a role in what we call "clinical judgment." Once the proper choice is made, this *Encyclopedia* will refresh knowledge of the clinical aspects of flap execution, as well as the blood supply and the safeguards.

This *Encyclopedia* tends to encompass defects throughout the body and is divided into three volumes. For the reader who wants an increased knowledge of a particular flap, selected references are included at the end of each chapter.

We hope that this work will be helpful to all, including the most experienced surgeons, reinforcing with certainty that a good number of options have been considered and that the best were chosen.

Dr. William Grabb dreamed of a sequel to his book on skin flaps. He had organized and outlined the book and had chosen an initial group of contributors. His foresight encompassed the tremendous influence that microvascular and musculocutaneous flaps would have on the availability of usable flaps. He asked Berish Strauch and Luis O. Vasconez to join him as associate editors, to guide the sections on microvascular and musculocutaneous flaps, respectively. The decision to go forward with the *Encyclopedia* was made in 1981 during the annual meeting of the American Society of Plastic and Reconstructive Surgeons in New York.

Dr. Grabb's untimely death in 1982 halted progress on the work for over nine months. The two associate editors finally decided that the concept of the *Encyclopedia* was too important to plastic surgery for the project not to be completed.

Advice was sought from Lauralee Lutz in Ann Arbor. Lauralee had served as Dr. Grabb's administrative secretary and in-house editor. Her advice resulted in bringing aboard Dr. R. D. (Lee) Landres in New York to help with the editing of the *Encyclopedia*. All the contributors were contacted, and the chapters began to be produced.

The enormity of the task soon became apparent, and Dr. Elizabeth Hall-Findlay, who had worked previously with Drs. Strauch and Vasconez, was asked to join the two editors.

Multiauthored textbooks are often disorganized and repetitive. Faced with well over 400 chapters written in several languages and with various styles, we made a decision: Each chapter was to be reorganized into a similar format—with an introduction, a section on anatomy, and a section on flap design and dimensions, followed by operative technique and clinical results. In general, line drawings were to be the main figures, with some case illustrations. Details of history and research results were to be be omitted. Interested readers would be encouraged to refer to original publications, with each chapter followed by a relevant but not overbearing list of references. We knew we were into at least three volumes and did not want the work to be burdened with unnecessary detail. Despite the rewriting and uniform organization, there was a serious attempt to keep the authors' information unchanged.

This work has already traveled extensively. It has originated from all over the world. The chapters were initially rough-edited and placed on computer disks by Dr. Landres. The disks were sent to Dr. Hall-Findlay in Banff, Alberta, in the Canadian Rocky Mountains. There they were edited directly off the disks, and appropriate illustrations and references were chosen. Most of the chapters spent some time deep in the mountains at one of the most beautiful sites in the world—Lake O'Hara Lodge. There, care had to be taken not to lose any of the text or "work in progress" if the electric generator failed. Further work and refinements always seemed to take ten times longer than expected.

Drs. Vasconez and Strauch reviewed the editorial changes as they progressed and, as well, solicited and received new chapters as delays became prolonged. Meetings were held in Banff, where we closeted ourselves away with "the book," reviewing text and illustrations and discussing editorial comments.

The editors at Little, Brown and Company in Boston have been invaluable in seeing the project to completion. Fred Belliveau had organized and supervised the project from its inception. Curtis Vouwie helped during the seemingly never-ending delays, and Susan Pioli has both encouraged and prodded the work to completion.

Although the delays resulted in criticisms of being out of date, we felt that many of these chapters have stood and will stand the test of time. We tried to keep up with the chapters, without adopting the unproven. Of necessity, we stopped inclusions of new chapters in 1987. We hope that the book will not only be comprehensive, but also useful to surgeons in reviewing options when faced with routine or unusual problems or defects.

We can never thank everyone who has been involved in helping, directly or indirectly, with the *Encyclopedia*. Drs. Strauch, Vasconez, and Hall-Findlay wish to express in com-

mon their appreciation to Dr. Lee Landres, who has worked tirelessly for the past seven years on this work. Dr. Hall-Findlay wishes to recognize and thank Cheryl Low and Lynn Enderwick, who helped with many endless secretarial chores while, at the same time, handling patients and managing the office. Checking references accurately would not have been possible without the help of Merle Duncan, librarian at the medical library of the University of Calgary. Patricia Velasquez, Elke Berthold, Doris Freytag, Liesbeth Heynen, and Vickilynn Norton have all helped by being loving and devoted nannies to Jamie, David, and Elise. Dr. Hall-Findlay's mother, Betty Hall, and her in-laws, Jim and Edith Findlay, helped immeasurably with child care during their many visits to Banff, so that work on the *Encyclopedia* could go on. Don Findlay cannot be thanked enough for his understanding and patience.

B. S.
L. O. V.
E. J. H.-F.

INTRODUCTION: THE HISTORY OF VASCULARIZED COMPOSITE-TISSUE TRANSFERS

R. A. CHASE

The compelling drive of human beings to reconstruct deficient or missing parts and the desire of victims to undergo such reconstruction are best appreciated by recognizing the early development and use of pedicle-flap transfers long before the advent of anesthesia. Imagine the tolerance a patient must have had to undergo nasal reconstruction using a forehead pedicle flap without anesthesia. The seminal work of Sushruta (1) in the pre-Christian era must have resulted in meager success; however, the basic principle behind the "Indian flap" is so sound that the procedure is still used in contemporary surgery.

From those early developments, at first slowly, and then like a wild fire in the last four decades, the world has witnessed enormous progress in tissue-transfer surgery. The latter-day developments in anesthesia, antibiotics, hematology, instrumentation, and wound-healing research have given surgeons devoted to reconstruction the opportunity to achieve results that would have been considered miraculous only four decades ago. When immunologic barriers to risk-free transplantation are breached, a whole new wave of applications of existing and developing reconstructive strategies will break upon the world.

PEDICLE TRANSFERS

It is interesting to note, at least from what can be gleaned from recorded history (2), that the first successful transfer of human tissues to heterotopic sites was done by what we now call pedicle techniques. Such transfers are never even transiently, deprived of blood supply. Thus, on a trial-and-error basis, it should not be a surprise that the success of the Hindu Sushruta (1) during the pre-Christian era depended on the use of pedicle flaps of tissue in the face and forehead.

The designation of "Indian flap" for nasal reconstruction has survived, and its use in contemporary surgery testifies to its practicality. It appears to have taken centuries for the principle and procedure itself to travel from its origin in India to Europe—first to the Brancas in Italy, who became known in the fifteenth century for use of the technique and the principle to develop new and imaginative reconstructive procedures. Tagliacozzi in the sixteenth century made use of the printing press to disseminate knowledge of the techniques abroad through his celebrated *De Curtorum Chirurgia* (3) published in 1597.

Nonetheless, the procedures lay dormant for about 200 years until a newspaper, the *Madras Gazette,* and the *Gentleman's Magazine* (4) reported the Indian method for nose reconstruction in 1794. Among others, Carpue (5) in England and von Graefe (6) in Germany further developed the technique in Europe. Zeis, in his 1830 description of the procedure (7), displayed illustrations suggesting the dusky appearance of the flap early after surgery. Warren was the first in the United States to publish this technique in 1837 (8). It appeared in the *Boston Medical and Surgical Journal* (now the *New England Journal of Medicine*).

The pedicle flap principle, initiated by trial and error in pre-Christian history, was established and refined in the nineteenth century and formed the fundamental basis for the spectacular developments in the modern decades of surgery.

I shall mention a few landmarks in the development of tissue transfers during the nineteenth and twentieth centuries. In 1829, Fricke of Hamburg published a book describing many alternate facial flaps (9). Shortly thereafter, Tripier, Malgaigne (10), Burrow, Estlander, von Graefe (6), Abby, Denonvilliere, Rosenthal, Dieffenbach, and Zeis (2)—to name the principals—added further innovations in the shift of tissues to adjacent areas within the face for reconstruction.

Hamilton of Buffalo reported the first successful cross-leg flap in 1854 (12). He also was the first to apply the principle of delay to flap transfer. In 1868, Prince published *A New Classification and a Brief Exposition of Plastic Surgery* (12) with examples of applications of pedicle-flap techniques in plastic surgery. At the Practitioner's Society of New York in 1891, Shrady used an open jump flap cut from one arm and carried after vascularization by the contralateral index finger to fill a cheek contour defect (13). Shortly thereafter, in 1896, the renowned William Stewart Halsted (14) first "waltzed," by end-over-end transfer, a flap from the abdomen up to the neck of a burn victim. He was the first to use the term *waltzed.*

In pedicle-transfer surgery, aside from studies of the delay phenomenon (11,15,16), effects of drugs and radiation (17), and thinning of the flap (18), the refinements during this era were confined largely to the carrying pedicle itself. In 1849, Jobert of Paris, in his two-volume textbook *Chirurgie Plastique* (19), described "the temperature changes in skin flaps and the reinnervation of flaps" and noted that "the size of the pedicle should be proportional to the size of the flap."

The renowned Sir Harold Gillies stated, "In general, a flap should not be larger than the width of its carrying pedicle." In 1920, he added a rider: "A longer flap could be raised if the flap contained in its base a larger vascular pedicle such as the superficial temporal artery" (20).

Gillies' book, *Plastic Surgery of the Face* (21), is a classic in the field and, together with that of John Staige Davis, ushered in the modern era of plastic surgery. Both were based on lessons learned from current works and publications early in the twentieth century, such as those of Vilray Blair (22), and experiences during World War I. Gillies himself had been stimulated and influenced by Morestin, whom he had visited in France. The war experience was very influential on many great contributors to plastic surgery—V. H. Kazanjian, Ferris Smith, R. H. Ivy, Eastman Sheehan, and Sterling Bunnell, to name a few.

As noted by Khoo Boo-Chai (23), John Wood in 1863 had described a flap that, in 1869 (24), he called a "groin flap." He commented on the importance of incorporating known vessels—in his patients, the superficial epigastric vessels.

John Staige Davis, reporting World War I experiences, expanded the uses of pedicle flaps (2,25) and later with William German et al. (26) explored the vascular anatomy of the skin and subcutaneous tissues important in designing such flaps.

John Roberts of Philadelphia pointed to lessons learned in the war and applicable to reparative surgery using pedicle flaps on the hand (27). In 1919, Albee described the surgical construction of an osteoplastic finger substitute using a pedicle flap and a bone graft (28). Also in 1919, at the clinic day of the American Orthopaedic Association at Jefferson Hospital in Philadelphia, P. G. Skillern presented a patient from Polyclinic Hospital in whom a double-pedicle "strap" flap was used for coverage of the dorsum of the right hand (29). Steinler's books appeared in 1923 and 1925 (30,31), at the same time Allen Kanavel's book (32) was published, and later Marc Iselin's *Atlas* (33,34) and Cutler's *The Hand* (35).

In 1931, Jacques Joseph, using illustrations of Manchot from 1889, justified and published illustrations of deltopectoral flaps as vascular-pattern flaps (36,37). The deltopectoral flap was later popularized and used imaginatively by V. Y. Bakamjian, as described in his papers starting in 1965 (38,39). McGregor and Jackson showed its use in hand surgery (40).

A debate between S. H. Milton (41) and P. M. Stell (42) raged in the early seventies on the appropriate base for random flaps. By then, the classification of flaps according to the nature of the pedicle had begun to crystallize. McGregor and Morgan had hinted at it in 1960 (43). Ten years later, McGregor and Jackson proposed that one could outline self-contained vascular territories (44). They referred to work by Shaw, who, together with Payne, had described such a flap based on the superficial epigastric arterial and venous system (45). The technique was developed for care of the wounded during World War II. Other developments in tissue transfer in hand surgery were described in the volumes on hand surgery in World War II (see below).

General plastic surgery as a discipline made enormous strides during this war. For example, at the beginning of the war, there were only four fully experienced plastic surgeons in Great Britain: Gillies, McIndoe, Mowlem, and Kilner. This nucleus of surgeons and their trainees established plastic surgical centers throughout Great Britain, and each made major contributions to the field.

In the United States, Fomon's 1939 *The Surgery of Injury and Plastic Repair* (46) and Barsky's *Principles and Practice of Plastic Surgery* (47) appeared at the beginning of World War II. During the war, Ivy and a group of plastic surgical luminaries wrote two manuals on plastic and maxillofacial surgery for use by military surgeons (48). Plastic surgical centers such as the one at Valley Forge General Hospital were spawning grounds for consolidation of reconstructive strategies. James Barrett Brown, Sheehan, McDowell, Tanzer, Littler, and Cannon exemplify what could be an enormous list of contributors. Books by Sheehan (49), Ivy (50), Kazanjian and Converse (51), May (52), New and Erich (53), Padgett and Stephenson (54), Pick (55), and Smith (56), among others, were published after experiences during the war.

McGregor et al. described the anatomic basis for a flap based on the superficial circumflex iliac vessels (57), the classic McGregor or groin flap. The groin flap has been a mainstay in reconstructive hand surgery (58,59). The terms *random* and *axial* were applied to flaps in McGregor and Morgan's paper in 1973 (60,61).

Early in the twentieth century, the carrying pedicle for random or chance axial pedicle flaps was large and flat. It was refined to a closed tube independently by the Russian Filatov in 1917 (62) and by Gillies at about the same time (20,63,64). Pedicle flaps with identifiable blood vessels had become the rule wherever possible.

Sterling Bunnell's second edition of *Surgery of the Hand* (65) drew heavily from experiences in hand centers during World War II. It was filled with a variety of types of pedicle flaps, as well as his additional technical modifications of the tubed-pedicle flap technique.

William L. White put together an organized review of flap grafts (66) for a meeting that he organized and chaired in Pittsburgh in 1959.

With waltzing, jumping, and tubing, the transfer of tissues from place to place in endless combinations (67), including composites of skin, fascia, muscle (68), and bone, was firmly established (69).

ISLAND PEDICLE FLAP

Since the turn of this century, further refinement of the carrying pedicle had reached the point where flaps are transferred regularly on vascular and neurovascular bundles. The principle of transfer without an intact epithelialized skin pedicle was initiated by Robert Gersuny, of Vienna. In 1887, he published a description of the transfer of a composite flap of soft tissue from the neck to the oral lining of the cheeks (70) carried on a very narrow pedicle of dermis and subdermal vessels from the periosteum of the mandible. This was a one-stage transfer of a pedicle flap without an intact skin pedicle and without specifically identifiable blood vessels.

In August of 1882, Theodore Dunham, of New York, excised a large epidermoid cancer of the cheek and eyelid. He raised a flap from the forehead, and in his publication (71) said, "This flap was so cut as to contain traversing its pedicle and ramifying in it, the anterior temporal artery." Three days after the first procedure, Dunham dissected out the vascular pedicle and buried it beneath the skin of the cheek. The skin pedicle was returned to its donor site. This was the first recorded two-stage island pedicle flap preserving the transferred blood supply intact.

However, it was Monks in 1898 who repaired the defect resulting from an excision of a lower eyelid epithelioma and who first reported a one-stage island pedicle flap (72). He illustrated the procedure that same year in the *Boston Medical and Surgical Journal*. Shelton Horsely beautifully illustrated the use of a forehead flap carried on temporal vessels in a paper in the *Journal of the American Medical Association* in 1915 (73).

J. F. S. Esser, publishing in the *New York Journal of Medicine* in 1917 (74), pointed out that during his care of wounded soldiers in Austria, he often used flaps from the neck directly under the jawline near the external maxillary artery. These flaps had no skin pedicle, but a carrying arm consisting of soft tissue that contained the external maxillary artery. Said Esser, "I called them 'island flaps' because after being placed in the facial defect resulting when scars are removed, they give the effect of a free transplantation."

There was renewed interest in the island pedicle flap for a variety of uses in the sixties (75–80). For example, temporal arterial island flaps found a place in eyebrow reconstruction and for coverage of difficult areas requiring a permanently transferred blood supply.

In this contemporary period of hand surgery, the biologic or island pedicle flap described earlier was first applied to the hand. Erik Moberg (81), discussing a paper by Donal Brooks on nerve grafting (82) at the annual meeting of the American Orthopaedic Association at Bretton Woods, New Hampshire, in 1954, suggested that neurovascular flap techniques were useful in restoring stereognosis to the hand. He showed some exemplary cases. Littler discussed uses of the neurovascular island 2 years later, and Tubiana et al. (79,80), Frackelton and Teasley (83), Holevich (84), Hueston (85), O'Brien (86), Lewin (87), Peacock (78), Winsten (88), and many, many others (89) published ingenious applications of the versatile techniques. Littler reviewed the development in detail during his Monk's Lecture delivered in Boston in 1982 (90).

The versatile island flap (91) could be used as part of a carrier for a nerve transfer to innervate an intact but anesthetic digit tip. It could be used to bring cover and blood supply to a badly damaged devascularized finger. It was useful in transferring composite parts of useless digits to restore others, including whole joints. Many hand surgeons have pointed to its efficacy in the restoration of protective and useful sensibility and blood supply in osteoplastic thumb reconstruction (92–100).

MUSCLE AND MUSCULOCUTANEOUS FLAPS

The first published, planned muscle flap was that of Louis Ombredanne of Paris in 1906 (101). He described a pectoralis minor flap for breast reconstruction, turning down the humeral insertion of the pectoralis minor to recreate a breast mound following mastectomy.

Tanzini introduced a latissimus dorsi muscle flap for breast reconstruction in 1906 (102). The first true musculocutaneous flap was that described in detail in 1912 by Professor Stefano d'Este and published in a monumental paper on chest-wall reconstruction after mastectomy (103). He used the latissimus dorsi and showed the anatomy of both a musculocutaneous flap and an axial flap of skin alone from the same area. Illustrated examples were shown.

The roots, then, were well set at the beginning of the century for refinement of the principles of the modern muscular and musculocutaneous flaps that have become so popular and important in the current era. The interest in muscle and musculocutaneous flaps was renewed when Neal Owens in 1955 suggested the use of a compound neck pedicle composed of the sternocleidomastoid muscle overlying platysma, subcutaneous tissue, and skin in the reconstruction of major facial defects (104).

Ralph Ger, of Capetown, showed the virtue of muscle transfer for coverage of difficult areas in the distal lower limb in a seminal paper in 1966 (105). Shortly thereafter, Miguel Orticochea, of Bogota, Columbia, described the musculocutaneous flap method (106). He presented the technique, using a gracilis musculocutaneous flap as a cross-leg flap with success.

Typically, the empirical but logical use of muscle alone (107) and muscle with overlying skin led to possible application of that principle throughout the body (108–113). For example, after sporadic reports of muscle flaps and musculocutaneous flaps, McCraw and Dibbell outlined possible independent myocutaneous flaps (114); then, fasciocutaneous flaps (115,116) were launched (117–119). Muscles with nutrient vessels are usable as pedicles to carry substantial skin and soft tissue. As an example, the rectus abdominis muscle with its superior epigastric vascular leash may be used to carry a large transverse segment of soft tissue (120), that is axial on its ipsilateral and random on its contralateral side, from the lower abdomen to the breast area.

Credit goes to Elliott and Hartrampf for championing this remarkable transfer of tissue (121). Muscle and musculocutaneous flaps have found multiple uses in upper limb surgery, and even intrinsic muscles are useful as muscle or musculocutaneous carriers (122). Hentz et al. (123) showed the use of the abductor digiti minimi as a musculocutaneous flap within the hand.

FREE COMPOSITE-TISSUE TRANSFER WITH IMMEDIATE REVASCULARIZATION

Once the pedicle for transfer was refined to require only blood vessels with or without sensory nerves, the only remaining deterrent to unlimited anatomic transfer of composite tissues was the length of vascular tether. It followed predictably that the next advance would be an assault on that deterrent. The answer would come from refinements of techniques described by Carrell at the turn of the century (124,125), made possible by the advent of the operating microscope.

Stimulated by the possibilities offered by microsurgery reported by Jacobson and Suarez from Burlington, Vermont (126), Buncke and Schultz (127) worked tirelessly with methods to improve sutures and instruments. Their influence on Berish Strauch, Avron Daniller, Donald Murray, and others in our Stanford laboratories resulted in rat renal transplant developments and rat limb replants.

Clinically, Komatsu and Tamai's thumb replantation in 1968 (128) ushered in the new era of digit replantation (129–132). Buncke et al. reported their one-stage Nicoladoni thumb reconstruction, transferring a big toe to the thumb position in monkeys (133), and Cobbett soon thereafter reported a successful clinical case of such a free digital toe-to-hand transfer (134). The procedure is now well established in hand surgery (135–137).

Berish Strauch and Donald Murray (138), stimulated by the work of Harry Buncke, worked out and reported the transfer of groin skin flaps to the neck in rats.

With that background, and with knowledge of Goldwyn, Lamb, and White's experiments (139) and the vascularized island experiments of Krizek et al. (140), Kaplan, Buncke, and Murray attempted and reported a free flap from the groin to an intraoral site in 1971 (141). The flap survived for 2½ weeks, but it failed to heal to the poorly vascularized recipient bed. Rollin Daniel, after hearing the paper reporting the case, was stimulated to persevere. When the opportunity arose, he and Ian Taylor tried again and reported the first successful free-flap transfer in 1971 (142).

There followed a rash of reports of free groin flap transfers in hand surgery (143–149). The clear advantages of such free flaps are that they supply skin and soft-tissue cover with permanent arterial blood supply and sometimes sensibility in a single stage. Subsequent tendon grafts then may restore extension function. The flap may be a composite of skin and soft tissue with tendons to eliminate the need for later tendon grafting, or it may carry bone as well (150). Morrison et al. have introduced us to the wraparound free composite flap in thumb reconstruction (151)—a modification that Lister, Steichen, and others have used to restore a thumb tip and nail. Free microvascular transfers apply to any part or composite of parts whose viability may be maintained by isolated vessels (152–154).

FREE FUNCTIONAL MUSCLE AND MUSCULOCUTANEOUS FLAPS WITH IMMEDIATE REVASCULARIZATION

The first reported attempts to free transfer skeletal muscle were those of Noel Thompson (155), who startled those attending the Fifth International Congress of Plastic and Reconstructive Surgery in Melbourne in 1971 by showing a technique of free transfer of the palmeris longus or intrinsic foot muscles (the extensor digitorum brevis) to the face (156) without surgical revascularization. After transfer, the patients regained function through muscular neurotization. In 1975, Gerhard Freilinger, of Vienna, did similar free muscle grafts (157), innervating them with nerve grafts from the contralateral facial nerve.

Meanwhile, Tamai and colleagues had been experimenting with free muscle transfers with microvascular and microneural anastomoses in dog rectus femoris muscles (158). They showed survival of the transferred muscles with an interval of denervation atrophy followed by recovery of innervation at about 3 months. They suggested the use of such transfers in humans.

Harii et al. reported free gracilis muscle transfers to the face using microvascular and microneural revascularization and innervation techniques with success (159). They suggested that the principle of free revascularized and reinnervated muscle transfers "would find broad use in recontructive surgery."

Ralph Manktelow, of Canada, having seen some examples of free vascularized muscle transfers at the Sixth People's Hospital in Shanghai and having carried out some animal experiments in his laboratory, started to build a series of free, revascularized, and reinnervated muscle transfers in the upper limb of selected patients. In 1978, at the annual meeting of the American Society for Surgery of the Hand, Manktelow and McKee reported their experience with free musculocutaneous transfers, using a gracilis muscle in one patient and a pectoralis muscle in another, transferred to restore finger flexion (160). The feasibility and growing reliability of these free muscle and musculocutaneous transfers (161–163), as prophetically stated by Harii et al. (159), obviously will have a "wide range of applications in reconstructive surgery."

It has taken the perseverance and faith of a Harry Buncke (164), the energetic aggressiveness of a Bernie O'Brien (165), the patience and technical expertise of Tamai and Harii (166), the organization of the Kleinert (167), Kutz (168), and Lister groups, and the ever-growing list of young microsurgeons (169) to take the early work of Jacobson and Suarez and to place it firmly in the armamentarium of reconstructive surgeons. These pioneers found their greatest pleasure in doing what people said could not be done (170).

Work with venous flaps and arteriovenous flaps is moving from the laboratory to clinical application, one more step toward broadening the armamentarium of the reconstructive surgeon.

There appear to be inexhaustible imaginations among surgeons developing new and innovative flaps for use in every part of the body. Progressive liberation from the large carrying pedicle to the refined vascularized and innervated island flaps to vascularized free flaps has opened the way for near-infinite variations in flap design. New additions to these volumes cover the broad spectrum of composite-tissue transfers in reconstructive surgery. The elders in the field look with a mixture of amazement and envy at surgeons active in the development of new strategies to deal with old problems. In facial, neck, intraoral, esophageal, breast, upper and lower limb, abdominal-wall, genital, and anal reconstruction, there have been new reconstructive techniques added to those in the first edition of this encyclopedia.

The advent of anesthesia opened the way for a flood of new operative procedures in the second half of the 19th century. The evolution of microsurgery in this century has been responsible for the current plethora of new techniques. It is my firm belief that the next wave of innovations will emerge as a result of progress in the related field of transplantation. Solutions for the residual immunologic problems in transplantation will prepare the way for a torrent of procedures based on knowledge of techniques developed by surgeons devoted to the field of composite-tissue transfer.

Meanwhile, exhaustive studies of gross and microscopic vascular anatomy, exemplified by Taylor's mapping of neurovascular territories (171), coupled with anatomic studies to clarify the spectacular advances in imaging, feed into the growing armamentarium available to today's reconstructive surgeons.

References

1. Wallace AF. History of plastic surgery. *J R Soc Med* 1978;71:834.
2. Zies E. *The Zeiss index and history of plastic surgery, 900 B.C. to 1863 A.D.,* Vol. 1. Baltimore: Williams & Wilkins, 1977.
3. Tagliacozzi G. *De curtorum chirurgia per institione,* Vol. 2. Venice: 1597.
4. *Gentleman's Magazine.* London, October 1974;891.
5. Carpue JC. An account of two successful operations for restoring a lost nose from the integuments of the forehead. London: 1816.
6. von Graefe CF. *Rhinoplastik.* Berlin: 1818.
7. Zeis E. *Handbuch der Plastischen Chirurgie.* Berlin: 1818.
8. Warren JM. *Boston Med Surg J* 1837.
9. Fricke JCG. *Die Bildung neuer Augenlider (Blepharoplastik) nach Zerstorungen und dadurch hervorge-brachten Auswartswendungen derselben.* Hamburg: 1829.
10. Malgaigne JF. *Manuel de médecine operatoire.* Brusells: 1834.
11. Hamilton FH. Elkoplasty: on ulcers treated by anaplasty. *NY J Med* 1854.
12. Prince D. *Plastics: a new classification and a brief exposition of plastic surgery.* Philadelphia: Lindsay and Blakiston, 1868.
13. Shrady G. The finger as a medium for transplanting skin flaps. *Med Rec* 1891.
14. Halsted W. Plastic operation for extensive burn of neck. *Johns Hopkins Hosp Bull* 1896.
15. Blair VP. The delayed transfer of long pedical flaps in plastic surgery. *Surg Gynecol Obstet* 1921;3:261.
16. Hoffmeister FS. Studies on timing of tissue transfer in reconstructive surgery. *Plast Reconstr Surg* 1957;19:283.
17. Patterson TIS, Berry RJ, Wiernik G. The effect of x-radiation on the survival of skin flaps in the pig. *Br J Plast Surg* 1972;25:17.
18. Colson P, Houot R, Gangolphe M, et al. Utilisation des lambeaux degraisses (lambeaux-greffes) en chirurgie reparatrice de la main. *Ann Chir Plast* 1967;12:298.
19. Jobert AJ. (de Lamballe). *Traité de chirurgie plastique.* Paris: Bailliere, 1849.
20. Gillies HD. Present-day plastic operation of the face. *J Natl Dent Assoc* 1920;1:3.
21. Gillies HD. *Plastic surgery of the face.* London: Frowde, 1920.
22. Blair VP. *Surgery and diseases of the mouth and jaws.* St. Louis: Mosby, 1912.
23. Boo-Chai K. John Wood and his contributions to plastic surgery: the first groin flap. *Br J Plast Surg* 1977;30:9.
24. Wood J. Fission and extroversion of the bladder with epispadias with the results of 8 cases treated by plastic operations. *Med Chir Trans* 1869;2:85.
25. Davis JS. The use of the pedunculated flap in reconstructive surgery. *Ann Surg* 1918;68:221.
26. Germany W, Finesilver EM, Davis JS. Establishment of circulation in tubed skin flaps. *Arch Surg* 1933;26:27.
27. Roberts JB. Salvage of the hand by timely reparative surgery. *Ann Surg* 1919;70:627.
28. Albee FH. Synthetic transplantation of tissues to form a new finger. *Ann Surg* 1919;69:379.
29. Skillern PG Jr. A surgical clinic at Polyclinic Hospital. *Int Clin* 1919;3:75.
30. Steindler A. *Reconstructive surgery of the upper extremity.* New York: Appleton, 1923.
31. Steindler A. *A textbook of operative orthopedics.* New York: Appleton, 1925.
32. Kanavel AB. *Infections of the hand,* 5th ed. Philadelphia: Lea & Febiger, 1925.
33. Iselin M. *Chirurgie de la main: plaies, infections, chirurgie reparatrice.* Paris: Masson, 1933.
34. Iselin M. *Surgery of the hand, wounds, infections and closed tramata.* Philadelphia: Blakiston, 1940.
35. Cutler CW Jr. *The hand: its disabilities and diseases.* Philadelphia: Saunders, 1942.
36. Gibson T, Robinson DW. The mammary artery pectoral flaps of Jacques Joseph. *Br J Plast Surg* 1976;29:370.
37. Joseph J. *Nasenplastik und sonstige Gesichtsplastik nebst einem Anhang ueber Mammaplastik und einige weitere Operationem aus dem Gebiete der ausseren Korper Plastik.* Leipzig: Verlag von Curt Kapitzsch, 1931.
38. Bakamjian VY. A two-stage method for pharyngoesophageal reconstruction with a primary pectoral skin flap. *Plast Reconstr Sutg* 1965;36:173.
39. Bakamjian VY, Long M, Rigg B. Experience with the medially based deltopectoral flap in reconstructive surgery of the head and neck. *Br J Plast Surg* 1971;24:174.
40. McGregor IA, Jackson IT. The extended role of the deltopectoral flap. *Br J Plast Surg* 1970;23:173.
41. Milton SH. Pedicled skin flaps: the fallacy of the length-width ratio. *Br J Surg* 1970;57:502.
42. Stell PM. The viability of skin flaps. *Ann R Coll Surg Engl* 1977;59:236.
43. McGregor I. Flap reconstruction in hand surgery: the evolution of presently used methods. *J Hand Surg* 1979;4B:1.
44. McGregor IA, Jackson IT. The groin flap. *Br J Plast Surg* 1972;25:3.
45. Shaw DT, Payne RL. One-stage tubed abdominal flaps: single-pedicle tubes. *Surg Gynecol Obstet* 1946;83:205.
46. Fomon S. *The surgery of injury and plastic repair.* Baltimore: Williams & Wilkins, 1939.
47. Barsky AI. *Principles and practice of plastic surgery.* Philadelphia: Saunders, 1938.
48. Ivy RH. *Manual of standard practice of plastic and maxillofacial surgery.* Philadelphia: Saunders. 1942.
49. Sheehan JE. *General and plastic surgery with emphasis on war injuries.* New York: Hoeber and Harper, 1945.

50. Ivy RH, Curtis L. *Fractures of the jaws.* Philadelphia: Lea & Febiger, 1945.
51. Kazanjian VH, Converse JM. *The surgical treatment of facial injuries.* Baltimore: Williams & Wilkins, 1949.
52. May H. *Reconstructive and reparative surgery.* Philadelphia: Davis, 1947, 1958.
53. New GB, Erich JB. *The use of pedicle flaps of skin in plastic surgery of the head and neck.* Springfield, Ill.: Charles C. Thomas, 1950.
54. Padgett EC, Stephenson KL. *Plastic and reconstructive surgery.* Springfield, Ill.: Charles C. Thomas, 1948.
55. Pick JF. *Surgery of repair: principles, problems, procedures,* Vols. 1 and 2. Philadelphia: Lippincott, 1949.
56. Smith F. *Plastic and reconstructive surgery.* Philadelphia: Saunders, 1950.
57. Smith PJ, Foley B, McGregor IA, et al. The anatomical basis of the groin flap. *Plast Reconstr Surg* 1972;49:41.
58. Heath PM, Jackson IT, Cooney WP, et al. Simultaneous bilateral staged groin flaps for coverage of mutilating injuries of the hand. *Ann Plast Surg* 1983;11:462.
59. Lister GD, McGregor IA, Jackson IT. The groin flap in hand injuries. *Injury* 1973;4:229.
60. McGregor IA, Morgan G. Axial and random pattern flaps. *Br J Plast Surg* 1973;26:202.
61. Smith PJ. The vascular basis of axial pattern flaps. *Br J Plast Surg* 1973;26:150.
62. Filatov VP. Plastic procedure using a round pedicle. *Surg Clin North Am* 1959;39:277.
63. Gillies HD. The tubed pedicle in plastic surgery. *NY Med J* 1920;11:1.
64. Webster JP. The early history of the tubed pedicle flap. *Surg Clin North Am* 1959;39:261.
65. Bunnell S. *Surgery of the hand,* 2d ed. Philadelphia: Lippincott, 1948.
66. White WL. Flap grafts to the upper extremity. *Surg Clin North Am* 1960;40:389.
67. Holevich J. Our technique of pedicle skin flaps and its use in the surgery of the hand and fingers. *Acta Chir Plast* 1960;24:271.
68. Hokin JAB. Mastectomy reconstruction without a prosthetic implant. *Plast Reconstr Surg* 1983;72:810.
69. Gilles H. Autograft of amputated digit. *Lancet* 1940;1:1002.
70. Gersuny R. Plastischer Ersatz der Wangenschleimhaut. *Zentralbl Chir* 1887;14:706.
71. Dunham T. A method for obtaining a skin flap from the scalp and a permanent buried vascular pedicle for covering defects of the face. *Ann Surg* 1893;17:677.
72. Monks GH. The restoration of a lower eyelid by a new method. *Boston Med Surg J* 1898;139:385.
73. Horsley JS. Transplantation of the anterior temporal artery. *JAMA* 1915;64:408.
74. Esser JFS. Island flaps. *NY Med J* 1917;106:264.
75. Chase RA. Expanded clinical and research uses of composite tissue transfers on isolated vascular pedicles. *Am J Surg* 1967;114:222.
76. Kuei SJ, Chen EC, Li SY. The use of temporal artery pedicle skin flaps in the repair of facial burns and other deformities. *Chin Med J* 1964;83:65.
77. Murray JF, Ord JVR, Gavelin GE. The neurovascular island pedicle flap: an assessment of late results in sixteen cases. *J Bone Joint Surg* 1967;49A:1285.
78. Peacock EE. Reconstruction of the hand by the local transfer of composite-tissue island flaps. *Plast Reconstr Surg* 1960;25:298.
79. Tubiana R, DuParc J. Restoration of sensibility in the hand by neurovascular skin island transfer. *J Bone Joint Surg* 1961;43B:474.
80. Tubiana R, DuParc J, Moreau C. Restauration de la sensibilité au niveau de la main par transfert d'un transplant cutané heterodigital muni de son pedicule vasculo-nerveux. *Rev Chir Orthop* 1960;46:163.
81. Moberg E. Nerve-grafting in orthopedic surgery. *J Bone Joint Surg* 1955;37A:305.
82. Brooks DM, Seddon HJ. Pectoral transplantation for paralysis of the flexors of the elbow. *J Bone Joint Surg* 1959;41B:36.
83. Frackelton WH, Teasley JL. Neurovascular island pedicle: extension in usage. *J Bone Joint Surg* 1962;44A:1069.
84. Holevich J. A new method of restoring sensibility to the thumb. *J Bone Joint Surg* 1973;45B:496.
85. Hueston J. The extended neurovascular island flap. *Br J Plast Surg* 1965;18:304.
86. O'Brien B. Neurovascular pedicle transfers in the hand. *Aust NZ J Surg* 1965;35:1.
87. Lewin ML. Sensory island flap in osteoplastic reconstruction of the thumb. *Am J Surg* 1965;109:226.
88. Winsten J. Island pedicle to restore stereognosis in hand injuries. *N Engl J Med* 1963;268:124.
89. Rose EH. Local arterialized island flap coverage of difficult hand defects preserving donor digit sensibility. *Plast Reconstr Surg* 1983;72:848.
90. Littler JW, George H. Monks lecture: man's thumb, nature's special endowment. Harvard Medical School, October 2, 1982.
91. Chase RA. *Atlas of hand surgery,* Vol. 1. Philadelphia: Saunders, 1973.
92. Chase RA. An alternate to pollicization in subtotal thumb reconstruction. *Plast Reconstr Surg* 1969;44:412.
93. Dykes ER. Reconstruction of the thumb. *Hawaii Med J* 1967;27:33.
94. Floyd WE. Reconstruction of the thumb. *J Med Assoc Ga* 1968;57:425.
95. Greeley PW. Reconstruction of the thumb. *Ann Surg* 1946;124:60.
96. McGregor IA, Simonetta C. Reconstruction of the thumb by composite bone-skin flap. *Br J Plast Surg* 1964;17:37.
97. Reid DAC. The neurovascular island flap in thumb reconstruction. *Br J Plast Surg* 1966;19:234.
98. Suzuki T, Takahashi T, Chang S, et al. Reconstruction of the thumb. *Jpn Med J* 1967;41:1013.
99. Woudstra ST. Reconstruction of the thumb. *Arch Chir Med* 1967;19:29.
100. Murray JF, Ord JVR, Gavelin GE. The neurovascular island pedicle flap: an assessment of late results in sixteen cases. *J Bone Joint Surg* 1967;49A:1285.
101. Teimourian B, Adham MN. Louis Ombredanne and the origin of muscle flap use for immediate breast mound reconstruction. *Plast Reconstr Surg* 1983;72:905.
102. Tanzini. Sporo il nito nuova proceso di aupertozione della menuelle. *Riforma Med* 1906;22:757.
103. d'Este S. La technique de l'amputation de la mamelle pour carcinome mammaire. *Rev Chir* 1912;45:164.
104. Owens N. A compound neck pedicle designed for the repair of massive facial defects: formation, development and application. *Plast Reconstr Surg* 1955;15:369.
105. Ger R. The operative treatment of the advanced stasis ulcer. *Am J Surg* 1966;111:659.
106. Orticochea M. The musculocutaneous flap method: an immediate and heroic substitute for the method of delay. *Br J Plast Surg* 1972;25:106.
107. Minami RT, Hentz VR, Vistnes LM. Use of vastus lateralis muscle flap for repair of trochanteric pressure sores. *Plast Reconstr Surg* 1977;60:364.
108. Carroll RE, Kleinman WB. Pectoralis major transplantation to restore elbow flexion to the paralytic limb. *J Hand Surg* 1979;4A:501.
109. Chase RA, Nage DA. Cosmetic incisions and skin, bone, and composite grafts to restore function of the hand. In: *American academy of orthopaedic surgeons instructional course lectures.* Chap. 6. St. Louis: Mosby, 1974.
110. Hovnanian AP. Latissimus dorsi transplantation for loss of flexion or extension of the elbow. *Ann Surg* 1956;143:493.
111. Jackson IT, Pellett C, Smith, JM. The skull as a bone graft donor site. *Ann Plast Surg* 1983;11:527.
112. Stern PJ, Neale HW, Gregory RO, et al. Latissimus dorsi musculocutaneous flap for elbow flexion. *J Hand Surg* 1982;7:25.
113. Zancolli E, Mitre H. Latissimus dorsi transfer to restore elbow flexion. *J Bone Joint Surg* 1973;55A:1265.
114. McCraw JB, Dibbell DG. Experimental definition of independent myocutaneous vascular territories. *Plast Reconstr Surg* 1977;60:212.
115. Barclay TL, Sharpe DT, Chisholm EM. Cross-leg fasciocutaneous flaps. *Plast Reconstr Surg* 1983;72:843.
116. Fonseca JLS. Use of pericranial flap in scalp wounds with exposed bone. *Plast Reconstr Surg* 1983;72:786.
117. Grabb WC, Myers MB, eds. *Skin flaps.* Boston: Little, Brown, 1975.
118. Mathes SJ, Nahai F. *Clinical atlas of muscle and musculocutaneous flaps.* St. Louis: Mosby, 1979.
119. McCraw JB, Dibbell DG, Carraway JH. Clinical definition of independent myocutaneous vascular territories. *Plast Reconstr Surg* 1977;60:341.
120. Bunkis J, Walton RL, Mathes SJ, et al. Experience with the transverse lower rectus abdominis operation for breast reconstruction. *Plast Reconstr Surg* 1983;72:819.
121. Elliott LF, Hartrampf CR. Tailoring of the new breast using the transverse abdominal island flap. *Plast Reconstr Surg* 1983;72:887.
122. Reisman NR, Dellon AL. The abductor digiti minimi muscle flap: a salvage technique for palmar wrist pain. *Plast Reconstr Surg* 1983;72:859.
123. Chase RA, Hentz VR, Apfelberg D. A dynamic myocutaneous flap for hand reconstruction. *J Hand Surg* 1980;5A:594.
124. Carrel A. La technique operatoire des anastomoses vasculaires et la transplantation des viscere. *Lyon Med* 1920;98:859.
125. Carrel A. Results of the transplantation of blood vessels, organs and limbs. *JAMA* 1908;51:1662.
126. Jacobson JH, Suarez EL. Microsurgery in the anastomosis of small vessels. *Surg Forum* 1960;11:243.
127. Buncke HJ, Schulz WP. Total ear reimplantation in the rabbit utilizing microminiature vascular anastomoses. *Br J Plast Surg* 1966;19:15.
128. Komatsu S, Tamai S. Successful replantation of a completely cut-off thumb. *Plast Reconstr Surg* 1968;42:374.
129. Chen ZW, Meyer VE, Kleinert HE, et al. Present indications for replantation as reflected by long-term functional results. *Orthop Clin North Am* 1981;12:849.
130. Gelberman RH, Urbaniak JR, Bright DS, et al. Digital sensibility following replantation. *J Hand Surg* 1978;3A:313.
131. Weiland AJ, Daniel RK, Riley LH. Application of the free vascularized bone graft in the treatment of malignant or aggressive bone tumor. *Johns Hopkins Med J* 1977;140:85.
132. Vilkki S. Replantation studies on clinical replantation surgery with reference to patient selection, operative techniques and postoperative control. *Acta Univ Tamperensis (A)* 1983;156.
133. Buncke HJ, Buncke CM, Schulz WP. Immediate Nicoladoni procedures in the rhesus monkey, or hallux-to-hand transplantation, utilising microminiature vascular anastomoses. *Br J Plast Surg* 1966;19:332.
134. Cobbett JR. Free digital transfer: report of a case of transfer of a great toe to replace an amputated thumb. *J Bone Joint Surg* 1969;51B:677.

135. Buncke HJ, McLean DH, Geroge PT, et al. Thumb replacement: great toe transplantation by microvascular anastomosis. *Br J Plast Surg* 1973;26:194.

136. O'Brien BM, MacLeod AM, Sykes PJ, et al. Microvascular second toe transfer for digital reconstruction. *J Hand Surg* 1978;3A:123.

137. Ohtsuka H, Torigai K, Shioya N. Two toe-to-finger transplants in one hand. *Plast Reconstr Surg* 1977;60:51.

138. Strauch B, Murray DE. Transfer of composite graft with immediate suture anastomosis of its vascular pedicle measuring less than 1 mm in external diameter using microsurgical techniques. *Plast Reconstr Surg* 1967;40:325.

139. Goldwyn RM, Lamb DL, White WL. An experimental study of large island flaps in dogs. *Plast Reconstr Surg* 1963;31:528.

140. Krizek TJ, Tani R, Desprez JD, et al. Experimental transplantation of composite grafts by microsurgical vascular techniques. *Plast Reconstr Surg* 1965;36:538.

141. Kaplan EN, Buncke HJ, Murray DE. Distant transfer of cutaneous island flaps in humans by microvascular anastomoses. *Plast Reconstr Surg* 1973;52:301.

142. Taylor GI, Daniel RK. The free flap: composite tissue transfer by vascular anastomosis. *Aust NZJ Surg* 1973;43:1.

143. Ohmori K, Harii K, Sekiguchi J, et al. The youngest free groin flap yet? *Br J Plast Surg* 1977;30:273.

144. Daniel RK, Terzis JK. *Reconstructive microsurgery*. Boston: Little, Brown, 1977.

145. Daniel RK, Weiland AJ. Free tissue transfers from upper extremity reconstruction. *J Hand Surg* 1982;7A:66.

146. Taylor GI, Townsend P, Corlett R. Superiority of the deep circumflex iliac vessels as the supply for free groin flaps: experimental work. *Plast Reconstr Surg* 1979;64:595.

147. Taylor GI, Townsend P, Corlett R. Superiority of the deep circumflex iliac vessels as the supply for free groin flaps: clinical work. *Plast Reconstr Surg* 1979;64:45.

148. Baudet J, LeMaire JM, Guimberteau JC. Ten free groin flaps. *Plast Reconstr Surg* 1976;57:577.

149. Brent B, Byrd HS. Secondary ear reconstruction with cartilage grafts covered by axial, random, and free flaps of temporoparietal fascia. *Plast Reconstr Surg* 1983;72:141.

150. Swartz WM. Immediate reconstruction of the wrist and dorsum of the hand with a free osteocutaneous groin flap. *J Hand Surg* 1984;9A:18.

151. Morrison WA, O'Brien BM, MacLeod, AM. Thumb reconstruction with a free neurovascular wrap-around flap from the big toe. *J Hand Surg* 1980;5A:575.

152. Van Genechten F, Townsend PLG. Free composite-tissue transfer in a compound hand injury. *Hand* 1983;15:325.

153. Taylor GI, Corlett R, Boyd JB. The extended deep inferior epigastric flap: a clinical technique. *Plast Reconstr Surg* 1983;72:751.

154. Fisher J, Cooney WP. Designing the latissimus dorsi free flap for knee coverage. *Ann Plast Surg* 1983;11:554.

155. Thompson N. Treatment of facial paralysis by free skeletal muscle grafts. In: *Transactions of the fifth international congress of plastic and reconstructive surgery*. Melbourne: Butterworth, 1971.

156. Smith JW. A new technique of facial animation. In: *Transactions of the fifth international congress of plastic and reconstructive surgery*. Melbourne: Butterworth, 1971.

157. Freilinger G. A new technique to correct facial paralysis. *Plast Reconstr Surg* 1975;56:44.

158. Tamai S, Komatsu S, Sakamoto H, et al. Free muscle transplants in dogs with microsurgical neurovascular anastomoses. *Plast Reconstr Surg* 1970;46:219.

159. Harii K, Ohmori K, Torii S. Free gracilis muscle transplantation with microvascular anastomoses for the treatment of facial paralysis. *Plast Reconstr Surg* 1976;57:133.

160. Manktelow RT, McKee NH. Free muscle transplantation to provide active finger flexion. *J Hand Surg* 1978;3A:416.

161. Ikuta Y, Kubo T, Tsuge K. Free muscle transplantation by microsurgical technique to treat severe Volkmann's contracture. *Plast Reconstr Surg* 1976;58:407.

162. Manktelow RT, Zuker RM, McKee NH. Functioning free muscle transplantation. *J Hand Surg* 1984;9A:32.

163. Terzis JK, Dykos RW, Williams HB. Recovery of function in free muscle transplants using microneurovascular anastomoses. *J Hand Surg* 1978;3A:37.

164. Bunke HJ. Cobbett JR, Smith JW, et al. *Techniques of microsurgery*. Sommerville, NJ: Ethicon, 1969.

165. O'Brien BM, Miller GDH. Digital reattachment and revascularization. *J Bone Joint Surg* 1973;55A:714.

166. Tamai S, Hori Y, Tatsumi Y, et al. Hallux-to-thumb transfer with microsurgical technique: a case report in a 45-year-old woman. *J Hand Surg* 1977;2A:152.

167. Kleinert HE, Kasdan ML, Romero JL. Small blood vessel anastomosis for salvage of severely injured upper extremity. *J Bone Joint Surg* 1963;45A:788.

168. Kutz JE, Dimond M. Replantation in the upper extremity. *Surg Rounds* 1982;14:9.

169. Strauch B. Microsurgical approach to thumb reconstruction. *Orthop Clin North Am* 1977;8:319.

170. Ikuta Y. Free flap transfer: historical review, surgical procedures and some clinical cases. *Hiroshima J Med Sci* 1976;25:29.

171. Taylor GI, Gianoutsos MP, Morris SF. The neurovascular territories of the skin and muscles: anatomic study and clinical implications. *Plast Reconstr Surg* 1994;94:1.

CONTENTS

VOLUME I: HEAD AND NECK

SECTION 1: HEAD AND NECK RECONSTRUCTION

PART A ■ SCALP, FOREHEAD, AND NAPE OF NECK RECONSTRUCTION

PART B ■ EYELID AND ORBITAL RECONSTRUCTION

Lower Eyelid

PART C ■ NASAL RECONSTRUCTION

Nasal Tip, Dorsum, and Alae

Nasal Columella

PART E ■ CHEEK AND NECK RECONSTRUCTION

Cheek and Neck

PART F ■ LIP RECONSTRUCTION

PART G ■ INTRAORAL RECONSTRUCTION

PART H ■ PHARYNGOESOPHAGEAL

VOLUME II: UPPER EXTREMITIES

SECTION II: UPPER EXTREMITY RECONSTRUCTION

PART A ■ FINGER AND THUMB RECONSTRUCTION

Fingertip

Finger

Thumb Tip

PART B ▪ HAND

VOLUME III: TORSO, PELVIS, AND LOWER EXTREMITIES
SECTION III: BREAST, CHEST WALL, AND TRUNK RECONSTRUCTION
PART A ■ BREAST RECONSTRUCTION

Breast Mound

Nipple

PART B ■ AXILLA AND CHEST WALL RECONSTRUCTION

SECTION IV: ABDOMINAL WALL AND PELVIC-REGION RECONSTRUCTION

PART A ABDOMINAL WALL AND GROIN RECONSTRUCTION

PART B ■ VAGINAL, VULVAR, AND PERINEAL RECONSTRUCTION

PART C ■ PENILE, SCROTAL, AND PERINEAL RECONSTRUCTION

PART D ■ ANAL RECONSTRUCTION

PART E ■ LUMBOSACRAL RECONSTRUCTION

SECTION V: LOWER EXTREMITY RECONSTRUCTION

PART A LOWER LEG AND KNEE RECONSTRUCTION

PART B ■ FOOT AND ANKLE RECONSTRUCTION

HEAD AND NECK RECONSTRUCTION

CHAPTER 1 ■ SCALP FLAPS AND THE ROTATION FOREHEAD FLAP

E. F. WORTHEN

The table of contents for this text reveals a dizzying array of skin flap titles. Names ascribed to flaps over the years have resulted in a confusing adulteration as each designer seeks to single out a particular flap from all the rest. In this preliminary chapter, an attempt is made to define the true distinctions in the nomenclature of skin flaps.

"A flap is a flap is a flap," as one might well paraphrase Gertrude Stein. All skin flaps share the common feature of a transferable segment of skin with a pedicle of continuing blood supply. Flaps may be *local* or *distant* (depending on the proximity of the donor site to the defect), random or axial (a distinct vascular stem is identifiable in the axial as opposed to an anastomosing dermal network in the random), *peninsular* or *island* (the skin bridge is preserved over the pedicle in the peninsular). Anatomic location may identify a flap [groin, scapular, transverse rectus abdominus myocutaneous (TRAM), and so on]. Imaginative and picturesque names have been used to describe the shape of flaps like clouds in the sky (e.g., banana peel, seagull, pinwheel). Flaps may be designated by ethnic origin (Indian flap); others, perhaps with a thought toward posterity, bear the name of the designer.

Scalp flaps, whenever possible, should be local flaps because of the singularity of the hair-bearing surface. Massive defects may require the use of distant skin, but a compromised aesthetic result is inevitable. For this reason, the remainder of this chapter is confined to consideration of local flaps (Fig. 1). While axial and island flaps may be used for specialized needs, only basic peninsular flaps are discussed.

INDICATIONS

The choice between use of a transposition flap or a rotation flap is most often influenced by the size and nature of the defect. When the defect is large enough, a simple transposition flap ensures the greatest margin of safety because of direct, straight-line flow of the blood supply. A skin graft will be needed to close the flap donor site. When the defect is small and closure of the secondary wound by primary suture is possible, the rotation flap facilitates the adjustment of tension and uneven wound margins.

ANATOMY

A *peninsular* scalp flap is a segment of cutaneous cover composed of a full thickness of epidermis and dermis with an independent territory of vascularity consisting of a subdermal plexus with afferent arterial supply and efferent venous drainage. The scalp is a unique and specialized integument in which hair shafts penetrate a thick dermis into a highly vascular subcutaneous layer densely bound to a base of flat, rigid aponeurosis. This base, the galea aponeurotica, is the tendinous apparatus through which the frontalis and occipitalis muscles activate the scalp. This motion is a gliding action of the galea over the underlying pericranium allowed by a gossamer webbing of loose areolar strands in the subaponeurotic layer. This latter plane is essentially avascular, rendering the scalp independent of the pericranium beneath it and thereby facilitating flap transfer.

The arteries of the scalp and their accompanying veins originate peripherally and ascend to the dome in bilateral fashion (1) (Fig. 2); thus, it is preferable to base scalp flaps peripherally. In the younger patient, there is widespread anastomosis of the end vessels at the vertex, which provides greater latitude of safety in flap design, even permitting retrograde flaps based on this rich vascularity at the vertex. This latter advantage is not

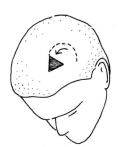
Rotation flap

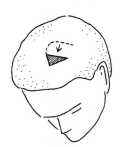
Transposition flap

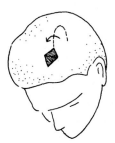
Interpolation flap

FIG. 1. Types of local scalp flaps.

3

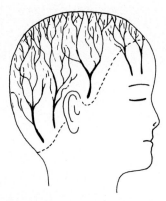

FIG. 2. Pattern of blood supply of the scalp with points of penetration from the deeper tissues located at the lower end of each vessel. These vessels from anterior to posterior are supratrochlear, supraorbital, superficial temporal, posterior auricular, and occipital.

enjoyed by the older patient in whom arteriosclerosis diminishes these end vessels. One may surmount even this obstacle by including a large artery in the base of the flap together with delay of the flap. This has been demonstrated with the transfer of postauricular skin on a pedicle extending across the dome to the contralateral superficial temporal vessels (2). Successful microvascular replantation in which the entire scalp and one ear survived on a singular artery and vein reanastomosis has been reported (3,4).

DESIGN OF THE PENINSULAR FLAP

The forehead and scalp constitute a single anatomic unit differentiated only by the location of the hairline. Preservation of this hairline in a normal configuration is a primary consideration because it creates the frame of the upper face in the frontal and temporal areas. Disruption and asymmetry of this frame are to be avoided.

The rigidity of the scalp does not lend itself to some of the more popular and useful flaps, such as the rhomboid flap, which require plasticity of the surrounding tissue for closure of the donor site. For this reason, one is limited to transposition, interpolation, or rotation flap design (see Fig. 1). During the following discussion, one must bear in mind that although geometry offers a worthwhile foundation for understanding basic flap design, it is best replaced with an artistic eye once the basic tenets have been mastered.

Transposition Flaps

This design offers the simplest and safest form of peninsular flap in that the axis of blood supply is compromised minimally (Fig. 3B). After the site of origin for a transposition flap has been determined, the recipient defect should be converted to an appropriate form, usually a triangular line of excision outside the borders of the defect (Fig. 4A). This triangle should be right-angled wherein the hypotenuse becomes the near margin of the flap. The right angle of the defect assumes a position opposite the flap. The apex C should be directed toward the periphery of the scalp. The pivot point D will be located on a linear extension across the base of the flap parallel to AB at a distance from the apex at least equal to AB. From point D, a linear projection is developed parallel to AC (Fig. 4B). With point D as the axis, an arc is drawn from point A to the intersection with DE. The area ABF (Fig. 4C) is excised after seating the flap in place (Fig. 4D).

The disadvantage of the traditional transposition flap is the inability to close the donor area. As shown in Fig. 4D, closure of the donor defect would result in a force in the same direction as the flap movement, which is not possible. Thus, the defect requires supplemental coverage, usually in the form of a skin graft.

Interpolation Flaps

These flaps are similar to the transposition flap but differ in that the axis of blood supply rotates to a greater degree (Fig. 3C). Although this may introduce the question of vascular compromise, the interpolation flap offers the opportunity to close the donor site primarily, particularly if preceded by skin expansion. The interpolation flap may be cut in any form and rotated through any arc desired, but it is characterized by "skipping over" normal scalp during the transfer.

Rotation Flaps

Preparation of the rotation flap again requires conversion of the defect to triangular form. In this case, the triangle must be isosceles with its apex C directed toward the base of the future pedicle of the flap (Fig. 5A). Apex C should be limited to an angle of 30 degrees to minimize "buckling" at this point after closure. Pivot point D will be located on a projection of line AC. Line CD must be at least 50% longer than AC. Midway between A and D, a point is designated, which becomes the center for an arc drawn from B to D that completes the outline for the flap (Fig. 5B). This flap offers primary closure of the

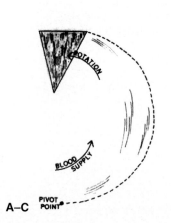

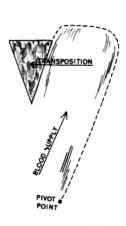

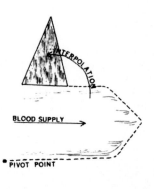

FIG. 3. A–C: Relationship between direction of flap transfer and arterial blood flow.

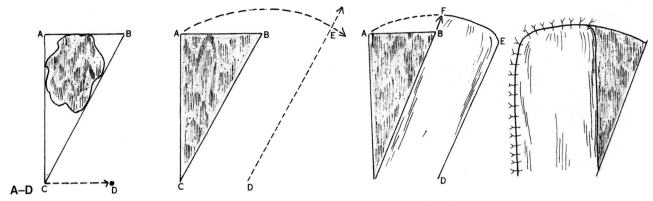

FIG. 4. **A–D:** Design and transfer of the transposition flap.

secondary defect by distributing tension over a wide and linear area.

OPERATIVE TECHNIQUE

Preoperative shaving of the hair is unnecessary. As opposed to most skin incisions, scalp incisions should be beveled at an angle parallel to the hair shafts to avoid a linear hairless scar. As shown in Fig. 6, a traditional vertical incision ab will interrupt the hair follicles in segment c. The resulting hairless scar becomes an artificial "part" that may be unsatisfactory to the patient.

As the incision is continued through the galea, the avascular subaponeurotic layer affords quick and easy separation by blunt dissection. Although bleeding from the wound margin is frequently profuse, it can be controlled readily by pressure and plastic clips without the need for ties or cautery. Definitive hemostasis is accomplished later with closure of the wound. Relaxing or "gridiron" incisions in the rigid galea are used frequently but will permit only 1 mm of extension for each incision. Scalp expanders may be used to good advantage to facilitate scalp closure in larger defects. The lack of elasticity in the scalp will create a buckling effect or dog-ear at the base of a flap with rotation greater than 30 degrees. Smaller redundancies will diminish with time, but larger ones may require secondary excision. Closure of the scalp should be performed in two layers beginning with suture of the galea aponeurotica followed by closure of the integument.

Forehead Rotation Flap

The entire forehead is available as an arterialized flap based on the superficial temporal artery to reconstruct forehead defects involving up to 40% of the surface area. As illustrated in Fig. 7A, the superior border of a forehead rotation flap is developed in the hair-bearing scalp and traverses the frontal scalp to the preauricular crease (5).

Elevation of the flap is accomplished easily down to the supraorbital rim, resulting in a "free-swinging" extensile segment of tissue. After mobilization is complete, back-cutting of the base is permissible but rarely necessary. Once the flap has been rotated to the desired position, the hairline on the distal margin of the flap is aligned with and sutured to the temporal hairline on the lateral margin of the defect (Fig. 7B).

The forehead defect is closed without tension, often with a suture line oriented transversely, to minimize the only portion of scar that will be visible on the exposed forehead. The secondary frontal scalp defect extends across the entire width of the frontal scalp but is relatively narrow and amenable to primary closure by relaxation and advancement of the scalp posterior to the defect (Fig. 7C). The effectiveness of this flap is shown in Fig. 8.

CLINICAL RESULTS

Because of the great vascularity of the forehead rotation flap, necrosis and infection rarely pose a significant problem. The

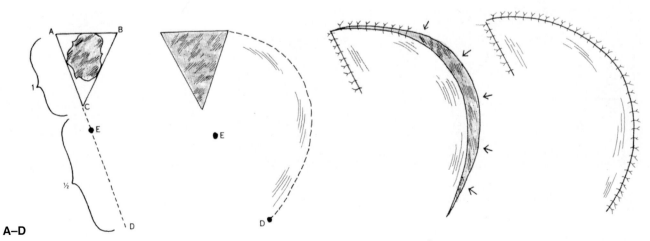

FIG. 5. **A–D:** Design and transfer of the rotation flap.

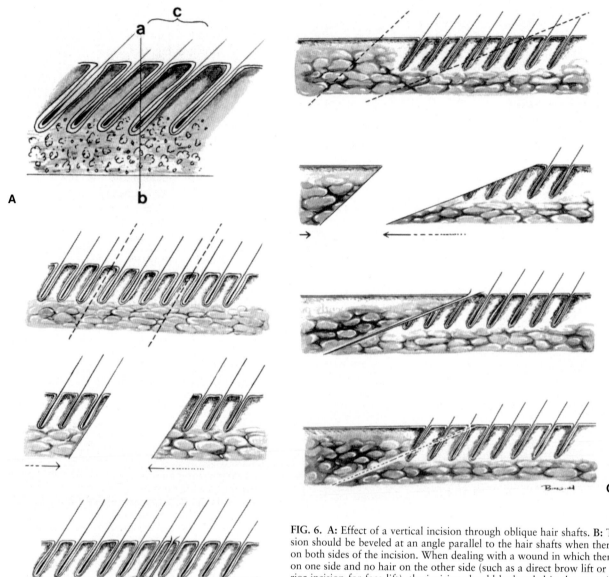

FIG. 6. **A:** Effect of a vertical incision through oblique hair shafts. **B:** The incision should be beveled at an angle parallel to the hair shafts when there is hair on both sides of the incision. When dealing with a wound in which there is hair on one side and no hair on the other side (such as a direct brow lift or an anterior incision for face lift), the incision should be beveled in the opposite direction. This cuts the hair shafts and leaves the follicles intact. **C:** The hairless skin then is brought over the cut hair shafts. When the wound heals, the hair shafts grow out through the overlying intact skin and help disguise the incision.

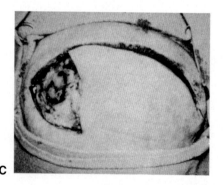
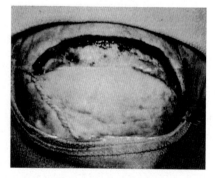
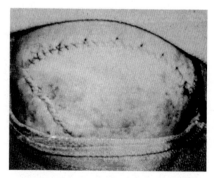

FIG. 7. **A:** Incision for forehead rotation flap. **B:** Reestablishment of temporal hairline and closure of original defect. **C:** Completion of wound closure.

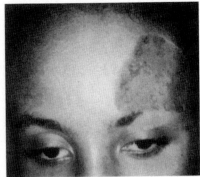 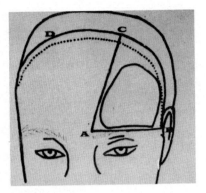 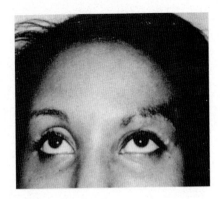

A–C

FIG. 8. A: Unsightly split-thickness skin graft of forehead. An area as large as 40% of the forehead can be reconstructed with a forehead rotation flap. B: Outline of forehead rotation flap within the scalp and area of excision. C: Final result. (From Worthen, ref. 5, with permission.)

only disadvantages encountered are lateral displacement of a prominent widow's peak, which is easily minimized by hairstyling, and temporary asymmetry of the forehead furrows when these are deep and prominent.

SUMMARY

The basic principles involved in transposition and rotation flaps are described and can be applied to scalp defects. The rotation flap can be used effectively to close large forehead defects. Cosmetic results are excellent.

References

1. Corso PF. Variations of the arterial, venous and capillary circulation of the soft tissues of the head by decades, as demonstrated by the methacrylate injection technique, and their applications to the construction of flaps and pedicles. *Plast Reconstr Surg* 1961;27:160.
2. Galvao MSL. A postauricular flap based on the contralateral superficial temporal vessels. *Plast Reconstr Surg* 1981;68:891.
3. Miller GDH, Anstee EJ, Snell JA. Successful replantation of an avulsed scalp by microvascular anastomoses. *Plast Reconstr Surg* 1976;58:133.
4. Nahai F, Hurteau J, Vasconez L. Replantation of an entire scalp and ear by microvascular anastomoses of only one artery and one vein. *Br J Plast Surg* 1978;31:339.
5. Worthen EF. Repair of forehead defects by rotation of local flaps. *Plast Reconstr Surg* 1976;57:204.

CHAPTER 2 ■ MULTIPLE PINWHEEL SCALP FLAPS

T. R. VECCHIONE

The removal of scalp lesions with primary closure can tax the imagination and ingenuity of the surgeon. Lesions greater than 3.0 cm in diameter sometimes require extensive mobilization of surrounding tissues and/or elaborate flap designs for closure. The literature is filled with variations of transposition and rotation flaps for these situations (1–3).

This is not a new method, but a practical variation on a well-established theme. This application is a multiflap closure, and it takes on a pinwheel or camera-shutter configuration.

INDICATIONS

This method takes advantage of a full 360° of mobilization of the surrounding tissues. Excision and linear closure move tissue in only two directions. There is essentially no elasticity of the scalp, and complete mobilization of flaps of surrounding tissue is necessary even for short tissue advancement. If the lesion is simply removed and closed in a

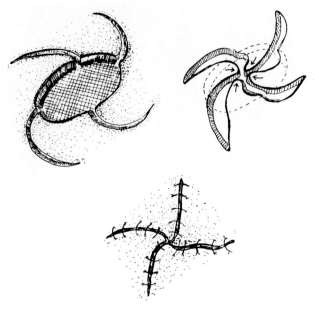

FIG. 1. The inscription of the four arcs can be geometrically constructed using the technique described in the text.

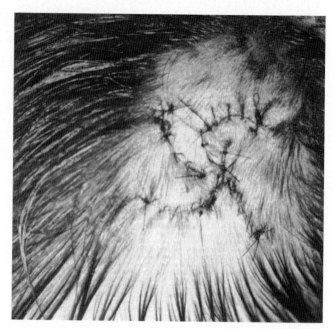

FIG. 2. An infiltrating squamous cell carcinoma was excised resulting in a 4.5- to 3.8-cm defect to periosteum. The four rotational flaps close the lesion without excessive overhang. The apices of all the flaps are held at the midpoint by one subcuticular suture. The minor change in direction of hair follicles has not been a significant problem.

straight line, a significant amount of normal tissue must be removed.

The advantages of this pinwheel method are as follows:

1. Minimal undermining
2. Ease in design
3. No excessive excision of normal tissue (apart from minimal recontouring of small dog-ears)
4. The distribution of tension over four radiating suture lines instead of one.

ANATOMY

The multiflap closure in a pinwheel fashion can be used anywhere on the scalp, since the mobility and blood supply are relatively uniform (see Chap. 1).

FLAP DESIGN AND DIMENSIONS

Limberg's extensive studies of transposed triangular flaps have been used for many years in the closure of 60° rhomboid defects (1,4,5). The use of multiple Limberg flaps for closure has been described (2). This basic principle is the point around which many variations have been built. This presentation is one of those variations.

The two coordinated movements, a lateral movement and a rotation, are the basics of this plastic surgical principle. The "standing cones" or dog-ears at the flap bases have to be trimmed, but these are not large because four flaps are rotated, thus dissipating the cervical distortion at the flap base.

In constructing the spiral arms of the pinwheel, what is needed is a simple, yet accurate, geometric method that does not require tedious calculations or complex templates. Most spirals, including the spiral of Archimedes and the logarithmic spiral, require construction using a polar-coordinate system. However, the curve of an involute of a circle is easily constructed and seems ideal for a practical solution to the pinwheel flap arms.

This is most easily done by unwinding a thread wrapped around a cylinder of a diameter that is approximately twice the diameter of the excised lesion. If a marking pencil tip is placed in a loop at the distal end of the string as the taut string

is unwound from the cylinder, the curve of an involute of a circle is produced that is ideal for producing the arms of the pinwheel flap. By repeating the procedure four times starting at 0°, 90°, 180°, and 270° on the excised circle, the four arms are created (Fig. 1). Once the principle of flap design is mastered, free-hand flap construction can be equally effective. The diameter of twice the excised lesion diameter was chosen because a smaller diameter produced too small a flap pedicle and a diameter greater than twice the excised diameter produced too small an arc for proper rotation.

CLINICAL RESULTS

The rounded edges, broad base, and smaller arc of rotation make this method relatively free of complications. Edge necrosis has been encountered only in a very small percentage of cases. The vascularity of the scalp, along with the integrity, inelasticity, and thickness of the tissue, accounts for the clinical success of this procedure (Fig. 2).

SUMMARY

A pinwheel variation in design of multiflap closure in the inelastic scalp tissue is presented.

References

1. Limberg AA. Design of local flaps. In: Gibson T, ed. *Modern trends in plastic surgery,* 2d Ed. London: Butterworth, 1966.
2. Lister GD, Gibson T. Closure of rhomboid skin defects: the flaps of Limberg and Dufourmental. *Br J Plast Surg* 1972;25:300.
3. Brobyn T, Cramor L, Hulnick S, Rodsi M. Facial resurfacing with the Limberg flap. *Clin Plast Surg* 1976;3:481.
4. Limberg AA. *Mathematical principles of local plastic procedures on the surface of the human body.* Leningrad: Medgis, 1946.
5. Jervis W, Salyer KE, Vargas-Busquets MA, Atkins RW. Further applications of the Limberg and Dufourmentel flaps. *Plast Reconstr Surg* 1974;54:335.

CHAPTER 3 ■ "BANANA PEEL" SCALP, FOREHEAD, AND NAPE OF NECK FLAPS

M. ORTICOCHEA

The forehead and the nape of the neck have a surgical unity with the rest of the scalp, thus enabling reconstructive procedures to be carried out from one area to the other without separation between them (1–4).

ANATOMY

The cutaneous covering of the skull (Fig. 1) includes not only the hair-bearing skin, but also the forehead and the nape of the neck. The scalp itself is composed of (1) the hairy skin that covers the skull, (2) the subcutaneous adipose cellular tissue, (3) the underlying epicranial aponeurosis, (4) the subaponeurotic layer of loose connective tissue, and (5) the pericranium (external periosteum).

The location of vascular pedicles of the cutaneous covering of the skull is divided into three groups on the basis of which vessels they contain (Fig. 2).

Anterior Orbital Pedicle

The anterior orbital pedicle is made up of arteries and veins that reach the skin of the forehead from the orbital cavity and are collateral branches of the ophthalmic vessels. In the middle, they consist of the *supraorbital vessels*, the most important elements of this group. These vessels reach the forehead via the supraorbital foramen or supraorbital notch of the middle part of the supraorbital border. The notch is easily palpable. This pedicle also includes the *supratrochlear vessels* that reach the skin on the forehead through the medial part of the supraorbital border. When planning scalp flaps, one should take advantage of the fact that the vessels in this group are located in the central and medial part of the supraorbital border (Fig. 2A).

Lateral Pedicle

The lateral pedicle contains the *superficial temporal vessels*, terminal branches of the external carotid vessels, that reach the scalp after passing in front of the external ear (Fig. 2). In front of the superior pole of the ear, they divide into two branches: the frontal branch that proceeds forward, anastomosing with the supraorbital vessels, and the parietal branch that runs upward and backward and ends by anastomosing with the terminal branches of the occipital and posterior auricular arteries.

The superficial temporal vessels are the most important vascular elements to reach the cutaneous covering of the skull because (1) they are the longest vessels of the scalp and thus irrigate a large area of it, and (2) their easy mobilization allows them to be included in a variety of flaps (see Fig. 6).

The *posterior auricular vessels*, collateral branches of the external carotid vessels, reach the scalp just behind the external ear (Fig. 2B). These vessels pass the mastoid process of the temporal bone, branching through the scalp in back and above the external ear. They anastomose with the parietal branch of the superficial temporal vessels and with the occipital vessels. The posterior auricular pedicle is less important than the superficial temporal one, because it is of smaller caliber and has shorter branches that are mobilized with difficulty during surgery, since they are firmly attached in the mastoid auricular region.

Posterior Pedicle

The posterior vessels are made up of two groups. The upper group (Fig. 2B) corresponds to the two lateral and medial branches of the occipital vessels. These vessels, after running a horizontal trajectory under the insertion of the trapezius and

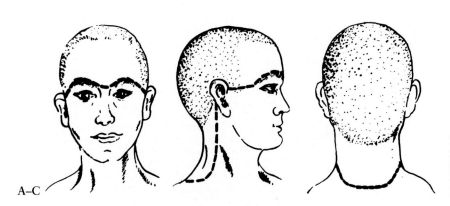

FIG. 1. Schematic representation of the external limits of the cutaneous covering of the skull. **A:** Anterior view. **B:** Lateral view. **C:** Posterior view. (From Orticochea, ref. 1, with permission.)

A–C

9

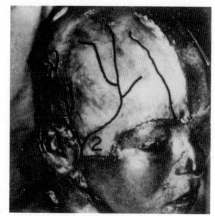
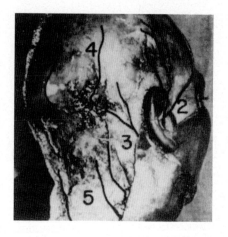

A,B

FIG. 2. A,B: Schematic representation of the circulation of the cutaneous coating of the skull: *(1)* supraorbital and supratrochlear vessels; *(2)* superficial temporal vessels; *(3)* posterior auricular vessels; *(4)* lateral and medial branches of occipital vessels; *(5)* multiple perforating vessels, which are collateral branches of the occipital, vertebral, and superficial cervical arteries. (From Orticochea, ref. 1, with permission.)

splenius muscles, come to the surface, crossing the trapezius muscle and rising to the scalp at a point above the superior nuchal line. The lower group (Fig. 2B) contains multiple perforating vessels that supply the skin that covers the neck muscles. These vessels reach the skin on the nape of the neck after running through the trapezius and splenius muscles. These multiple perforating vessels are collateral branches of (1) the occipital artery, (2) the posterior branches of the vertebral artery, and (3) the superficial cervical artery. They are of small caliber and short length. Thus, the skin on the nape of the neck has little circulatory autonomy in comparison with the scalp.

When a dissection is carried caudally, the scalp vessels course into a deeper layer—a fact of importance in the raising of scalp flaps. On reaching the external limits of the forehead and of the scalp dissection, the epicranial aponeurosis thins and disappears, and these vascular elements leave the cutaneous covering and pass to a deeper plane. The supraorbital and supratrochlear vessels follow the supraorbital margin and then enter the orbital cavity. The superficial temporal vessels reach the parotid region and go deeper, entering the parotid gland.

The posterior auricular vessels enter the scalp in a cephalic direction at the retroauricular space, and the occipital vessels enter the scalp under the insertions of the trapezius muscle. This is important to the surgeon, since a careful dissection with a blunt instrument must be made when lifting and dissecting the flaps of the scalp caudally in order not to damage the vessels where they pass from the forehead and the scalp to a deeper level, where they are firmly attached (Fig. 3).

Considering the cutaneous covering of the skull as a unity, there are five possible zones of raw surface to be reconstructed

and, therefore, five different applications of the three-flap technique: (1) forehead, (2) right temporal region, (3) left temporal region, (4) central region of the skull, and (5) nape of the neck.

FLAP DESIGN AND DIMENSIONS

To repair a very large defect of the cutaneous covering of the skull, we mobilize the entirety of what is left of the scalp, forehead, and nape of the neck, including these structures within three flaps. Each flap must have its own vascular pedicle as far as possible to ensure circulation. An exact knowledge of the anatomy of the cutaneous covering of the skull and the possible distribution of the vascular pedicles is extremely important in carrying out this operation.

Three-Flap Technique for a Central Scalp Defect

In cases of large defects in the central part of the scalp (Fig. 4), the rest of the cutaneous covering of the skull can be used to form three flaps—two anterior ones that are placed in the front part of the defect and a transverse flap that is placed in the back. In this way, we take advantage of two important aspects of the anatomy of the forehead, scalp, and nape of the neck: First, the secondary defect from the two anterior flaps can be covered with small split-thickness skin grafts (Fig. 5) that give the forehead an anatomic continuity. Second, the posterior transverse flap (3 in Fig. 2B) placed in back and

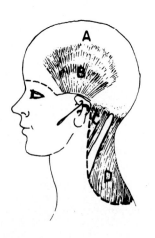
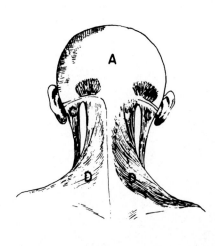

FIG. 3. Constitution of the osteomuscular sphere of the skull. *Left.* Lateral view: *(A)* osseous structures: frontal, parietal, and occipital bones; *(B)* temporal muscle covered by the temporal fascia; *(C)* sternocleidomastoid muscle; *(D)* trapezius muscle. *Right.* Posterior view: *(A)* occipital bone; *(C)* sternocleidomastoid muscle; *(D)* trapezius muscle. (From Orticochea, ref. 1, with permission.)

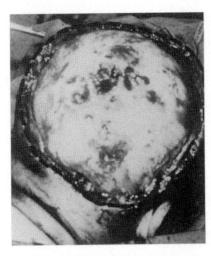

FIG. 4. After surgical extirpation of a large tumor, a broad surface in the central scalp remains to be reconstructed. The diameter of the raw surface is 24 cm, and its area is 452 cm². The pathologic specimen, when it contracted, was 18 cm in diameter. The diameter of the section of occipital bone that was removed was 10 cm. (From Orticochea, ref. 3, with permission.)

under the central defect allows us to use the abundant skin of the nape of the neck (Figs. 6 and 7).

The posterior transverse flap is situated at the nape of the neck and has its pedicle located in the retroauricular region, through which the occipital or posterior auricular vessels enter. This pedicle should be placed on the side opposite the raw surface to be reconstructed. Flap dimensions vary, depending on the size both of the patient's head and of the raw surface to be reconstructed.

The anteroposterior midline of the scalp is a place where vascular territories converge from both sides of the skull. It constitutes a physiologic barrier that limits the frontiers of these territories. This is why caution is necessary and why the posterior transverse flap should not be made too long.

Since the circulation in the skin of the nape of the neck is less than that in the scalp, and since this flap crosses the midline, necrosis at the end of the flap can occur. To avoid this, the surgeon should design the flap with a wide pedicle (Fig. 5D).

OPERATIVE TECHNIQUE

The epicranial aponeurosis is thick, resistant, and not very elastic. This is why the surgeon must make multiple shallow longitudinal incisions parallel to the longer axis in the epicranial

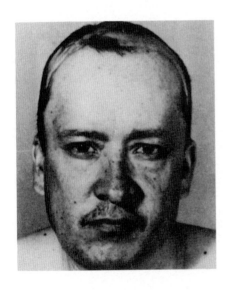

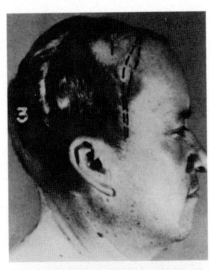

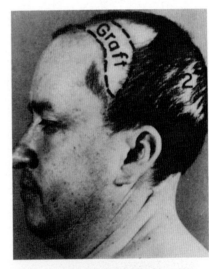

A–C

FIG. 5. Final result of surgery. It was necessary to place a small skin graft in the region adjoining the forehead. From an aesthetic viewpoint, this gives a very good result. (From Orticochea, ref. 3, with permission.)

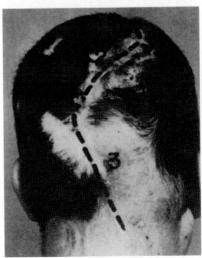

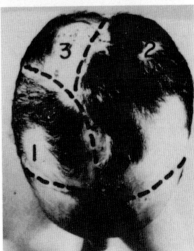

D,E

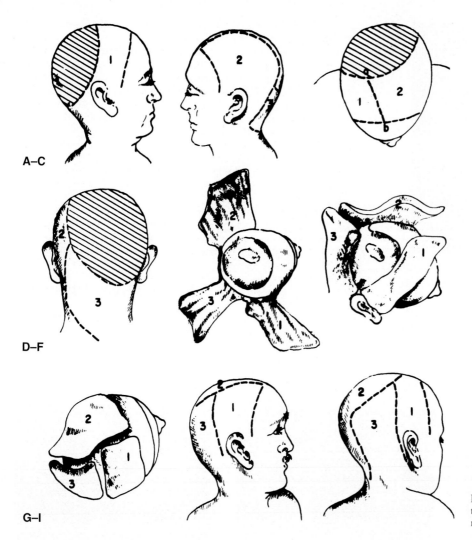

FIG. 6. A–I: Schematic development of the three-flap technique. (From Orticochea, ref. 3, with permission.)

aponeurosis of each of the flaps to facilitate their increased width (Fig. 6), making it possible for these multiple flaps to cover large defects. When doing this, the surgeon must be very careful not to section or damage the vessels that are very closely attached to the epicranial aponeurosis. The veins are of large caliber and have thin walls and thus can be easily damaged.

When incising the epicranial aponeurosis, it is easier to interrupt the venous circulation than the arterial circulation. Damaging the veins produces greater and more serious circulatory disturbances than damaging the arteries.

The vessels in the flap pedicles are very vulnerable for two reasons: (1) the epicranial aponeurosis becomes thin and dis-

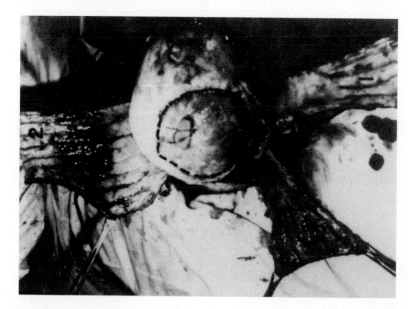

FIG. 7. The three flaps are stretched out. The epicranial aponeurosis has been divided with multiple shallow longitudinal incisions. The dotted line shows the zone of occipital bone that was removed. Inside the circle is that area that corresponds to the dura mater. (From Orticochea, ref. 3, with permission.)

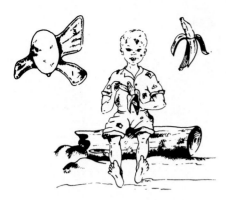

FIG. 8. The surgeon must move the cutaneous covering of the skull with the same facility with which a boy peels a banana. (From Orticochea, ref. 3, with permission.)

appears, and (2) the vessels pass from a superficial plane (scalp) to a deeper plane.

Three-Flap Technique for a Central Scalp Defect

The incision (Fig. 5C) that separates the two anterior flaps along the midline should be oblique, so that when the flaps are rotated and slid back, they will fit up against the posterior transverse flap (3 in Fig. 2B) when it is moved up and forward. The anterior flaps should be carefully undermined with blunt instruments, and great caution should be used when dissecting their pedicles, because the superficial temporal vessels and the posterior auricular vessels pass deeply and can be easily damaged.

The anterior flaps (1 and 2 in Fig. 2) and the posterior transverse flap (3 in Fig. 2B), once mobilized, should be interpolated and sutured without being submitted to exaggerated tension. When extensive surfaces of the scalp are being reconstructed, it will be necessary to cover small raw zones with free skin grafts.

SUMMARY

Large defects of the scalp can be closed using a three-flap technique that peels the skin off the skull as one would peel a banana (Fig. 8). This takes advantage of the excess skin that can be mobilized from the neck. The epicranial aponeurosis is also incised parallel to the vessels to allow many defects to be closed primarily. If the defect is large, however, a skin graft will be required.

References

1. Orticochea M. Flaps of the cutaneous covering of the skull. In: Grabb WC, Myers MB, eds., *Skin flaps*. Boston: Little, Brown, 1975:155–183.
2. Orticochea M. Four-flap scalp reconstruction technique. *Br J Plast Surg* 1967;20:159.
3. Orticochea M. New three-flap scalp reconstruction technique. *Br J Plast Surg* 1971;24:184.
4. Orticochea M. A pneumatic cranial tourniquet to control haemorrhage during operations on the scalp. *Br J Plast Surg* 1977;30:223.

CHAPTER 4 ■ TEMPOROPARIETO-OCCIPITAL AND TEMPOROPARIETO-OCCIPITOPARIETAL SCALP FLAPS

J. JURI

In the treatment of frontal or frontoparietal alopecias, the temporoparieto-occipital flap is the method of choice, since it provides enough hair to cover the alopecic area up to the contralateral region (1–6). The flap can be extended if necessary as the temporoparieto-occipitoparietal scalp flap (7–9).

INDICATIONS

These flaps have the valuable advantage that the donor area is closed by approximation of its edges, at the expense of a large retroauricular advancement flap.

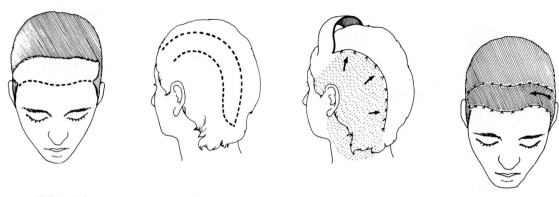

A–D

FIG. 1. Schematic representation of the temporoparieto-occipital flap. **A:** Design of the anterior implant line and recipient area. **B:** Flap design. **C:** Flap transposition and closure of the donor area with a large advancement flap (*arrows*). **D:** Flap in its final position and sutured to the recipient site. (From Juri et al., ref. 6, with permission.)

When the alopecia affects the frontal area (Figs. 1 and 2), only one flap will be required to close the defect. If the alopecia also involves the parietal region, a second flap from the contralateral zone is placed behind the first one a month later.

When a large area of central alopecia cannot be covered completely, an extended flap (Figs. 3 and 4) can be used not only to cover part of the defect, but also to help camouflage the remaining defect with an appropriate hairstyle.

ANATOMY

Both flaps are based on the superficial temporal vessels. The temporoparieto-occipitoparietal scalp flap, called the *encircling flap*, is made possible by the wide anastomotic net of the temporal vessels with the ipsilateral occipital ones and of the latter with the contralateral occipital vessels.

FLAP DESIGN AND DIMENSIONS

Temporoparieto-Occipital Scalp Flap

The glabrous surface to be resected is marked, taking the measurements of the flap to be designed (Fig. 1A). The flap base will be determined by the pulse of the superficial temporal artery, which is either palpated or marked using a Doppler probe 2 to 3 cm over the zygomatic arch. Then two points are marked, one on each side of the base point at a distance of 2 cm. These will indicate the width of the flap (4 cm), from which two parallel lines are drawn in an upper direction, along the parietal region, and down the occipital area (Fig. 1B). Although the viability of this flap is supported by its temporal pedicle, it is best to do one or two delays, especially if it is noted that the flap will suffer a slight torsion in the base during its transposition.

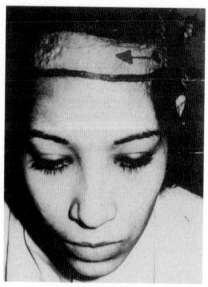
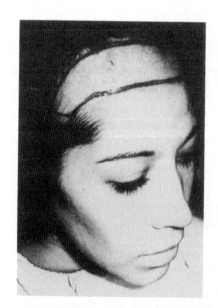
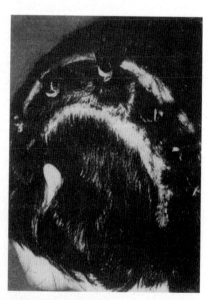

A–C

FIG. 2. **A:** Preoperative view. Design of the glabrous surface, which is going to be resected. (The *arrow* shows the direction of the flap.) **B:** Preoperative view. The extension of the glabrous surface that reaches the contralateral temporal region is observed. **C:** Design of the temporoparieto-occipital flap that is going to be transferred. (*continued*)

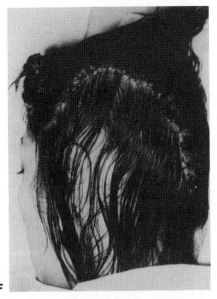
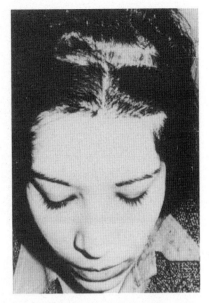
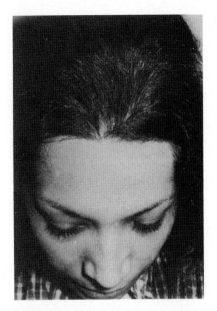

D–F

FIG. 2. *Continued.* **D:** Intraoperative view. Closure in two layers without tension in the donor site. **E:** Appearance of the flap after a week. **F:** Postoperative frontal view 5 years later. (From Juri et al., ref. 6, with permission.)

Temporoparieto-Occipitoparietal Scalp Flap

When the glabrous surface that extends from one temporal zone to the contralateral one is more than 25 cm long, the temporoparieto-occipital flap does not have enough length to reach the opposite hair-bearing region. In this case, a larger flap that will reach the contralateral parietal zone is required. Therefore, we employ the temporoparieto-occipitoparietal flap that is 30 to 32 cm long and 4 cm wide. The design of this flap is based on that of the preceeding flap, and it uses the remaining hair-bearing regions of the parietal, occipital, and contralateral parietal regions (Fig. 3B, C).

OPERATIVE TECHNIQUE

Temporoparieto-Occipital Scalp Flap

Once the flap is raised and before suturing it to the recipient site, a large retroauricular flap up to the base of the neck is made to take advantage of the elasticity of this region and to allow closure of the donor area without tension (Fig. 1C). Subsequently, the anterior edge of the flap is sutured to the frontal skin in only one layer. The skin of the forehead is brought over a de-epithelialized surface of 2 mm in the anterior

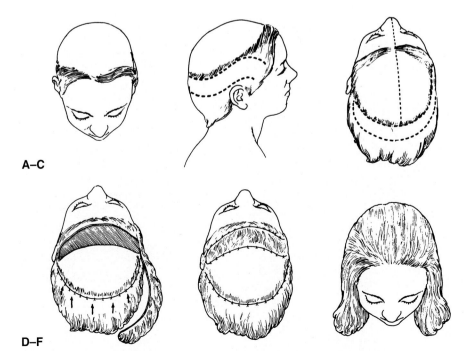

A–C

D–F

FIG. 3. Schematic representation of the temporoparieto-occipitoparietal flap. **A:** Extensive frontoparieto-occipital alopecia. **B:** Lateral view of the donor site and flap design. **C:** Superior and posterior views of the flap design. **D:** Raising of the flap, closure of the donor site, and resection of the frontal glabrous surface. **E:** Flap in its new position. **F:** Final appearance of the flap. (From Juri et al., ref. 6, with permission.)

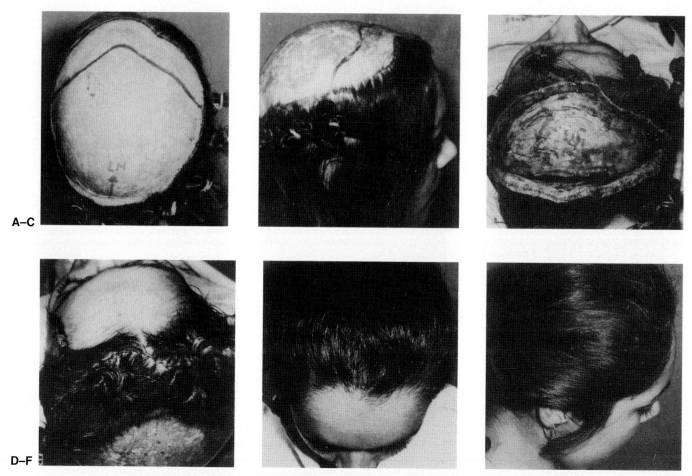

FIG. 4. A, B: Preoperative views. Preparation of the flap and the recipient site. **C:** Intraoperative view. Preparation of the frontal recipient site. **D:** Intraoperative view. Final suture of the flap in its new position. **E, F:** Postoperative frontal and lateral views 1½ years later. (From Juri et al., ref. 6, with permission.)

edge of the flap so as to avoid an uneven suture line. Then the remaining glabrous area is resected, and the posterior edge of the flap is sutured (Fig. ID).

Temporoparieto-Occipitoparietal Scalp Flap

Because of the great extension of this flap, we prefer to do two delays. The first delay includes both edges of the flap up to the contralateral occipital region, and the second delay, done a week later, involves the end of the flap (contralateral parietal region). A week later, the flap is raised from its bed and closure is done with a large advancement flap that contours all the donor area (Fig. 3D). The glabrous recipient zone is resected (Fig. 3D), and the flap is placed in its new position (frontal region), where it is sutured in only one dermal plane. In this manner, hair that was of little aesthetic value is transferred to the frontal region, which is aesthetically more important. This hair hides the remaining central alopecia.

SUMMARY

Both the temporoparieto-occipital flap and its extended counterpart, the temporoparieto-occipitoparietal flap, can be effec-

tively used to treat frontal and parietal alopecia in both male and female patients.

References

1. Juri J. Use of parieto-occipital flaps in the surgical treatment of baldness. *Plast Reconstr Surg* 1975;55:456.
2. Juri J, Juri C, de Antueno J, Gonzalez Otharan A. Surgical treatment of baldness. In: Sisson G, Tardy M, eds., *Plastic and reconstructive surgery of the head and neck*. (Proceedings of the Second International Symposium). New York: Grune & Stratton, 1977;221.
3. Juri J, Juri C, Arufe H. Use of rotation scalp flaps for the treatment of occipital baldness. *Plast Reconstr Surg* 1978;61:23.
4. Juri J. Use of pedicled flaps in the surgical treatment of alopecias. In: Unger WP, ed., *Hair transplantation*. New York: Marcel Dekker, 1979;143.
5. Juri C, Juri J, Colnago A. Monopedicled transposition flap for the treatment of scalp alopecias. *Ann Plast Surg* 1980;4:349.
6. Juri J, Juri C, Colnago A. Reconstruction of scalp hemicircumference. *Ann Plast Surg* 1980;4:304.
7. Juri J, Juri C. Aesthetic aspects of reconstructive scalp surgery. *Clin Plast Surg* 1981;8:243.
8. Juri J, Juri C. Two new methods for treating baldness: temporoparieto-occipitoparietal pedicled flap and temporoparieto-occipital free flap. *Ann Plast Surg* 1981;6:38.
9. Juri J, Juri C. Use of flaps in the surgical treatment of baldness. In: Vallis CP, ed., *Hair transplantation for the treatment of male pattern baldness*. Springfield, Ill.: Charles C. Thomas, 1982;545–556.

CHAPTER 5 ■ DIAGONAL FRONTOPARIETO-OCCIPITAL SCALP FLAPS

J. JURI

EDITORIAL COMMENT

The oblique flap does not ensure the inclusion of a known arterial pedicle or a way to extend it beyond its known blood supply. Consequently, the need for increasing care and delays is clear.

When alopecia affects the scalp hemicircumference, the only monopedicled flap that allows reconstruction of this region is a diagonal flap on a frontal pedicle (1–3).

ANATOMY

The diagonal frontoparieto-occipital scalp flap, which we call a *diagonal flap*, receives its blood supply from the frontal vessels. The area of convergence of the frontal branch of the superficial temporal artery and the supraorbital branches, because of their numerous connections with the contralateral vessels, allows the design of this flap across the midline (Fig. 1B, C). A second delay is performed at the end of the flap because of the perforating vessels in the occipital region.

FLAP DESIGN AND DIMENSIONS

This flap has a width of 3.5 to 4 cm, and its base is located in the frontal area next to the beginning of the alopecia (Fig. 1B). It extends over all the cranial vault, crossing the midline, and up to the hair-bearing retroauricular region (Fig. 1C). A flap is obtained with a length of 30 to 32 cm.

OPERATIVE TECHNIQUE

We do two delays. The first involves the flap edges, and the other, a week later, includes the last 3 cm at the end of the flap. A week after the second delay, the flap is raised from its bed and transposed to the recipient zone that has been designed to reconstruct the alopecic hemicircumference (Fig. 1D), an area of great aesthetic value. The donor site is closed by approximation of its edges (Fig. 1E), hiding the extensive alopecic surface in its central portion (Fig. 1F). Partial

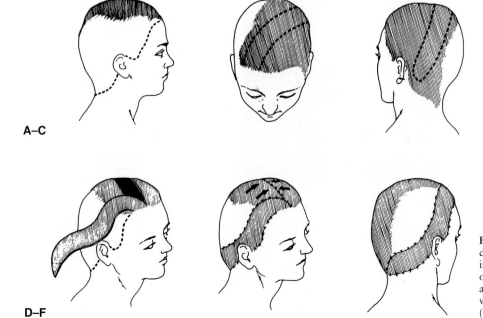

A–C

D–F

FIG. 1. Schematic representation of the diagonal flap. A: Alopecia and frontal implant line. B,C: Flap design. D: Raising of the flap. E: Closure of the donor site and final suture of the flap. F: Posterior view of the flap in its final position. (From Juri et al., ref. 2, with permission.)

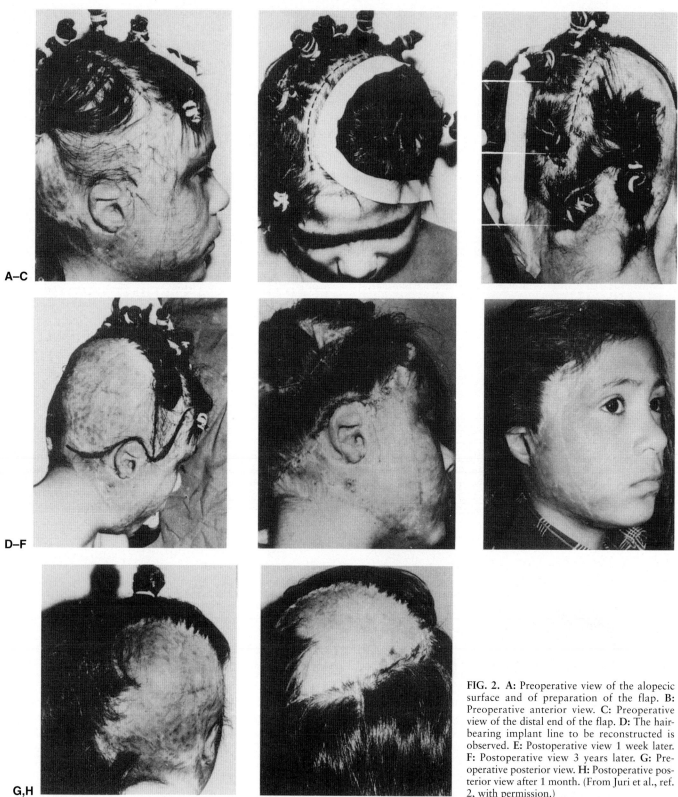

A–C

D–F

G,H

FIG. 2. **A:** Preoperative view of the alopecic surface and of preparation of the flap. **B:** Preoperative anterior view. **C:** Preoperative view of the distal end of the flap. **D:** The hair-bearing implant line to be reconstructed is observed. **E:** Postoperative view 1 week later. **F:** Postoperative view 3 years later. **G:** Preoperative posterior view. **H:** Postoperative posterior view after 1 month. (From Juri et al., ref. 2, with permission.)

successive resections of the residual alopecic area can be performed at later stages.

SUMMARY

The diagonal frontoparieto-occipital flap can be used to reconstruct the hairline from the frontal to the occipital region along one side of the scalp (Fig. 2).

References

1. Juri C, Juri J, Colnago A. Monopedicled transposition flap for the treatment of scalp alopecias. *Ann Plast Surg* 1980;4:349.
2. Juri J, Juri C, Colnago A. Reconstruction of scalp hemicircumference. *Ann Plast Surg* 1980;4:304.
3. Juri J, Juri C. Aesthetic aspects of reconstructive scalp surgery. *Clin Plast Surg* 1981;8:243.

CHAPTER 6 ■ TEMPOROPARIETAL (SUPERFICIAL TEMPORAL ARTERY) FASCIAL FLAP

H. S. BYRD

EDITORIAL COMMENT

Detailed studies of the temporoparietal area have resulted in some controversy over the number of layers. For clinical purposes, the author's description and guidelines are accurate and clinically safe.

The superficial temporal artery fascial flap is derived by dissecting the scalp away from its underlying subcutaneous fascia and the contained axial (superficial temporal) vessels, thereby creating a vascularized fascia that can be transferred about a single vascular pedicle.

INDICATIONS

This flap is useful in reconstructing defects of the forehead, eyebrow, eyelid, and ear (1–4) (see also Chap. 95). It also has been used to provide a vascular cover for bone grafts where an adequate soft-tissue bed does not exist.

ANATOMY

The temporoparietalis is a thin sheet arising from the temporal fascia above and anterior to the ear. It is divided into three parts that spread out like a fan over the temporal fascia. There is a temporal part anteriorly, a parietal part superiorly, and a triangular part between. The temporoparietalis inserts into the lateral border of the galea aponeurotica. The auricularis anterior and superior are recognized as small but inconstant muscle bellies that contribute to this layer.[1]

[1] The name of this layer was determined at the International Nomenclature Committee in Paris in July 1995 and was submitted under "Nomina Anatomica" to the Sixth International Congress of Anatomists in Paris, also in July 1955.

The key to the anatomy of the temporoparietal fascial flap is an understanding of the relationship of the superficial temporal vessels to the layers of the scalp (Fig. 1). The specific fascia carried by the superficial temporal vessels is the temporoparietalis fascia with its upper galeal aponeurotic extension. The temporoparietalis fascia must be distinguished from the denser and anatomically deeper temporalis fascia, which invests the temporalis muscle. Confusion arises at the level of zygoma, where both the temporalis and temporoparietalis fasciae attach.

At the level of the ear, the vessels are found deep to the subdermal fat and on the surface of the temporoparietalis fascia. At a level approximately 10 cm above the crus helix, the vessels take a more superficial course, penetrating the subdermal fat and eventually entering the subdermal plexus. While there is some variance in the level at which the axial vessels become contiguous with the subdermal plexus, generally this occurs 12 cm above the crus helix. At this level, a subdermal dissection violates the blood supply and thereby describes the limit of the fascial vascular domain.

FLAP DESIGN AND DIMENSIONS

The courses of the frontal branch, parietal branch, and posterior ramifications of the superficial temporal artery are identified with the Doppler probe. The axis of rotation is taken at a point in the preauricular fold anterior to the crus helix and overlying the tubercle of the zygomatic process of the temporal bone. A flap of sufficient length to reach the defect is obtained by measuring from the axis along the underlying vessels. If a flap length of more than 10 cm is required, the flap is extended by following the posterior branches of the temporal artery that communicate with the occipital vessels (Figs. 1 to 4).

OPERATIVE TECHNIQUE

An incision is made over the course of the superficial temporal vessels, just to the level of the dermis. The dissection is then

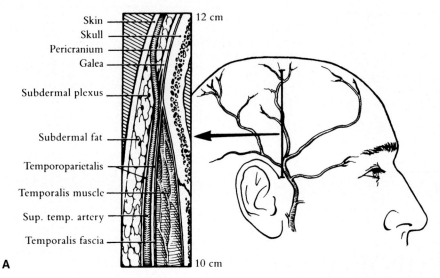

Skin
Skull
Pericranium
Galea
Subdermal plexus
Subdermal fat
Temporoparietalis
Temporalis muscle
Sup. temp. artery
Temporalis fascia

12 cm

10 cm

A

FIG. 1. A: Relationship of temporoparietal fascial flap to the layers of the scalp. Cross section of temporal scalp in the area between 10 and 12 cm above the crus helix. At the 10-cm point, the vessels are still on the surface of the temporoparietal fascia, but by the 12-cm point, the vessels have entered the more superficial subdermal plexus. **B:** Frontal and parietal branches of the superficial temporal artery and vein lying on the temporoparietal fascia. **C:** Layers of tissue in the temporal region. **D:** Arc of anterior rotation of the temporoparietal fascial flap. **E:** Posterior extension of the flap.

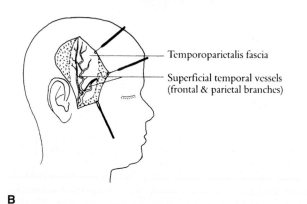

Temporoparietalis fascia

Superficial temporal vessels
(frontal & parietal branches)

B

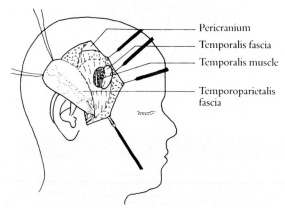

Pericranium
Temporalis fascia
Temporalis muscle
Temporoparietalis fascia

C

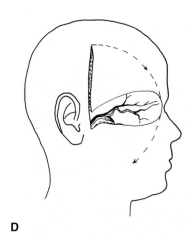

D

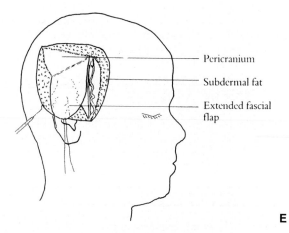

Pericranium

Subdermal fat

Extended fascial flap

E

carefully deepened through the subdermal fat in a plane that leaves the temporal vessels exposed on the surface of the temporoparietalis fascia. The subdermal fat remains on the skin. Numerous small perforating branches from the main axial vessels to the subdermal plexus must be divided and cauterized. Care should be taken not to interrupt the course of the primary vessels, either by a plane of dissection that is carried too deep or by imprecise cauterization.

A superior extension of the flap, requiring a transition in the plane of dissection through the subdermal fat to the base of the hair follicles, is now avoided. When greater flap lengths

are required, dissection is carried posteriorly (Fig. 1E), following the anastomotic arc between the occipital and superficial temporal vessels in a plane deep to the subdermal fat.

The posterior dissection is begun at approximately 5 cm above the ear and is continued to approximately 10 cm above the ear, creating a base 5 cm wide. The extended portion of the flap generally widens from this point in order to maximize the contribution of the vascular arcade. Scalp elevation sufficient to provide the necessary width and length is accomplished, and the subcutaneous fascia (galea and temporoparietalis fascia) is divided distally and along its lateral margins. Elevation

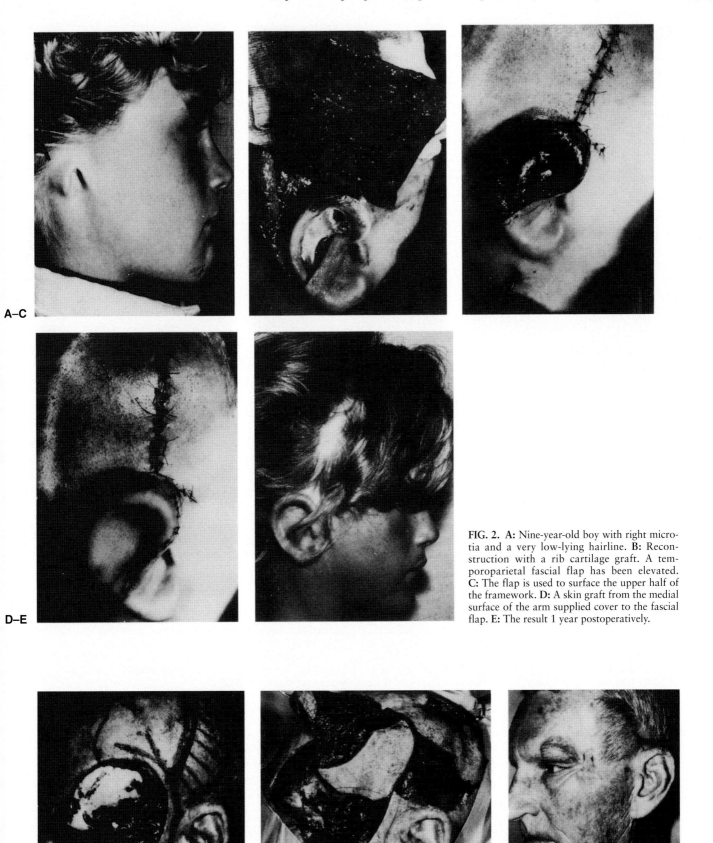

A–C

D–E

FIG. 2. A: Nine-year-old boy with right microtia and a very low-lying hairline. B: Reconstruction with a rib cartilage graft. A temporoparietal fascial flap has been elevated. C: The flap is used to surface the upper half of the framework. D: A skin graft from the medial surface of the arm supplied cover to the fascial flap. E: The result 1 year postoperatively.

A–C

FIG. 3. A: A large basal cell epithelioma was chemosurgically excised, resulting in exposed frontal bone and loss of the left eyebrow. B: An extended temporoparietal flap carrying an island of hair-bearing skin from the parieto-occipital area to serve as eyebrow and a segment of temporal scalp skin to replace sideburn was rotated into the defect. C: The result 4 months postoperatively. Note that the extended flap allows one to carry an island of skin from the posterior parieto-occipital scalp, affording hair growth in an upward and outward direction when transferred to the brow.

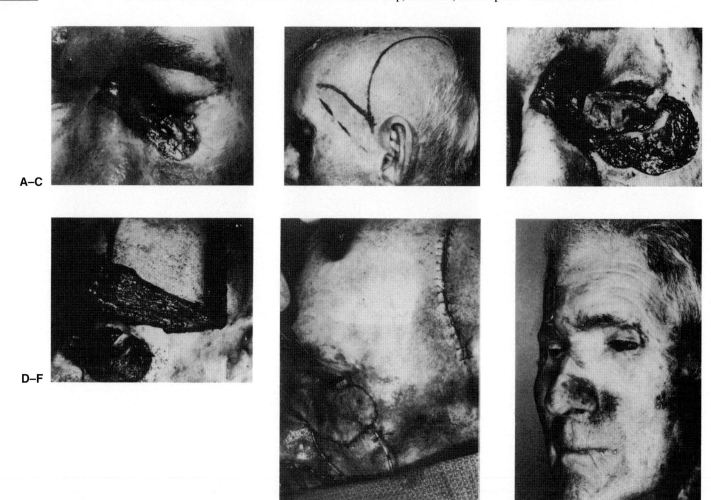

FIG. 4. A: Chemosurgical excision of a recurrent basal cell epithelioma resulted in total full-thickness loss of the lower eyelid and the medial 25% of the upper eyelid. **B:** Design of the incisions used to elevate the flap. **C:** Reconstruction consisted of replacement of lining and support with a septal cartilage-mucosa graft. **D:** The graft was vascularized by an extended temporoparietal fascial flap. **E:** A supraclavicular full-thickness skin graft has been applied. **F:** The result 1½ years postoperatively demonstrates good central support with a well-defined lid. A small lateral symblepharon exists where the lining graft was folded onto itself in the area of the lateral fornix.

of the fascia in a plane superficial to the pericranium and anterior to the fascia of the temporalis muscle is achieved. Division of the temporoparietalis fascia near the posterior base of the pedicle should hug the cartilaginous margin of the crus helix in order to avoid injury to the primary vessels. The branch to the ear will be divided with this back cut, and careful hemostasis to avoid injury to the main vessels is mandatory.

A subcutaneous plane of dissection from the axis of the flap to the defect is accomplished. The fascial flap is then tunneled into position, and the desired covering grafts are applied. The flap also may be lined with appropriate grafts, if needed. The donor scalp wound is closed, and suction catheters are employed.

CLINICAL RESULTS

Twenty-three superficial temporal artery fascial flaps have been used. Five of these flaps were of the extended variety. One flap was used as a free microvascular transfer. No total flap loss has occurred, although three partial losses were seen when attempts were made to extend the flap in a superior direction beyond the 12-cm limit. Flaps extended posteriorly have remained viable with lengths of 16 to 18 cm. While

greater flap lengths may be possible, the predictable clinical limits of this extended flap have not been determined.

Donor wounds have generally been acceptable. Neither scalp loss nor alopecia has occurred when the subdermal fat was preserved with the skin.

SUMMARY

The temporoparietal fascial flap can be used to provide thin, vascularized tissue to the forehead, eyebrow, eyelid, and ear. This flap can support underlying cartilage grafts and an overlying skin graft.

References

1. Ohmori S. Reconstruction of microtia using the Silastic frame. *Clin Plast Surg* 1978;5:379.
2. Tanzer RC. Total reconstruction of the auricle: a 10-year report. *Plast Reconstr Surg* 1967;40:547.
3. Tettmeier RE, Gooding RA. The use of a fascial flap in ear reconstruction. *Plast Reconstr Surg* 1977;60:406.
4. Byrd HS. The use of subcutaneous axial fascial flaps in reconstruction of the head. *Ann Plast Surg* 1980;4:191.

CHAPTER 7 ■ MICROVASCULAR FREE TRANSFER OF TEMPORO-OCCIPITAL SCALP FLAPS

K. OHMORI

EDITORIAL COMMENT

The application of methods of scalp reduction, as well as the use of expanders, has facilitated the treatment of large areas of alopecia. There is still a place for microvascular transfer of hair-bearing tissue, however, even though the risk and magnitude of the procedure are increased.

I have developed four types of microsurgical scalp flaps, viz., free temporo-occipital, free occipitotemporal, free temporo-occipitoparietal, and free occipito-occipital flaps (1,2) (Fig. 1).

INDICATIONS

The temporo-occipital scalp flap has been employed in the treatment of cicatricial alopecia (Juri type I) and male pattern baldness (Juri type II) with excellent results, especially in producing an anterior hairline with natural hair direction (3). Advantages of microsurgical free temporo-occipital scalp flaps include the one-stage creation of a frontotemporal hairline with natural hair direction, the achievement of a minimal and inconspicuous donor scar, and only a short period of hospitalization.

ANATOMY

The superficial temporal artery arises from a branch of the external carotid artery and turns beneath the parotid gland. This artery then runs superficially, approximately 1 cm below the level of the ear tragus. Subsequently, it routinely gives off four branches: the zygomatic branch, a branch to the auricle, an anterior branch, and a posterior branch. There are many variations in the positions of these branches. The zygomatic artery becomes a branch of the anterior branch when the latter leaves the superficial temporal artery at a more proximal point. However, even the size of the auricular branch, which is usually located just over the small mimic muscle of the auricle, varies.

The main trunk of the superficial temporal artery usually makes a wide curve between the level of the ear tragus and 2 cm above it. After giving off its anterior branch, it then runs toward the top of the head, where it provides a posterior branch. Along the latter it gives off a branch posteriorly, that is usually not evident in the angiography of the external carotid artery, but is easier to see when it is dissected out clinically. This branch is located about the distance of two to three fingerbreadths from the hairline, just over the auricle. This small branch and the posterior branch of the superficial temporal artery may have multiple anastomoses between them

and the posterior auricular artery and the occipital artery itself. The arterial supply of the free temporo-occipital flap is based on these two branches (Fig. 2).

Routinely, the vein runs posterior and superior to the superficial temporal artery, but it can often be seen wrapped around the artery, especially at the level of the tragus. Then it usually receives two tributaries that are accompanied by the anterior and posterior branches of the superficial temporal artery. A tributary from the auricle joins either the posterior part of the superficial temporal vein or its common trunk. There are venae comitantes accompanying the superficial temporal artery, but they are usually quite small in caliber. The main drainage of the free temporo-occipital flap appears to be the posterior tributary of the superficial temporal vein.

FLAP DESIGN AND DIMENSIONS

Since the scalp tissue is well vascularized by a tight network of vessels, one can design the flap in almost all directions and for more than 20 cm in length, as long as the flap is more than 4 cm in width and has a good vascular pedicle. Despite this advantage, closure of the donor defect becomes difficult to achieve without leaving a visible area of alopecia. To overcome this problem, the inferior border of the free temporo-occipital flap is designed almost parallel to the parieto-occipital hairline, and the distance between the latter and the inferior border of the flap should remain less than 6 cm. Extensive undermining of the neck can then be done to slide the inferior margin of the scalp defect upward. The superior border of the flap is also designed parallel to the inferior border, and the width of the flap kept less than 5 cm.

After the distal two-thirds of the flap are marked, its central axis is bent approximately 90° where the pulsating path of the posterior branch of the superficial temporal artery can be felt. This point should be located about 2 cm above the origin of the small posterior branch that originates from the posterior branch of the superficial temporal artery.

The design is then completed about 1 to 2 cm above the hairline, bringing both parallel lines together at this point. With such a plan, this free flap can be employed easily in the treatment of baldness (Fig. 3).

OPERATIVE TECHNIQUE

Donor Site

Because of the numerous variations seen in the pedicle of the flap, dissection of the pedicle vessels should be carried out

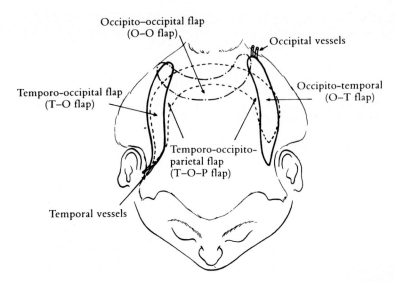

FIG. 1. Four types of microsurgical scalp flaps.

before raising the flap completely. All the arterial and venous branches should be dissected out first, while keeping intact the posterior branch of the superficial temporal artery and the small branch arising from it, together with the posterior tributary of the superficial temporal vein.

To perform this operative procedure more easily, it is better to include all the superficial temporal fascia with these vessels, that are raised together en bloc from the deep temporal fascia to provide a pedicle for the free flap. All the vessels that do not supply the flap are coagulated or ligated. Then the remaining portion of the flap is raised from the pericranium by incising both sides, so that the galea is left attached to the flap (Fig. 4).

Recipient Site

To give a natural direction to the anterior hairline, the superficial temporal vessels on the opposite side are exposed (Fig. 5).

In cases of temporofrontal alopecia, the recipient vessels can be prepared as proximally as possible, to produce the sideburn and the temporofrontal hairline in one piece. However, when the flap is used in cases of baldness, the hair-bearing portion of the flap should be started at the frontotemporal junction. The recipient vessels are therefore prepared inside the scalp, about 2 cm above the hairline of the auricle. In some cases, however, the caliber of the superficial temporal vein may be too small, necessitating a more proximal dissection and the use of a vein graft. In all my patients, one artery and one vein were anastomosed.

CLINICAL RESULTS

Sixty-eight free scalp flaps have been performed in the Tokyo Metropolitan Police Hospital, and 39 free temporo-occipital flap transfers have been done in the Juri Clinic of Plastic Surgery, Buenos Aires, Argentina. In this combined series of 107 free scalp flap transfers, only two flaps underwent necrosis.

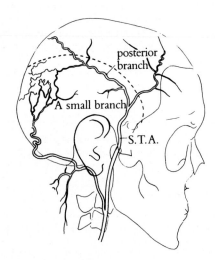

FIG. 2. The branches of the external carotid artery to the scalp. A small branch of the superficial temporal artery (STA) can be easily identified along with the posterior branch and preserved with the flap.

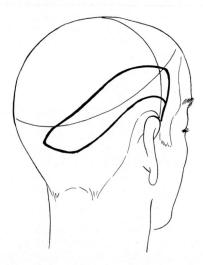

FIG. 3. Design of the free temporo-occipital flap.

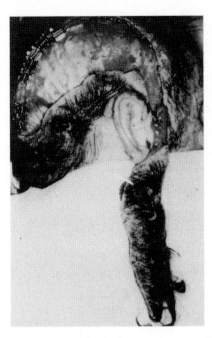

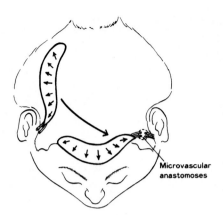

FIG. 5. The donor and recipient sites can be designed so that a natural anterior hairline can be formed.

FIG. 4. The temporo-occipital scalp flap raised on its pedicle.

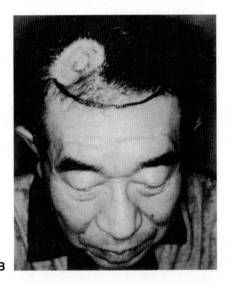
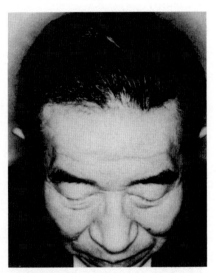

A,B

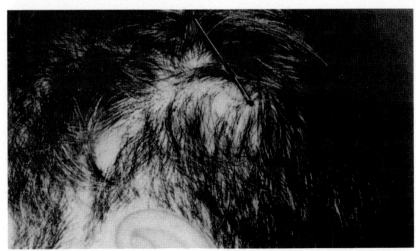

C

FIG. 6. A: A patient with cicatricial alopecia. B: Postoperative appearance. C: Minimal donor deformity.

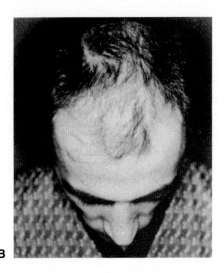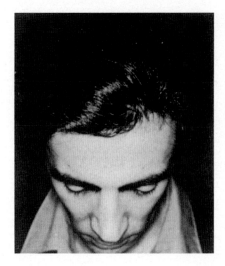

A,B

FIG. 7. **A:** Male pattern baldness. **B:** Post-operative appearance.

SUMMARY

The microsurgical transfer of a temporo-occipital scalp flap has been described as a treatment for baldness. Both cicatricial alopecia (Juri type I) and male pattern baldness (Juri type II) can be treated with this flap. However, such a procedure should be restricted to selected patients (Figs. 6 and 7).

References

1. Ohmori K. Free scalp flap. *Plast Reconstr Surg* 1980;65:42.
2. Ohmori K. Free scalp flap surgery. *Ann Plast Surg* 1980;5:17.
3. Juri J, Juri C. Aesthetic aspects of reconstructive scalp surgery. *Clin Plast Surg* 1981;8:243.

CHAPTER 8 ■ GALEA FRONTALIS MYOFASCIAL FLAP FOR CRIBRIFORM AND PARACRIBRIFORM AREAS

H. COSTA AND A. CEREJO

EDITORIAL COMMENT

This chapter and the one following (Chap. 9) demonstrate a reliable and accessible method of covering defects in the cribriform area, which may prevent cerebrospinal fluid leaks.

The galea frontalis flap (1–5) is highly vascularized and versatile. The flap may be used on either a wide or narrow pedicle for a variety of craniofacial problems.

INDICATIONS

Reconstructions using this flap are primarily applicable for defects of the cribriform and paracribriform areas, orbital roof, and frontal sinus. The flap also can be used for defects after various craniofacial-defect corrections, maxillofacial injuries (such as Le Fort II and III fractures), cerebrospinal fluid (CSF) leaks, and tumor ablation of the anterior cranial fossa (3–5).

ANATOMY

The occipitofrontalis is a broad, musculofibrous layer that covers the dome of the skull from the nuchal lines to the eye-

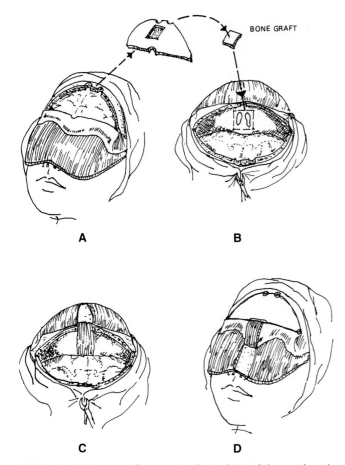

FIG. 1. A–D: Diagram of anatomic relationships of the myofascial frontalis galeal flap, with and without calvarial split-bone grafts, for treatment of anterior fossa cerebrospinal fluid leaks.

brows. The two frontal bellies are thin, quadrilateral, and adherent to the superficial fascia, with no bony attachments; the medial fibers are continuous with those of the procerus. The fibers are directed upward to join the galea aponeurotica in front of the coronal suture. Between the bellies, there is a variable interval occupied by an extension of the galea aponeurotica.

The galea flap is anteriorly based on the supratrochlear and supraorbital vessels, allowing transfer from an extracranial to an intracranial position, thus creating a vascularized myofascial barrier between cranial, orbital, and nasal cavities. In some cases, repair of an anterior cranial-base bone defect has been performed with split calvarial bone grafts harvested from the frontal craniotomy bone (Fig. 1) and covered with the flap.

FLAP DESIGN AND DIMENSIONS

The flap is raised from the deep aspect of the bicoronal flap, which is frequently used in craniofacial surgery (see Fig. 1). It may be based on either or both supraorbital and supratrochlear vessels and has a trapezoidal or rectangular shape. The larger trapezoidal flaps can cover all the anterior to cranial fossa. The pedicle width can range between 2 and 10 cm, and a flap length of 6 to 7 cm easily reaches the greater wings of the sphenoid bones, providing a vascularized myofascial barrier between cranial, orbital, and nasal cavities.

OPERATIVE TECHNIQUE

The operative approach has several stages: (a) a bicoronal flap and a bifrontal craniotomy are used for the surgical approach to the anterior fossa; (b) the bony defect is explored through an extradural approach; (c) the dural tear is defined through an intradural approach and prepared; (d) the galeal flap is used to reinforce the dural repair; and (e) if required, the bony defect is corrected using an inner- or outer-table calvarial bone graft.

The galeal flap is raised from the deep aspect of the bicoronal flap (see Fig. 1C). Two longitudinal myogaleal incisions are taken about 6 to 8 cm apart until the subcutaneous tissue is visualized. By sharp knife dissection, the myofascial flap is carefully raised, including the supraorbital and supratrochlear vessels. After careful hemostasis, the muscle flap is ready for transfer to the anterior cranial base, normally through a slit-type bone window created in the frontal bone flap (Fig. 1D).

If the anterior fossa cranial bone defect is small, a galeal frontalis myofascial flap is raised from the deep aspect of the bicoronal flap and transferred (see above text). If the anterior cranial-base bone defect is larger (more than 5 mm wide), however, a split-thickness bone graft is harvested from the frontal craniotomy bone flap. After careful modeling of the bone graft, fixation is usually possible by finger pressure. Then the frontalis myofascial flap is carried out as described (see Fig. 1A–D). Although an outer-table cranial bone graft has been used, contour defect of the frontal bone has not been a problem. The transverse dural incision is closed with continuous nonabsorbable suture: transcutaneous intradural and extradural drains are inserted; the frontal-bone flap is repositioned and fixed; and all wounds are closed.

CLINICAL RESULTS

The procedure was used with complete success in 12 patients with anterior fossa CSF leaks after trauma. In all patients, an intracranial-intradural approach was used, with transfer of a myofascial frontalis galeal vascularized flap. Repair of skull-base defects with calvarial bone grafts also was performed in seven of these patients. Follow-up has been between 6 months and 6.5 years. In all patients, neither recurrence of CSF leakage nor postoperative meningitis or its recurrence were observed.

SUMMARY

The galea frontalis myofascial flap is easy and quick to elevate, provides adequate size for nasal-cranial separation in most cases, and leaves an inconspicuous donor defect. It also can be used successfully after resection of skull-base tumors and frontofacial advancements.

References

1. Schramm VL, Myers EN, Maroon JC. Anterior skull base surgery for benign and malignant disease. *Laryngoscope* 1979;89:1077.
2. Ousterhout DK, Tessier P. Closure of large cribriform defects with a forehead flap. *J Maxillofac Surg* 1981;9:7.
3. Jackson IT, Adham MN, Marsh WR. Use of the galeal frontalis myofascial flap in craniofacial surgery. *Plast Reconstr Surg* 1986;77:905.
4. Costa H, Cerejo A, Baptista A, et al. The galea frontalis myofascial flap in anterior fossa CSF leaks. *Br J Plast Surg* 1993;46:503.
5. Rinehart CG, Jackson IT, Potparic Z, et al. Management of locally aggressive sinus disease using craniofacial exposure and the galeal frontalis fascia-muscle flap. *Plast Reconstr Surg* 1993;92:1219.

CHAPTER 9 ■ GALEAL FRONTALIS MYOFASCIAL FLAP

I. T. JACKSON AND Z. POTPARIC

The galeal frontalis myofascial flap is a distally based flap that contains the deep subcutaneous tissues of the forehead. It is usually elevated from the coronal flap by subcutaneous dissection, thereby creating a vascularized myofasciodisposal flap that is either placed intracranially, or used for coverage of the orbits or the nose or both. Recently, as a result of careful injection studies, the pericranium also has been included, as to do so increases the vascularity of the flap.

INDICATIONS

The goals in intracranial reconstruction with the galeal frontalis flap are to provide separation between the nasopharynx and brain, to obliterate dead space, to prevent cerebrospinal fluid (CSF) leakage (particularly if the dura is lacerated), and to provide vascularized coverage for bone grafts. The flap is used for reconstruction of defects after resection of anterior skull-base malignancies, trauma involving the anterior cranial fossa, and when a Le Fort III advancement is combined with frontal advancement. In the case of an old CSF leak, the flap is used in precisely the same way. Together with a skin graft, it also can be used as a vascularized soft-tissue bed for coverage of the orbits and the nose. Finally, it is an excellent material for packing the frontal sinus following trauma. In this situation, bone can be packed on top of it to fill this area completely (1). The flap should not be taken from a previously irradiated area or from an area to be irradiated.

ANATOMY

The key to the anatomy of the galeal frontalis myofascial flap is an understanding of the layers of the forehead skin and the scalp. These are histologically composed of the following five layers: (a) skin, (b) subcutaneous tissue, (c) frontalis muscle and its aponeurotic extension, (d) subgaleal fascia, and (e) cranial periosteum.

The subcutaneous fat tissue as well as the subgaleal loose connective tissue are called the *subgaleal* fascia; these layers vary considerably in thickness in different areas of the forehead as well as in different persons. The subgaleal fascia consists of several well-vascularized parallel connective tissue sheets that glide over one another. Histologically, three superimposed layers may be distinguished: a well-vascularized superficial layer underlying the galea frontalis muscle, a middle relatively avascular layer, and a deep loose areolar layer overlying the cranial periosteum. The layers that were originally included in the galeal frontalis myofascial flap are (a)

partial-thickness subcutaneous fat, (b) galeal frontalis muscle, and (c) superficial layers of subgaleal fascia (2). As mentioned, the pericranium has now been added (3).

The blood supply to the galeal frontalis flap is entirely from the supratrochlear and supraorbital vessels (Fig. 1). Both divide into larger superficial and smaller deep branches, either within or shortly after exiting from the orbit around the supraorbital rim. Deep branches have a short axial course in the cranial direction, traveling just on top of the periosteum and within the layers of the subgaleal fascia. As the larger superficial branches exit from the orbit, they first pierce the orbicularis oculi and corrugator muscles. For a short distance, they travel within the substance of these muscles and the frontalis muscle. They then pierce the frontalis muscle and become superficial to it and to the galea, coursing within the subcutaneous fat.

As they course toward the crown of the scalp, they become more superficial, travelling just below the dermis and hair follicles. Only a few anastomoses between the paired vessels cross the midline. At the level of subcutaneous tissue, dissection of the flap violates the axial blood supply and determines distal flap viability. Continuous axial vessels within the flap may range from 3 to 7 cm (4). The supraorbital artery provides the major blood supply, as the supratrochlear artery is transected more proximal to the flap because of its more superficial course. Volumes of galeal frontalis flaps, with sizes in the 9- × 14-cm range, vary from 15 to 30 cc (3).

Supratrochlear and supraorbital nerves provide sensory supply to the forehead and anterior scalp. Their course is similar, but not identical, to the course of the blood vessels. Harvest of the galeal frontalis flap unavoidably results in the transection of these nerves. The loss of sensation occurs approximately at the same level as the loss of the axial blood supply to the flap.

FLAP DESIGN AND DIMENSIONS

The flap is designed with its base at the level of the supraorbital rim, including the mid-forehead area, 1.0 to 1.5 cm lateral to the supraorbital notch on both sides. Extending the lateral border of the flap toward the frontotemporal ridge allows inclusion of well-vascularized lateral forehead tissue and provides additional axial length to the supraorbital vessels. The width of the flap base is 8 to 10 cm. A unilaterally based flap should be avoided because it causes asymmetry of the frontalis muscle and a noticeable deformity of the forehead (5).

The extent of distal random extension of the flap depends on the available axial blood supply. About 50% of

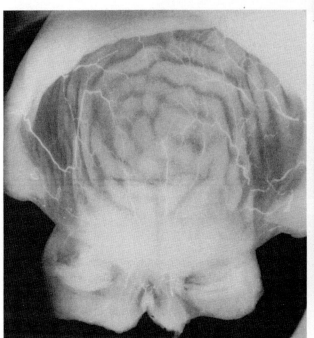
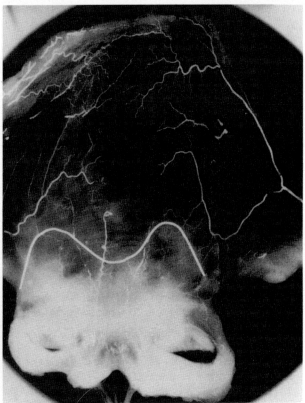

FIG. 1. Vascular anatomy of the galeal frontalis myofascial flap. **A:** Intact scalp shows numerous anastomoses between the temporal and supraorbital and supratrochlear vessels; blood supply is far superior in the scalp. **B:** Galea dissected from the full-thickness scalp with wire placed to show where most of the blood supply is in the galeal frontalis area. (This has been shown to be extended if the pericranium is included in the flap.)

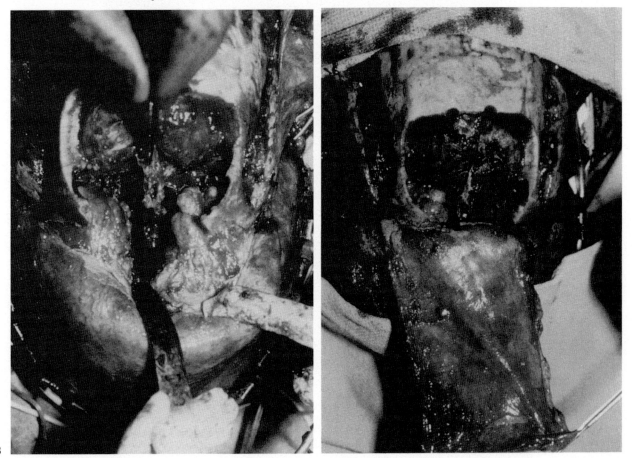

FIG. 2. A: Removal of ethmoid sinuses and their contents together with sphenoid sinus and clivus. The frontal and maxillary sinuses also had their contents resected. **B:** Galeal frontalis flap elevated. Note that this flap is very thick and includes a generous portion of tissue removed with the galea; this is taken down to the hair roots and is especially thick at the supraorbital region.

29

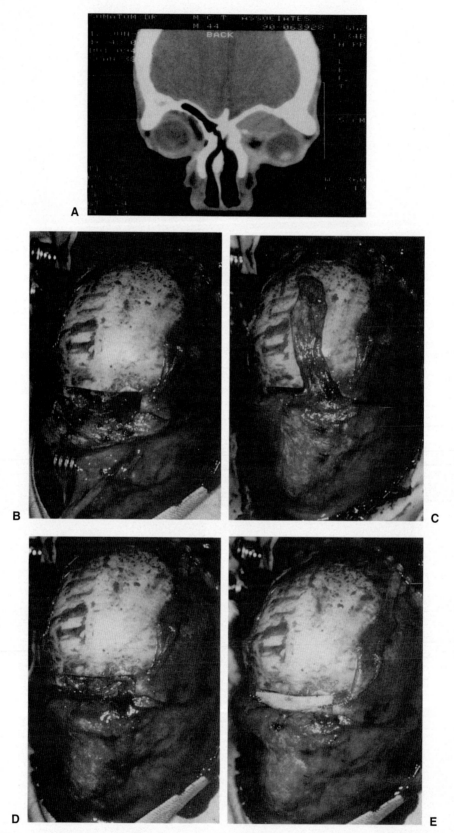

FIG. 3. A: CT scan shows mucocele of left frontal sinus, with erosion of sinus floor and displacement of left globe. **B:** Removal of anterior wall of frontal sinus with removal of the mucocele. Note the contents of the orbit seen through the orbital roof on the left. **C:** Narrow, one-sided galeal frontalis flap elevated on supraorbital vessels. **D:** The flap has been used to pack into the frontal sinus. **E:** Supraorbital rim replaced and held in place with microplates.

the axial length may be added as a random portion to provide for a well-vascularized flap. A distal flap portion larger than that should be considered a nonvascularized graft and should not be used for coverage of bone grafts or exposed areas.

To compensate for vascular and volume shortcomings of the galeal frontalis myofascial flap, consideration should be given to using the composite galeal frontalis pericranial flap. By including the pericranium and intact subgaleal fascia within the flap, a significant increase in blood supply and volume is achieved. The volume of this flap is about 50% greater than that of the galeal frontalis flap.

OPERATIVE TECHNIQUE

Most frequently, the coronal flap dissected in the subgaleal plane is used to approach the anterior cranial fossa. Occasionally, a midline incision is made in the frontal area; this is related to excision of tumor or skin resection in hypertelorism. The flap is dissected carefully from the skin by subcutaneous dissection just below the hair follicles in the hair-bearing scalp and just below the dermis in the forehead. The dissection includes most of the subcutaneous fat in the flap but also leaves some fat tissue on the skin side. Dissection through the subcutaneous tissue, instead of the top of the galeal and frontalis muscle, provides additional vessel length and supplies more volume. Care is taken not to injure the hair follicles superiorly or to go too deeply and miss the frontalis muscle. The flap is taken based on where the supratrochlear and supraorbital vessels enter its base. Transillumination of the flap or use of the hand-held Doppler may help to estimate continuous axial blood supply (2) (Figs. 2 and 3). Harvesting of the composite galeal frontalis pericranial flap requires elevation of the coronal flap in the subpericranial plane, followed by elevation of the composite flap in the subcutaneous plane.

CLINICAL RESULTS

We have used more than 500 flaps in the past 12 years. They were used for cranial-base reconstruction, frontal sinus obliteration, soft-tissue augmentation, or soft-tissue cover with an overlying skin graft. There was no problem with intracranial infection in any of the cases in which the flap was used intracranially. Breakdown of forehead skin, with underlying necrosis of the frontal bone, occurred in two patients. In one, the flap necrosed completely and, although there was no resulting infection, a free rectus abdominis flap was used to fill the intracranial dead space that occurred (6). Both patients received preoperative and postoperative irradiation.

Frontal contour irregularities, sensory deficit, and frontalis muscle dysfunction occurred in 75% of the patients. Those who had a wide flap based bilaterally in the forehead presented with weakness of eyebrow movement. Flaps based unilaterally caused eyebrow weakness on the affected side and asymmetric deformity of the forehead that was more conspicuous than the bilateral deformity. A narrow flap based in the midline is more likely to preserve frontalis muscle function.

All patients developed hypesthesia or anesthesia of the forehead. None of the patients had any problems related to sensory deficit. Half of the patients did not notice this to be a problem until they were asked specifically about it and examined for sensory deficit (5).

SUMMARY

The galeal frontalis myofascial flap provides vascularized tissue for reconstruction of the anterior cranial fossa. It is the flap of choice wherever there is intracranial/nasopharyngeal connection and concern about infection ascending from the nasopharynx into the extradural area and from there into the meninges or brain.

References

1. Rinhart GC, Jackson IT, Potparic Z, et al. Management of aggressive sinus disease using craniofacial exposure and the galeal frontalis fascia-muscle flap. *Plast Reconstr Surg* 1993;92:1219.
2. Jackson IT, Adham MN, Marsh WR. Use of the galeal frontalis myofascial flap in craniofacial surgery. *Plast Reconstr Surg* 1986;77:905.
3. Potparic Z, Fukuta K, Colen LB, et al. Galeo-pericranial flaps in the forehead: a study of blood supply and volumes. *Br J Plast Surg* 1996;49:519.
4. Fukuta K, Potparic Z, Sugihara T, et al. A cadaver investigation of blood supply to the galeal frontalis flap. *Plast Reconstr Surg* 1994;94:794.
5. Fukuta K, Avery C, Jackson IT. Long-term complications of the galeal frontalis myofascial flap in craniofacial surgery. *Eur J Plast Surg* 1993;16:174.
6. Jackson IT, Webster HR. Craniofacial tumors. *Clin Plast Surg* 1994;21:633.

CHAPTER 10 ■ MICROVASCULAR FREE TRANSFER OF OMENTUM

Y. IKUTA

If the scalp has been avulsed, the obvious first choice is replantation, when feasible (1). If the injury is old or results from other defects such as tumor excision or burns, other methods must be sought (2).

If the periosteum is still intact, split-thickness skin grafts can readily survive but do not provide stable coverage (3). Ulcerations are frequent, especially when the area is covered with a wig. The situation is even worse if a split-thickness skin graft is applied to a skull that has been decorticated of its outer table. Full-thickness skin grafts are more stable but do not take well, and the available donor sites are often not adequate (4).

The availability of local and distant flaps is limited. Instead, free vascularized skin, muscle, or omental flaps can be used with good results (5–8).

INDICATIONS

There are several advantages to the vascularized omental flap. It can be used, in association with a skin graft, to treat large defects. It can be easily shaped to any desired size, and it can be used to improve the circulation of a suitable recipient site. It is generally used when there is an extensive tissue defect, the surface of the defect is irregular in shape or narrow and deep, the circulation is poor, or infection is present.

However, since the omental tissue must be obtained by abdominal laparotomy, consideration must be given to the fact that its original function will decrease, with the risk of causing panperitonitis (9). The possibility of employing other procedures, such as a skin flap, a musculocutaneous flap, or a muscle flap with skin graft, must be seriously considered.

ANATOMY

The greater omentum is attached to the greater curvature of the stomach and transverse colon and covers most of the colon, ileum, and jejunum. It consists of a double layer of fused peritoneum, with the blood supply interposed between the two layers. There are five major variations in the routes of omental vessels (10). Usually, the right and left gastroepiploic arteries form an arterial arch along the greater curvature of the stomach, with the omentum nourished by three large branches that arise from the arch. As shown in Fig. 1, the right, middle, and left omental vessels that arise from the gastroepiploic arch form vascular arcades near the lower end of the omental apron. The accessory omental vessel is located on the right end of the omentum.

OPERATIVE TECHNIQUE

Donor Site

The greater curvature of the stomach is exposed by an upper midline abdominal incision, and the right and left gastroepiploic arteries and omental arcades are confirmed. The numerous vessels that enter the greater curvature from the gastroepiploic arch are ligated into several groups. The omentum is then detached from the greater curvature and transverse colon. After selecting which of the two gastroepiploic arteries to anastomose to the artery of the recipient site, the other artery is ligated and cut. Finally, the artery selected for use is severed. In most cases, the right gastroepiploic artery is used, because the left gastroepiploic artery is slightly smaller. If the length of the normal omentum is not sufficient, a lengthening procedure may be used (11).

It is advisable to introduce heparinized saline solution into the artery to be anastomosed and to confirm outflow from veins on the same side. This also makes it possible to ascertain whether the ligatures are secure, that there is no impairment of circulation within the omentum itself, and that lengthening has been properly achieved.

Recipient Site

The choice of arteries to be used at the recipient site depends on the extent and degree of avulsion. In the forehead, the supraorbital or supratrochlear vessels can be chosen. In the temporal region, the superficial temporal or posterior auricular vessels can be selected. In the occipital region, the occipital vessels can be used.

A split-thickness skin graft is then placed over the omentum and secured by the compression provided by the tieover method (Fig. 2).

SUMMARY

Vascularized omental transplantation should be considered in cases of extensive loss of skin, subcutaneous tissue, and periosteum of the skull and when replantation by microvascular anastomosis of vessels or other composite grafts may be inadequate. Indications must be sufficient to justify an abdominal laparotomy and removal of the omentum.

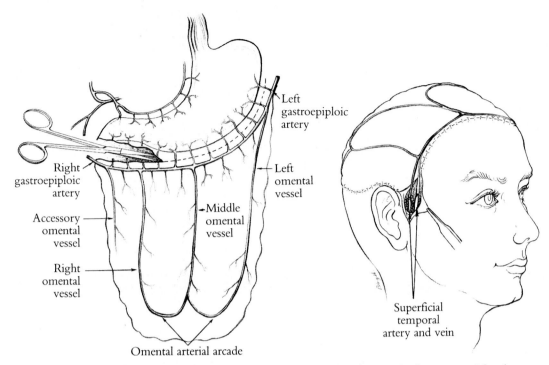

FIG. 1. The routes of omental vessels. The right and left gastroepiploic arteries form an arterial arch along the greater curvature of the stomach. There are three large omental vessel units. The right, middle, and left omental vessels form vascular arcades near the lower end of the omental apron. The accessory omental vessel is located on the right end of the omentum.

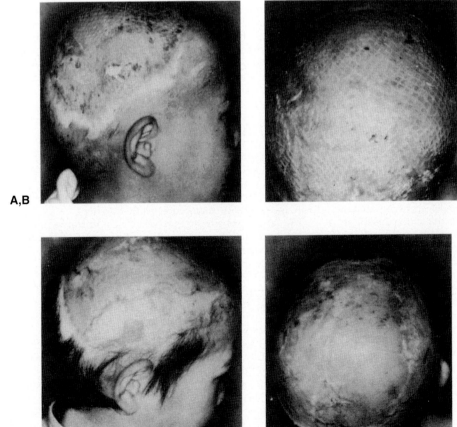

A,B

C,D

FIG. 2. A, B: A 5-year-old girl was attacked by a dog and had her scalp bitten off. Outer cortex of skull was removed to induce ingrowth of granulation tissue, and it was initially covered with an unstable meshed split-thickness skin graft. C, D: Three months postoperatively, the omentum provides a satisfactory cushion and the condition of the overlying skin graft is good. (From Ikuta, ref. 7, with permission.)

References

1. Miller GDH, Anstee J, Snell JA. Successful replantation of an avulsed scalp by microvascular anastomoses. *Plast Reconstr Surg* 1976;58:133.
2. Koss N, Robinson MC, Krizek TJ. Scalping injury. *Plast Reconstr Surg* 1975;55:439.
3. Lu MM. Successful replacement of avulsed scalp. *Plast Reconstr Surg* 1969;43:231.
4. Nummi P, Arppe A. Replacement of the avulsed scalp. *Scand J Plast Reconstr Surg* 1971;5:67.
5. Harii K, Ohmori K, Ohmori S. Transplantation with free scalp flaps. *Plast Reconstr Surg* 1974;53:410.
6. McLean DH, Buncke HJ. Autotransplant of omentum to a large scalp defect, with microsurgical revascularization. *Plast Reconstr Surg* 1972;49:268.
7. Ikuta Y. Autotransplant of omentum to cover large denudation of the scalp. *Plast Reconstr Surg* 1975;55:490.
8. Banzet P, LeQuang C. Free transplant of the greater omentum into the vault of the skull: three cases with vascular microanastomosis. *Chirurgie* 1976;102:457.
9. Hakelius L. Fatal complication after use of the greater omentum for reconstruction of the chest wall. *Plast Reconstr Surg* 1978;62:796.
10. Ninghsia Medical College, Department of Anatomy. Types of greater omentum arterial distribution and their clinical significance. *Chin Med J* 1978;4:127.
11. Alday ES, Goldsmith HS. Surgical technique for omental lengthening based on arterial anatomy. *Surg Gynecol Obstet* 1972;135:103.

CHAPTER 11 ■ TISSUE EXPANSION IN FOREHEAD AND SCALP RECONSTRUCTION

L. C. ARGENTA

EDITORIAL COMMENT

In the discussion following Radovan's pioneering article (1982) (1) on tissue expansion, Grabb stated, "I predict that over the next 5 years, the technique of tissue expansion will be of equal importance to the impact of microsurgery techniques in muscle flaps. Heaven only knows the principle of skin expansion has been staring us in the face."

The skin of the forehead and scalp differs considerably in color, texture, thickness, and hair-bearing qualities from tissue elsewhere on the body. Reconstruction of defects of this area is best accomplished with the use of similar tissue. Expansion of facial and scalp tissues is a relatively painless, well-tolerated procedure that can be accomplished over a period of several months (2).

Tissue expanders are available in multiple sizes and shapes from various manufacturers; custom prostheses can be produced if necessary. All prostheses presently available require periodic percutaneous injection of saline.

INDICATIONS

Because visits are required at 2- to 3-week intervals, skin expansion should be carried out only on reliable individuals who will conform to the required schedule and will modulate their activities appropriately during the expansion process. Expansion of facial and scalp tissues, in most cases, can be done only in well-healed injuries. Although the procedure has been used in subacute trauma, there is insufficient experience at this time to recommend this.

There is no tissue on the body that can cosmetically reproduce the qualities of the scalp. Expansion is particularly useful in individuals who have lost full-thickness hair-bearing tissue of the scalp secondary to burns or trauma.

PLANNING AND DESIGN

Careful planning is necessary so that the tissue to be expanded is compatible in physical nature to the area where tissue is needed. All incisions should take into account previous scars or should be at the margin of the tissue to be advanced. In the scalp, the prosthesis is placed beneath the galea.

The largest prosthesis that will fit comfortably into the pocket is selected. It must be adequate enough to develop the necessary expansion without being so large as to develop folds that may precipitate extrusion.

OPERATIVE TECHNIQUE

In prostheses with distant inflation reservoirs, the reservoirs should be placed away from the prostheses by at least 2 inches. The prosthesis is placed beneath the galea, with the reservoir over the mastoid.

A minimal amount of saline is placed in the prosthesis at the time of surgery. Inflation is then begun 2 or 3 weeks after the procedure. The patient returns to the office at weekly or biweekly intervals for inflation. Meticulously sterile procedures are required. The inflation is then carried out to the

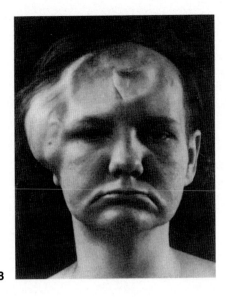 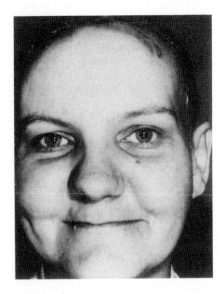

A,B

FIG. 1. A,B: A 34-year-old woman who had undergone frontal craniotomy for a meningioma with loss of the forehead skull secondary to infection. A previous attempt at cranioplasty had been abandoned because of the extreme tightness of the skin. An expander was placed in the right temporal area and expanded to 300 cc. The patient's forehead flap was then taken down, and a large methyl methacrylate cranioplasty was used to close the defect. The expanded skin allowed an adequate amount of tissue for closure over the cranioplasty.

point of pain until the overlying tissue becomes tense. If excessive pain or tension develops, some fluid can be removed.

The scalp may be difficult to expand initially. Approximately 2 weeks after expansion commences, the resistance of the galea seems to diminish and expansion proceeds more rapidly. The overlying skin becomes loose, and the prosthesis can be felt moving within the underlying pocket. The overlying tissue characteristically becomes ruberous and remains so until the prosthesis has been removed. Some pressure discomfort is usually described after inflation, but this rapidly subsides after the overlying tissue softens.

If insufficient scalp is generated to cover the entire defect, the expanded tissue may be advanced as far forward as possible, leaving the prosthesis beneath the flap. Within several weeks, reexpansion can be accomplished. The hair follicles are more distantly separated from one another than in normal skin, but the result is usually more than adequate for cosmetic improvement.

CLINICAL RESULTS

Skin of the face, neck, and scalp has been successfully expanded in patients as young as 3 and as old as 57 years of age. In head and neck reconstruction, the development of a capsule adjacent to the prosthesis more than compensates for the loss of tissue.

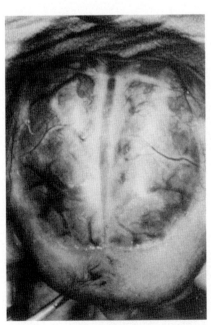 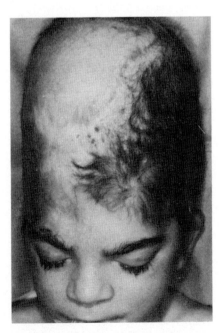 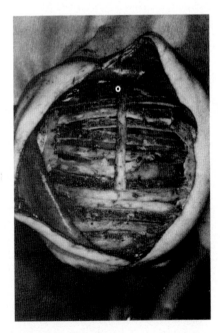

A–C

FIG. 2. A: A newborn with a large defect of the skull with exposed brain. Large flaps were developed on either side, one based anteriorly and the other posteriorly. Both closed over the brain. B: The patient at age 6. The flaps have been dissected from the brain, a reinforced silicone sheet was tented from the edges of the cranium over the brain, and the scalp was expanded over a period of 8 weeks. C: Intraoperative photograph of split-rib cranioplasty within the expanded scalp. Bone graft consolidation was achieved in 6 weeks.

Furthermore, the dense vascular network within the capsule and adjacent to it makes the expanded tissue extremely robust for the development of flaps. Several patients have successfully undergone bone grafting to reconstruct facial bones or cranium within the capsule. All have gone on to rapid consolidation of the bone graft. Also, synthetic prostheses may be placed beneath expanded tissue (Figs. 1 and 2).

Provided that there is sufficient underlying supportive structure, there will be minimal or no contracture of expanded skin. Frequently, dog-ears that have resulted from the rotation of flaps necessitate resection months later.

Infection occurs less commonly in the head and neck than elsewhere in the body, partly because of the dense vascular network in this area. Perioperative antibiotics are employed, but long-term antibiotics are not. The development of late infection complications has almost always been secondary to breaks in inflation technique, with contamination of the injection reservoir, or the development of an intraoral communication.

Erosion of the prostheses through the suture line may occur if inflation is begun prematurely or if the prostheses are inflated at an excessively rapid rate. It is critical that the surgeon be judicious in the expansion process. Once extrusion has occurred, the prosthesis should be removed within 48 hours; however, the expanded tissue can still be rotated. The inflation reservoir is constructed of a harder and less flexible silicone and is particularly prone to extrusion if improperly situated.

In almost all cases, the overlying skin is slightly ruberous and occasionally mottled during the expansion process. This may persist for several days after removal of the prostheses, but it quickly subsides.

SUMMARY

Tissue expansion can be used effectively to reconstruct scalp and forehead defects.

References

1. Radovan C. Breast reconstruction after mastectomy using a temporary expander. *Plast Reconstr Surg* 1982;69:195.
2. Argenta LC, Watanabe MJ, Grabb WC. The use of tissue expansion in head and neck reconstruction. *Ann Plast Surg* 1983;11:31.

CHAPTER 12 ■ TRANSPOSED (MCGREGOR) FLAP IN EYELID RECONSTRUCTION

I. A. MCGREGOR

This flap consists of an inferiorly based transposed flap raised on the skin area below and lateral to the outer canthus, and it is moved medially to close V-shaped full-thickness defects of the lower eyelid. Transfer of the flap leaves a triangular secondary defect laterally, and this is closed using a Z-plasty.

INDICATIONS

The reconstruction that uses this flap is primarily applicable to full-thickness defects of the lower eyelid that can be created in the form of a V, although, as discussed later, the principle also can be applied to comparable defects of the upper eyelid (1,2). This flap can be used for defects of up to two-thirds of the breadth of the lower lid, canthus to canthus, but defects greater in breadth are unsuitable. The technique is one of the triad of reconstructions used to treat full-thickness V-shaped defects of increasing breadth (Fig. 1). With the narrow V, the defect can be closed directly; where the defect is broader and direct closure would be under tension, reduction of tension can be provided by dividing the slip of the lateral canthal ligament to the lower eyelid—lateral canthotomy. It is when the defect is still too broad for lateral canthotomy alone that the transposed flap has to be advanced medially to bring together the two limbs of the V and close the defect.

The method is easiest to carry out technically when an element of tarsal plate is present on both sides of the defect. The presence of the plate provides a good base for suturing the two margins of the V together, and while the method can be used for defects that abut on one or the other canthus, the absence of tarsal plate on one side of the defect makes secure closure of the defect more difficult.

FLAP DESIGN AND DIMENSIONS

Before raising the flap, the lines along which the various incisions will be made are drawn out on the skin. With the V-shaped defect outlined on the eyelid, the line that indicates the upper border of the transposed flap extends laterally from the outer canthus, continuing the upward curve of the margin of the lower eyelid, to just short of the temple hairline. The upward curve is required to provide an adequate vertical height of the reconstructed eyelid segment and to avoid ectropion.

From the lateral extremity of this line, a further line is drawn in a generally downward direction parallel to the lateral limb of the V on the eyelid, the angle between the two lines being approximately 60°. The effect is to outline a flap with the overall shape of a parallelogram. As already indicated, transfer of the flap medially leaves a triangular defect that is closed by a Z-plasty. This is designed at this stage, before any skin incisions are made, constructed around the lateral part of the line representing the upper margin of the flap. This acts as the common limb of the Z, it and the line representing the lateral margin of the flap together forming one of the Z-plasty flaps. Design of the Z-plasty is completed with the drawing of a line that runs upward and laterally from the upper margin of the flap, outlining the second Z-plasty flap.

OPERATIVE TECHNIQUE: LOWER EYELID DEFECTS

With the V excision of the full thickness of the eyelid completed, the flap, as outlined, is raised at the face lift level lateral to the orbicularis oculi. When the orbicularis is reached, the plane of elevation becomes deep to the muscle, the muscle being advanced as part of the flap. In the process of elevating the flap, the slip of the lateral canthal ligament to the lower eyelid is divided. This division can be carried out as a formal step, but the ligament can just as effectively be felt as a resistance to medial flap advancement and be divided.

With a skin hook to gently pull the flap medially, sites of resistance to advancement can be identified with the finger and divided with scissors. In the process, much of the lower border of orbicularis is divided, as well as the orbital septum, neither structure being divided as a formal, visualized step, but rather felt as a focus of resistance to medial advancement. The amount of tissue that must be divided in this way depends very much on the breadth of the V and the amount of flap advancement required to approximate its two limbs. A broad V necessitates more extensive soft-tissue division; a narrow V, less. Division must be continued until the flap can be advanced to close the defect with a minimum of tension. The extent of mobilization required also depends to some extent on the preexisting laxity of the eyelids and local tissues generally. When the amount of soft-tissue division is considerable, the flap may ultimately appear to be attached inferiorly by little more than the skin and immediately subcutaneous tissues superficially and the conjunctiva deeply. There should be no particular concern about this. In contrast to the cheek rotation

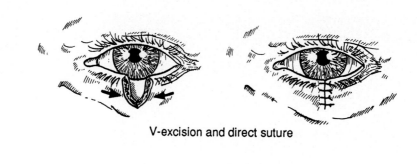

V-excision and direct suture

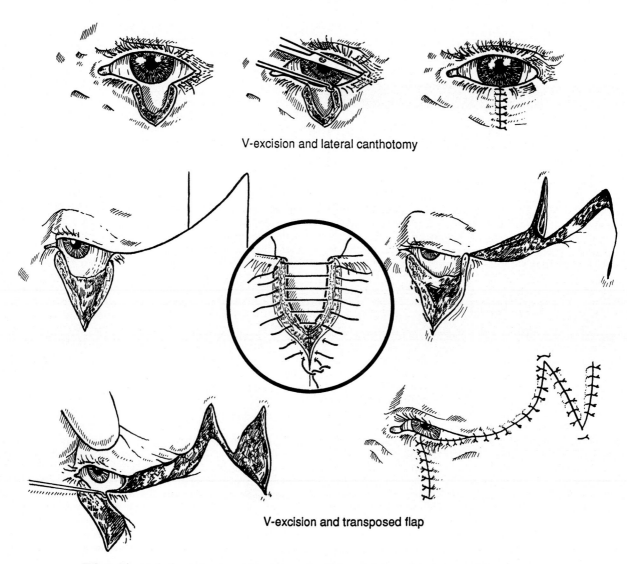

V-excision and lateral canthotomy

V-excision and transposed flap

FIG. 1. The triad of techniques used in reconstructing V-shaped defects of the lower eyelid of increasing width: V excision and direct suture, V excision and lateral canthotomy, and V excision and transposed flap. Also shown is the method of closing the V without exposing suture material in the conjunctival sac (*inset*).

flap used in lower eyelid reconstruction, with its recognized vulnerability to necrosis, the ratio of length to breadth and the relative smallness of the transposed flap make it safe.

Management of the Conjunctiva

When the lateral canthotomy has been carried out, the conjunctiva provides no resistance to medial advancement and does not need to be formally divided. There is an abundance of lax conjunctiva in the lateral fornix that allows unimpeded lateral movement of the eyeball. As the flap is drawn medially, the conjunctiva spreads out to line the skin and muscle that are being advanced to form the reconstructed segment of the eyelid. Their free margins lie side by side and, when sutured together, will form the margin of the reconstructed lid.

Method of Suture

The method used to close the V defect is designed to avoid exposing suture material within the conjunctival sac. With the margins of the V approximated, suturing is carried out in two layers, the tarsal plate and the conjunctiva behaving as a single structure. When the tarsal plates have been accurately approximated, the conjunctiva heals quickly and without incident. The plates can be effectively sutured together with interrupted 6–0 chromic catgut on an atraumatic needle, placing the knots on the muscle side of the tarsal plate. As part of this approximation, it is essential to match the lid margins carefully, and care in this respect is continued in the skin closure, using identification points such as the gray line and the eyelashes. The reconstruction is completed by suturing together the free margins of the flap and the conjunctiva. The sutures used to approximate the tarsal plates have a very low tensile strength, and it is important to make sure that there is no tension on the suture line.

Completion of the Z-Plasty

At the time of initial elevation of the transposed flap in preparation for its transfer, the triangular flap designed as part of the Z-plasty is also elevated, in readiness to be rotated downward into the triangular secondary defect that opens up when the transposed flap is advanced medially. When this triangular flap has been rotated into the defect and sutured in position,

suturing of the skin is completed lateral to the outer canthus. In most elderly patients there is considerable laxity in the tissue above the suture line, and some adjustment in tension and trimming of the upper margin may be required to make the suture line lie neatly.

The point has been made that in designing the flap its upper margin runs upward as well as laterally to give the reconstructed eyelid segment adequate height and prevent ectropion. When the reconstruction has been completed, the lateral tip of the transposed flap ends up at a significantly higher level than preoperatively, so that the final suture line lateral to the outer canthus is steeper than before, an advantageous change in direction, since any scar contracture will pull the eyelid upward as well as laterally.

OPERATIVE TECHNIQUE: UPPER EYELID DEFECTS

As in the lower eyelid, the three methods of closing V-shaped defects as the V increases in breadth—direct suture, direct suture with lateral canthotomy, and advancement medially of the transposed flap with Z-plasty—are applicable to comparable defects of the upper eyelid (Fig. 2). In the case of the

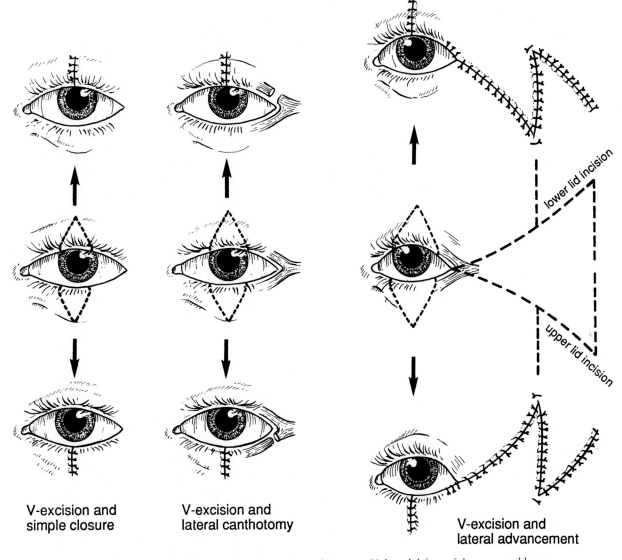

V-excision and simple closure

V-excision and lateral canthotomy

lower lid incision

upper lid incision

V-excision and lateral advancement

FIG. 2. Application of the triad of reconstructive techniques to V-shaped defects of the upper and lower eyelids. (From McGregor, ref. 1, with permission.)

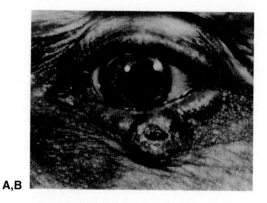

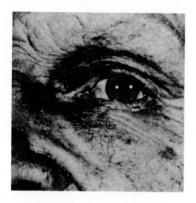

A,B

FIG. 3. A,B: Examples of the technique of V excision and flap transposition as applied to defects of the lower eyelid.

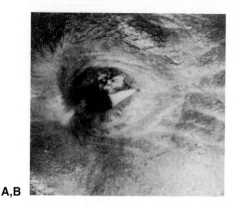

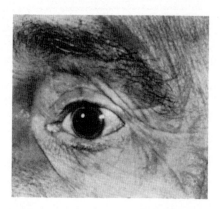

A,B

FIG. 4. A,B: Examples of the technique of V excision and flap transposition as applied to defects of the upper eyelid.

transposed flap, the design and technique mirror those used for the lower eyelid, with the flap based superiorly and the skin incision following the downward curve of the upper eyelid. Division of the slip of the lateral canthal ligament to the upper eyelid allows the flap to be advanced medially, and the secondary defect is closed with the Z-plasty designed over the lateral end of the transposed flap. Mobilization to allow advancement of the flap involves division of orbicularis muscle fibers and the orbital septum in addition to the upper eyelid slip of the lateral canthal ligament. The upper fornix, into which the lacrimal ducts open, lies behind the orbicularis and the orbital septum and should escape injury, although awareness of their presence is likely to add to the natural caution of the surgeon dissecting in that area. In practice, no deficit in tear production has been seen. Removal of a wedge of the levator muscle as part of the resection results in less functional deficit than one might expect. Although the main insertion of the levator tendon is central, it has extensions on both sides that reach each of the canthi. These extensions seem to retain sufficient attachment to the remnant of the tarsal plate on each side of the V resection to provide adequate function. As with the lower eyelid, the method works best and is technically easier if tarsal plate is present in both sides of the defect, but it is still possible to use this method when the defect is close to a canthus, although with a little more difficulty. The main fault in design is likely to be failure to plan the flap to provide adequate vertical height in the reconstructed lid.

Patients requiring this reconstruction frequently have considerable laxity in the upper eyelid, and this reconstruction is likely to add to it because of the dog-ear that develops at the apex of the V with transfer of the flap medially. If necessary, the reconstruction can be revised subsequently.

The amount of mobilization required in reconstructing a defect that approaches two-thirds of the breadth of the lower eyelid is considerable. In view of the much greater anatomic complexity of the upper eyelid and the major contribution played in function by the levator muscle, it is probably wise to restrict the reconstruction to defects of less than half the width of the upper lid rather than the two-thirds possible when the lower lid is involved.

SUMMARY

Probably the greatest virtues of this technique are its simplicity, safety, and reliability, as well as the fact that it is applicable to either eyelid (Figs. 3 and 4). Provided the flap is designed correctly and the reconstruction is not pushed beyond its proper limits, particularly as used in the upper eyelid, it gives little trouble.

References

1. McGregor IA. Eyelid reconstruction following subtotal resection of upper or lower eyelid. *Br J Plast Surg* 1973;26:346.
2. McGregor IA, McGregor FM. *Cancer of the face and mouth.* Edinburgh: Churchill Livingstone, 1986.

CHAPTER 13 ■ CHEEK ROTATION SKIN (MUSTARDÉ) FLAP TO THE LOWER EYELID

J. C. MUSTARDÉ

Reconstruction of the full thickness of an eyelid requires two basic layers: a skin-covering layer and a mucous-secreting layer. One of these layers can be a free graft, but at least one must be in the form of a flap with a continuous blood supply.

INDICATIONS

Eyelid tissues, including the tarsal plate and margin, will stretch to some degree, and a defect of about a quarter of the lower lid width can be closed directly. Closure of a defect only a few millimeters greater than a quarter of the lower lid width can usually be obtained by dividing the lower crus of the lateral canthal ligament. Where this does not allow sufficient relaxation to permit closure, a cheek rotation flap can then be used.

In defects involving from one-quarter to one-half of the eyelid, a comparatively small cheek rotation is required. Because of the stretch of tissues just alluded to, the dimension of the actual full-thickness lid reconstruction that must be carried out will be only about a quarter of the original width of the lid, i.e., about 6 to 7 mm. It is probable that adequate lining for the reconstructed segment will be available from the tissues of the lower fornix (Fig. 1).

This does not provide a very defined, stable margin, but such a small sector of the lid is involved, lying in an area where the cornea is unlikely to be affected, that the instability of the reconstructed margin may be of little importance. If adequate conjunctiva is not available, however, or if the reconstructed area is wider than about 6 mm, it is best to line the reconstructed part of the lid with a small composite nasal septal graft.

Where a defect greater than half the eyelid exists and the width of the reconstructed lid part is greater than one-quarter of the lid width, a much larger cheek rotation skin flap must be used. This presents no great problem in itself, but the instability of the weak reconstructed *margin*, both with respect to the possibility of it turning outward (which will produce epiphora) or turning in (where the squamous epithelium may come to rub on the cornea), as well as the lack of permanent support to the reconstructed lid segment, must be taken into account.

A mucus-secreting lining for the skin flap can be provided by using a graft of any mucosal surface. However, there will be no orbicularis muscle in the reconstructed lid segment, and because of the constant lifting action of the orbicularis muscle, skin flaps, mucosal grafts, and even tarsal plate from another eyelid will slowly stretch under the influence of gravity and time (witness the end result in seventh nerve palsy affecting a completely *normal* lower eyelid). It is therefore necessary in a reconstruction of any extent in a lower eyelid to provide not

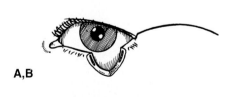
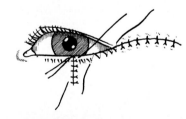

A,B

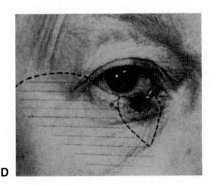
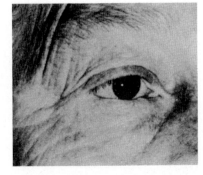

C,D

FIG. 1. Reconstruction of a quarter to a half of the lower lid. A small rotation of the cheek is sufficient to provide skin cover, while lining can often be obtained from the conjunctiva in the lower fornix. (From Mustardé, ref. 1, with permission.)

41

only a mucus-secreting lining, but also some supportive material that will permit the fashioning of a permanently stable margin and that also will give constant positive support to the reconstructed segment of the lid (1).

FLAP DESIGN AND DIMENSIONS

I believe that the best foundation for lower eyelid reconstruction is to use a flap for the skin layer. Skin for this purpose may be obtained from almost any region around the orbit, but one of the simplest and most logical techniques is to use a cheek rotation flap to carry the thin skin that lies lateral to the lateral canthus into the region of the reconstructed eyelid. The incision line of the flap should curve upward and outward from the lateral canthus. The length of the cheek incision, as well as the amount of undermining to be carried out, is determined on a trial-and-error basis by constantly checking whether the flap can be rotated across to fill the defect.

Rotation of the cheek flap is facilitated by resecting a skin triangle below the eyelid defect (Fig. 1C).

OPERATIVE TECHNIQUE

The ideal material that produces the desired effects in reconstruction of defects greater than half the eyelid is a graft of nasal septal cartilage that still retains mucous membrane on one surface. Such a composite graft can be obtained easily if the alar base is temporarily detached to allow greater access to the nasal septum. The cartilage layer may be thinned carefully to about 1-mm thickness (Fig. 2). This also will result in a tendency for the remaining cartilage to curve concavely toward the mucosal layer and hence conform to the eyeball.

In carrying out the reconstruction (Fig. 3), the cheek rotation flap will probably have to be carried down in front of the ear for some distance, and it must be thoroughly undermined in the subcutaneous layer (as in a face lift) to permit easy rota-

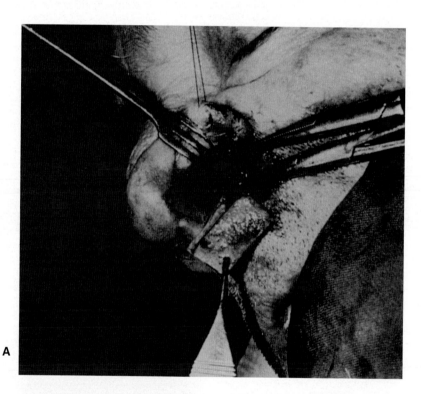

A

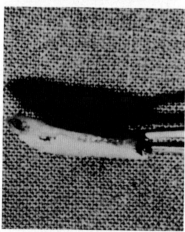

B,C

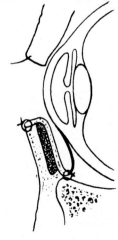

FIG. 2. Composite graft of nasal septal cartilage, along with mucosa on one side. Note excess mucosa, which will form the lid margin. **A:** Cartilage surface outward. **B:** On edge with mucosa above. **C:** When the graft is covered by a skin flap, it produces a lining layer for the reconstructed lower lid, permanent support to the lid, and a stable mucosa-covered margin. (From Mustardé, ref. 1, with permission.)

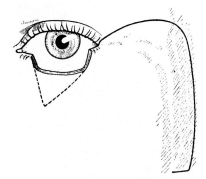 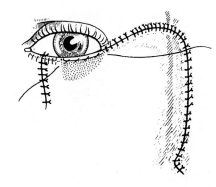

FIG. 3. Reconstruction of lower eyelid defects of greater than half the lid width, showing rotation of skin flap after resection of "relaxing" triangle and use of a composite nasal septal graft to line and support the reconstructed lid segment. (From Mustardé, ref. 1, with permission.)

tion without tension. The composite septal graft is held in position using running 6–0 Prolene sutures to coapt the nasal mucosal edges to conjunctiva, and a similar over-and-over suture should be used to fix the top edge of the mucosal fringe to the skin, after the mucosal fringe has been turned forward over the upper edge of the cartilage (Fig. 4). A light pressure dressing should be applied over the reconstructed lid segment to prevent a hematoma formation, that might separate the overlying skin flap from the composite graft. The pull-out sutures may be left for 1 week, but the 6–0 sutures should be removed in 5 days.

When resection of a tumor involves the medial side of the lid and the canaliculus is divided, the medial wall of the canaliculus that remains should be slit for 3 to 4 mm and a

small 1-mm tube should be left in situ for 10 days in hopes that it will produce a passageway to drain tears (Fig. 4F).

The technique for total reconstruction of the lower lid is merely an extension of the technique just described. All the dimensions are increased to produce a reconstruction of the required size (Figs. 5 and 6). The incision line of the skin flap will almost certainly benefit from the use of a back cut, and it is important that the cartilage in the graft should be of sufficient size to rest on the lower orbital margin, thus avoiding later drooping of the reconstructed lid. The sheer weight of the large cheek flap will call for the insertion of one or even two permanent sutures of 5–0 Prolene, hitching subcutaneous flap tissue to the periosteum of the orbital margin.

A–C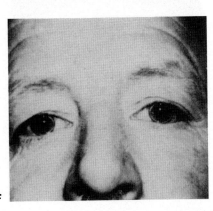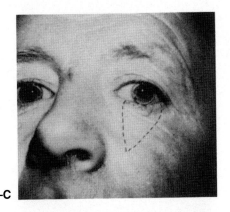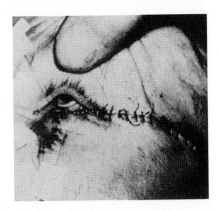

D–F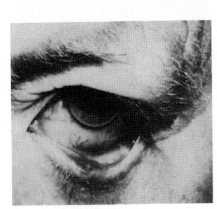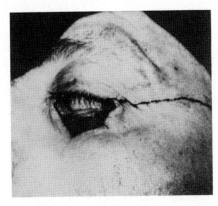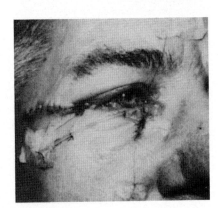

FIG. 4. Reconstruction of lower eyelid defects of greater than half the lid. **A–C:** Stages of the reconstruction along the lines described in Fig. 3. **D,E:** Postoperative result, showing well-supported, stable, lower eyelid margin with mucosa-lined fornix. **F:** Another patient, showing tube placed in remnant of lower canaliculus (see text). (From Mustardé, ref. 1, with permission.)

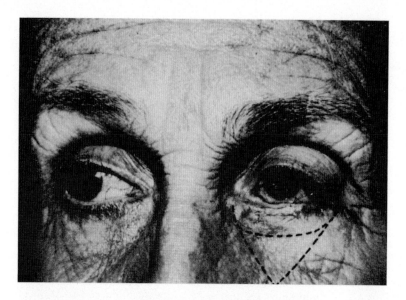
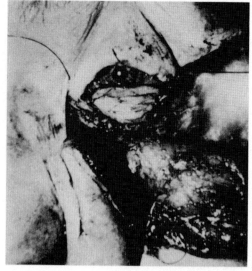

A,B

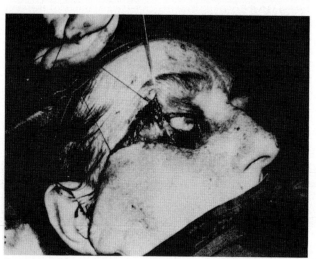
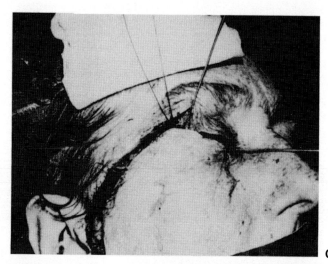

C,D

FIG. 5. Total reconstruction of the lower lid. A: Preoperative appearance, showing design of resection of tumor and triangle of skin below tumor that needs to be excised. B: Composite nasal septal graft in position. Note fringe of mucosa along top edge of cartilage to form lid margin. C,D: Insertion of 5–0 Prolene suture to hitch subcutaneous flap tissue to periosteum of orbit. E: Postoperative appearance 1 year after surgery. Note absence of drooping lid. F: As in part E, but showing support given to lid by cartilage of graft and the stable mucosa-covered margin with deep inferior fornix. (From Mustardé, ref. 1, with permission.)

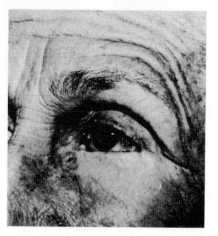
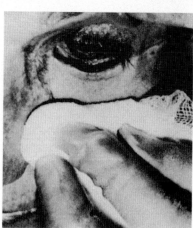

E,F

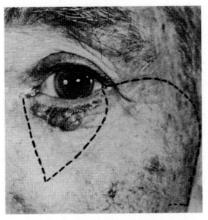 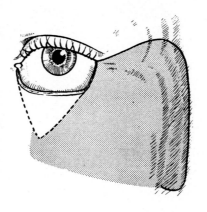 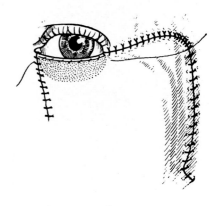

FIG. 6. A–C: Total reconstruction of the lower lid. This figure demonstrates the extent of resection and the amount of cheek to be rotated to cover the large composite nasal septal graft. (From Mustardé, ref. 1, with permission.)

SUMMARY

One of the best ways to reconstruct the lower eyelid is to use a cheek rotation flap lined with a septal chondromucosal graft when needed.

Reference

1. Mustardé JC. *Repair and Reconstruction in the Orbital Region*, 2d ed. Edinburgh: Churchill Livingstone, 1980; Chap. 7.

CHAPTER 14 ■ CHEEK ROTATION SKIN (IMRE) FLAP TO THE LOWER EYELID

G. S. PAP

During the years before World War I, Professor Imre designed the cheek-skin flap that now bears his name (1–7). The area of the Imre flap can be extended to embrace all tissue from the lower lid downward and from the nasolabial crease laterally (4). This flap uses local tissue similar in texture to that of the defect site, and it avoids a secondary defect. Incisions are placed along the natural wrinkle lines, and repair of a simple or composite defect can be achieved in one operation.

INDICATIONS

The Imre skin flap is indicated for reconstruction of partial or total defects of the lower lid, defects below the lower lid, defects at or below the medial canthus, cicatricial ectropion, and avulsion of the lower lid at the medial canthus. It also can be used, in conjunction with other local skin flaps, for repair

of defects in the periorbital region. These include defects at or above the medial canthus, where the Imre flap is used in conjunction with a sliding flap of skin from the forehead at the medial end of the brow; defects at or below the medial canthus, where the Imre flap is used with the adjacent nasal skin as an advancement flap along the nasolabial fold; for correction of an uneven palpebral fissure; or for repositioning of the medial canthal ligament in trauma patients (8).

FLAP DESIGN AND DIMENSIONS

The Imre flap is a sliding flap. It uses advancement along a curved incision, with a Burow's triangle raised at its distal end. The flap consists of skin and subcutaneous tissue and is of equal thickness throughout its length. In composite defects, it may be lined with remnants of conjunctiva from the lower

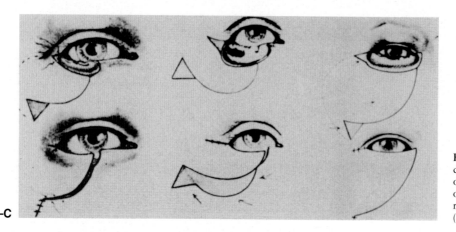

A–C

FIG. 1. Imre flap design for various defects of the lower lid. **A:** For repair of one-third of the lower lid. **B:** For repair of two-thirds of the lower lid. **C:** For repair of total loss of the lower eyelid. (From Pap, ref. 8, with permission.)

fornix of the eyelid or with a composite mucosa and cartilage graft from the nasal septum (see Chap. 13). The excision of Burow's triangle is a constant and pivotal feature. The design of the flap varies with the location and size of the defect.

OPERATIVE TECHNIQUE

Suturing of the flap donor site is always begun at the end farthest from the primary defect. Sutures are placed in such a fashion that they first transfix the lower wound margin. The sutures then advance the flap and simultaneously push and raise it upward, to make it rest in its new location after seven to eight sutures.

For repair of the lateral half of the lower lid, the skin margin below the curved incision is not undermined (Fig. 1A). For repair of oval or round defects on the lower eyelid, the flap should be equal in width to the vertical height of the defect. The flap and all wound margins and incisions need to be widely undermined. While suturing, the flap is advanced

upward and medially, and the opposite margin of the cheek is shifted in a temporal direction (Figs. 2 and 3B).

For repair of a defect below the lateral lid, the cheek flap resembles the design in Fig. 3B. The flap is again of equal width with the diameter of the defect, and the flap base almost reaches a horizontal line that extends from the upper margin of the defect. It is imperative that all wound margins be generously undermined. Occasionally, redundant skin at the end of the flap near the defect needs to be excised.

For total reconstruction of the lower lid, the length of the incision is about five times the distance from the tip of the flap to the new lid margin. The original Burow's triangle is converted into a crescent-shaped skin defect at the base of the flap. The flap is widely undermined beyond the line extending from the lateral canthus to the temporal side of the crescent-shaped defect (Figs. 1C and 2). If there is enough conjunctiva available, it can be used to line the upper margin of the flap (9). In patients in whom there is not enough conjunctiva, the margin of the flap can be lined with a tarsoconjunctival flap from the upper lid (Fig. 4).

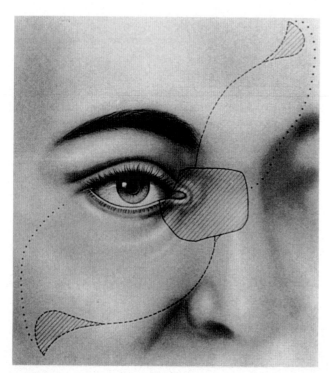

FIG. 2. The flap is undermined to the end of the *dotted line*. The excess is excised and the flap is advanced to fill the defect. A second flap may be used in a similar manner. (From Imre, ref. 1, with permission.)

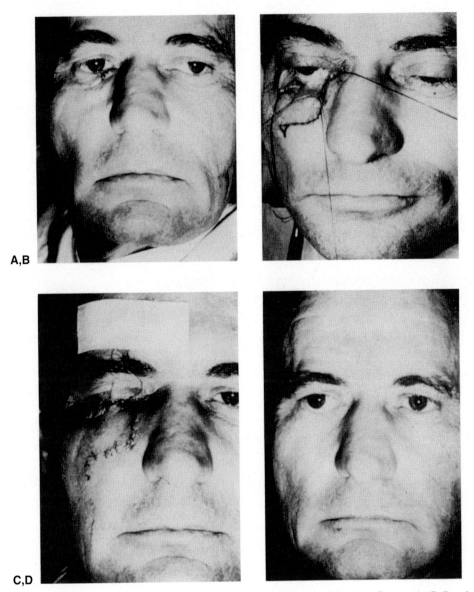

FIG. 3. **A:** Basal cell carcinoma of the medial canthus. **B:** Design of the Imre flap repair. **C:** Repair is completed with a Frost suture to help support the lid. **D:** Final result. The lid margin is a little lower than normal. (Courtesy of Dr. M. Spira.)

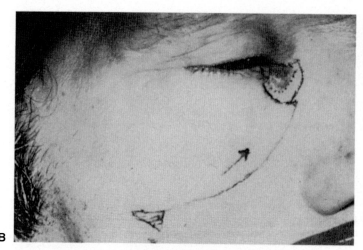
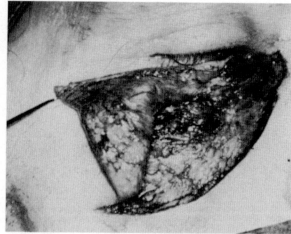

A,B

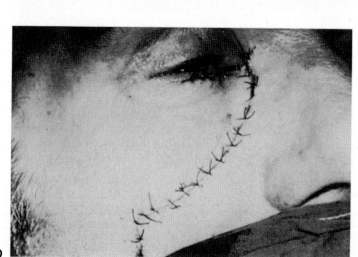
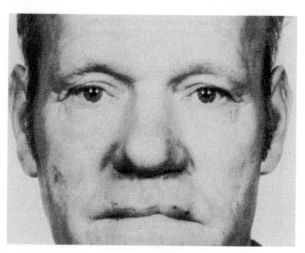

C,D

FIG. 4. **A:** Basal cell carcinoma overlying the lower lacrimal canaliculus. Design of the Imre flap, with the margins of the excision outlined. **B:** Flap dissected. **C:** Repair completed. The anterior edge of the canalicular gutter is sutured to the superior border of the flap. **D:** Final result. (From Bennett and Werb, ref. 9, with permission.)

SUMMARY

The Imre flap can be used to reconstruct partial or complete defects of the lower eyelid.

References

1. Imre J Jr. *Lidplastik*. Budapest: Studium Kiadasa, 1928.
2. Imre J Jr. New principles in plastic operations of the eyelids and face. *JAMA* 1921;76:1293.
3. Imre J Jr. In: Thiell R. ed., *Ophtalmologische Operationslehre*. Leipzig: Thieme-Verlag, 1942;87–108.
4. Metzger JT, Imre J Jr. The Imre flap. *Plast Reconstr Surg* 1959;23:501.
5. Stades FC. Tijdschrit voor Diergeneeskunde (Dutch). *Reconstr Eyelid Surg (Suppl)* 1987;1:586.
6. Borges AF. W-plasty rotation flap to cover nasal defect. *Ann Plast Surg* 1990;24:303.
7. Hoffman K, Stadler R. Imre modified bilobed flap rotation graft (Ger). *Hautarzt* 1993;44:148.
8. Pap GS. A comparison of three methods of eyelid reconstruction. *Plast Reconstr Surg* 1972;49:513.
9. Bennett JP, Werb A. The preservation of lachrymal drainage following excision of basal cell carcinoma of the lower eyelid. *Br J Plast Surg* 1981;38:385.

CHAPTER 15 ■ SUPERIORLY BASED TARSOCONJUNCTIVAL ADVANCEMENT (HUGHES, LANDHOLT, KÖLLNER) FLAP FOR RECONSTRUCTION OF THE LOWER EYELID

M. A. CALLAHAN

This is one of the oldest, time-tested flaps for eyelid reconstruction. It will result in a reconstructed eyelid of excellent color match, thickness, and function (1–5) (Fig. 2). The tarsoconjunctival flap for lower eyelid reconstruction supplies the deficient lower lid with conjunctiva for lining and tarsus for structural support. This posterior lamella flap should be combined with a free skin graft (or skin flap) to create the new anterior lamella of the lower lid.

Note that, as originally described, the upper eyelid was split along the gray line. Because of associated complications, this flap achieved a bad reputation. It is no longer performed as originally described, and even Dr. Hughes warns against splitting the upper eyelid (6).

INDICATIONS

Application of this technique is limited, in that the vertical height of the upper lid tarsal plate measures 10 to 12 mm, and if more than 7 mm of this tarsal plate is removed, the upper lid may itself become crippled and deformed. Therefore, this technique is most useful for repair of lower lid defects that are no more than 5 to 7 mm in vertical height. The best results are obtained when the horizontal extent of the defect is less than the distance from the inner to outer canthus. If necessary, however, the technique can be used to reconstruct the entire margin of the lower lid.

Defects of the lower lid that extend horizontally the full length of the lid and vertically to the inferior orbital rim are better repaired by the bipedicle or bucket-handle flap (Tripier) technique, as described in Chap. 17. When the lower lid defect exceeds 7 mm vertically and half the horizontal lid length has been resected, the Tenzel semicircular flap gives excellent results. The Tenzel flap also can be used in certain patients in whom a tarsoconjunctival flap is contraindicated.

When all the lower lid must be removed, including the base of the lid past the inferior orbital rim, the Mustardé cheek rotation flap, as described in Chap. 13, provides the best cosmetic and functional result.

Since the lids are closed for a significant period of time, this flap is not advisable when the patient has corneal or retinal disease that needs attention or when the lids cover the only seeing eye.

OPERATIVE TECHNIQUE

Fig. 1 illustrates resection of a lower lid tumor well below the lower lid tarsal plate, leaving a 5- to 7-mm vertical defect.

Two 4–0 silk sutures are placed along the upper lid margin, being careful to avoid the lash follicles, to evert the lid and expose the inner tarsal surface (Fig. 2B). The sutures are anchored to the drapes with hemostats. A horizontal mattress "tension" suture is placed across the lower lid defect to hold the wound edges in position temporarily, so that the width of the tarsoconjunctival flap can be estimated. The tension of the suture should be adjusted to approximate that of the normal lid. Alternatively, the width of the tarsoconjunctival flap can be estimated before the malignant lesion of the lower lid is resected.

A horizontal incision is made through the conjunctiva and tarsus of the upper lid 3 to 3.5 mm from the lid margin down to the submuscular fascia of the orbicularis muscles. The vertical limbs of the incision are extended in this same plane into the superior conjunctival cul-de-sac. Dissection in this area is best accomplished with a moistened cotton-tipped applicator, because Müller's muscle bleeds quite profusely unless the lid has been infiltrated with epinephrine.

Many authorities believe that retraction of the upper lid results primarily from the incorporation of Müller's muscle and the levator aponeurosis in the flap. These authors stress that it is important to form only a tarsoconjunctival flap and not to include the upper lid retractors. Of course, this leaves the flap tip and skin graft solely dependent on the conjunctival blood supply. Inclusion of the upper lid retractor muscles, whose blood supply is derived from branches of the dorsal nasal, frontal, supraorbital, and lacrimal arteries in the flap pedicle, largely obviates any chance of slough. As a result, slight retraction of the upper lid must be accepted as a trade-off. As described below, retraction of the upper lid can be dealt with by recessing the upper lid retractor muscles at the time of flap revision.

The profile illustration in Fig. 1C shows a 3- to 3.5-mm marginal strip of tarsus along the upper lid margin. The tarsoconjunctival flap has been advanced and sutured into the lower lid defect to form the new posterior lamella. As illustrated, the most superior extent of the dissection is carried out in such a way that no special attempt is made to separate Müller's muscle and the levator aponeurosis from the base of the flap.

Interrupted absorbable 5–0 catgut sutures are placed between the flap and the lower lid defect, so that neither suture loop nor knot protrudes posteriorly to irritate the globe (Fig. 1D). A retroauricular full-thickness skin graft is sutured on top of the flap to form the new anterior lamella of the lower lid. As an alternative, if the patient possesses abundant lower lid skin, a horizontal advancement flap of skin can be brought in either medially or laterally to cover the tarsocon-

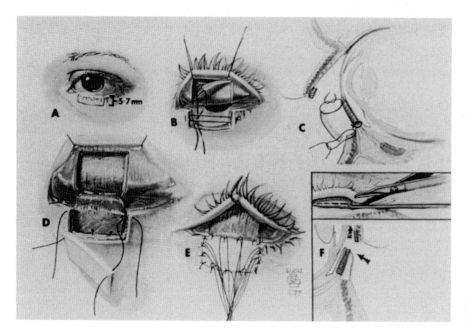

FIG. 1. Superiorly based tarsoconjunctival flap reconstruction of a lower lid.

junctival flap. Reconstructing the anterior lamella by a vertical advancement flap from below is to be avoided at all costs, because the lower lid will surely retract after the pedicle is divided.

The skin graft is sutured in place with a tie-over bolster soaked in an ophthalmic antibiotic solution to help inhibit bacterial growth during the first few postoperative days. A light pressure patch is applied for 48 hours and is changed on the first postoperative day. If a skin graft has been used, the cotton bolster is left in place for 10 to 14 days.

After the flap has been sutured in place, the patient is committed to a second procedure 2 to 6 months later, at which time the pedicle is divided. Collateral circulation from the recipient lid is sufficient to support the skin graft and the flap 6 weeks following reconstruction. However, more time should elapse to allow for scar maturation and suppleness of the lid, so that the tendency toward retraction of the lower lid will be decreased. In general, the wider the flap, the longer the pedicle should be left before division. When dividing the pedicle, a drop of topical anesthetic is placed in the cul-de-sac and the lid margins and base of pedicle are infiltrated with a local anesthetic. To protect the globe, two muscle hooks or a grooved director (shown in the upper frame of Fig. 1F) should be placed behind the flap, which is then divided with straight

scissors, so that a 1- to 2-mm stump of tarsus and conjunctiva remains above the new lower lid margin (Fig. 1F). This will compensate for inward rotation of the skin surface, which is often accompanied by entropion and trichiasis. If any excess tissue remains on the posterior lamella after 1 month, it can be trimmed under topical anesthesia.

After the pedicle is divided, the upper lid margin is examined for peaking or retraction. If these signs are present, the posterior aspect of the base of the upper lid is infiltrated with a local anesthetic. The stump of the pedicle (conjunctiva, Müller's muscle, and levator aponeurosis) is recessed toward its original position in the upper cul-de-sac (upward smaller arrow in Fig. 1F) until the height of the upper lid is 2 to 3 mm below the contralateral side. The upper lid will remain ptotic for a few days, but this will correct itself with the slight retraction that occurs as healing progresses. The missing segment of tarsus and conjunctiva in the center of the lid will be replaced by epithelialized fibrous tissue, and no suturing in the upper lid should be done. The orbit's excellent blood supply lessens the risk of flap necrosis and slough of the skin graft.

At the end of the procedure, an antibiotic ointment (gentamicin) is instilled and the eye is patched for a few hours, until oozing subsides. The eye should not be patched for a longer period because a readherence of the raw surfaces may occur.

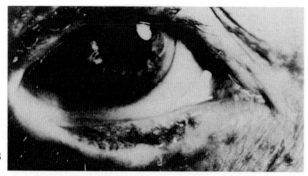
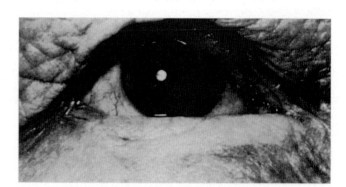

A,B

FIG. 2. A: Preoperative appearance of a right lower lid demonstrating a sclerosing basal cell carcinoma. The lid margin has been everted slightly by a cotton-tipped applicator. B: Reconstructed lower lid 2 years following tarsoconjunctival advancement flap and a retroauricular skin graft.

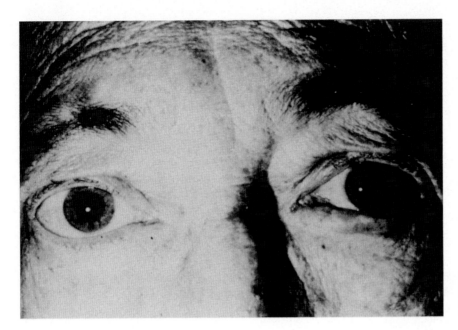

FIG. 3. Complications of Hughes tarsoconjunctival flap showing slight retraction of left upper lid and notching of the lateral aspect of the lower lid.

During eyelid reconstruction, the cornea should be adequately protected by a large contact lens or scleral shell. The cornea and conjunctiva should be moistened frequently with balanced salt solution (BSS) as the operation progresses to prevent desiccation. Alternatively, absorbable gelatin sponge, softened by BSS, can be placed over the cornea and conjunctiva.

If suture keratitis occurs postoperatively, the offending suture should be removed immediately, if possible, because keratopathy, pannus formation, and irreversible scarring of the cornea may occur. Occasionally, keratitis may be temporarily managed by a soft contact bandage lens. If a crucial suture in the repair seems to be the culprit, replace it as soon as possible, in the operating room, if necessary.

CLINICAL RESULTS

Unless a 3-mm bridge or strut of normal tarsus is left along the upper lid margin, notching, loss of lashes, or upper lid retraction may occur. Retraction and peaking of the upper lid also may occur if the Müller's muscle–levator aponeurosis complex is advanced inferiorly or resected during the reconstruction. This complication may be treated by recession of Müller's muscle and the levator palpebral muscle at the time of pedicle division.

The complications of notch formation and retraction of the upper lid (Fig. 3) were corrected by recession of the upper lid retractors and pentagonal resection of the obtrusive lower lid notch present laterally. This patient also suffered from kerati-

tis sicca postoperatively and had to wear a soft contact bandage lens for 1 year to allay her ocular discomfort.

If tear secretion is borderline, as documented by Schirmer testing, and the patient has keratitis sicca, an alternative technique should be considered, since the accessory lacrimal glands, which are concentrated in the upper cul-de-sac, are disrupted by this operation.

SUMMARY

The tarsoconjunctival flap for lower eyelid reconstruction supplies the deficient lower lid not only with conjunctiva for lining, but also with tarsus for structural support.

References

1. Czermak W. *Die Augenarztlichen Operationen.* Vol. 1, 2nd Ed. Berlin: Urban und Schwarzenberg, 1908;253–254.
2. Dupuy Dutemps L. Autoplastie palpébro-palpébrale integrate. Réfection d'une paupière, détruite dans toute son epaisseur, par greffe cutanée et tarso-conjonctivale prisé a l'autre paupière. *Monde Med* 1928;38:705.
3. Dupuy Dutemps L. Autoplastie palpébro-palpébrale integrate. Refection d'une paupière détruite dans toute son epaisseur par greffe cutanée et tarso-conjonctivale prisé a l'autre paupière. *Bull Med (Paris)* 1929;43:935.
4. Hughes WL. *Reconstructive surgery of the eyelids.* St. Louis: Mosby, 1943.
5. Köllner O. Verfahren fur den plastischen Ersatz des Unterlides. *Munchen Med Wochenschr* 1911;58:2166.
6. Hughes WL. A new method for rebuilding a lower lid. *Arch Ophthalmol* 1966;17:1008.

CHAPTER 16 ■ LATERAL TARSOCONJUNCTIVAL FLAP FOR LID TIGHTENING

S. A. LAUER

The lateral tarsoconjunctival flap is designed to restore horizontal tension in the lower eyelid. As soft tissues of the face stretch with age, the tarsoligamentous sling becomes weakened and lax, due primarily to stretching of the canthal tendons. Constant pulling and stretching of the eyelid eventually can produce an involutional ectropion, which occurs when horizontal laxity is sufficient for gravity to pull the eyelid away from the eye.

Restoration of tension in the tarsoligamentous sling can be accomplished in a number of ways, some of which threaten the underlying lacrimal drainage apparatus and the stability of the tear film. Tightening the lateral canthal tendon (1) with the lateral tarsoconjunctival flap has become the preferred means of restoring horizontal tension in the lower eyelid.

INDICATIONS

The primary indications for use of the flap are correction of an involutional ectropion or, in some instances, to provide corneal protection in cases of seventh-nerve paralytic ectropion that do not resolve spontaneously. In the latter case, the flap is usually employed in combination with implantation of an upper-lid gold weight to restore upper-lid mobility. Where additional protection of the corneal epithelium is required, such as with tumors at the cerebellopontine angle that produce fifth- and seventh-nerve palsies, the lower lid is not only tightened by a lateral tarsoconjunctival flap, but is concurrently elevated with a sling such as a fascial sling, or by inserting spacer material beneath the tarsus.

The flap can also be utilized to prevent vertical lid retraction after skin excision during a lower-lid blepharoplasty. In addition, it can be used to correct an entropion, or in-turning,

of the lower lid; although this condition, resulting from a combination of forces, may require additional surgery, the flap alone may be used to reverse horizontal lid laxity.

Cicatricial ectropion or vertical lid retraction can be produced by scarring and shortening of the skin in the lower eyelid. The lateral tarsoconjunctival flap can then be used, in combination with skin augmentation with a full-thickness skin graft or regional skin flap (2,3) (Fig. 1A-C).

ANATOMY

It is now generally accepted that the lateral canthal tendon is a fibrous connective tissue arising from the lateral ends of the superior and inferior tarsal plates (1,4). It inserts at the lateral orbital tubercle within the orbit, approximately 1.5 mm posterior to the lateral orbital rim. The tendon averages 10.6 mm in length from the lateral canthal angle to its bony insertion and 6.6 mm in width, with the distance from the midpoint of the tendon to the frontozygomatic suture averaging 9.7 mm. Superiorly, the tendon is contiguous with the lateral horn of the levator palpebrae superioris; posteriorly, it is contiguous with the check ligament of the lateral rectus muscle. Both of these structures also insert at the lateral orbital tubercle. Anteriorly, there is a small pocket of fat (Eisler's fat pad), which is situated between the orbital septum and the lateral canthal tendon.

There are slips of striated muscle that pass from the overlying pretarsal orbicularis oculi muscle and intermingle with the connective tissue of the lateral canthal tendon.

FLAP DESIGN AND DIMENSIONS

The lateral tarsoconjunctival flap is created by transecting the inferior crus of the lateral canthal tendon, and then using the tarsus to resuspend the lid, approximating the attachment to the lateral orbital tubercle. The flap should be made slightly longer than the distance between the lateral canthus and the lateral orbital rim. Epithelium-bearing tissues must be removed from the flap before resuspension of the lid to avoid the development of an inclusion cyst.

OPERATIVE TECHNIQUE

The procedure can be done under local anesthesia. Injection of the anesthetic is at the lateral canthus and beneath the conjunctiva of the lateral inferior fornix. A lateral canthotomy

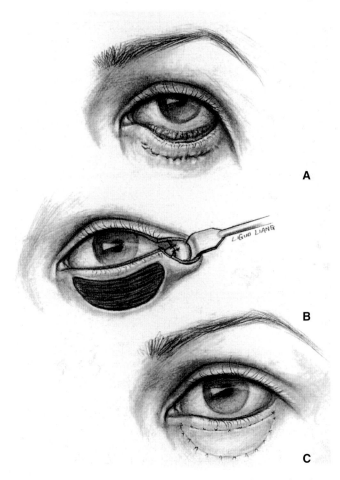

FIG. 1. A: Eyelid with vertical lid retraction due to skin loss. **B:** Release of skin contracture of lid and suture of lateral canthus to a higher position on the orbital rim. **C:** Postcorrection of vertical lid retraction with lateral tarsoconjunctival flap and full-thickness skin graft.

attention to restoring the lid margin at the lateral canthal angle (5–7) (Fig. 2E).

CLINICAL RESULTS

Although this flap has now been used for many years in lower-eyelid surgery with excellent clinical results, there are some points to bear in mind. First, the goal of the surgery is to create tension at the lateral anastomosis of the lid to the orbital rim. Care must be taken when suturing the lid to the periosteum, because dehiscence can occur. Steri-strips are helpful in the early postoperative period, to aid in supporting the lid while the wound is maturing. Second, as with any wound at the lid margin, care must be taken when suturing the lateral canthal edge, because the eye is very sensitive to disruption of the lid margin. Finally, it is best to create more tension in the lower lid than is immediately necessary, because the soft tissues can be expected to relax with time.

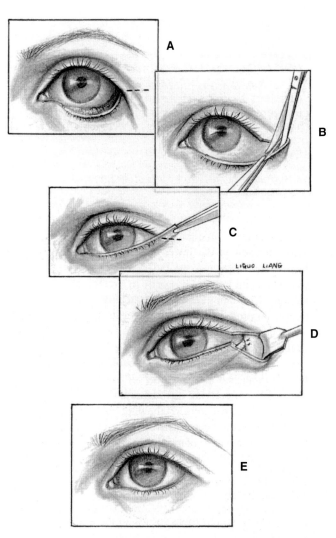

FIG. 2. A: A lateral canthotomy is planned dividing the fornix. **B:** The inferior crus of the lateral canthal tendon is selectively cut. **C:** The lid will move up easily if the tendon has been cut. **D:** The lid is sutured by placing a suture in the tarsal plate and anchored to the medial surface of the orbital rim laterally. **E:** The skin is closed, restoring the lateral canthal angle.

is performed with scissors or blade (Fig. 2A). The inferior crus of the lateral canthal tendon is selectively cut to avoid horizontal shortening of the lid; it is easiest to identify the inferior crus by stretching the lid and feeling for areas of resistance on attempted lid elevation (Fig. 2B, C).

The cut edge of the lid margin is then pulled laterally until horizontal tension has been restored; a mark is placed along the margin at the point chosen to be the new edge of the lateral canthus. Epithelium-bearing tissue at the margin lateral to this point is resected. The tarsus is then separated from the overlying pretarsal orbicularis. A blade is used to scrape conjunctival epithelial cells from the posterior surface of the tarsus. The flap of tarsus and palpebral conjunctiva remains attached to the capsulopalpebral fascia inferiorly. The flap is measured so that it is just longer than necessary for reattachment to the lateral orbital rim, and excess tissue is excised (Fig. 2C). The last step in the procedure is to resuspend the tarsus to the lateral orbital rim. This is generally accomplished with a double-armed, permanent, monofilament suture passed in a horizontal mattress fashion. The suture should be passed several times through the tarsus, because cheese-wiring is common. With the last pass, the suture should exit the anterior surface of the tarsus. The suture is passed through the orbital periosteum in a posterior-to-anterior direction, making sure that the path of the needle begins behind the lateral orbital rim (Fig. 2D). The skin is then closed, with special

SUMMARY

The lateral tarsoconjunctival flap, originally designed for the correction of involutional ectropion, has evolved into a multipurpose flap that is useful whenever horizontal tightening of the lower eyelid is desired.

References

1. Gioia VM, Linberg JV, McCormick SA. The anatomy of the lateral canthal tendon. *Arch Ophthalmol* 1987;105:529.
2. Lauer SA. Ectropion and entropion. In *Focal Points,* vol. 12, no. 10. San Francisco: American Academy of Ophthalmology, 1994.
3. Jordan DR, Anderson RL. The lateral tarsal strip revisited: the enhanced tarsal strip. *Arch Ophthalmol* 1989;107:604.
4. Whitnall SE. On a tubercle on the malar bone, and on the lateral attachments of the tarsal plates. *J Anat Physiol* 1911;45:426.
5. Rathbun JE. *Eyelid Surgery.* Boston: Little, Brown, 1994.
6. Hornblass A, Chanig CJ. *Oculoplastic, orbital and reconstructive surgery.* Baltimore: Williams and Wilkins, 1988.
7. Putterman AM. *Cosmetic oculoplastic surgery.* Philadelphia: WB Saunders, 1993.

CHAPTER 17 ■ BIPEDICLE UPPER EYELID FLAP (TRIPIER) FOR LOWER EYELID RECONSTRUCTION

C. D. BUCKO

The bipedicle upper eyelid flap has been used to repair horizontally oriented losses of the lower eyelid, both marginal and nonmarginal, of less than 10 to 15 mm in vertical height. Usually, when repairing a marginal loss, a composite chondromucosal graft is used on the undersurface.

INDICATIONS

This flap is useful in replacing the absent central two-thirds of the lower eyelid that results from trauma, tumor excision, or congenital colobomas. It can be used to replace a horizontal marginal loss in the central two-thirds of the lower lid, to replace skin loss in the central two-thirds of a lower lid, or to fill in after release and elevation of the lower lid (cicatricial lesions) where vertical height is less than 10 to 15 mm.

The flap is relatively simple to design and execute and is also a safe flap with a good blood supply. It is composed of eyelid skin and muscle and is therefore of good texture and color match. If a composite graft is included, the flap can be used for full-thickness lid replacement (marginal loss). The donor scar is invisible, and there is no functional loss of the donor lid, since the flap tissue is usually in excess in adults. The flap can be used to replace the entire central two-thirds of the eyelid.

Disadvantages of the flap include the following: The width of the flap is limited to 10 to 15 mm in adults and even less in children, and the flap cannot be used for defects of the extreme medial or lateral eyelid. Upper lid tissue is used to reconstruct the lower lid, and this may cause functional loss if

incorrectly used. There are no eyelashes present in the flap. Two stages are required to complete the reconstruction.

FLAP DESIGN AND DIMENSIONS

The flap is outlined with the inferior edge corresponding to the supratarsal fold from point *A* to point *B* (Fig. 1A). These two points are located above the medial and lateral canthi, respectively, where the fold disappears. The superior incision (*CD*) is made parallel to line *AB* (Fig. 1A), creating a bipedicled flap approximately 10 to 15 mm wide, depending on the amount of redundant tissue present in the preseptal area. A wider flap may be used, but this will require a skin graft to close the donor area.

OPERATIVE TECHNIQUE

Complete reconstruction requires at least two stages separated by 1 to 2 weeks, since both bases must be transected in the second stage, after the flap has secured vascularization from its new bed in the lower lid.

The flap is incised and undermined deep to the orbicularis oculi muscle in the areolar plane between the muscle and the orbital septum. The donor defect is closed directly with 6-0 nylon skin sutures from the medial base to the lateral base.

The flap is swung inferiorly into the lower lid defect and sutured into place (Fig. 1B). In nonmarginal defects, a one-layer closure of the skin with interrupted 6-0 nylon sutures is

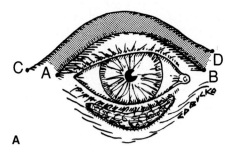

A

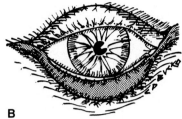

B

FIG. 1. **A:** Bipedicle flap has been outlined, with inferior edge and supratarsal crease from point *A* to point *B*. Superior edge is 10 to 15 mm above crease. **B:** Flap is sutured into central defect, leaving bases in canthal areas intact. Donor area is closed up to bases.

sufficient. It is not possible to close the skin at the medial and lateral edges during this primary stage because of the flap bases. These bases usually become tubed and will be excised in a second stage.

When closing a marginal defect, the undersurface of the flap must be grafted with a composite chondromucosal graft (Fig. 2A). Neither advancement of the remaining conjunctiva nor use of a superior lid tarsoconjunctival flap for lining (Köllner or reverse Landholt-Hughes technique) should be used (1), unless the vertical loss is less than 5 mm (usual width

of the inferior tarsal plate). Mucosal advancement may result in entropion and retraction of the lower lid with scleral "show" (1), and the Köllner technique, if misused, can cause severe upper lid retraction and lagophthalmos (2).

The chondromucosal graft can be taken from the nasal septum (Fig. 2B) or from the upper lateral nasal area. A lateral alar rhinotomy facilitates taking the graft. Closure of the nasal incision is rapid and simple and leaves minimal scar. If the septal cartilage is used, it must be thinned before it is sutured into the lower lid. The graft is trimmed along the superior edge, so

A,B

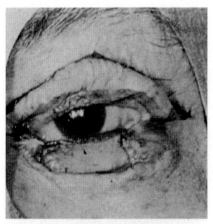

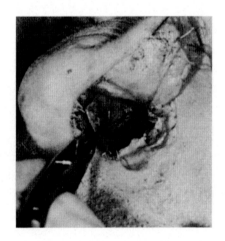

C,D

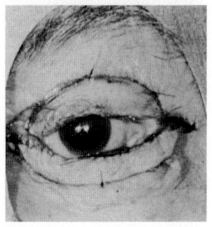

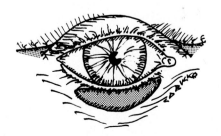

FIG. 2. **A:** Chondromucosal graft forms internal lamella. **B:** Chondromucosal graft is obtained from septum through lateral rhinotomy. **C:** Flap covers composite graft. **D:** Bases are transected, and excess is discarded. Flap is inset into medial and lateral edges of defect. Donor area closure is completed.

that the mucosa extends 2 to 3 mm beyond the edge of the cartilage, to allow the mucosa to be turned over the edge of the cartilage and meet the skin flap at the new gray line. The cartilage should extend well below the defect inferiorly to give support to the reconstructed lid. Excision of additional conjunctiva may be necessary.

The flap is then used to form the anterior surface of the reconstructed lid (Fig. 2C). A tie-over bolster to prevent tubing of the flap has been suggested (2). However, this may interfere with the circulation in the flap.

An eye patch may be applied, but no pressure should be exerted. The bandage can be changed as needed over the ensuing 10 to 14 days prior to division of the pedicles. Division of the pedicles is usually safe after 10 days. The upper and lower lid are infiltrated with plain Xylocaine, and the two bases are transected at the margins of the defect. The ends of the flap are trimmed and inset with 6-0 nylon. The remaining pedicles from the upper lid are excised, leaving

small triangles, rather than returned to the lid, because of the thickening and tubing of the pedicle tissues (Fig. 2D), that result in conspicuous scar.

SUMMARY

The bipedicle upper eyelid flap is a safe and reliable flap that can be used to reconstruct defects of the central two-thirds of the lower eyelid up to 15 to 20 mm in vertical height.

References

1. Mustardé JC. *Repair and reconstruction in the orbital region: a practical guide.* Edinburgh: Churchill Livingstone, 1980. Chap. 11, 122.
2. Callahan A. *Reconstructive surgery of the eyelids and ocular adnexa.* Birmingham, AL: Aesculapius, 1966.

CHAPTER 18 ■ SKIN ISLAND ORBICULARIS OCULI MUSCULOCUTANEOUS FLAP FOR LOWER EYELID RECONSTRUCTION

R. V. ARGAMASO

A substantial loss of lower eyelid tissue may result from trauma or surgery. Reconstruction by skin-flap transfer has been of particular interest to reconstructive surgeons.

INDICATIONS

In recent years, the introduction of musculocutaneous flaps has increased the survival rate of skin transfers. In many instances, the quality of results also has improved.

It is noteworthy that long before musculocutaneous flaps became popular, Tripier performed a transposition of an orbicularis oculi musculocutaneous flap from the upper to the lower eyelid in 1889 (1). The same concept was elaborated on for repair of lower lid defects after tumor ablation (2). The Tripier flap was further modified by converting the skin component into an island on a bipedicled orbicularis oculi muscle that was then transferred to the lower lid for correction of severe ectropion (3).

Described below is a skin island orbicularis oculi musculocutaneous flap obtained from the suprabrow area and used for reconstruction of the lower eyelid. The upper eyelid was not a suitable donor, since it was also partially damaged.

ANATOMY

The orbicularis oculi is a flat, circular muscle arising from the nasal part of the frontal bone, frontal process of the max-

illa, and anterior surface of the medial palpebral ligament. The pretarsal and preseptal sections occupy the eyelids, while the orbital portion surrounds the orbits, spreading to the temple and down to the cheeks. The muscle layer is relatively thinner within the eyelids than that which surrounds the orbits. The latter forms a complete ellipse without interruption. Its upper fibers blend with those of the frontalis and corrugator muscles.

The blood supply comes from three main sources. Branches of the facial artery penetrate the muscle from its inferomedial aspect. The superficial temporal artery sends several branches approaching the lateral side. The internal maxillary artery also contributes by way of the supraorbital and infraorbital arteries. These vessels interlace with one another within the muscle to form arcades that give out branches to the overlying skin. The veins follow the locations of the main arteries.

Filaments of the temporal and zygomatic branches of the facial nerve innervate the orbicularis oculi muscle.

FLAP DESIGN AND OPERATIVE TECHNIQUE

A lenticular island of skin is outlined adjacent to the eyebrow (Fig. 1). The inferior boundary is along the full extent of the follicular line. Skin and subcutaneous fat are incised. Below the bulbs of the hair follicles, the knife is beveled in

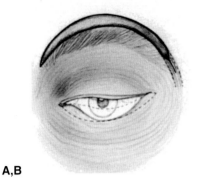
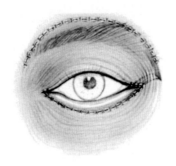

A,B

FIG. 1. **A:** Diagram of the skin island outlined above the eyebrow. The flap should be as wide as the defect of the lower lid. *Broken lines* delineate the muscle pedicle. **B:** The skin island is sutured in place. The muscle pedicle, actually wider than the width of the skin island, lies in a subcutaneous tunnel.

order to cut a wider strip of muscle than the overlying skin island.

At the lateral angle of the skin incision, muscle continuity is kept intact so that a pedicle can be developed for the musculocutaneous flap. This is a critical area where the skin is undermined very superficially to prevent injury to the blood vessels entering the muscle. Skin undermining is continued inferiorly in the same superficial plane above the orbicularis ring.

The skin-muscle flap is then elevated starting medially from its tip toward its base near the temple. The pivot point should be at the same horizontal level as the outer canthus or palpebral fissure. An arc of rotation is established that will allow the flap to sweep over the entire territory of the lower lid.

A tunnel is made beneath the lateral canthal skin for the entry of the flap toward its final destination. There should be ample space for the pedicle to settle in without undue compression. The apex of the flap should reach the medial canthus. The muscle layer of the flap is spread out by sutures over the orbital fibers of the recipient bed and tied over bolsters on the skin.

The flap is lined either by advancing conjunctiva at the inferior sulcus or by a free graft of mucosa obtained from the inside of the cheek.

CLINICAL RESULTS

The use of upper lid skin in the patient illustrated in Fig. 2 was not feasible because this was also traumatized and somewhat deficient. Rotation of a Mustardé flap (4) would have sacrificed normal facial skin and produced unwanted scars on the face. A free-flap transfer to restore lower lid form is a formidable undertaking, and therefore, a skin island orbicularis oculi musculocutaneous flap was designed.

Since the skin and muscle components of the suprabrow area are thicker than those of normal eyelids, the island flap would appear bulkier than when upper lid tissues are employed. Also, pigmentation of the suprabrow skin seems lighter than that of most lid skin. In other patients, some eyebrow hair may be present within the area of the skin island. For these reasons, this flap should be considered and recommended only when other more ideal flaps are not available.

Dissection of the muscle pedicle should be restricted to a limited area to avoid injury to the zygomatic and temporal fibers of the facial nerve. Transient weakness in eyelid closure has been observed. Loss of elevation of the eyebrow is more common because of complete transection of the frontalis muscle insertion into the orbicularis, but this may be a small price to pay for the correction of functional and aesthetic deformities of the lower eyelid.

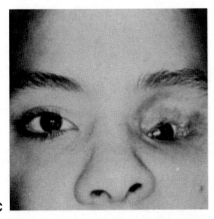
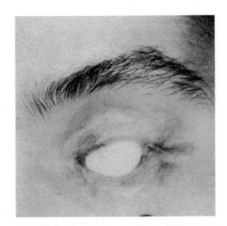
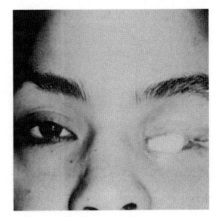

A–C

FIG. 2. **A:** A 20-year-old woman who sustained a gunshot wound to her face. The injury involved comminuted fractures of the floor and rim of the left orbit, total disruption of the left globe, subtotal destruction of the lower eyelid, and partial avulsion of the upper eyelid. Initial treatment consisted of debridement of the contents of the left socket and wound closure using the remnants of lid skin to cover the concavity of the orbit. Reconstruction of the orbital floor and rim was performed with rib grafts. The cavity was resurfaced with mucosal grafts obtained from the cheeks. **B:** Close-up of skin island flap. **C:** Moderate inversion of the reconstructed lid margin secondary to contracture of the mucosal graft requires additional surgery. Eyebrow scar is comparable to that following a direct brow lift procedure.

SUMMARY

A one-stage transfer of a skin island musculocutaneous flap of orbicularis oculi from its supraorbital segment is described as an alternate method for reconstruction of the lower eyelid.

References

1. Tripier L. Lambeau musculo-cutané en forme de point. *Gaz Hopitaux* 1889;62:1124.
2. Goldstein MH. Orbiting the orbicularis: restoration of muscle ring continuity with myocutaneous flaps. *Plast Reconstr Surg* 1983;92:294.
3. Siegel RJ. Severe ectropion: repair with a modified Tripier flap. *Plast Reconstr Surg* 1987;80:21.
4. Mustardé JC. The use of flaps in the orbital region. *Plast Reconstr Surg* 1970;45:146.

CHAPTER 19 ■ CHEEK V-Y ADVANCEMENT SKIN FLAP TO THE LOWER EYELID

I. J. PELED AND M. R. WEXLER

EDITORIAL COMMENT

This procedure is probably not the best choice among the various alternatives available. To be successful, the V-Y advancement must overcompensate. The medial and lateral extent of the Y limbs should be the canthal ligaments, to prevent retraction and possible ectropion.

Several methods of lower eyelid reconstruction have been reported, including rotation cheek flaps (1–3), musculocutaneous orbicularis flaps (4), partial- or full-thickness upper eyelid flaps (5–9), nasolabial and supraorbital flaps (10), and full-thickness skin grafts for coverage (11). These have been combined with conjunctival flaps and chondromucosal grafts for lining (11,12).

Using the reliable V-Y advancement principle described by Gillies (13) [later modified to an island subcutaneously based by Kutler (14) in fingertip reconstruction] and the triangle of cheek skin discarded during reconstruction in the Mustardé cheek rotation skin flap (3), the lower eyelid can be reconstructed by covering a chondromucosal graft with a V-Y advancement cheek flap (15).

INDICATIONS

Lower eyelid reconstruction is performed fairly often following tumor ablation, trauma (avulsion, burns), or when using a lower eyelid flap for reconstruction of the upper lid. When the remaining defect is wider than one-third of the lower eyelid, direct suturing should not be attempted, and local or distant tissue is necessary.

This technique involves only one stage. There is no dog-ear to revise later, no discarding of healthy tissue, and the upper eyelid remains intact. Use of the technique

does not preclude later use of the rotation cheek flap, if necessary.

ANATOMY

The V-Y cheek flap is a random one that is subcutaneously based in the nasolabial area, which is very richly supplied by branches of the facial artery. Wide lateral undermining between the dermis and the subcutaneous tissue allows upward

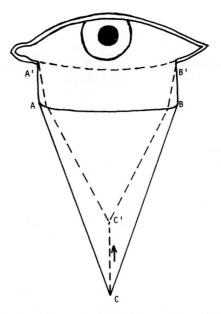

FIG. 1. Schematic drawing of lower eyelid defect and subcutaneous-based triangular cheek skin flap (*A'B'BA*, eyelid defect; *ABC*, triangular cheek skin flap; *A'B'C'*, sutured flap; *CC'*, V-Y advancement).

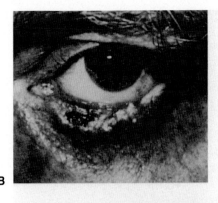
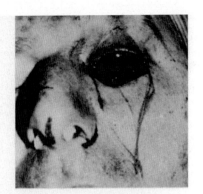

A,B

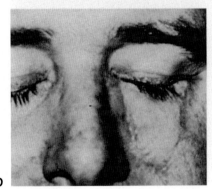
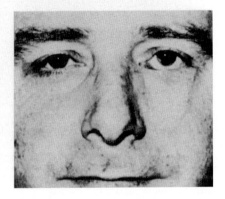

C,D

FIG. 2. A: Extensive basal cell carcinoma of the left lower eyelid. **B:** Defect following tumor ablation. Note the lines drawn for the V-Y flap. **C,D:** Good cosmetic and functional results 6 months following operation. (From Peled et al., ref. 15, with permission.)

advancement without tension and does not jeopardize the blood supply of the flap.

FLAP DESIGN AND DIMENSIONS

The triangular flap is drawn in the cheek under the defect (Fig. 1). The width of the flap is the same as the width of the defect, and the height of the flap is 1½ times greater.

OPERATIVE TECHNIQUE

After design of the flap in the cheek below the defect, the skin of the V-Y flap is incised to the subcutaneous plane and is undermined laterally, carefully preserving all the subcutaneous tissue attachments.

The flap is advanced upward until it reaches the desired position of the eyelid border without tension. It is anchored medially and laterally to the orbital periosteum with two nonabsorbable sutures. This maneuver compensates for gravity and avoids ectropion. The flap donor area is closed in a Y fashion. Lining of the defect is obtained with a nasal chondromucosal graft taken from the nasal septum (12) or lateral nasal wall (16) and it is then sutured to the remaining conjunctiva (see Chap. 13).

CLINICAL RESULTS

The only disadvantage in the technique occurs in defects with a vertical height greater than 12 mm, where the skin that is advanced upward is thicker and may be hairy in males. No complications were encountered, and cosmetic and functional results have been satisfactory as seen in the patient in Fig. 2 (17).

SUMMARY

The cheek V-Y advancement skin flap can be effectively used for wide defects of the lower eyelid.

References

1. Hagerty RF, Smoak RD. Reconstruction of the lower eyelid. *Plast Reconstr Surg* 1966;38:52.
2. McGregor IA. Eyelid reconstruction following subtotal resection on upper or lower lid. *Br J Plast Surg* 1973;26:346.
3. Mustardé JC, Jones LT, Callahan A. *Ophthalmic plastic surgery up-to-date.* Birmingham, AL: Aesculapius, 1970.
4. Anderson RL, Edwards JJ. Myocutaneous flaps for major eyelid and canthal reconstruction. In: Bernstein L, ed., *Plastic and reconstructive surgery of the head and neck,* Vol. 11. New York: Grune & Stratton, 1981;306.
5. Gorney M, Falces E, Jones H, et al. One-stage reconstruction of substantial lower lid margin defects. *Plast Reconstr Surg* 1969;44:592.
6. Jones HM. One-stage composite lower lid repair. *Plast Reconstr Surg* 1966;37:349.
7. McCoy FJ, Crow ML. Adaptation of the switch flap to eyelid reconstruction. *Plast Reconstr Surg* 1965;35:633.
8. Orticochea M. Total reconstruction of the eyelid. *Br J Plast Surg* 1977;30:44.
9. Pollock WL, Colon GA, Ryan RF. Reconstruction of the lower eyelid by a different lid-splitting operation. *Plast Reconstr Surg* 1972;50:184.
10. Paletta FX. Lower eyelid reconstruction. *Plast Reconstr Surg* 1973;51:653.
11. Macomber WB, Wang MK. Total reconstruction of upper and lower eyelids in the treatment of cancer. *Clin Plast Surg* 1978;5:501.
12. Mustardé JC. Reconstruction of the upper lid and the use of nasal mucosal grafts. *Br J Plast Surg* 1969;21:367.
13. Gillies H. *Plastic surgery of the face.* London: Frowdes, Hodder & Stoughton, 1920;20.
14. Kutler W. A new method for fingertip amputation. *JAMA* 1947;133:29.
15. Peled I, Kaplan H, Wexler MR. Lower eyelid reconstruction by V-Y advancement cheek flap. *Ann Plast Surg* 1980;5:321.
16. Paufique L, Tessier P. Reconstruction totale de la paupiere superieure. In: Troutman RC, Converse JM, Smith B, eds., *Plastic and reconstructive surgery of the eye and adnexa.* Melbourne: Butterworth, 1962.
17. Peled IJ, Wexler MR. The usefulness and versatility of V-Y advancement flaps. *J Dermatol Surg Oncol* 1983;9:12.

CHAPTER 20 ■ LATERALLY BASED TARSOCONJUNCTIVAL TRANSPOSITION FLAP TO THE LOWER EYELID

C. BEARD AND J. H. SULLIVAN

In this method of up to total lower eyelid reconstruction, the tarsoconjunctiva and skin are obtained from separate, rather than contiguous, areas (1,2). The procedure was developed to be used in place of the popular Hughes operation (3), the latter requiring occlusion of the eye for several weeks (see Chap. 15). This visual deprivation was troublesome to many patients, particularly those with less than good vision in the unoperated eye.

INDICATIONS

This operation can be used for almost any lower lid reconstruction when the defect is too large for direct closure. Since it is based laterally, this flap is ideally suited for defects that extend to the lateral canthus. If the most lateral portion of the lower lid is intact, it must either be transferred to the nasal side of the defect as a full-thickness, inferiorly based pedicle flap or simply excised to allow space for the proximal portion of the transposition flap. Since the operation works well for total lower lid reconstruction, we have found it simpler to excise the normal temporal lid tissue.

ANATOMY

We believe that the tarsoconjunctival flap retains much of its vascularity through its conjunctival plexus. In most instances, the pedicle contains terminal branches of the superficial temporal and transverse facial arteries. Despite its narrow base, the flap blanches with pressure, recolors with release of pressure, and oozes blood from its raw surface. It is possible, however, that the tip of the flap acts as a free graft.

FLAP DESIGN AND DIMENSIONS

The flap contains tarsus and conjunctiva from the upper lid, is based at the lateral canthal tendon, and is transposed to the lower lid on a narrow pedicle. The length of the flap is determined by applying lateral traction on the nasal remnant of the lower lid to narrow the defect and then marking the upper lid opposite the cut nasal edge of the lower lid defect. The flap is taken from the upper portion of the tarsus. The width of the flap to be developed is about 4 mm, or slightly less than half the tarsal width.

OPERATIVE TECHNIQUE

The operative technique is illustrated in Fig. 1. The lower lid tumor is removed under frozen-section control. The upper lid is everted on a Desmarres retractor. A vertical incision is first made at the predetermined mark defining the length of the flap. The incision is made into an L shape by a horizontal extension parallel to the lid margin. The L is converted to a U by a parallel horizontal incision through conjunctiva and Müller's muscle along the upper tarsal border. It extends into the palpebral conjunctiva beyond the lateral extent of the tarsus. The upper incision is continued laterally to a point above the canthus, and the inferior incision is carried into the lateral fornix.

The tarsoconjunctival flap thus outlined is elevated at first along the anterior tarsal surface and then posterior to the lateral canthal tendon until the lateral wall of the orbit can be felt with the dissecting scissors. A small triangle of conjunctiva below the lateral canthal tendon is excised to create a bed for the proximal end of the flap (Fig. 1B).

The flap is rotated 180° (from the everted upper lid) on its horizontal axis until its conjunctival surface faces the globe. It is stretched into position to fill the posterior aspect of the lower lid defect. It should hug the globe firmly. Insufficient tension may result in ectropion. If the flap is lax, it must be shortened appropriately. The tip of the flap is sutured to the free edge of the lower lid tarsus with interrupted 6–0 plain catgut. The inferior edges are approximated with a running suture. It is not necessary to close the donor site in the upper lid. We initially sutured conjunctiva and Müller's muscle to tarsus, but occasionally we observed upper lid retraction. By allowing the wound to granulate, we have seen no ill effects.

We have not attempted to cover the flap with a full-thickness skin graft, but we believe a split-thickness graft could be used if necessary. In most instances, skin cover can be accomplished by an advancement flap from below. If skin cannot easily be elevated to the lid margin, a horizontal relaxing incision can be made over the orbital rim. The resulting defect can be covered with a full-thickness retroauricular or supraclavicular skin graft. We have, on one occasion, successfully provided skin cover by a transposition flap from the upper lid, forming back-to-back flaps.

CLINICAL RESULTS

The complications that have been observed are entropion and deformity of the canthal angle. Ectropion has been the result of transposing too long a tarsoconjunctival flap and not the result of vertical skin shortage. Correction has been made by horizontal lid shortening.

The canthal deformity consists of a visible band of tarsoconjunctiva behind the angle. Lysis of the band, after lid heal-

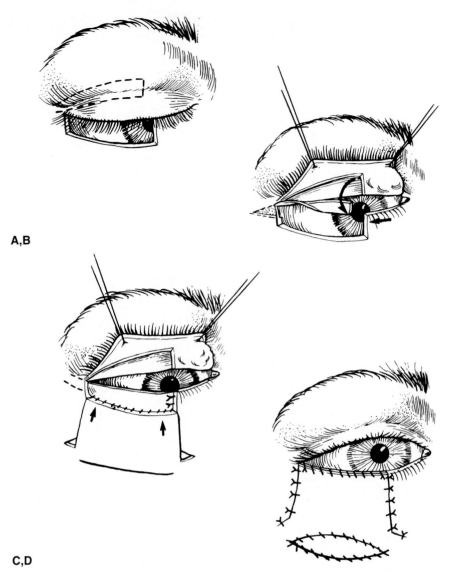

A,B

C,D

FIG. 1. A: The tumor is excised. The *dotted line* shows the extent of the tarsoconjunctival flap. **B:** The lid is everted. (Note that the lid is actually everted with a Desmarres retractor and not sutures, as shown in the illustration.) Lateral traction is placed on the remaining nasal lid. The extent of the flap is marked. The flap is elevated and rotated 180° on its horizontal axis and into position in the lower lid. A triangle of conjunctiva is excised beneath the lateral canthal tendon. **C:** The flap is sutured into position with 6–0 plain catgut. An inferior skin advancement flap is prepared. If necessary, a relaxing incision is made at its base. **D:** The skin is advanced. The lid margin is sutured with 6–0 plain catgut; the skin, with 6–0 silk. If necessary, a full-thickness skin graft is used to fill the defect over the orbital rim.

ing, has relieved this condition. We have not seen damage to the lacrimal secretory function. Necrosis of the tarsoconjunctival flap or skin coverage has not been observed in any of our patients.

SUMMARY

A one-stage tarsal transposition procedure is useful for repair of lower eyelid defects too large for simple closure. The posterior layer of the reconstructed lid is furnished by a laterally based tarsoconjunctival flap from the upper lid. The anterior layer is supplied by skin flaps and grafts as needed.

References

1. Hewes EH, Sullivan JH, Beard C. Lower eyelid reconstruction by tarsal transposition. *Am J Ophthalmol* 1976;81:512.
2. Gomey M, Falces E, Jones H, Manis JR. One-stage reconstruction of substantial lower eyelid margin defects. *Plast Reconstr Surg* 1969;44: 592.
3. Hughes WL. *Reconstructive surgery of the eyelids*, 2d Ed. St. Louis: Mosby, 1954;135.

CHAPTER 21 ■ NASOLABIAL SKIN FLAP TO THE LOWER EYELID

C. E. PALETTA AND F. X. PALETTA, SR.

Over the course of my career, I (F.X.P.) have used many different techniques to reconstruct the lower eyelid (1–4). Some of these techniques include (1) the nasolabial flap, (2) the upper eyelid skin flap, (3) the supraorbital skin flap, (4) the midforehead skin flap, (5) the cervical tube skin flap, (6) the full-thickness skin flap, and (7) the Hughes procedure (Fig. 1). I have found each of these procedures to be successful (5–8). Some are obviously more appropriate in selected patients. Donor site morbidity and scarring are often determining factors in technique selection.

When I first used the nasolabial skin flap for lower eyelid reconstruction, I felt that it would be necessary to perform secondary procedures such as an additional mucous membrane graft for lining (9), a fascial sling for support, and reconstruction of the lacrimal apparatus for tear drainage. Follow-up on these patients, however, has demonstrated that additional procedures are rarely necessary.

INDICATIONS

Based on my experience, the nasolabial flap can be used for partial or total lower eyelid reconstruction. In the older patient, the primary indication is reconstruction following resection for carcinoma. In younger individuals, loss of tissue in this area was usually from traumatic avulsion or following surgical excision of tumors. There have also been occasional cases of lower eyelid tissue loss from infectious causes. Finally, in the neonatal population, congenital defects of the lower eyelid can present for reconstruction.

FLAP DESIGN AND DIMENSIONS

The nasolabial flap is easily elevated under local anesthesia in the adult patient. General anesthesia is required in the younger patient. This flap is usually performed directly following tumor excision. Free tumor margins are determined by frozen section. If there is uncertainty about whether all the margins are free of tumor, the lower eyelid defect is covered with a sterile dressing (such as Biobrane, sterile saline gauze, or Xeroform) until permanent sections confirm that all margins are free of tumor. The outline of the skin flap is in the adjacent nasolabial fold (Fig. 2). The flap is based superiorly, so that it can easily be rotated to the lower eyelid position. A small dog-ear is usually created during the transposition of the flap. This can either be excised primarily, or, if there is concern over compromise to the blood supply of the flap, the dog-ear can be removed as a secondary procedure 6 to 12 weeks later. These flaps can readily be elevated without delay because of their excellent blood supply. The width of the flap is usually 1.5 to 2.0 cm, and the length depends on the width and loca-

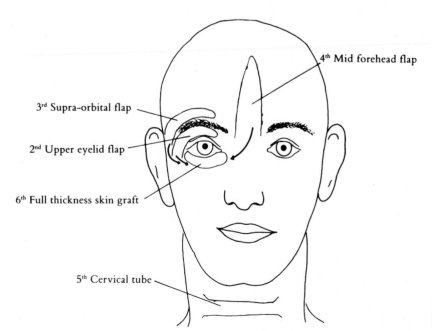

4ᵗʰ Mid forehead flap

3ʳᵈ Supra-orbital flap

2ⁿᵈ Upper eyelid flap

6ᵗʰ Full thickness skin graft

5ᵗʰ Cervical tube

FIG. 1. Diagrammatic outline of several neighboring regional area flaps used to reconstruct the lower eyelid. (From Paletta, ref. 8, with permission.)

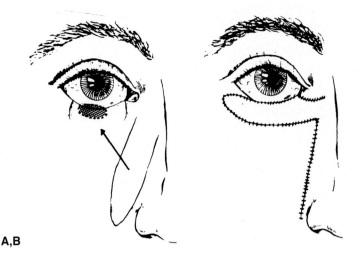

A,B

FIG. 2. Technique of nasolabial flap reconstruction of lower eyelid. **A:** Outline of the area to be excised in the lower eyelid and the nasolabial flap to be elevated. **B:** The flap is transferred to the lower eyelid, and the donor site is closed. (From Paletta, ref. 8, with permission.)

tion of the lower eyelid defect. While rarely necessary for lower eyelid reconstruction, the superiorly based nasolabial flap can extend as far as the ipsilateral oral commissure.

OPERATIVE TECHNIQUE

When dealing with a skin malignancy such as basal cell carcinoma of the lower eyelid, surgical resection may require full-thickness excision of the palpebral margin, skin, tarsal plate, and conjunctiva. Following resection or creation of the lower eyelid defect, the soft tissue requirements are either measured or a template is made of the defect. The nasolabial flap is then designed with its proximal base adjacent to the medial aspect of the lower eyelid defect. The nasolabial flap is then infiltrated with a local anesthetic (usually 1% Xylocaine with epinephrine 1:100,000). The flap is raised beginning distally in a soft-tissue plane approximately two-thirds the depth between the deep dermis and the underlying facial musculature. This plane of flap elevation ensures adequate vascularity of the flap without adding excessive fatty tissue in the lower eyelid region. The soft tissue of the cheek is then widely undermined and advanced toward the nose for closure in the nasolabial line. The superior portion of the flap is sutured to the bulbar conjunctiva with a 5–0 absorbable suture (either chromic catgut or polyglycolic acid suture). The knots of these sutures are buried to avoid irritation of the globe or cornea. To provide a sling effect, it is best to inset the flap under a slight amount of tension. The inferior portion of the nasolabial flap is sutured to the upper cheek skin with either 6–0 nylon or silk. Either a light dressing or no dressing may be used, but care must be given to postoperative eye care and wound cleansing with hydrogen peroxide and antibiotic ointment (Figs. 3 to 5). The nonabsorbable sutures are removed in 5 to 7 days (4).

CLINICAL RESULTS

In our series of over 100 lower eyelid reconstructions utilizing the superiorly based nasolabial flap, there has been no case of complete or partial flap necrosis. There have been minor complications in 5% of patients. These include slight ectropion, excess fat in the skin flap in some of the young patients, and some scleral exposure below the limbus of the eye. One patient required a fascial sling to correct excessive scleral exposure. Epiphora was seen occasionally, but rarely persisted in the majority of patients. In cases where the lower canaliculus was excised or obstructed by scar, the upper canaliculus appeared adequate to control tearing. In male patients, hair growth in the transposed flap did not present itself as a problem. This was primarily because the flap's design rarely required including the lowermost portion of the nasolabial flap where facial hair is more prominent.

SUMMARY

The superior nasolabial flap is an excellent choice in the reconstruction of major lower eyelid defects. Its main advantages are that it can be done easily under local anesthesia; it is a one-stage

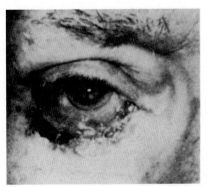
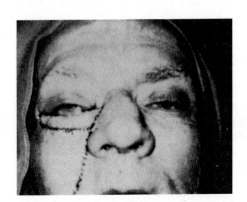
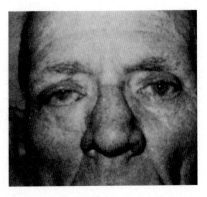

A–C

FIG. 3. **A:** A 65-year-old man with an extensive basal cell carcinoma of the lower eyelid. **B:** Excision of the lower eyelid and immediate repair with a nasolabial flap. **C:** Reconstructed lower eyelid 3 weeks following operation. (From Paletta, ref. 8, with permission.)

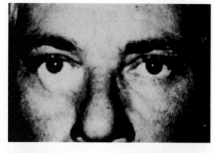
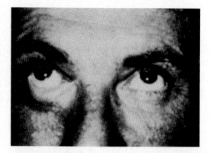
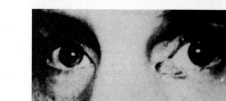
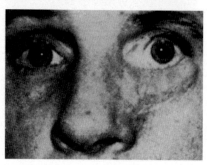

A,B

A,B

FIG. 4. **A:** Right lower eyelid 6 years following reconstruction with a nasolabial flap of the entire lower eyelid for melanoma in a 34-year-old man. **B:** No restriction of upward gaze. (From Paletta, ref. 8, with permission.)

FIG. 5. **A:** Recurrent basal cell carcinoma of the left medial canthus and lower eyelid in a 38-year-old woman. **B:** Six months following repair with a nasolabial skin flap, there is drooping of the reconstructed lid margin. (From Paletta, ref. 8, with permission.)

procedure; the donor site is usually adequate and presents little donor-site morbidity; and it provides an adequate amount of local tissue for large defects of the lower eyelid.

References

1. Paletta FX. Early and late repair of facial defects following treatment of malignancy. *Plast Reconst Surg* 1954;13:95.
2. Hughes WL. A new method for rebuilding a lower lid. *Arch Ophthalmol* 1966;17:1008.
3. Berkeley R. Total lid reconstruction with plastic repair. *Am J Surg* 1969; 118:741.
4. Hecht SD. An upside-down Cutler-Beard bridge flap. *Arch Ophthalmol* 1970;84:760.
5. Smith B, English FP. Techniques available in reconstructive surgery of the eyelid. *Br J Ophthalmol* 1970;54:450.
6. Fox SA. A procedure for lower lid reconstruction. *Arch Ophthalmol* 1971; 85:79.
7. Pap GS. A comparison of three methods of eyelid reconstruction. *Plast Reconstr Surg* 1972;49:513.
8. Paletta FX. Lower eyelid reconstruction. *Plast Reconstr Surg* 1973;51:653.
9. Millard DR. Eyelid repair with chondromucosal graft. *Plast Reconstr Surg* 1962;30:267.

CHAPTER 22 ■ LATERALLY BASED TRANSVERSE MUSCULOCUTANEOUS FLAP FOR LOWER EYELID RECONSTRUCTION

C. D. BUCKO

One of the best flaps that can be used to reconstruct the lower eyelid is a laterally based transverse musculocutaneous flap from the upper eyelid.

INDICATIONS

This flap can be used to replace tissue loss from the lateral two-thirds of the lower lid resulting from trauma, tumor excision, and congenital colobomata. More specific applications

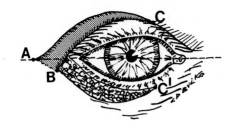

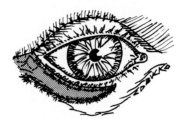

A,B

FIG. 1. **A:** Triangular flap is outlined using point *A* at lateral orbital rim, point *B* at edge of defect, and point *C* at apex on supratarsal crease. **B:** Flap has been transposed and sutured into recipient bed. Suture at lateral canthus gives support to lid. Donor site is closed along supratarsal crease.

are (1) to replace lost skin and muscle of the lateral two-thirds of the lower lid and cheek of up to 15 to 20 mm in vertical height, (2) to replace a full-thickness loss of the lateral two-thirds of the lower lid of up to 15 to 20 mm in vertical height, (3) to reconstruct lost lateral canthal soft tissue, and (4) to fill in the defect when raising the position of the lateral lower lid margin (as a result of congenital or severe senile ectropion or Treacher Collins syndrome) (1–4).

The flap is simple to design and execute; it is a safe flap with a good blood supply. Texture and color are similar to that of lost tissue, and the flap can be used as a full-thickness replacement, if a graft is included on the undersurface. The donor site is invisible, and there is no functional loss in the donor area, since tissue is usually in excess in adults.

FLAP DESIGN AND DIMENSIONS

The flap is usually elevated in the submuscular plane to include innervated and vascularized preseptal orbicularis muscle and the overlying skin. The tarsal plate is located beneath the flap and is not included. The orbital septum and levator aponeurosis are left intact deep to the preseptal orbicularis layer.

A simple, easy to execute, safe flap can be designed. The flap can be raised as a random flap, as a musculocutaneous flap, or as a composite flap in conjunction with a chondromucosal graft on its deep surface for replacement of a full-thickness lid loss.

The base of the flap is located at the lateral orbital rim (*AB* in Fig. 1A), and the apex is located on the medial supratarsal fold corresponding to the medial edge of the lower lid defect (*C* and *C'* in Fig. 1A). Primary closure of the donor site can be obtained if the flap is less than 15 to 20 mm wide at the central portion and base, depending on the amount of redundant donor skin and muscle (less in children). A wider flap could be used, but skin grafting of the donor site would be required.

The inferior edge of the flap (*CB* in Fig. 1A) corresponds to the supratarsal fold and extends from the apex (point *C*) to point *B*, located at the most inferolateral edge of the lower lid defect. Point *A*, at the base, lies over the orbital rim at the level of a horizontal line connecting the medial and lateral canthi. The distance between points *A* and *B*, the base of the flap, can be up to 15 to 20 mm in adults. The superior edge of the flap begins at point *A*, at the base, and tapers to point *C*, at the apex. If additional flap length is needed to extend to the medial third of the lower lid, point *C* can be moved into the medial canthal area or even onto the lateral nose without fear of flap necrosis if the flap is used as a musculocutaneous flap.

OPERATIVE TECHNIQUE

The flap is pivoted into the lower lid defect and sutured with 6-0 nylon skin sutures (Fig. 1B). If the full thickness of the lower lid needs reconstruction, the posterior lamellar defect is closed by using a chondromucosal composite graft (Fig. 2A)

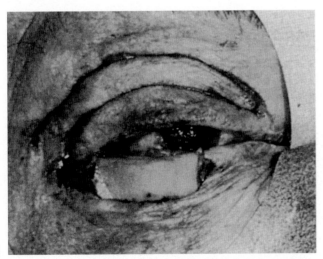

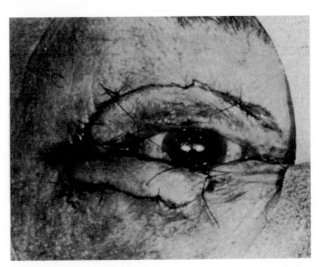

A,B

FIG. 2. **A:** Chondromucosal composite graft is used for posterior lamella in marginal defect. **B:** Flap covers anterior defect.

and the anterior defect is covered by the flap (Fig. 2B). This graft can be taken from the nasal septum (see Chap. 17) or from the upper lateral nasal cartilage through a lateral rhinotomy. The graft should extend from the free margin down to the orbital rim in order to create a stable lid if more than two-thirds of the lid is being reconstructed.

The lateral canthus can be reinforced with a 4-0 mattress suture from the lateral orbital rim periosteum slightly above the lateral canthus to the undersurface of the flap at the lateral canthus (Fig. 1B). The donor area is closed with 6-0 nylon sutures (muscle sutures are not needed).

CLINICAL RESULTS

See Chap. 17.

SUMMARY

The laterally based transverse musculocutaneous flap is a safe, reliable, simple flap that can be used to reconstruct defects of the lateral two-thirds of the lower lid of up to 15 to 20 mm in vertical height.

References

1. Callahan A. *Reconstructive surgery of the eyelids and ocular adnexa.* Birmingham, AL: Aesculapius, 1966; 293–296.
2. Fricke JCG. *Die Bildung neuerAugenlider (Blepharoplastik) nach Zerstorungen und dedurch hervorgebrachten Auswartswendungen derselben.* Hamburg: Perthes & Brasser, 1829.
3. Mustardé JC. *Repair and reconstruction in the orbital region: a practical guide.* Edinburgh: Churchill Livingstone, 1980;55–56.
4. Soll DB. Entropion and ectropion. In: Soll DB, ed., *Management of complications in ophthalmic plastic surgery.* Birmingham, AL: Aesculapius, 1976;194.

CHAPTER 23 ■ SKIN-MUSCLE-TARSOCONJUNCTIVAL (ESSER) FLAP FROM THE LOWER TO THE UPPER EYELID

J. C. MUSTARDÉ

While two basic layers of skin and mucosa must always be provided in reconstructions of the upper eyelid, a permanent stiffening layer to counter the effects of gravity and time is not needed, as it is in lower lid reconstruction. However, there is an even greater need to provide a stable margin because of possible damage to the cornea if the squamous epithelium of the outer layer should come in contact with the cornea during the constant upward and downward excursions of the lid.

Any technique that relies solely on providing the two basic layers, joined along their free edges by a scar, ignores the fact that in a normal upper lid the skin of the lid immediately above the margin is fixed, albeit indirectly, to the extension of the levator aponeurosis. This prevents the skin from sliding down over the eyelid margin. It is an anatomic entity virtually impossible to reproduce in a reconstructed upper lid whose basis has been the provision of a skin layer and a lining layer that are not already adherent to each other by natural means.

INDICATIONS

To overcome the tendency for the covering layer to slide down under the force of gravity while the levator muscle tends to pull the lining layer upward, an ideal solution is to rotate a flap of the full thickness of the lower lid into the upper lid defect. Such a flap has its own stable, *normal* margin and its own built-in adhesion of the area of skin immediately proximal to the margin to the underlying structures of the lid (albeit to a lesser extent than in the upper lid). This flap, which is actually the reverse of the flap described by Esser, will preserve the marginal eyelid vessels in its base, and after a 2-week interval, they can be divided. At that stage, the problem is resolved by closure of the resulting lower eyelid defect (see Chap. 13) (1).

ANATOMY

Since the marginal vessels are relatively large for such a small flap, its viability is extremely good, despite 180° rotation of the flap. It is important to realize that the marginal eyelid vessels lie about 3 mm from the lid margin and immediately beneath the layer of the orbicularis muscle.

OPERATIVE TECHNIQUE

Defects of up to Half the Upper Eyelid

Because of the degree of stretch in eyelid tissues (that permits defects of up to a quarter of the lid to be closed directly), it is necessary to take a flap from the lower lid of not more than one-quarter of its width (approximately 6 to 7 mm). Hence the lower lid can be closed directly (Fig. 1) after the division of the vascular pedicle 2 weeks later.

The marginal vessels should not be damaged. Moreover, the pedicle width should not be less than 5 mm, and the various wounds must not be closed under tension. For reconstructions of this size, the hinge of the flap should lie directly below the center of the upper lid defect. It can be placed on either side, whichever is more suitable, always remembering that the lower lid punctum should never be sacrificed.

Defects Between Half and Three-Quarters of the Upper Eyelid

If the defect in the upper lid is a few millimeters greater than half the upper lid width, the lower lid flap will be a few millimeters larger than a quarter of the width of the lower lid (Fig. 2). This small additional segment of lower eyelid must be reconstructed by moving a small lateral cheek rotation flap lined with conjunctiva or with a composite nasal septal graft of cartilage and mucosa (see Chap. 13).

It should be noted that where a defect of more than half the upper lid is present, the cut edge of the levator palpebral muscle must be sutured to the connective tissue of the lower lid flap. No great care is required to judge exactly at what level this attachment should be made, since the patient will balance the level of the two upper eyelids to obtain equal light appreciation (Fig. 3).

Subtotal and Total Defects of the Upper Eyelid

Unless the defect is only 2 to 3 mm greater than half the width of the upper eyelid, the preceding technique should not

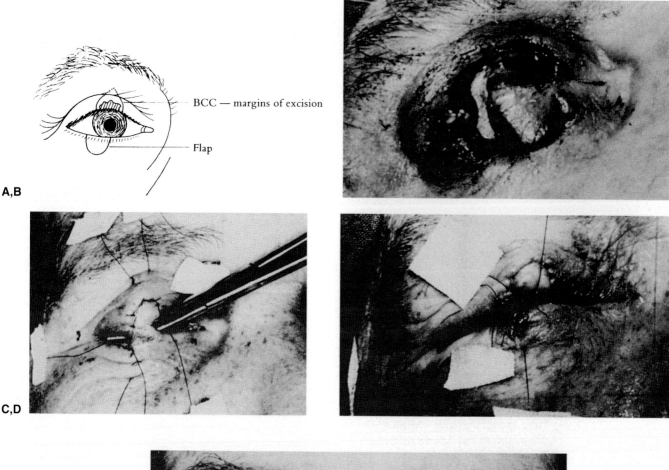

BCC — margins of excision

Flap

A,B

C,D

E

FIG. 1. **A–D:** Reconstruction of defects of up to half the width of the upper eyelid. Because of the stretch of lid tissues, a small flap of only a quarter of the width of the lower lid needs to be rotated into the upper lid defect. **E:** Postoperative result. Note the stable margin in the reconstructed upper lid, with no tendency for the skin to roll down over the margin. (From Mustardé, ref. 1, with permission.)

be used. A more balanced two-stage procedure is required (Fig. 4). Stage 1 consists of designing a full-thickness flap of the lower eyelid that has a broad pedicle (7 to 8 mm) and that is large enough to fill the upper lid defect. If there is any remnant of the upper lid, then the pedicle should be designed on that side so that the wound to be closed primarily along the upper lid margin will be the most central one, closest to the pupil.

In subtotal and total defects of the upper lid (Fig. 5), the end of the flap is turned up and sutured into the upper lid defect in layers (including suturing the levator muscle to the connective tissue) as far as can be done without putting the tissues under tension. In the nonunited areas, skin may be joined

temporarily to conjunctiva to minimize infection and the formation of granulation tissue.

Stage 2 consists of dividing the base of the lower eyelid flap, setting it completely in place in the upper lid, and reconstructing the resulting lower lid defect by using a cheek rotation flap lined with a composite nasal septal graft of mucosa and cartilage (see Chap. 13).

SUMMARY

The best tissue for reconstruction of the upper eyelid is that obtained from the lower eyelid. The upper eyelid is the most

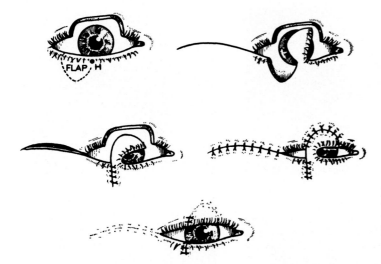

FIG. 2. Defects between half and three-quarters of the width of the upper lid. Reconstruction of the upper lid is carried out by transferring a flap slightly larger than one-quarter the width of the lower lid. This necessitates bringing in a small cheek flap to reconstitute the lower lid when the pedicle on the full-thickness flap is divided. (From Mustardé, ref. 1, with permission.)

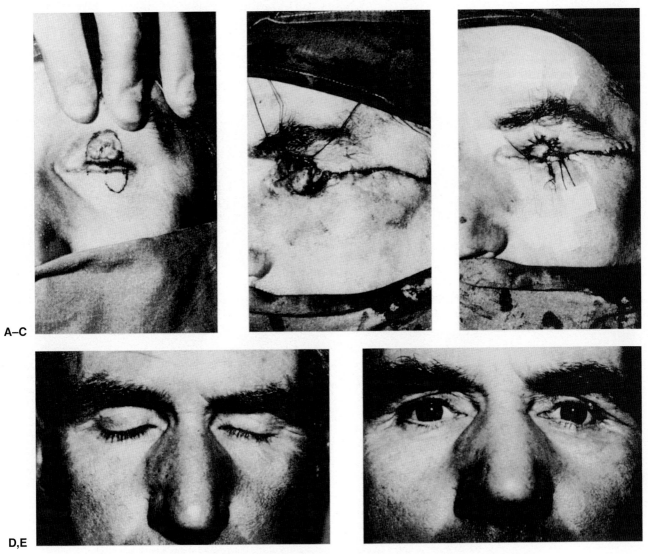

FIG. 3. Tumor of the upper eyelid that left a defect of over half the width of the upper eyelid after resection. A–C: First stage of the surgery. D, E: Postoperative appearance showing stable margin in the upper lid reconstruction. Lower lid reconstruction was carried out by lining the cheek flap with conjunctiva. It would have been advisable to have used a small composite nasal septal graft to obviate the postoperative droop of the reconstructed segment of the lower eyelid. (From Mustardé, ref. 1, with permission.)

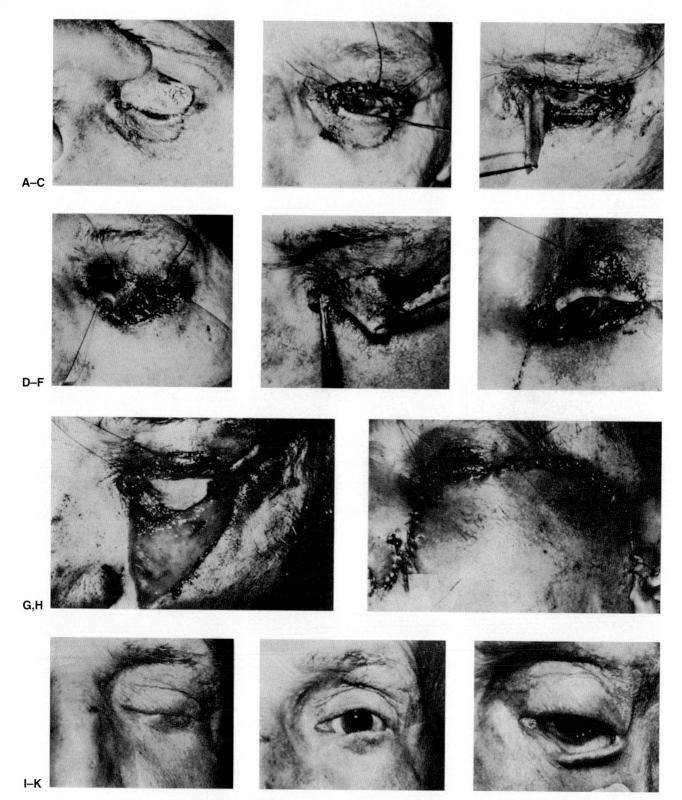

FIG. 4. Subtotal reconstruction of the upper lid. A small remnant of upper lid is preserved on the medial side, and thus the hinge of the lower lid flap that will be used is designed on the medial side to ensure good primary union in the upper lid scar that will be closest to the cornea. **A–D:** Resection of upper lid tumor, design and raising of full-thickness lower lid flap, and insertion of free end into upper lid defect. **E, F:** Division of the base of the lower lid flap and completion of the flap insertion into upper lid defect. **G:** Reconstruction of the lower lid with a composite nasal septal graft in situ. **H:** Rotation of the cheek flap to complete reconstruction of lower lid. **I–K:** Postoperative views showing functioning upper lid with a stable margin. The reconstructed part of the lower lid also can be seen, and the support given to this segment by the composite graft is well demonstrated. (From Mustardé, ref. 1, with permission.)

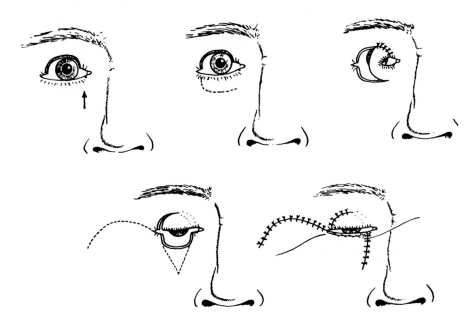

FIG. 5. Reconstruction of large defects of the upper lid (see text for details of technique). Note that where a remnant of the upper lid is left, the base of the flap to be raised from the full thickness of the lower lid should be on the side of the largest remnant. Where no upper lid remains, the base of the lower lid flap should be placed on the lateral side to establish lymphatic drainage as quickly as possible in the reconstructed upper lid. (From Mustardé, ref. 1, with permission.)

difficult to reconstruct, since it must be movable. The first principle of sound eyelid reconstruction is to use the lower lid to reconstruct the upper lid, but use other sources to reconstruct the lower lid.

Reference

1. Mustardé JC. *Repair and reconstruction of the orbital region*, 2d Ed. Edinburgh: Churchill Livingstone, 1980; Chap. 11.

CHAPTER 24 ■ INFERIORLY BASED SKIN-MUSCLE-CONJUNCTIVAL ADVANCEMENT (CUTLER-BEARD) FLAP FROM THE LOWER TO THE UPPER EYELID

C. BEARD AND J. H. SULLIVAN

EDITORIAL COMMENT

In using so much of the full-thickness skin and conjunctiva of the lower lid to recreate the upper lid, the danger of a significant portion of patients developing ectropion is something to be considered before selecting this procedure for use.

The upper eyelid is far more important functionally than the lower lid, since it is responsible for almost all the protection of the cornea. Without an adequate upper lid, the globe cannot survive long as a useful organ. Reconstructive procedures for major upper eyelid repair are few and complex. The inferiorly based skin-muscle-conjunctival advancement flap has with-stood the test of time. This two-stage procedure can be used for total lid replacement, yet it is one of the simplest of the upper eyelid reconstructive operations.

INDICATIONS

The advantages of this procedure are its usefulness in correcting large upper lid defects, its simplicity, and the surprising freedom from deformation of the lower lid (1). The necessity for prolonged visual obstruction with this procedure may be a problem in an occasional patient. A much shorter period of occlusion is possible with the Mustardé "switch flap" (2). It may be possible to reduce the period of occlusion thought to be necessary with the Cutler-Beard flap, but we have not attempted to do so.

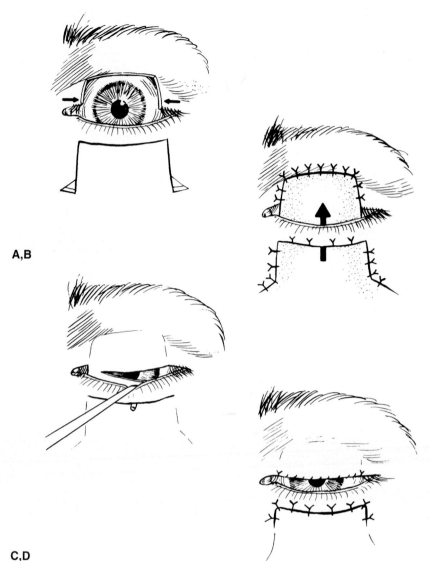

A,B

C,D

FIG. 1. A: The tumor is excised. Moderate traction is placed on the lid remnants to narrow the width of the defect. A full-thickness incision is made through the lower lid at the tarsal edge. Vertical full-thickness incisions are made to a depth of the fornix. Relaxing skin triangles are excised. B: The flap is advanced upward behind the marginal bridge and sutured in two layers into the upper lid defect. The lower edge of the bridge can be loosely closed. C: After 6 to 8 weeks, the lid fissure is recreated by a full-thickness scissor cut arched downward about 2 mm. This cut should be beveled forward in order to have the conjunctiva slightly lower than the skin. D: The base of the flap is returned to its anatomic position and sutured in two layers. The skin and conjunctiva are approximated with a running suture of 6–0 catgut.

ANATOMY

This flap consists of an inferiorly based full-thickness lower lid flap (skin, orbicularis muscle, orbital septum, lower lid retractors, and conjunctiva) advanced beneath the lower lid margin to replace the upper lid.

OPERATIVE TECHNIQUE

The procedure (Fig. 1) begins with complete removal of the upper lid tumor under frozen-section control or freshening of the margins of traumatic or congenital defects. Remnants of the remaining lid are held under moderate traction to lessen the width of the defect. The measurement of this width is used to determine the width of the full-thickness lower lid flap. A horizontal skin incision of the same distance is made. It is deepened at one end into the inferior fornix. Using scissors, a full-thickness horizontal incision is completed immediately below the tarsus to the width of the skin incision. Full-thickness vertical scissor cuts are made from the ends of the horizontal cut to the extreme depths of the inferior fornix, forming a rectangular flap. The flap is mobilized by undermining the skin inferiorly over the orbital rim.

It is then advanced posterior to the bridge of the lower lid margin into the upper eyelid defect, where it rests without tension.

A two-layered closure of the upper lid to the lower lid is sufficient; 6–0 plain catgut is used to approximate the conjunctiva, and 6–0 silk is used for the skin. It is possible to identify the levator aponeurosis and secure it to the flap as an intermediate layer, but ptosis has not resulted from failure to do this. It is our practice to attach conjunctiva loosely to the skin of the lower lid bridge. Others have postulated that the marginal arcade may thereby be seriously compromised and have allowed the inferior edge to heal by secondary intention.

In dressing the wound, it is important to avoid pressure over the marginal bridge. An eye patch, cut in half, is placed above and below the bridge and covered with fluffed gauze held firmly with tape.

Six to 8 weeks are felt to be necessary for the tissues to heal and vascularize. The second stage of the repair is then carefully performed. The flap is divided with scissors in a downward arch, anticipating retraction of approximately 2 mm. The absence of tarsus not only causes the lid to retract, but also favors development of entropion. For this reason, the dividing incision should be beveled forward, leaving excess conjunctiva to be rotated over the new lid margin and secured to the skin with a running 6–0 plain catgut closure.

The base of the flap is freed from its medial and lateral adhesions, and the flap is allowed to retract to its anatomic position in the lower lid. The junction of skin and conjunctiva at the inferior margin of the bridge is freshened. Conjunctival and skin surfaces are sutured, and a simple dressing is applied.

CLINICAL RESULTS

Disadvantages of the procedure are the necessity for obstructing vision for 6 to 8 weeks; the lack of a skeleton (tarsus) in the new lid margin, resulting in a tendency to entropion; the potential for damage to the lower lid margin; and the absence of lashes in the reconstructed lid.

The functional results of this procedure are excellent. The main objection to the cosmetic result has been the absence of eyelashes. If this is troublesome to the patient, a cilia graft may be considered as a third stage. The best donor site is from the eyebrow, but lash grafts are notoriously unsatisfactory. The usual result is unruly and stubble-like hairs. The patient should understand the uncertainties of lash grafts before, rather than after, the procedure is done. Artificial lashes are often a superior substitute.

We are aware of one instance where the marginal bridge became necrotic and was lost. This is believed to be a complication of the pressure dressing rather than a result of the surgical closure of the margin of the lower lid bridge. Edema of the transplanted tissue has occurred, but it has always subsided with time. We have seen no failures of the flap to thrive.

Entropion of the reconstructed upper lid margin is not rare. When present, it is often symptomatic and may result in keratitis. It can usually be corrected by a buccal mucous membrane graft to the lid margin.

SUMMARY

The Cutler-Beard inferiorly based skin-muscle-conjunctival flap from the lower to the upper eyelid is a simple two-stage operation for the reconstruction of large upper lid defects. It uses a subtarsal full-thickness flap of the lower lid to fill the upper lid defect.

References

1. Cutler NL, Beard CA. Method for partial and total upper lid reconstruction. *Am J Ophthalmol* 1955;39:1.
2. Mustardé JC. *Repair and reconstruction in the orbital region.* Edinburgh: Churchill Livingstone, 1980;140.

CHAPTER 25 ■ MODIFIED TESSIER FLAP FOR RECONSTRUCTION OF THE UPPER EYELID

J. J. HURWITZ

EDITORIAL COMMENT

This flap accomplishes the objective of total upper eyelid reconstruction, particularly because it utilizes skin and underlying muscle, which actually improves the viability of the flap, as well as providing sufficient tissue for restoring the entire horizontal diameter of the upper eyelid.

There are a number of options available for major upper eyelid reconstruction. The flap originally described by Tessier (1) was a nasojugal flap used in the reconstruction of a total defect in the lower eyelid. However, a modified Tessier flap (skin-muscle nasojugal flap), combined with a buccal mucous membrane graft, allows for total reconstruction of an upper eyelid defect. This includes the anterior and posterior lamella, attachment to the levator aponeurosis so that the eyelid can move up and down, and provision of an adequate blood supply to the reconstructed eyelid, especially in patients previously irradiated (2).

INDICATIONS

The modified Tessier flap is especially indicated for major reconstruction of the upper eyelid when the lower lid cannot be utilized for a bridge graft, if the upper lid has been sacrificed in removing a large tumor, or if it has been lost due to trauma. The skin-muscle flap described should be lined with mucosa to help form the posterior lamella of the eyelid. Mucosa is taken from the mouth in the buccal region, but may also be taken from inside the lip. Alternatively, conjunctiva may be taken from the upper fornix of the contralateral eye, but this may not be appropriate if the patient has disease in that area, or does not want the uninvolved eye approached surgically.

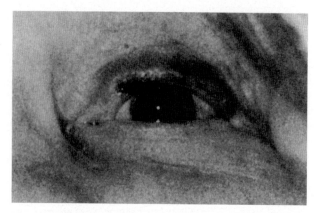

FIG. 1. Preoperative upper eyelid with basal cell epithelioma.

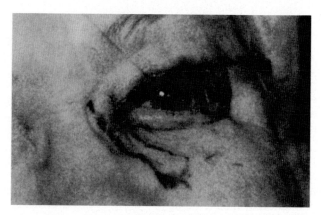

FIG. 3. The nasojugal flap has been outlined. Note that the base extends to the nasal skin.

ANATOMY

Because the thickness of a flap from the nasojugal area is greater than that of upper eyelid skin and orbicularis, more stability is provided to the reconstructed lid and this decreases the need for tarsal replacement. Also, the excellent medial canthal blood supply, particularly the angular artery and some of its tributaries, allows for an increased length-to-width ratio of the flap. The flap will be rotated to the upper lid to cover a buccal mucosal flap.

The posterior lamella of the eyelid consists of conjunctiva; in this reconstruction, buccal mucous membrane is chosen for replacement. Buccal mucous membrane is somewhat thicker than conjunctival mucous membrane; therefore it provides stability to the lid, to a certain extent decreasing the need for any tarsal replacement. For the anterior lamella, both the skin and muscle of the flap that lie on the superficial aspect of the mucosal graft afford an adequate replacement.

FLAP DESIGN AND DIMENSIONS

After conjunctival replacement, the modified Tessier flap is developed. An almost vertical flap is marked out in the orbitonasal angle and nasojugal region. Its base is centered over the angular vessels and lies above the level of the medial canthal ligament, allowing the flap to reach 90° of transposition. To rotate the flap into the upper lid, more torsion is necessary than in rotation to the lower lid; this is achieved by

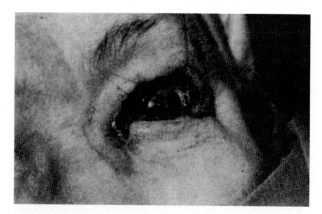

FIG. 2. A major portion of the eyelid has been resected.

having the upper arm of the flap base extend more onto the surface of the nose, allowing for rotation into the upper lid and decreasing the potential for compromise of the circulation due to kinking (see Fig. 3).

The length of the flap is determined by the length of the defect to be filled; it is useful to have a slightly longer flap, to allow for potential horizontal shrinkage; extra vertical length will allow for vertical shrinkage as well. It is suggested that the subciliary incision extend all the way from the flap base to the lateral canthus.

OPERATIVE TECHNIQUE

The malignant tumor is removed under frozen-section control until clear margins are obtained, leaving a virtual full-thickness total upper eyelid defect (Figs. 1 and 2). Outlining with a scalpel and then undermining with scissors, and taking care to avoid the parotid duct opening, conjunctival replacement is first performed with a posterior lamella graft from the buccal mucosa.

Depending on the size of the graft taken, the cheek may be left open or sutured with 5–0 absorbable material with a knot buried within the defect. The graft is then harvested and thinned, and secured with 5–0 running sutures from the upper border to the levator aponeurosis (Fig. 3), which can be identified with the patient opening and closing the eyes, with the white sheet of aponeurosis moving. If the aponeurosis is difficult to locate, one can dissect to the preaponeurotic fat pad, incise the septum, reflect the fat superiorly, and the cut end of the levator aponeurosis will then lie directly beneath; 5–0 Dexon sutures can be used to secure the graft to the lateral and medial edges of the conjunctiva.

A lid-crease incision is made from underneath the punctum (4 mm below), extending laterally to the lateral canthus. An inferolateral incision is made from the most medial aspect of the subciliary incision; this lateral flap edge will be the superior edge of the flap in the upper lid. Another incision is made in, or close to, the nasojugal fold; this medial flap edge will be the lid margin (lower edge) in the upper lid. The two inferolateral incisions are then joined, the flap undermined, and then rotated into the lid defect (Fig. 4). The flap donor site may be closed with either an advancement flap from the cheek or a free full-thickness skin graft.

If there is lagophthalmos and incomplete closure of the eye, too much of the levator aponeurosis has been removed. It is then an excellent idea to perform a marginal aponeurotomy before flap placement, by grasping the levator aponeurosis

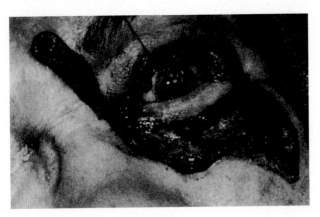

FIG. 4. The flap has been elevated. The mucosal graft is shown sutured into the defect.

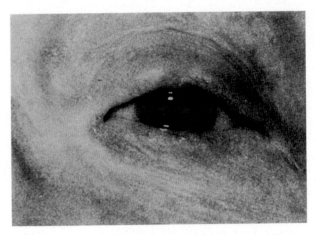

FIG. 6. Eyelid healed.

and placing horizontal incisions in it approximately 3 mm above the cut edge. Then, horizontal incisions superior to the initial set, but 3 to 4 mm higher, are made. This makes the aponeurosis similar to an accordion, lengthens it, and allows for better eyelid closure.

The modified Tessier flap is rotated into the upper lid and sutured along its superior and lateral borders (Fig. 5). With opening and closing of the patient's eyes, exact determination of the mucocutaneous junction is possible. The inferior aspect of the mucosal graft can now be trimmed, and the lower edge of flap skin sutured to the lower edge of graft. Again, it is important that skin does not overhang mucosa, or corneal irritation will result.

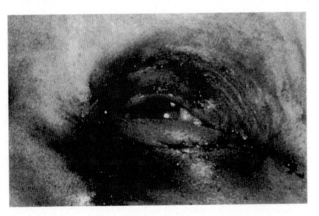

FIG. 5. Flap inset. Mucosal graft is in excess.

Antibiotic-steroid ointment can be placed on the graft and into the palpebral aperture, and a pressure dressing placed over upper and lower lids, with no undue pressure over the medial canthus area. A protective shield at night is useful, so that sutures are not disrupted by the patient (Fig. 6).

CLINICAL RESULTS

Initially, there may be a small amount of tip ischemia in the flap, but necrosis does not develop. An anterior conjunctival overhang of the mucocutaneous junction is desirable but, with mucosa shrinking more than the skin-muscle flap, this overhang tends to decrease with time.

Among the advantages of the modified Tessier flap are that it is a one-stage procedure, scarring occurs along normal lid folds, the skin is more supple than that of the forehead, and no surgery on the other eyelid is necessary.

SUMMARY

The flap, combined with a buccal mucous membrane graft, allows for major reconstruction of an upper eyelid defect, without using the ipsilateral lower lid or the contralateral eye.

References

1. Tessier P. *Eyelid reconstruction or blepharopoesis in plastic surgery of the orbit and eyelids.* New York: Masson, USA Inc., 1981.
2. Avram DR, Hurwitz JJ, Kratky V. Modified Tessier flap for reconstruction of the upper eyelid. *Ophthal Surg* 1988;22:470.

CHAPTER 26 ■ V-Y-S-PLASTY FOR CLOSURE OF A CIRCULAR DEFECT OF THE MEDIAL CANTHAL AREA

R. V. ARGAMASO

EDITORIAL COMMENT

This is a most helpful flap, most reliable for defects in the medial canthal area, although it is also applicable for areas around the lateral aspect of the nose and upper lip. It is superior to the pure advancement flaps.

The V-Y-S-plasty, first reported in 1974 (1), is a simple procedure that conserves tissues and avoids skin undermining in the repair of round skin defects.

INDICATIONS

Closure of a round skin defect may be accomplished in several ways. When there is laxity in the surrounding skin, the wound edges are simply approximated in a straight-line closure. More often, some undermining of skin margins is necessary to reduce tension at the suture lines; dog-ears that form on either extremity of the line of closure are excised and discarded.

A straight-line scar contracture crossing the valley of the medial canthal area is more likely to bowstring and simulate an epicanthal fold. In some instances, therefore, a small skin defect in this region is allowed to heal secondarily. The residual scar may not appear too distracting. In other instances, wound contraction and spontaneous epithelialization are protracted events, and there is always some risk of displacing the lacrimal punctum or everting the eyelid. A split-thickness skin graft or a forehead transposition flap may be acceptable alternatives, despite differences in color match or thickness of skin.

I prefer the V-Y-S-plasty as a procedure for repair of round skin defects that do not lend themselves to direct approximation of the skin margins without disturbing the neighboring structures of the eyelids. It is a simple procedure that conserves tissue and avoids skin undermining.

This technique also has been employed in other areas of the face and has been found to be effective in avoiding disfigurement of symmetrical or paired structures. In addition, this technique has been adapted for the extremities, where the integument tends to be tense.

FLAP DESIGN AND DIMENSIONS

The lesion is outlined with ink to include a rim of normal skin for tumor clearance. The somewhat circular area to be extirpated is encompassed by another skin marking, lenticular in configuration and similar to that which one would use in excision for direct linear closure of the wound (Fig. 1A). The axis of this spindle-shaped figure parallels a natural fold or wrinkle crease.

OPERATIVE TECHNIQUE

The initial incision follows the outline along the rim of normal tissue surrounding the lesion to be removed. Upon removal of the lesion, two triangular outlines remain, with a circular defect intervening between. These triangles represent skin that converts into dog-ears if and when the round defect is repaired in linear fashion by drawing the opposite wound edges together. Skin advancement at the medial canthal site should be minimized. Tension affecting the lid skin is more likely to cause eversion of its margin or medial displacement of its punctum.

Additionally, the caruncle may be further exposed. While this outcome may appear to be a minor anatomic derangement, it can be a source of serious aesthetic concern for the patient. The V-Y-S-plasty resolves this issue by reserving the dog-ears and developing them into flaps that can be conveniently rotated and advanced toward each other in the following manner.

A side of one triangle is totally incised, and a short back cut is added at the apex along the skin marking on its other side. A triangular flap is created, based on one partially intact side. The other triangle is dealt with in a similar manner, but the relative positions of the incisions are reversed (Fig. 1B).

Even with only slight undermining, these flaps will rotate readily to approximately 45° and simultaneously advance toward each other when their apposing margins are sutured together. It is stressed that *no undermining should be performed on skin beyond the areas demarcated*. This point is the essence of the operation.

The sides of the triangles are then sutured to their new positions, and finally, the small secondary defects at the sites of the back cuts are closed simply by direct skin approximation (Fig. 1C).

A single case has been reported (2) in which the dog-ears were saved to fill a round defect. In contrast to the technique reported here, the triangular flaps were based on the same side (mirror image) and turned over 90° before they were sutured to each other.

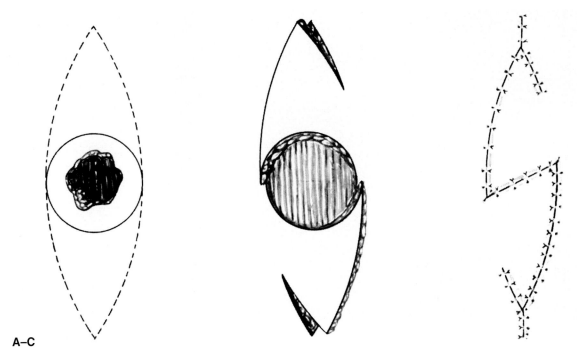

A–C

FIG. 1. **A:** Skin markings for skin excision and sites of the triangular flaps. **B:** Triangular flaps and intervening defect. Note that there is no undermining of skin other than the flaps. **C:** Final closure.

CLINICAL RESULTS

Although one major drawback of the procedure is that some segments of the scar cannot be directed for camouflage in a wrinkle crease, the result is still superior to a thin split-thickness skin graft or the thick glabellar flap. Incorporated in this technique are well-established principles of wound closure in plastic surgery. The procedure is simple, conserves tissue, and avoids skin undermining (Figs. 2 and 3). The description "dollar plasty" has been suggested by colleagues, who envision the scar line as having some resemblance to a stylized dollar sign.

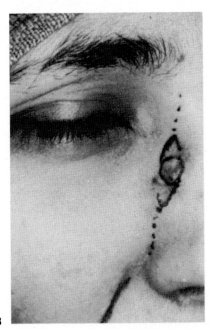
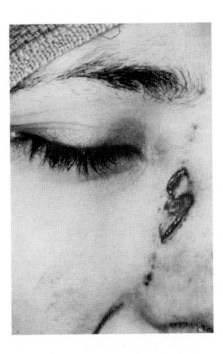

A,B

FIG. 2. **A:** Preoperative skin markings around a pigmented basal cell carcinoma. **B:** Lesion removed and flaps prepared. *(Continued)*

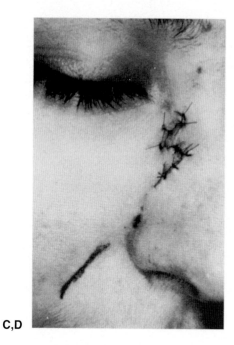
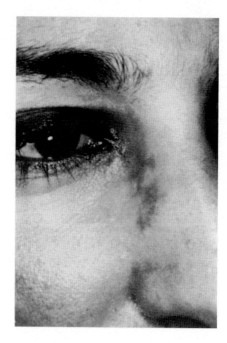

C,D

FIG. 2. *Continued.* **C:** Repair completed.
D: Early result at 2 weeks.

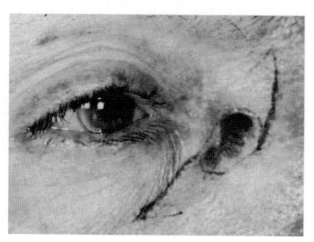
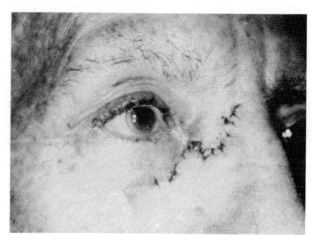

A,B

FIG. 3. **A:** Preoperative skin markings on an elderly man with two adjacent lesions (basal cell carcinoma). **B:** One week postoperatively immediately prior to suture removal. Note no demonstrable alteration in position of canthal structures.

SUMMARY

The melding of the V-Y advancement with the double rotation flaps of the S-plasty enhances the reparative efficacy of treatment of circular defects, with particular relevance in the medial canthal territory.

References

1. Argamaso RV. V-Y-S-plasty for closure of a round defect. *Plast Reconstr Surg* 1974;53:99.
2. Fischl RA. A flap for nasolabial defects, or "save the dog-ear." *Br J Plast Surg* 1969;22:351.

CHAPTER 27 ■ V-Y GLABELLAR SKIN FLAP TO THE MEDIAL CANTHAL REGION

J. C. MUSTARDÉ

EDITORIAL COMMENT

This is a very good flap; however, the reader should understand that the forehead glabellar skin is much thicker than the eyelid skin.

Tumors at the medial canthus are generally basal cell carcinomas, as they are elsewhere on the eyelids, and they are comparatively slow growing. In the early stages of their development, they may be relatively superficial, and it may be possible to resect such lesions, along with sufficient normal tissue without the need for deep dissection. The defect can then be covered by a full-thickness skin graft. An estimate of the depth of the tumor and the possible involvement of the underlying canaliculi and tear sac may be obtained by injecting a local anesthetic beneath the tumor to see whether it "balloons" off readily from the deep tissue and by the passage of a lacrimal probe.

INDICATIONS

In patients in whom it has been determined that the medial canthal lesion cannot be resected superficially, the degree of hollowing that would be left after an adequate resection would give a poor aesthetic result with skin graft coverage alone. Indeed, if periosteum and even bone are involved, a skin graft would probably not survive. A skin flap with a substantial layer of subcutaneous tissue must be used.

FLAP DESIGN AND DIMENSIONS

One of the simplest and most satisfactory techniques for doing such reconstructions is to bring down the thick glabellar skin as a V-Y flap in a one-stage operation. Depending on the width of skin available between the eyebrows, a flap designed in the form of an inverted V can be used to cover a defect at the medial canthus of up to 15 mm in diameter (Fig. 1). In conjunction with other flaps, such a flap may be employed to cover even larger areas. The flap is incised down to the galea aponeurotica, leaving an adequate pedicle on the bridge of the nose. The vertical dimension of the flap should be about three times the breadth at its lowest part. Once the flap has been slid down to cover the defect, it will be found that the forehead wound can be closed in the form of an inverted Y.

V-Y Forehead Flap Combined with Lower Eyelid Reconstruction

Where resection at the medial canthus is carried out with resection of part of an eyelid, it is usually the lower eyelid that is more involved. If it is not possible to close the lower lid defect by direct approximation of the cut surface of the tarsal plate to periosteum, a formal cheek rotation flap reconstruction of the lower lid can be carried out in the manner described in Chap. 13 (Fig. 2) (1).

V-Y Flap Combined with Upper Eyelid Reconstruction

Where a medial canthal resection involves a part of the upper lid, and where the upper lid cannot be closed by direct approximation to periosteum, a V-Y flap can be combined with a cheek rotation flap that carries a small full-thickness flap of the lower lid. This small flap is rotated 180° to fill the defect in the upper lid, and the base of the flap will form the new medial canthus (Fig. 3).

OPERATIVE TECHNIQUE

If the resection at the medial canthus has to be laterally extended to include a few millimeters of either or both eyelids (Fig. 4A), the cut surface of the tarsal plates should be sutured to the periosteum at the site of the medial canthal tendon using a 5–0 Prolene suture. Loss in one or the other eyelid, up to a quarter of eyelid width, can be dealt with by this technique. Full-thickness loss of more than a quarter of either eyelid, however, will require additional reconstructive procedures specific to the eyelid or eyelids involved.

In many patients in whom resection at the medial canthus has to be carried out to a depth that will require resurfacing by means of a V-Y flap, a part or all of the lacrimal sac also may have to be sacrificed. Provided that sufficient conjunctiva exists in the fornices, an anastomosis may be done between the upper open end of the lacrimal sac and the conjunctiva. This is kept patent by a 3-mm-diameter tube of soft plastic, that is left in situ for 2 weeks (Fig. 4B).

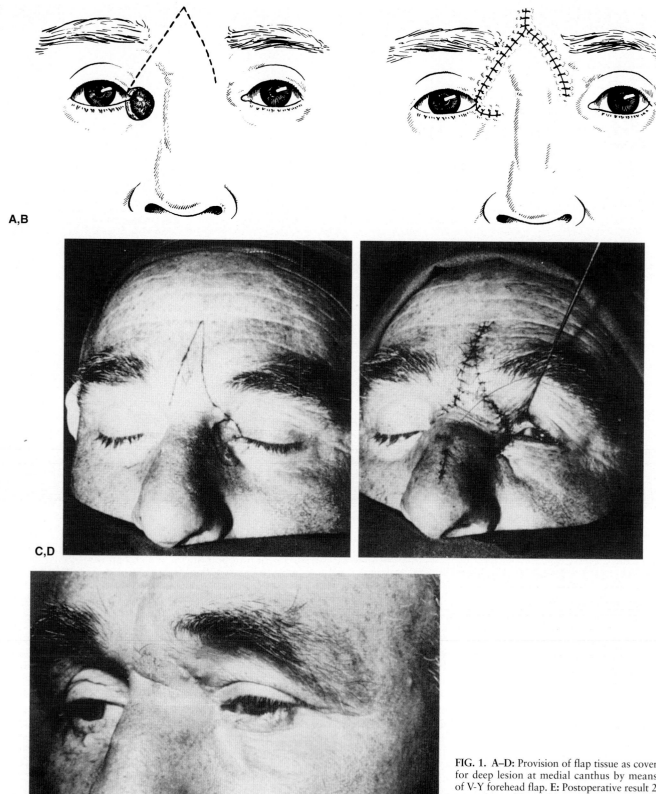

A,B

C,D

E

FIG. 1. **A–D:** Provision of flap tissue as cover for deep lesion at medial canthus by means of V-Y forehead flap. **E:** Postoperative result 2 years later. (From Mustardé, ref. 1, with permission.)

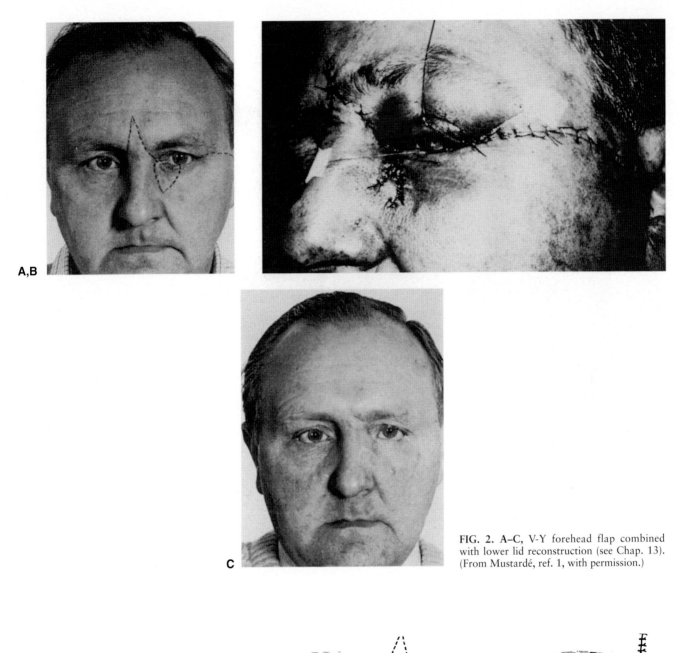

FIG. 2. A–C, V-Y forehead flap combined with lower lid reconstruction (see Chap. 13). (From Mustardé, ref. 1, with permission.)

FIG. 3. V-Y flap combined with upper lid reconstruction using a "switch" flap of full-thickness lower lid rotated into the upper lid (see Chap. 23). (From Mustardé, ref. 1, with permission.) *(Continued)*

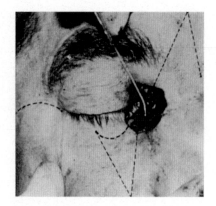
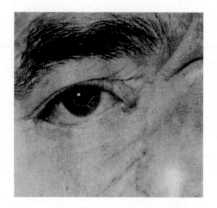
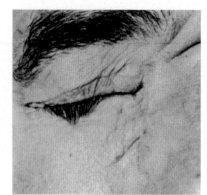

FIG. 3. *Continued.*

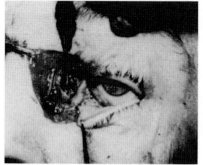
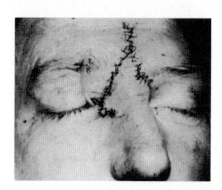

A,B

FIG. 4. Deep resection of the medial canthus and resection of the medial end of the upper and lower lids. **A:** A probe is inserted into the medial cut end of the nasolacrimal duct. **B:** Immediate postoperative result. The defect has been closed by advancing the upper and lower lids toward the midline and by bringing down a V-Y flap from the glabella. A 3-mm plastic tube keeps the anastomosis between the conjunctiva and the nasolacrimal duct patent. (From Mustardé, ref. 1, with permission.)

SUMMARY

The V-Y glabellar flap is an excellent choice for reconstruction of deep lesions of the medial canthal area.

Reference

1. Mustardé JC. *Repair and reconstruction of the orbital region,* 2d Ed. Edinburgh: Churchill Livingstone, 1980; Chap. 11.

CHAPTER 28 ■ FOREHEAD SKIN FLAP FOR TOTAL UPPER AND LOWER EYELID RECONSTRUCTION

J. C. MUSTARDÉ

Total simultaneous reconstruction of both upper and lower eyelids is rarely required. Technically, the lower eyelid could be reconstructed by means of a cheek rotation flap lined by a composite graft of nasal septal mucosa and cartilage. The main problem, however, is reconstruction of the upper lid, because the ideal materials for carrying out the operation are no longer available. Skin for upper lid reconstruction must inevitably be brought in as a flap from the periphery of the orbit, and this means skin of a much thicker type than normal eyelid skin. Lining can be obtained either from the remaining conjunctiva in the fornices or as a free graft of mucosa. However, the chief difficulty is the absence of muscular activity in the new eyelid, particularly the closing activity of the orbicularis muscle, but also, to a lesser extent, the lifting action of the levator palpebrae muscle (1).

INDICATIONS

All instances of simultaneous upper and lower eyelid reconstruction reported to this author have been the result of trauma. The damage to the surrounding tissue, beyond the confines of the lids themselves, has usually been extensive enough to rule out the immediate use of a cheek rotation flap, even for reconstructing the lower lid. The problem of producing eyelids that not only will open sufficiently wide to provide useful vision, but also will close adequately enough

to afford a sufficient degree of protection to the cornea is, indeed, grave in the absence of adequate muscle function. Options open to the surgeon faced with the problem of having to totally reconstruct both eyelids at one time may be extremely limited.

In such circumstances, and provided a useful eye is still present, the main consideration is the preservation of the sight in that eye, even if this means occluding it for some considerable time. This is, in effect, "banking" the affected eye against the possibility that some day the patient will have only one seeing eye. It can then be exposed and lids constructed that will afford some degree of protection, as well as permitting the use of the eye itself, even if only to a limited degree.

OPERATIVE TECHNIQUE

The remains of the conjunctiva are dissected from both fornices toward the limbus, so that these thin flaps can be turned over the cornea and united by a pull-out running suture. Skin cover can then be obtained by the use of a midline forehead flap (see Fig. 2). A flap of this thickness will provide reasonably adequate support for the lower lid at a later date and will serve to nourish the conjunctival flaps in the initial stage of the surgery. Two and a half weeks later, the unused portion of the forehead flap is divided and returned to its normal position (Fig. 1A–F).

If the patient has sound vision in the other eye, it may be that no further surgery should be done and the affected eye can be "banked" against future use, because of the considerable problems encountered in an attempt to fashion eyelids.

In children who appear to tolerate a greater degree of corneal exposure better than adults, and in adults who have poor or absent vision in the other eye, the further management of eyelid reconstruction could commence 3 to 4 weeks after division of the flap pedicle.

A semicircular area of skin and subcutaneous tissue should be excised from the upper half of the flap covering the eye, down to—but not including—the conjunctival layer, and over an area corresponding to what would have been the tarsus and preseptal part of the upper lid. The exposed deep surface of the conjunctiva should then be covered by a full-thickness skin graft taken from behind the ear (Fig. 1G), inserting as much excess as possible. The thinner upper "lid" can be separated from the thicker, stiffer lower "lid" along the line of junction of the skin graft and flap some 8 to 10 weeks later, when any contraction of the graft that might

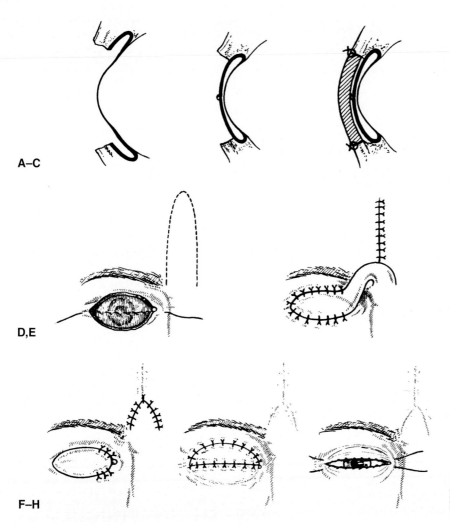

A–C

D,E

F–H

FIG. 1. A–H: Simultaneous reconstruction of both eyelids (see text for details).

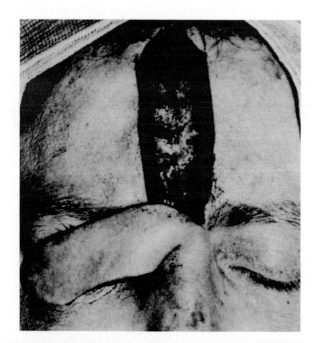

FIG. 2. Forehead flap that could be used to provide primary cover for both lids. The forehead defect can be closed directly, and the base of the flap can be returned in 2 weeks. (From Mustardé, ref. 1, with permission.)

have developed should have settled down (Fig. 1H). At the same time, the shallow fornices might have to be deepened using grafts of nasal or buccal mucosa sutured in place between the eyeball and the "lid" as a double layer. Such an addition to the fornix would almost certainly be necessary to free the globe from the upper lid and allow it to rotate upward under the lid for protection of the cornea during sleep.

Any remnant of levator palpebrae muscle that was preserved and hitched forward at the time of the original surgery might produce some slight elevation in the lid, but the probability of this is very slight. A certain amount of upward lift of the eyelid might be imparted by the action of the frontalis muscle, as in the grossly scarred lids that result from very deep burns. This, combined with a slight tilting of the head backward, would probably enable the patient to look out from under the rather inert upper lid and yet allow coverage of the cornea during sleep. The thick forehead skin on the lower lid should not be interfered with, since this will impart a degree of stiffness to the lid that will prevent it from drooping.

CLINICAL RESULTS

From my personal knowledge, this procedure has actually been used, with at least some degree of success, by three surgeons.

SUMMARY

In the very rare circumstance where both upper and lower eyelids need reconstruction, a midline forehead flap can be used either to "bank" the eye for later use or to create some semblance of eyelids.

Reference

1. Mustardé JC. *Repair and reconstruction of the orbital region,* 2d ed. Edinburgh: Churchill Livingstone, 1980; Chap. 9.

CHAPTER 29 ■ SECONDARY SUPERFICIAL TEMPORAL ARTERY–NECK FLAP FOR ORBITAL RECONSTRUCTION

H. P. LABANDTER AND B. GUYURON

EDITORIAL COMMENT

This is an excellent technique for eye socket reconstruction. However, there are two limiting factors: (1) the length of the temporal artery, and (2) the size of the defect. If the defect is too far medial or too large, the procedure may not be able to line the eye socket completely.

Eye socket reconstruction using skin or mucosal grafts and flaps has been notoriously difficult because of scarring, contracture, and donor deformities (1,2). The ideal reconstruction should be done with hairless tissue, cause minimal donor-site deformity, and provide sufficient tissue for adequate prosthetic reconstitution.

Experimental work has demonstrated the possibility of vascularizing tissue such as skin flaps and even composite flaps by the introduction of known axial vessels using omentum (3,4). Experimental and clinical work has shown that a random-pattern flap can be converted into a "secondary" axial-pattern skin flap on a known vascular supply (5). The superficial temporal artery can be placed beneath the hairless skin below the ear. Once vascular connections have been established, the flap can be transferred to cover various areas of the face within the arc of flap rotation.

INDICATIONS

Advantages of the procedure not only include the use of a known axial-pattern flap of hairless skin, but there is also no flap contracture, donor-site deformity is minimal, and a deep reliable sulcus for prosthetic placement can be established.

ANATOMY

The area to be used as lining for the eye socket is situated below and posterior to the tragus of the ear and is a patch of hairless skin. A site is selected where the donor area scars can be hidden, if possible, by hairstyling. In the adult male, the area of skin is limited to the space between the beard and the hairline, approximately 3.5 × 4 cm in width. Vertically, the distance can be extended as needed.

The superficial temporal artery, which is a terminal branch of the external carotid, begins in the parotid gland behind the neck of the mandible and crosses over the posterior root of the zygomatic arch. About 5 cm above the arch, it divides into an anterior and posterior branch. The frontal anterior branch runs upward and forward in a tortuous fashion, supplying muscle, skin, and pericranium in that area. The posterior parietal branch is larger than the anterior branch, curving upward and backward on the side of the head, lying superficial to the temporal fascia, and anastomosing with the opposite artery and the posterior auricular and occipital arteries. Variations in the superficial temporal arteries include differences in the relative sizes of the frontal and parietal branches. Either of these may be absent. The maximum length of the posterior parietal branch will be used as "donor" vessels for this flap.

FLAP DESIGN AND DIMENSIONS

The pivot point of the flap lies at the superior end of the tragal notch, at about the level of the zygomatic arch. The vascular pedicle extends superiorly for a distance of 8 to 10 cm. From this point, extending across the face to the medial end of the orbit would be approximately the same distance (Fig. 1A). The vessels are lifted together with a fascial envelope to protect the microvasculature and are inserted inferiorly under a trapdoor of skin measuring approximately 3.5 × 4 cm (Fig. 1B). Variations in the exact site and size of the skin disk can be tailored according to the amount of skin required to line the socket, the amount of hairless skin readily available, and how much can be removed and still allow direct closure of the donor site (Fig. 1C).

The arc of rotation for practical use is 180° to 200° extending superiorly to 3 to 4 cm above the helix of the ear, medially

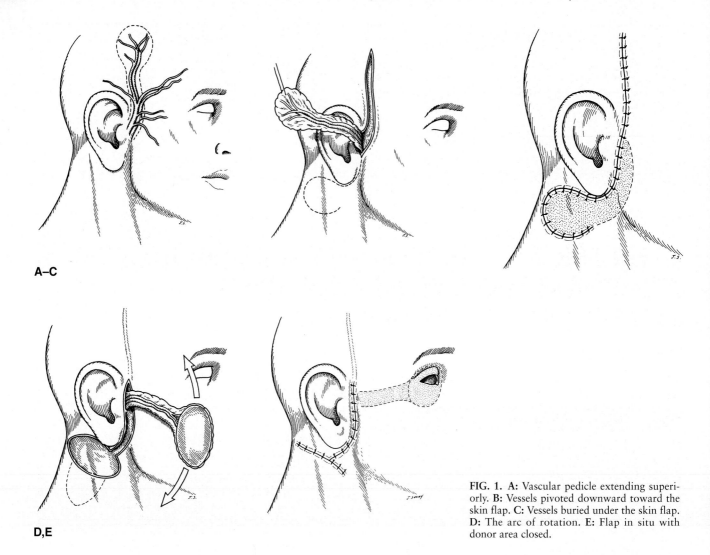

A–C

D,E

FIG. 1. A: Vascular pedicle extending superiorly. B: Vessels pivoted downward toward the skin flap. C: Vessels buried under the skin flap. D: The arc of rotation. E: Flap in situ with donor area closed.

to the medial canthus, and inferiorly down to the upper part of the sternocleidomastoid and postauricular area (Fig. 1D).

OPERATIVE TECHNIQUE

Donor Site

Measurement is made from the medial canthus to the pivot point of the superficial temporal vessels just above the zygomatic arch to determine the length required. The skin is opened through a preauricular incision at face lift level, and an anterior flap is developed. The incision is extended upward superiorly for 6 to 8 cm to identify the superficial temporal artery and vein under the fascia.

By careful dissection using magnifying loupes, the artery and vein are traced up superiorly and posteriorly as far as possible, maintaining a good connective-tissue sheath. Above the top of the helix, the area around the vessels is expanded into a fascial paddle (Fig. 1B) so that the proximal half of the buried portion of the vessels is encased in a protective fascial layer together with the microvasculature surrounding the vessels. This paddle may be made as large as 2 × 2 cm.

The entire fascial paddle and vessels are then carefully raised and pivoted downward to see how comfortably they lie over the proposed skin area on the side of the neck. The desired ellipse of skin is tested for ease of direct closure by

moving the head and palpating between fingers. The appropriate area is marked out in a transverse or vertical direction. Three sides of the skin may be raised as a trapdoor to join the preauricular incision (Fig. 1C).

Three weeks following this procedure, the entire skin paddle is raised carefully to subcutaneous level and freed together with the vascular pedicle. The preauricular incision is opened, and using face lift scissors, a wide tunnel is created toward the lateral aspect of the eyelid commissure.

Recipient Site

The lining tissue is opened transversely, and the sulcus is deepened by sharp and blunt dissection superiorly and inferiorly. When this has been completed, there may be sufficient mucosa to serve as adequate lining to the lids, or the inner parts of the upper and lower lids can be lined with a full-thickness skin graft from behind the ear. The pedicle is then tunneled subcutaneously, and the skin is laid into the posterior aspect of the socket (Fig. 1E). Care must be taken not to constrict the vessels and to avoid kinking. The use of fluorescein and a Doppler probe helps to verify the viability of the flap and the patency of the vessels. A drain is used throughout the cheek, emerging in the neck area. The face is closed in layers, and the flap in the posterior aspect of the socket can be tacked down loosely or fitted superiorly and inferiorly with tie-over bolsters coming through the superior and inferior sulcus of the eyelids (Fig. 2).

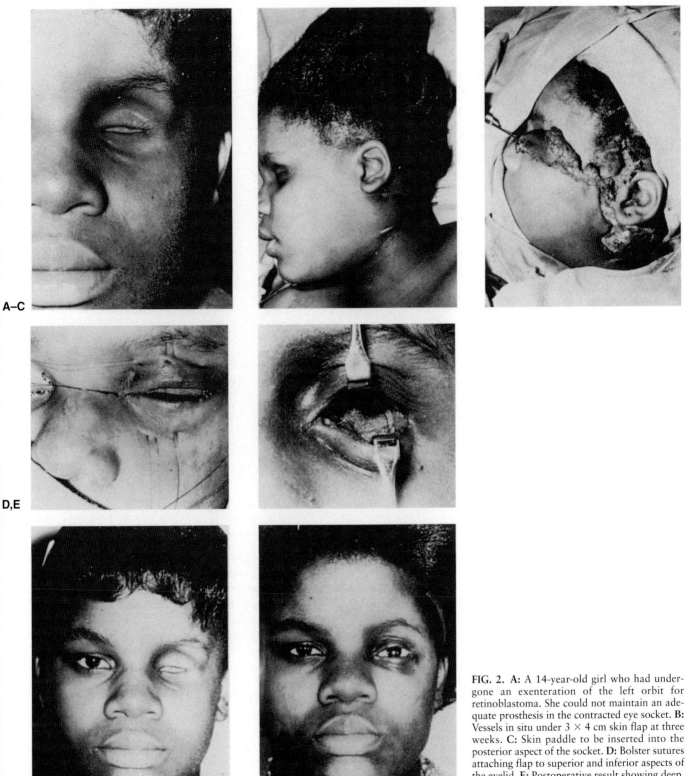

FIG. 2. A: A 14-year-old girl who had undergone an exenteration of the left orbit for retinoblastoma. She could not maintain an adequate prosthesis in the contracted eye socket. **B:** Vessels in situ under 3 × 4 cm skin flap at three weeks. **C:** Skin paddle to be inserted into the posterior aspect of the socket. **D:** Bolster sutures attaching flap to superior and inferior aspects of the eyelid. **E:** Postoperative result showing deep, well-lined socket. **F,G:** Preoperative (*left*) and postoperative (*right*) views of patient revealing a functional eye socket with reasonable symmetry.

A–C

D,E

F,G

CLINICAL RESULTS

That this is a two-stage procedure, that in some cases limited skin is available in adult males, and that visible scars may be a problem, are among the disadvantages of this procedure. In addition, extremely careful dissection of vessels is required. The second stage at 2 to 3 weeks must be done with care, and any kinking or hematoma may compromise the vascularity of the flap. Extended musculofascial flaps, free flaps, and even tubed pedicle flaps have been used, but all have multiple disadvantages.

SUMMARY

This is a useful technique for acquiring hairless skin from the neck and postauricular areas when a deep permanent eye socket is needed for prosthetic placement.

References

1. Mustardé JC. The orbital reconstruction. In: Mustardé JC, ed. *Plastic surgery in infancy and childhood,* 2d ed. Edinburgh: Churchill Livingstone, 1979.
2. Soll DB. Anophthalmic socket surgery. *Int Ophthalmol Clin* 1978;18:169.
3. Erol OO, Spira M. Development and utilization of composite island flap employing omentum: experimental investigation. *Plast Reconstr Surg* 1980;65:405.
4. Erol OO. The transformation of a free skin graft into a vascularized pedicled flap. *Plast Reconstr Surg* 1976;58:470.
5. Yao S. Vascular implantation into skin flap: experimental study and clinical application. A preliminary report. *Plast Reconstr Surg* 1981;68:404.

CHAPTER 30 ■ POSTAURICULAR FASCIOCUTANEOUS ISLAND FLAP

B. GUYURON AND H. P. LABANDTER

Dissatisfaction with the available modalities for eye socket reconstruction, particularly in an irradiated and previously operated field, prompted us to look for another alternative. Following much preplanning influenced by Washio's work (1,2), and after considerable cadaver dissections, clinical trials, and staged procedures, we came to the conclusion that a postauricular fasciocutaneous island flap can successfully be transferred for the correction of certain difficult defects (3).

INDICATIONS

The postauricular fasciocutaneous flap can be used for defects of the forehead, eye socket, lateral nose, cheeks, and commissure area. It can even be used for intraoral defects in the buccal sulcus area or the palatal region. An invaluable indication for this flap is the Treacher Collins syndrome, which usually represents a very difficult reconstructive challenge.

Hematoma, infection, partial flap loss, and injury to the temporalis branch of the facial nerve are all theoretical complications of this flap. However, in our experience, there were only two small superficial losses of the distal portions of the flaps, and both healed without further difficulties. The disadvantages of this flap include tedious dissection and a limited amount of available skin, which make it unsuitable for large defects. Occasionally, a split-thickness skin graft is needed to cover the donor-site defect.

This flap provides an adequate amount of skin and soft-tissue bulk for reconstruction of a missing eye socket and orbital area. The color match is close to the facial color for extended reconstruction. Being non–hair-bearing, the skin can be used to replace missing conjunctiva or mucosa. The donor defect can usually be closed primarily or with a small skin graft, which is usually not visible.

ANATOMY

Even though the useful cutaneous portion of the flap receives a random-pattern circulation from the posterior branch of the superficial temporal vessel, the whole flap, including the triangular piece of dermis and the temporalis fascia, is raised as an island flap. Therefore, the arterial supply comes from the superficial temporal artery and the posterior branch of this vessel and then through the subdermal plexus reaching the cutaneous portion, which after passing through the capillary returns through the posterior branch to the superficial temporal vein.

FLAP DESIGN AND DIMENSIONS

This flap has three distinct anatomic components: the skin, dermis, and fascial portion, which encompasses the postauricular vessels. The cutaneous portion of the flap is the non–hair-bearing skin of the postauricular area. This portion can be as large as 5 × 6 cm. The dermis portion is a triangular-shaped area located cephalad to the upper pole of the helix at

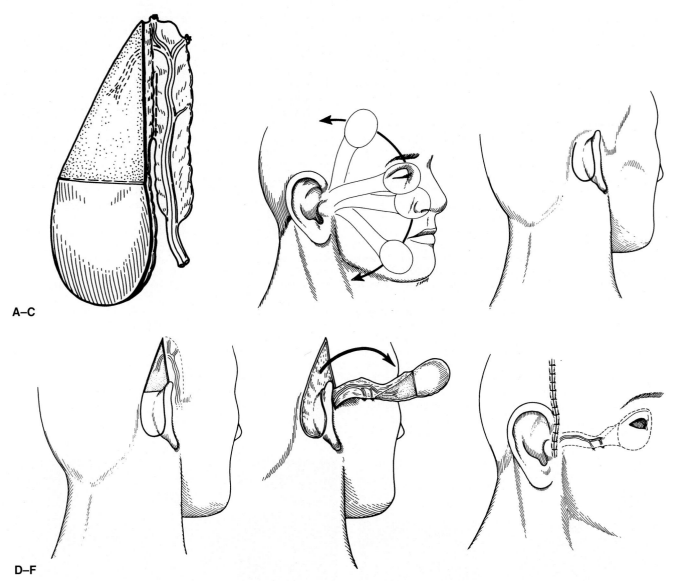

FIG. 1. A: The three different portions of the postauricular island flap: postauricular skin, de-epithelialized supra-auricular scalp, and temporalis fascia encompassing the superficial temporal vessels. **B:** The arc of rotation of the postauricular flap. **C:** The incision in the postauricular area, which includes the non–hair-bearing skin of the retroauricular region. **D:** The triangular portion of the flap is designed by connecting the most superior and posterior portions of the skin flap to a point about 6 cm cephalad to the upper pole of the ear. A vertical line from this point to the upper pole of the ear will then outline the anterior limb of the triangle. **E:** The mobilized flap and donor effect. Please note the cutback incision that has been made between the triangular flap and the vascular pedicle to augment the reach of the flap. **F:** The donor-site and preauricular skin closure with the flap delivered to the orbit through a subcutaneous tunnel. (From Guyuron, ref. 3, with permission.)

the base of the triangle positioned caudally (Fig. 1A). The base of this triangle is attached to the upper border of the postauricular skin to be transferred as a flap. This triangular deepithelialized area is approximately 6 cm long in a cephalocaudal direction, and it contains the posterior arterial and venous branches of the superficial temporal vessels. The third portion of the flap is the temporalis fascia just anterior to the triangular de-epithelialized skin of the scalp encompassing the superficial temporal artery and vein. This fascia is rectangular in shape, and its anterior boundary is about 5 to 10 mm anterior to the superficial temporal vessels. The posterior limits are de-epithelialized triangular skin, which extends cephalad up to 6 or 7 cm from the upper pole of the helix. The caudal limit is at the upper border of the zygoma, where it is often detached to allow freedom of movement for the vascular pedicle.

This flap can be rotated 360°, the pivot point being located at the level of the tragus. This flap will have a radius of about 14 cm. However, the useful rotation of the flap extends from the forehead area down to the mandibular angle, including the oral commissure and the lateral nasal area. This flap can be used for reconstruction of palatal defects (Fig. 1B). The postauricular portion of the flap includes non–hair-bearing skin of the retroauricular region, leaving 6 to 7 mm of skin along the ear margins (Fig. 1C). To design the posterior limb of the triangular flap, a line is drawn 6 cm cephalad to the upper pole of the ear to the most cephalad portion of the postauricular skin flap. The base of the triangular flap will be the superior edge of the cutaneous flap, and the anterior limit is a line 1 cm anterior to the palpable superficial temporal vessels.

OPERATIVE TECHNIQUE

A postauricular incision is made, and the skin flap is raised, including the underlying superficial fascia. Extreme care is exercised to leave the perichondrium intact. Inferior, anterior, and posterior outlines of the skin flap are included in this incision, leaving the superior portion attached to the triangular flap. The incision along the anterior border of the triangular portion is carried through the skin with great caution to avoid injury to the superficial temporal vessels just beneath the skin. This incision is continued along the preauricular fold much like a face lift incision. Next, the posterior incision is made through the skin as well as the fascia.

The identification and separation of the superficial temporal vessels from the overlying skin are now undertaken. The temporalis fascia, encompassing the superficial temporal vessels, is left attached to the vessels. To ensure vessel safety, the fascia is incised 10 mm anterior to the vessels. The triangular temporalis fascia flaps are raised off the temporalis muscle together. The vessels are dissected proximally to the point where they enter the parotid gland. These tortuous vessels can be dissected to give considerable length to the pedicle.

If the flap is being used for an eye socket reconstruction, a subcutaneous tunnel is then created carefully to preserve the integrity of the temporalis branch of the fascial nerve. When the dissection reaches the lateral orbital wall, it should be continued in a subperiosteal plane to preserve the lateral canthal attachments to the skin and upper portion of the periosteum.

The triangular portion of the flap is then de-epithelialized, and the reach of the flap is measured (Fig. 1E). If further length to the pedicle is needed to allow the flap to reach the medial canthal region, a cutback incision is made between the pedicle and the triangular flap starting caudally, close to the origin of the vascular pedicle. As much as an inch of the pedicle can be separated safely from the triangular flap, leaving from 3.5 to 4 cm of the pedicle attached to the triangular portion of the flap (Fig. 1E).

Although the flap often looks slightly congested, it usually recovers in a few hours. The flap donor area in the postauricular region is covered with a split-thickness skin graft if necessary, and tie-over sutures are used. The rest of the donor-site incision is closed by approximation of the skin (Fig. 1F).

CLINICAL RESULTS

This flap has been used successfully in 15 patients to reconstruct missing or contracted eye sockets (Fig. 2). It has been used in two Treacher Collins patients to reconstruct the soft-tissue deficiency in the malar area, for reconstruction of a palatal deformity in one patient, and for the reconstruction of a total lower eyelid in another patient.

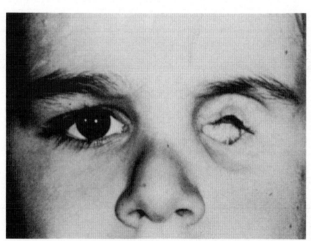

A

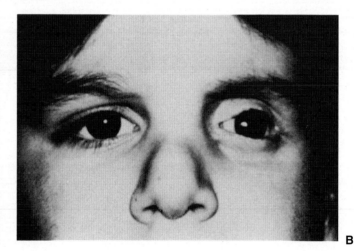

B

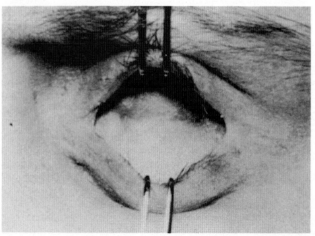

C

FIG. 2. A: Preoperative photograph of a 10-year-old boy following enucleation and radiation of the left orbit and a previously failed attempt at eye socket reconstruction. B: Two years following eye socket reconstruction using the postauricular fasciocutaneous technique. C: After reconstruction, the eye socket is supple and functional. (From Guyuron, ref. 3, with permission.)

SUMMARY

A flap of postauricular skin based on the superficial temporal vessels and surrounding fascia is described. This flap is excellent for reconstruction of missing or contracted eye sockets or for small to medium-sized facial defects such as on the eyelids or for internal defects.

References

1. Washio H. Retroauricular-temporal flap. *Plast Reconstr Surg* 1969;43:162.
2. Washio H. Further experiences with the retroauricular temporal flap. *Plast Reconstr Surg* 1972;50:160.
3. Guyuron B. Retroauricular island flap for eye socket reconstruction. *Plast Reconstr Surg* 1985;76:527.

CHAPTER 31. Arm Skin Flap for Orbital Socket Reconstruction

M. R. Wexler and I. Peled

www.encyclopediaofflaps.com

CHAPTER 32 ■ REVERSE TEMPORALIS FLAP FOR RECONSTRUCTION AFTER ORBITAL EXENTERATION

N. MENON AND R. SILVERMAN

EDITORIAL COMMENT

The temporalis muscle is an excellent local flap to fill the exenterated orbit. The authors' suggestion of making an adequate orbitotomy to pass the muscle has the advantages of shortening the arc of rotation and avoiding an osteotomy of the lateral orbital rim. The secondary depression in the temple can be filled as the authors indicate with either AlloDerm or dermal-fat grafts.

Orbital exenteration usually involves the resection of the entire contents of the orbits, with or without resection of the eyelids. Techniques to replace the orbital contents with vascularized tissue have involved multiple stages or have included the use of microvascular techniques. This chapter introduces the reader to a single-stage pedicled transposition of the temporalis muscle into the orbital cavity through a window created in the lateral orbital wall.

INDICATIONS

Techniques to replace the orbital contents with vascularized tissue have included pedicled flaps (retroauricular island flap, cheek flap, pectoralis flap) (1–3) and free flaps (radial forearm, dorsalis pedis flap) (4–6). A single-stage pedicled transposition of the entire temporalis muscle as a pedicled flap into the orbital cavity, through a window created in the lateral orbital wall, can be accomplished in any patient who has undergone orbital exenteration and has an intact ipsilateral temporalis muscle. This single-stage technique provides the

muscle bulk needed to obliterate the orbital cavity, and provides a vascularized soft-tissue cover around the exposed bone and subjacent sinus cavities.

ANATOMY

The temporalis muscle is a fan-shaped muscle located on the lateral aspect of the skull. It originates along the inferior temporal line on the cranium. The deep temporal fascia covers both the superficial and the deep (cranial) aspects of the muscle. The deep temporal fascia joins the periosteum of the cranium along the superior temporal line (temporal crest). The muscle lies in the temporal fossa and inserts on the mandible after passing along the deep surface of the zygomatic arch (7). The muscle inserts on the coronoid process and along the anterior ramus of the mandible. The muscle is innervated by the mandibular branch of the trigeminal nerve (cranial nerve V). Contraction of the muscle causes retraction and elevation of the mandible (7).

The muscle is supplied by two dominant vascular pedicles and a minor pedicle, making it a type III muscle (Mathes and Nahai classification) (7). The dominant pedicles are the anterior and posterior deep temporal arteries, both of which are branches of the internal maxillary artery. The deep middle temporal artery (branch of the superficial temporal artery) forms the minor vascular pedicle (2). The venous drainage of the muscle is through the venae comitantes that accompany the arterial supply.

Both dominant vascular pedicles are located on the deep surface of the muscle at the level of the zygomatic arch within a centimeter of each other. On the other hand, the minor pedicle is located on the superficial surface of the muscle in the preauricular region just cephalad to the zygomatic arch (7).

FLAP DESIGN AND DIMENSIONS

The temporalis muscle can be transposed as a pure muscle flap or as a musculocutaneous flap. It is best to use the temporalis as a pure muscle flap, as taking the skin paddle along with the muscle would leave an unacceptable donor scar with a significant amount of alopecia (7). The vascular supply configuration allows the muscle to be split coronally (into anterior and posterior halves) or sagittally (into deep and superficial halves) (8). In this application, transposition of the muscle en bloc provides total fill of the orbital cavity in a safe, expedient manner. Furthermore, with muscle-splitting techniques, there is a real risk that the pedicles could be damaged during the dissection.

In a limited cadaver study, three parameters were measured to quantify the crucial dimensions involved in the operation: (a) the height of the temporalis from the zygomatic arch to the point most superior on the inferior temporal line, (b) the width of the temporal fossa from the point most anterior to the point most posterior on the inferior temporal line, and (c) the dimensions of the bony window in the lateral orbital wall needed to pass the muscle without compression (9). The mean height was determined to be 8.45 cm, whereas the mean width was determined to be 10.5 cm (9). The mean dimensions of the bony window in the cadaver study were found to be 3.3 cm × 1.9 cm (9).

OPERATIVE TECHNIQUE

Tissue Planes and Anatomic Landmarks

The coronal or hemicoronal incision provides the most access and exposure of the temporalis muscle. A stealth incision can camouflage the postoperative scar on the scalp. It is better to use Raney clips for hemostasis along the scalp edges rather than electrocautery, so as to minimize alopecia along the scar edges. Electrocautery can be used to dissect through the subcutaneous tissue until a loose areolar plane is reached. The subsequent plane over the temporal region will be the superficial temporal fascia (also called the temporoparietal fascia); the corresponding plane over the cranium would be the galeal plane. Dissection through the superficial temporal fascia reveals the glistening white, deep, temporal fascia that envelops the temporalis muscle; division of the galeal plane should reveal the periosteum of the cranium.

After exposure of the deep temporal fascia inferolaterally and the periosteum of the skull medially, the scalp can be mobilized anteriorly, to provide exposure to the zygomatic arch and the lateral orbital rim. The periosteum is incised medial to the temporal crest, and a subperiosteal dissection is performed inferolaterally, to elevate the temporalis muscle from the temporal fossa and to detach the muscle from its origin. Care must be taken to ensure that the dissection remains in a subperiosteal plane (especially laterally around the region of the zygomatic arch), as the two major pedicles to the muscle flap lie on the deep (cranial) surface of the muscle. The insertion of the muscle on the coronoid process of the mandible is maintained, as it provides a convenient point of rotation; greater mobility and range of transposition can be achieved if the insertion is taken down, but in most instances this is unnecessary. Furthermore, because both dominant pedicles are located on the deep (cranial) surface of the muscle very close to its insertion, the risk of damaging the pedicles may not justify the gain in mobility.

A burr is used to make a window in the lateral wall of the orbit (orbital surface of the zygomatic bone), and rongeurs can be used to make the window large enough to pass the entire temporalis muscle. The window should be made large enough to pass the muscle without causing any compression.

One alternative to a lateral wall orbitotomy is to transpose the temporalis muscle over the lateral orbital rim and into the orbital cavity. However, we believe this option is less desirable, as it is more difficult to fill the entire orbit and to secure the muscle inside the orbit. Furthermore, on closure, the transposed muscle can be compressed between the skin flap and the lateral orbital rim, which could potentially cause arterial or venous insufficiency.

Distorting of the transverse dimension and the upper face contour is an additional drawback of this technique. Another alternative to the lateral wall orbitotomy is a lateral rim osteotomy. An osteotomy can be made on either side of the zygomaticofrontal suture, and after transposition of the temporalis into the orbit, the bony rim fragment can be fixed with a miniplate and screws. The drawback of this technique is that the periosteum and microvasculature within the cortex of the lateral rim are disrupted on performing the osteotomy. Because patients who undergo orbital exenteration are likely to receive or have already received radiation therapy, disrupting the vasculature increases the risk of developing osteoradionecrosis of the lateral rim, with concomitant exposure of the fixation system.

CLINICAL RESULTS

Depicted here is an example of a 74-year-old man who presented 6 months after orbital exenteration for ocular melanoma (Fig. 1). At presentation, he had exposed bone, with communication into the paranasal sinuses and chronic drainage from the orbit. After thorough debridement of the

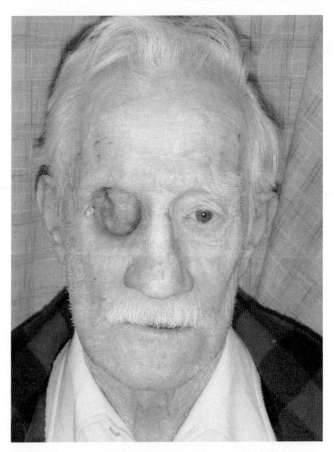

FIG. 1. Preoperative right orbital defect after orbital exenteration.

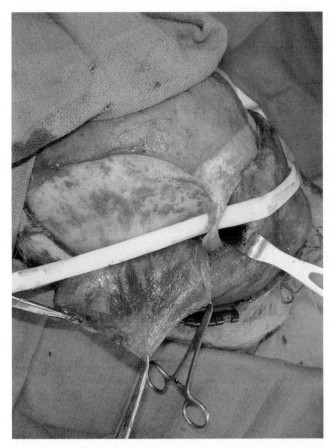

FIG. 2. The temporalis muscle has been reflected laterally to expose the deep surface of the muscle. The Penrose drain passes through the window created in the lateral orbital wall.

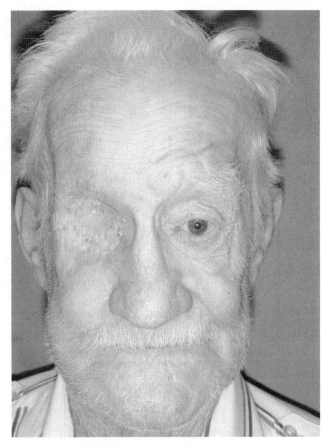

FIG. 3. Anteroposterior (AP) view at 7 months postoperatively, showing well-healed reconstruction.

orbit, the temporalis muscle was exposed, using a coronal incision up to the lateral orbital rim and zygomatic arch (Fig. 2). After creation of a window in the lateral orbital wall, the temporalis was then detached from its origins and transposed into the orbit through the window in the lateral orbital wall. The muscle flap was inset into the orbit, sutured to the surrounding skin edges, and covered with a nonmeshed split-thickness skin graft.

Postoperatively, the patient had a well-healed right orbit with no drainage (Fig. 3). The patient reported no problems with mastication or motion of the mandible. A contour defect in the right temporal fossa was noticeable, and the patient underwent placement of a porous polyethylene implant to fill in the contour defect 9 months after the original operation. The patient has subsequently done well. At this time, the authors prefer the immediate use of layered AlloDerm (LifeCell Corp., Branchburg, NJ) in order to fill in the donor-site defect. This can be done at the time of the initial operation, due to the ability of AlloDerm to become revascularized and therefore to resist infection (10). The donor-site contour defect can also be addressed with the use of dermal-fat grafts.

SUMMARY

The temporalis muscle can be used as a pedicled flap for reconstruction after orbital exenteration in a one-stage operation. After transposition, the entire muscle can be used to fill the orbit and to provide a vascular bed for an onlay split-thickness skin graft. Preservation of the lateral orbital rim allows for retention of the transverse width and anterior projection of the upper face. Transposition of the temporalis has minimal effect on mastication, as the other muscles of mastication compensate adequately. The contour defect in the temporal fossa can be corrected by either AlloDerm or synthetic implant, depending on the risk of infection.

References

1. Ariyan S. Pectoralis major, sternomastoid and other musculocutaneous flaps for head and neck reconstruction. *Clin Plast Surg* 1980;7:89.
2. Matsumoto K, Nakanishi H, Urano Y, et al. Lower eyelid reconstruction with a cheek flap supported by fascia lata. *Plast Reconstr Surg* 1999; 103:1650.
3. Guyuron B. Retroauricular island flap for eye socket reconstruction. *Plast Reconstr Surg* 1985;76:527.
4. Weng CJ. Periorbital soft tissue and socket reconstruction. *Ann Plast Surg* 1995;34:457.
5. Tahara S. Eye socket reconstruction with free radial forearm flap. *Ann Plast Surg* 1989;23:112.
6. Thai KN, Billmire DA, Yakuboff KP. Total eyelid reconstruction with free dorsalis pedis flap after deep facial burn. *Plast Reconstr Surg* 1999; 104:1048.
7. Mathes SJ, Nahai F. *Reconstructive surgery: principles, anatomy and technique*, vol. I. St. Louis: Quality Medical Publishing, 1997;386–396.
8. Holmes A, Marshall K. Uses of the temporalis muscle flap in blanking out orbits. *Plast Reconstr Surg* 1979;63:336.
9. Menon NG, Girotto JA, Goldberg NH, Silverman RP. Orbital reconstruction after exenteration: use of a transorbital temporal muscle flap. *Ann Plast Surg* 2003;50:38.
10. Menon NG, Rodriguez ED, Byrnes CK, et al. Revascularization of human acellular dermis in full-thickness abdominal wall defects in the rabbit model. *Ann Plast Surg* 2003;50:523.

CHAPTER 33 ■ MICROVASCULAR FREE TRANSFER OF A FIRST WEB SPACE SKIN FLAP OF THE FOOT TO RECONSTRUCT THE UPPER AND LOWER EYELIDS

L. A. CHAIT

The reconstruction of both upper and lower eyelids when their total loss accompanies orbital exenteration is difficult (1,2). This deformity may result from tumor excision or trauma. For this reason, the use of a prosthesis that is either applied directly over the cavity or attached to spectacles is often advised. However, patients sometimes request reconstruction (Fig. 1).

INDICATIONS

The neurovascular free flap from the first web space of the foot has been invaluable in reconstructing both upper and lower eyelids in these instances (3,4). The texture of the dorsal skin of the toes and the color match are found to be acceptable. The web itself forms a natural lateral canthus, and the thicker plantar skin gives enough support to maintain a light prosthesis. Crude sensation returns to the outer part of the flap. At first, this is referred to the temporal region, but later it tends to reorient to the eyelid itself. Both skin cover and lining for each of the upper and lower lids are provided in a single operation, and much of the scarring that results from local flap reconstruction can be avoided.

ANATOMY

See Chap. 323.

FLAP DESIGN AND DIMENSIONS

The flap includes the skin of the first web space of the foot, with extensions running onto adjacent toes as far as their tips. Enough skin must be removed from each toe to allow it to be folded on itself to provide both lid cover and lining. A small area of dorsal foot skin proximal to the web is included (Fig. 2). The flap must be taken from the foot on the ipsilateral side, because the web has to provide the lateral canthus and the dorsal skin must be external.

OPERATIVE TECHNIQUE

After marking the specific design on the first web space, a lazy S incision is made proximally over the dorsum of the foot. The dorsal veins from the flap are identified and traced to the greater saphenous vein. Other tributaries are ligated, and the saphenous vein is isolated to the midfoot level. The dorsalis pedis artery and its venae comitantes are located just lateral to the extensor hallucis longus tendon. This artery is traced distally, and its continuation as the first dorsal metatarsal artery is identified passing into the first web space flap. The artery is freed, and all branches, including the large proximal perforating artery, are ligated. The extensor hallucis brevis tendon is divided during this procedure. The venae comitantes are left intact, since they may be needed as a backup venous drainage system. The deep peroneal nerve that accompanies the dorsalis pedis artery and its extension is identified and preserved.

At the recipient site, a vertical preauricular incision is made, and the superficial temporal artery and vein and the temporal nerve are identified. These are freed proximally and distally for a short distance, and minor branches and tributaries are ligated. A skin incision is then made around the orbital margin at the junction of normal skin and the cavity lining. A strip of skin graft or conjunctiva measuring at least 1.5 cm in width is removed circumferentially from just within the bony rim to create a recipient bed for the flap. A horizontal incision is then made connecting the lateral side of the orbital incision to the preauricular one.

If perfusion to the isolated flap is found to be adequate, the vessels are clamped and ligated and the flap transferred. (For closure of the donor site, see Chap. 323.) The flap is sutured into place with the dorsal skin outward and the web on the lateral side to form a lateral canthus. The skin from each toe (the great toe is superior) is folded on itself to provide both lid cover and lining. The thicker plantar skin is sutured first to the edge of the orbital cavity lining, and the outer rim is sutured next. End-to-end anastomoses are then carried out between the dorsalis pedis artery and the saphenous vein and the superficial temporal artery and vein, respectively. The deep peroneal nerve extension is sutured to one or two branches of the temporal nerve.

The horizontal skin wound may be closed directly over the pedicle, but if there is any tension as a result of excess fatty tissue around the distal pedicle, a temporary skin graft may be used for closure.

When the initial edema and scarring have settled down, the flap and its pedicle will have to be defatted and trimmed. A strip of conchal cartilage may be inserted along the new lower lid for additional support. A very thin hair-bearing Wolfe graft inserted just below the rim of the lower lid has proved useful to provide lower lid lashes (Fig. 3).

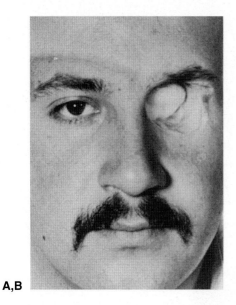
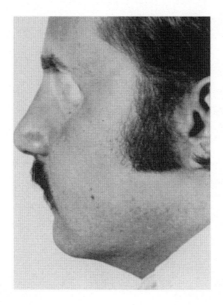

A,B

FIG. 1. A,B: Patient 10 years after orbital exenteration for rhabdomyosarcoma. Socket was lined with a split-thickness skin graft.

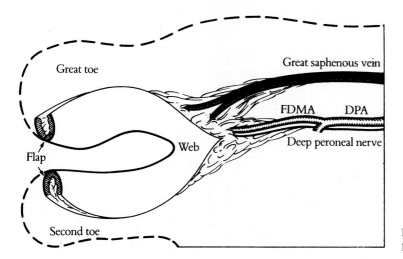

FIG. 2. The flap and its vascular supply (DPA, dorsalis pedis artery; FDMA, first dorsal metatarsal artery).

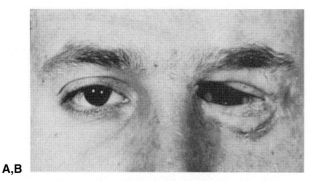
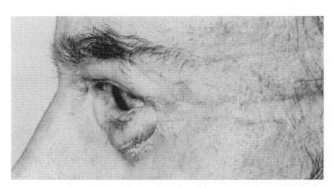

A,B

FIG. 3. A,B: The flap 4 months after initial surgery. A hair-bearing Wolfe graft has provided lower lid lashes.

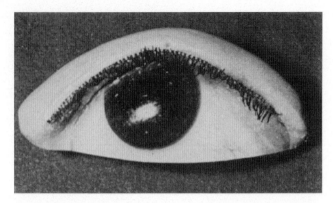

FIG. 4. The eye prosthesis with a flesh-colored eyelid-bearing attachment along its upper rim.

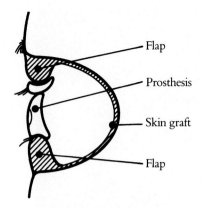

FIG. 5. Diagrammatic cross section through the orbit showing how the prosthesis rests between the two parts of the flap.

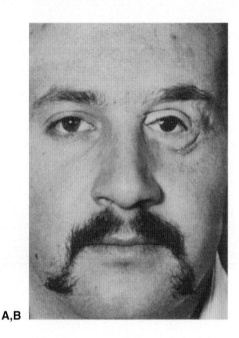
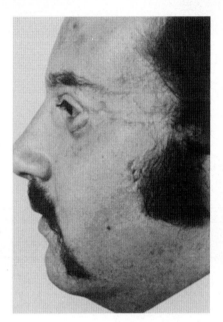

A,B

FIG. 6. A,B: Final result with prosthesis in place.

The prosthesis should be designed to fit between (not behind) the newly created upper and lower eyelids. A small flesh-colored segment that includes upper lashes is fashioned and attached to the upper rim of the eye prosthesis (Fig. 4). The prosthesis should be light and should rest securely between the two lids (Fig. 5). A small additional flange will hook behind either the upper or the lower lid and may obviate the use of glue as a means of fixation. The prosthesis should be easy to remove and replace in order to allow adequate cleansing of the orbital cavity.

CLINICAL RESULTS

The junction between the flesh-colored upper segment of the prosthesis and the upper lid flap provides a very pleasing tarsal fold (Fig. 6).

SUMMARY

A free first web space flap can be effectively used to reconstruct upper and lower eyelids after complete orbital exenteration.

References

1. Carraway JH, Horton CE, Adamson JF, Mladick RA. Reconstruction after extended orbital exenteration. In: Tessier P, Callahan A, Mustardé J, Salyer KE, eds., *Symposium on plastic surgery in the orbital region*, vol. 12. St. Louis: Mosby, 1976.
2. Meyer R. Eyelid reconstruction following enucleation and exenteration. In: Hueston JT, ed., *Transactions of the Fifth International Congress of Plastic and Reconstructive Surgery*. Melbourne: Butterworth, 1971;991–1000.
3. May JW, Chait LA, Cohen BE, O'Brien BMcC. Free neurovascular flap from the foot in hand reconstruction. *J Hand Surg* 1977;2:387.
4. Morrison WA, O'Brien BMcC, Hamilton RB. Neurovascular free foot flaps in reconstruction of the mutilated hand. *Clin Plast Surg* 1978;5:265.

CHAPTER 34 ■ DORSALIS PEDIS FREE FLAP FOR EYE SOCKET RECONSTRUCTION

B. GUYURON AND H. P. LABANDTER

Contracted or missing eye sockets, especially in an irradiated orbit, represent a major reconstructive task for the orbital surgeon. Failure of simple eye socket reconstruction requires complex procedures. Most grafts are doomed to failure, and local flaps may leave undesirable donor-site scars. Distant flaps require many stages and leave visible scars, and the patient is placed in an uncomfortable position for 2 or 3 weeks. In selected patients, we have transferred the dorsalis pedis flap to reconstruct the missing or contracted eye socket.

INDICATIONS

This procedure should be used only if simpler techniques of eye socket reconstruction fail. The procedure of choice for eye socket reconstruction is the application of a full-thickness skin graft. If this fails, the next choice is a postauricular fasciocutaneous flap (see Chap. 30) or a secondary axial-pattern flap (1). If the clinical examination indicates a diminished or absent superficial temporal pulse and the local condition supports this finding, a vascularized dorsalis pedis flap can be chosen for eye socket reconstruction.

ANATOMY

For details of the anatomy of the flap (2,3), see Chaps. 304 and 518.

FLAP DESIGN AND DIMENSIONS

We use the central portion of the dorsalis pedis flap, the size of the flap depending on the size of the defect (Fig. 1A). Although the short and long saphenous veins can be used for the venous anastomosis, we prefer to use one of the venae comitantes of the anterior tibial artery because of its length and ease of dissection. The flap is designed with adequate dimensions to reconstruct the socket, as well as an additional de-epithelialized portion of the margin of this flap which is used to correct the periorbital deficit.

OPERATIVE TECHNIQUE

Donor Site

Flap dissection is similar to what is described in Chaps. 304 and 518. We expose the anterior tibial vessels proximally, and the flap is dissected from proximal to distal and from medial to lateral, keeping the main vessels attached to the overlying skin.

Recipient Site

If the superficial temporal vessels are absent or unsuitable, which is usually the indication for this procedure in preference to a fasciocutaneous flap, the facial artery and external jugular vein are dissected free through a small transverse cervical incision, and a subcutaneous tunnel is created to connect this area to the preauricular incision.

If the superficial temporal vessels are still available, one team exposes them through a preauricular incision. The vein is usually found anterior to the artery. However, as the vein nears the parotid gland, it is closer to the superficial temporal artery. At this point, the lumen sizes of both vein and artery are most closely matched, although exposure is not ideal. The vessels are isolated carefully.

A subcutaneous tunnel is then created directly from the upper pole of the parotid gland to the lateral orbital area, preserving the temporal branch of the facial nerve. The upper and lower eyelids are then separated from the orbit, and an attempt is made to keep the eyelids as thin as possible. Meticulous hemostasis is critical to avoid a collection of blood under the flap.

The flap is then placed in position (Fig. 1B), and an adequate amount of full-thickness skin graft is harvested from the portion of the flap that is to be de-epithelialized and is used to augment the periorbital area. The graft is used to line the posterior aspect of each eyelid to create a sulcus. The flap is not folded under the eyelid because of its thickness. The full-thickness skin graft is sutured to the palpebral margin or to the remnant of the palpebral conjunctiva on one side and to the junction of the de-epithelialized and epithelial portions of the flap on the other side (Fig. 1C).

A few darts along the junction of the full-thickness skin graft with the flap are advisable in order to avoid circular contracture. Through-and-through 4-0 Prolene sutures on a Keith needle are used to anchor the sulcus to the skin of the supraorbital and infraorbital regions. These stitches are then tied over bolsters, and the cavity is packed (Fig. 2).

CLINICAL RESULTS

Along with the usual complications associated with free flaps and the dorsalis pedis donor site, injury to the temporal branch of the facial nerve may occur.

SUMMARY

Achievement of a functional eye socket in a single-stage operation is the main advantage of this procedure. This

97

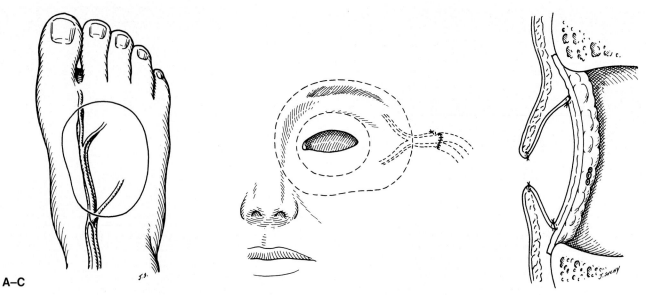

A–C

FIG. 1. A: Design of the dorsalis pedis flap on the dorsum of the foot. B: The dorsalis pedis flap in position, with vascular anastomoses and extension of the de-epithelialized portion over the supraorbital and infraorbital rim, for augmentation of this area. C: Sagittal view of the orbit with dorsalis pedis flap in position covering the posterior wall of the orbit and the superior and inferior orbital rim, and full-thickness skin graft lining the posterior aspects of the eyelids.

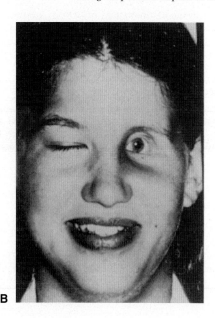
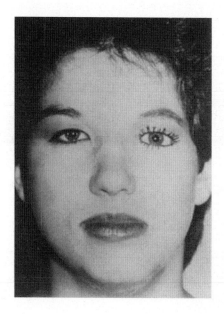

A,B

FIG. 2. A: A 17-year-old-girl who underwent enucleation of the eye and radiation to the left orbit 12 years previously. Two previous skin grafts failed to reconstruct an adequate eye socket. She also had a persistent infection requiring removal of the silicone implant used to augment the left orbit. A free-vascularized dorsalis pedis flap and full-thickness skin graft were used to rebuild the eye socket. B: Although a functional eye socket was reconstructed in one stage, this flap did not provide adequate tissue to augment the periorbital region because of the significant bony and soft-tissue deficit. The patient underwent a second operation to reconstruct the left supraorbital rim and augment the orbital content with rib cartilage grafts.

operation provides an adequate amount of healthy skin with excellent blood supply and little or no chance of contraction. The thinness of the flap is a desirable advantage. Two to three weeks later, a temporary prosthesis can be placed in the sulcus.

References

1. Guyuron B, Labandter HP, Berlin AJ. Fasciocutaneous flap: secondary axial pattern flap and microvascular free flap in socket reconstruction. *Ophthalmology* 1984;91:94.
2. McCraw JB, Furlow LT, Jr. The dorsalis pedis arterialized flap: a clinical study. *Plast Reconstr Surg* 1975;55:177.
3. Ohmori K, Harii K. Free dorsalis pedis sensory flap to the hand with microneurovascular anastomoses. *Plast Reconstr Surg* 1976;58:546.

CHAPTER 35 ■ BILOBED NASAL SKIN FLAPS

A. MATARASSO AND B. STRAUCH

The bilobed nasal flap is a useful and time-honored technique for reconstructing defects of the nose and various other regions of the body (1–4). It is a transposition flap consisting of two lobes of skin and subcutaneous tissue based on a common pedicle (5).

INDICATIONS

This flap is most commonly used for patients following removal of basal-cell cancers. Bilobed nasal flaps are appropriate for partial-thickness losses of less than 1.5 cm of the lateral aspect of the nose, ala, and tip area. It is feasible in situations where sufficient laxity exists in surrounding nasal tissue, to allow the excess to be transposed for wound coverage, while permitting primary closure of the final donor site. The concept of transferring tissue laxity from the upper to the lower nose or "robbing Peter to pay Paul," allows losses of tissue to be replaced in kind (6). A bilobed flap may also be used in conjunction with other flaps to reconstruct more complex contour defects in the nasal area (7). For example, it may be used to cover a full-thickness nasal-tip defect, where lining and support are provided by a composite graft to the underside of the bilobed nasal flap.

ANATOMY

This flap is essentially a rotation flap divided into two transposition flaps. The bilobed flap has a random-pattern blood supply. However, there is evidence that, when the flap is designed near the level of the inner canthus, a portion has a direct axial blood supply (angular and supraorbital arteries) (8). The flap is composed of full-thickness nasal skin and subcutaneous tissue. A readily apparent cleavage plane is established between the flap and the underlying muscular elements.

FLAP DESIGN AND DIMENSIONS

Approaches to the bilobed flap have changed over time from consideration of two flaps alike in size and form to the utilization of a smaller secondary flap, more triangular in shape, facilitating closure of the donor deformity (9). Esser (10), the first to describe the use of bilobed rotation flaps for the repair of nasal tip defects, believed that 90° was the optimal angle between the two flaps; however, it could vary between 95° and 180° (11). The greater the angle, the larger is the resultant dog-ear that must be adjusted. This should be considered when planning the flap, because trimming the excess tissue can compromise the vascular pedicle.

Flap design and planning takes place from the defect backward to the donor site. An often stated good rule is to measure twice and cut once. When the defect is created, the appropriate flaps are designed for resurfacing. A useful technique involves drawing a perpendicular line through the defect and connecting the ends to form a semicircle; two flaps are then designed within the arc. When designing the flaps, careful attention should be given to preserve the natural borders of the nose, to prevent flap transposition from obliterating normal nasal-cheek contours.

The primary flap used for reconstructing the defect usually lies within the mid-access at 45° or less to the defect, and it is slightly smaller than the defect. The laxity in the surrounding skin is assessed by pinching the skin. A secondary flap, somewhat triangular in shape, is designed to achieve closure of the donor defect. The flaps are raised concurrently on a common base and rotated (Fig. 1). After final insetting of the flap, it is frequently necessary to adjust the base and distal edges of the flap.

OPERATIVE TECHNIQUE

In patients who do not present with an already open wound from Mohs' micrographic surgery, the tumor can be excised under pathologic frozen-section control and the defect repaired in one stage. Flaps are not irreversibly demarcated until negative wound margins are obtained. When dealing with recurrent or aggressive basal-cell carcinomas, allowing the wound to granulate or using a temporary closure with a skin graft for a sufficient period of time (e.g., 1 year) are advisable to ensure tumor eradication before a flap is fabricated. This avoids distortion of the normal architecture in the event of recurrence.

The final defect is outlined and wound edges pared, if indicated. The two flaps are designed and raised simultaneously, with wide undermining as necessary to allow easy rotation into position, without tension. The primary flap closes the tumor defect and the secondary flap is used to close the donor site. At this time, final tailoring and backcuts are judiciously performed, and the flap inset. The wounds are closed in a single layer with 5–0 nylon suture, and the secondary donor site is closed by direct advancement (Fig. 2).

CLINICAL RESULTS

Flaps should be designed with a sufficient length-to-width ratio, the tip handled gently, and closure performed with

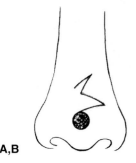
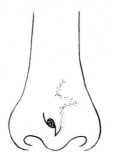

A,B

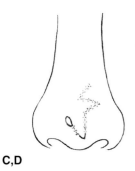
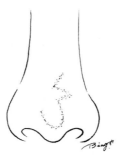

C,D

FIG. 1. Operative steps in closure of a nasal defect with the bilobed flap. **A:** Design for rotation in a semicircle; commonly, each flap is capable of up to 90° rotation, as indicated. **B:** Flaps are widely elevated to and beyond their bases, and transposed; the secondary defect is smaller than the primary, and is closed directly. **C:** Insetting, final tailoring, and backcutting. **D:** Final results.

minimal tension. Tension should be avoided, as it often affects the most distal aspect of the flap, which is already in the most precarious blood-supply situation. If flap ischemia occurs, it should be promptly recognized and treated. If tension is a factor, sutures can be removed; if fluid collection is the etiology, it should be evacuated. Other methods to treat venous occlusion (e.g., leeches) or arterial compromise (e.g., steroids, nifedipine, etc.) can be considered.

As with all reconstructive cases, patients should have been previously counseled about the aesthetic limitations, since many expect to achieve the same appearance they had prior to extirpation. The flap also requires additional incisions that leave permanent scars in adjacent tissues.

As with all circular flaps, "pin cushioning" is a potential disadvantage of this technique. During surgery, flaps can be thinned to the extent that the subdermal plexus is maintained. Flaps that do swell should be digitally massaged after initial healing. Ultimately, they can require corticosteroid injections, secondary revisions, or ancillary techniques.

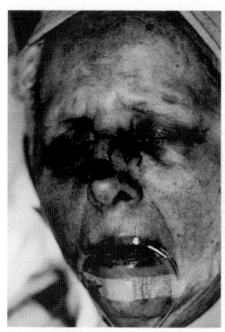
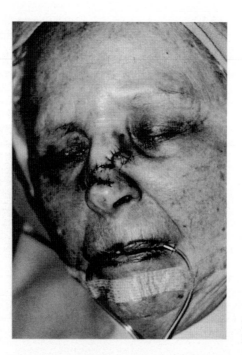

A,B

FIG. 2. **A,B:** Flap design, transposition, and insetting.

SUMMARY

The bilobed nasal flap is a versatile flap that is useful for the repair of defects of the lateral nose, ala, and nasal-tip area. It is a single-staged procedure that takes advantage of the laxity in the surrounding skin of the upper nose, thereby providing a close color and texture match for resurfacing of nasal defects.

References

1. Elliot RA. Rotation flaps of the nose. *Plast Reconstr Surg* 1969;44:147.
2. Converse JM. *Reconstructive plastic surgery*, 2nd ed. Philadelphia: Saunders, 1977;439.
3. McGregor JC, Soutar DS. A critical assessment of the bilobed flap. *Br J Plast Surg* 1981;8:587.
4. Bennett JE. Reconstruction of the nose: reconstruction of lateral nasal defects. *Clin Plast Surg* 1981;8:587.
5. Grabb WC, Smith JW, eds., *Plastic surgery*, 3rd ed. Boston: Little, Brown, 1979;49–50.
6. Millard DR, Gillies H, eds., *The principles and art of plastic surgery*. Boston: Little, Brown, 1957;52.
7. Jackson IT. *Local flaps in head and neck reconstruction*. St. Louis: Mosby, 1985;109–117.
8. Marchac D, Toth B. The axial frontonasal flap revisited. *Plast Reconstr Surg* 1985;76:686.
9. Dean RK, Kelleher JC, Sullivan JG, Barbak GJ. Bilobed flaps and skin flaps. In: Grabb WC, Smith JW, eds., *Plastic surgery*, 3rd ed. Boston: Little, Brown, 1979;289–296.
10. Esser JFS. Gestielte locale nasonplastik mit zweizipfligem lappen: dekung des sekundaren detekes vom ersten zipfel durch den zweiten. *Dtsch Z Chir* 1918;385:143.
11. Zimany A. The bilobed flap. *Plast Reconstr Surg* 1953;11:424.

CHAPTER 36 ■ V-Y FLAP RECONSTRUCTION FOR NASAL ALAE DEFECTS

S. L. EISENBAUM AND M. P. BARNETT

EDITORIAL COMMENT

This is an attractive idea, in that it replaces skin similar to what has been lost. However, this flap has the limitations of just about every V-Y type of advancement flap in that mobility is limited, depending on the looseness of the skin that is being mobilized.

Sliding, subcutaneous V-Y advancement flaps for the reconstruction of nasal defects have been gaining in popularity, especially in nasal dorsum reconstruction (1–4) and, with certain precautions (see below), in lateral nostril reconstruction. The flaps have been used for small defects of the ala nasi that do not involve the rim.

INDICATIONS

The advantages of having like tissue in the same operative field, with an excellent blood supply, make the V-Y flap a good choice for nasal reconstruction. It can also be used in reconstructions of the ala nasi, for defects generally limited to less than 1.5 cm in diameter and not involving the rim. V-Y flap reconstructions for ala defects due to basal cell carcinoma excision have been used in an outpatient setting in a small series of patients (5).

ANATOMY

The flap described is based totally on subcutaneous connections and depends on the blood supply in this tissue for its sur-

vival. The amount of advancement is limited mainly by the vertical depth of subcutaneous tissue between the skin and the underlying bone or cartilage and, to a lesser extent, on the looseness of the tissue distal to the defect. This distal tissue "back-slides" into the defect as the advancement flap pedicle applies a force in the direction whence it came (6). The skin of the nostril is relatively unyielding, and therefore most of the mobility rests in the flap itself.

FLAP DESIGN AND DIMENSIONS

In areas on the lateral surfaces of the nose where the subcutaneous tissue is relatively thick, large subcutaneously based flaps can be developed and advanced with excellent results. Because of the excellent blood supply of the nose, undermining of these flaps can be performed to a significant extent, without injuring or compromising the flap. Most of these flaps in the lateral nose and medial face are, in actuality, musculocutaneous flaps fed by vessels from small underlying facial muscles (6).

The closer to the alar margin one approaches, the thinner and more densely adherent the subcutaneous tissue becomes. If an attempt is made to cut down to the surface of the cartilage along the rim, the blood supply becomes compromised, and, essentially, no blood comes through the cartilage. The thin subcutaneous pedicle of such flaps transposed along the alar margin provides a force that may lead to notching at the alar rim (6).

OPERATIVE TECHNIQUE

In a series of nine patients with basal cell carcinoma, the procedure was done under local anesthesia in an outpatient setting.

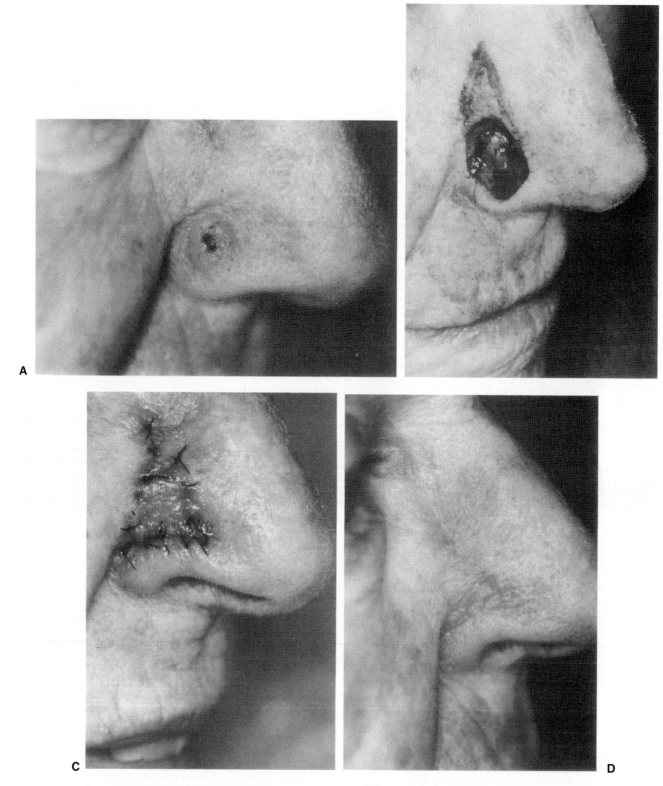

FIG. 1. A 75-year-old woman with a basal cell carcinoma of the right nostril and a 1.6 × 1.3 cm defect. **A:** Preoperative lesion. **B:** Intraoperative defect. **C:** Immediately postoperative. **D:** Results 3 months postoperatively. (From Eisenbaum, Barnett, ref. 5, with permission.)

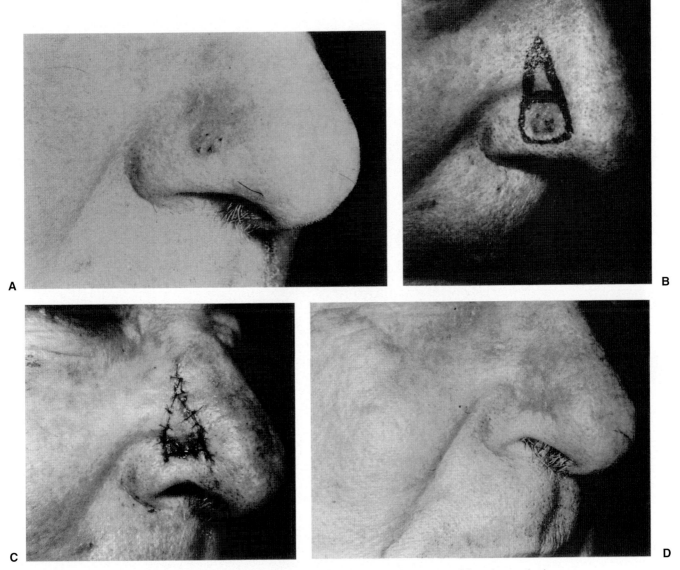

FIG. 2. A 74-year-old man with mixed basal cell and squamous cell carcinoma of the right nostril, who sustained a 1.5-cm defect. **A:** Preoperative lesion. **B:** Flap markings. **C:** Immediately postoperative, with small area of vascular compromise. **D:** Results 5 months postoperatively. (From Eisenbaum, Barnett, ref. 5, with permission.)

The area of lesion excision and the flap are marked preoperatively. After excision of the lesion, the specimen is tagged with a suture for pathologic orientation and usually sent for frozen section. Once all margins are known to be clear, the V-Y flap is dissected out and moved inferiorly on a subcutaneous pedicle to repair the defect; 5-0 and 6-0 interrupted nylon sutures are used. The closer the resected margin is to the alar rim, the greater is the tendency for retraction of the nostril margin; in particular, peaking and notching of the alar rim should be avoided (5) (Figs. 1 and 2).

CLINICAL RESULTS

This flap has limitations, particularly in instances involving the inferior margins of the nose near the nares. Some notching along the alar rim may occur and, in younger individuals, would probably be severe. When using the flap for lateral nostril reconstruction, attempts to use a poorly designed or small flap may result in retraction or peaking of the nostril. For repair of the nostril rim, other more suitable techniques have been described (1,7–11). The higher the defect is located on the nostril away from the rim, the easier is the reconstruction and the better the result.

SUMMARY

The advantages of having like tissue in the same operative field, with an excellent blood supply, make the V-Y flap a good choice, with certain precautions necessary when it is used for lateral nostril reconstruction.

References

1. Cronin TD. The V-Y rotation flap for nasal tip defects. *Ann Plast Surg* 1983;11:282.
2. Dreyer TM. The stair-step flap for nasal alar reconstruction. *Plast Reconstr Surg* 1984;74:704.
3. Hardin JC, Jr. Alar rim reconstruction by a dorsal nasal flap. *Plast Reconst Surg* 1980;66:293.
4. Strauch B, Fox M. V-Y bipedicle flap for resurfacing the nasal supratip region. *Plast Reconstr Surg* 1989;83:899.
5. Eisenbaum SL, Barnett MP. V-Y flap reconstruction for nostril defects. *Ann Plast Surg* 1991;26:488.
6. Argenta LC. Invited comment. *Ann Plast Surg* 1991;26:493.
7. Hauben DJ, Sagi A. A simple method for alar rim reconstruction. *Plast Reconstr Surg* 1987;80:839.
8. Jackson I. Nose reconstruction. In: Berger K, ed., *Local flaps in head and neck reconstruction.* St. Louis: Mosby, 1985;87–188.
9. Zook EG, Beck AL, Russell RC, et al. V-Y advancement flap for facial defects. *Plast Reconstr Surg* 1980;65:786.
10. Rieger RA. A local flap for repair of the nasal tip. *Plast Reconstr Surg* 1967;49:147.
11. Marchac D. Lambeau de rotation fronto-nasal. *Ann Chir Plast Esthet* 1970;15:48.

CHAPTER 37 ■ CATERPILLAR NASAL SKIN FLAP FOR NASAL TIP RECONSTRUCTION

T. D. CRONIN

EDITORIAL COMMENT

This is a two-stage operation to restore the projection of the tip of the nose. The advanced flap is bunched up just above the scar, and in a second procedure, the extra skin is brought down to resurface the scar. It is not clear whether or not this procedure is applicable to freshly excised wounds. The tip of the nose also can be resurfaced with a local "banner" flap, and projection of the tip can be obtained with a cartilage graft, if necessary.

Small losses of the nasal tip may be repaired by a caterpillar flap, which consists of a V-Y advancement as the first stage (1).

INDICATIONS

The caterpillar flap is suitable for repairing small losses of the nasal tip. If nasal lining is required, this method would probably not be adequate unless small flaps could be turned in from the margins for lining. Thick, sebaceous, or excessively scarred nasal skin might be too thick or stiff to fold properly.

ANATOMY

The blood supply to this flap follows a random pattern.

OPERATIVE TECHNIQUE

First Stage

A triangular flap is elevated, taking care to carry the apex no higher than or only slightly higher than the inner canthi to avoid difficulties in closure owing to fixation of the skin at the latter points. The flap is advanced downward and folded onto itself. A shift of 1 to 1.5 cm can be accomplished readily.

The skin edges are widely undermined, and the upper end of the wound is closed for a distance equal to the advancement required. In closing the remainder of the wound, it is wise to draw the skin edges medially from one skin edge to the other by the use of buried sutures to prevent tension from side to side on the flap. Furthermore, so as not to lose any of the length of the flap, it should be kept completely extended while it is being sutured. In this way, a maximum amount of tissue is folded onto itself near the tip.

Second Stage

Three to 6 weeks later, the skin is unfolded and brought down to form the new tip—its rounded shape forms an admirable tip. If an increase in the prominence of the new tip is desired, a small piece of septal or ear cartilage can be inserted (Figs. 1 and 2).

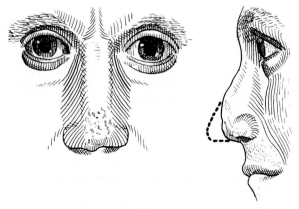

A

FIG. 1. **A:** Small loss of nasal tip. *(Continued)*

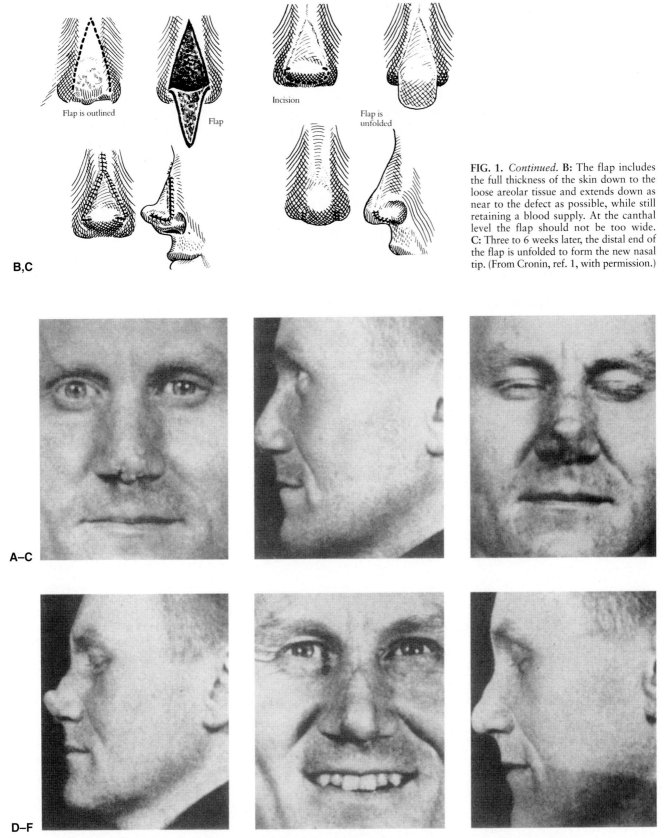

FIG. 1. *Continued.* **B:** The flap includes the full thickness of the skin down to the loose areolar tissue and extends down as near to the defect as possible, while still retaining a blood supply. At the canthal level the flap should not be too wide. **C:** Three to 6 weeks later, the distal end of the flap is unfolded to form the new nasal tip. (From Cronin, ref. 1, with permission.)

FIG. 2. **A,B:** Small loss of nasal tip. **C,D:** Appearance after elevation, advancement, and folding of the flap. **E,F:** Appearance 27 days after the second stage. Avoidance of notching at the canthal level on profile is avoided by not making the flap too wide at that level. (From Cronin, ref. 1, with permission.)

SUMMARY

A two-stage caterpillar flap can be used to reconstruct small defects of the nasal tip.

Reference

1. Cronin TD. A new method of nasal tip reconstruction utilizing a local caterpillar flap. *Br J Plast Surg* 1951;4:180.

CHAPTER 38 ■ V-Y BIPEDICLE FLAP FOR RESURFACING THE NASAL SUPRATIP REGION

B. STRAUCH AND M. FOX

For resurfacing the nasal supratip region, use of the V-Y bipedicle flap allows the concealment of the lower incisions in the normal alar creases and of the upper incisions in the glabellar folds (1).

INDICATIONS

The supratip area of the nose lies between the tip area and the nasal dorsum, overlying the septal angle of the cartilaginous septum. Supratip nasal skin has a distinctive texture, contour, and color. Techniques used for resurfacing this area include skin and composite grafts and local and distant flaps (1–7). If the incisional lines are so placed as to be hidden in the natural creases, a local flap would appear to be the most satisfactory choice, since it provides for restoration of both normal contour and skin color.

FLAP DESIGN AND OPERATIVE TECHNIQUE

The lesion in the supratip area is marked for appropriate excision. Two lateral triangular areas are then drawn to the nasolabial folds, defining an elliptical defect, the lower borders of which conform to the upper borders of the alar crease. A V is then planned, starting high in the glabellar area, coming down the side of the nose, and extending out on the cheek in the border between the cheek and the eyelid skin (Fig. 1A).

The lesion and the triangular areas are then excised, and the upper part of the flap is incised. The nasal skin is completely undermined over the entire surface of the nose, extending to the nasolabial fold laterally on each side. The distal tip skin is undermined slightly to provide easier closure.

The bipedicle flap can then be advanced distally for up to 1.0 cm, and the point of closure of the Y can be determined. The tip of the nose is brought up to meet the leading edge of the flap (Fig. 1B). The defects are closed (Fig. 1C). Resection of a segment of the lower lateral cartilages may facilitate this maneuver. A surgical defect of up to 1.5 cm may be corrected in this manner (Figs. 2 and 3).

CLINICAL RESULTS

Resurfacing the nasal supratip area with a local flap yields attractive results, since it provides tissue of normal color, contour, and texture in a single stage. Skin grafts may result in a

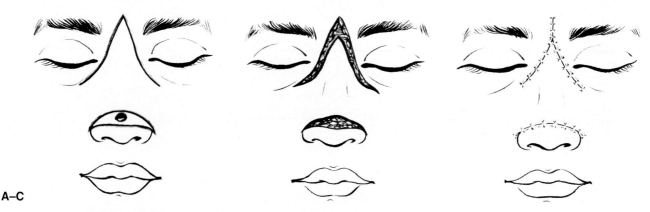

A–C

FIG. 1. A: Outline of supratip excision, with high V planned, beginning in the glabellar area. B: Bipedicle flap mobilized and shifted distally. Distal tip is elevated to meet the leading edge of the flap. C: Closure of defects. (From Strauch, Fox, ref. 1, with permission.)

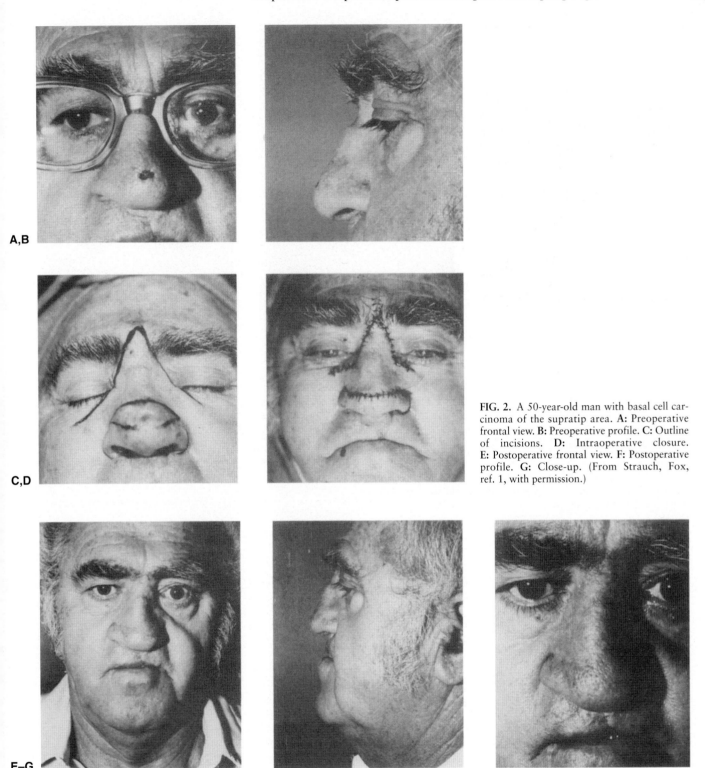

FIG. 2. A 50-year-old man with basal cell carcinoma of the supratip area. **A:** Preoperative frontal view. **B:** Preoperative profile. **C:** Outline of incisions. **D:** Intraoperative closure. **E:** Postoperative frontal view. **F:** Postoperative profile. **G:** Close-up. (From Strauch, Fox, ref. 1, with permission.)

contour defect, as well as pigmentary changes. Although a composite graft may minimize contour defects, pigmentary changes may still occur. Nasolabial flaps do not provide sufficient length for cross-midline coverage and tend to interrupt the normal flow of the nasolabial fold.

Bilobed flaps (2,3) provide coverage for the supratip area; however, the multiple incisions necessary on the leading surface of the nose, as well as the trapdoor tendency of small flaps in this area, make this procedure less attractive. The unipedicle flap (4–6) imposes an additional scar along the length

of the nasolabial area. In addition, fullness results in the area of pedicle rotation. An advantage of the unipedicle flap is that it can resurface the area distal to the supratip.

The V-Y bipedicle flap allows for easy closure in the glabellar area and a suture line that is well hidden in the alar creases (1). It provides tissue of optimal match for color, texture, and contour. The bipedicle attachment also provides for an extremely hardy circulation (7). The flap advances distally for 1.0 cm, and the mobility of the nasal tip provides an additional 0.5 cm of advancement. The elevated tip descends to a

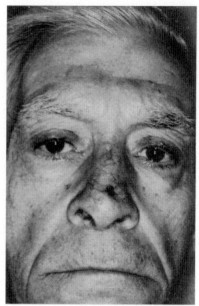
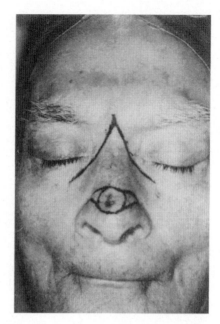
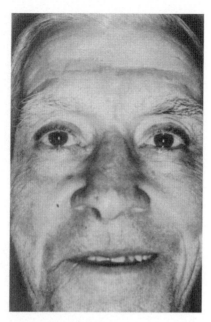

A–C

FIG. 3. A 72-year-old man with basal cell carcinoma of the supratip area. **A:** Preoperative frontal view. **B:** Intraoperative drawing. **C:** Late postoperative view. (From Strauch, Fox, ref. 1, with permission.)

more normal location in the postoperative period. This technique should not be used for surgically created defects greater than 1.5 cm in diameter.

SUMMARY

A procedure for the coverage of surgically created supratip defects up to 1.5 cm in diameter is described using a V-Y bipedicle flap of nasal skin.

References

1. Strauch B, Fox M. V-Y bipedicle flap for resurfacing the nasal supratip region. *Plast Reconstr Surg* 1989;83:899.
2. Zimany A. The bilobed flap. *Plast Reconstr Surg* 1953;11:423.
3. Elliot RA Jr. Rotation flaps of the nose. *Plast Reconstr Surg* 1969;44:147.
4. McGregor I. *Fundamental techniques of plastic surgery.* Edinburgh: E&S Livingston, 1965;171.
5. Rieger R. A local flap for repair of the nasal tip. *Plast Reconstr Surg* 1967;40:147.
6. Marchac D, Toth B. The axial frontonasal flap revisited. *Plast Reconstr Surg* 1985;76:686.
7. Furnas DW, Furnas H. Angular artery flap for total reconstruction of the lower eyelid. *Ann Plast Surg* 1983;10:322.

CHAPTER 39 ■ BANNER-SHAPED NASAL SKIN FLAP

J. K. MASSON AND B. C. MENDELSON

Most defects on the lower two-thirds of the nose are best closed with what Elliott (1) named a "banner flap," presumably because the triangular shape of the flap resembles a banner or pennant. Although described by Elliott as a rotation flap, it is essentially the larger of two unequal flaps transposed as a type of Z-plasty (2).

INDICATIONS

The main indications for the frequent use of the banner flap are its versatility and safety, which are more recognized with increased use of the flap. Frequently, defects that are 1.5 to 2 cm in diameter have been closed, and on several occasions, defects as large as 2.5 cm in diameter have been managed. In

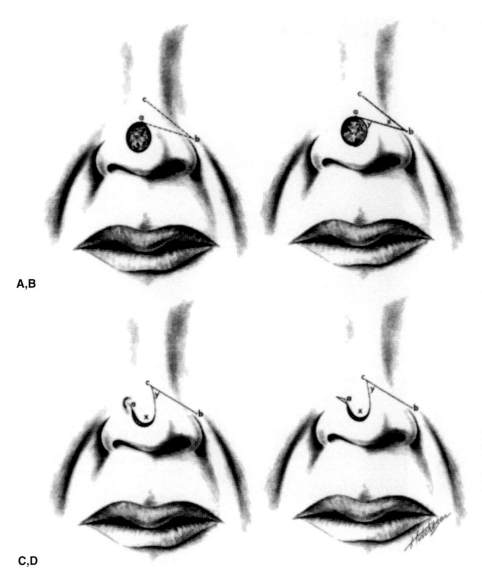

A,B

C,D

FIG. 1. Principles of the banner flap procedure. **A:** Triangular flap is outlined by points *a*, *b*, and *c*. **B:** Larger flap *x* and smaller flap *y*. Each may be transposed as a modified Z-plasty. **C:** Flap *y* is inset, and tip of flap *x* is trimmed to fit the residual defect. **D:** The resultant dog-ear at point *a*, if excessive, may be reduced by a triangular excision (leaving the base untouched). (From Masson and Mendelson, ref. 2, with permission.)

some circumstances, the flap has been taken from below the defect or extended onto the cheek or has been converted into a bilobed flap.

Skin grafts may have a good color match, but they leave an obvious depression. Nasolabial flaps provide an excellent color match, but the amount of subcutaneous fat and the possibility of a second stage to divide the pedicle limit their usefulness. Even then, one-fourth of the patients have required a separate defatting procedure to improve the appearance of the flap.

We believe that the larger flaps described by Rieger (3) and Lipshutz and Penrod (4) have no inherent advantage over banner flaps. In fact, they share the risks involved, in that they require more extensive mobilization of the skin. Situations requiring more complicated flaps, such as island pedicle flaps from the forehead or subcutaneous pedicle flaps from the forehead or nasolabial region, are infrequent.

ANATOMY

The terminations of the external maxillary artery form the main arterial supply and allow the successful use of many kinds of random flaps. The veins of this region empty into the anterior facial vein and also communicate through the ophthalmic vein with the cavernous sinus. The lymphatic vessels drain to the submaxillary and deep cervical lymph channels.

FLAP DESIGN AND DIMENSIONS

Time spent on initial outline of the best flap design is most worthwhile. The flap is outlined with a marking pen at a tangent to the edge of the defect, merging at point *a* (Fig. 1A,B). Point *b* is marked well out laterally and, if convenient, is placed in the alar crease, where the scar will tend to be camouflaged. However, for other than small defects, point *b* must be placed higher than the alar crease to minimize subsequent elevation of the nostril rim (Fig. 2A).

The length *ab* is significantly longer than the diameter of the defect, since the flap will be long and narrow, allowing easier closure of the secondary defect. The tip of the banner flap *x* will be excised later. Point *c* is placed above the defect, but not necessarily out to the lateral extent of the defect; this point can be extended later, if needed, to allow a better fit of the base of the flap into the defect.

The base of the flap *ac* is made narrower than the diameter of the defect, because during closure the defect can be narrowed in its transverse diameter to fit the slightly narrower flap.

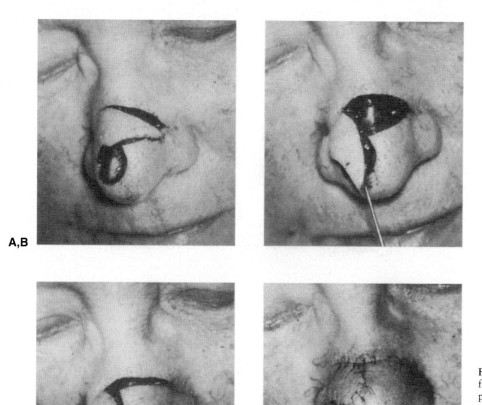

A,B

C,D

FIG. 2. Operative steps in the banner flap procedure. **A:** For a larger defect, point *b* is placed higher than the alar crease, to reduce elevation of the nostril rim. **B:** Elevation and mobilization of both flaps *x* and *y*. **C:** Elevation of the nasal tip advances flap *y* upward and closes the donor area. This is held with a few buried catgut sutures. **D:** Flap *x* is then tailored to fit the operative defect, and the skin incision is closed with skin sutures.

OPERATIVE TECHNIQUE

The flap is outlined and elevated (Fig. 2B) with wide undermining of the nasal skin using blunt dissection on the cartilaginous plane (especially under the base of the flap *x*) to allow ease of rotation. Flap *y* is also elevated (Fig. 1C,D).

The smaller flap *y* is transposed toward point *c* (Fig. 1C) and set in position with two or three buried chromic catgut sutures on side *bc*. Once flap *y* is inset, the final size and shape of the defect are apparent.

The larger flap *x* is inset by laying it down over the defect, and with the scalpel, the flap is trimmed across the redundant tip, curved to the shape of the defect (Fig. 2C). The flap is then secured. Starting at the distal end of the flap, 6-0 silk skin sutures are carefully placed to even out the discrepancy in length between the two sides being sutured. No buried catgut sutures are used on the flap because they tend to cause distortion. The closure toward point *a* is performed last, because there is usually the need to excise a small triangle in this area (Fig. 1D).

CLINICAL RESULTS

Fortunately, older patients who are the ones most likely to have epitheliomas are also the most favorable candidates for a local flap, since aging skin leads to laxity with redundance to the point of drooping of the nasal tip.

With the transposition of a banner flap to close a defect on the external nose, there is some resultant shortening as the donor area of the flap is closed. In such a situation, the shortening provides some definite cosmetic improvement and also often results in functional improvement by enhancing the airway.

Asymmetrical elevation of the alar rim tends to occur when the banner flap is taken primarily from one side of the nose. This can be minimized by taking the flap from across the bridge of the nose, so that the donor defect involves both sides of the nose. With closure, therefore, a more symmetrical shortening is produced than if the flap were taken primarily from one side of the nose (Fig. 3). Some asymmetrical elevation of the nostril rim can be tolerated because, as with the incision, the defect will all but disappear within a period of months (Fig. 4).

The safety of the banner flap was demonstrated several years ago in our first report on 100 such flaps. Of this group, only three were not satisfactory. There was partial necrosis in one, which healed by secondary intention; another flap dehisced after suture removal, requiring resuturing; and a third flap left unsatisfactory scars, which required a surgical revision at a later date. Since that report in 1977, we have continued to use and to be satisfied with the results that this flap offers in repairing many surgical defects of the external nose (Fig. 5).

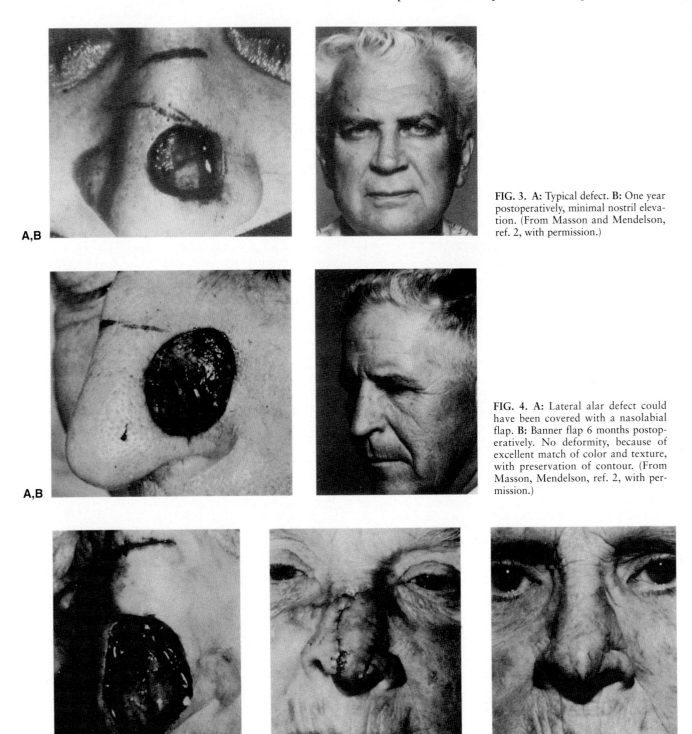

A,B

FIG. 3. **A:** Typical defect. **B:** One year postoperatively, minimal nostril elevation. (From Masson and Mendelson, ref. 2, with permission.)

A,B

FIG. 4. **A:** Lateral alar defect could have been covered with a nasolabial flap. **B:** Banner flap 6 months postoperatively. No deformity, because of excellent match of color and texture, with preservation of contour. (From Masson, Mendelson, ref. 2, with permission.)

A–C

FIG. 5. **A:** Very large defect. **B:** Fifth day after operation. Moderate alar rim distortion could have been reduced with bilobed flap; note how the defect has narrowed transversely to a vertical ellipse. **C:** Result 3 years after surgery. Symmetry improved. (From Masson, Mendelson, ref. 2, with permission.)

SUMMARY

Wide experience with the banner flap for closure of postoperative defects of the nasal dorsum shows that it is not only a predictably safe and versatile procedure, but also that its use permits a superior cosmetic result.

References

1. Elliott RA, Jr. Rotation flaps of the nose. *Plast Reconstr Surg* 1969;44:147.
2. Masson JK, Mendelson BC. The banner flap. *Am J Surg* 1977;134:419.
3. Rieger RA. A local flap for repair of the nasal tip. *Plast Reconstr Surg* 1967;40:147.
4. Lipshutz H, Penrod DS. Use of complete transverse nasal flap in repair of small defects of the nose. *Plast Reconstr Surg* 1972;49:629.

CHAPTER 40 ■ NASOLABIAL AND CHEEK SKIN FLAPS

R. R. CAMERON

Nasolabial and cheek skin flaps can be ideal sources for partial nasal reconstruction (1–19). Exact duplication is impossible because of the unique features of the skin covering the nose: thin, resilient, and clear cephalad; thicker, less mobile, and sometimes with prominent pores and blood vessels caudally. The cheeks and forehead are the best color matches, and their proximity simplifies transfer. Flaps from both these areas can be developed in superficial planes so that bulk is diminished.

There is an area of relative redundancy that extends from the inner canthus of the eye to the inferior margin of the mandible, especially in older patients. Most smaller flaps are drawn from the outpouching of redundant tissue from the ala of the nose to the crura of the mouth. This area is generally free of hair growth, except for the lower cheek in males.

Medially, superiorly, and laterally based flaps are best used for reconstruction of the nose, while inferiorly based flaps lend themselves to transfer to the upper lip and nasal floor.

INDICATIONS

Flap tissue is necessary for coverage when there is a full-thickness defect of the nose or when bone or cartilage are exposed. Nasolabial cheek tissue can be used for coverage of defects of any part of the nose. The more cephalad portion, however, is usually best covered by forehead tissue.

Coverage of the lateral wall is often possible by direct advancement with wide undermining (Fig. 6) or by rotation of a subcutaneous pedicle flap from the nasolabial fold (see Chap. 44).

The alae of the nose also can be reconstructed using nasolabial flaps. Local turnover flaps or the addition of cartilage within the flap may be necessary for support. Narrow flaps may be used to reconstruct losses in the alar rim or to correct retraction of the rim, such as is seen with severe facial burns. The rim may be released and restored to its normal position, and the defect so created can be filled with a small nasolabial flap (Fig. 4).

Reconstruction of the columella presents a problem because of its small size and the difficulty of duplicating the gentle flare at its junction with the upper lip. Passage of a superiorly based flap through an incision in the alar crease allows placement of the flap about the columella and also provides for septal and nasal floor reconstruction (Fig. 3).

Nasolabial flaps can be turned over and used for lining. Coverage can be achieved using a variety of methods (Fig. 2).

ANATOMY

Blood supply to the nasolabial and cheek skin is from the angular artery (a branch of the anterior facial artery), the infraorbital artery, the transverse facial artery, and the infratrochlear artery (20).

Nasolabial cheek flaps are random flaps, since no attempt is usually made to include any specific arterial supply. Because of the rich vascularity and free anastomoses of arterial supply and venous drainage, superior, medial, lateral, and inferior pedicles are possible. Subcutaneous pedicles are, however, more reliable if based laterally or inferiorly. This is so because the development of the subcutaneous pedicle interrupts the rich subdermal network of vessels. Development of a nasolabial flap on an arteriovenous pedicle using the facial artery and vein has been described.

While the sensory supply of these flaps is rarely critical, these flaps are often fortuitously included with superior or lateral pedicles because of the orientation and arborization of the infraorbital nerve.

FLAP DESIGN AND DIMENSIONS

Flap size is limited by the redundancy of tissue and the ability to close the donor site primarily without deformity. Within these parameters, size is determined by the need for lining of the nose or for inclusion of bone, cartilage, or alloplastic support. If such requirements are present, the flap may need to be doubled on itself or lined by a second flap or skin graft.

Superiorly and medially based flaps are limited in width. Rarely, as much as 5 cm has been used. The flap may be up to 10 to 12 cm in length, as long as appropriate delay procedures are used. Shorter flaps rarely require a delay, unless there is questionable vascularity of the tissues. Rotation of superiorly based flaps usually occurs about a point just medial to the superior end of the lateral incision (point *B* in Fig. 1A).

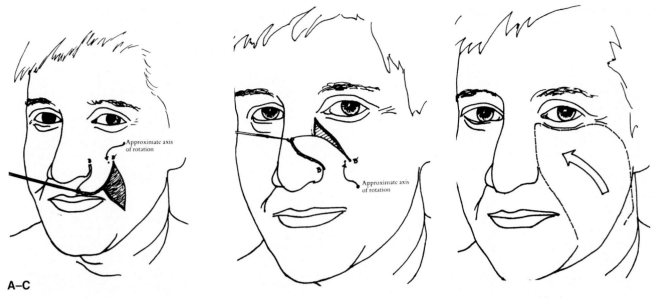

A–C

FIG. 1. **A:** Superiorly based nasolabial flap indicating point of rotation. **B:** Inferiorly based nasolabial flap indicating point of rotation. **C:** Large inferiorly based nasolabial cheek flap.

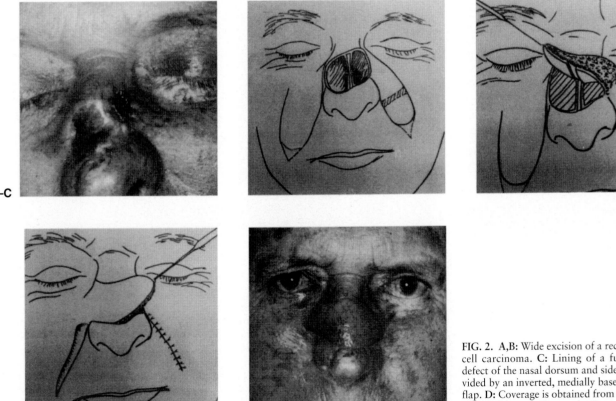

A–C

D,E

FIG. 2. **A,B:** Wide excision of a recurrent basal cell carcinoma. **C:** Lining of a full-thickness defect of the nasal dorsum and side wall is provided by an inverted, medially based nasolabial flap. **D:** Coverage is obtained from the opposite side. **E:** Postoperative result. (From Cameron et al., ref. 11, with permission.)

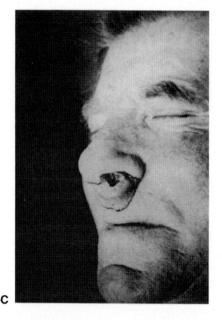
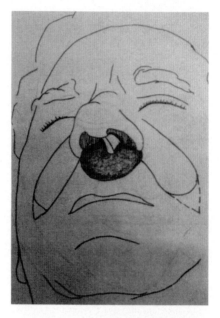
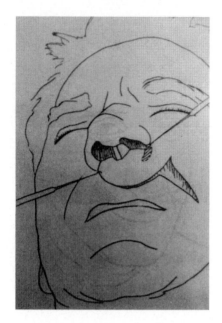

A–C

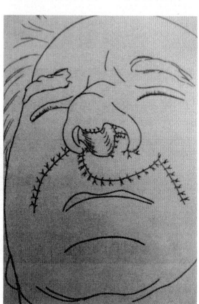
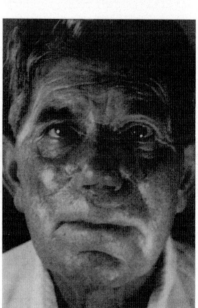

D,E

FIG. 3. A,B: Resection of a large basal cell carcinoma requiring reconstruction of the columella, upper lip, and nasal floor using bilateral nasolabial flaps. C: The left nasolabial flap was used to resurface the lip and nostril floors. D: The right nasolabial flap was brought through an incision in the top of the right ala and used to reconstruct the columella. Later, the pedicle was severed and returned. E: Postoperative result. (From Cameron et al., ref. 11, with permission.)

Inferiorly and laterally based flaps are more limited in available length. Tissue based laterally and advanced onto the nose is most restricted by the available redundancy between the inner canthus of the eye and the nasolabial fold. Much more tissue is available, however, if rotation-advancement techniques are used with cheek tissues, much as Mustardé has demonstrated for lower eyelid reconstruction (21). The point of rotation for these flaps will be just medial to the inferior extent of the lateral incision (point *B* in Fig. 1B).

OPERATIVE TECHNIQUE

Orientation of the pedicle will be determined by the location of the defect and the requirements for rotation and/or advancement of appropriate amounts of tissue to the defect with the least amount of torsion and tension on the pedicle. Flap thickness is partly determined by the needs of the defect,

but it is limited by the thickness of the donor tissues. In most cases, the requirements are for a thin flap, and elevation is made in the subdermal plane. In all cases, elevation should protect the muscles of facial expression and the nerves that supply them.

In many instances, secondary revisions are required to obtain the best aesthetic result. The reduplication of nasal contours is difficult at best, so some patients may be disappointed with the results. Proper initial design, precise estimate of size, and careful insetting of the flap, combined with segmental replacement of tissue, when practical, will frequently obviate extensive secondary revision.

CLINICAL RESULTS

Use of nasolabial cheek tissues loses much of its advantage if significant donor deformities result. For this reason, the

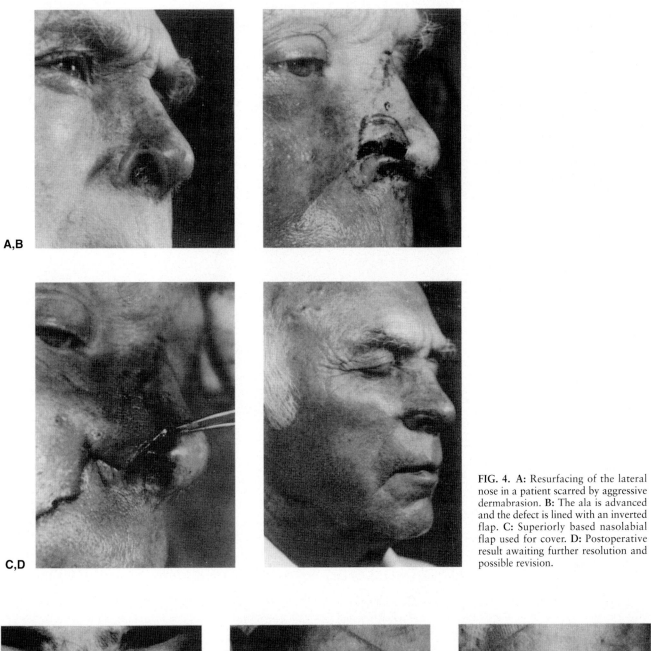

FIG. 4. A: Resurfacing of the lateral nose in a patient scarred by aggressive dermabrasion. **B:** The ala is advanced and the defect is lined with an inverted flap. **C:** Superiorly based nasolabial flap used for cover. **D:** Postoperative result awaiting further resolution and possible revision.

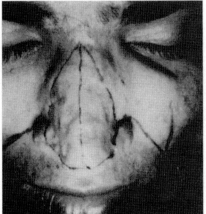
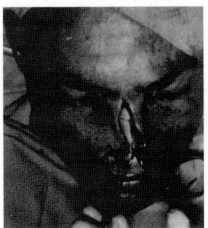
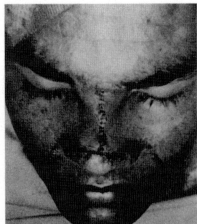

FIG. 5. Resurfacing of the nasal dorsum with bilateral nasolabial cheek flaps. (From Cameron et al., ref. 11, with permission.)

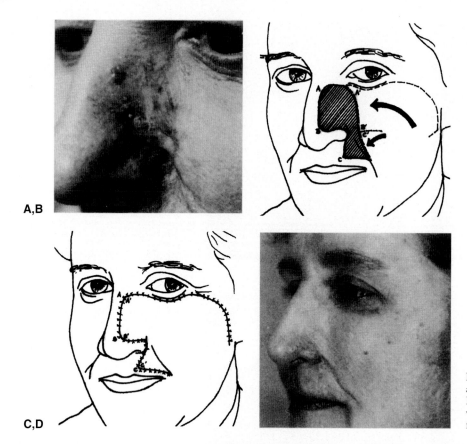

A,B

C,D

FIG. 6. **A:** Patient with radiation change and secondary neoplastic lesions. **B,C:** Resurfacing of the lateral nose and upper lip with rotation-advancement nasolabial cheek flap. **D:** Postoperative result.

mechanics of transfer must consider primary donor-site closure without irreparable secondary deformity. If the procedure is ill-conceived, ectropion of the lower eyelid or upper lip can occur.

Placement of a donor incision in the midface is abhorrent to many reconstructive surgeons. However, the scars resulting from transfer of this tissue can be quite acceptable if care is taken with donor-site closure. Such scars are often preferable to the deformities sometimes seen with forehead donor sites.

Z-plasties, W-plasties, scar revisions, and replacement of bulky flaps with full-thickness grafts may all have a place in secondary revisions (Fig. 6). There are particular problems in using nasolabial tissue in elderly males with thick nasal and adjacent skin—a procedure that may result in bulky, contracted flaps (22).

SUMMARY

Nasolabial and cheek skin can be used to reconstruct the various areas of the nose. Superiorly, inferiorly, medially, and laterally based flaps have their particular applications and limitations.

References

1. Hagerty RF, Smith W. The nasolabial cheek flap. *Am Surg* 1958;24:506.
2. McLaren LR. Nasolabial flap repair for alar margin defect. *Br J Plast Surg* 1963;16:234.
3. DaSilva G. A new method of reconstruction of the columella with a nasolabial flap. *Plast Reconstr Surg* 1964;34:63.
4. Pers M. Cheek flaps in partial rhinoplasty. *Scand J Plast Reconstr Surg* 1967;1:37.
5. Reginata LE, Belda W. Correction of scaphoid facies and restoration of nasal foundation with bilateral nasolabial flaps. *Rev Paul Med* 1968;72:130.
6. Wynn SK, Wiviott W. Resurfacing the nose with bilateral cheek flaps. In: *Transactions of the 4th International Congress of Plastic and Reconstructive Surgery*. Amsterdam: Excerpta Medica, 1968;590.
7. Georgiade NG, Mladick RA, Thorne FL. The nasolabial tunnel flap. *Plast Reconstr Surg* 1969;43:463.
8. Wesser DR, Burt GB, Jr. Nasolabial flap for losses of the nasal ala and columella. *Plast Reconstr Surg* 1969;44:300.
9. Climo MS. Nasolabial flap for alar defect. *Plast Reconstr Surg* 1969;44:303.
10. Heybrook G. Some applications of the nasolabial flap in reconstruction of the nose and lips. *Br J Plast Surg* 1970;23:26.
11. Cameron RR, Latham WD, Dowling JA. Reconstructions of the nose and upper lip with nasolabial flaps. *Plast Reconstr Surg* 1973;52:145.
12. Fryer MP. Subtotal nose reconstruction with a cheek flap. *Plast Reconstr Surg* 1974;53:436.
13. Cameron RR. Nasal reconstruction with nasolabial cheek flaps. In: Grabb WC, Myers MB, eds. *Skin flaps*. Boston: Little, Brown, 1975.
14. Millard DR, Jr. Reconstructive rhinoplasty for the lower two-thirds of the nose. *Plast Reconstr Surg* 1976;57:722.
15. Jackson IT, Reid CD. Nasal reconstruction and lengthening with local flaps. *Br J Plast Surg* 1978;31:341.
16. Orticochea M. Reconstructing one-half of the nose with a combined cheek and upper lip flap. *Br J Plast Surg* 1979;32:217.
17. Antia NH, Daver BM. Reconstructive surgery for nasal defects. *Clin Plast Surg* 1981;8:535.
18. Bennett JE. Reconstruction of lateral nasal defects. *Clin Plast Surg* 1981;8:587.
19. Guerrerosantos J, Dicksheet S. Nasolabial flap with simultaneous cartilage graft in nasal alar reconstruction. *Clin Plast Surg* 1981;8:599.
20. Corso PF. Variations of the arterial, venous and capillary circulation of the soft tissues of the head by decades as demonstrated by the methyl methacrylate injection technique, and their application to construction of flaps and pedicles. *Plast Reconstr Surg* 1961;27:180.
21. Mustardé JC. *Repair and reconstruction in the orbital region*, 2d Ed. Edinburgh: Churchill-Livingstone, 1980.
22. Walkinshaw MD, Caffee HH. The nasolabial flap: a problem and its correction. *Plast Reconstr Surg* 1982;69:30.

CHAPTER 41 ■ ZYGOMATIC FLAP FOR RECONSTRUCTION OF THE LIP AND NOSE

A. GARDETTO AND C. PAPP

Reconstruction of soft-tissue defects of the upper lip and the nose, especially of the tip and the columella, is still one of the most difficult tasks for a plastic surgeon. Numerous possibilities, such as a composite graft, transposition flaps, and local flaps, have been described in the literature.

INDICATIONS

Although full-thickness skin grafts or transposition flaps may satisfy the requirements of the reconstruction, their aesthetic outcome is often not quite satisfactory. Color match and contour irregularity may be problems in grafts; also, conventional transposition flaps, such as the nasolabial flap, often retain a "bulky" appearance, even many years later (1). However, in many cases, a primary reconstruction with a final good result is not always possible because of the limited advancement. For these reasons, we consider the zygomatic flap as a new and promising approach for a one-stage procedure (2). The donor defect is quite similar to the nasolabial flap and therefore cosmetically inconspicuous. As an island flap, the zygomatic flap offers a big arc of rotation. Usually, there is no destruction of muscle and nerve tissue, and because of the central vessel, the arc of rotation is essentially larger.

ANATOMY

The zygomatic flap is supplied by the cutaneous zygomatic branch, a branch of the facial artery (3). It runs upward over the buccinator muscle and divides into two branches at the major zygomatic muscle's inferior border. One ascends laterally and branches out in the subcutaneous fatty tissue. The second one continues through the major zygomatic muscle and penetrates the subcutaneous tissue above the muscle, similar to the first branch.

FLAP DESIGN AND DIMENSIONS

The zygomatic flap is an island axial pattern flap, and when properly designed, it can follow naturally existing contour lines, thus respecting and preserving the normal facial topography

and leaving the patient with minimal surgical deformity. For the design of the flap, it is very important to mark the origin of the cutaneous zygomatic branch. The measurements based on the auxiliary lines proposed by the authors make the dissection of the vessel's origin relatively easy (Fig. 1).

The point of origin from the facial artery is defined by using the mean-distance calculation of 10 mm lateral from the vertical line and 28 mm below the transverse line. The flap has to be designed directly over the origin of the cutaneous zygomatic branch. The size of the flap has been demonstrated by selective injection of the cutaneous zygomatic branch, indicating the supplied skin territory. The length of the flap is extended from 1 to 1.5 cm distal to the vessel's origin until the

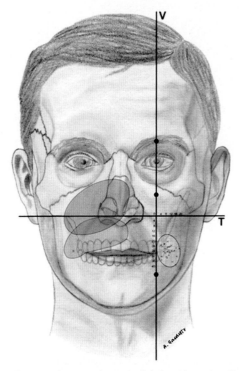

FIG. 1. Schematic diagram depicting left hemiface. Auxiliary lines proposed by the authors: V, vertical line through the three pressure points of the trigeminal nerve branches; T, transverse line through the most caudal parts of the zygomatic processes of the maxilla. Topogram shows the distance of the described cutaneous zygomatic branch origin. The right and left hemifaces are shown together, and the distances are measured in millimeters in relation to the auxiliary vertical line and transverse line: *crosses*, left side; *rhomboids*, right side; *spot*, mean distance (n = 34). The ellipsoid visualizes the radius of the potential branch origin. Right hemiface: Arc of rotation of the zygomatic flap by orthograde (upper lip) and retrograde (nose) pedicles is shown.

117

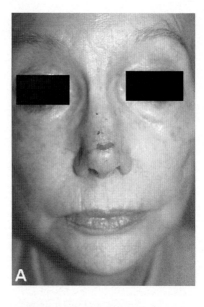

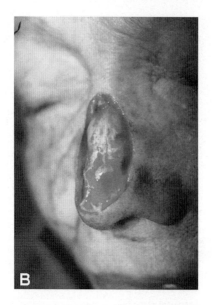

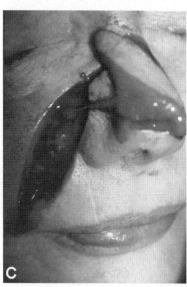

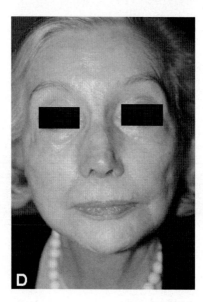

FIG. 2. A: Preoperative: A 70-year-old woman with a recurrence of a basal-cell carcinoma extending from the tip to the bridge of the nose. B: Intraoperative: The area of the wide resection of the tumor is shown. C: Intraoperative: The elevated zygomatic flap pedicled on the cutaneous zygomatic branch and transposed into the defect. D: Postoperative: Appearance at 6 months.

transverse line, for a total length of 4 cm. However, the width of the flap is extended strictly from the nasolabial fold, its medial border, until 2 cm toward the cheek area. The width especially should not be designed too large, to ensure a tension-free wound closure. Because of the presented anastomosis with other cutaneous branches from the facial artery and the infraorbital artery, the maximum potential length reaches to 6 cm (2,3). In this way, an enlargement of the axial skin flap is possible, and the arc of rotation can be extended by orthograde and retrograde pedicles (Fig. 1). Thus, the flap can be designed to abut the ala of the nose, and reconstruction of nasal defects can be achieved without conspicuous scars.

OPERATIVE TECHNIQUE

After skin incision, the flap is elevated from the medial border in the subcutaneous plane, always keeping in mind that the goal is tension-free advancement, with maximum preservation of the underlying subcutaneous pedicle. After identification of the facial artery and the origin of the cutaneous zygomatic branch, a careful preparation of the pedicle is necessary to allow a maximum arc of rotation.

Once selected, the skin paddle is dissected by incising down to the underlying muscle without cutting it. It is very important to dissect the flap strictly above the fascia of the mimic musculature, to prevent injuries of the buccal branches of the facial nerve. As soon as the island flap is circumscribed, it can be raised and carefully transposed into the defect, exercising caution to not twist the pedicle. If the defect lies at the tip of the nose, the flap should be transferred through a subcutaneous tunnel, and the pedicle positioned underneath the alar groove incision. The long pedicle of this flap allows a reconstruction without bulking. The donor area is sutured primarily in the nasolabial fold, and a drain is inserted for 24 hours (Fig. 2).

SUMMARY

The zygomatic flap can follow naturally existing contour lines while retaining color match and texture. The advantage of the nasolabial flap as a transposition flap is the long axial pedicle, which enables transposition of the island flap at the base, allowing for adequate tissue replacement as well as its use for deep defects without bulking. The procedure relies on the fact that the cutaneous zygomatic branch is a constant branch of the

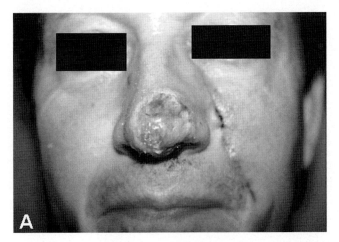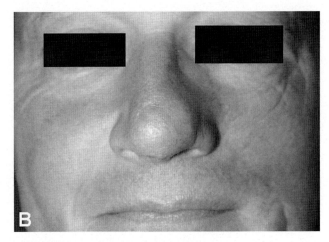

FIG. 3. A: Preoperative: A 57-year-old man with a soft-tissue defect on the tip of the nose following a dog bite and previously unsuccessful surgery. **B:** Postoperative: View of an excellent result following reconstruction with the zygomatic flap 8 months after operation.

facial artery. It is always present and its position can be easily marked preoperatively, simplifying the surgical technical effort.

The existence of anastomosis between the zygomatic branch and cutaneous branches from the infraorbital artery allows the extension of the arc of rotation by orthograde and retrograde pedicles. Because of this enlargement, the axial skin island flap is a good possibility, and reconstruction of nasal tip defects can be performed without considerable scars (Figs. 2 and 3). Therefore, it can be considered by every plastic surgeon as an option in reconstruction of soft-tissue defects of the nasal and perinasal regions. Our experience with the new island axial pattern flap has been good, and we can recommend this technique. However, we must emphasize

that exact anatomic knowledge, combined with careful dissection, is the basis for successful dissection and application.

References

1. Kalus R, Zamora S. Aesthetic considerations in facial reconstructive surgery: the V-Y flap revisited. *Aesthetic Plast Surg* 1996;20:83.
2. Gardetto A, Erdinger K, Papp C. The zygomatic flap: a further possibility in reconstructing soft tissue defects of the nose and upper lip. *Plast Reconstr Surg* 2004;113:485.
3. Gardetto A, Moriggl B, Maurer H, et al. Anatomical basis for a new island axial pattern flap in the perioral region. *Surg Radiol Anat* 2002; 24(3–4):147.

CHAPTER 42 ■ CHEEK ADVANCEMENT FLAP FOR PARANASAL RECONSTRUCTION

G. KRONEN, T. BENACQUISTA, AND B. STRAUCH

EDITORIAL COMMENT

This is an excellent and reliable flap for defects in the paranasal area. One should always remember not to extend the flap into the nose; by doing so, the rules of the aesthetic unit will be broken, resulting in an unacceptable outcome that will require secondary revision.

The cheek enjoys an obvious prominence in the architecture of the face. In older patients, there is an area of relative redundancy of tissue extending from the medial canthus of the eye to the inferior border of the mandible, providing for more available skin for the reconstructive procedures often required in this age group. With the use of cheek advancement flaps for paranasal reconstruction, important considerations include the anatomic complexity of the region (1–3), the avoidance of excess skin excision and resultant scarring and contracture, and careful flap design to avoid the transfer of hair-bearing skin (2). It is also important to match flap thickness as closely as possible to that of the original defect to achieve the most pleasing aesthetic outcome (4).

INDICATIONS

Cheek advancement flaps are useful for coverage of the paranasal region, when there is a full-thickness defect in this area, or when bone is exposed at the nasomaxillary junction or maxilla. Split-thickness skin grafts do not usually provide satisfactory coverage, since the contraction associated with wound healing tends to pull the lower-eyelid margin inferiorly. Full-thickness skin grafts taken from the postauricular, preauricular, or supraclavicular region will provide excellent texture, color match, and resilient skin; however, they will be noticeable as patches in an otherwise unscarred face (4), when applied to defects greater than 5 mm in depth.

ANATOMY

There is a rich vascular anastomotic network supplying the cheek skin, which is based on branches of the external carotid artery, with a smaller contribution from the internal carotid artery. The facial artery, which courses superomedially from the lower border of the mandible toward the modiolus near the buccal angle, constitutes the main blood supply. Other contributions are received from the transverse facial artery (a branch of the superficial temporal artery), the buccal and infraorbital branches of the internal maxillary artery, and the zygomatic branch of the lacrimal artery (a branch of the ophthalmic artery).

Venous drainage of the cheek parallels the arterial system. Lymphatic drainage is achieved via the superficial and deep parotid nodes, the buccal nodes surrounding the facial vein, and the submandibular nodes, ultimately to empty into the cervical chain of lymph nodes (5–8).

Cheek flaps are usually designed as random pattern flaps. Because of the rich anastomotic network of arterial supply and venous drainage, there is little concern as to their cutaneous viability, and no attempt is made to incorporate an axial vascular supply. This allows for great freedom when planning random-pattern flaps for reconstruction, as flaps that are based superiorly, medially, laterally, and inferiorly are all possible. However, caution must be exercised when elevating these flaps, so that a layer of subcutaneous tissue is raised with the flap, to preserve the subdermal vascular plexus.

FLAP DESIGN AND DIMENSIONS

The cheek advancement flap can be utilized to reconstruct defects of various sizes in the paranasal region. Advantages of the flap are that it is very extensile because excess skin in the neck and preauricular regions can be mobilized as necessary, to close the defect, and closure of the donor site is effected without residual deformity (2). Flap design is therefore limited primarily by the amount of redundant tissue present that can pose a challenging problem in younger patients because of the reduced amount of donor tissue possible.

When designing cheek flaps, incisions should be preferably placed within lines of relaxed skin tension or in wrinkle lines; the end results will then be a fine scar that is well camouflaged (9). The limiting factor is the cheek-nasal junction. The flap should not be used to cover or replace nasal skin.

OPERATIVE TECHNIQUE

The excision is planned as a square or rectangle (2). From the side of the defect, two incisions are drawn—one along the nasolabial fold medially, and another superiorly along the lower eyelid–cheek junction where the thin skin of the lower eyelid begins to thicken. Flap dissection then proceeds in the subcutaneous plane, to preserve the subdermal vascular plexus, extending inferiorly and laterally as far as necessary, to mobilize the flap enough to close the paranasal defect.

As dissection proceeds inferiorly along the nasolabial fold and approaches the inferior border of the mandible and midcervical region, elevation is maintained within a plane superficial to the platysma muscle, to avoid injury to the marginal mandibular branch of the facial nerve (10). When proceeding laterally, one must stay superior to the superficial musculoaponeurotic system (SMAS), to further avoid facial nerve injury (11).

Once the cheek flap has been elevated, there are several key points for successful insetting of the flap, not only to achieve the desired aesthetic result, but also to minimize the risk of postoperative complications. As the skin of the paranasal region is somewhat thin, careful defatting of the subcutaneous tissue may be performed without risk of damaging the subdermal vascular plexus, so that when the flap is inset, it will have the same thickness as the original premorbid recipient site. Because of gravitational effects and flap weight relative to the lower eyelid skin, suturing the flap

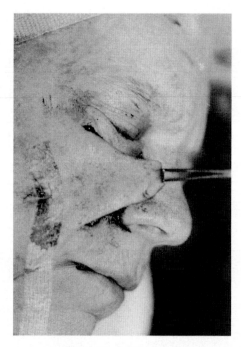

FIG. 1. Cheek flap elevated.

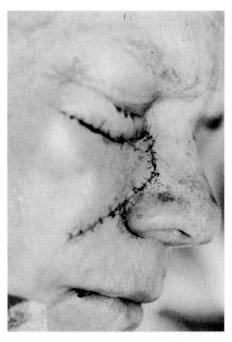

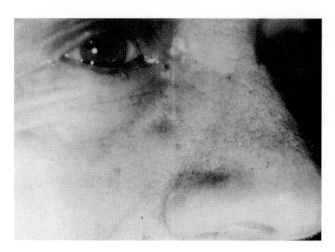

FIG. 3. Flap heals with minimal evidence of scarring.

FIG. 2. Flap inset; the anterior border closes the defect, which does not extend into the nasal skin.

undersurface to the periosteum of the zygoma is recommended, to prevent sagging of the cheek and resultant ectropion of the lower eyelid.

As the flap is sutured, skin excesses may appear on either side of the flap base. These can be excised as Burrow's triangles or can be left and revised secondarily. The flap should not violate the side of the nose (Figs. 1–3).

CLINICAL RESULTS

Use of the cheek advancement flap for closure of superomedial defects has several advantages. First, flap elevation requires a more limited dissection than rotation flaps to obtain the amount of skin advancement necessary to effect defect closure. The defect is reconstructed with tissue that is similar in color, texture, and thickness. However, male patients must be advised that the advancement flap may elevate the facial hair line. The scars situated in the nasolabial fold are not particularly noticeable.

The development of postoperative ectropion can be minimized by suturing the flap undersurface to the periosteum of the zygoma.

SUMMARY

The cheek advancement flap can be utilized to close moderately sized defects of the paranasal region. With careful planning, design, and execution, excellent function and aesthetic results can be achieved.

References

1. Friedman M. *Operative techniques in otolaryngology—head and neck surgery: facial flaps and facial reconstruction,* vol. 4. Philadelphia: Saunders, 1993;31–34.
2. Jackson IT. *Local flaps in head and neck reconstruction.* St. Louis: Mosby, 1985;223.
3. Zide BM, Jelks GW. *Surgical anatomy of the orbit.* New York: Raven, 1985;36.
4. McCarthy JG. *Plastic surgery.* Philadelphia: Harcourt Brace Jovanovich, 1990;2038.
5. Williams PL, ed. *Gray's anatomy.* New York: Churchill Livingstone, 1989;736–746.
6. Cameron RR. Nasolabial and cheek skin flaps. In: Strauch B, Vasconez L, Hall-Findlay E, eds. *Grabb's encyclopedia of flaps.* Boston: Little, Brown, 1990;146–147.
7. Gunter JP, Sheffield RW. Transposition cheek skin flaps: the rhombic flap and its variations. In: Strauch B, Vasconez L, Hall-Findlay E, eds. *Grabb's encyclopedia of flaps.* Boston: Little, Brown, 1990;337.
8. Corso PF. Variations of the arterial, venous, and capillary circulation of the soft tissues of the head by decades as demonstrated by the methyl methacrylate injection technique and their application to construction of flaps and pedicles. *Plast Reconstr Surg* 1961;27:180.
9. Crow ML, Crow FJ. Resurfacing large cheek defects with rotation flaps from the neck. *Plast Reconstr Surg* 1976;58:196.
10. Kaplan I, Goldwyn RM. The versatility of the laterally based cervicofacial flap for cheek repairs. *Plast Reconstr Surg* 1978;61:390.
11. Mitz V, Peyronie M. Superficial musculoaponeurotic system (SMAS) in the parotid and cheek area. *Plast Reconstr Surg* 1976;58:80.

CHAPTER 43 ■ NASAL PLUS NASOLABIAL SKIN FLAPS FOR RECONSTRUCTION OF THE NASAL DORSUM

J. W. SNOW

The use of an L-shaped skin flap with its base straddling the midline at the root of the nose and its distal aspect overlying the lateral aspect of the nasal pyramid has been found effective for reconstruction of the caudal half of the nasal dorsum following tumor excision. The donor site is closed with an L-shaped nasolabial skin flap.

Both these flaps have good vascularity, as well as the proper skin color match and thickness. The lines of inset fall within the natural lines of the nose and nasolabial region. This technique is different from a bilobed flap, which shares a mutual base (see Chap. 35).

A lateral nasal defect remains where the tip of the nasal flap originated, and this can be closed by an adjacent nasolabial skin flap that is tailored to fit the defect. The nasolabial flap donor site can be closed by approximation of the wound edges.

The flaps have to be drawn with relative precision. The plane of dissection must be kept at a deep level, so that the flap thickness corresponds to that of the defect and the blood supply is maintained. Two small fragments of skin need to be excised (Fig. 1) to facilitate adaptation of the flap to the defect.

OPERATIVE TECHNIQUE

The underlying cartilage and bone may be planed if a hump is present in order to decrease the length of the basic flap; i.e., the shortest distance between two points is a straight line. Removal of part of the cartilage and bone may be done with impunity.

CLINICAL RESULTS

Over the last few years, six patients have presented appropriate defects for this method of reconstruction. It has worked well in all six. If the defect is relatively large (2 cm), the nasal tip might be elevated somewhat as a result of

A–C

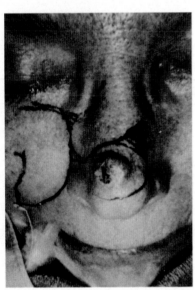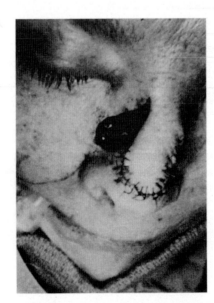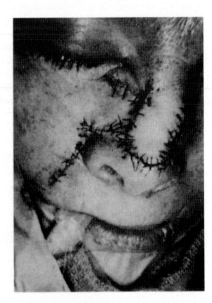

FIG. 1. A: The double L-shaped skin flaps have been outlined. A triangle of skin will be excised on the left lateral nose, in order to accommodate the nasal flap. **B:** The L-shaped nasal skin flap has been rotated into the dorsal nasal defect. **C:** The L-shaped nasolabial skin flap has been rotated into the lateral nasal defect and its distal end trimmed. *(Continued)*

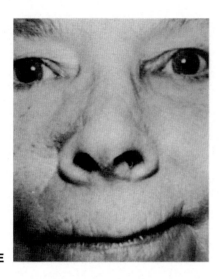
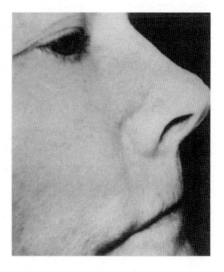

D,E

FIG. 1. *Continued.* D,E: Result 4 months postoperatively.

tension on the flap, but it gradually returns to its former position.

Care must be taken to prevent ectropion if the flap lies too near the lower lid. Slight shifting of the columella toward the nasolabial flap side has occurred, but this gradually decreases with time.

SUMMARY

Reconstruction of the distal half of the nose can be accomplished using an L-shaped nasal flap for the defect and an L-shaped nasolabial flap for the donor site.

CHAPTER 44 ■ SUBCUTANEOUS PEDICLE SKIN FLAPS

J. N. BARRON* AND M. N. SAAD

EDITORIAL COMMENT

The Pers technique (Fig. 4) is a most elegant method using the nasolabial flap for reconstruction of nasal rim defects. It is much safer when the subcutaneous pedicle is based on a known arterial blood supply. The assurance of blood supply when performing the Pers technique for reconstruction of the alar rim is not as precise when compared to the use of a flap with a definite vessel.

The subcutaneous pedicle skin flap consists of a skin paddle and a pedicle containing only subcutaneous tissue (1–3). Three donor sites are available for nasal reconstruction: (1) the nose itself, (2) the nasolabial area, and (3) the frontoglabellar region.

In the open technique, the donor and recipient sites are joined by an incision, and the flap is transferred under direct vision. In the closed technique, the skin lying between the donor and recipient sites is undermined, and the flap is transferred through a tunnel.

INDICATIONS

The nose, the nasolabial area, and the frontoglabellar region are all ideally suited for nasal reconstruction because they

---

* Deceased.

provide good color and texture matches. Although subcutaneous pedicle flaps are less robust than standard flaps, this is more than amply compensated for by their greater mobility and the small (but obvious) advantage of avoiding an unsightly dog-ear at the base of the flap. Also, scarring that results from the dissection of a subcutaneous pedicle is less than that which follows the use of a standard flap.

It is not advisable to repair very small defects with subcutaneous pedicle flaps, since there is the danger of mushrooming. In such instances, a graft or standard flap is preferable.

Nasal skin itself is particularly useful for the repair of lining defects. Because the nose has very little skin to spare, however, nasal skin defects alone are best reconstructed with flaps from the other two regions.

Subcutaneous pedicle flaps from the check adjacent to the nose can be used for the replacement of nasal lining, as well as for repair of skin defects of the lower part of the nose, especially the alae. Coverage of upper nasal, canthal, lower eyelid, and adjacent cheek defects is ideally performed with flaps from the frontoglabellar region. Although standard forehead flaps can be used, they have the disadvantages of limited mobility and the need for secondary correction of contour abnormalities at the base of the flap.

ANATOMY

It is not necessary to include an anatomically designated axial vascular system in the pedicle, although, if available, this is an advantage. Many subcutaneous pedicle flaps rely on a random capillary circulation, and because this is a low-pressure flow, it demands an ultra-atraumatic technique for dissection. We believe that the unilateral subcuticular suture disturbs the flap margin much less than ordinary interrupted sutures.

A direct vascular supply can be included with some subcutaneous pedicle skin flaps (4). Superiorly based nasolabial flaps derive their blood supply from the supraorbital and supratrochlear anastomoses, and the inferiorly based flap is nourished by the terminal branches of the facial artery or the superior labial vessels. Flaps from the frontoglabellar region can include blood supply from the supratrochlear vessels.

FLAP DESIGN AND DIMENSIONS

The function of the pedicle is to transmit blood, lymph, and nerve supply to the flap. Thus a good pedicle design is essential (Fig. 1). The pedicle should be long enough to allow the flap proper to reach the recipient site without the slightest tension. The pedicle also should contain sufficient vascular elements to sustain the viability of the flap and, if possible, provide adequate sensation. The design should be such that kinking is avoided, and whenever possible, gravity should help venous and lymphatic drainage.

It is important that the skin paddle be designed to fit the defect accurately, so that when suturing is completed, no more tension exists than occurred in the original position. One should bear in mind that the size of a defect could be larger than anticipated, as in the case of fibrosis in recurrent basal cell carcinoma following radiotherapy (Fig. 2).

The width of the pedicle should be as generous as possible, and the pedicle certainly should not be narrower than that of the skin paddle. It is obvious that the shorter the length of the pedicle, the better. However, under no circumstances should the pedicle be so short that the skin flap has to be sutured into position under tension.

The design of the subcutaneous pedicle skin flap is usually that of a transposition or advancement flap. Its thickness will depend on local factors and vascularity.

OPERATIVE TECHNIQUE

After the flap and the subcutaneous pedicle have been outlined, the flap is incised through skin and subcutaneous tissue along its distal and lateral margins and through skin only along its proximal margin. The subcutaneous pedicle is then liberated in the subdermal plane by sharp dissection over its full length. At this stage it is advisable to create a tunnel through which the flap and the pedicle will eventually reach the recipient site. This tunnel should be generous in size and made by blunt dissection.

The deeper part of the flap and pedicle are then raised off the deep fascia, starting with sharp dissection and then proceeding more proximally with blunt dissection. Finally, the two sides of the pedicle are divided with scissors, thus

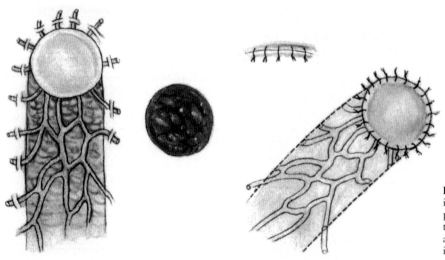

A,B

FIG. 1. A, B: Design of the flap showing skin paddle and subcutaneous pedicle (closed technique). Note that the circulation is random pattern, although axial vessels may be included in the pedicle in certain cases.

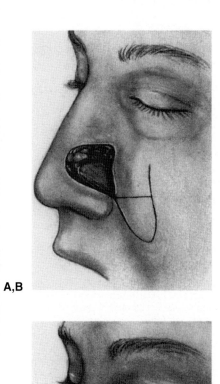
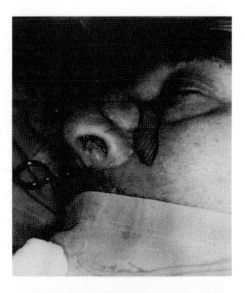

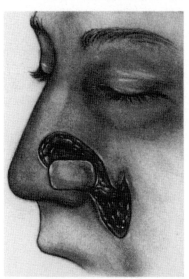
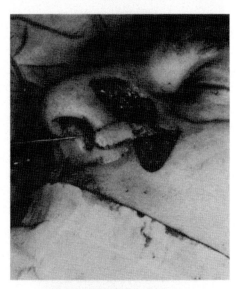

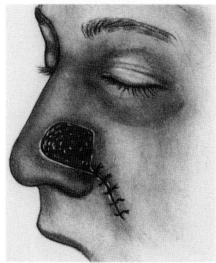
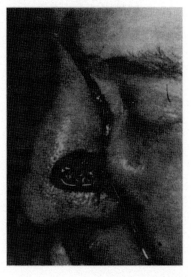
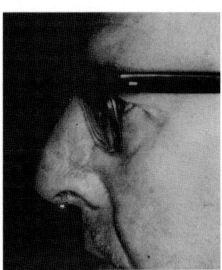

A,B

C,D

E–G

FIG. 2. A–G: Recurrent basal cell carcinoma on the left side of the nose, invading mucosal lining. Full-thickness excision, using subcutaneous nasolabial skin flap for lining. Gillies' "bishop's miter flap" was used for cover.

completing the mobilization of the flap and pedicle. The flap is then picked up with skin hooks and passed through the tunnel into the defect. Any tension at this stage can be released by further dissection of the pedicle.

Meticulous hemostasis is imperative, and if necessary, suction drainage should be established. The donor area is then sutured, avoiding any tension across the pedicle, and if required, a free graft is applied.

tissue base near the margin of the defect, and inverted into the cavity, where it is sutured to the mucous membrane. Skin cover can be provided by nasolabial, frontoglabellar, or forehead flaps.

These small lining flaps have good viability, but they need an intranasal pack for 48 hours to support them and to prevent a hematoma from forming between the two layers.

Flaps from the Nose

When used for lining, the flap is taken from the region immediately adjacent to the defect, dissected up on a subcutaneous

Flaps from the Nasolabial Area

Especially in elderly patients, fairly large flaps can be taken from the nasolabial area, leaving a linear inconspicuous scar

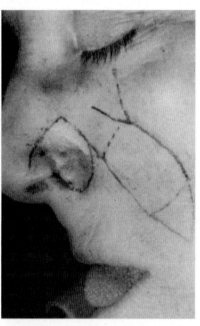
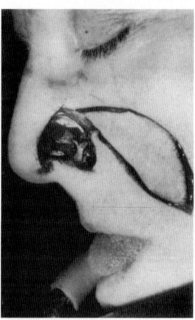
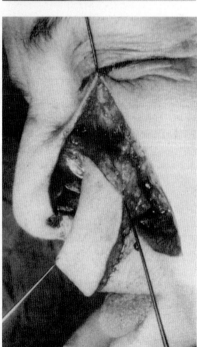
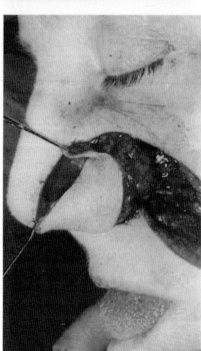
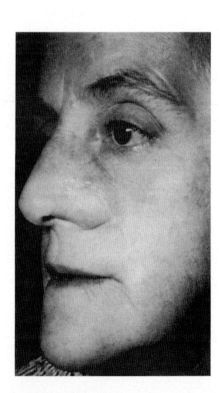

A,B

C–E

FIG. 3. A–E: Full-thickness defect of alar margin. Superiorly based subcutaneous nasolabial skin flap (open technique) was used for lining and then folded for external cover. Note that the base of the pedicle is up toward the medial canthus.

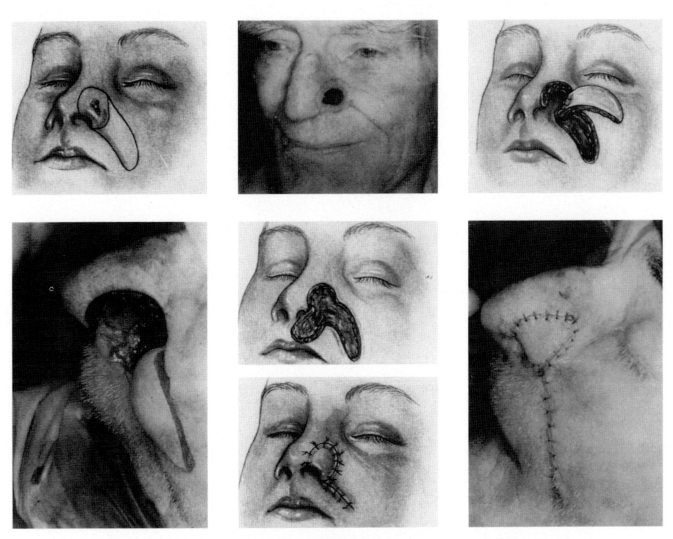

FIG. 4. Pers technique for alar defect. Proximal portion of nasolabial subcutaneous pedicle flap was used for lining. Remainder of flap was folded for external cover.

at the donor site. These flaps can be based superiorly or inferiorly (4–9).

The nasolabial pedicle can sometimes cause a noticeable fullness in the nasofacial groove, and occasionally, this may require a later adjustment. However, if this is evident at the time of operation, an excision of the paranasal subcutaneous tissue will allow the pedicle enough room to lie without causing an obvious bulge.

Nasolabial flaps can be raised from the region immediately adjacent to the defect, and in these cases, the pedicle is designed so that the flap slides directly into its new position. This technique is particularly suitable for defects of the alar base and margin (Fig. 3). A particularly elegant technique for repairing combined skin and lining defects of the alar margin and alar base using nasolabial pedicle flaps was described by Pers in 1967 (9) (Fig. 4).

Flaps from the Frontoglabellar Region

There is a considerable amount of tissue available in this area for nasal reconstruction. With adequate mobilization of the forehead skin and frontalis muscle, quite extensive secondary defects can be closed leaving minimal, inconspicuous scarring (8,10,11) (Figs. 5 and 6).

CLINICAL RESULTS

Most flaps retain good color during the operation if the design is satisfactory. Some flaps become pale, particularly if vasoconstrictors have been used with the local anesthetic. These pale flaps usually recover and behave well unless a hematoma occurs.

Congested flaps result from improper technique that causes kinking or tension, and experience has shown that congested flaps are those that will give the most trouble postoperatively. If a flap becomes congested after insetting and suture, it is necessary to investigate, find the cause, and take corrective measures.

SUMMARY

Subcutaneous pedicle skin flaps can be ideal for nasal reconstruction, both for lining and cover. Flaps can be taken from nasal skin itself (lining), the nasolabial area (lining and cover), and the frontoglabellar region (cover).

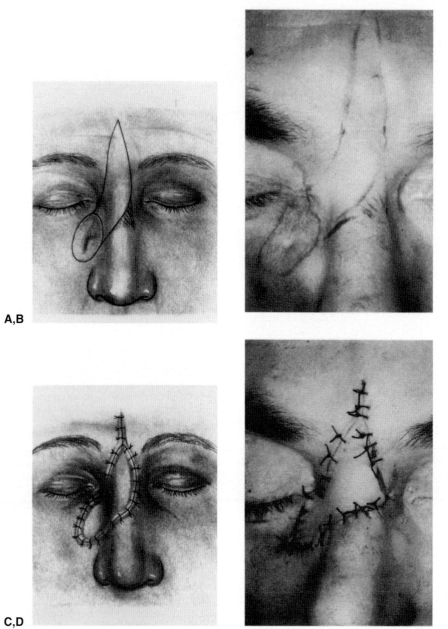

A,B

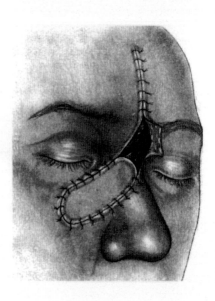

C,D

FIG. 5. A–D: Basal cell carcinoma on the left side of the nose and lower eyelid. A sliding (advancement) frontonasal subcutaneous pedicle flap based on the contralateral supratrochlear vessels was used.

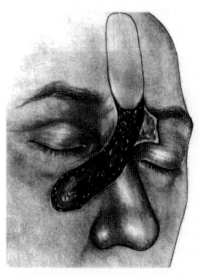

A,B

FIG. 6. A,B: A similar, but larger defect repaired by transposition of a frontonasal subcutaneous pedicle flap.

References

1. Andrews EB. Island flaps in facial reconstruction. *Plast Reconstr Surg* 1969;44:49.
2. Barron JN, Emmett AJJ. Subcutaneous pedicle flaps. *Br J Plast Surg* 1965;18:51.
3. Zook EG, Van Beek AL, Russell RC, Moore JB. V-Y advancement flap for facial defects. *Plast Reconstr Surg* 1980;65:786.
4. Herbert DC, Harrison RG. Nasolabial subcutaneous pedicle flaps. *Br J Plast Surg* 1975;28:85.
5. Grate MR Jr, Hicks JN. Nasolabial subcutaneous pedicle flap. *South Med J* 1973;66:1234.
6. Herbert DC, DeGeus J. Nasolabial subcutaneous pedicle flaps. *Br J Plast Surg* 1975;28:90.
7. Herbert DC. A subcutaneous pedicled cheek flap for reconstruction of alar defects. *Br J Plast Surg* 1978;31:79.
8. Lejour M. One-stage reconstruction of nasal skin defects with local flaps. *Chir Plast* 1972;1:254.
9. Pers M. Cheek flaps in partial rhinoplasty. *Scand J Plast Reconstr Surg* 1967;1:37.
10. Converse JM, Wood-Smith D. Experiences with the forehead island flap with a subcutaneous pedicle. *Plast Reconstr Surg* 1963;31:527.
11. Spira M, Gerow FJ, Hardy SB. Subcutaneous pedicle flaps on the face. *Br J Plast Surg* 1974;27:258.

CHAPTER 45 ■ NASALIS MUSCULOCUTANEOUS SLIDING FLAPS FOR NASAL TIP RECONSTRUCTION

F. J. RYBKA

Projecting like a masthead from the surface of the face, the nasal tip is subjected to more than its share of skin cancers and trauma. Subcutaneous sliding flaps, including V-Y flaps, have been described for reconstruction of a great number of areas about the face, almost to the exclusion of the nasal tip (1–7). These flaps are generally based on a random-pattern subcutaneous blood supply, unlike the flap described herein.

INDICATIONS

The alar flap has some aesthetic advantages over vertical flaps, in that it follows the lines of the alar groove, the natural crease line leading to the tip. Also, most tip lesions are not squarely midline, but paramedian, and they are usually reconstructed using a lateral flap (Fig. 1).

Sliding flaps offer distinct aesthetic advantages over rotation flaps, because of the absence of both redundant tissue (dog-ears) and chronic edema (8,9).

ANATOMY

The facial muscles are unique in human anatomy, in that they have as their insertion the skin of the face. This insertion may be more aponeurotic than muscular, as it is with the nasalis muscle.

The nasalis muscle originates, with several other facial muscles, from a common fibrous band in the nasolabial fold. As it approaches the alar groove, the nasalis muscle is separated from the skin by subcutaneous fat, but as it continues medially toward the tip (as an aponeurosis), it becomes intimately associated with the dermis of the tip skin, with no layer of subcutaneous fat in between.

The nasalis muscle, like the tensor fasciae latae, is not much of a muscle, and it can be best demonstrated by sniffing. This flap is one of the smallest musculocutaneous flaps described, and one might question if we are not stretching terminology to classify it as a musculocutaneous flap at all.

However, similarities are readily found when we compare it with the tensor fasciae latae flap. Like the tensor fasciae latae, its fascia is very long, with a ratio of perhaps one-fifth muscle to four-fifths muscle fascia. The fascia of both muscles carries the axial blood supply with it, just as dependably as if the muscle were present.

Often, a distinct blood vessel, a perforating branch of the alar artery, can be identified as it penetrates into the muscle base near the piriform process of the maxilla. The alar branch of the superior labial artery has been determined to give off 7 to 12 branches every 2 mm or so as it courses around the base of the ala, following closely the piriform aperture.

The nasalis branches penetrate this muscle and then follow it up the side of the nose, parallel with the alar groove. In the aponeurosis, they finally anastomose with the branches of the alar artery from the opposite side.

FLAP DESIGN AND DIMENSIONS

Separation of the nasal skin from the cheek skin next to the alar base will allow a teardrop-shaped island, anchored only by nasalis muscle and subcutaneous tissues, to advance up to

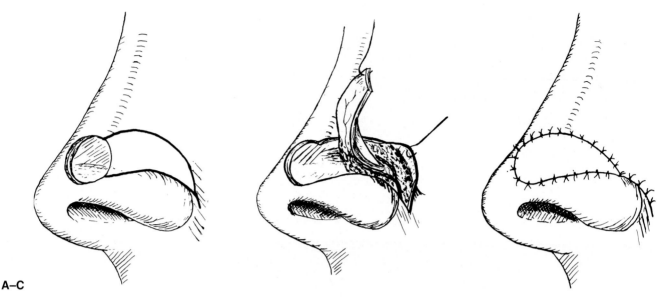

A–C

FIG. 1. **A:** The typical defect is in a paramedian position on the nasal tip. The nasalis musculocutaneous flap is designed with its caudal line right at the alar groove and the cephalad line determined by the width of the defect. **B:** The flap is elevated down to the muscular attachments at the base of the piriform fossa. **C:** The flap is advanced. Any small dog-ears resulting from the concave flap merging against a convex recipient area can be excised. (From Rybka, ref. 8, with permission.)

1.5 cm without risk. Bilateral nasalis musculocutaneous sliding flaps can be used to close defects up to 2.25 cm wide.

OPERATIVE TECHNIQUE

The caudal incision of the teardrop-shaped flap is right in the alar groove; hence it blends in very well with natural crease lines. The width of the flap is determined by the width of the defect. Thus the cephalad incision is made from the upper pole of the defect to join the caudal incision adjacent to the alar base. It is important that the flap extend all the way to the level of the alar base, since only there can the separation of skin from its muscle and blood supply take place. More distally, this is all fused with the dermis of the skin flap.

At the base, only the skin is completely divided, creating the island. The soft tissues are teased with a hemostat, and the restraining fibrous bands are cut until the island is attached only by the deeper muscle, which includes the blood supply. The nasalis muscle is wider than the usual flap base, and it

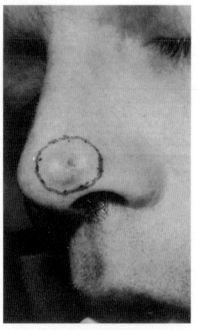
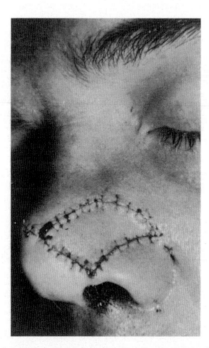
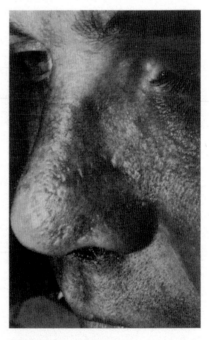

A–C

FIG. 2. **A:** A 32-year-old man with nodular basal cell carcinoma. Outline of planned resection. **B:** Immediate reconstruction with the nasalis musculocutaneous flap. **C:** Result 3 months postoperatively. (From Rybka, ref. 8, with permission.)

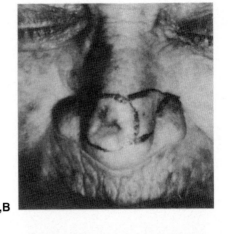
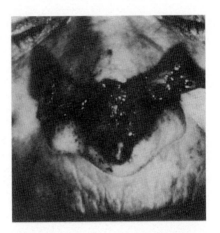

A,B

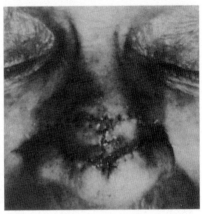
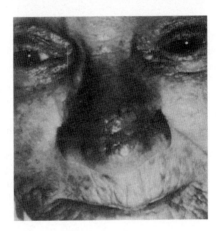

C,D

FIG. 3. A: An 80-year-old woman with a large basal cell carcinoma. The areas of resection and bilateral nasalis flaps are outlined. B: The bilateral nasalis musculocutaneous flaps are elevated. C: The immediate closure. D: Result 3 weeks postoperatively. (From Rybka, ref. 8, with permission.)

must therefore be dissected away from the cephalad part of the flap. Advancement up to 1.5 cm should be accomplished without much difficulty (Fig. 2).

CLINICAL RESULTS

Over the past 10 years, 47 patients have had the nasal tip reconstructed with this flap. The majority of these followed the excision of a basal cell carcinoma (40 of 47).

The maximum diameter of the defect reconstructed by the single flap was 1.25 cm. In six patients, a bilateral flap was used, and this allowed reconstruction of a defect 2.0 cm in diameter (Fig. 3). In a few patients, a limited rhinoplasty was performed to diminish the size of the defect. In such cases, one must be absolutely certain that all tumor has been completely removed.

SUMMARY

An alar island sliding flap that is ideally suited to nasal tip reconstruction is described. It is actually a small musculocuta-neous flap based on the nasalis muscle. Tip defects up to 1.5 cm in diameter can be reconstructed with a unilateral flap, and defects up to 2.25 cm in diameter can be reconstructed with a bilateral flap.

References

1. Herbert DC, Harrison RG. Nasolabial subcutaneous pedicle flaps: I. Observations on their blood supply. *Br J Plast Surg* 1975;28:85.
2. Herbert DC, DeGeus J. Nasolabial subcutaneous pedicle flaps: II. Clinical experience. *Br J Plast Surg* 1975;28:90.
3. Herbert D. A subcutaneous pedicled cheek flap for reconstruction of alar defects. *Br J Plast Surg* 1978;31:79.
4. Trevaskis AE, Rempel J, Okunski W, Rea M. Sliding subcutaneous pedicle flaps to close a circular defect. *Plast Reconstr Surg* 1970;46:155.
5. Esser FJS. Island flaps. *NY State J Med* 1917;106:264.
6. Kubacek V. Transposition of flaps on the face on a subcutaneous pedicle. *Acta Chir Plast* 1965;2:108.
7. Zook E, Van Beek A, Russell R, Moore J. V-Y advancement flaps for facial defects. *Plast Reconstr Surg* 1980;65:786.
8. Rybka FJ. Reconstruction of the nasal tip using nasalis myocutaneous slid-ing flaps. *Plast Reconstr Surg* 1983;71:40.
9. Staahl TE. Nasalis myocutaneous flap for nasal reconstruction. *Arch Otolaryngol Head Neck Surg* 1986;112:302.

CHAPTER 46 ■ WRAPAROUND CARTILAGE FLAP FOR CORRECTION OF CLEFT-LIP NASAL DEFORMITY

I. J. PELED, Y. RAMON, AND Y. ULLMANN

EDITORIAL COMMENT

This is another technique that attempts to obtain symmetry of the normal alar cartilage with a slanted one from a cleft-lip deformity. A satisfactory and similar result can be obtained with the free use of a cartilage graft as an onlay procedure.

A turnover contralateral lower lateral alar cartilage flap is suggested for the correction of cleft nose alar deformity. The flap wraps around the deficient medial crus and acts as a pulley, repositioning and augmenting the affected alar cartilage.

INDICATIONS

Cleft-lip nasal deformity includes lateral displacement of the medial crus, as well as depressed and laterally deflected lower lateral alar cartilage. In addition, there is a relatively larger, retrodisplaced naris, with deviation of the nasal tip to the noncleft side. Definitive correction of cleft-lip nasal deformity is difficult to achieve, and there is no ideal surgical procedure for all deformities (1–4). The technique presented repositions the affected lower lateral cartilage and augments and suspends the medial crus to make the nasal tip as symmetrical as possible.

OPERATIVE TECHNIQUE

Under local or general anesthesia with local infiltration, an open nasal approach is carried out with a V-shaped columellar incision. This enables direct visualization and appreciation of the degree of deformity. In cases of a short columella, the V-to-Y closure of the incision offers a 2 to 3 mm increase in columellar length. After the incision has been completed and the medial crura identified, the cartilage is exposed with bilateral rim incisions. Horizontal markings determine the proposed height of the alar cartilage (Fig. 1A).

The cephalic portion of the contralateral alar cartilage is incised up to the medial dome, and is completely released from the mucosal side as a medially based alar cartilage flap (Figs. 1B and 2A). The marked cephalic portion of the alar dome on the cleft side is resected and put aside for a tip graft, if additional tip projection is necessary. The remaining alar dome is released from the mucosal side only in the medial portion of the dome, and the flap is brought under it (Figs. 1C and 2B), turned around in front, and finally sutured to the contralateral side with 5–0 nylon (Figs. 1D and 2C).

The flap pulls the alar cartilage of the cleft side medially, and gives additional projection to the depressed dome. When additional tip projection is necessary, a tip graft is placed above both domes and secured into position with 5–0 nylon. When necessary, other procedures are performed on the upper cartilage, nasal bones, and septum. On completion, skin incisions are sutured with 6–0 nylon.

CLINICAL RESULTS

Satisfactory and long-lasting results were obtained in our small series, justifying this approach for the improvement of

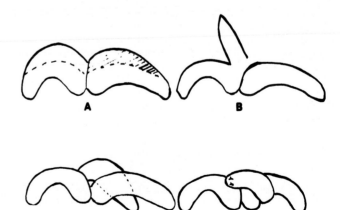

FIG. 1. A: Normal (*left*) and deformed (*right*) alar cartilages. *Broken line* marks flap incision and hatched area is portion to be excised. B: Medially based alar cartilage flap. C: The flap is tunneled between the medial crus and nasal mucosa. D: The flap wraps around the medial crus and is sutured to the normal side.

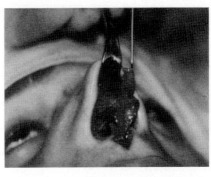
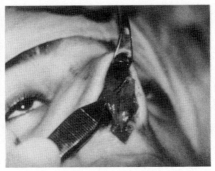
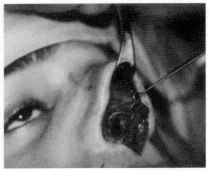

A–C

FIG. 2. **A:** Left cartilage flap suspended with hook. **B:** Forceps tunneled behind the medial crus for grasping the flap. **C:** The flap wraps around the right medial crus and is sutured to the left alar cartilage.

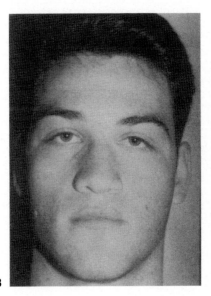
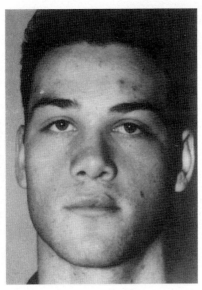

A,B

FIG. 3. **A:** Preoperative frontal view. **B:** One year following surgery.

cleft nasal deformities. Patients were satisfied with the procedure and pleased with the cosmetic result (Fig. 3).

SUMMARY

The turnover contralateral cephalic alar cartilage flap is a good solution for the correction of cleft nose alar deformity.

References

1. Humby, G. The nostril in secondary harelip. *Lancet* 1938;1:275.
2. Barsky, AJ. *Principles and practice of plastic surgery.* Baltimore: Williams and Wilkins, 1950.
3. Whitlow DR, Constable, JD. Crossed alar wing procedure for correction of late deformity in the unilateral cleft lip nose. *Plast Reconstr Surg* 1973;52:338.
4. Ribeiro, L. Revising the nasal tip: a new approach. *Plast Reconstr Surg* 1989;84:671.

CHAPTER 47 ■ COLUMELLA AND NASAL SEPTUM SKIN-CARTILAGE FLAP TO NASAL ALA

M. ORTICOCHEA

EDITORIAL COMMENT

This is an elegantly conceived procedure that is applicable to smaller defects, but there are several problems, including wound contraction and retraction, the possibility of producing asymmetry with the opposite side, the lack of color match, the unpredictability of the alar roll, and retraction of the columella.

Defects of the ala nasi are common, and many methods have been proposed for their repair. The following technique provides a repair of good shape, color, and texture and supplies sufficient cartilage to prevent the ala from collapsing during inhalation (1).

OPERATIVE TECHNIQUE

An anteriorly based flap is raised that consists of half the columella and the membranous septum, the medial crus of the alar cartilage, and as much of the skin lining from the cartilaginous septum as may be required (see Figs. 2 and 4). The medial crus of the alar cartilage is divided, producing a mobile flap that can be transposed readily and sutured into the alar defect.

The donor area is covered with a skin graft. The tissues are fairly stiff, and little deformation occurs. With smaller defects, the raw surface of the flap (inside the nostril) may be allowed to heal by secondary intention, and this may impart a natural roll to the reconstructed alar margin. With larger defects (Figs. 1 to 5), the flap as well as the donor area is skin-grafted.

Three weeks postoperatively, the patient is fitted with an intranasal prosthesis and continues to wear it for 3 to 6 months or until all contraction has ceased.

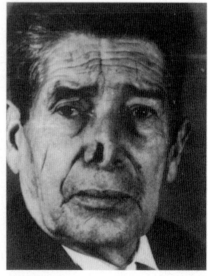 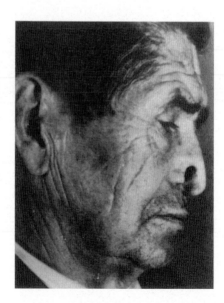

A,B

FIG. 1. A,B: The alar defect. (From Orticochea, ref. 1, with permission.)

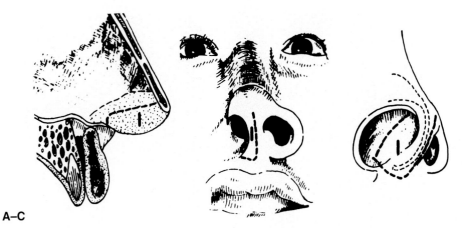

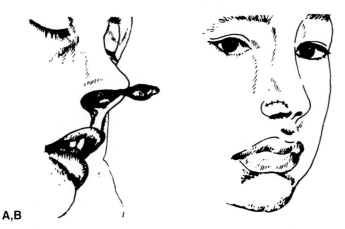

FIG. 2. A–C: The flap is outlined. The incision passes along the midline of the columella and then into the nasal vestibule and back toward the nasal tip. The exact size and shape depend on those of the defect. (From Orticochea, ref. 1, with permission.)

FIG. 3. A: The flap includes the medial crus of the alar cartilage, and when this is divided, the flap is readily mobilized. **B:** The transposed flap used to reconstruct the right ala. (From Orticochea, ref. 1, with permission.)

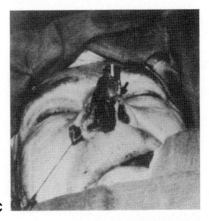
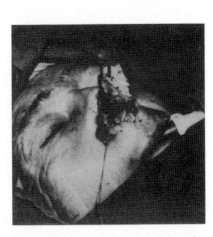
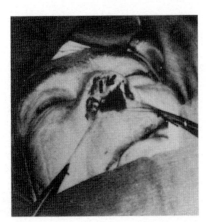

FIG. 4. A: The flap has been raised, and the *arrow* marks the site where the medial crus of the alar cartilage has been sectioned. **B:** The flap and the donor site have been covered with a skin graft held in place with small quilting sutures. **C:** The flap is transposed into the alar defect. The *arrow* indicates the vascular pedicle. (From Orticochea, ref. 1, with permission.)

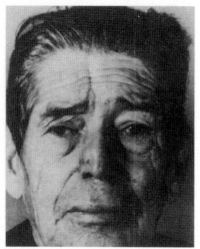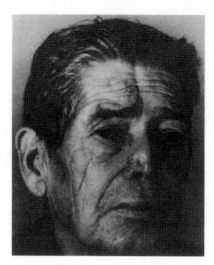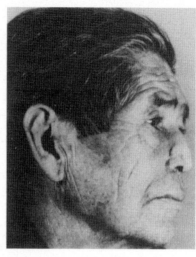

A–C

FIG. 5. **A–C:** The final result. (From Orticochea, ref. 1, with permission.)

SUMMARY

The nasal ala can be reconstructed with a columella and nasal septum skin-cartilage flap.

Reference

1. Orticochea, M. Repair of defects of the ala nasi with a flap from the columella and nasal septum. *Br J Plast Surg* 1978;31:176.

CHAPTER 48 ■ TISSUE EXPANSION IN NASAL RECONSTRUCTION

L. C. ARGENTA

EDITORIAL COMMENT

The attractiveness of expansion of the forehead skin for nasal reconstruction should be weighed against the following difficulties: loss of *pliability* of the skin flap owing to capsular formation, increasing *thickness* of the flap, and the need for a multistaged procedure. In most nasal reconstructions, the secondary forehead defect can be closed primarily, or if a small raw area is left open, it will heal by contracture with an acceptable scar.

See Chapter 11 for a detailed description of the indications, flap design, operative technique, and clinical results of tissue expansion for scalp and forehead defects.

CLINICAL RESULTS

In one patient who underwent expansion of forehead skin for total nasal reconstruction, there was some mild tissue contraction because of inadequate structural support. Once the cantilever bone graft was placed, no further contraction was observed (Fig. 1).

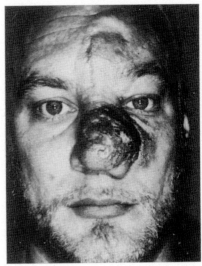
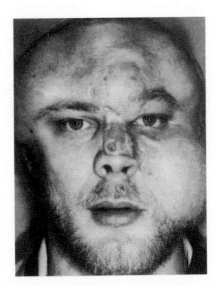
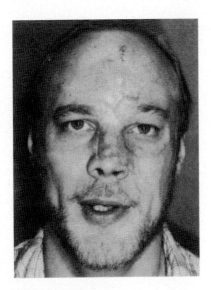

A–C

FIG. 1. **A:** A 34-year-old man with a cavernous hemangioma of the central third of the face. The nose was debrided to periosteum, and a split-thickness skin graft was used for initial closure. **B:** Multiple expanders were placed in the face and expanded over 10 weeks. **C:** The patient 1 year after completion of the excision and advancement of the flaps. The sutures in the forehead are in an area where a small dog-ear required resection after 1 year when it did not subside.

CHAPTER 49 ■ LATERAL NASAL (MITER) SKIN FLAP

R. A. RIEGER

Nasal skin is difficult to match in color, texture, and thickness. It is therefore desirable to repair nasal defects with nasal skin. Since nasal skin is relatively inelastic, it takes a relatively large nasal skin flap to reconstruct a small nasal defect.

A glabellar flap has been described by Gillies, who noted that it should be used only for defects in the upper half of the nose. A similar but more extensive flap can be devised to close defects in the lower third of the nose, particularly on the tip and either side of the midline (1).

INDICATIONS

The flap is indicated for reconstruction of defects up to 2 cm in diameter on or near the nasal tip and similar defects on the dorsum of the nose near the midline. Defects near the cheek are better closed with other methods.

The nasal tip area has always been a difficult one to reconstruct, and available methods of repair have their limitations. Full-thickness skin grafts commonly become too red and are cosmetically unacceptable. There are many problems with island flaps.

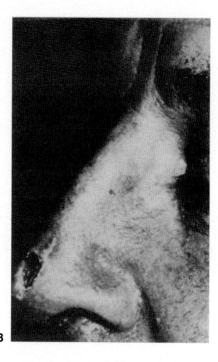
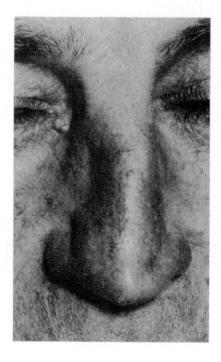

A,B

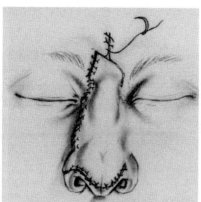

FIG. 1. A: This patient had radionecrosis of the nasal tip. B: Six months after closure of the central nasal tip defect with a lateral nasal flap. Note the minimal scarring. (From Rieger, ref. 1, with permission.)

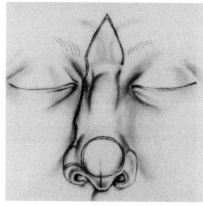
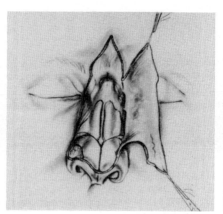

A–C

FIG. 2. A: Initial incisions for the circular removal of a nasal tip lesion and the raising of a lateral nasal skin flap. B: Flap lifted off the nose. C: Flap sutured in place. Note the combination V-Y and Z-plasty closure in the glabellar region. (From Rieger, ref. 1, with permission.)

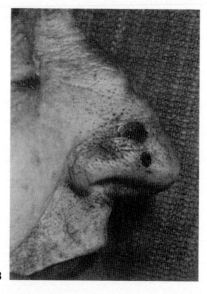
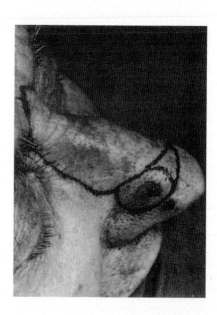

A,B

FIG. 3. A: Patient with two basal cell carcinomas on the side of the nasal tip. B: Lateral nasal flap marked out. The smaller and inferior basal cell carcinoma was excised and the wound edges approximated. The flap was used to close the defect resulting from excision of the larger tumor.

(Continued)

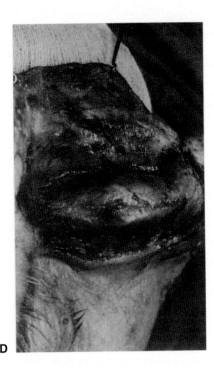
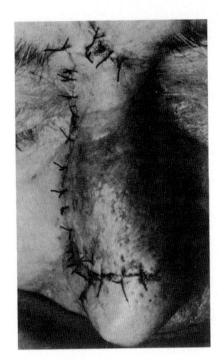

C,D

FIG. 3. *Continued* **C:** The flap includes almost all the skin of the nose. **D:** The flap has been moved and the wounds sutured.

Although the lateral nasal flap appears to introduce extensive nasal scarring, the resultant scar is very acceptable (Fig. 1B), and although the nasal tip is elevated, this is not obvious when the flap has healed.

ANATOMY

The blood supply to the flap is through the base along the lateral side of the nose, and since no specific vessels are included in the base, it is a random-pattern flap (see Chap. 50 for axial modifications (2)).

FLAP DESIGN AND DIMENSIONS

The lateral nasal flap is designed as a transposition flap with a broad base and extensive undermining of the flap to allow freedom of movement.

OPERATIVE TECHNIQUE

The incision of the distal end of the flap for the repair of central tip defects should lie well down on the lateral side of the nose, close to the cheek. It may be necessary to free the flap down to the medial canthal tendon (Fig. 2A, B). The cephalic end of the flap extends up onto the forehead in the glabellar region, where a back cut is made. Closure of the resultant secondary glabellar defect can then be achieved in a V-Y fashion, with or without an added Z-plasty (Fig. 2C).

Although a limited transposition of nasal skin is possible, the flap works because the nasal tip is elevated at the time of wound closure, effectively reducing the distance the flap has to be moved.

CLINICAL RESULTS

A minor problem has been the different thicknesses of skin in the flap. The thin skin of the epicanthal region is moved downward into the thicker skin of the nasal area. Thick forehead skin also may have to be sutured to thin epicanthal eyelid skin. If careful skin approximation is undertaken, there should be no great problem. In fact, the resultant scar in the upper part of the nose is very acceptable (Fig. 1B).

It requires some fortitude to virtually lift the skin from the whole dorsum of the nose (Fig. 3B, C). However, the cosmetic results are well worthwhile. There have been very few cases in which any flap loss has occurred. Excessive tension is usually the main cause of trouble, and it was felt that the use of epinephrine may have contributed to small losses at the flap tip in one or two patients. Epinephrine certainly causes prolonged pallor of the flap, which can be quite worrisome.

SUMMARY

The lateral nasal flap can be effectively used to close defects up to 2 cm in diameter at or near the nasal tip.

References

1. Rieger RA. A local flap for repair of the nasal tip. *Br J Plast Surg* 1967;40:147.
2. Marchac D, Toth B. The axial frontonasal flap revisited. *Plast Reconstr Surg* 1985;76:686.

CHAPTER 50 ■ AXIAL FRONTONASAL FLAP

D. MARCHAC AND B. TOTH

This flap is a modification of the flap described by Rieger (Chap. 49) (1) with one fundamental difference. The flap described, rather than being a random-pattern flap, is an axial flap with a well-defined vascular pedicle. This allows for a much narrower pedicle and consequently more radical sliding and rotation of the nasal skin located above the defect.

INDICATIONS

The axial frontonasal flap can be adjusted more precisely with what we feel is a better cosmetic result. The donor site can be closed in a V-Y manner with the donor scar lying in a glabellar frown line. The flap is not only ideal for reconstruction of defects at the base of the nose, but more important, it is able to provide a sizable amount of skin of similar texture and color for the nasal tip as well. The scars are well hidden at the sides of the nose or in the glabellar area. The flap is not recommended when the alar margin is involved (2–4).

ANATOMY

This flap is based on a vascular pedicle located at the level of the inner palpebral ligament (Figs. 1 and 2). This pedicle is a branch of the angular artery, joining with the supraorbital arteries. It is well visualized on arteriographic studies and cadaver dissections.

FLAP DESIGN AND DIMENSIONS

Because of its axial nature, the flap can be transferred either with a narrow skin bridge or even as an island if located on the side opposite to the defect (Fig. 3). A curved line is drawn from the defect along the side of the nose passing medial to the canthal ligament and curving upward to follow a glabellar frown line. One should go rather high on the glabella to avoid a dog-ear when closing and then go down in a frown line on the opposite side toward the pedicle. When the defect is not centrally located, it is generally best to use the pedicle on the side of the pedicle defect since this gives the greatest flap length for reconstruction.

OPERATIVE TECHNIQUE

The dissection is best begun by undermining upward from the defect in the deep plane used in rhinoplasties, below the muscle layer. The flap should initially be elevated on the side opposite to the pedicle. The contralateral vascular pedicle will be seen during this stage and cauterized. In the glabellar region, only the skin is lifted as the flap. One should then carefully dissect the pedicle side. If more laxity is needed, the skin incision can be lengthened and the muscles tenting above and medial to the canthal ligament can be carefully separated.

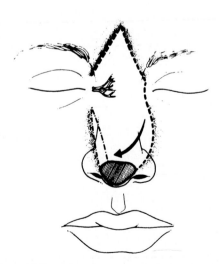

FIG. 1. The axial flap is based on vessels emerging at the level of the inner canthus. This allows increased mobility and precise adjustment. (From Marchac, Toth, ref. 6, with permission.)

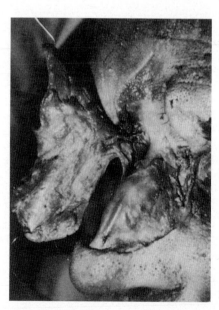

FIG. 2. Fresh cadaver dissection showing the pedicle of the frontonasal flap. (From Marchac, Toth, ref. 6, with permission.)

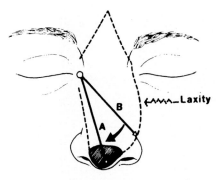

FIG. 3. The axis of rotation should be considered and the incision taken rather low on the lateral side of the nose. (From Marchac, Toth, ref. 6, with permission.)

Undermining is performed at the periphery of the skin incisions, especially at the level of the tip and on the lateral side of the nose opposite to the pedicle. The flap can then be adjusted to fit the defect. Especially when the defect is on the lower part of the nose, one should carefully evaluate the axis of rotation of the flap and include enough skin laterally on the side of the nose opposite to the pedicle to ensure closure without distortion.

The thickness of the edges of the flap must be adjusted at the lateral side of the nose and the inner canthal regions. If too thick, the flap can be carefully thinned on its periphery. Careful approximation of the edges is important. The resection of the dog-ear created by the rotation at the lateral side of the nose is the final stage and should be generous (Figs. 4 and 5).

The wide exposure obtained through this approach permits modification of the framework. If a patient has a large dorsal hump, the flap will often fit better if the hump is reduced in size.

CLINICAL RESULTS

Between 1969 and 1995, 150 patients underwent frontal nasal flap reconstruction for soft-tissue defects of the nose. Half of the procedures were performed for defects of the upper half of the nose, while an equal number were done for reconstruction of the nasal tip. Most of these flaps were performed for reconstruction following excision for basal cell carcinoma (5,6).

The survival rate of the flap was 100%; there was not even a partial loss at the tip. Only one recurrence was noted 3 years following initial excision of a recurrent lesion after x-ray therapy. Following wide reexcision, the same flap was able to be readvanced.

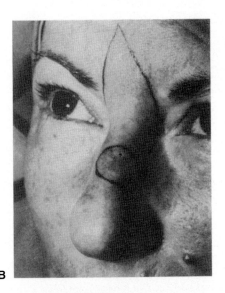
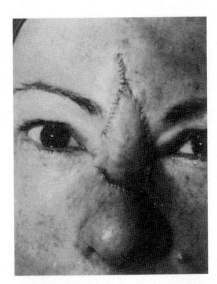

A,B

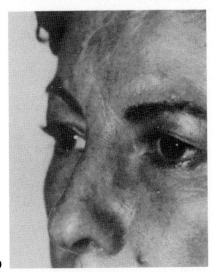
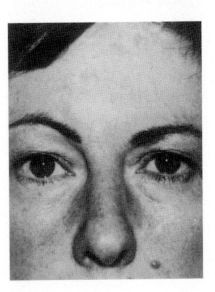

C,D

FIG. 4. A: A 52-year-old woman with a basal cell carcinoma of the dorsum of the nose. Note how high the frontal incision goes to avoid a dog-ear. **B:** After flap rotation and adjustment. **C,D:** Appearance 1 year postoperatively. (From Marchac, Toth, ref. 6, with permission.)

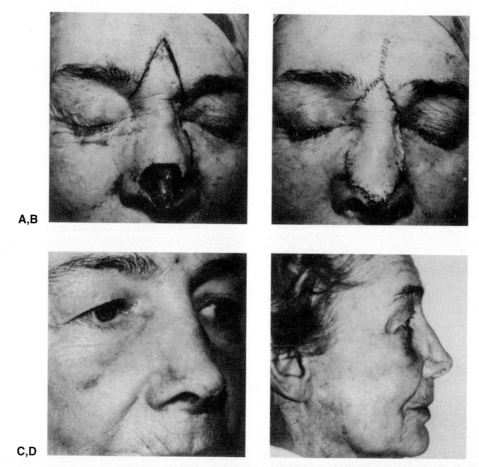

FIG. 5. A: After excision of a recurrent basal cell carcinoma on a 61-year-old woman, the flap has been incised. **B:** After rotation and adjustment. **C,D:** Two weeks postoperatively. There is moderate shortening. (From Marchac and Toth, ref. 6, with permission.)

The aesthetic results were excellent. The most visible scar was on the lateral side of the nose up to the inner canthus, mainly caused by the difference in skin thickness at this level. Some patients presented with occasional redness of the tip of the flap. Since the frontonasal flap comes down with no tension, bringing similar skin to the edge of the defect, the final lower scar is hardly visible, and there is no distortion.

SUMMARY

The axial modification of the fronto-nasal flap has expanded and refined its application in nasal defects.

References

1. Rieger RA. A local flap for repair of the nasal tip. *Br J Plast Surg* 1967; 40:147
2. Marchac D. Lambeau de rotation fronto-nasal. *Ann Chir Plast Esthet* 1970;15:44.
3. Marchac D, Al Khatib B. Les résultats à distance du lambeau fronto-nasal. *Ann Chir Plast Esthet* 1974;19:335.
4. Rigg BM. The dorsal nasal flap. *Plast Reconstr Surg* 1973;52:361.
5. Marchac D, Papadopoulos D, Duport G. Curative and aesthetic results of surgical treatment of 138 basal cell carcinomas. *J Dermatol Surg Oncol* 1982;8:379.
6. Marchac D, Toth B. The axial frontonasal flap revisited. *Plast Reconstr Surg* 1985;76:686.

CHAPTER 51 ■ FRONTOTEMPORAL FLAP

R. MEYER

This extremely versatile flap was introduced in 1952 (1) and was subsequently adapted by me for a variety of reconstructive functions in the middle third of the face as well as in the orbital and periorbital areas (2–9).

INDICATIONS

In experienced hands, the main advantages of the flap are (1) easy adaptability to the requirements of shape and structure of the recipient site, (2) good color match, and (3) inconspicuous scarring at the donor site. In my opinion, these advantages outweigh the fact that the procedure requires three stages.

With the addition of ear cartilage and split-thickness skin grafts to the flap, the tip, columella, septum, and ala can be rebuilt to reproduce the external shape and internal structures of the defect. The most frequent defect I have repaired with the frontotemporal flap is the loss of the tip and one ala caused by an animal or human bite, trauma, or tumor excision.

For repair of the tip, columella, and both alae, either the frontotemporal flap or a composite flap from the ear on a frontoparietal carrier flap is indicated (10–13). I have also found the frontotemporal flap adaptable for subtotal reconstruction of the nose.

FLAP DESIGN AND DIMENSIONS

The frontotemporal flap consists of two parts: a horizontal superciliary, or carrier, flap and a temporal portion that represents the composite part of the flap used to replace the missing structures at the recipient site. The carrier flap can be cut as narrow as 5 mm in the cutaneous layer, but by beveling the incision on both sides, a subcutaneous flap width of approximately 10 mm is possible.

A defect of the *entire ala* extending to the upper lateral cartilages, as well as to the lower border of the nasal bone, requires a broad triangular flap at the temple that has to be lined over nearly its entire inner surface.

The *lobulocolumellar loss* of tissue can include the anterior part of the septum with the lamina quadrangularis, in addition to the columella and the membranous septum. In such instances, the prefabrication at the temple must be composed of a three-layered quadrangular, rectangular, or trapezoidal plate destined to rebuild the septum, as well as of an anterior pillar simulating the columella and tip (Fig. 1).

In cases of loss of the *tip and one ala* as a result of animal or human bite, trauma, or tumor excision, I outline the flap at the temple in the shape of a crescent. On its concave side, a pocket is formed in the subcutaneous tissue and lined with a split-thickness skin graft. To obtain a prominent tip, the cartilage graft inserted in the very superficial subcutaneous pocket at the temple is shaped with a pronounced convexity.

For filling a defect limited to the *ala*, I usually choose a composite graft from the concha or the crus helicis of the ear. However, where I want to be absolutely sure that the consistency and color of the reconstructed part of the ala will be the same as the other nostril, I use the frontotemporal flap (Fig. 2).

For repair of the *tip, columella, and both alae*, the reconstructive complex at the temple has to be outlined as a flap in the shape of a trefoil, with a sheet of auricular cartilage extending into all three divergent lobes. Beneath each of the two lateral lobes, a pocket is formed and lined with a split-thickness skin graft.

OPERATIVE TECHNIQUE

Because the thin bridge flap between the glabella and the temple cannot be rolled, it is covered on its raw side with split-thickness skin graft (Figs. 1C and 2B,C). The superciliary defect can easily be closed by undermining the frontal skin. Multiple horizontal incisions in the frontal fascia may facilitate approximation, and deep anchoring sutures to the periosteum of the orbital rim minimize upward pull of the eyebrow. Since the suture line runs parallel to the wrinkle lines, an acceptable scar can be expected in most cases. Atraumatic technique and intradermal running sutures help to make the scar inconspicuous.

In the first stage, the part of the nose to be reconstructed is virtually prefabricated in the temporal area. Be it tip, ala, columella, anterior septum, or part or all of the four, the missing feature can be outlined, with or without the inner lining but practically always with cartilaginous support, and prepared with its inherent structures in the temporal area.

The cartilaginous support, which is taken from the auricular concha and has already been trimmed to the appropriate shape, is placed between the external skin and the vestibular lining in a superficial subcutaneous pocket at the temple. In a deeper pocket, I place a split-thickness skin graft that will provide the recipient site with vestibular lining. In cases of reconstruction of the tip and both nares, I prepare two independent pockets on each side of the outlined flap. These become the vaults of the two nares. Small split-thickness skin grafts are applied to these pockets and held in place with ointment gauze bolus dressings.

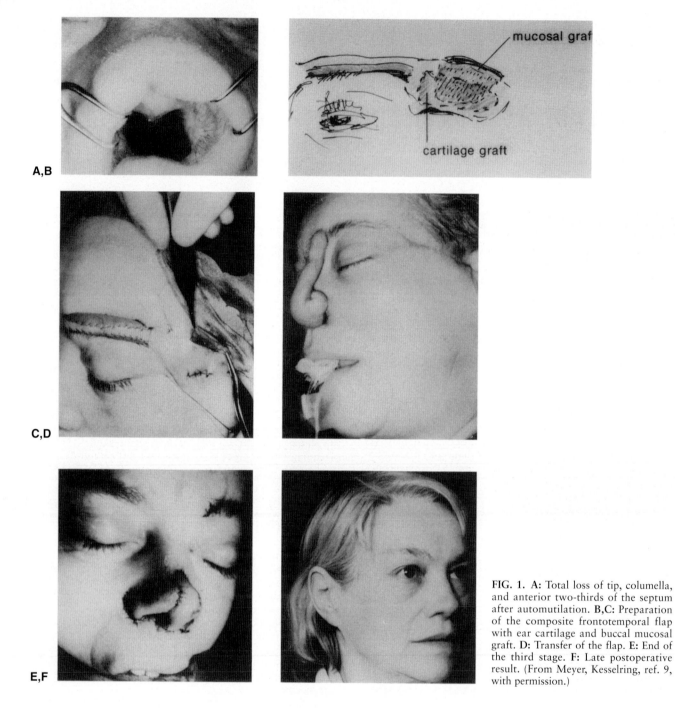

FIG. 1. A: Total loss of tip, columella, and anterior two-thirds of the septum after automutilation. **B,C:** Preparation of the composite frontotemporal flap with ear cartilage and buccal mucosal graft. **D:** Transfer of the flap. **E:** End of the third stage. **F:** Late postoperative result. (From Meyer, Kesselring, ref. 9, with permission.)

Two to 3 weeks later, the prefabricated tip–ala complex is transferred to the recipient site by means of the carrier flap. The pedicle is sectioned or occasionally used for retouches at the recipient site, in a third stage, another 2 to 3 weeks later.

Although the donor site in the temporal area can, on occasion, be closed primarily by advancement of the undermined skin edges, it is usually necessary to close the defect with a preauricular rotation flap. If there is persistent traction of the lids or a distortion of the temporo-orbital region, a supplementary correction can be performed during the third stage of the reconstruction.

A defect of the *entire ala* extending to the upper lateral cartilages, as well as to the lower border of the nasal bone, requires a broad triangular flap at the temple that has to be lined over nearly its whole inner surface. Thus a pocket deep

under the cartilage graft is developed and lined with a split-thickness skin graft (Fig. 3).

If only the *columellar and lobular skin* are lost, I use the composite graft mentioned earlier. However, such a graft would not be sufficient if the membranous septum is also involved, In the latter case, I prefer to perform the reconstruction using the frontotemporal flap, which is a simple, second bipedicle flap beside the superciliary carrier flap in the same direction.

When the *lobulocolumellar loss of tissue includes the anterior part of the septum,* with the lamina quadrangularis in addition to the columella and the membranous septum, the upper border of the nasal defect is incised in the midline in a second stage, and the wound margins, as well as both alae, are spread laterally to facilitate insertion of the compound flap

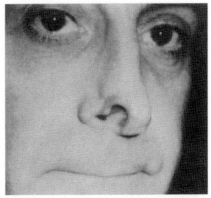
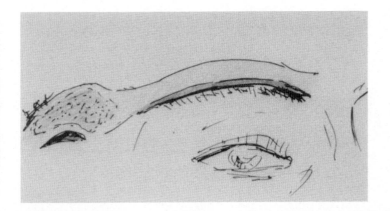

A,B

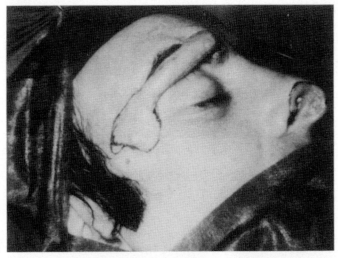
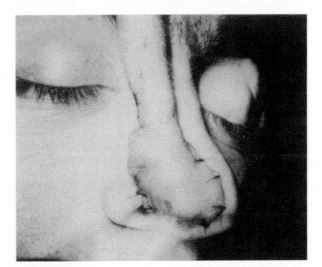

C,D

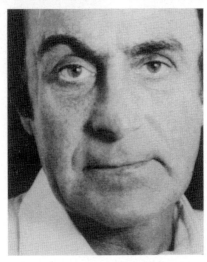

E,F

FIG. 2. A: Tip-ala defect after dog bite. B,C: Reconstructive complex in the right temporal region. D: Transfer of the flap. E: Early postoperative result. F: Late postoperative result.

into the nasal cavity. The anterior cut edge of the nostrils is sutured on both sides to the apicocolumellar pillar in a third stage. The level of this insertion will determine the appropriate triangular shape of the lower pyramid and the height of the nasal tip.

In nearly all cases of septocolumellar reconstruction, I have had to defat the septal component of the flap, which must be thick enough primarily to ensure a sufficient blood supply. Since it seems to be too broad at the end of the repair and represents a partial obstruction of the nares, the neoseptum

has to be narrowed by resection of subcutaneous tissue in a fourth stage.

The lining for the septal plate can be provided by mucosal graft from the cheek instead of a split-thickness skin graft to obtain a mucosal wall at least on one side. When a large amount of septal tissue has to be removed (as in the case of tumor) and the columellar skin can be left intact, a flap from the temple may be brought to the septum and interposed between the columella and the posterior edge of the perforating defect to push the tip and columella in an anteroinferior

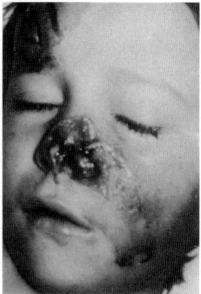 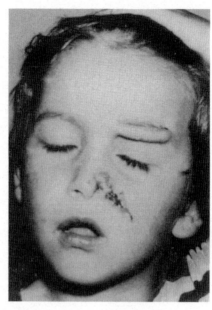 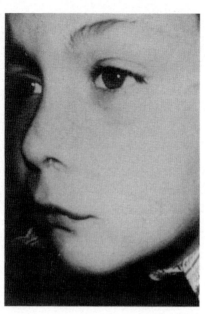

A–C

FIG. 3. **A:** Fresh dog bite injury in a child. **B:** Frontotemporal flap prepared after the first stage. **C:** Postoperative result. (From Mendelson BC, et al., ref. 13, with permission.)

direction. At a third stage, the divided carrier flap is inserted into the cavity to fill an eventual remaining septal defect. This procedure allows the construction of a desirable straight profile and prevents secondary retraction.

There are *sequelae of multiple rhinoplasties* in which progressive inelasticity from scarring of the covering tissues precludes the insertion of cartilage or bone grafts. I have had to enlarge the cutaneous cover and, for this purpose, choose the frontotemporal flap as the last resort for correction of such crucified noses. The temporal portion of the flap is shaped as a trefoil, similar to that used for tip-ala-columella defects. At a second stage, the scarred nasal skin is incised in the midline and spread to receive the flap. Since the scarred tissue at the recipient site has a poor blood supply, the pedicle should not be severed for 3 to 5 weeks.

For *subtotal reconstruction of the nose*, a trapezoidal flap is outlined on both temples at a first stage. It is reinforced with conchal cartilage graft and lined with a split-thickness skin graft. When the two frontotemporal flaps are detached from the temple at a second stage, they are transferred to the defect and form both lateral walls of the nasal pyramid. There they are sutured to the edge of the defect at the lateral border of the piriform aperture and also are sutured together in the midline. If the septum is present, as in most cases of subtotal loss of the nose, it will be incorporated as a supporting strut beneath the two joined flaps. One of the two superciliary carrier flaps is used at a third stage for building the missing columella and for giving a better contour to the dorsum of the nose. This three-stage procedure is valuable for subtotal repair, but it is not sufficient for total reconstruction of the nose.

SUMMARY

The frontotemporal flap can be used to reconstruct various types of partial nasal defects.

References

1. Schmid E. Ueber die Haut-Knorpel-Transplantationen aus der ohrmuschel und ihre funktionelle und aesthetische bedeutung bei der deckung von gesichtsdefektenn. *Fortschr Kiefer Gesichtschir* 1961;7:48.
2. Meyer R. Rekonstruktion der nasenfluegel mit zusammengestztem ohrmuscheltransplantat. *Monatsschr Ohrenheilkd* 1955;89:27.
3. Meyer R. Rinoplastica parziale con lembo frontale e frontotemporale. *Minerva Chir* 1960;15:1.
4. Meyer R. Die partielle ersatzplastik der nase. *Helv ChirActa* 1964;31:304.
5. Denecke HL, Meyer R. *Plastic surgery of the head and neck, vol. 1: corrective and reconstructive rhinoplasty.* New York: Springer-Verlag, 1967.
6. Meyer R. Total nasal reconstruction. In: Conley J, Dickinson JT, eds. *Plastic and reconstructive surgery of the face and neck.* New York: Grune & Stratton, 1972.
7. Meyer R. Nasal-septal perforation and nostril stenosis. In: Goldwyn R, ed. *The unfavorable result in plastic surgery.* Boston: Little, Brown, 1972.
8. Meyer R, Kesselring UK. Reconstructive surgery of the nose and orbit. In: Sisson GA, Tardy EM, eds. *Plastic and reconstructive surgery of the face and neck,* vol. 2. New York: Grune & Stratton, 1977.
9. Meyer R, Kesselring UK. Reconstructive surgery of the nose. *Clin Plast Surg* 1981;8:435.
10. Haas E, Meyer R. Konstruktive und rekonstruktive chirurgie. In: Gohrbandt E, Gabka J, Berndorfer A, eds. *Handbuch der plastischen chirurgie.* Berlin: W de Gruyter, 1968.
11. Washio H. Retroauricular-temporal flap. *Plast Reconstr Surg* 1969;43:162.
12. Orticochea M. A new method for total reconstruction of the nose: the ears as donor areas. *Br J Plast Surg* 1971;24:225.
13. Mendelson BC, Masson JK, Arnold PG, Erich JB. Flaps used for nasal reconstruction: a perspective based on 180 cases. *Mayo Clin Proc* 1979;54:91.

CHAPTER 52 ■ MIDLINE FOREHEAD SKIN FLAP (SEAGULL FLAP)

D. R. MILLARD, JR.

In ancient India, many centuries before Christ, the Kumas caste of potters cut forehead flaps for nasal reconstruction following punishment mutilations. Since then, there have been many modifications of the original design, but the seagull-shaped forehead skin flap has advantages that most of the other flaps do not enjoy.

INDICATIONS

The midline forehead skin flap (and its variations) can serve as cover for any nasal reconstruction from a severe tip and alae loss to a total nasal defect (1–4). Using this flap, an aesthetic and functional reconstruction can be achieved by creating a nose that blends well with the face and enjoys patent bilateral airways. It is important that the bridge and tip stand proudly, that the alae and columella contours are sculptured, and that the scars are unnoticeable. An advantage of the seagull-shaped forehead flap is that it is cut to cover regional units, thus hiding its tracks in light and shadows by camouflage.

ANATOMY

Since some glabellar and frontalis muscle fibers are included in this flap, it could be considered a type of musculocutaneous flap. Its main vascular supply is the supratrochlear bundle based on the medial aspect of one brow. The circulation to the distal portions of the flap is primarily random pattern.

FLAP DESIGN AND DIMENSIONS

The flap is best suited to a forehead of ample height (3 inches from brow to hairline). If the forehead is too narrow, the flap can be set at an oblique angle. The design is created with the body of the seagull placed in a midvertical position on the forehead (Fig. 1A). The tail, which is the base of the flap, is placed over one of the supratrochlear vascular bundles.

The wings are spread out perpendicular to the axis of the body along the natural transverse lines of the forehead. They are tapered at each end, and they are shaped wide enough to

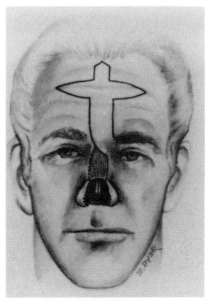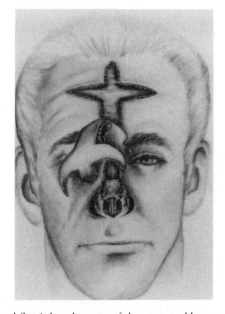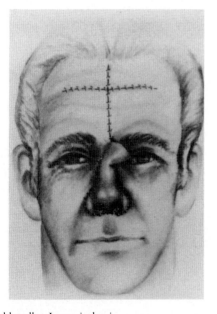

A–C

FIG. 1. **A:** The seagull-shaped flap is based on one of the supratrochlear vessel bundles. Its vertical axis is placed over the midline of the forehead, and the wings are designed to lie in natural transverse creases. **B:** Local flaps are turned over and carried down to septal support for lining. The forehead flap is elevated and transposed 180° to cover the new nose. **C:** The body of the seagull lies along the bridge, the wings curl at the alae and turn into the nostril sills, and the seagull head and neck area creates the tip and columella. Because tissue is taken from two planes, the donor site can be closed in a T.

construct alae and long enough to curl into the nostril floor as alar bases and nostril sills. The neck, head, and beak end of the flap are destined for the nasal tip and columella. When local tissue is used for lining, this specific seagull pattern serves as ideal cover in regional units for the bridge, tip, alae, and columella (Fig. 1B).

Designing the flap in both the horizontal and vertical axes reduces the amount of forehead taken in any one plane. This facilitates primary closure in an inconspicuous midline T scar (Fig. 1C).

OPERATIVE TECHNIQUE

Although the flap could probably be transposed without delay, a surgical delay by incisions is advocated. This can be accomplished when the local turnover flaps, which are usually based on scars, are delayed. If needed, an L-shaped septal chondromucosal flap can be advanced for support at this initial stage (see Chap. 69).

The local flaps used for lining are turned over and carried down to the septal support. The midline forehead skin flap is then elevated, transposed 180°, and sutured into position (Fig. 1B,C).

Division of the pedicle is safe after 3 weeks. As Sir Harold Gillies noted (5), division of the entire pedicle leads to edema

of the reconstructed nose. If the vascular supply is left intact, however, edema does not occur as readily. Therefore, only the skin portion is divided. Deep tissue is removed, if necessary, in order to preserve the vascular pedicle. The skin pedicle is transposed back to the glabellar area to reseparate the brows and to complete the bridge reconstruction as a unit.

SUMMARY

A midline forehead skin flap designed in the shape of a seagull is an excellent method of reconstructing both severe nasal tip losses and total nasal defects.

References

1. Millard DR Jr. Reconstructive rhinoplasty for the lower half of a nose. *Plast Reconstr Surg* 1974;53:133.
2. Millard DR Jr. Aesthetic aspects of reconstructive surgery. *Ann Plast Surg* 1978;1:533.
3. Millard DR Jr. Aesthetic reconstructive rhinoplasty. *Clin Plast Surg* 1981;8:169.
4. Millard DR Jr. Reconstructive rhinoplasty of the nose tip. *Clin Plast Surg* 1981;8:507.
5. Gillies HD. *Plastic surgery of the face.* London: Oxford University Press, 1920.

CHAPTER 53 ■ ISLAND FOREHEAD SKIN FLAP

R. V. ARGAMASO

The superiority of forehead skin for nasal reconstruction is unquestioned. For a full-thickness skin replacement of a sizable defect at the distal part of the nose, the island skin flap deserves practical consideration (1).

INDICATIONS

Distally, the skin of the nose is thick and contains numerous sebaceous glands. It drapes over the alar and upper lateral cartilages that support the lobule and give definition to the nasal tip. Full-thickness skin loss through trauma or disease results in a diminution of tip projection. Cicatricial contractures and secondary deformities from skin-graft replacement with poor color match and thickness can become sources of great embarrassment.

ANATOMY

A convenient pedicle for a forehead flap is supplied by the orbital branches of the ophthalmic artery. The supraorbital artery is a branch of the ophthalmic vessel as it crosses over the optic nerve. It exits with the supraorbital nerve through the supraorbital foramen and divides into superficial and deep branches. The supratrochlear artery, a terminal branch of the ophthalmic artery, leaves the orbit at its medial angle and ascends to the forehead near the midline.

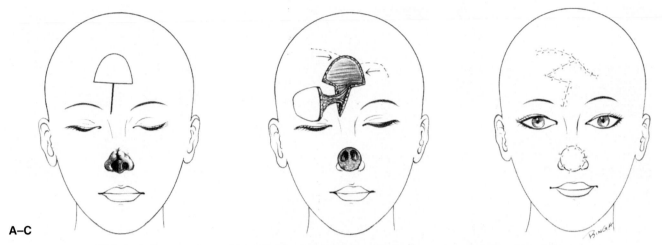

FIG. 1. A: Preoperative markings. **B:** Island pedicle incompletely dissected toward the origin of the supratrochlear artery. **C:** Flap inset and donor area closed. (From Argamaso and Bautista, ref. 1, with permission.)

These vessels anastomose freely with each other, with the frontal branch of the superficial temporal artery, and with vessels from the opposite side of the forehead. This rich network of anastomoses ensures an adequate circulation to a large skin island through a relatively narrow subcutaneous pedicle supplied by either one of these orbital arteries.

FLAP DESIGN AND DIMENSIONS

The vertical dimension of the donor area of the forehead should be of sufficient length to provide a flap for easy transposition and reach to the nasal tip. An outline of the nasal defect is drawn on paper and transposed downside-up to the forehead donor area. The size of the outline transferred to the skin is slightly exaggerated to increase the area, allowing for tissue shrinkage. Hair follicles are avoided.

Before the skin incision is made, a mock transfer is executed using a piece of gauze to simulate the pedicle. With the inferior portion fixed at the point of rotation, the gauze is turned to the nasal defect to test the extent of the arc of rotation.

From the midpoint of the inferior border of the skin island, a perpendicular line is drawn to the medial angle of the orbit in the direction of the supratrochlear artery. This line will represent the direction in which a superficial skin incision is made in order to develop the subcutaneous pedicle of the island skin flap (Fig. 1).

OPERATIVE TECHNIQUE

The superior and lateral borders of the skin island are deeply incised down to, but excluding, the galea. However, the inferior border is incised down to dermis only. This superficial incision is extended in a vertical direction to the medial orbital rim, following the skin marking. A subcutaneous pedicle approximately 2 cm wide is developed by sharp dissection and elevated from the underlying galea. The pedicle base is extended as closely as possible to the origin of the supratrochlear vessel as it emerges from the rim of the orbit.

The nasal dorsal skin is elevated through the forehead incision, creating a tunnel through which the island skin flap is introduced to reach the recipient site, where it is sutured in place. This tunnel should be wide enough to contain the pedicle without strangulating its vessels.

The forehead donor site is closed by widely undermining the forehead skin, rotating a flap from one side of the defect, and complementing it with an advancement flap from the opposite side (Fig. 2).

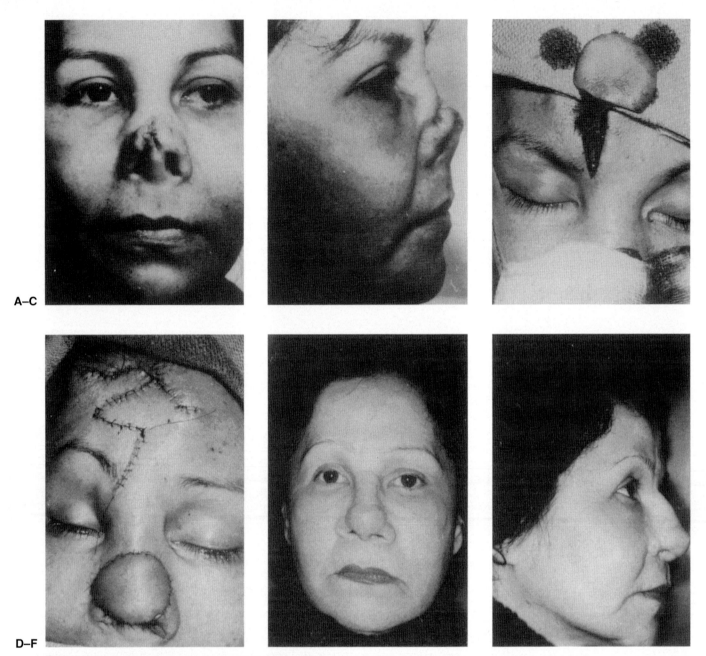

A–C

D–F

FIG. 2. **A,B:** A 45-year-old Filipina woman was referred for reconstruction of her nose. She had a history of multiple silicone injections for augmentation of her nasal dorsum three years previously. A year later, the skin of her nose became erythematous. Soon thereafter, despite surgical intervention, frank infection ensued, resulting in skin necrosis in the alar regions. Subsequently, the patient underwent several reconstructions that were complicated by infections and graft failures. These areas eventually healed with severe scarring. **C:** The scarred areas were excised and the skin defect was repaired with an island flap from the paramedian area of the forehead. **D:** Flap inset and donor site closed. **E,F:** The introduction of a subcutaneous pedicle on the dorsum of the bony pyramid of the nose elevated the overlying skin and obliterated the frontonasal angle. However, this drawback, inherent in the method, was welcomed by the patient, for it served to augment the low profile of her Asian nose. A small bone graft eventually was added to enhance the reconstruction. Scar revisions also were performed. (From Argamaso and Bautista, ref. 1, with permission.)

SUMMARY

An island skin pedicle flap of the forehead is a reliable and direct method for reconstruction of nasal defects. It offers tissue of similar texture and color to the skin of the distal portion of the nose.

Reference

1. Argamaso RV, Bautista BN. Partial and total nose reconstruction. *Phil J Surg Spec* 1981;36:17.

CHAPTER 54 ■ SUPRATROCHLEAR ARTERY (OFF-MIDLINE) FOREHEAD SKIN FLAP

I. K. DHAWAN AND N. C. MADAN

A forehead flap that is located to one side of the midline and that extends to the hairline recess can be based on one supratrochlear artery (1–4).

INDICATIONS

This flap can provide enough skin to cover the nasal tip and two-thirds of the alae and the columella.

ANATOMY

The supratrochlear artery is a branch of the ophthalmic artery, and it leaves the orbit at its superomedial aspect. In the forehead, it runs vertically, accompanied by its vein, into the hairline recess.

FLAP DESIGN AND DIMENSIONS

The base of the flap, that includes the supratrochlear vessels, is at the orbital margin, near the medial end of the eyebrow. The carrier segment is between 0.5 and 1.0 cm wide. When the flap is turned to cover nasal defects, the pivot point is at the lateral side of the base, and the flap arcs through 180°. The length of the flap depends on the height of the browline and the depth of the hairline recess. The paddle is designed to fit the defect and can be "flagged" to one side of the carrier segment. The position of the paddle is determined by the hairless skin available on either side of the vessels (Fig. 1).

OPERATIVE TECHNIQUE

The supratrochlear artery is marked preoperatively either by palpation or by use of a Doppler flowmeter. The flap is raised in the loose areolar plane above the periosteum down to the orbital rim, taking care not to damage the vessels at the base. The defect left by the carrier segment is closed in two layers, and that left by the paddle, if large, is covered by a postauricular full-thickness skin graft. The raw surface of the carrier segment is covered by a split-thickness skin graft, since it is too narrow to be tubed.

It is not advisable to carry the flap on a subcutaneous pedicle, since this leaves a ridge on the nasal bridge and produces venous compression and flap edema. The carrier

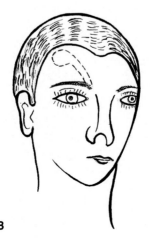
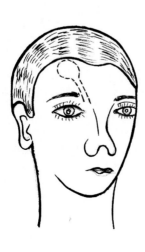

A,B

FIG. 1. **A:** The flap paddle may be "flagged" on one side if the artery is close to the hairline. **B:** Alternatively, the paddle may be placed uniformly on either side of the vessel. *(Continued)*

151

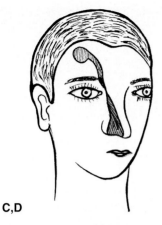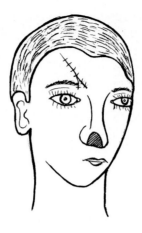

C,D

FIG. 1. *Continued.* **C:** For nasal defects, the arc of rotation is 180°. **D:** A small donor site defect can be closed by direct approximation of the wound edges, larger donor site defects may require a postauricular skin graft.

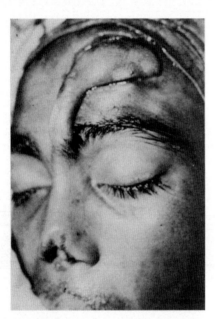

FIG. 2. A partial defect of the nasal tip, alae, and columella with the supratrochlear artery skin flap raised.

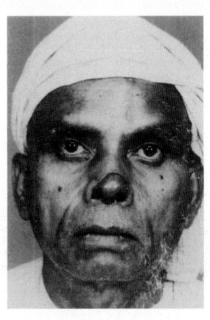

FIG. 3. Postoperative view of a patient.

segment is sectioned between 18 and 21 days, reinserting only the proximal portion as a triangle to restore eyebrow alignment.

CLINICAL RESULTS

The supratrochlear artery forehead skin flap has been used to repair 17 defects of the nose. There has been no loss of the flap, and it has provided well-matched skin of good texture. The defect has been satisfactorily reached, and the residual defect in the hairline recess has been minimal (Figs. 2 and 3). The flap is not suitable for reconstruction of the entire nose, nor can it be used in individuals with a very low hairline.

SUMMARY

An off-midline forehead flap based on one supratrochlear artery and vein has been described for reconstruction of partial nasal tip defects.

References

1. Dliawan IK, Aggarwal SB, Hariharan S. Use of an off-midline forehead flap for the repair of small nasal defects. *Plast Reconstr Surg* 1974;53:537.
2. Kazanjian VH. The repair of nasal defects with the median forehead flap: primary closure of the forehead wound. *Surg Gynecol Obstet* 1946;83:37.
3. Richardson GS, Hanna DC, Gaisford JC. Midline forehead flap: nasal reconstruction in patients with a low browline. *Plast Reconstr Surg* 1972;49:130.
4. Sawhney CP. Use of a longer midline forehead flap for rhinoplasty, with new design of closure of the donor site. *Plast Reconstr Surg* 1979;63:395.

CHAPTER 55 ■ AXIAL PARAMEDIAN FOREHEAD FLAP

G. C. BURGET

A vertical, axial paramedian forehead flap is the donor tissue of choice for nasal reconstruction. However, in some situations it is not ideal. It is thicker than the normal skin of the nasal dorsum, and when it is used to resurface this subunit it produces a greater aquiline hump than the original nose possessed. Because it is somewhat rigid, forehead skin is not an ideal replacement for the alar lobule. The soft skin of a nasolabial flap more easily forms itself into a blob, which resembles the normal convexity of the alar subunit. In children, the upper half of the forehead is covered with fine lanugo hairs. These hairs become thick when they are denervated causing the forehead flap nose to be fuzzy during the first year following reconstruction. Nevertheless, the paramedian forehead skin is the ideal replacement for nasal tip skin, and may be used successfully to restore any part of the nose.

ANATOMY

As shown by McCarthy and associates (1), vertical branches of the angular and supratrochlear arteries cross the superior orbital rim in the region of the wrinkle line that lies perpendicular to the corrugator muscle. They cross the orbital rim deep to the frontalis and corrugator muscles and rapidly enter the subcutaneous layer as they ascend the forehead. In the upper half of the forehead, many fine branches of the arteries lie in the subcutaneous fat close to the dermis. The entire frontalis muscle and some of the subcutaneous fat may be removed from the distal end of a paramedian forehead flap without injuring its axial arteries.

FLAP DESIGN AND DIMENSIONS

The many modifications of the forehead flap have been designed to increase its length, so that columellar defects may be covered, or to enlarge its surface area, so that the total nose may be resurfaced. Nonvertical variations, such as New's sickle flap or Gillies' up-and-down flap, deprive the forehead flap of its axial quality. Converse's scalping flap is large enough to cover the entire nose, but as the name implies, it increases the patient's morbidity. In truth, the classical vertical paramedian forehead flap will cover the entire nose from radix to columellar base without the necessity for extravagant variations or mechanical forehead tissue expansion.

After millennia of experience, new principles continue to emerge:

1. The flap is designed vertically and axially. This makes it vascularly robust, so that it may be radically thinned and depilated.
2. The base of the flap is made no wider than 1.5 cm for easy mobility without strangulation.
3. The base of the flap is positioned to include a branch of the angular-supratrochlear arteries, which is located with the Doppler pulse amplifier.
4. Additional length is attained by extending the flap's proximal end across the orbital rim or its distal end into the hair-bearing scalp.
5. The flap is not designed to fit the nasal defect, for the nasal defect, distorted by edema, scar contraction, and local injections, does not represent what is missing from the nose.
6. An exact three-dimensional pattern of nasal surface subunits taken from the contralateral normal side of the nose or from an ideal model is used as a template for the flap's design.
7. No marginal excess of skin is included when the flap is incised. This minimizes centripetal flap contraction, which obliterates surface contour.
8. Distal portions of the flap are thinned to the thickness of nasal tip skin and are depilated where necessary.
9. The base of the flap is excised and discarded, not replaced on the forehead.
10. The upper half of the donor defect is allowed to close by biologic wound contraction and forehead skin autoexpansion. There is no necessity for skin grafts, local flaps, or mechanical tissue expansion to close this secondary defect.

It requires the talents of a tailor to fashion a forehead flap. A flap cut too small collapses the cartilage framework of the nose. A flap cut too full allows centripetal contraction to pull the excess skin into a blob, obscuring nasal surface contour. The pattern for a made-to-measure forehead flap may be fashioned from heavy aluminum foil such as that used to pack sutures.

There is a strong impulse to make the flap fit the nasal defect, as Millard has said (2), "to fill the hole." However, the defect that exists at the time of nasal reconstruction does not reflect the amount of skin missing from the nose. It has been enlarged by edema and distorted by wound contraction and intraoperative lidocaine injections. The shape of the defect is not the shape nor size of the missing part of the nose. Therefore, one should turn to the remaining normal contralateral parts of the nose for a pattern. The nasal defect is sketched in mirror image with methylene blue dye on the normal contralateral side of the nose, which is undistorted by inflammation or injections. If the entire nose is missing, then a model of an ideal nose may be used to create a pattern for the flap. The defect may be

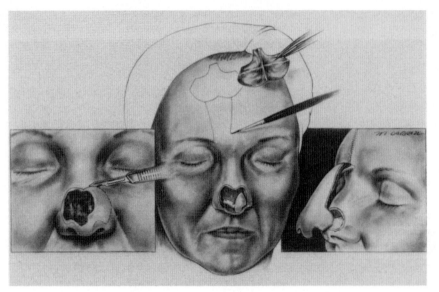

FIG. 1. It is sometimes wiser to replace an entire surface subunit with forehead flap tissue than merely to patch the hole. Here the remaining normal skin of the tip subunit is excised following the borders of the alar cartilages. A three-dimensional foil pattern is flattened to two dimensions and traced just below the hairline. No marginal excess skin is taken with the exact-pattern flap. As postoperative centripetal (trapdoor) contraction occurs, the bulge of the flap will not disrupt the surface contour but will, in fact, resemble the normal bulge of the nasal tip subunit.

enlarged to cover entire topographic surface subunits of the nose (Fig. 1), especially when convex regions such as the alar lobule, dorsum, hemitip, or tip subunits are to be replaced. A trapdoor contraction occurs in the transplanted forehead tissue and the bulge of the entire subunit comes to resemble the normal bulge of an ala, dorsum, hemitip, or tip.

The forehead flap is designed vertically to preserve its axial quality. Branches of the supratrochlear and angular vessels are located with the Doppler pulse amplifier, and the base of the pedicle is then centered on these vessels. This allows the proximal two-thirds of the pedicle to be designed very narrow without compromising its blood supply. Assured of an axial blood supply, the flap may be thinned and depilated and thus may include up to 1.5 cm of hair-bearing scalp tissue for replacement of the columella. If the flap is designed on an angle as slight as 15° off the vertical, it will cut across branches of the axial vessels, in which case thinning and depilation become risky. It is better to maintain the vascular robustness of an axial flap and obtain the needed flap length from the hair-bearing scalp than to gain length with an eccentric flap design. A vertical forehead flap in a non–cigarette smoker will easily bear the rough treatment of thinning and depilation, while an oblique random forehead flap may not be thinned and must therefore be applied to the surface of the new nose with all its redundant layers of tissue.

The pattern of the missing surface subunits is designed in three dimensions from the remaining normal side of the nose (or from an ideal model). After the exact location of vascular branches has been confirmed with the Doppler pulse amplifier, the pattern is flattened to two dimensions and traced with methylene blue near the hairline in axis with the supratrochlear vessels on the side of the nasal defect. A 1.5 cm columellar extension of hair-bearing scalp may be included distally.

OPERATIVE TECHNIQUE

The base of the pedicle is traced 1.2 to 1.5 cm wide, and no wider, to allow axial rotation (twisting) without strangulation. The proximal two-thirds of the pedicle may be quite narrow and then expand suddenly to incorporate the pattern. When the flap is incised, the cuts are made on the inside of the blue lines so that not even a half millimeter of excess skin is included. In its distal 2 cm, the flap is elevated superficial to the frontalis muscle. Proximally, the frontalis muscle is elevated off the periosteum with the pedicle to protect the axial vessels. If extra length is needed, corrugator muscle fibers are

divided using magnifying loupes so that vascular branches are preserved while restricting bands of muscle are released. If the flap still proves short, then the pedicle is extended across the orbital rim, including a bit of the eyebrow if necessary. Again, it is helpful to mobilize the pedicle by dividing corrugator muscle fibers while preserving vascular branches.

After the flap is elevated, its borders and its distal 2 cm are thinned using curved Joseph's scissors. Hair follicles remaining in the distal part of the flap are clipped off with fine scissors under 2.5× magnification. During the thinning, axial branches of the supratrochlear-angular arteries visible in the subcutaneous tissue very close to the dermis are preserved. During thinning close attention is given to the nasal defect, since some of its regions require more subcutaneous tissue than others, and the flap may be thinned accordingly. The thinned flap is transported to the nasal defect. Right-sided flaps rotate clockwise; left-sided flaps rotate counter-clockwise. Key sutures fix the flap in position. Fine sutures adjust its edges.

Suturing may be done in such a way as to enhance nasal contour. At the junction of the upper lip, the cheek, and the alar groove, the flap is pulled inferiorly before the key stitch is placed (3). This forces the alar tissues to bulge in a normal convexity and stretches the tissues of the lateral side wall so that they do not bulge. A no. 19 suction drain may be placed under the forehead flap and hooked to a vacuum tube. The negative pressure created pulls the various layers of the nose together during the postoperative phase.

The secondary forehead defect continues to vex surgeons. It has not been generally recognized that the forehead is a forgiving donor surface. Although frequently it cannot be closed with sutures, nevertheless, skin grafts, local flaps, or mechanical tissue expanders are not needed. In fact, they compound the deformity and increase patient morbidity. The forehead defect that remains after local advancement of tissues will close biologically by the process of wound contraction and forehead autoexpansion. These processes require neither further incisions, pain, hospitalization, inconvenience, nor expense. They are performed without compensation by the myofibroblasts. Any frontalis muscle remaining in the donor defect is removed. Then the forehead and scalp surrounding the donor site are elevated from the periosteum of the frontal bone for 7 cm bilaterally and superiorly. Two to four heavy simple sutures tied under moderate tension pull the limbs of the defect together. These key sutures are placed close to the wound edge to minimize their stitch marks, since they will remain in place for 10 days. Distal dog-ears are excised laterally and superiorly. The limbs of the defect are closed in layers. Exposed periosteum in the central open region of the donor wound is protected from desiccation with petrolatum gauze and ointment. No contraction occurs in the open defect for about 3 weeks. Then, during the fourth and fifth postoperative weeks, the wound rapidly contracts, autoexpanding the adjacent skin and producing a surprisingly forgiving result. Mechanical tissue expansion, local rotation or advancement flaps with their necessary scars, or the postage-stamp application of a skin graft is unnecessary. These adjunctive procedures actually increase patient discomfort, scarring, or contour deformities.

The raw posterior surface of the forehead pedicle may be left open. However, a thin split-thickness skin graft applied to the back of the flap minimizes the problems of an open wound and the need for postoperative office visits. The patient is instructed not to place spectacles on the flap, but rather to suspend them from the forehead. A commercially available device known as Frame-Ups (Arox Company, P.O. Box 24740, Los Angeles, CA 90024) allows the weight of the spectacles to rest on the cheeks. Nearly all skin sutures are removed between the second and fourth postoperative days. The incisions are supported with 1/8-inch-wide skin tapes. The several key tension-bearing forehead sutures remain until the tenth day, but since they have been placed close to the skin edge, their stitch marks are minimal. The petrolatum gauze is removed from the open donor wound around the fifth postoperative day. After that, a small bandage is kept over the defect until closure occurs in the fifth postoperative week.

Postoperative complications of flap necrosis have been rare, except in patients who smoke cigarettes. Long-term cigarette smoking appears to affect the arterial circulation of the forehead skin. Even cessation of smoking for several weeks before surgery does not seem to change the vascular frailty of the skin flap. In operations on patients who smoke, the Doppler pulse amplifier is used to identify and trace the course of distinct axial vessels for inclusion in the forehead pedicle. Patients who have had facial radiation therapy for acne or hair removal many years before are also likely to have wound problems. Patients with rhinophyma or numerous comedones are at high risk for infection. In these patients, the use of benzoyl hydroxide and antibiotics preoperatively is helpful. In severe cases, a preliminary dermabrasion of the forehead and nasal skin is done to reduce sebaceous hypertrophy or the cystic nature of the skin.

An Intermediate Operation

In complex reconstructive cases, it is helpful to elevate the flap at an intermediate stage and shape the underlying tissues. In 1974, Millard (4) advocated leaving the pedicle in place while making

adjustments to the nasal contour. At such an intermediate operation, the entire forehead flap is lifted off the subsurface framework of the nose but remains attached along the nostril margin and at the columella distally, as well as to its pedicle proximally. The elevated flap is thinned, additional cartilage grafts are added to the nasal framework as necessary, and the subsurface structures are shaped to create an ideal nasal contour. In general, such an intermediate operation has been necessary only in large restorations that involve more than half the nose.

Excision of the Pedicle

Twenty-one days after the nose was assembled, the skin pedicle is excised and discarded. If it were replaced on the forehead, it would remain permanently as a visible lump. Because of its narrow design, the pedicle may be excised without fear that the eyebrows will be pulled together. Sufficient glabellar skin remains to ensure satisfactory eyebrow separation. The proximal stump of the pedicle is thinned of fat and frontalis muscle. It is inset as a small inverted V 8 to 10 mm high, just medial to the eyebrow. The distal part of the flap has an increased vascular efficiency that allows it to be elevated off the nasal defect for 1.5 cm caudally. The cephalic portion of the nasal flap is thinned, and the underlying nasal defect shaped to an ideal contour. Then the transplanted forehead skin is trimmed to size and inset along the superior edge of the nasal defect. The nasal flap, made rigid by subcutaneous scar, is subject to postoperative hematoma and resultant abscess. For this reason, loosely tied quilting or basting sutures of 5–0 or 6–0 material are placed through the flap to cause the donor skin to adhere to its recipient bed. These sutures are removed within 48 hours. This has proven more effective than a vacuum drain placed beneath the flap.

A CLINICAL CASE

One case is presented to demonstrate how lining flaps and hard-tissue grafts combine in one stage to form a subsurface architecture over which a thin forehead flap is fitted to create the visual impression of a nose. The patient (Fig. 2) was a 39-year-old woman who had a deeply invading basal cell carcinoma excised and was referred for immediate reconstruction. There had been a full-thickness loss of the right nasal ala and hemitip and a more superficial loss of parts of the left hemitip, nasal dorsum, and right lateral side wall.

The first of three surgical stages was undertaken on the day following surgical excision. At this first operative sitting, the nasal lining sleeve was assembled, a framework of hard-tissue

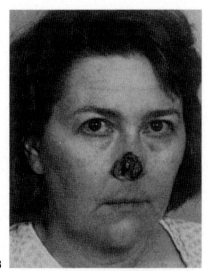
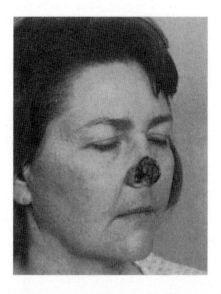

A,B

FIG. 2. A,B: A basal cell carcinoma has been excised resulting in loss of the right hemitip and parts of the left hemitip, dorsum, right side wall, and right ala.

grafts was fused to its submucosal surface, and a forehead flap was tailored and fitted over the framework.

The Nasal Lining Sleeve

Thin, flexible, vascular nasal lining flaps are in short supply. Thick lining flaps of skin and subcutaneous fat, such as nasolabial flaps, are readily available, but they bulge inward and outward, destroying the nasal airway and the nasal shape. Nasal lining flaps with poor vascularity, such as marginal turnover flaps, may themselves survive but will not nourish the primary cartilage grafts required to impart contour and support to the rebuilt nose. Rigid lining flaps, such as the composite grafts of skin and cartilage placed under a forehead flap weeks before it is formed into a nose, become stiff and maintain whatever form they have assumed while on the forehead. The shape of the new nose is then dictated by these preplaced lining grafts. The only nasal lining flaps that are at once thin, supple, and highly vascular are intranasal flaps from the vestibule, the middle vault, and the nasal septum.

The present case demonstrates the use of such ideal lining material. A bipedicled flap was designed on the nasal lining just above the margin of this patient's defect (Fig. 3). The flap, 8 mm wide by 2.5 cm long, had its medial base at the membranous septum where the medial and lateral crura of the alar cartilage meet. The lateral base of the flap was located on the nostril floor, just behind the alar base. The flap, with an attached fragment of alar cartilage, was freed with blunt scissors dissection from the overlying skin and nasal subcutaneous tissue.

The junction of the lateral and medial cartilaginous crura was divided preserving the bridge of vestibular skin, which was the medial base of the flap. As this supple ribbon-like strip of tissue was brought down to the level of the nostril margin, it formed folds and kinks. Nevertheless, it was a robust flap that could support the primary cartilage grafts needed to splint the nostril margin and create the normal contour of a nasal tip and an alar lobule.

A secondary lining defect then existed above the nostril margin flap. A second lining flap, of contralateral mucoperichondrium based on the dorsum of the septum and presumably receiving branches of the ethmoidal arteries, was employed to line the middle nasal vault. (The ipsilateral mucoperichondrium was reflected caudally and posteriorly.) The exposed cartilage and bone of the septum were left attached to the contralateral mucoperichondrium in this case, but they might safely have been removed and replaced as a free graft. The contralateral mucoperichondrial lining flap was incised on three sides but remained attached along the septal dorsum. It was then hinged laterally and sutured to the lateral edge of the piriform aperture, as first described by DeQuervain (5).

The cartilage remaining attached to this flap was scored vertically so that the flap could be arched into a vault for the nasal airway (see Fig. 5). When sutured together with 5–0 catgut, the two lining flaps created a highly vascular, thin, and pliable lining sleeve. Such a lining sleeve will provide neither rigidity nor contour to the new nose until primary grafts of cartilage carved to resemble specific nasal topographic subunits are fused to its submucosal surface. The technique employed in the present case, using ipsilateral and contralateral septal flaps, results in a

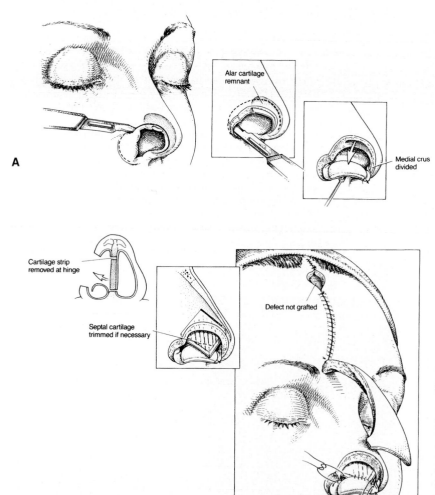

A

B

FIG. 3. A,B: The lining sleeve is assembled from a bipedicled alar margin flap mobilized from just above the defect and a composite flap of septal cartilage and contralateral mucoperichondrium. This results in a septal fistula. Primary bone and cartilage grafts added to this thin, supple, and highly vascular lining will give it rigidity and a nasal shape. The vertical paramedian forehead flap is custom-fitted to the internal hard-tissue scaffold and thinned until it is no thicker than normal nasal tip skin. (From Burget, ref. 8, with permission.)

septal fistula. Although careful follow-up of many such fistulae has found that they become self-cleaning and asymptomatic, nevertheless, another lining technique is now preferred for small unilateral full-thickness losses of the lower part of the nose.

Using the new technique (Fig. 4), the entire anterior septal mucoperichondrium, designed as a flap with a narrow pedicle just over the nasal spine, can be employed as lining for the nasal vestibule and alar margin. Such a flap consistently survives if it is based on a 1.3-cm pedicle located in a zone between the anterior plane of the upper lip and the lower edge of the piriform aperture—the zone containing the septal branch of the superior labial artery. The flap may extend from the nasal floor below to the level of the medial canthus above and posteriorly to the ethmoid perpendicular plate.

Here are details of the technique (Fig. 4). The entire anterior septal mucoperichondrium is injected with 1:50,000 epinephrine solution, and after a few minutes, it is elevated off the septal cartilage and bone. The flap is designed with a septal component and bipedicled component, which give it the shape of a hatband (the bipedicled portion) into which a press card (the septal portion) has been stuck. When pivoted into position and fixed there with 5–0 catgut sutures, this oddly shaped flap lines the new vestibule of the nose. The exposed cartilage and bone of the septum are removed as in a submucous resection. The contralateral septal perichondrium remains exposed in the donor defect and soon covers itself with transitional epithelium.

This two-component flap lines the lower one-third of the nose without creating a septal fistula.

A Shapely and Rigid Chassis

The flimsy vestibular lining sleeve is converted into a composite flap (Fig. 4). Cartilage and bone grafts are carved with precision to mimic in microform the shapes of the surface subunits of the nose. When these contoured grafts are fused to the submucosal-perichondral surface of the lining sleeve, they cause it to expand, become stiff, and take on an ideal nasal shape (reduced by 2.5 mm in all dimensions) (Fig. 5). The lining sleeve depends on the grafts for its rigidity and shape; the grafts depend for their life on contact with the vascular lining. It is the shape of this fabricated composite flap that gives normality or beauty to the final visual impression. Four different hard-tissue grafts are required for a major nasal restoration: a strut, a buttress, a brace, and a batten. Each piece serves to fix the underlying mucosal lining in position. Each piece imparts a shape to a specific surface subunit of the nose.

Here is how the internal scaffold was constructed:

1. *The columellar strut.* Cartilage from the wall of the concha measuring 4 mm by 3.5 cm was removed through an anterior incision. This graft material was formed into

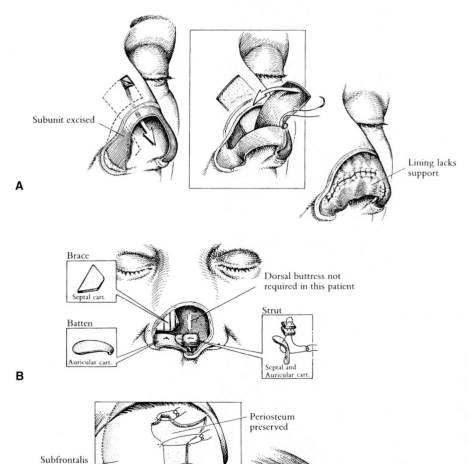

FIG. 4. A–C: An alternate method for assembling lining is the use of the septal pivot flap. A rectangular septal mucoperichondrial component and a bipedicled nostril margin component are both based medially on a pedicle containing the septal branch of the superior labial artery. As they pivot forward, the exposed cartilage and bone of the septum are removed for graft material. The contralateral septal perichondrium is left bare in the donor site. Three of the four hard-tissue grafts were used in the present case. Each graft was modeled to resemble in microform a nasal surface subunit.

a new alar arch incorporating the columellar-lobular rotation angle of 50°. The strip of cartilage was sutured to the stump of the medial crus. Then it was scored, bent, and sutured to the submucosa of the new right vestibular dome and to the medial crus of the normal contralateral alar cartilage. A piece of septal cartilage was shaped into a small chamfered tip graft measuring 4 × 9 mm and sutured in an appropriate position to give optimal tip projection. It is not surprising that this whole complex resembles the umbrella graft described by Peck (6), for it serves an identical purpose.

2. *A flying buttress for the nasal bridge.* A piece of septal cartilage may be needed to supply a replacement for the lower nasal bridge. It acts as a flying buttress between the distal septum and nasal tip to prevent snubbing of the nose. In the present case, the nasal bridge was intact, and a flying buttress was not necessary.

3. *A brace for the middle vault.* There must be a continuous sheet of hard tissue extending from the nasal bones down to the nostril margin to prevent the biologic force of wound contraction from notching the alar margin upward. In the present case, the necessary brace of septal cartilage was left attached to the contralateral septal flap as it hinged laterally. It could have been removed

safely, carved, and replaced on the lining sleeve in order to prevent collapse of the middle vault or upward contraction of the nostril rim.

4. *An alar batten.* Much as a thin strip of wood stiffens a sail, a thin, curved strip of cartilage stiffens the alar margin against constriction, collapse, or upward notching. In the present case, a strip of chonchal wall cartilage was carved to resemble the convex alar lobule subunit and was fastened along the lower edge of the lining sleeve from the alar base to the apex of the new nostril.

When complete, the bone and cartilage scaffold of the nose enveloped the mucosal lining sleeve, stood erect by itself, felt rigid to the touch, and had the external shape of a normal nose, although it was somewhat smaller (Fig. 5). An axial paramedian forehead flap was designed to fit over the internal framework of the new nose like a tailor-made garment. As described earlier in this chapter, the flap was thinned, depilated, and sutured into position. The gaping upper one-third of the forehead donor site healed by biologic wound contraction over a 6-week period. Twenty-one days after the nose was assembled, the pedicle was excised. Ten months later, a single operative revision was done (Figs. 6 and 7; see Fig. 8 for result four months after secondary revision).

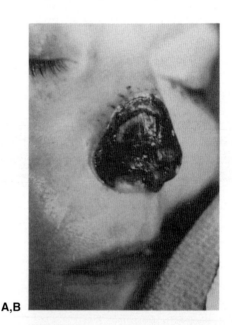
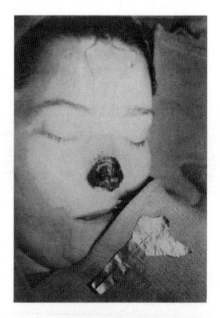

A,B

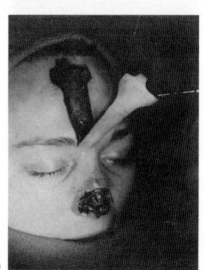
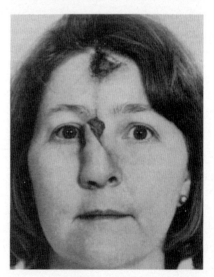

C,D

FIG. 5. A–D: The subsurface nasal architecture is complete. It is rigid and has the desired nasal shape reduced in all dimensions by 2.5 mm. An exact-pattern axial forehead flap is incised on the forehead on the inside of the methylene lines. The distal 2 cm of the flap are radically thinned and depilated. The upper one-third of the donor site heals by biologic wound contraction.

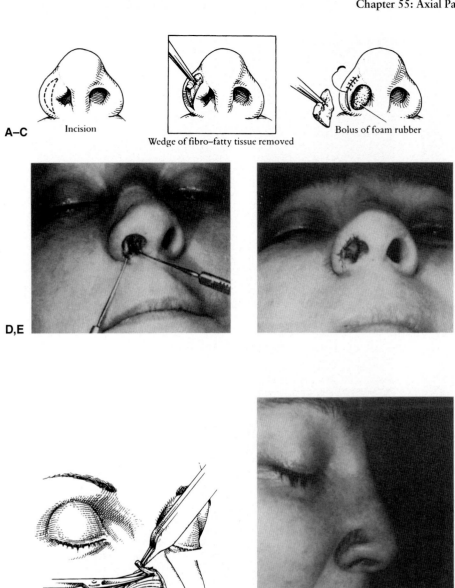

A–C

Incision

Wedge of fibro–fatty tissue removed

Bolus of foam rubber

D,E

FIG. 6. A–E: Ten months after pedicle division, a secondary revision was done. The nostril margin was thinned by excising a wedge of fibrofatty tissue. No skin should be excised unless the alar margin is to be elevated. (From Burget, ref. 8, with permission.)

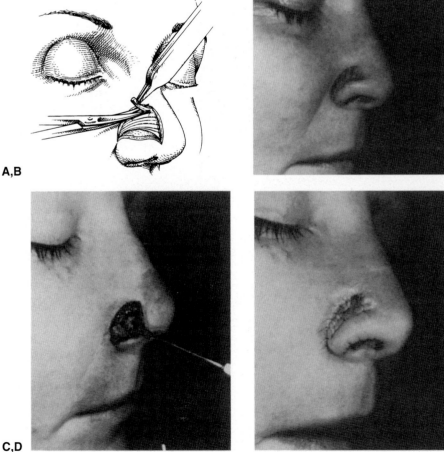

A,B

C,D

FIG. 7. A–D: At the revisionary operation, the forehead flap tissue was elevated and the underlying fibrofatty layer was shaped by excising thin strips of tissue. Loosely tied mattress sutures were employed to hold the flap in its contoured bed. (From Burget, ref. 8, with permission.)

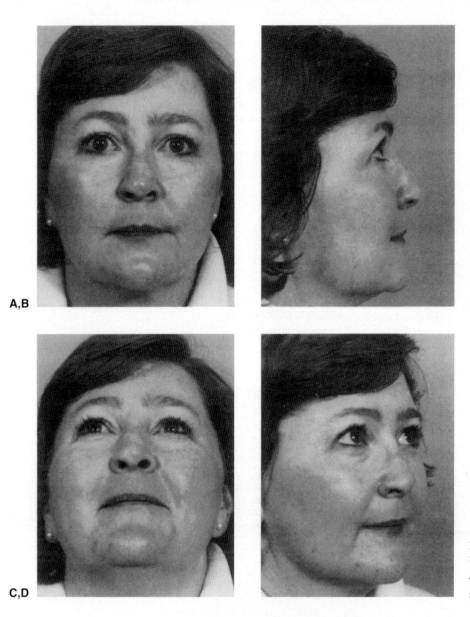

A,B

C,D

FIG. 8. A–D: Final photographs taken 4 months after the secondary revision and 15 months after the nose was assembled. The patient wears no makeup on her nose.

SUMMARY

A reconstructed nose is nothing more than a lump of transplanted tissues. The contoured surface of the lump reflects lines and patches of light and casts lines and patches of shadow. If a plastic surgeon respects the principle of subunits, and is assured of proper contour by the creation of a modeled hard-tissue chassis on thin, compliant, vascular lining, and anticipates the inexorable force of the myofibroblasts, and is guided by careful measurement and a good eye, he or she can cause this modeled lump of transplanted tissues to impart from the outset the visual impression of a nose.

References

1. McCarthy JG, Lorenc ZP, Cutting C, et al. The median forehead flap revisited: the blood supply. *Plast Reconstr Surg* 1985;76:866.
2. Millard DR. Preface to Aesthetic aspects of reconstructive surgery. *Clin Plast Surg* 1981;8:164.
3. Garst WP. Personal communication, 1976.
4. Millard DR. Reconstructive rhinoplasty for the lower half of the nose. *Plast Reconstr Surg* 1974;5:33.
5. DeQuervain F. Veber partielle seitliche rhinoplastik. *Zentrabl Chir* 1902;29:297.
6. Peck G. *Techniques in aesthetic rhinoplasty.* New York: Gower, 1984; 153–163.
7. Millard DRM. Numerous personal communications, 1969–1977.
8. Burget GC. Aesthetic restoration of the nose. *Clin Plast Surg* 1985;12:463.

CHAPTER 56 ■ SCALPING FOREHEAD FLAP

J. G. MC CARTHY

EDITORIAL COMMENT

This is one of the best techniques for total nasal reconstruction. The editors caution the surgeon to have all preliminary reconstructions completed, so that the only defect left to reconstruct is the nose itself. The skin-grafted defect left in the forehead may be eliminated with tissue expansion of the forehead at a later time.

The scalping forehead flap, described by Converse in 1942 (1,2), represents the logical extension of the classical (Indian) forehead flap in nasal reconstruction. This flap satisfies requirements for length and, in addition, delivers a large area of forehead skin of satisfactory color and texture match for nasal reconstruction.

INDICATIONS

The scalping flap is a reliable technique for reconstructing large nasal defects. The flap skin is supple enough to be folded to recreate the lobular portion of the nose. The flap design provides the desired length for reconstruction of the columella, and the reconstructed nose thus has adequate size and projection.

The main disadvantage of this flap is the residual forehead donor defect. This is easily camouflaged in females, however, by an appropriate hairstyle. The skin graft can be reduced in size by serial excision or by replacement with local skin transferred either as a Schimmelbusch (3) or Juri (4) flap.

ANATOMY

The forehead scalping flap includes the forehead skin, the scalp and galea, and a major portion of the vasculature of the forehead and anterior portion of the scalp.

The frontalis muscle, the galea, and their overlying integument are vascularized by an extensive anastomotic network from the supraorbital, supratrochlear, and superficial temporal vessels (Fig. 1). All these vessels, with the exception of the superficial temporal system on the ipsilateral side of the flap, ensure a rich blood supply to the flap.

The venous drainage is remarkably efficient. The supraorbital veins, which run superficial to the frontalis muscle, communicate with the anterior branch of the superficial temporal vein. The superficial temporal vein drains the upper portion of the flap into the posterior facial vein. The supraorbital vein joins with the supratrochlear vein at the medial angle of the orbit to form the angular vein.

The frontalis muscle, which is not included in the flap (see Fig. 5), is a thin quadrilateral muscle intimately adherent to the superficial fascia. Its vertically oriented fibers are pale in color. The medial margins, joined above the root of the nose, gradually diverge from each other, leaving a muscular gap in the central portion of the forehead.

FLAP DESIGN AND DIMENSIONS

In planning the procedure, the surgeon must first define the nature and extent of the nasal defect to be resurfaced by the flap. A wool or flannel cloth pattern of the defect is made and transferred to the lateral aspect of the selected side of the forehead. In the male with a receding hairline, the donor area on the forehead should be positioned as far laterally as possible to camouflage the donor site when the patient's full face is observed.

It must be emphasized that if the residual stump is that of a large nose, its size should be reduced, because it is technically simpler to build a smaller nose than a large one (Fig. 2). When the lobular portion of the nose, including the columella and alar rims, is to be replaced, the distal end of the flap is folded on itself (see Fig. 10). Consequently, the working portion of the flap should be of sufficient size to allow such a degree of flap fashioning.

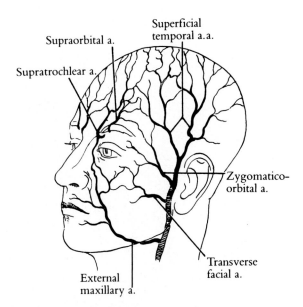

FIG. 1. Blood supply of the forehead. Most forehead flaps are axial-pattern flaps based on the superficial temporal, supraorbital, and supratrochlear vessels. (From Converse, ref. 8, with permission.)

161

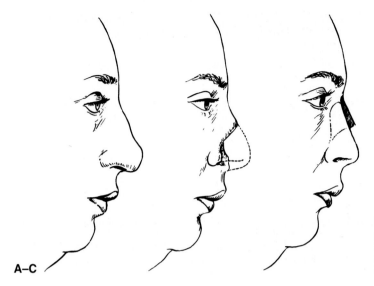

FIG. 2. Reduction of the residual nasal stump prior to subtotal nasal reconstruction. If the nose was large prior to amputation (**A**), it is advantageous to reduce the projection of the residual stump (**B**) to facilitate nasal reconstruction (**C**). (From Converse, ref. 8, with permission.)

While the shape of the pattern had been roughly triangular in the past (narrower above than the wider distal portion), a rectangular design has been employed in recent years.

When reconstructing the lobular portion of the nose, it is a good rule to be able to advance the flap to the lower lip without tension in order to have a columella of adequate length and a nasal tip of sufficient projection (Fig. 3).

While the lining flaps maybe multiple in origin, the covering cutaneous flap should ideally restore the entire aesthetic unit. In resurfacing the nose, the surgeon should strive to design the flap so that it extends from the most distal portion of the nasal tip and the borders of the alae to the root of the nose. This is especially important along the dorsum of the nose, where a transverse junction line (scar) between the flap and the dorsal skin is obvious. The junction scars between a central flap and the adjacent lateral aspect of the nose (or cheek) are less conspicuous.

Occasionally, it is necessary to resect the skin over the tip of the nose or a unilateral alar remnant in order to reconstruct a satisfactory aesthetic unit. The distal end of the flap can be folded on itself to give a satisfactory lobule and alar rim (usually after a secondary defatting procedure).

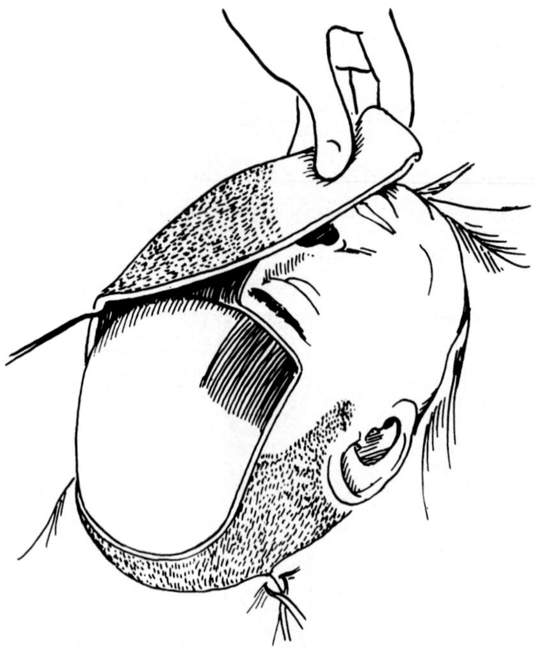

OPERATIVE TECHNIQUE

First Stage

An outline in ink should extend approximately 2 mm beyond the border of the pattern to allow for slight shrinkage of the detached flap. The forehead or donor portion of the incision extends through the skin and subcutaneous tissues, sparing the frontalis muscle (Fig. 4).

A plane of dissection is established between the light-colored fibers of the frontalis muscle and the donor forehead skin (Fig. 5). Avoidance of a local anesthetic solution with epinephrine is helpful, since the solution tends to blanch the underlying muscle and make its identification more difficult. It is imperative that the frontalis muscle not be raised with the flap, since its preservation on the forehead provides expressive movements to the skin graft and gives more satisfactory donor-site contour.

When the area of junction with the frontalis muscle and the galea is reached, the latter is incised and the remainder of the flap is raised along the plane between the galea and the pericranium (Fig. 5).

The incision extends in a cephalic direction from the lateral border of the skin flap that has been dissected from the frontalis muscle. The flap incision is continued posteriorly to the level of a line extending across the scalp from the tip of one auricle to the apex of the contralateral helix (coronal incision; Fig. 4A). The incision is then extended along this line and across the midline to a point usually at the superior pole of the opposite helix. In this way, the incision preserves the contralateral superficial temporal vessels. Laterally, the temporal fascia is raised with the flap. The dissection is carried caudally to a point above the nasofrontal angle medially and the supraorbital arches laterally, care being taken to preserve

FIG. 3. To reconstruct the tip of the nose, columella, and alae, the flap must be sufficiently long to reach the lower lip prior to inserting. (From Converse and McCarthy, ref. 2, with permission.)

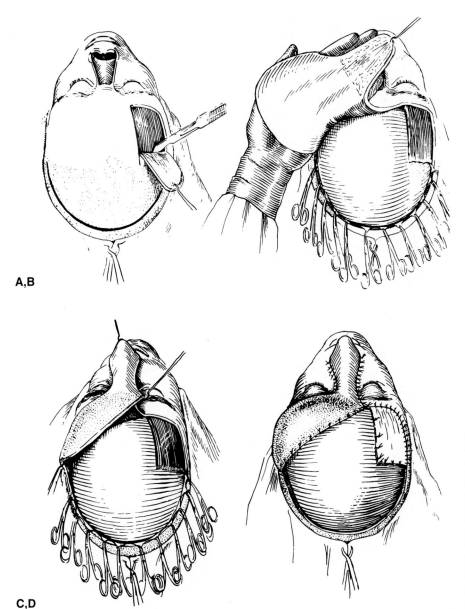

A,B

C,D

FIG. 4. The scalping forehead flap (1). **A:** The working portion of the flap represents forehead skin that is elevated superficial to the frontalis muscle. Note that the incision within the scalp extends across the calvaria on a line between both auricular helices. **B:** The carrier portion of the flap is elevated at the subgaleal level. **C:** The flap is transferred to the nasal defect. **D:** The donor defect is resurfaced with a full-thickness skin graft, either at the time of the initial procedure or at the second stage (division of flap). The pericranium is covered with a Telfa dressing. (From Converse and McCarthy, ref. 2, with permission.)

the supratrochlear and supraorbital vessels, as well as the supraorbital nerve (Fig. 4C). A large flap that can be folded on itself without tension or twisting is raised.

It has been my experience that the larger the scalp portion of the flap, the easier is its return to the original site over the calvaria. Once the flap pedicle is folded on itself, it requires little postoperative care. A small raw area between the flap and its attachment to the nose can be covered by a dressing or a

small upturned flap from the root of the nose. This area requires cleaning with a cotton-tipped applicator whether it is left uncovered or is resurfaced with a small flap.

The donor defect is resurfaced with a full-thickness skin graft, which is taken either from the postauricular region or from the supraclavicular area if the defect is large. The quality of the healed skin graft is superior when the grafting technique is deferred until the second stage.

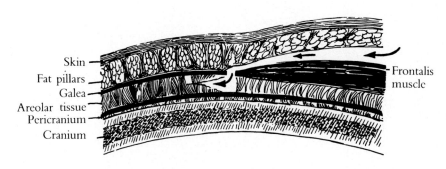

Skin
Fat pillars
Galea
Areolar tissue
Pericranium
Cranium

Frontalis muscle

FIG. 5. The working portion of the flap (forehead skin) is elevated superficial to the frontalis muscle (*arrows*). The carrier portion is raised at a deeper level (deep to the galea).

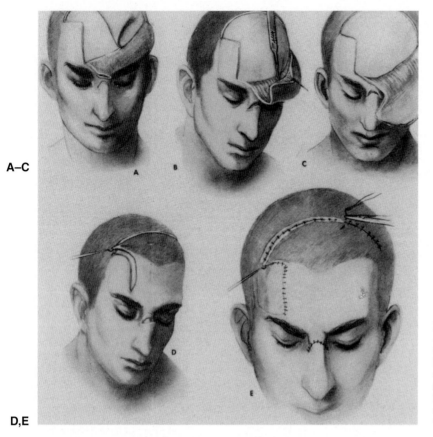

A–C

D,E

FIG. 6. The second stage (division of the flap). **A:** The temporary dressing (Telfa, skin allograft, or porcine xenograft) is removed after the flap has been divided at the appropriate level at the root of the nose. **B:** The flap is then unfolded by simple incising. **C:** The flap is then distended to its former size. **D,E:** The flap is returned and sutured to the posterior scalp border. (From Converse, ref. 8, with permission.)

Second Stage (Flap Division)

The flap is usually divided and returned to the calvaria between the fourteenth and eighteenth days (Fig. 6), unless the nasal recipient site is poorly vascularized, such as after radiotherapy. Further delay renders the task of approximating the margins of the flaps to the edge of the coronal incision a difficult one.

At the time of division and final inset of the flap, it is essential that the pedicle be divided at a level that will leave sufficient flap tissue to resurface the more cephalic portion of the nasal defect.

Secondary Defatting Procedures (Fig. 7)

Earlier attempts at nasal reconstruction resulted in noses that were smaller in volume than desired, because adequate nasal lining had not been provided. With the passage of time, there was a shrinkage of the reconstructed nose. In his 1920 text (5), Gillies stated: "The author had recognized that all noses must be skin lined, but on digesting Keegan's written work, one was absolutely convinced that this was the right principle" (6,7).

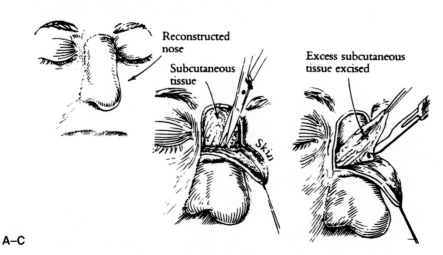

A–C

FIG. 7. **A–C:** A major portion of the flap can be incised and elevated, and the undersurface defatted, in order to give a more sculpted appearance to the nose. (From Converse, ref. 8, with permission.)

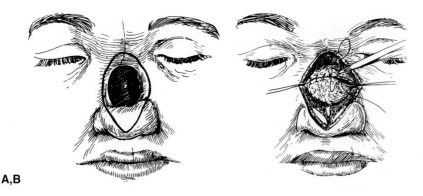

FIG. 8. Local turnover flaps for nasal lining. **A:** Outline of flaps. **B:** Following elevation, closure is accomplished with absorbable sutures.

A common mistake in the past had been to line a forehead flap with a skin graft in order to furnish a lining, as in subtotal nasal reconstruction. The skin graft caused stiffness of the flap and difficulty in adapting the flap to the shape of the nose. Another major disadvantage was the technical difficulty in finding a surgical plane of cleavage between the flap and skin graft in order to insert a bone or cartilage graft for skeletal support in subtotal nasal reconstruction.

Lining should therefore be provided by flaps—preferably local turnover flaps (Fig. 8). If the latter are not available, a median forehead flap with a subcutaneous pedicle is an alternative method of providing lining (Fig. 9). Infolding of the distal aspect of the flap provides a nasal tip and columella with vestibular lining (Fig. 10).

I prefer to reconstruct the nose by first restoring cutaneous coverage and lining, waiting until postoperative edema has subsided, and furnishing skeletal support at a later stage. In many situations (especially smaller defects), there is no need for skeletal support. If the bony structures (platform) in the root of the nose are present, cantilever bone grafting is the method of choice (Fig. 11). However, if the bony platform has been destroyed, a cartilage graft removed from the core of a costal cartilage is the preferred technique for achieving nasal skeletal support.

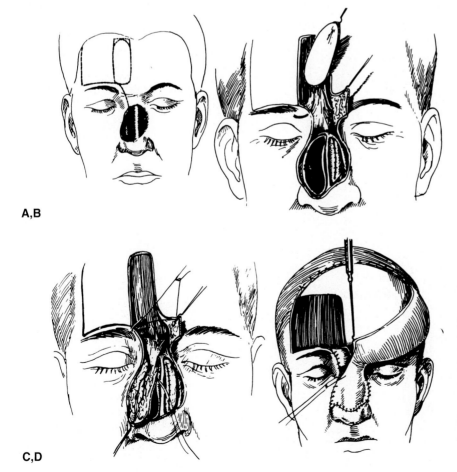

FIG. 9. Reconstruction of a full-thickness defect of the nose by a combination of a scalping flap and an island forehead flap. **A:** Respective positions of the forehead flaps, which will provide the covering and the lining tissue. **B:** The island flap is raised on a subcutaneous pedicle. Mucous membrane from the septum provides lining tissue over the left nasal fossa. **C:** The island flap furnishes the lining for the remainder of the defect. **D:** The scalping flap transfer is being completed. (From Converse, ref. 9, with permission.)

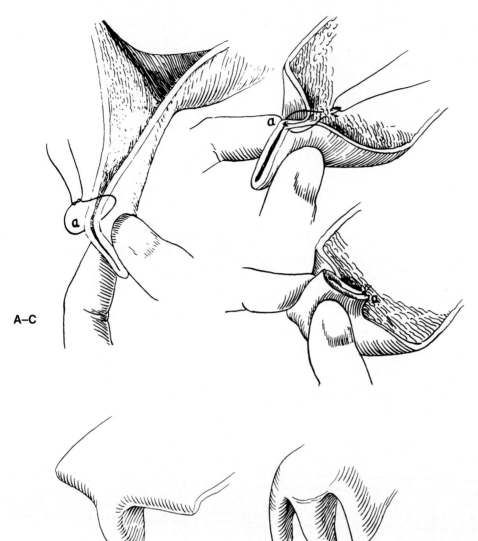

A–C

D,E

FIG. 10. Reconstruction of the nasal tip, columella, and alar rims with the distal portion of the scalping forehead flap. **A:** A suture (*a*) is inserted in the distal portion of the flap. **B:** The suture (*a*) is then placed through a more proximal portion of the undersurface of the flap. **C,D,E:** In this way, the nasal tip, columella, and alar rims are reconstructed. (From Converse, ref. 10, with permission.)

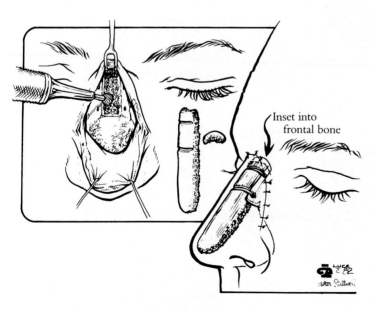

Inset into frontal bone

FIG. 11. Cantilever insert bone graft (ilium) maintained by wire fixation to the bony stump.

SUMMARY

The scalping flap is a reliable technique for providing a relatively large area of forehead skin of satisfactory color, texture, and thickness for resurfacing nasal defects.

References

1. Converse JM. New forehead flap for nasal reconstruction. *Proc R Soc Med* 1942;35:811.
2. Converse JM, McCarthy JG. The scalping forehead flap revisited. *Clin Plast Surg* 1981;8:413.
3. Schimmelbusch C. Ein neues verfahren der rhinoplastik und operation der sattelnase. *Verh Dtsch Ges Chir* 1895;24:342.
4. Juri J, Juri C, Cerisola J. Contribution to Converse's flap for nasal reconstruction. *Plast Reconstr Surg* 1982;69:697.
5. Gillies HD. *Plastic surgery of the face*. London: Oxford University Press, 1920.
6. Gillies HD. The development and scope of plastic surgery. *Northwest Univ Bull* 1935;35:1.
7. Keegan DR. *Rhinoplastic operations, with a description of recent improvements in the Indian method*. Paris: J. Baillere, 1900.
8. Converse JM, ed. *Reconstructive plastic surgery*, 2nd ed. Philadelphia: Saunders, 1977.
9. Converse JM. Clinical applications of the scalping flap in reconstructive surgery of the nose. *Plast Reconstr Surg* 1969;43:247.
10. Converse JM. Reconstruction of the nose by the scalping technique. *Surg Clin North Am* 1959;39:335.

CHAPTER 57 ■ RETROAURICULAR-TEMPORAL FLAP

H. WASHIO AND V. C. GIAMPAPA

The retroauricular-temporal flap can be used to transfer tissues from behind the ear for reconstruction of limited defects of the nose, forehead, cheek, and lower eyelid (1,2).

INDICATIONS

Available donor tissue should be carefully weighed against the size of the defect. The procedure is not recommended for patients with known vascular problems, such as arteriosclerosis, hypertension, or uncontrolled diabetes. It is also not indicated for elderly or obese patients. Two retroauricular-temporal flaps can be elevated at the same time. This flap also can be used in conjunction with other local flaps, such as a forehead flap.

ANATOMY

There are ample anastomoses between the superficial temporal artery and the retroauricular (postauricular) artery (Fig. 1A). By incorporating these two vessel systems in a temporal scalp flap, a flap has been designed that can be elevated without delay.

FLAP DESIGN AND DIMENSIONS

The superficial temporal and retroauricular arteries are identified with a Doppler flowmeter. Selection of points *A*, *B*, *C*, and *D* in Fig. 1A is the key. Point *A* is the point around which the entire flap turns; it is a fixed point just in front of the anterior end of the helix and behind the superficial temporal artery.

The next step is the selection of point *C*. For the flap to reach a defect, line *AC* must be approximately half the length of the distance between point *A* and the defect. In an average-sized adult, the nose is about 14 cm away from point *A*. This means that for nasal reconstruction, line *AC* will have to be approximately 7 cm in length. To avoid injury to the superficial temporal artery and also to facilitate effective design of the flap, line *AC* is directed 10° to 15° posteriorly from an imaginary vertical line drawn through point *A*.

The selection of point *B* is important, since line *AB* forms the base of the pedicle. The length of line *AB* should be about 8 cm, and angle *CAB* should be about 60°. Ordinarily, one can select this point near to or at the hairline. Obviously, this is not possible in an individual who is bald or has a receding hairline.

Point *D* is marked in such a way that the two triangles *ABC* and *DBC* are symmetrical (Fig. 1A,B) and form a rhombus *ABDC*. The advantage of having this rhombus is that the raw surfaces of the two triangles will rest on each other when the flap is transferred, thus eliminating this raw surface (Fig. 1C).

The margin for the rest of the flap is drawn in a curve from point *D* in order to include the retroauricular vessels and the postauricular skin (Fig. 1A).

OPERATIVE TECHNIQUE

The outer incision of the flap is made first. It is essential to include the galea aponeurotica in the flap. Then the postauric-

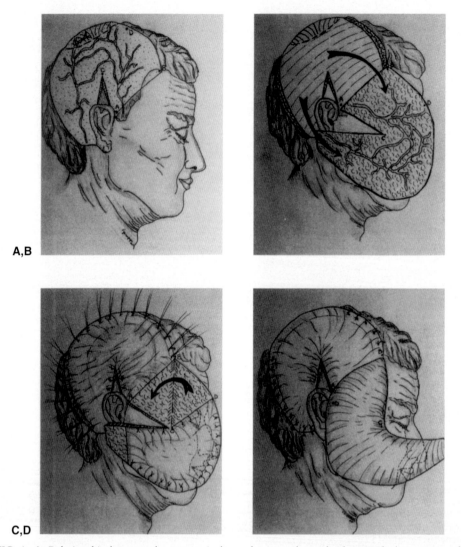

A,B

C,D

FIG. 1. **A:** Relationship between the retroauricular and temporal vessels along with the position of key points in the flap. **B:** Elevation of the flap. The central cut *AC* should be made last while looking directly at the major vessels through the galea on the underside of the flap. **C:** The raw surfaces are covered with a split-thickness skin graft. The two triangles *ABC* and *DBC* will fold onto each other. **D:** Transfer of the flap.

ular skin is incised and elevated. The central cut *AC* is made last under direct vision. Major branches of the artery can be identified easily by looking through the translucent galea from underneath (Fig. 1B).

Hemostasis is accomplished by electrocoagulation and direct suture. The raw surfaces of the flap donor site and the flap are covered by split-thickness skin grafts (Figs. 1C and 2D).

The next step is preparation of the recipient area. This is the time to add additional structural support or to rearrange the tissues of the recipient area. Any attempt to do this after the flap has been transferred is not recommended. The flap is then transferred and sutured securely in place (Fig. 2D). The thickness of the flap will allow sharp bending along lines *AB* and *BC* without compromising the circulation. However, any undue tension on the flap must be avoided. Elevation and transfer of the flap are carried out in one stage.

The flap is divided between 7 and 14 days, depending on the size of the raw surface of the recipient site. The carrier portion of the flap is then returned to its donor area.

CLINICAL RESULTS

There was one tip necrosis in a series of 16 patients. This was believed to be due to arterial spasm subsequent to an attempted arteriogram. There was one case of infection of the scalp after the flap was returned to the donor site.

SUMMARY

The retroauricular temporal flap can be used without a delay to reconstruct areas of the face using the skin and cartilage from behind the ear.

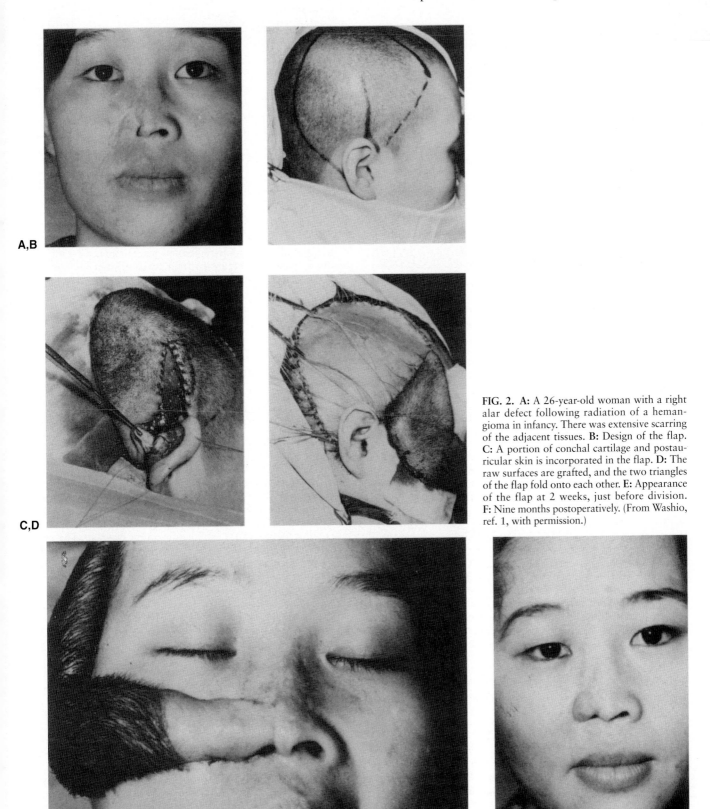

A,B

C,D

E,F

FIG. 2. A: A 26-year-old woman with a right alar defect following radiation of a hemangioma in infancy. There was extensive scarring of the adjacent tissues. **B:** Design of the flap. **C:** A portion of conchal cartilage and postauricular skin is incorporated in the flap. **D:** The raw surfaces are grafted, and the two triangles of the flap fold onto each other. **E:** Appearance of the flap at 2 weeks, just before division. **F:** Nine months postoperatively. (From Washio, ref. 1, with permission.)

References

1. Washio H. Retroauricular-temporal flap. *Plast Reconstr Surg* 1969; 43:162.

2. Washio H. Further experiences with the retroauricular-temporal flap. *Plast Reconstr Surg* 1972;50:160.

CHAPTER 58 ■ TEMPOROPARIETAL FASCIAL FLAP FOR NASAL RECONSTRUCTION

G. H. SASAKI

EDITORIAL COMMENT

This chapter presents another source of tissue for reconstruction of the ala nasi. Obviously, it is not a first or second choice. If used at all, it would be most applicable for patients with male pattern baldness.

An axial subcutaneous fascial flap based on the superficial temporal vessel and its major branches has provided an alternative method for reconstruction of full-thickness defects of the ear and anterior upper half of the face (1–3). The development and use of this flap for nasal reconstruction are logical extensions of its potential.

Stimulated by Corso's demonstration (4) of a paucity of venous drainage within the terminal areas of arterial branching, I have modified the design of the axial subcutaneous fascial flap to achieve both a longer pedicle and improved viability.

INDICATIONS

Nasal defects can often be reconstructed from local tissue sources. However, further experience will determine the reliability and applicability of the temporoparietal fascial flap for these defects. Advantages of this flap include (1) transposition of a well-vascularized, thin, and pliable flap that accepts grafts on either side as needed, (2) reconstruction in a single stage, and (3) transposition of tissue outside the area of trauma, radiation, or tumor.

Potential difficulties with this flap are (1) variability in vascular distribution, (2) paucity of venous drainage, (3) inadequate pedicle length, and (4) loss of hair at the donor site.

ANATOMY

From injected cadaver dissections, the temporoparietal fascia appears to represent a distinct, separate layer superficial to both the fascia of the temporalis muscle and the contiguous galea aponeurotic extensions superior to the crest of the temporal fossa. At the level of the condylar process of the mandible, the superficial temporal artery passes between the mandibular condyle and the external auditory canal and then insinuates over the zygomatic arch to lie on the temporoparietal fascia. Within the confines of anatomic variation, the main superficial temporal artery divides at the level of the apex of the ear into its frontal and parietal branches. Further cephalad, the parietal segment generally divides into two or three terminal branches (Fig. 1).

In injected and noninjected specimens, the main superficial temporal artery and its frontal and parietal branches can be visualized easily from the level of the tragus to about 12 cm in a cephalad direction. At about 14 cm, the terminal branches of the parietal segment take a more superficial route, blending into the subdermal plexus. Further dissection to create a vascularized paddle of subcutaneous fascia may be unsafe unless deep dermis is incorporated into the fascial flap. Venous collaterals coursing parallel with the arteries or within the arterial domain of the flap can be identified easily.

FLAP DESIGN AND DIMENSIONS

The course of the superficial temporal artery and its major tributaries is traced by Doppler probe to achieve a flap of sufficient length to reach the nasal defect (Fig. 2). At about 12 cm above the tragus, a mark is made to designate the unsafe level for dissection. The axis of rotation is taken at a pivot point in the preauricular fold anterior to the tragus. In general, a flap 15 to 16 cm in length which may accept grafts on either surface and/or incorporate a skin paddle can be elevated. The arc of rotation provides sufficient length to reconstruct a nasal defect on the contralateral side extending from the radix to the lobule.

OPERATIVE TECHNIQUE

The initial incision is made along the preauricular fold in a cephalad direction, following the course of the selected arterial branch whose arc of rotation is best suited for the defect. This incision is terminated at a level about 12 cm above the tragus.

Dissection and undermining of the preauricular skin and scalp flap are begun proximally, staying in a plane immediately over the major vessels to expose the subcutaneous fascial tissue and the easily visualized major tributaries of arteries and veins.

Measuring cephalad a distance of 12 cm above the tragus from this point, a dermal paddle (or skin paddle in a bald zone) is designed on the scalp to provide an adequate pedicle length and a suitable template for the nasal defect. At this point, the incision around the paddle is made to the level of the dermis. Starting from the inferior border of the paddle, the dissection is carried cephalad in a plane either in the deep dermis or just as deep as hair follicles of the dermis. The level of dissection depends on the depth of the underlying vessels.

The temporoparietal fascia is now divided at the level of the tragus on each side of the pedicle, which is at least 2.5 cm

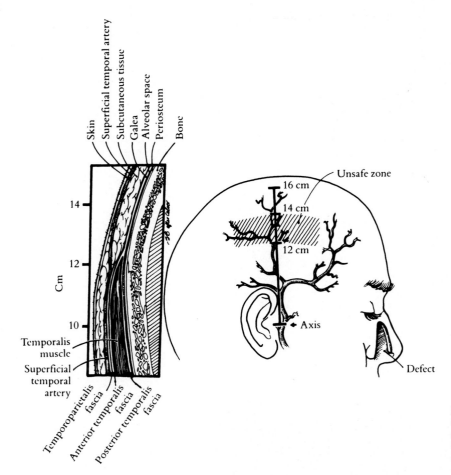

FIG. 1. Schematic representation of the superficial temporal artery and its main frontal and parietal branches in relationship to the distinct temporoparietal fascia and the galea aponeurotica.

across. The fascial flap is then elevated with relative ease off the anterior fascia of the temporalis muscle and more cephalad, superficial to the pericranial tissues and deep to the galea aponeurotica (Fig. 3). Every attempt must be made to incorporate as many venous channels as possible within the flap to facilitate drainage.

After a large subcutaneous tunnel at the axis of the flap is created to the nasal defect, the flap is passed unhindered and may be lined or covered with simple or composite grafts as needed. Alternatively, the flap paddle may be prelined with grafts 4 to 6 weeks prior to transfer. The donor wound is approximated primarily over closed suction drainage.

CLINICAL RESULTS

The temporoparietal fascial flap has been used in four patients with nasal defects of durations ranging from 2 months to 2 years. The vascularized fascial flap has provided stable coverage, allowing a suitable graft for cover or lining (with or without cartilaginous support) to suit the defect.

The full-thickness nasal deformities included one subtotal nasal loss and three partial lobular defects. Immediate skin grafting for cover and lining was performed in three patients, while the remaining patient is shown in Fig. 4. In this patient, a 5-mm rim of ischemia was noted at the reconstructed alar margin, but it resulted in no loss of tissue or exposed cartilage.

Moderate hair loss was noted at the donor site in two of three patients, but this presented no significant cosmetic problem. Sensation to the ear was preserved in all patients.

SUMMARY

Partial nasal reconstruction can be accomplished in a single stage using the temporoparietal fascial flap.

FIG. 2. Schematic depiction of the axial subcutaneous fascial flap, indicating the axis of rotation, the unsafe zone of dissection, and the distal dermal segment, with the potential for incorporation of a skin paddle in the design.

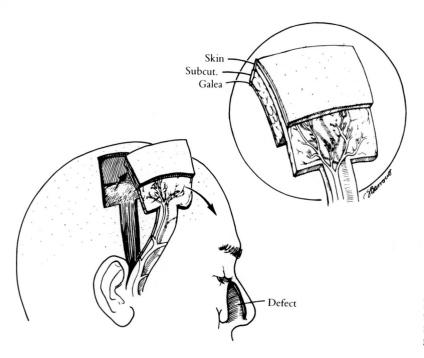

Skin
Subcut.
Galea

Defect

FIG. 3. Schematic drawing of the flap elevation off the anterior fascia of the temporalis muscle and, more cephalad, the pericranial tissue deep to the galea aponeurotica.

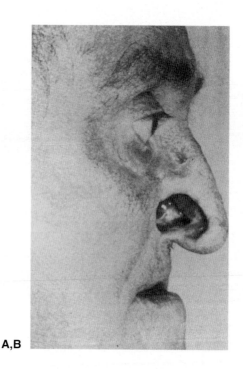
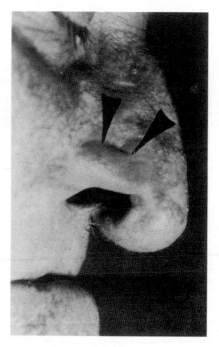

A,B

FIG. 4. A: A 2.5 × 3.0 cm defect after full-thickness resection of the reconstructed ala and entire cartilaginous septum and partial excision of the ipsilateral primary palate and upper lip for persistent basal cell carcinoma. A forehead flap had been used in a previous reconstruction, and another basal cell carcinoma had been removed in the area of the right nasolabial fold. A conchal-cutaneous graft from the ear was allowed to mature for 6 weeks under a skin paddle in a bald spot based on the parietal branch of the superficial temporal artery. **B:** Reconstruction at 1 year postoperatively using prelined conchal-cutaneous ear graft transposed on the fascial flap through a subcutaneous pocket. *Arrows* indicate the cephalad border of the conchal graft under the skin paddle taken from a bald spot.

References

1. Tegtmeier RE, Gooding RA. The use of a fascial flap in ear reconstruction. *Plast Reconstr Surg* 1977;60:406.
2. Byrd HS. The use of subcutaneous axial fascial flaps in reconstruction of the head. *Ann Plast Surg* 1980;4:191.
3. Kernahan DA, Littlewood AHM. Experience in the use of arterial flaps about the face. *Plast Reconstr Surg* 1961;28:207.
4. Corso PF. Variations of the arterial, venous, and capillary circulation of the soft tissues of the head by decades as demonstrated by methyl methacrylate injection technique, and their application to the construction of flaps and pedicles. *Plast Reconstr Surg* 1961;27: 160.

CHAPTER 59 ■ REVERSED SUPERFICIAL TEMPORAL ARTERY POSTAURICULAR COMPOUND SKIN AND CARTILAGE FLAP

M. ORTICOCHEA

EDITORIAL COMMENT

The principle of reversal of flood described in this chapter, both arterial and venous, has taken on considerable importance over the past several years, both in this and other sites of the body. The innovative technique of nasal reconstruction is a relatively complicated one, and the goal might be achieved more simply with some of the other techniques described.

The three anatomic structures of skin coverage, nasal framework, and nasal lining can be found in the external ear. The retroauricular skin and that of the mastoid region will cover the nasal surface. The conchal cartilage and, occasionally, a long, thin portion of the mastoid and temporal bone will provide the framework. The thin skin firmly adhering to and covering the lateral surface of the cartilage of the conchal cavity will form the internal lining of the reconstructed nose.

INDICATIONS

Bilateral reversed superficial temporal artery postauricular compound skin and cartilage flaps can be used for total nasal reconstruction (1–4). The advantages are that coverage, lining, and framework can be provided at the same time. The skin is the same color, texture, and thickness as that of a normal nose. The patient can breathe normally, since the nostrils are of a good size.

The ears from which the conchae have been removed keep their normal shape, size, and appearance and are only slightly flatter than normal. Replacement of the concha by a skin graft does not change its cosmetic appearance.

ANATOMY

The technique depends on the transfer of each concha on a flap with its base on the temple and including the superficial temporal vessels. To make this feasible, the natural flow of blood in these vessels must be reversed.

This is accomplished by dividing the vessels in front of the ear and transplanting the cut end into the substance of the flap behind the ear (see Fig. 4). The retrograde blood supply then comes from the natural anastomoses with the branches of the

ophthalmic vessels in the lateral forehead (supraorbital, supratrochlear, and lacrimal).

This principle of reversal of blood flow is applicable to many flaps in facial and body reconstruction and makes new flap designs possible.

FLAP DESIGN AND DIMENSIONS

The flap base must be fairly high in the frontal area to ensure sufficient flap length. Otherwise, there may be difficulty in bringing the concha far enough to reconstruct the alae, nostrils, and columella. Vascular impairment of the upper pole of the remaining portion of the ear may occur if the crus of the helix pedicle is too narrow. It is important to include all the skin adjacent to the triangular fossa with the pedicle. Postoperative edema of the reconstructed nose may persist for some months, but later resolves. Tissue contraction occurs postoperatively at all stages. For this reason, all the postauricular skin is included in the flap. Hairy skin, however, is avoided.

OPERATIVE TECHNIQUE

Total nasal reconstruction using this technique requires four stages:

1. The flaps are delayed on each side of the head.
2. The lower pedicle of each flap is delayed (see Fig. 6).
3. The auricular ends of the flaps are sutured to their new site in the nasal region (see Fig. 7).
4. The carrier pedicles are returned to their donor sites, and any revisions of the new nose are carried out (see Fig. 8).

Stage 1

The patient is placed in the Trendelenburg position to engorge the superficial temporal vessels, and the flaps that overlie these vessels are marked. Each flap measures 4 × 12 cm (Figs. 1 and 2). The patient is returned to the Fowler position before the flaps are incised.

The frontal portion of the flap is dissected at the level of the loose areolar tissue between the galea aponeurotica and the pericranium. The posterior branch of the superficial temporal vessels and other collaterals are sectioned and tied (Fig. 1).

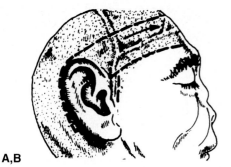

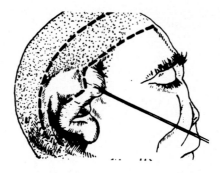

FIG. 1. A: The flap is 4 cm wide and it overlies the superficial temporal vessels. The preauricular incision allows exposure of the vessels, which are ligated at the level of the tragus and subsequently transplanted beneath the flap. **B:** On the posterior ear, the incision is made 1 cm from the helical rim. (From Orticochea, ref. 4, with permission.)

The auricular portion of the flap includes the full thickness of the concha. The preauricular skin and the cartilage are sectioned along the anterior, superior, and posterior borders of the concha. A small inferior pedicle (2 cm wide) should be left intact to ensure a blood supply to the thin preauricular skin (Fig. 3). On the medial aspect of the ear, the lower incision continues parallel to the helix and about 1 cm from the rim of the ear as far as the retroauricular groove. The upper incision is carried along the hairline to the lower margin of the mastoid process (Fig. 2). The posterior incision limiting this flap should reach the level of the earlobe in its lower end.

A 4-cm-wide pedicle over the mastoid is retained to ensure the blood supply of the medial auricular skin, for at this stage the supply still comes from below and not from above. It will be noted that the flap includes all the skin covering the medial aspect of the concha plus the glabrous skin over the temporal bone and the mastoid process (Fig. 2). When separating this skin from the underlying structures, the posterior auricular vessels are divided. The skin of the mastoid region and that of the upper end of the sternocleidomastoid region should be raised to improve their blood supply. This procedure will ensure cutaneous vascular continuity. At this stage, a strip of cortex from the temporal and mastoid bones may be included in the flap for support of the nasal skeleton.

Transplantation of the Superficial Temporal Vessels

The thin skin at the upper end of the postauricular sulcus, which connects the auricular portion of the flap to the scalp pedicle, has few blood vessels and constitutes a vascular barrier (M in Fig. 4B; also see 2 in Fig. 6). Transplantation of the superficial temporal vessels is essential to overcome this barrier and to ensure adequate blood supply to the auricular end of the flap.

Through a vertical preauricular incision 1.5 cm in front of the ear, the superficial temporal vessels are dissected free, with the fatty tissue surrounding them retained. They are ligated at the level of the lower border of the tragus (Figs. 4 and 5). A tunnel is then made with scissors through the substance of the flap at the upper end of the concha, and the divided vessels are passed through and sutured to the posterior border of the flap. The raw undersurface of the carrier portion of the flap above the ear is covered with a split-thickness skin graft.

Finally, the flap donor area is resurfaced with a split-thickness skin graft. This graft covers the pericranium of the frontal bone, the temporal fascia, the musculoskeletal surface

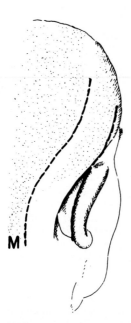

FIG. 2. The incision marking the posterior limit of the frontoauricular flap should extend to the level of the lower end of the earlobe (M). (From Orticochea, ref. 4, with permission.)

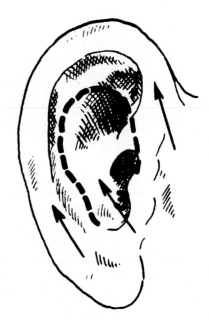

FIG. 3. Diagram of the incision on the lateral surface of the ear. The preauricular skin and cartilage are divided as shown. Three vascular bridges are retained (*arrows*); the skin covering the concha is supplied through that marked *3*, while the remainder of the ear is nourished by the pedicles at the crus of the helix and at the lobule. (From Orticochea, ref. 1, with permission.)

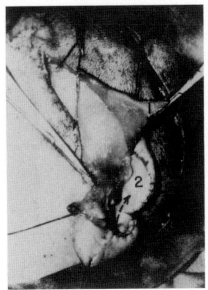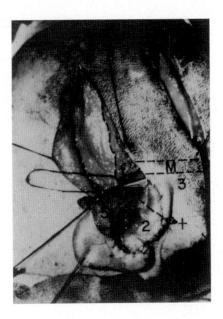

A,B

FIG. 4. **A:** The flap is partly raised. The superficial temporal vessels (*1*) are dissected in such a way that a cuff of subcutaneous tissue remains around them. Note the hemostats on the cut end of the vessels. **B:** The region *M* has few blood vessels and constitutes a vascular barrier, which is by-passed by transposing the vessels to the point +. (From Orticochea, ref. 3, with permission.)

of the temporal bone and mastoid process, and the site where the concha was in contact with the bone. The same procedure is carried out on each side of the head.

Stage 2

Before transplantation of the lower end of the frontoauricular flap (containing preauricular and retroauricular skin, conchal cartilage, and temporal bone) to the nasal region, the delay of the lower pedicle of the flap is carried out (Fig. 6). This delay will avoid vascular insufficiency by sectioning the skin between the two vertical incisions and raising the lower end of the flap.

Stage 3

The auricular end of each flap is detached from the inferior skin attachment of the concha. The flaps are then sutured in place to the lateral borders of the nasal defect and to each

other in the midline (Fig. 7). A two-layer closure of both lining and skin is made in each case, but the cartilage is not sutured. Finally, the remaining portion of the ear is returned to its normal position and sutured to the neighboring tissues.

Stage 4

The pedicle of the flap is divided at the desired level in the nasal region. When this is done and the lower ends of the superficial temporal vessels are divided, an abundant flow of blood from the artery results, thus demonstrating that reversal of flow has been achieved. The pedicles are returned to their donor site, and the necessary trimming of the nasal flaps is carried out (Fig. 8).

SUMMARY

Bilateral reversed superficial temporal artery postauricular compound skin and cartilage flaps can be used for total nasal

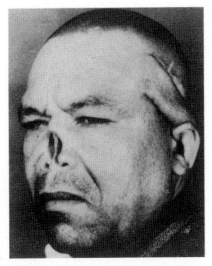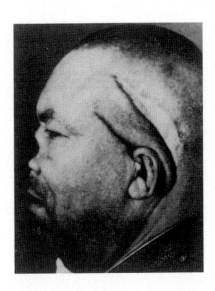

A,B

FIG. 5. **A,B:** The reversed superficial temporal artery compound skin and cartilage flap before it is moved. (From Orticochea, ref. 4, with permission.)

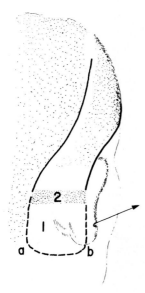

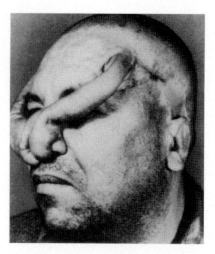

FIG. 7. The flaps have been moved to the nose. The donor areas and the underside of the carrier portion of the flaps have been skin grafted. (From Orticochea, ref. 3, with permission.)

FIG. 6. The final delay. An incision (*ab*) joins the lower ends of the vertical incisions. The lower end of the flap (*1*) is raised as far as the narrow zone (*2*) before being resutured to its original site. The blood supply from the transposed superficial temporal artery through the narrow zone is sufficient to nourish the flap. (From Orticochea, ref. 4, with permission.)

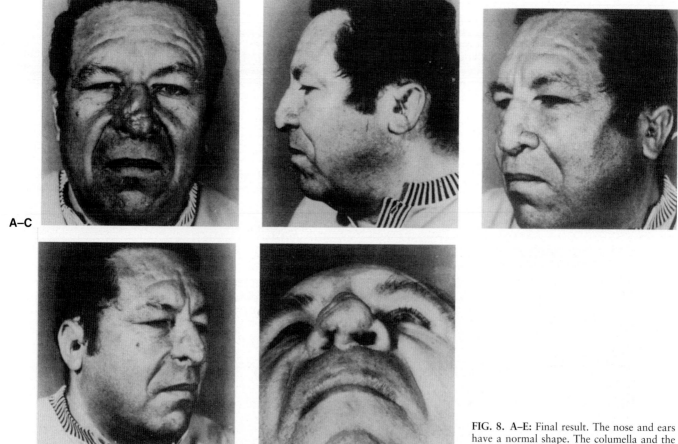

A–C

D,E

FIG. 8. A–E: Final result. The nose and ears have a normal shape. The columella and the size of the nostril openings are normal. (From Orticochea, ref. 4, with permission.)

reconstruction. The flaps are transferred on long pedicles based on each temple, and the success of the operation depends on two biological phenomena: (1) the ability of the blood flow in the superficial temporal vessels to be reversed, and (2) the revascularization of the inferior part of the flap (normally supplied by the postauricular vessels) by the reversed flow in the superficial temporal vessels.

References

1. Orticochea M. A new method for total reconstruction of the nose: the ears as donor areas. *Br J Plast Surg* 1971;24:225.
2. Orticochea M. Méthode pour la reconstruction totale du nez. *Ann Chir Plast* 1977;22:181.
3. Orticochea M. Refined technique for reconstructing the whole nose with the conchas of the ears. *Br J Plast Surg* 1980;33:68.
4. Orticochea M. A new method for total reconstruction of the nose: the ears as donor areas. *Clin Plast Surg* 1981;8:481.

CHAPTER 60 ■ CERVICAL AND CLAVICULAR TUBED SKIN FLAPS

B. C. MENDELSON AND J. K. MASSON

These flaps are predominantly of historical significance (1). The current management of skin malignancies occurs earlier and is more appropriate and the indications for radiotherapy are stricter than in the past. These facts have dramatically reduced the need for nasal reconstructions. During the years when major nasal reconstruction was more common, clavicular and cervical tubed pedicle flaps were used frequently. That era corresponded to the time in which tubed pedicle flaps were in general use by plastic surgeons.

INDICATIONS

Both cervical and clavicular tubed skin flaps provide skin of quite good color match with facial skin (second only to that of forehead flaps), but the texture is softer and finer than either forehead or nasal skin.

In general, forehead flaps provide the best nasal reconstructions (2), but where such flaps are prohibited because of preexisting scarring or extensive facial radiation, the healthy tissue provided by distant flaps may be required (3).

The major advantage of these distant flaps over forehead flaps is the avoidance of further facial scarring. The clavicular flap, unlike the cervical flap, has the advantage of not leaving any visible scarring when the patient is clothed (4).

Because these flaps require initial attachment to the nasal bridge, there is some difficulty in molding the details of columella and nostrils satisfactorily when the distal end is later transected (5). Accordingly, their best use is for coverage. The clavicular flap, without the size limitation of forehead or cervical flaps, can provide sufficient tissue for much larger defects extending onto the adjacent cheek and lip.

The major limitation of these flaps is the need for multiple operations and a long time for completion. While some of the cervical flaps can reach directly to the nose, most of these distant flaps have insufficient reach and require migration via an intermediate attachment, with several weeks extra preparation time (6). There is a real risk of major com-

plications in the use of these, as well as other, tubed pedicle flaps.

Both flaps are contraindicated in the presence of heavy scarring of the skin of the neck or clavicular region. In males, a heavy growth of hair in these regions is also a contraindication.

ANATOMY

Both these flaps are based on a random pattern of circulation.

FLAP DESIGN AND DIMENSIONS

Clavicular Tubed Flap

The flap is usually designed parallel to and just below the clavicle (7). Its dimensions are determined by the size of the nasal defect and the distance to the nose. Traditional teaching strongly advises a maximum length-breadth ratio of 3:1 (6).

At least four surgical procedures are necessary for transfer of one end of the clavicular tube to the nose. Previously, either end of the flap was used for nasal coverage, but it is now known that the acromial skin of the lateral end can be safely transferred to the nose without delay, carried on the medially based deltopectoral flap (see Chap. 124).

The only use of this flap at present is when the skin of the medial end of the flap in the sternoclavicular joint region is preferred over the lateral skin. Since it is not usually possible for the flap to reach the nose directly, the lateral end is migrated by means of an intermediate stage on the neck (Fig. 1).

Cervical Tubed Flap

Cervical flaps can be used in several different ways. Small nasal defects (e.g., heminasal, columella) can be corrected using a narrow tubed cervical flap. The flap can be created in

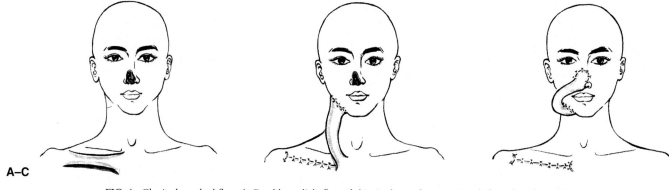

A–C

FIG. 1. Clavicular tubed flap. A: Double-pedicle flap of skin is elevated over or just below clavicle and is tubed. A delay of the lateral end is performed 4 weeks later. B: Three weeks later, the lateral end is migrated via an intermediate attachment to the neck. One or two delay operations on the medial end are performed. C: Three weeks after its delay, the medial end is transposed to the cephalad end of the defect. Three weeks later, the unused portion is discarded. (From New and Erich, ref. 4, with permission.)

the line of the neck skin folds, and the upper end (postauricular skin) can be used for the definitive repair (2).

A larger area of skin is obtained by the more obliquely placed cervical flap (Fig. 2). The pedicle essentially parallels the sternomastoid muscle and carries the paddle of skin situated over the lower neck sternoclavicular joint region. The traditional operation, performed as a tube pedicle, was, by definition, a multistaged procedure. It is now recognized that the same paddle of skin can be carried to the nose using the sternomastoid muscle as the carrier pedicle, i.e., the sternomastoid musculocutaneous flap (see Chap. 190). Since this is a two-stage procedure, with the reduced risk associated with an axial-pattern flap, there is no current indication for using the oblique cervical flap.

If the neck skin itself is used for the repair, the flap must be situated low on the neck, especially in men, to avoid hair-bearing skin. As a consequence, the flap is too short for direct reach to the defect, and migration by means of an intermediate attachment is required (Fig. 3). The nasolabial region is a more comfortable temporary attachment for the patient than the mucosa of the lower lip.

The transverse cervical flap is usually 15 × 4 cm (8).

OPERATIVE TECHNIQUE

Clavicular Tubed Flap

At the first stage of the operation, the pedicle is tubed in the traditional manner (4). At the second operation some 4 weeks

later, a delay of the lateral end of the flap is performed, and 3 weeks later, the lateral end is attached to the neck.

One or even two delay operations on the medial end, 4 weeks apart, are advised (especially if the nasal recipient bed has been radiated) before finally attaching the medial end to the nasal defect.

Three weeks later, the final inset is performed, and the residual pedicle is either discarded (if not required) or else the neck attachment is brought onto the face for further coverage (Fig. 1). Usually several touch-up procedures are subsequently necessary.

Cervical Tubed Flap

The skin flap is tubed, and the donor wound edges are undermined and approximated behind the bipedicle. Three weeks later, a delay is performed on one end, and that end is transferred 3 weeks after the delay procedure, usually to a temporary recipient site on the nasolabial fold.

Three weeks later, the remaining neck attachment is delayed, and a further 3 weeks later, the definitive transfer to the nose is achieved.

Three weeks after that, the excess pedicle tissue is removed, and the final inset is performed. Usually, several touch-up procedures are necessary.

CLINICAL RESULTS

Despite producing some excellent results, there has been a significant complication rate associated with use of the clavicular

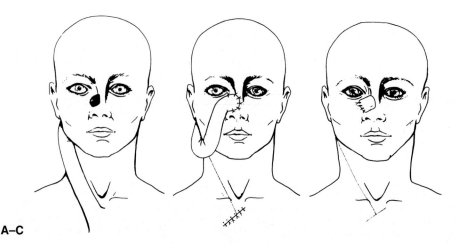

A–C

FIG. 2. Oblique cervical tubed flap. A: The tubed pedicle is formed obliquely parallel to the sternomastoid muscle. B: The distal end is transposed to a partial nasal defect. C: The residual flap is finally detached and inset after previous partial severance of the pedicle.

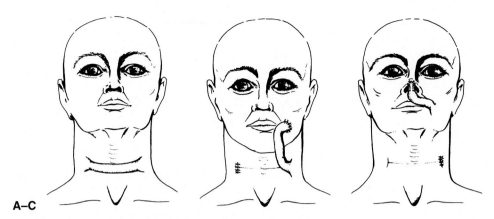

FIG. 3. Transverse cervical tubed flap. **A:** The tubed pedicle is formed transversely across the lower neck. Delay of one end is performed 3 weeks later. **B:** The delayed end is transferred to the nasolabial region. The neck end is delayed 3 weeks later. **C:** The neck end of the flap is transferred to a partial nasal defect.

flap. In a report on 56 clavicular tubed flaps from the Mayo Clinic (1) (only six of which were for total nasal reconstruction), there was a median of six operations required (range 4 to 11) over a median 4-month period for basic completion of the reconstruction. A median number of three touch-up procedures was later performed.

The clavicular flap had the highest complication rate of the various flaps used. Eleven percent underwent a major ischemic event, requiring debridement and later reattachment. In addition, 15% developed minor necrosis and 17% had other minor complications.

SUMMARY

Clavicular and cervical tubed flaps have been described for use in nasal reconstruction. The clavicular flap is best for nasal coverage, and the cervical flap is appropriate for smaller defects such as the columella. However, advances in plastic surgical techniques, such as axial-pattern and musculocutaneous flaps, have largely supplanted random-pattern tubed flaps.

References

1. Mendelson BC, Masson JK, Arnold PG, Erich JB. Flaps used for nasal reconstruction: a perspective based on 100 cases. *Mayo Clin Proc.* 1979;54:91.
2. Young F. The repair of nasal losses. *Surgery* 1946;20:670.
3. Blocksma R, Innis CO. Reconstruction of the amputated nose: report on 30 cases. *Plast Reconstr Surg* 1955;51:390.
4. New GB, Erich JB, eds. *The use of pedicle flaps of skin in plastic surgery of the head and neck.* Springfield, Ill.: Charles C Thomas, 1950.
5. Erich JB. Traumatic defects of the nose and cheeks. *Surg Clin North Am* 1949;29:1009.
6. Erich JB. A survey of skin grafts and pedicle flaps for repair of nasal defects. *Ann Otol Rhinol Laryngol* 1963;72:808.
7. Aymard JL. Nasal reconstruction. *Lancet,* 1917.
8. Paletta FX, Van Norman RT. Total reconstruction of the columella. *Plast Reconstr Surg* 1962;30:322.

CHAPTER 61 ■ UPPER ARM (TAGLIACOZZI) SKIN FLAP

B. C. MENDELSON AND J. K. MASSON

EDITORIAL COMMENT

This is a classic plastic surgery flap; although it has been supplanted by a host of other options, the advantage of having medial arm skin which is a reasonable color and texture match for this location still remains. However, the use of a free flap is probably a preferable choice.

The Tagliacozzi flap serves as a symbol in the tradition of plastic surgery. Tagliacozzi's portrait is on the logo of the American Board of Plastic Surgery, and his flap is centered in the emblem of the American Association of Plastic Surgeons. The only major advance in the use of this flap since it was first reported by Gaspare Tagliacozzi in 1597 (1,2) has been the introduction of anesthesia. Several variations of this pedicled arm flap have been described (3–8).

INDICATIONS

In current practice, pedicle flaps from the arm have limited application in nasal reconstruction. The skin color is often a poor match with facial skin, certainly less satisfactory than that of forehead and clavicular skin flaps. The texture of the hairless skin of the anteromedial surface is too fine and the dermis too thin for effective total nasal reconstruction without the provision of additional support at a subsequent operation. The thinness of the skin, however, can be an advantage for coverage of an exposed nasal skeleton. The immobilization required is a most trying position for the patient and can result in permanent stiffness of the shoulder (9). The major advantage of the flap is that less time is required for a nasal reconstruction than with any of the other distant pedicle flaps, e.g., clavicular. Also, further facial scarring associated with forehead flaps can be avoided.

The Tagliacozzi flap is still the preferred flap in several situations (8). This flap should be used for total nasal reconstruction in children, preserving the forehead for definitive rhinoplasty later in life. It is also preferred for those in whom the forehead is not available, either because of a low hairline or because of the unacceptable aesthetic result of a skin graft on the residual forehead donor site. This is a real factor in darker-skinned patients (African-American, Latino, Indian), in whom hyperpigmentation of the graft is anticipated.

ANATOMY

There is an arterial axis in the upper arm between the deltoid branches of the thoracoacromial artery and the recurrent branches of the radial and ulnar arteries of the elbow (10). On this basis, the Tagliacozzi flap may be partly an arterialized rather than a true random-pattern tubed pedicle flap. This may account for its good vascularity compared to other distant pedicle flaps, e.g., clavicular. The classically located flap ignores the adjacent arterialized skin of the lateral arm used in the cervicohumeral flap (see Chap. 131).

FLAP DESIGN AND DIMENSIONS

The size of the flap, ultimately limited by the dimensions of the arm, depends on the size of the nasal defect, but with allowance for subsequent shrinkage of 25%. Planning is done in reverse, locating and orienting the flap so that it is sited adjacent to the nose when the arm is raised into position for immobilization.

An average flap is constructed with parallel incisions 15 cm long and about 8 cm apart on the anteromedial aspect of the arm and is tubed in the manner illustrated in Fig. 1. In most cases, a skin graft is required to cover the donor area.

OPERATIVE TECHNIQUE

The bipedicle is traditionally left for 3 weeks. In practice, either end of the flap could be transposed to the nose first. Maintenance of antegrade circulation into the proximal end, with severance of the distal end, would seem logical, but Tagliacozzi and others successfully severed the proximal end first (10,11).

A second delay procedure of simply incising and resuturing the third side some 2 to 3 weeks before transposition may be performed (10). This is probably not necessary under ordinary circumstances, but it is usually done "for security."

When the flap is attached to the nasal bridge, its area of contact with recipient nasal tissue is augmented considerably if turndown flaps of local nasal skin have been used to line the defect. At this stage, satisfactory fixation of the arm to the head is most important for patient comfort and for preventing traction of the tube from its nasal attachment.

Tagliacozzi's method of fixation—using a preformed leather vest, hood, and series of straps to hold the palm onto the scalp—was possibly more comfortable for the patient than the more expedient current method of adhesive strappings or plaster of Paris headcap with arm splints and reinforcing struts.

After 3 weeks, the remaining brachial attachment is severed and the flap is left hanging from the nose for about 10 days, like an elephant trunk (9). This period allows an improvement of circulation and so permits a safer and more radical defatting at the time of final shaping and insetting of the tip. This step reduces the number of subsequent touch-up procedures required. Tagliacozzi advised flap severance at 14 to 20 days and shaping of the tip 14 days later (Fig. 2).

Methods in which the alae and columella are shaped first are more dangerous and require an additional delay procedure

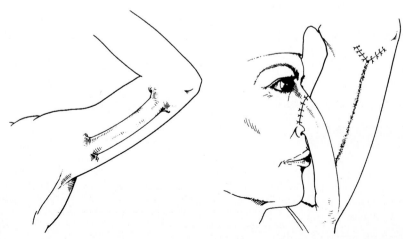

A,B

FIG. 1. **A:** The flap is prepared by creating a double-ended tube based on parallel incisions on the anteromedial arm. The donor area can occasionally be closed directly, but usually requires a skin graft. **B:** The distal end is severed and attached to the nasal bridge.

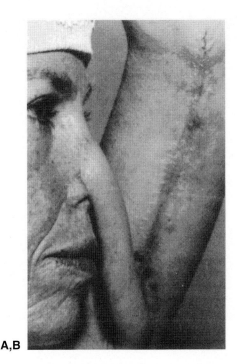
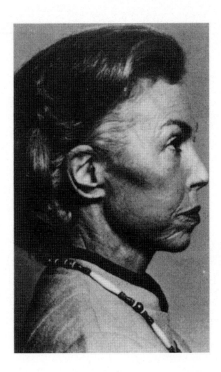

A,B

FIG. 2. **A:** The proximally based flap is attached to the nasal bridge following a previous delay procedure. **B:** The final result. There is no forehead deformity. The skin has a fine texture but does not have a good color match. (From Mendelson et al., ref. 12, with permission.)

(9,12). However, such methods do have the advantage of facilitating fashioning of the tip region.

Further revisions are deferred until edema and induration resolve, usually between 3 and 6 months.

CLINICAL RESULTS

In the Mayo Clinic review of 180 nasal reconstructions (12), 10 Tagliacozzi flaps were used. There were no flap losses and only one case of minor necrosis. The most frequent complication was infection (30%), mostly at the donor site.

The median number of operations required was four over a 2-month period. The least number was four over a 6-week period. An average of two subsequent touch-up procedures was required. Tagliacozzi's description was of six operative steps over a period of 91 to 136 days.

An objective analysis of the quality of color match shows a marked disparity between the results achieved in Caucasians and in those with pigmented skin. In a group of 14 Caucasian patients, half had excellent color matches and all were satisfactory (9). In 10 Pakistani patients, most of the flaps developed increased pigmentation, which often appeared after the delay prior to the flap transfer. Half the results were regarded as poor matches (11).

No flap losses were reported in the 44 patients listed in the three published series reviews (9,11,12), an impressive record for tubed pedicle flaps.

SUMMARY

The upper arm (Tagliacozzi) skin flap has been described for use in nasal reconstruction. It is one of the oldest skin flaps in use, and it still has some application in present-day plastic surgical practice.

References

1. Tagliacozzi G. *De curtorum chirurgia per insitionem (icones)*. Venice: Bindoni, 1597.
2. Gnudi MT, Webster JP. *The life and times of Gaspare Tagliacozzi*. New York: Herbert Reichner, 1950.
3. Nelaton C, Ombredanne L. *La Rhinoplastie* 1904.
4. Reneaume de la Garanne. *Histoire de l'Academie Royale des Sciences*. Paris, 1712;29.
5. Von Graefe O. *Rhinoplastik*. Berlin, 1818.
6. Dieffenbach IF. *Operative Chir* 1845;1:327.
7. Fabrizi O. *Gaz Hop* 1841.
8. Ortiz-Monasterio F, Olimedo A, Barrera G. A modified Tagliacotian rhinoplasty. *Br J Plast Surg* 1978;31:66.
9. Arregui K, Murray JE, Cannon B. The use of arm flaps for "facial defects." In: *Transactions of the 3rd International Congress of Plastic Surgery*. Amsterdam: Excerpta Medica, 1963.
10. Conway H, Stark R, Nieto Cano G. The arterial vascularization of pedicles. *Plast Reconstr Surg* 1953;12:348.
11. Blocksma R, Innis CO. Reconstruction of the amputated nose: report on 30 cases. *Plast Reconstr Surg* 1955;15:390.
12. Mendelson BC, Masson JK, Arnold PG, at al. Flaps used for nasal reconstruction: a perspective based on 180 cases. *Mayo Clin Proc* 1979; 54:91.

CHAPTER 62 ■ TRAPEZIUS MUSCULOCUTANEOUS ISLAND FLAP

W. R. PANJE

EDITORIAL COMMENT

The trapezius musculocutaneous flap, as outlined, is supplied by the branches of the transverse cervical artery. It would be difficult for the flap to consistently reach the glabellar area for a secure attachment. A wide area of attachment would allow more effectively for greater circulation than the so-called training technique. This particular method of nasal reconstruction should be considered after other simpler and more effective methods have been discarded.

Surgical reconstruction of a total nasal defect can be effectively accomplished by using the trapezius musculocutaneous extended island flap.

INDICATIONS

This flap provides the abundant cutaneous tissue required for total nasal reconstruction without the need for delay. It also offers an excellent color match. The procedure can be accomplished in a two-staged operation, leaving a relatively hidden donor site. No external cast immobilization is required in the transfer of this regional flap to the face.

ANATOMY

For the first stage of this procedure, an extended trapezius musculocutaneous island flap is developed based on the transverse cervical vessels. The accessory nerve innervation to the remaining trapezius muscle can be preserved. Once the flap is divided prior to insetting, it has, of course, a random-pattern circulation.

FLAP DESIGN AND DIMENSIONS

As with other methods of total nasal reconstruction, the initially reconstructed nose should be 20% to 30% larger than the desired final goal because of shrinkage. A cutaneous segment of flap 16 cm long by 10 cm wide is elevated onto the trapezius muscle carrier, which is 16 × 5 cm.

OPERATIVE TECHNIQUE

Initially, a triangular incision (the apex located over the acromion) is made lateral to medial along the clavicle and the anterior border of the trapezius muscle to allow identification of the transverse cervical vessels into the posteroinferior part of the neck. This incision provides access to the lower neck for identification of the posterior belly of the omohyoid muscle (crucial for convenient location of the transverse cervical vessels) and dissection of the trapezius muscle and eleventh nerve. It also allows external delivery of the vascular pedicle from the neck to increase the arc of the flap. In dissecting the transverse cervical vascular pedicle, overzealous exposure of the vessels should be avoided.

The distal cutaneous portion of the flap, dissected caudal to the scapular spine, is tubed onto itself. The end is attached to a cephalic-based half-circle flap developed over the glabella (Fig. 1). The length of the half-circle or trapdoor flap should equal the radius of the tubed portion of the flap. The muscle portion of the flap is not rolled onto itself because of bulkiness and the risk of compressing the vascular pedicle.

The patient's head should be positioned to avoid tension, and the flap should be allowed to heal in place for about 18 days. Since the flap is relatively heavy, it will need additional support during the healing phase. This can be provided, in part, by suturing the flap to the edges of the defect. External support also may be necessary.

Side view

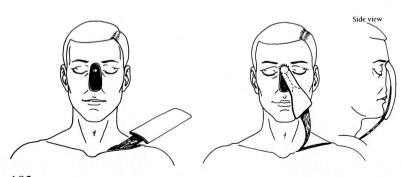

FIG. 1. Trapezius musculocutaneous island flap elevated and attached to the glabella. (From Panje, ref. 1, with permission.)

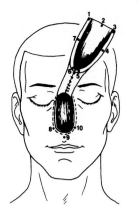
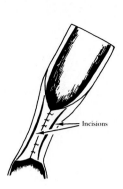
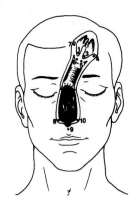

Incisions

FIG. 2. The undersurface of the flap. By making the incisions shown in the tubed portion, lining is provided for the internal surface of the nose. Infolding the distal portion of the flap not only forms the alae and columella, but also lines the nasal vestibules. (From Panje, ref. 1, with permission.)

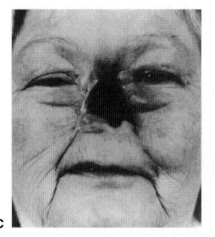
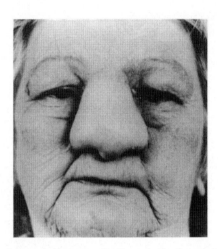
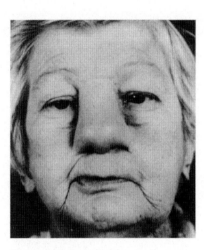

A–C

FIG. 3. A: One year following total rhinectomy. **B:** One month after total nasal reconstruction using the trapezius musculocutaneous island flap. **C:** One year postoperatively. (From Panje, ref. 1, with permission.)

The skin portion of the flap should measure at least 12 cm. This should allow the end of the flap (now the distal portion) to reach the level of the mental crease. Training of the flap is begun with intermittent clamping as tolerated. The flap is then severed from its shoulder attachment. Excess muscle and fat are removed from the distal part of the flap. It is important not to damage the subdermal plexus during this maneuver, since the flap has become completely randomized and depends on the plexus for nutrition. The proximal part (5 cm) of the flap is not debulked.

The undersurface of the tubed portion of the flap is incised to leave some skin for lining (Fig. 2). The flap is then sutured to the nasal defect using a two-layered closure. The distal part of the flap is then folded on itself, as shown in Fig. 2. The distal corners of the flap will approximate each other at a midpoint about 5 to 7 cm from the flap's distal edge. This infolding creates the columella and nasal alae while providing the lining for the nasal vestibule. The nares are packed for 5 to 7 days in order to obliterate the dead space.

The reconstructed nose will usually undergo shrinkage within 3 or 4 months. During this period, the nares should be supported. Further minor procedures, such as debulking, refashioning, or adding dorsal support, may be required. The patient should start shoulder exercises within the first week to prevent stiffness (Fig. 3).

CLINICAL RESULTS

A significant muscle paralysis can occur if care is not taken to prevent injury to the accessory nerve. It should be remembered that there are several distally located eleventh nerve branches that innervate the trapezius. Frequently, the most distal branch will be cut in isolating the transverse cervical vessel pedicle. However, the proximal branches to the trapezius can be preserved with maintenance of muscle function.

SUMMARY

A trapezius musculocutaneous island flap can be used to reconstruct the total nasal defect.

Reference

1. Panje WR. A new method for total nasal reconstruction: the trapezius myocutaneous island paddle flap. *Arch Otolaryngol* 1982;108:156.

CHAPTER 63 ■ MICROVASCULAR FREE TRANSFER OF A RETROAURICULAR SKIN FLAP

T. FUJINO AND M. WADA

This would appear to be an exceptionally difficult flap to transfer successfully, because of the variability of the blood supply and the disparity in size between donor and recipient vessels. The success of this flap may, in fact, depend on inosculation of the thin flap.

Retroauricular skin, located at the back of the ear, provides a good color match for facial cover. A free skin flap based on the retroauricular vessels can be designed in this area (1).

ANATOMY

The retroauricular artery usually arises from the external carotid artery (in 93% of cases) and runs relatively deep, passing through the parotid gland. It emerges in front of the anterior surface of the mastoid process behind the auricle. Because this artery lies 3 cm beneath the skin near the mastoid process, one might anticipate problems when preparing it for transfer. Inasmuch as the external diameter of this artery near the mastoid process is about 1.2 mm, however, we found that preparation was not difficult. Furthermore, the retroauricular artery rises upward abruptly at the mastoid process to a position 1 cm below the skin surface in the central portion of the posterior aspect of the auricle. It is therefore possible to expose this artery through careful dissection. It should be kept in mind that in 7% of cases, the retroauricular artery also arises from the occipital artery (Fig. 1A) (2,3).

The retroauricular artery distributes some branches behind the auricle and supplies the flap area. The artery runs lateral and slightly posterior to the facial nerve trunk. Thus, with care, injury to this nerve during preparation of the flap can be avoided.

The relationship of the artery to the greater auricular nerve is not uniform. The retroauricular vein does not always accompany the artery. It courses in a more superficial zone, usually 1.5 cm below the skin surface of the mastoid region and 0.3 cm below the surface behind the auricle. The mean external diameter of the vein behind the auricle is 1.4 mm; it appears abruptly as it ascends above the auricle. The vein is situated in a posterosuperior position to the artery.

FLAP DESIGN AND DIMENSIONS

A free retroauricular skin flap 5 × 7 cm in average size can be fashioned. The flap can be extended further by taking into account the anastomosis between the retroauricular artery and the superficial temporal artery. The proposed flap design is marked along the area just behind the helix distally, along the hairline proximally, at the tip of the helix cranially, and at the lowest part of the earlobe caudally (Fig. 1).

OPERATIVE TECHNIQUE

The incision is started just behind the helix and proceeds deep and above the perichondrium toward the concha. At the junction of the mastoid process and concha, a paired perforating artery and vein 1 mm in diameter, respectively, are found. To obtain a long vessel axis, the perichondrium is incised, and dissection is further carried out deep along the mastoid process (Fig. 2) (1,4).

CLINICAL RESULTS

In a single attempt at resection of a large hemifacial cavernous hemangioma and resurfacing of the nose with a retroauricular skin flap, the flap survived and there was no functional deficit. Unless the concomitant vein is anastomosed, vascular circulation might be impaired temporarily, because of an incompletely closed vascular circuit. In this situation, undue tension after microvascular anastomosis is contraindicated.

SUMMARY

A good color match can be obtained by using a free retroauricular flap to resurface facial defects.

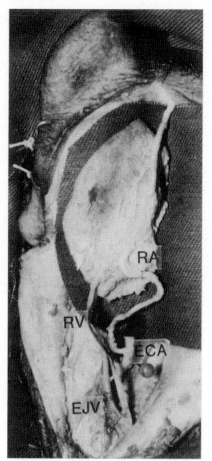

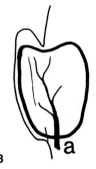 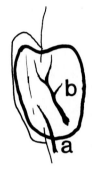

A,B

FIG. 1. A: Diagram of the free retroauricular flap. On the left, the retroauricular artery (a) originates from the external carotid and supplies the entire flap region. On the right, the retroauricular artery (a) originates from the external carotid artery and supplies the lower portion of the flap. A second artery (b) originates from the occipital artery and supplies the upper portion of the flap. B: An example of a free retroauricular skin flap (RA, retroauricular artery; RV, retroauricular vein; ECA, external carotid artery; EJV, external jugular vein).

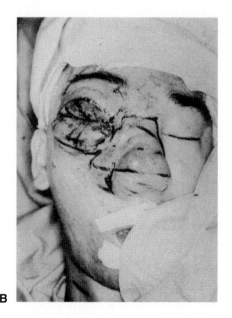 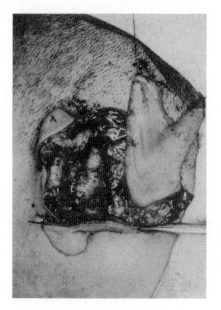

A,B

FIG. 2. A: A 24-year-old man with a huge cavernous hemangioma with bleeding from the lower eyelid every other day and a progressive decrease in vision. The patient had received radiation therapy at the age of 4 years. Bilateral carotid angiograms showed extensive involvement of the right orbit and maxillary sinus, with some abnormal patterns in the left orbit and maxillary sinus. B: Design of the flap on the back of the ear. (Continued)

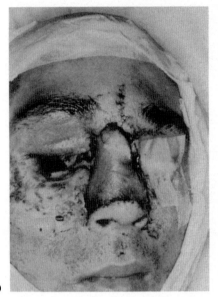

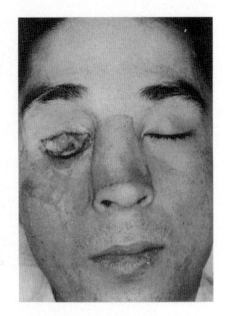

C,D

FIG. 2. *Continued*. **C:** On the first postoperative day it was necessary to remove all sutures from the flap edges. This was followed by good bleeding from all edges. **D:** Eleven months after the free flap to the nose and 10 months after the combined procedure on the cheek. (From Fujino et al., ref. 1, with permission.)

References

1. Fujino T, Harashina T, Nakajima T. Free skin flap from the retroauricular region to the nose. *Plast Reconstr Surg* 1976;57:338.
2. Wada M. A contribution to the study of the topographic relationships between blood vessels and nerves. *Jpn Keio Med Soc.* 1978;55:149.
3. Wada M, Fujino T, Terashima T. Anatomic description of the free retroauricular flap. *J Microsurg* 1979;1:108.
4. Fujino T, Ikuta Y, Harashina T. Technique of microsurgery. In: Fujino T, ed. Tokyo: Igakushoin, 1977;72–76.

CHAPTER 64 ■ MICROVASCULAR FREE TRANSFER OF A RETROAURICULAR FLAP

S. KOBAYASHI

EDITORIAL COMMENT

This chapter extends Washio's technique of a pedicled retroauricular flap using microvascular techniques. The flap is a good one, but the anatomy is variable and therefore not always totally reliable.

A skin flap from the retroauricular area can be elevated on the posterior auricular vessels. The flap provides thin skin that matches facial skin in color and texture, with minimal donor-site deformities, and with the donor site easily hidden by hair.

This flap has not been too widely used as a free flap, because the involved vessels are sometimes too small.

INDICATIONS

A retroauricular skin flap can be used in the treatment of medium-sized defects of the intraoral mucosa, nose, eyelid, and eye socket (1–4). It can also be used to correct composite defects which include hair, such as skin defects in the hair-bearing area of the temporal hairline, preauricular sideburns, and upper eyelid-eyebrow region. The transitional zone from skin to hair can be naturally restored through the incorporation of hair in the flap, particularly when compared to conventional two-stage techniques (5).

ANATOMY

The retroauricular mastoid skin is supplied mainly by the posterior auricular artery (PA). This vessel usually branches off from the external carotid artery, and it ascends between the parotid gland and the styloid process of the temporal bone, to the groove between the cartilage of the auricle and the mastoid process. The PA supplies the skin located in the posterior aspect of the auricle. The posterior auricular vein does not always run along with the artery; instead, it may be located in a more superficial and posterior position vis-à-vis the artery. Anatomic variations of the posterior auricular vessels have been reported in the literature (4,6,7). The diameter of these vessels is sometimes too narrow for use in free-flap transfer (Fig. 1).

Flaps can be elevated from the retroauricular area based on the tributaries of the superficial temporal artery (STA), i.e., the posteriorly running branch of the parietal branch of the STA, or the anterior auricular branches of the STA; the posterior auricular vessels have a vascular network running between these STA tributaries (3,8). A flap based on the STA sometimes tends to become congested (5).

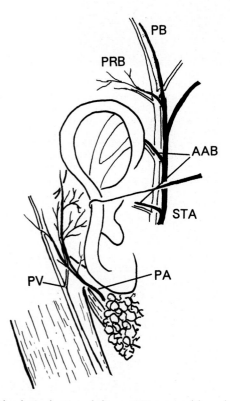

FIG. 1. Blood supply around the ear (*PB,* parietal branch of *STA; PRB,* posteriorly running branch of parietal branch of *STA; AAB,* anterior auricular branches of the *STA; PA, PV,* posterior auricular artery and vein).

FLAP DESIGN AND DIMENSIONS

Retroauricular mastoid skin, measuring up to about 6 × 6 cm, can be safely elevated in adult patients, based on the posterior auricular vessels and transferred when the vessels have a reliable diameter of approximately 1 mm, and when a reliable vein can be included in the flap. The retroauricular skin located at the helical margin must be preserved to prevent auricular deformities after flap harvesting. When it is necessary to transfer the retroauricular hairline, a hairline of about 1 to 2 cm in width can be added to the flap.

Since the diameter of the posterior auricular vessels varies between individuals, preoperative assessment of the vessels is recommended, using a color Doppler flow imager. Without invasive techniques, this device can be used to determine the approximate diameter of the vessels and the direction of the blood flow.

OPERATIVE TECHNIQUE

The skin incision line on the lower flap edge is extended along the anterior margin of the sternocleidomastoid muscle; the artery and vein are identified. Great care should be taken at this point, because the diameter of these vessels may be less than 1 mm. Since the vessels run deep between the sternocleidomastoid muscle and the posterior surface of the parotid gland, the vessels should be carefully dissected, to avoid damage to the neighboring facial nerve. The posterior auricular artery increases in diameter in the proximal area close to the branching of the stylomastoid artery. When a retroauricular flap is used as a free flap, the artery must be dissected from at least this branching point to the proximal region. Once vessel dissection is completed, the flap is elevated down to the subaponeurotic area. If the posterior auricular vessels are too narrow for transfer as a free flap, the flap should be elevated based on the tributaries of the STA.

CLINICAL RESULTS

In the transfer of seven retroauricular free flaps based on the posterior auricular vessels, we have had no flap losses (Fig. 2). In an additional two cases, preoperative planning had involved raising the flap with the same vessels, but we decided to switch to an STA pedicle flap. This was based on an intraoperative assessment that the posterior auricular vessels were too narrow for microvascular anastomosis, especially the posterior auricular vein.

SUMMARY

This flap is extremely useful in reconstructing facial skin defects. It provides a good skin color and texture match, and hairline defects can be managed in one stage. However, when this flap is raised, careful attention must be paid to anatomic variations in the blood vessels and vascular network around the ear.

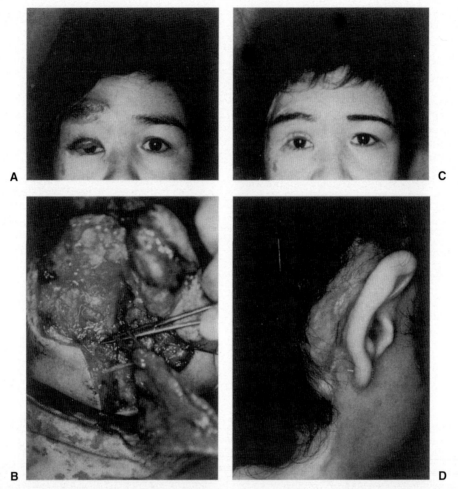

FIG. 2. A: A 41-year-old woman had a hemangioma on the upper eyelid, temporal and forehead region. The entire area, with the exception of the eyebrow, had been treated with a split-thickness skin graft at another hospital; ectropion of the lid occurred. Texture and color of skin grafts did not match the surrounding skin. **B:** A retroauricular hairline flap was transferred to reconstruct the upper eyelid and eyebrow in one stage. The posterior auricular vessels were anastomosed to the anterior branch of the superficial temporal vessels. The resulting upper eyelid was too bulky; although the transferred skin was thin, subcutaneous tissue in the flap included fascia and loose areolar tissue that increased total flap thickness. **C,D:** Two secondary revisions were performed, including excision of subcutaneous structure of the transferred flap, to correct bulkiness in the upper eyelid. Results obtained were satisfactory, with a natural-appearing hair transitional zone achieved from the eyebrow to the upper eyelid. Skin color and texture of the transferred flap matched the facial skin, with minimal donor-site defect.

References

1. Fujino T, Harashina T, Nakagima T. Free skin flap from the retroauricular region to the nose. *Plast Reconstr Surg* 1976;57:338.
2. Leonard AG, Kolhe PS. The posterior auricular flap: intra-oral reconstruction. *Br J Plast Surg* 1987;40:570.
3. Guyuron B. Retroauricular island flap for eye socket reconstruction. *Plast Reconstr Surg* 1985;76:527.
4. Park C. The chondrocutaneous postauricular free flap. *Plast Reconstr Surg* 1989;84:761.
5. Kobayashi S, Yoza S, Kakibuchi M, et al. Retroauricular hairline flap transfer to the face. *Plast Reconstr Surg* 1995;96:42.
6. Wada M, Fujino T, Terashima T. Anatomic description of the free retroauricular flap. *J Microsurg* 1979;1:108.
7. Kolhe PS, Leonard AG. The posterior auricular flap: anatomical studies. *Br J Plast Surg* 1987;40:562.
8. Song R, Song Y, Qi K, et al. The superior auricular artery and retroauricular arterial island flaps. *Plast Reconstr Surg* 1996;98:657.

CHAPTER 65 ■ NASAL RECONSTRUCTION WITH AURICULAR MICROVASCULAR TRANSPLANT

J. J. PRIBAZ AND D. L. ABRAMSON

EDITORIAL COMMENT

This technique extends the use of the procedure of selecting appropriate portions of the ear for nasal reconstruction. By accomplishing microvascular anastomosis, assurance of the survival of the segments is far more likely.

The ascending helix of the ear is a laminated structure composed of cartilage surrounded by a thin, tightly adherent layer of skin. This composite tissue provides all that is necessary for reconstruction of full-thickness defects of the ala and columella. Composite grafts are frequently used to repair defects of the nasal ala (1–4). Although technically relatively easy to perform, they are limited by problems with viability, dimension, and atrophy. A free-tissue transfer harvested from the ascending helix can be used to repair defects of the distal part of the nose, including nasal sill, ala, tip, and columella (5–7).

INDICATIONS

Patients with full-thickness defects of the nasal tip, sill, ala, and columella, which would yield suboptimal results with a composite graft, should be considered for the procedure. Selection should include those patients with major concerns about further scarring of the midface or forehead. In addition, those who have undergone reconstructive attempts with more conventional techniques that have failed, are candidates for this procedure. Advantages of this flap include possible modifications of flap dimensions and orientation, to allow replacement of any portion of the distal hemi-nose. The flap is supplied by branches arising from the superficial temporal vascular pedicle, making microvascular transfer technically feasible. The size of the flap is limited only by the resulting donor deformity.

ANATOMY

Nose and auricular cadaver specimens were compared and, when superimposed, the unfolded nostril is very similar to the ascending helical rim (Fig. 1). Both the ascending helix and the nostril consist of laminated cartilage surrounded by a skin envelope. If the nostril sill is to be reconstructed, the crus of the helix can be included in the flap (Fig. 2). Microfil radiopaque dye was used to assess the vascularity of this region. One to three branches arising from the superficial temporal artery supplied this portion of the ear.

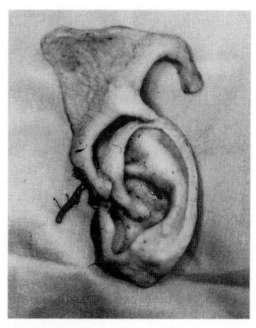

FIG. 1. The "unfolded" nose is superimposed over the ascending helix of the ear in a cadaver specimen.

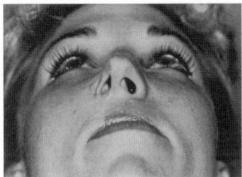
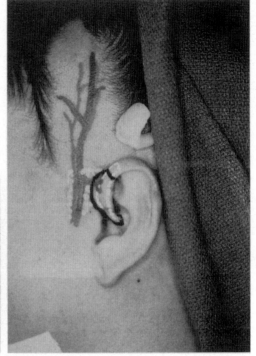

FIG. 2. **A:** A 28-year-old woman with deficiency of the right ala and nostril sill, despite multiple reconstructive attempts after sarcoma excision. **B:** A wax model has been made of the defect, then transferred to the contralateral ear, and the flap marked along the crus of the helix and the ascending helical rim. The superficial temporal vessels have been marked out after Doppler examination. The anatomy of this flap is depicted. White dots from the vessels to the outline of the flap represent the subcutaneous tissue that is harvested with the flap.

FLAP DESIGN AND DIMENSIONS

The first step in designing the flap is to define the defect. Bone wax can be used to fashion a three-dimensional model. The model can be transferred to the ascending helix and used to determine the amount of skin and cartilage required, as well as the orientation of the tissue to be included in the flap (Fig. 2).

OPERATIVE TECHNIQUE

As stated above, a small model of the defect should be made. The flap should then be designed on the ascending helix to provide a symmetric reconstruction. For alar and nostril-sill reconstruction, the contralateral ear is used; for columella reconstruction, either ear can be used.

A preauricular incision is made, and the superficial temporal vessels are isolated above the ear. When harvesting this flap, no effort is made to dissect the individual small branches of the superficial temporal artery that supply the upper third of the ear. Instead, subcutaneous tissue in the preauricular area is harvested in continuity with the superficial temporal vessels and ascending helical rim. The appropriate recipient vessels, usually the facial artery and vein, are isolated through an incision in the nasolabial fold.

The flap is then transferred, inset, and anastomoses performed. Cases with multiple previous surgical procedures may require the use of vein grafts to reach recipient vessels in the upper neck. The facial artery is usually of good caliber, but sometimes the facial vein, which is usually located more laterally, may be quite small. If it is deemed unsuitable, then a vein

graft will be needed to the upper neck. The donor defect is closed through a combination of advancement of the helical rim, as described by Antia and Buck (8), and a cheek advancement or postauricular flap.

CLINICAL RESULTS

The ascending helix can be used as a microvascular transfer to correct many defects of the distal hemi-nose. Our experience includes reconstruction of the nasal tip, ala, columella, and sill, or combinations of these. Defects were created following excision of arteriovenous malformations, basal cell carcinoma (BCC), small-cell carcinoma (SCC), and sarcoma, as well as a single case following a human bite. This procedure was performed in patients ranging from 7 to 76 years of age.

The flap is versatile in reconstructing a variety of nasal defects, with size limited only by the donor deformity of the ear. In our experience, patients usually undergo a secondary procedure, either minor scar revisions or debulking of the flap pedicle (Figs. 2 and 3).

SUMMARY

The use of the auricular free flap requires a substantial effort, but can provide an elegant and predictable result for selected patients with defects of the distal nose. The ideal candidate for this procedure would be a patient who desires excellent color and contour match, but wishes to avoid cheek or forehead donor morbidity.

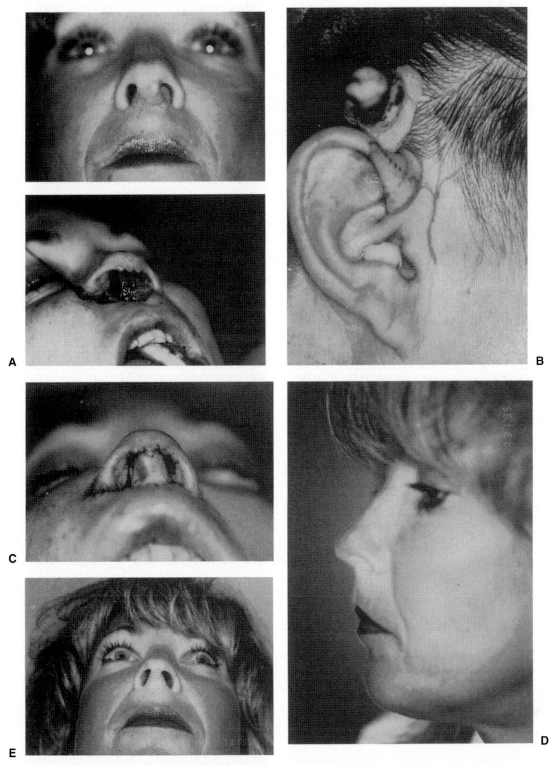

FIG. 3. A: A 42-year-old woman with an arteriovenous malformation involving the columella and upper lip. The lesion was radically resected. **B:** Planned flap marked on the ascending helix of the right ear. **C:** Immediate postoperative result. **D,E:** Long-term result 3 years postoperatively.

References

1. Joseph J. *Nasenplastic und sonstige Gesichtsplastik*. Leipzig: Kabitzsch, 1931.
2. Brown JB, Cannon B. Composite free grafts of skin and cartilage from the ear. *Surg Gynecol Obstet* 1946;82:253.
3. Dupertuis SM. Free ear lobe grafts of skin and fat. *Plast Reconstr Surg* 1946;1:135.
4. Converse JM. Reconstruction of nasolabial area by composite grafts from concha. *Plast Reconstr Surg* 1950;5:247.
5. Lin SD, Lin GT, Lai GS, et al. Nasal alar reconstruction with free "accessory auricle." *Plast Reconstr Surg* 1984;73:827.
6. Parkhouse N, Evans D. Reconstruction of the ala of the nose using composite free flap from the pinna. *Br J Plast Surg* 1985;38:306.
7. Pribaz JJ, Falco N. Nasal reconstruction with auricular microvascular transplant. *Ann Plast Surg* 1993;31:289.
8. Antia NH, Buck VI. Chondrocutaneous advancement flap for the marginal defect of the ear. *Plast Reconstr Surg* 1967;39:472.

CHAPTER 66 ■ NASAL ALAR RECONSTRUCTION WITH AN EAR HELIX FREE FLAP

S. M. SHENAQ, T. A. DINH, AND M. SPIRA

EDITORIAL COMMENT

This procedure provides a very elegant reconstruction of the nasal alar region; however, the surgeon must be expert in microvascular techniques.

A vascularized chondrocutaneous free flap from the root of the auricular helix can serve as a solution to the problem of alar reconstruction. It is unlike local flaps that may result in additional facial scarring and bulky alae that require multiple thinning revisions. This flap produces satisfactory symmetry between the two alae and a good color match. The donor defect can be concealed with hair in female patients (1–10).

INDICATIONS

The structural similarities between the alae and the auricular helices have allowed the use of free helical composite grafts to repair small nasal defects of less than 2.0 cm (11–16). More recent delineation of the vascular territories of the ear has allowed the use of vascularized helical free flaps in the repair of large alar defects. With a chondrocutaneous microsurgical free flap from the root of the auricular helix, a successful reconstruction of a 3.2 × 3.0 cm full-thickness alar defect is possible.

This flap has several advantages: (a) The size of the flap can be easily tailored to the needs of reconstruction; this is especially important in large defects. (b) Similarities in the structure, contour, thickness, and color match between the helical rim and the nasal ala minimize the need for later revision and often provide superior reconstructive results over local flaps, especially for large defects. (c) The donor defect is acceptable and easily covered with temporal hair, especially in female patients. (d) When required, this flap facilitates the reconstruction of the base of the ala at the alar/cheek angle.

Disadvantages include the requirement for microsurgical expertise to perform this type of procedure, and the considerable additional time necessary, compared to more standard procedures.

ANATOMY

The ala nasi consists of external skin, cartilaginous support, and inner lining. The normal ala is thin, but contains enough cartilage to prevent its collapse. The helical rim of the ear and the alar rim are the only places in the body where "skin abuts skin," an important reason why reconstruction is so difficult.

The auricular helix contains a sufficient amount of supporting cartilage enveloped in thin skin, very similar to the structure of the natural ala nasi. The thin helical edge closely resembles the thin alar rim. That part of the helix is chosen that best approximates the contour of the ala, thus minimizing the need for secondary procedures. Microsurgical technique allows successful transference of a composite flap in a one-stage free-flap procedure, utilizing the root of the helix and adjacent preauricular skin.

FLAP DESIGN AND DIMENSIONS

For reconstruction of the left ala, the right auricular helix is chosen. The superficial temporal vessels of the flap are placed at the inferior lateral angle of the helix, thus allowing for better reach. The left anterior superficial temporal artery and vein are also preserved as a second backup vascular source.

OPERATIVE TECHNIQUE

The procedure is described in a 36-year-old woman with squamous-cell carcinoma involving the left alar rim, nostril, and lower alar cartilage that required excision. The residual defect measured 3.2 × 3.0 cm, and the septal mucosa was clearly visible through the defect (Fig. 1). One-year follow-up postexcision showed no sign of cancer recurrence.

The procedure was performed under general anesthesia. Intraoperatively, the margins of the defect were found on frozen

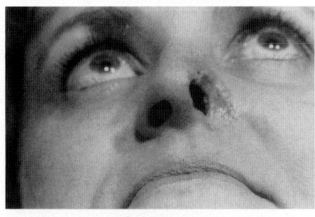

FIG. 1. Basal view of alar defect after cancer excision.

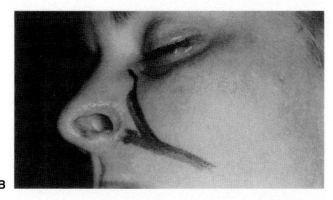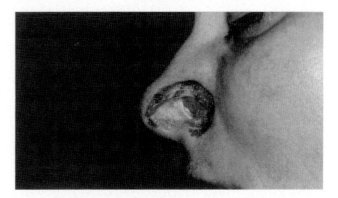

A,B

FIG. 2. Close-up intraoperative photographs showing defect (**A**) before and (**B**) after preparation for reconstruction.

section to be free of any malignancy (Fig. 2). The facial vein was isolated through an incision along the nasolabial crease. Because of sclerosis of the facial and superior labial arteries, the superficial temporal artery on the ipsilateral side was chosen to be the recipient artery via a 12-cm vein graft from the foot.

An appropriate outline of the left alar defect, measuring 3.5 × 3.0 cm, was marked on the superior helix of the right ear to include a portion of the preauricular skin. The proximal portions of the superficial temporal vessels were exposed and skeletonized for approximately 4 cm, to achieve an adequate pedicle length. The flap was elevated to include the root of the helix and adjacent preauricular skin (Fig. 3).

The flap was inserted into the defect, and restoration of the alar rim was achieved (Fig. 4). The free flap was revascularized by anastomosing its arterial vascular pedicle to the left superficial temporal artery, employing the vein graft previously mentioned. The vein was then anastomosed to the facial vein lying under the nasolabial fold. Standard microvascular techniques were employed, using simple interrupted sutures of 10-0 nylon for the anastomosis.

The donor defect on the right ear was covered by advancing skin over the exposed cartilage and closed with multiple interrupted sutures of 4-0 nylon. The vein-graft donor site was closed. The entire surgical procedure took approximately 7 hours.

CLINICAL RESULTS

There was an uncomplicated postoperative course, and no donor-site problems were encountered. A minor scar revision of the flap edges was performed 4 months later. One-year follow-up showed satisfactory symmetry between the two alae and a good color match. The donor site on the right ear could be concealed with hair (Fig. 5).

SUMMARY

The ear, because of its similar structure, color, texture, and contour, provides excellent tissue for reconstruction of the ala,

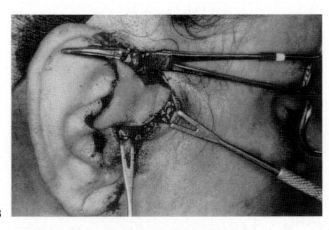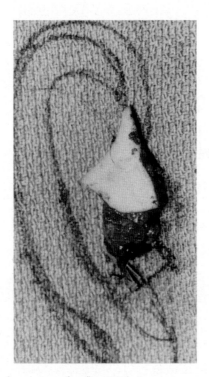

A,B

FIG. 3. Intraoperative photographs showing the helical composite chondrocutaneous free flap, (**A**) during and (**B**) after harvest, with its superficial temporal vessels.

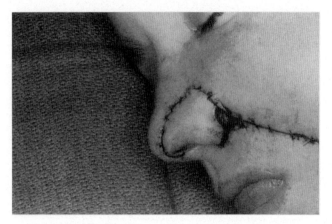

FIG. 4. Left ala immediately postinsertion of flap.

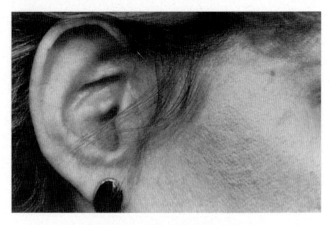

FIG. 5. Donor site at 1-year follow-up.

columella, and nasal tip. Vascularized helical free flaps provide a good solution to the problem of repairing large alar full-thickness defects.

References

1. Hallock GG, Dreyer TM. The stair-step flap for nasal alar reconstruction. *Ann Plast Surg* 1987;18:34.
2. Hirshowitz B, Kaufman T, Ullman J. Reconstruction of the tip of the nose and alar by load cycling of the nasal skin and harnessing of extra skin. *Plast Reconstr Surg* 1986;77:316.
3. Gliosci A, Sabbagh E, Hipps CJ. Reconstruction of the ala of the nose by local pedicle flap. *Plast Reconstr Surg* 1968;41:149.
4. Fox JW IV, Golden GT, Edgerton MT. Surgical correction of absent nasal alae of the Johnson-Blizzard syndrome. *Plast Reconstr Surg* 1976;57:484.
5. Hardin JC Jr. Alar rim reconstruction by a dorsal nasal flap. *Plast Reconstr Surg* 1980;66:2293.
6. Pers M. Cheek flaps in partial rhinoplasty. *Scand J Plast Reconstr Surg* 1967;1:37.
7. Herbert DC. A subcutaneous pedicled cheek flap for reconstruction of alar defect. *Br J Plast Surg* 1978;31:79.
8. Spear SL, Kroll SS, Romm S. A new twist to the nasolabial flap for reconstruction of lateral alar defects. *Plast Reconstr Surg* 1987;79:915.
9. Hauben DJ, Sagi A. A simple method for alar rim reconstruction. *Plast Reconstr Surg* 1987;80:839.
10. Washio H. Retroauricular-temporal flap. *Plast Reconstr Surg* 1969;43:162.
11. Konig F. Ueber nasenplastik. *Beitr Klinish Chir* 1914;94:515.
12. Dupertius SM. Free ear lobe grafts of skin and fat. *Plast Reconstr Surg* 1946;1:135.
13. Field LM. Nasal alar rim reconstruction utilizing the crus of the helix, with several alternatives for donor site closure. *J Dermatol Surg Oncol* 1986;12:253.
14. Lehman JA, Garrett WS Jr, Musgrave RH. Earlobe composite grafts for the correction of nasal defects. *Plast Reconstr Surg* 1971;47:122.
15. Lin SD, Lin GT, Lai CS, et al. Nasal alar reconstruction with free "accessory auricle." *Plast Reconstr Surg* 1984;73:827.
16. Parkhouse N, Evans D. Reconstruction of the ala of the nose using a composite free flap from the pinna. *Br J Plast Surg* 1985;38:306.

Online Chapter

CHAPTER 67. Microvascular Free Transfer of a Compound Dorsalis Pedis Skin Flap with Second Metatarsal Bone *K. Ohmori*

www.encyclopediaofflaps.com

CHAPTER 68 ■ NASAL VESTIBULAR CHONDROMUCOSAL FLAP

D. R. MILLARD, JR.

EDITORIAL COMMENT

The editors feel that correction of the retruded columella could be accomplished by shortening the nose as the author did, but it also could be achieved by judicious placement of cartilaginous grafts to the columella. In correcting notching of the alar rim, the described procedure is indicated when a shortage of nasal lining but an adequate amount of external nasal skin are present.

The chondromucosal flap for correction of columellar retraction after septal resection was first described in 1963 (1). This flap has several donor areas and great versatility, and it is available for unilateral or bilateral use (2,3).

INDICATIONS

When the columella is retracted, the nasal tip is depressed from lack of anterior septal support, and the lateral side walls

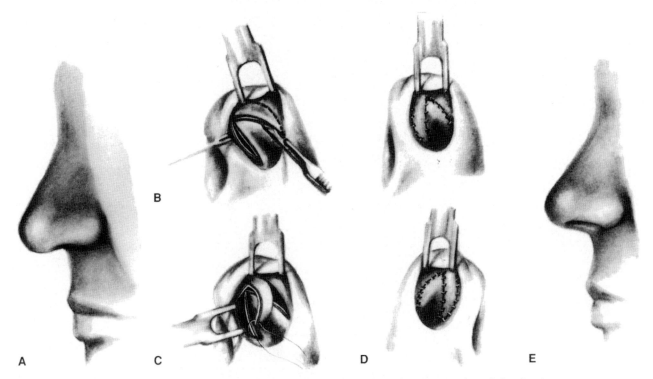

FIG. 1. A: Retracted columella, long side walls, and depressed nasal tip. **B:** Lateral vestibular chondromucosal flap marked and being cut with an anterosuperior base. **C:** Chondromucosal flap being transposed into membranous septal releasing incision. **D:** Bilateral transposition of these flaps, sutured into place. **E:** Side wall lifted as columella is released and nasal tip elevated slightly. (**B–D** from Millard, ref. 3, with permission.)

are relatively long, then lateral chondromucosal flaps, including portions of the lower lateral alar cartilage, are available (Fig. 1A). When there is a hanging columella that is exaggerated by retracted lateral side walls or even collapse of the alar margins and nasal obstruction, reverse chondromucosal flaps are available (Fig. 2A).

These flaps are also available for a unilateral deformity and can even be taken from one lateral vestibule and slid subcutaneously over the septum to supply the opposite side. (The temporary fistula can be closed after several weeks.)

During reconstruction of a columella or side wall, the chondromucosal flaps can be used to provide lining and support. These flaps also can be quite helpful in conjunction with a nasolabial skin covering flap.

ANATOMY

This is a compound flap containing lining and cartilage. The vascular dependability of this flap is remarkable, considering the hazardous width-to-length ratio. This is probably due to the fact that the flap is backed by cartilage, which acts as a splint to prevent collapse or kinking of the vessels within it.

FLAP DESIGN AND DIMENSIONS

The chondromucosal flap is relatively narrow (0.5 to 0.75 cm wide) and at least four to five times longer than it is wide. Viability and maneuverability depend on its base, which is superior and anterior high up under the tip and above the front point of the septum (Figs. 1B and 2B).

OPERATIVE TECHNIQUE

Retracted Columella and Depressed Nasal Tip

The membranous septal incision that releases the retracted columella should be extended laterally along the standard intercartilaginous line as far as the length of the flap (Fig. 1A). The incision then makes a sharp turn around at the end of the flap, coming back anteriorly and parallel to the first incision along an anterior vestibular line—fashioning a flap width of 0.5 to 0.75 cm (Fig. 1B).

As the columella is advanced forward, these bilateral chondromucosal flaps will ride forward with the tip and swing medially into the membranous septal gap (Fig. 1C). The flaps come together between the columella and the septum, with their cartilages touching and the lining facing out. Closure of the lateral donor areas will lift the relatively long side walls for additional correction of the deformity (Fig. 1D, E).

Hanging Columella and Retracted Lateral Side Walls

By taking the excess of chondromucosal tissue from between and including various portions of the columella and septum, this part of the deformity is corrected (Fig. 2B). Transposition of these flaps in a "wing spreading" maneuver places both support and additional lining into the defect produced by lateral relaxing incisions inside the vestibule parallel with the alar margins (Fig. 2C). Not only does this let the retracted alar rim down, but the added support opens the airway and maintains the improved aperture (Fig. 2D, E).

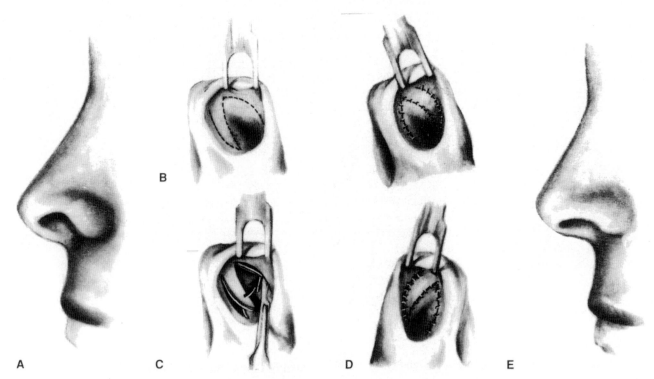

FIG. 2. **A:** Retracted alae and hanging columella. **B:** Chondromucosal flaps taken from membranous septum based anteriorly and superiorly. **C:** Flap being transposed into vestibular alar releasing incision. **D:** Bilateral transposition of these flaps, sutured into place. **E:** Simultaneous correction of hanging columella and retracted alae.

SUMMARY

Nasal vestibular chondromucosal flaps can be taken from the lateral side walls to correct a retracted columella and depressed nasal tip. Reverse chondromucosal flaps can be taken from the septum to correct a hanging columella that is exaggerated by retracted lateral side walls. Unilateral defects also can be corrected using this flap.

References

1. Millard DR Jr. The triad of columella deformities. *Plast Reconstr Surg* 1963;31:370.
2. Millard DR Jr. Secondary corrective rhinoplasty. *Plast Reconstr Surg* 1969;44:545.
3. Millard DR Jr. The versatility of a chondromucosal flap in the nasal vestibule. *Plast Reconstr Surg* 1972;50:580.

CHAPTER 69 ■ L-SHAPED SEPTAL CHONDROMUCOSAL FLAP

D. R. MILLARD, JR.

EDITORIAL COMMENT

This is an attractive idea, but it is extremely difficult to execute and still retain an adequate blood supply to the cartilage.

Nasal reconstruction requires the provision of support, as well as cover and lining (1). When the support normally provided by the septum has been lost, an L-shaped septal chondromucosal flap usually can be advanced from remaining septum. It can then be lifted out of the nasal cavity, so that its front prow rests on the nasal spine area, and it can be fixed at this point (2).

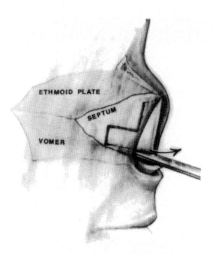

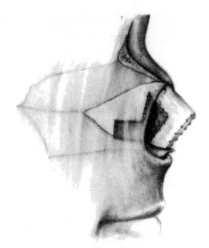

FIG. 1. The remaining septum is marked and cut as an L-shaped chondromucosal flap based superiorly. The chisel is seen freeing the anterior portion of the flap from the vomerine groove. The broken line at the base of the L (toward the dorsal tip of the nasal bones) is the area where the cartilage can be divided subperiosteally if release is needed.

FIG. 2. The L-shaped chondromucosal flap has been advanced out of the nasal vestibule and fixed on the nasal spine. The mucosa has been sutured to close off the cartilage posteriorly, and a split-thickness skin graft is placed to cover the anterior raw area of the septum temporarily. This scaffold offers excellent support for reconstruction of the nose.

INDICATIONS

The septum is the most important normal nasal support of two-thirds of the distal bridge, the tip, and the columella. When this portion of the septum has been lost by cancer ablation, trauma, burns, or infection, new support must be supplied. Usually, this has been accomplished by free grafts of costal cartilage or iliac bone after new lining and cover have been transported to the nasal defect.

In many cases, even though the actual effective bridge, tip, and columella support of the septum has been lost, there is still enough septum hidden back in the nasal cavity. The remaining septum has thin but strong cartilaginous support, and it is covered tenaciously with mucosa, which, of course, is ideal for reconstructing the distal half of the nose.

FLAP DESIGN AND DIMENSIONS

The superior base of the L, as well as its right angle, is maintained at least 1 cm wide to ensure adequate vascularity through the covering mucosa (Fig. 1).

OPERATIVE TECHNIQUE

If there is difficulty with rotation of the L component forward, careful subperichondrial division of a part or all of the septal cartilage at the proximal base of the chondromucosal flap (broken line in Fig. 1) will facilitate its deliverance out into the real world (Fig. 2).

The exposed cartilage of the underside of this flap is shaved back to allow closure of mucosa without tension, as a protected compartment. The raw front of the septal L is covered temporarily with a split-thickness skin graft (Fig. 2).

It is wise to advance this lined nasal framework and allow it to become established as a dependable scaffold for 1 month before cloaking it with the lining and cover of a nasal reconstruction.

SUMMARY

A septal chondromucosal flap can provide ideal support for a nasal reconstruction.

References

1. Millard DR Jr. Aesthetic reconstructive rhinoplasty. *Clin Plast Surg* 1981;8:169.
2. Millard DR Jr. Reconstructive rhinoplasty for the lower half of a nose. *Plast Reconstr Surg* 1974;53:133.

CHAPTER 70 ■ INTERNAL NASAL VESTIBULAR SKIN-MUCOSAL FLAPS

T. R. VECCHIONE

The columella is the cornerstone of naso-oral construction and is necessary for a pleasing balance. When it is destroyed by infection, trauma, or disease, its absence becomes glaringly obvious (Fig. 1A). The successful treatment of patients lacking the lower septum and columella with a simple one-stage flap is presented.

INDICATIONS

The difficulty in reconstructing this subtle aesthetic unit has stimulated many elaborate operative techniques requiring multiple stages (1). Various composite grafts from the ear and lip have been described, but these are of benefit only in the partially deficient columella with sufficient surrounding tissue

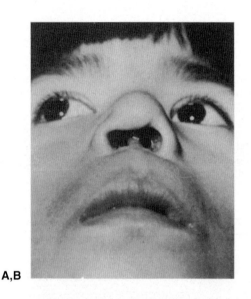
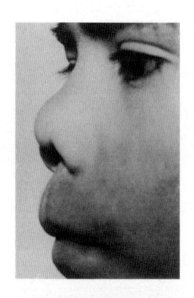

A,B

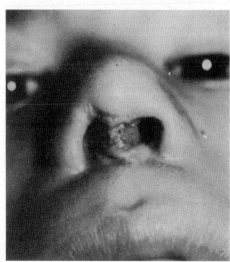
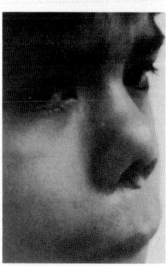

C,D

FIG. 1. A,B: An 8-year-old boy with absent columella secondary to severe infection at age 4. The columella, membranous septum, and 0.4 × 3.0 cm of cartilaginous septum were missing. C,D: The patient 2 years after local tissue columellar reconstruction.

198

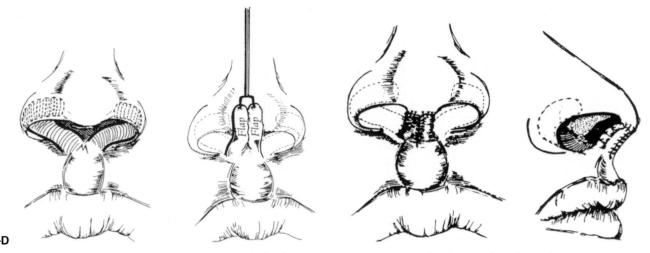

A–D

FIG. 2. **A:** The local skin-mucosal flaps are based just above the philtrum, extending out along the nasal vestibule and then upward to include mucosa lining the lateral alar cartilage. **B:** When the two flaps are brought together in the midline, they extend beyond the nasal tip. **C:** The flaps are sutured to the dissected nasal tip. The flap donor sites heal by epithelialization and wound contracture. **D:** On close inspection, the bucket-handle effect can be seen, but this is not readily recognized at conversational distances.

present for composite graft take. These grafted tissues also were noted to shrink and become "fibrotic lumps."

The mucosa of the upper lip followed by a split-thickness skin graft has been used, but wound contracture and fibrosis have detracted from the long-term results (2). A frontonasal flap based on the temporalis artery (3) has been refined (4) by using a median frontal flap tunneled subcutaneously to bring a pedicle to the columella. The versatile nasolabial flap has been transferred through the nasal mucosa passing between the ala and triangular cartilages in a three-staged procedure (5). The centrally based upper lip flap and an adjacent nasolabial flap have been used to reconstruct the columella in a one-stage procedure (6). The price paid is a bearded columella and facial scars.

The internal nasal vestibular flap presented here eliminates any external scars in the flap donor site.

ANATOMY

This flap consists mainly of nasal vestibular skin, but it may include some mucosa. The circulation is of a random-pattern type.

FLAP DESIGN AND DIMENSIONS

Bilateral skin-mucosal flaps are based on the nasal floor just superior to the philtrum and extend around the nasal cupola.

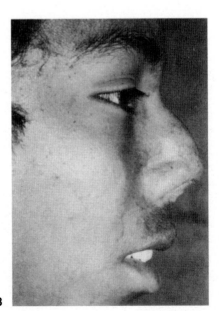

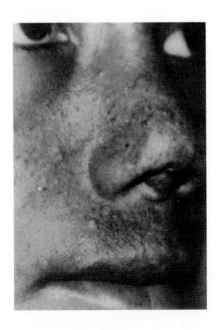

A,B

FIG. 3. **A:** A 17-year-old boy following columellar reconstruction with internal nasal vestibule skin-mucosal flaps. The columella and membranous septum were lacking. They had been involved with a hemangioma that had been managed by multiple resections. **B:** Same patient 6 months after a preauricular dermal overgraft to the newly reconstructed columella.

The flaps usually measure about 6 mm in width and extend parallel to the alar rim approximately 2 cm.

OPERATIVE TECHNIQUE

Once the vestibular lining is elevated off the lateral alar cartilage, the flaps are raised and rotated toward the midline to reconstruct the columella (Fig. 2A). A small anteriorly based flap under the nasal tip is elevated, providing a raw surface into which the distal tips of the flaps are inset. After the flaps are sutured, the nasal airways are packed with petrolatum gauze. The flap donor site is allowed to close by epithelialization and wound contracture.

CLINICAL RESULTS

The intact alar cartilage minimizes the distortion caused by contraction as the nasal vestibule reepithelializes. Resurfacing the caudal edges of the reconstructed columella with a non–hair-bearing skin graft may be necessary in some patients.

Occasionally, a dermal overgrafting procedure may be required to improve the color match (Fig. 3).

SUMMARY

A method is presented for using local internal nasal flaps in the reconstruction of an absent columella.

References

1. Paietta FX, Van Norman RT. Total reconstruction of the columella. *Plast Reconstr Surg* 1962;30:322.
2. Smith F. *Plastic and reconstructive surgery*. Philadelphia: Saunders, 1930. P. 506.
3. Heanley C. The subcutaneous tissue pedicle flap in columella and other nasal reconstruction. *Br J Plast Surg* 1955;8:60.
4. Cardoso D. The loss of columella after leishmaniasis: reconstruction with submucous tissue pedicle flap. *Plast Reconstr Surg* 1958;21:117.
5. DeSilva GS. A new method of reconstructing a columella with a nasal labial flap. *Plast Reconstr Surg* 1964;34:63.
6. Snow JW, Harris HW. One-stage columella reconstruction. *Plast Reconstr Surg* 1968;42:83.

CHAPTER 71 ■ MULTI-ISLAND FREE RADIAL FOREARM FLAP FOR RECONSTRUCTION OF THE NASAL LINING

R. L. WALTON

EDITORIAL COMMENT

Total nose reconstruction has reached a level of spectacular development (1–4), particularly with the clinical examples demonstrated by Walton and Burget. Nasal lining is a most important step prior to the placement of the cartilaginous framework and the overlying skin. The multi-island free radial forearm flap demonstrated here provides the nasal lining quite well. Obviously, it requires a considerable amount of planning.

The first stage for reconstruction of total and subtotal nasal defects is the microsurgical transfer and restoration of the nasal lining and adjacent cheek and upper lip elements, using a multi-island free radial forearm flap. Two months following microsurgical transfer of the nasal lining flap, nasal reconstruction proceeds with application of a cartilage framework and a paramedian forehead flap.

INDICATIONS

Restoration of major nasal loss involving overlying skin and underlying nasal passages including support and lining requires staged reconstruction. A microsurgical approach is used for restoration of the nasal lining prior to external nasal cover reconstruction. Following defect evaluation and careful discussion with the patient, the operative sequence is initiated (Figs. 1 to 3).

FLAP DESIGN AND DIMENSIONS

Preoperatively, an Allen test is performed to ensure adequate hand perfusion via the ulnar vascular pedicle. The nasal site is dissected first, with excision of the remnant scar and any skin grafts, to recreate the original defect (Fig. 4). Templates of the missing vestibular and adjacent lip and cheek defects are made of foil from surgical suture packets and then transferred to the forearm, where they are aligned to the radial vascular

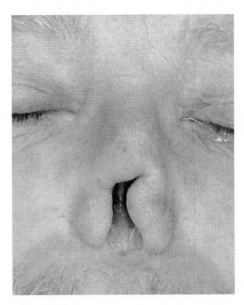

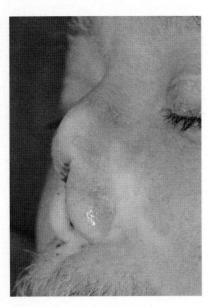

FIG. 1. Preoperative frontal view of subtotal nasal defect showing composite loss of nasal tip, columella, alae, anterior septum, and vestibular lining.

FIG. 2. Preoperative three-quarter view depicting subtotal nasal defect.

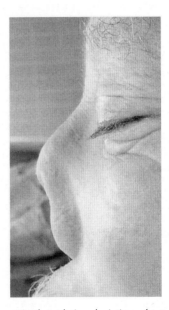

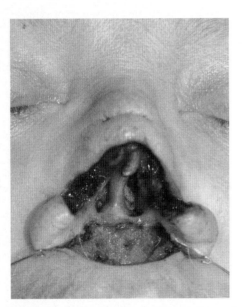

FIG. 3. Preoperative lateral view depicting subtotal nasal defect.

FIG. 4. Preparation of the nasal site. Contracted scar has been removed, and the wound and adjacent nasal elements are repositioned anatomically.

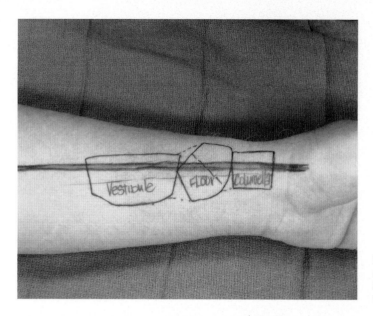

FIG. 5. Templates of the missing nasal lining elements are aligned to the radial vascular pedicle. In this case the multi-island flap will restore the nasal vestibular lining, the floor, and columellar elements.

pedicle as separate islands. The radial side of the flaps is positioned to overlap the vascular pedicle by no more than 5 mm, so as to place the pedicle out of harm's way during subsequent procedures. For the vestibular lining element, we have found it helpful to orient the vascular pedicle at the cephalic edge, so as to allow unsullied access to the nasal tip and vestibule for placement of the supporting cartilage grafts and for sculpting (Fig. 5).

Care is taken to provide sufficient skin island separation, to accommodate the three-dimensional positioning of these elements at the nasal site. For this purpose, in the planning stage, we have found it useful to attach each of the island templates with strips of paper tape, to duplicate the radial vascular pedicle, and then to determine the best three-dimensional configuration of the islands that duplicates the missing anatomy without kinking the vascular pedicle. The fine vascular perforators from the radial pedicle to the overlying skin islands cannot be identified via Doppler or contrast angiography preoperatively, thereby calling for a flap design and configuration based largely on confidence in the vascular anatomy. The distribution of these vessels in the distal forearm has proved to be fairly consistent in our experience, with adequate physiologic flow provided in more than 100 consecutive multi-island flaps without any loss.

OPERATIVE TECHNIQUE

The proximal pedicle should be at least 8 to 10 cm in length, to allow it to span the distance from the nasal defect site to the facial artery and vein at the inferior border of the mandible. This distance is measured intraoperatively so that adequate pedicle length is provided. A 2-cm incision is made just below and parallel to the inferior mandibular border at the site of the facial vessels. The platysmal fibers are dissected apart longitudinally, to expose the facial artery and vein. The marginal branch of the facial nerve is identified and protected. A submuscular aponeurotic system (SMAS) tunnel spanning the nasal site and the facial vessel site is then bluntly dissected with progressive surgical dilators.

The one- to three-island radial forearm flap is dissected under tourniquet control (Fig. 6). Each island is dissected from its ulnar margin above the level of the forearm fascia to the tendon of the flexor carpi radialis. Here, the dissection transitions to the subfascial plane to the radial vascular pedicle. On the radial side of the flap, the dissection proceeds through the subcutaneous tissue, with care taken to identify and protect the dorsal sensory branches of the radial nerve. Occasionally, one or two small branches of the radial sensory nerve may be found entering the radial forearm flap. These are

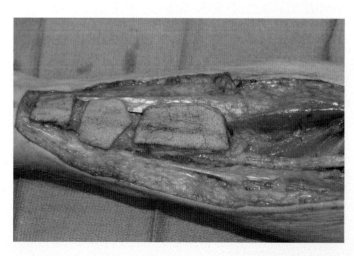

FIG. 6. The radial forearm flap has been dissected above the level of the deep forearm fascia and separated into three separate islands. Following debulking of the flap islands, the flap will be transferred to the nasal site, where it is revascularized to the facial vessels.

divided, and the proximal stumps are buried in the volar fore-arm musculature, to avoid painful neuroma formation.

The radial artery and its venae comitantes are dissected distal to the last skin island in the chain, ligated with fine polypropylene sutures, and divided. The dissection then proceeds deep to the radial vascular pedicle, where several large branches will be seen entering the dorsal musculature. These are ligated with fine monofilament sutures and divided. Using operative magnification, dissection of the island flaps is then performed, with identification and preservation of the multiple small filamentous branches from the radial vascular pedicle to each island. Despite their very small size, preservation of these branches is paramount to successful flap perfusion. The vascular pedicle is then dissected proximally to its appropriate length, with ligation and division of its multiple forearm muscular branches (Fig. 6).

The flap is allowed to perfuse at the forearm site for 30 minutes prior to transfer. During this time, the operating microscope is used to debulk selected elements of the flap (especially the vestibular lining element). This is accomplished by incising the fibrous interstitium between the fat lobules and gently suctioning the fat away directly by a process dubbed "liplplucksion." We have found this to be a very effective technique for performing the initial debulking of the acute flap, without compromising its blood supply.

After the flap pedicle is divided, the flap is transferred to the nasal site, where it is temporarily secured with 4–0 silk sutures. The vascular pedicle is gently directed through the subcutaneous tunnel in the cheek, using a 32 to 36 French-size chest tube guide lubricated with a continuous lactated Ringer solution drip, to avoid avulsion of any vascular branch ligatures or inadvertent twisting. The vascular repairs are performed end-to-end to the facial artery and vein. Although no systemic anticoagulation is used, we routinely employ high-concentration heparin irrigation (50,000 units heparin per 100 mL lactated Ringer solution) while performing the vascular anastomoses. Aspirin (81 mg) is also administered intraoperatively and for 21 days postoperatively for its prostacyclin and antiplatelet effects.

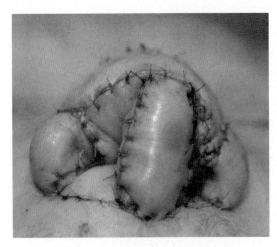

FIG. 8. Inset of the radial forearm flap (submental view). The separate flap islands have been articulated to duplicate the three-dimensional anatomy of the missing elements.

Following reestablishment of vascular inflow, the flap is inset anatomically with fine sutures. To avoid contraction of the nasal vestibular lining elements, we have found it useful to brace the flaps with small grafts of cadaver allograft cartilage placed in the midline and along the caudal edge of the vestibule and secured with 6–0 PDS suture prior to skin grafting (Fig. 7). When placed over the supporting cartilage allografts, the take of the full-thickness skin graft is not compromised, owing to its excellent capacity for bridging. The undersurface of the vestibular element, which now lies externally, is closed with a full-thickness skin graft from the inguinal region (Figs. 8 to 10). When the grafted area is large, a fine suction drain, fashioned from a 22-gauge butterfly intravenous needle, is placed beneath the skin graft, to facilitate graft adherence and to promote serous drainage. A simple Xeroform/ muropuracin dressing is applied to the grafted vestibular element. No internal nasal packing or stents are employed.

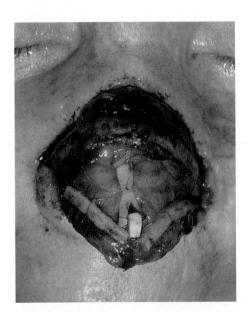

FIG. 7. Frontal view of the radial forearm flap inset prior to placement of the full-thickness skin graft. Note position of the vascular pedicle at the cranial edge of the flap. Cadaver cartilage allograft has been used to stent the vestibular lining element to stifle its shrinkage in the interim prior to placement of the definitive cartilage framework and the paramedian forehead flap. The cartilage allografts are secured with fine absorbable monofilament sutures. Skin graft "take" over the cartilage grafts occurs via bridging.

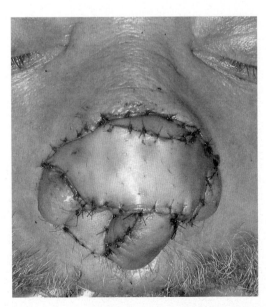

FIG. 9. Inset of the radial forearm flap (frontal view). The undersurface of the vestibular lining flap element is temporarily covered with a full-thickness graft from the inguinal region.

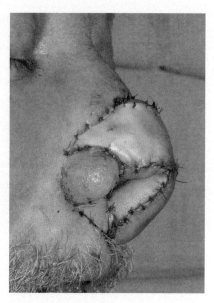

FIG. 10. Inset of the radial forearm flap (lateral view).

The forearm donor site is closed with a full-thickness skin graft from the inguinal region for optimal pliability and cosmetic appearance. The graft is secured with a stent dressing, and the forearm and hand are immobilized in a bulky dressing. The graft stent is removed at 7 days postoperatively, and the forearm is wrapped in an elastic compression sleeve for 6 weeks. Graded, active use of the hand is allowed at 10 days postoperatively.

When fully healed and edema has subsided, the external skin graft on the nose is removed, an autologous rib cartilage nasal framework is constructed, and a paramedian forehead flap is transferred for restoration of the external nasal cover.

SUMMARY

The radial forearm flap is an excellent option for use in restoration of nasal lining and adjacent cheek and lip defects for total and subtotal nasal reconstruction. The flap anatomy is consistent, allowing for configuration into multiple islands that can be articulated to duplicate the three-dimensional nasal lining anatomy. Flap dissection is superficial to the deep forearm fascia, using the venae comitantes for venous outflow. Revascularization is via the facial artery and vein. Cadaver allograft cartilage is used to stent the flap elements to prevent their shrinkage prior to definitive construction of an autologous cartilage framework.

References

1. Walton RL, Burget GC, Beahm EK: Microsurgical reconstruction of the nasal lining. *Plast Reconstr Surg* 2005;115(7):1812.
2. Burget GC, Walton RL: Optimal use of microvascular free flaps, cartilage grafts, and a paramedian forehead flap for aesthetic reconstruction of the nose and adjacent facial units. *Plast Reconstr Surg* 2007;120(5):1171.
3. Beahm EK, Walton RL: Nasal reconstruction. In: Butler CE, Fine NA, Eds., *Principles of cancer reconstructive surgery*. New York: Springer, 2006.
4. Walton RL, Beahm EK, Burget GC: Nasal reconstruction. In: Grotting JC, Ed., *Reoperative aesthetic and reconstructive plastic surgery*, 2nd Ed. St. Louis: Quality Medical Publishing, 2007;705–758.

CHAPTER 72 ■ FORKED FLAP

D. R. MILLARD, JR.

The forked flap was initially designed to lengthen a short columella in a secondary bilateral cleft. The forked flap is taken out of the lip continuous with the present short columella. This approach not only lengthens the columella, but also allows revision of bilateral lip scars and reduces the wide prolabium to a more natural philtrum dimension (1–4).

INDICATIONS

The forked-flap technique is of value in bilateral cleft patients when the columella is short and the upper lip is not tighter than the lower lip (Fig. 1). The procedure also has been found of value in primary bilateral cleft patients when the prolabium is extremely diminutive (Fig. 2), as well as when the prolabium is wide enough in the primary deformity to spare a forked flap from its sides and still leave enough central portion for a philtrum (Fig. 3).

In the unilateral cleft lip, the cleft side shortness of the columella is lengthened by flap C in the rotation-advancement operation. Flap C acts as a one-sided forked flap.

OPERATIVE TECHNIQUE

Short Columella and Wide Prolabium

This problem can be improved by a forked flap that includes the old bilateral cleft lip scars (Fig. 1).

Complete Bilateral Cleft Lip with Small Prolabium

The lateral elements are merely attached to the sides of the tiny prolabium in an adhesion procedure, and within a year, the muscle pull will have stretched the prolabium wide enough to give up a forked flap. This flap can then be taken out of the

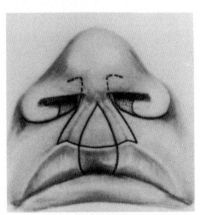
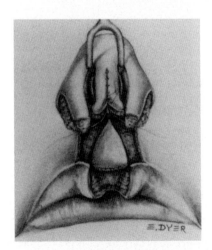
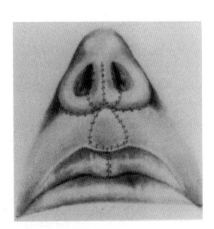

A–C

FIG. 1. **A:** Short columella and wide prolabium. Note that the forked flaps include the old bilateral cleft lip scars. Note also that the membranous septal incision is extended over the nasal tip, as indicated by the *broken line.* **B:** The forked flaps are sutured together and advanced along the septum. They are sutured together in front and then tubed behind to create a column. The distal tips of the fork are left free to spread at the columella base. The alar bases, with their tips denuded of epithelium, are sutured together at the nasal spine in a cinching procedure. **C:** The ends of the forked flaps are sutured to the alar bases to form the nostril sills. The lateral lip elements are sutured to the sides of the reduced prolabium, and the lateral mucocutaneous flaps are advanced to the midline below the prolabium to create a better cupid's bow and tubercle.

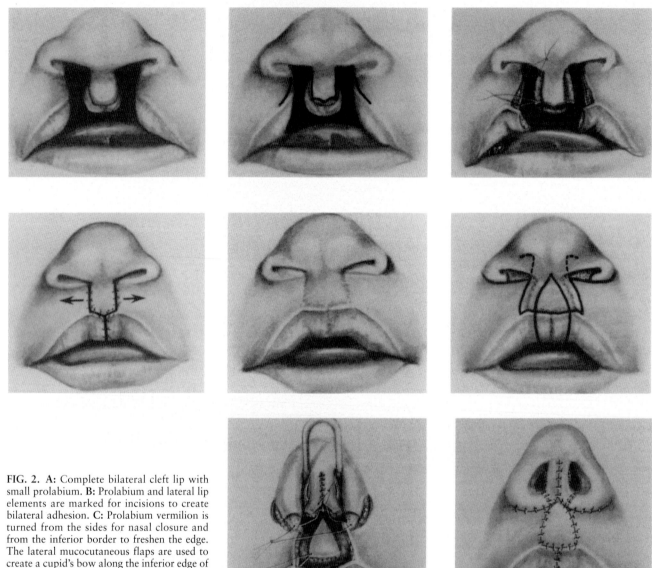

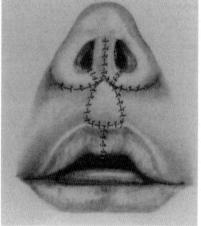

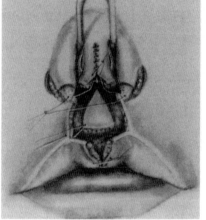

A–C

D–F

G,H

FIG. 2. **A:** Complete bilateral cleft lip with small prolabium. **B:** Prolabium and lateral lip elements are marked for incisions to create bilateral adhesion. **C:** Prolabium vermilion is turned from the sides for nasal closure and from the inferior border to freshen the edge. The lateral mucocutaneous flaps are used to create a cupid's bow along the inferior edge of the prolabium. **D:** After the adhesion is completed, the lateral muscle pull will stretch the prolabium. **E:** At 1 year, the prolabium is stretched enough to spare a forked flap. **F:** The forked flap and membranous septal incision are marked. **G:** The forked flap is sutured and advanced along the septum, the alar bases are cinched, and the lateral lip elements are advanced to the reduced prolabium. The lateral mucocutaneous flaps are advanced along the inferior edge of the prolabium. **H:** Final columella lengthening, nasal tip release, alar base narrowing, and lip closure.

lip and either banked in a whisker position below the alar bases or advanced into the columella (Fig. 2).

Complete Bilateral Cleft Lip with Wide Prolabium

If the prolabium is wide enough in the primary deformity to spare a forked flap from its sides and still leave enough central portion for a philtrum, then forks are banked in the whisker position. At the preschool age of 5 years or as soon as the premaxilla is in reasonably good alignment with the lateral maxilla and fixed, the forks are shifted out of the whisker position and advanced into the columella to release the depressed nasal tip (Fig. 3).

There are several points in the technique that may be helpful in achieving a natural effect: First, when cutting the forks in secondary cases, take as much prolabium on each side as necessary to shape it as a philtrum, and include the lip scars. Second, release the present short columella with a membranous septal incision that is carried well over the tip of the septum to ensure adequate release. Third, suture the skin of the forks together in front with 6–0 suture. Then roll this double flap into a column with subcutaneous sutures of 5–0 chromic catgut. Advance the new columella column along the membranous septum and fix it with 4–0 chromic catgut. Fourth, leave the distal ends of the forked flap free to spread sideways as the medial feet of the columella to form part of the nostril sill when sutured to the alar bases. Finally, subsequent septal or auricular cartilage grafts can be used in the columella to

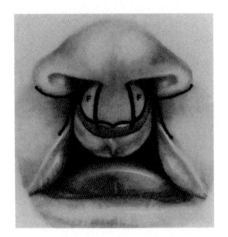
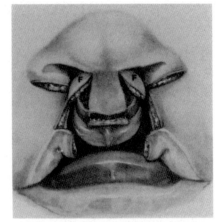
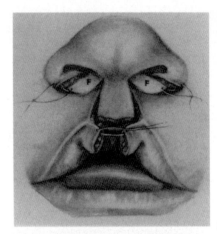

A–C

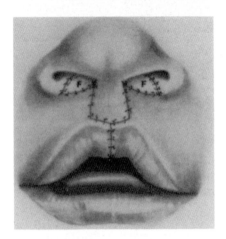
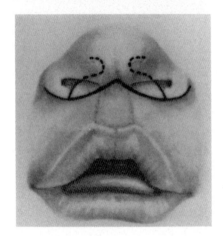

D,E

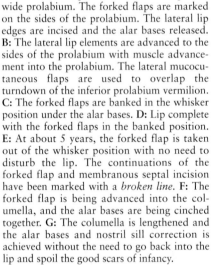
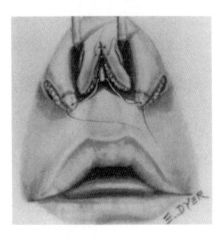
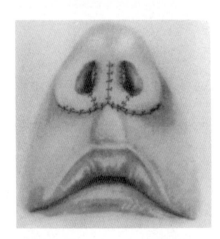

F,G

FIG. 3. A: Complete bilateral cleft lip with wide prolabium. The forked flaps are marked on the sides of the prolabium. The lateral lip edges are incised and the alar bases released. B: The lateral lip elements are advanced to the sides of the prolabium with muscle advancement into the prolabium. The lateral mucocutaneous flaps are used to overlap the turndown of the inferior prolabium vermilion. C: The forked flaps are banked in the whisker position under the alar bases. D: Lip complete with the forked flaps in the banked position. E: At about 5 years, the forked flap is taken out of the whisker position with no need to disturb the lip. The continuations of the forked flap and membranous septal incision have been marked with a *broken line.* F: The forked flap is being advanced into the columella, and the alar bases are being cinched together. G: The columella is lengthened and the alar bases and nostril sill correction is achieved without the need to go back into the lip and spoil the good scars of infancy.

improve the nasal tip support, which is severely lacking owing to the absence of septal projection in the tip in patients with bilateral clefts.

SUMMARY

In certain cleft lip deformities, forked flaps can be used to lengthen the columella both primarily and secondarily.

References

1. Millard DR Jr. Columella lengthening by a forked flap. *Plast Reconstr Surg* 1958;22:454.
2. Millard DR Jr. *Cleft Craft,* Vol. II. Boston: Little, Brown, 1977;359–374, 491–538.
3. Millard DR Jr. Closure of bilateral cleft lip and elongation of columella by two operations in infancy. *Plast Reconstr Surg* 1971;47:324.
4. Millard DR Jr. Earlier correction of the unilateral cleft lip nose. *Plast Reconstr Surg* 1983;70:65.

CHAPTER 73 ■ BILATERAL CHEEK ISLAND SKIN FLAPS

I. KAPLAN AND M. BEN-BASSAT

Many procedures for reconstruction of the columella have been described, but we have found that bilateral cheek island skin flaps have provided gratifying results (1).

INDICATIONS

These flaps are useful in patients in whom the columella alone is missing or in whom there is also a concomitant defect of the upper lip.

ANATOMY

Bilateral inferiorly based skin flaps are taken from the cheek area. The circulation of these flaps is based on the anterior facial vessels (Fig. 1B).

OPERATIVE TECHNIQUE

The flaps are raised as shown in Figure 1B. A rectangular skin paddle is carried on a subcutaneous pedicle. After a tunnel is formed under the skin of the upper lip, the flap is transferred to the defect. The two flaps are then sutured together to form the columella. The donor sites can usually be closed primarily.

If there is also a defect of the upper lip, it is repaired by including the skin from the base to the tip of the flap rather than by just using a skin paddle (Fig. 2).

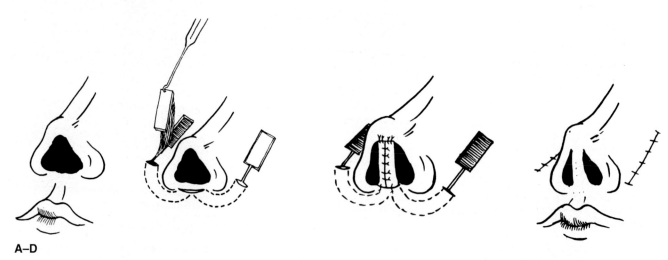

A–D

FIG. 1. A: Absence of the nasal columella. B: Bilateral island skin flaps are based on the anterior facial artery, which can be localized with a Doppler probe. C: The island flaps are tunneled through the upper lip and sutured together to form the columella. D: The flap donor-site wounds are closed by suturing the wound edges. (From Kaplan, ref. 1, with permission.)

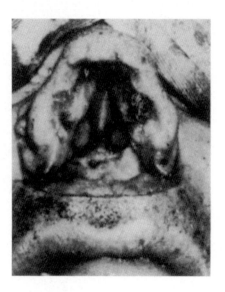
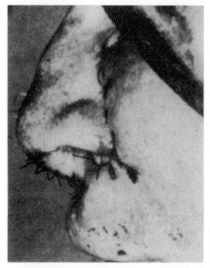

A,B

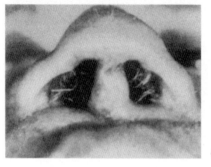

C

FIG. 2. A: Defect of the columella and the cephalad portion of the upper lip following radical excision of a skin cancer. **B:** Profile view at completion of the reconstruction of the columella and adjacent lip with bilateral cheek flaps. Note the sutured donor site of one of the flaps. **C:** Pyramidal view of the columella 3 weeks postoperatively. (From Kaplan, ref. 1, with permission.)

SUMMARY

Bilateral cheek island skin flaps can be used to reconstruct the columella. These flaps are especially useful when there is an associated defect of the upper lip.

Reference

1. Kaplan I. Reconstruction of columella. *Br J Plast Surg* 1972;25:37.

CHAPTER 74 ■ LABIAL MUCOSAL FLAPS FOR RECONSTRUCTION OF THE COLUMELLA

J. R. LEWIS, JR.

EDITORIAL COMMENT

The use of mucosal flaps to reconstruct the columella has two obvious disadvantages: (1) the lack of color match, and (2) the tendency of the mucosa to dry and crust. Both disadvantages are partly corrected by resurfacing of the mucosa with a skin graft.

A flap or flaps from the labial mucosa can be pulled through the lip at the proposed columella base and inserted into the nasal tip for reconstruction of the columella. This is a procedure that has been used on a number of occasions by the author.

INDICATIONS

Mucosal flaps may be used to supply bulk from the base of the lip up to the tip of the nose to form the columella. However, this gives a pink mucosal appearance that generally is secondarily grafted with a full-thickness graft from the back of the ear to give the desired skin color and texture.

The mucosal flap is an undesirable first choice unless there is no tissue available in the immediate area to use as a direct flap. This would be the case when there has been extensive surgery in the nasolabial areas for malignancy or injury or when there has been extensive radiation to the cheeks. However, in such instances, the mucosal flaps themselves may have a precarious blood supply.

ANATOMY

The anatomic basis of the labial mucosal flap that extends outward in the cheek and is based farther laterally would be the superior labial artery. The superior labial vein would complete the circulatory exchange. For bilateral labial flaps taken on the medial aspect of the lip, the circulation is more precarious and would depend on branches of the superior labial artery and a septal branch, unless this had been interrupted. The superior labial artery anastomoses with its counterpart on the opposite side, with the lateral nasal branches of the facial artery, and with the septal branch of the sphenopalatine artery. If the septum has not been resected with the columella for malignancy or has not been injured by trauma, the sphenopalatine artery may be used to give some additional circulation into this flap.

FLAP DESIGN AND DIMENSIONS

The flap based medially is a reverse flap (Fig. 1A). When using two such flaps brought together through a single opening at the base of the lip at the proposed base of the columella, they are sutured lightly together and brought up to the underside of the nasal tip (Fig. 1B). As with reverse flaps of any sort, circulation is more precarious and the length-to-width ratio is usually greater than ideal. One might wish to delay these flaps once or twice to ensure better circulation, although the author has accomplished direct transfer of these flaps in one stage.

A similar type of flap may be based more laterally on the labial branch of the facial artery. Such a flap would be brought upward and laterally with its mucosa and submucosa

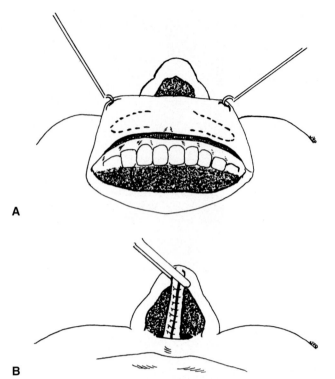

A

B

FIG. 1. **A:** Outline of medially based mucosal flaps. **B:** Labial flaps taken from the deep aspect of the upper lip are pulled through the base of the upper lip at the base of the proposed columella to be inserted into the tip of the nose. The two flaps are sutured together, although sometimes a small skin flap from beneath the tip of the nose may be turned downward on the anterior aspects of the flaps as a part of the reconstruction. Generally, these flaps require a later full-thickness skin graft from the postauricular area to give the skin color of the columella and, even later, a cartilage graft from the postauricular area to give contour and support to the columella.

from inside the cheek and then through the base of the lip in a fashion similar to the flaps described above.

If the flap is not too long in relation to its width (more than 3:1), and if the surgical outlining of the flap has been gentle and careful, one generally has enough vascular supply to salvage the flap. Delaying the flaps, of course, makes the circulation more secure.

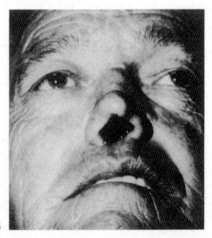

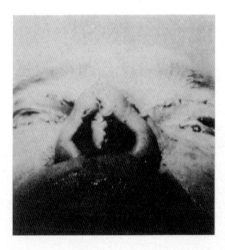

A,B

FIG. 2. **A:** Patient who has had a resection of the whole septum, a part of the base of the nose, and the whole columella for malignancy. **B:** Labial flaps being pulled through the base of the upper lip, to reconstruct the columella. Skin color to the columella is supplied by a secondary skin graft, since the mucosal flaps would give a pink, shiny appearance to the columella.

OPERATIVE TECHNIQUE

Generally, a short flap can be taken directly, by leaving a thick base for circulation into the flap. The venous return is likely to be satisfactory, since the patient lying on his or her back would naturally have good dependent drainage from the tip to the nose toward the lip. To be more secure, one could delay the flaps in the usual fashion, probably as a two-delay procedure, then bring the two flaps from either side of the lip toward the center, where they are based, and bring them out together through the base of the lip to the tip of the nose. Usually, these flaps do not have to be particularly long, but they should not be under tension or constricted by the opening through the lip skin.

Skin from the lip and from inside the nose may be turned onto the pedicle to give a better color match to the anterior aspect of the columella if this skin is available (Fig. 2). Also, an inlay skin graft may be used at a delay procedure to give skin cover. A conchal cartilage graft is usually inserted later for support and contour.

SUMMARY

A satisfactory columella can be constructed from labial mucosal flaps either from the lateral portion of the lip based on the labial branch of the facial artery or from the central portion of the lip as a reverse flap if they are properly delayed. Reverse mucosal flaps are not, however, the first choice for reconstruction of the columella.

CHAPTER 75 ■ NASOLABIAL SKIN FLAP FOR COLUMELLAR RECONSTRUCTION

C. PALETTA AND F. X. PALETTA, SR.

Reconstruction of the nasal columella using a variety of techniques including composite grafts and skin flaps have been described. Total columellar reconstruction requires a large volume of soft tissue that can be obtained through the use of an adjacent skin flap. A technique that is immediate, has a good color match, takes a small amount of time, and results in minimal scarring is the nasolabial flap.

INDICATIONS

Composite grafts from the outer helix of the ear have been used in columellar reconstruction, but they are best used for *partial* defects (1–3). Composite grafts are also limited because the tissue bed for columellar reconstruction is usually scarred or absent, thereby compromising the availability of a well-vascularized bed for adequate composite graft take. Various flaps have been described to lengthen the columella, especially in the bilateral cleft lip nasal deformity patient (4–6). When there is a complete loss of the columella, however, with exposure of the nasal septum, it is necessary to use a skin flap.

Tubed pedicle flaps from the neck and arm have been used successfully in the past. However, multiple stages are required to obtain the final result, and the flaps from these staged procedures tend to remain too thick and bulky in this region. The forehead flap is an excellent choice in total and partial nasal reconstruction, and it can also be useful in reconstruction of the columella. However, when the only defect is in the columella, the forehead flap is not the best first choice because of the distance of the flap from the defect and the potential wasted portion of the flap necessary in the transfer. The most accessible region for reconstruction of the *columella alone* is the nasolabial area (7). It provides an abundant amount of adjacent tissue with a good color match, and can easily be done under local anesthesia.

ANATOMY

See Chapter 40.

FLAP DESIGN AND DIMENSIONS

For coverage of the columellar region, a long nasolabial flap is preferred. The flap must curve around the adjacent alar base to reach its final destination. Because of this, the base of the pedicle should be 2 to 2.5 cm in width (Fig. 1). If possible in male patients, it may be advisable to base the pedicle inferiorly in order to avoid transferring hair-bearing skin to the newly constructed columella. If it is not possible to base this flap inferiorly due to prior scarring or if it is not preferable for any other reason, the hair-bearing portion of the nasolabial flap to be transferred to the columella should initially be replaced by a full-thickness skin graft. This graft should be taken either from the postauricular or supraclavicular region.

OPERATIVE TECHNIQUE

Design and elevation of the nasolabial flap for columellar reconstruction can easily be done under local anesthesia. When based superiorly, the nasolabial flap is elevated without delay

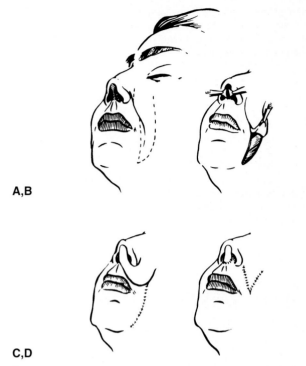

A,B

C,D

FIG. 1. A: Diagram of a superiorly based nasolabial flap. **B:** Elevation of the flap. **C:** Donor-site closure and transfer of the flap to the columellar defect. **D:** Detachment of the carrier portion of the flap 3 weeks later. (From Paletta and Van Norman, ref. 7, with permission.)

in the nasolabial groove, extending down to the inferior border of the mandible. The plane of dissection is just beneath the subcutaneous fat of the flap, superficial to the underlying facial musculature. The neighboring tissue on the cheek is widely undermined for closure of the donor site in the nasolabial fold.

When the tip of the nasolabial flap is transferred and inset, it is sutured to the mucous membrane of the remaining septum. An absorbable suture material such as 5–0 chromic catgut is used for the mucuous membrane. This mucous membrane must be carefully elevated off the septum for approximately 2 mm to allow for suture placement. After the tip of the flap has been aligned with the mucous membrane, the flap is rotated and inset to the appropriate segments on the nasal tip and upper lip. The flap is sutured to these adjacent points with a nonabsorbable suture such as 5–0 nylon or silk. Occasionally, when wide resection has been necessary to remove a cancer totally, the upper lip may need to be elevated in order to inset the flap to achieve complete closure of the defect. Under normal circumstances, upper lip skin elevation is to be avoided as it is not a fixed structure and this will lead to distortion of the upper lip.

daSilva (8) modified the classical superiorly based nasolabial flap by tunneling the flap transnasally for columellar reconstruction. Division of the flap was then performed at a second stage in 2 to 3 weeks. Kaplan (9) described a modification of the pedicled nasolabial flap. In one stage, he has used bilateral inferiorly based island nasolabial flaps for columellar reconstruction. This avoids a dog-ear and a second-stage procedure. Yanai et al. (10) further modified Kaplan's island technique by basing his nasolabial flaps superiorly.

When designed as a pedicle flap, the nasolabial flap can be detached at between 10 and 21 days. The remaining flap can be tailored and reinserted into the cheek. In patients with a lot of fatty tissue in this region of the face, defatting may be required to establish a smooth nasolabial line scar. A cartilage graft either from the septum or ear may be inserted at a later date if support is required (Fig. 2).

SUMMARY

When a nasal defect consists of total columellar loss, the nasolabial flap provides an excellent means of reconstruction.

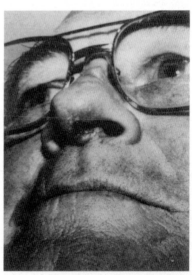
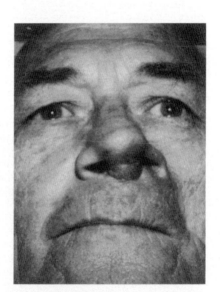
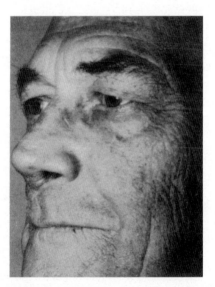

A–C

FIG. 2. A: A 62-year-old man with a basal cell carcinoma of the columella, nasal septum, and left nostril floor. **B:** Frontal view of the result of columella reconstruction with a nasolabial skin flap and a cartilage graft inserted secondarily. **C:** Oblique view of the final result.

References

1. Meade RJ. Composite ear grafts for reconstruction of the columella. *Plast Reconstr Surg* 1959;23:134.
2. Pegram M. Repair of congenital short columella. *Plast Reconstr Surg* 1954;14:305.
3. Pelliciari D. Columella and nasal tip reconstruction using multiple composite free grafts. *Plast Reconstr Surg* 1949;4:8.
4. Straith CL. Elongation of the nasal columella. *Plast Reconstr Surg* 1946;1:79.
5. Marcks KN, Trevaskis AC, Payne NJ. Elongation of columella by flap transfer and Z-plasty. *Plast Reconstr Surg* 1957;20:466.
6. Millard DR. Columellar lengthening by a forked flap. *Plast Reconstr Surg* 1958;22:454.
7. Paletta FX, Van Norman RT. Total reconstruction of the columella. *Plast Reconstr Surg* 1962;30:322.
8. da Silva G. A new method of reconstructing the columella with a nasolabial flap. *Plast Reconstr Surg* 1964;34:63.
9. Kaplan I. Reconstruction of the columella. *Br J Plast Surg* 1972;25:37.
10. Yanai A, Nagata S, Tanaka H. Reconstruction of the columella with bilateral nasolabial flaps. *Plast Reconstr Surg* 1986;77:129.

CHAPTER 76 ■ BIPEDICLED NASAL SEPTAL MUCOSAL FLAPS

D. N. F. FAIRBANKS AND G. R. FAIRBANKS

Medical folklore suggests nose picking to be a common cause of septal perforations, but septal operations appear to be the far more frequent offender at present. Intranasal cryosurgery and cautery for epistaxis, when performed bilaterally and simultaneously in corresponding areas, also can lead to perforations. Nasal septal abscess, which usually forms after untreated post-traumatic septal hematoma, syphilis, tuberculosis, Wegener's granulomatosis, and cocaine abuse, also can cause perforations.

A combined technique of bipedicled mucosal advancement flaps fortified with a temporalis fascia autograft is a good method of closing perforations (1).

INDICATIONS

The perforated nasal septum vexes both the patient and the physician (Fig. 1). It commonly causes intranasal crusting and epistaxis, and it occasionally causes whistling, particularly when the perforation is small. While these may be minor annoyances for some patients, for others they are major handicaps.

The nonoperative treatment of nasal septal perforations will not be discussed in this chapter (2,3). Surgical techniques reported in the literature for closure are varied and ingenious. However, advancement of viable tissue into a hole is indeed a difficult surgical challenge, one plagued by slough and reperforation often several months or years postoperatively. Many surgeons are still pessimistic regarding the probability of successful surgical closure.

Septal perforations can be closed with bipedicled advancement flaps of nasal mucosa designed to maximize the vascular supply of the septum (Fig. 2). The repair is then fortified by the submucosal insertion of a temporalis fascial or pericranial autograft. The graft increases the success of the repair, even when complete mucosal closure is difficult.

ANATOMY

A bipedicled flap of septal mucosa is designed so that the incisions along the nasal dorsum and nasal floor run parallel to the blood supply (4). The arteries that supply these flaps, through interconnecting anastomoses, are the anterior ethmoid, the posterior ethmoid, and the sphenopalatine (Fig. 2).

OPERATIVE TECHNIQUE

A graft of temporalis fascia (aponeurosis) is obtained from above the ear of the patient (Fig. 3). If the fascia is of poor

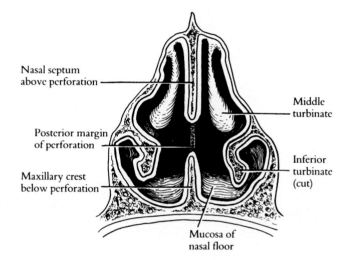

FIG. 1. Cross section of the nose through a perforation in the cartilaginous septum. (From Fairbanks, ref. 5, with permission.)

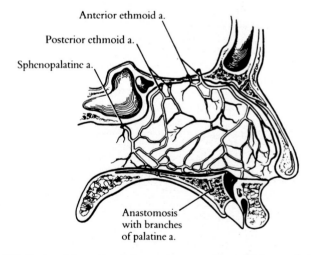

FIG. 2. Arterial supply of the nasal septum. (From Gollom, ref. 4, with permission.)

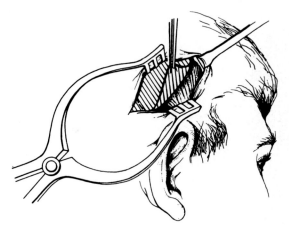

FIG. 3. Donor site for temporalis fascial autografts. [From Fairbanks (5), with permission.]

quality, or if a thicker graft is desired, the dissection is carried through the temporalis muscle to the pericranium, which can be used for the graft. Alternate donor material would be fascia lata or fascia from the external oblique muscle. The graft should be 2 cm larger in diameter than the perforation it is designed to cover.

The septal mucoperichondrium and mucoperiosteum are elevated on one side through a contralateral columellar incision (Fig. 4A). The perforation is incised circumferentially. One often finds the mucosa from opposing sides adhering together, since considerably more cartilage may be absent than the size of the perforation suggested. Tedious and patient dissection is required to incise the edges of the perforation without enlarging it.

The upper flap yields a considerable amount of redundant mucosa and is easy to advance; the lower flap is more difficult to advance. Its relaxing incision should be continued approximately 2 cm behind the posterior edge of the perforation at the angle where the vomer meets the nasal floor. From this point, it can be curved out onto the nasal floor, even beneath the inferior turbinate, to obtain extra mucosa, but it must then be curved back toward the septum anteriorly, where it ends in the floor of the nasal vestibule. The flaps should be made so as to advance and cover the perforation with no tension on the fragile leading edges.

On the contralateral side it may not be essential to raise another flap if closure on the first side is complete. However, bilateral flap closure will accelerate healing time and is therefore advisable. Nevertheless, only a lower flap should be developed on the second side, since advancement of an upper flap would result in cartilage being laid bare on both sides, and a new perforation would surely develop (Fig. 5).

Figure 6 depicts a lower flap designed similarly to the one on the opposite side, except that anteriorly the incision joins the columellar incision. Sometimes the lower flap can be advanced to cover the perforation completely. When it cannot, it should be made to cover at least any areas that were not completely covered on the opposite side, so that the graft, when it is inserted, will become vascularized from one side or the other.

Mucosal edges are brought together without tension and sutured with 5–0 ophthalmic plain catgut. A small piece of metal foil from the suture wrapper is temporarily inserted between the flaps of the right and left sides before the suturing, so that opposing flaps are not inadvertently sutured to each other. Then the graft, trimmed to size, is inserted through the columellar incision between opposing mucosal flaps (Fig. 7) so as to overlap the cartilaginous defect by a centimeter on all sides. The columellar incision is closed, and the nasal cavities are packed lightly with gauze packs impregnated with antibiotic ointment. The packs are left in place for 1 week.

When the nose is unpacked, any areas of the graft that were left uncovered will appear white and stringy, and crusts will form. They should not be debrided, for the graft gradually revascularizes and forms a sturdy base for mucosal epithelialization.

CLINICAL RESULTS

This combined technique has yielded more than a 90% success rate in the authors' experience with 35 patients over a 10-year period.

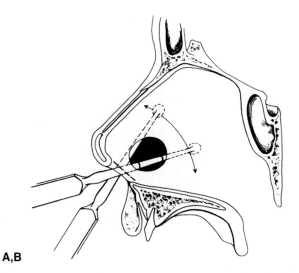

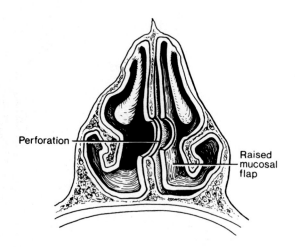

Perforation

Raised mucosal flap

A,B

FIG. 4. A: Elevation of mucosa from the left side of the septum around the perforation through a contralateral columellar incision. B: View of the elevated left septal mucosa on cross section. (From Fairbanks, ref. 5, with permission.)

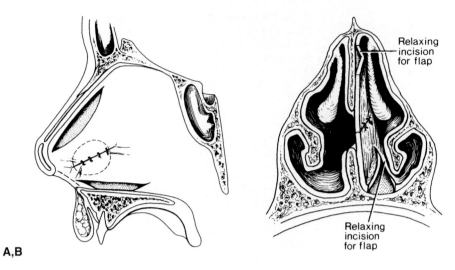

FIG. 5. **A:** Mucosal closure with bipedicled flaps on the left side. **B:** View of the
closure on cross section. (From Fairbanks,
ref. 5, with permission.)

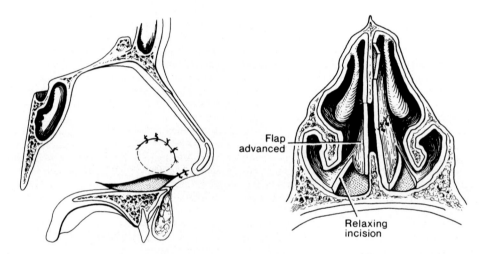

FIG. 6. **A:** Mucosal closure with a bipedicled flap from below only on the right side. **B:** The right-sided
mucosal closure on cross section. (From Fairbanks, ref. 5, with permission.)

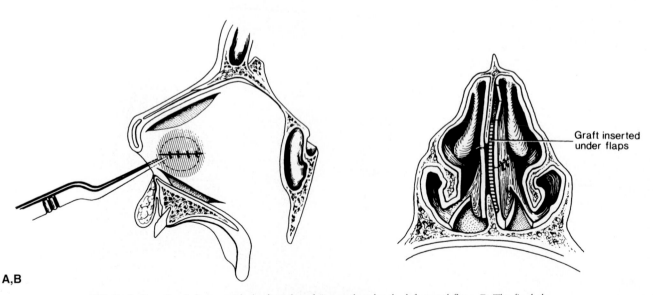

FIG. 7. **A:** Completed closure with the fascial graft inserted under the left septal flaps. **B:** The final closure on cross section. (From Fairbanks, ref. 5, with permission.)

SUMMARY

A bipedicled nasal mucosal flap to close septal perforations has been described. This flap is augmented by a temporalis fascial autograft.

References

1. Fairbanks DNF, Fairbanks GR. Surgical management of large nasal septum perforations. *Br J Plast Surg* 1971;24:382.
2. Kern EB, Facer GW, McDonald TJ, et al. Closure of nasal septal perforations with a Silastic button. *ORL Digest* 1977;39:9.
3. Fairbanks DNF, Fairbanks GR. Nasal septal perforations: prevention and management. *Ann Plast Surg* 1980;5:452.
4. Gollom J. Perforation of the nasal septum. *Arch Otolaryngol* 1968;88:518.
5. Fairbanks DNF. Closure of nasal septal perforations. *Arch Otolaryngol* 1980;106:509–513.

CHAPTER 77 ■ INFERIOR TURBINATE FLAP FOR CLOSURE OF SEPTAL PERFORATIONS

H. D. VUYK AND R. J. J. VERSLUIS

EDITORIAL COMMENT

Septal perforations are most difficult to close. The use of buccal mucosa or skin usually gives unsatisfactory results; consequently, the use of similar types of mucosa from the inferior turbinate is most advantageous. The limiting factor, as the authors indicate, is that two procedures may be required and there is only a small amount of tissue that can be mobilized safely.

The inferior turbinate flap, although not always successful, can be used to repair symptomatic septal perforations; specific symptoms such as epistaxis, whistling, and frontal headache appear to improve, even after partial closure.

INDICATIONS

Several methods for surgical closure of perforations of the nasal septum have been proposed (1–6). The inferior turbinate flap was introduced in 1980 by Masing and colleagues (1). Their concept was based on the assumption that symptoms such as crusting, obstruction, bleeding, and whistling are caused by the desiccating effects of the inspiratory airflow on the posterior rim of the perforation. Consequently, this technique aims at protection of the posterior rim from inspiratory airflow, not necessarily at complete closure of the perforation itself.

ANATOMY

The size of septal perforations in our series of 35 patients ranged from less than 0.5 cm to larger than 1.5 cm. The anterior margin of the perforation was localized in the vestibular or nasal-valve area in most patients and at the level of the anterior border of the inferior turbinate in a few patients. Apart from the symptomatic anterior perforation, only two patients had a second perforation more posteriorly that did not need treatment.

OPERATIVE TECHNIQUE

The procedure involves two stages (Fig. 1). In the first stage, a flap of the lateral nasal wall, which is centered around the inferior turbinate and includes vestibular skin, is raised and sutured anteriorly to the anterior, inferior, and superior edges of the septal perforation (Fig. 2). In the second stage, the pedicle of the flap is sectioned posteriorly, rotated into the perforation, and sutured in place to the posterior rim to close the defect. Silastic sheets are used to prevent adhesions with the lateral nasal wall, although not always successfully.

Some variations include a lateral alotomy for better exposure, an anterior mucosal flap, a retroauricular full-thickness graft, and a concomitant septal correction for a posterior deviation. A small anterior-superior-based septal rotation flap may be used to cover the anterior part of the inferior turbinate flap in the first stage. The mucosal defect on the lateral nasal wall may be covered with a full-thickness graft from the retroauricular skin. Fibrin glue in the first stage is helpful in fixing the flap and in its eventual coverage.

CLINICAL RESULTS

The procedure has the advantage of not disturbing the blood supply of the cartilage of the nose; however, multiple stages are involved, and sequelae may be difficult to treat. Although the perforation was closed by almost two thirds or more in 50% of the cases, postoperative scarring caused nasal

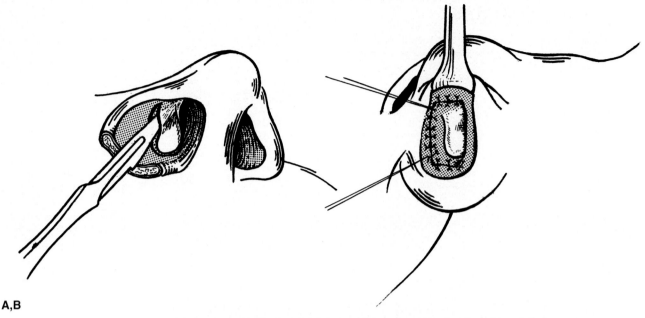

A,B

FIG. 1. Diagram of the two-stage (**A,B**) principle of closure of a nasal septal perforation with an inferior turbinate flap. (From Vuyk and Versluis, ref. 6, with permission.)

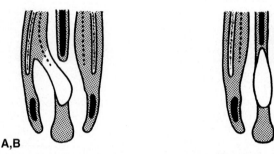

A,B

FIG. 2. A: Schematic development of an inferior turbinate flap. Alotomy is outlined for demonstration purposes. **B:** Diagram of inferior turbinate flap sutured to the mucosa on the opposite side of the septum anteriorly, inferiorly, and superiorly. Division of the pedicle of the flap posteriorly requires a second stage. (From Masing et al., ref. 1, with permission.)

obstruction or alar asymmetry in 21% of the cases; some patients required a third procedure, and many of the original symptoms did not improve. It was notable that the overall degree of patient satisfaction correlated with the degree of closure of the perforation.

SUMMARY

The inferior turbinate flap did not always prove totally satisfactory for closure of septal perforations. Complete reconstruction of this difficult problem remains a goal, however, even when some patients continue to have symptoms.

References

1. Masing H, Gammer C, Jaumann MP. Unsere Konzept zur operatieven Behandlung vom Septumperforationen. *Laryngol Rhinol Otol* 1980; 59:50.
2. Gollom J. Perforation of the nasal septum: the reverse flap technique. *Arch Otolaryngol* 1968;88:84.
3. Tardy ME. Septala perforations. *Otolaryngol Clin North Am* 1973; 6:711.
4. Fairbanks DNF. Closure of nasal septal perforations. *Arch Otolaryngol* 1980;106:509.
5. Karlan MS, Ossof R, Christu P. Reconstruction for large septal perforations. *Arch Otolaryngol* 1982;108:433.
6. Vuyk HD, Versluis RJJ. The inferior turbinate flap for closure of septal perforations. *Clin Otolaryngol* 1988;13:53.

CHAPTER 78 ■ ORAL MUCOSAL FLAPS FOR SEPTAL RECONSTRUCTION

M. FELDMAN AND Z. JABOURIAN

Repair of large septal perforations frustrates even the most experienced surgeon. This problem is exemplified by the myriad of procedures available for the repair of the perforated septum (1). Small and moderate-sized defects often can be closed with one of several standard mucosal advancement or rotation flaps; however, larger perforations (greater than 1.5 cm), once prepared intraoperatively with freshening of the margins, result in defects that are too formidable for reliable coverage using local flaps. One solution is to bring vascularized tissue from adjacent sites (2). The oral cavity provides an abundant supply of vascularized mucosa with virtually no donor-site deformity.

INDICATIONS

Nasal septal perforations may produce symptoms of nasal airway obstruction, dryness, crusting, whistling, and bleeding. If severe enough, these constitute indications for surgical correction; however, most perforations are small or very posterior and are usually asymptomatic. These need no intervention. Nonsurgical management consisting of nasal irrigation, ointments, or silicone buttons should be reserved for patients with few symptoms, those who refuse surgery, or those with a medical contraindication to surgery (3).

Each patient should undergo a detailed history with a thorough examination to determine the cause of the perforation. Before surgery is undertaken, it is critical to control whatever mechanism caused the initial perforation to prevent recurrence after repair (e.g., nose picking, cocaine abuse, Wegener's vasculitis).

ANATOMY

The oral mucosal flap is a random flap supplied primarily by the superior labial artery. This vessel is often tortuous, especially in the elderly, and runs in or behind the deeper fibers of the orbicularis oris muscle. It therefore may lie very superficially beneath the mucosa. A variably defined layer of connective tissue, the pharyngobasilar fascia, separates the mucosa from the overlying voluntary muscles and provides a surgical plane for dissection.

FLAP DESIGN AND DIMENSIONS

A medially based flap is outlined intraorally just adjacent to the frenulum in a horizontal fashion along the gingivolabial sulcus. The dimensions should be tailored according to the amount of mucosa needed for the repair. This depends on the size and location of the perforation and the distance the flap must travel from its pedicle (through the gingivolabial sulcus) into the nose.

Usually, the flap is 4 to 5 cm long and 1.5 to 2 cm wide. It is important to note that the flap usually shrinks to two thirds of its original length once it is mobilized. This flap should contain mucosa, subcutaneous tissue, and fascia, but not muscle.

OPERATIVE TECHNIQUE (4)

A lateral alotomy may be necessary for posterior or larger perforations (Fig. 1A). The scar tissue at the edges of the septal perforation is excised, and the surrounding mucoperichondrium and periosteum are elevated about the entire periphery for 5 to 10 mm (Fig. 1B).

A flap is outlined along the upper sulcus of the lip with its base adjacent to the superior labial frenulum. The long axis of the flap runs laterally and upward into the buccal sulcus, avoiding Stenson's duct (Fig. 1C). Flap size should be individualized according to the size and location of the perforation. In general, the flap will measure 1.5 to 2 cm wide and 4 to 5 cm long. Subcutaneous tissue and fascia are included to add bulk and to ensure adequate blood supply. The donor site can be either closed with chromic sutures or left to heal secondarily.

Using sharp scissors, a tunnel is made through a sublabial incision just cephalad to the flap base into the floor of the nasal vestibule (Fig. 1D). The size of this fistula is critical because flap necrosis will ensue from a tunnel that is too narrow. The flap is turned over 180 degrees and gently brought through the tunnel into the nasal cavity with the raw surface away from the perforation (Fig. 1E). The edges of the flap are tucked up under the elevated mucoperichondrium around the perforation. The flap is secured without tension to the septum with a minimum number of sutures (Fig. 1F). The opposite raw surface of the flap is covered with Gelfoam and left to epithelialize spontaneously. The alotomy incision is closed with subcutaneous and skin sutures, and the nasal cavity is lightly packed with petrolatum gauze that is removed the following day.

The flap base may be transected in 2 to 3 weeks and the oronasal fistula closed, or the flap may be left attached at its base and no closure performed.

CLINICAL RESULTS

Although many authors have published their operative technique of choice, few provide objective results. Three of three successful patients were reported (5), with perforations ranging from 1.5 to 2 cm in diameter; it has been stated (3), that for large perforations, "the only technique that has been successful in the author's experience has been the labial mucosal flap." Other surgeons also have had similar excellent results using this technique, although well-designed studies are lacking (6). Among the disadvantages of this procedure are that the oral

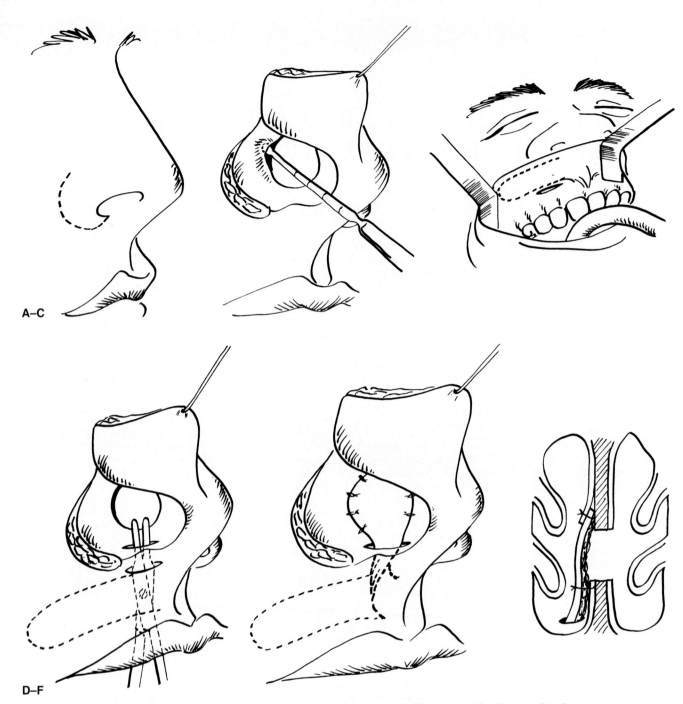

FIG. 1. A: Lateral alotomy incision made at the alar-facial crease. **B:** The mucoperichondrium at the edge of the perforation is elevated about the entire periphery for 5 to 10 mm. **C:** A medially based flap is outlined and sharply elevated. **D:** Creation of a sublabial-nasal fistula with scissor dissection. **E:** Flap turned over and brought into the nasal cavity through the tunnel. **F:** The edges of the flap are tucked up under the elevated mucoperichondrium; then sutures are placed.

mucosa does not contain respiratory epithelium and that a second procedure may be necessary to divide and inset the pedicle.

SUMMARY

Most septal perforations do not need surgical repair. If surgery is indicated, smaller perforations can be managed with local nasal flaps. The sublabial oral mucosal flap provides an uncomplicated yet reliable method for repair of large septal perforations with minimal patient morbidity.

References

1. Karlan MS, Ossoff RH, Sisson GA. A compendium of intranasal flaps. *Laryngoscope* 1982;92:774.
2. Converse JM, ed. *Reconstructive plastic surgery*, Vol. 2, 2d ed. Philadelphia: Saunders, 1977;1150–1152.
3. Kridel RWH, Appling WD, Wright WK. Septal perforation closure utilizing the external septorhinoplasty approach. *Arch Otolaryngol Head Neck Surg.* 1986;112:168.
4. Filiberti AT. Cited in Belmont JR. An approach to large nasoseptal perforations and attendant deformity. *Arch Otolaryngol Head Neck Surg* 1985;111:450.
5. Tipton JB. Closure of large septal perforation with a labial buccal flap. *Plast Reconstr Surg* 1970;46:514.
6. Tardy ME. Personal communication, 1987.

CHAPTER 79 ■ LOCAL MUCOSAL FLAPS FOR CLOSURE OF SEPTAL PERFORATIONS

T. ROMO III, A. D. PATEL, AND J. M. PEARSON

EDITORIAL COMMENT

This is a clear and useful approach to septal perforations surgery.

Perforations of the nasal septum can lead to symptoms such as whistling, obstruction, crusting, malodorous discharge, bleeding, and pain. Lasting surgical repair of such perforations can be a challenge, due to limited intranasal exposure, inelasticity, along with a possibly compromised blood supply to the residual nasal mucosa, and the desire to preserve mucosal functionality. Different surgical approaches, flaps, and grafts have been devised, with variable success regarding lasting closure and functionality. Presented here are local mucosal flaps that are available for use, and the senior author's (TR) graduated approach to nasal septal perforation repair.

INDICATIONS

Perforations that remain symptomatic, despite adequate medical management, are generally indicated for surgical closure. Etiologies include inflammatory processes, infections, neoplasms, intranasal substance abuse, and, most commonly, iatrogenic injury (1). The goal of surgery is to provide a multilayer, tension-free, physiologic closure while minimizing added morbidity. The appropriate selection of approach and flap depends on the location, shape, and size of the perforation, relative to the uninvolved nasal mucosa. Prior to surgical consideration, an extensive workup is paramount, because active disease or substance abuse generally results in surgical failure (2).

Intranasal mucosal pedicled flaps involve mobilizing and advancing mucoperichondrium or mucoperiosteum from any location in the nasal vault, including that overlying septum, nasal floor, or lateral wall. These flaps can be used for perforations of all sizes (1,3–5). Moderate-sized, caudal perforations can be closed with a two-staged transposition of an inferior turbinate flap. Advantages to this technique include abundant vascularity, wide arc of rotation, combined skeletal and epithelial support, and surgical ease (6,7). When adequate healthy nasal mucosa is not available, extranasal mucosal flaps can be used. Examples include the buccal mucosal flap (8) or the facial artery musculomucosal flap (FAMM) (9), in which the pedicle is tunneled into the nasal cavity. The disadvantages of these flaps are increased dryness and crusting.

Other approaches that have been described include endoscopic (10), endonasal (5), external rhinoplasty (11), midface degloving (12,13), and lateral rhinotomy (14). Greater surgical exposure facilitates more extensive advancement of healthy nasal mucosa. Generally, more invasive approaches allow greater exposure at the expense of increased accompanying morbidity.

ANATOMY

Nasal mucosa contains highly dynamic, pseudostratified, ciliated, columnar epithelium that is the basis of the mucociliary system. The mucosa lies atop perichondrium in the region of the cartilaginous septum, and atop periosteum over the bony septum and vault. In general, the periosteum is thicker and stronger than the perichondrium and so is thought to make a better substrate for repair (4). Between the perichondrium or periosteum, underlying cartilage or bone is an avascular region, which is the proper plane of dissection for the flaps. In the septal region, injuring the perichondrium on both sides at opposing locations will compromise the blood supply to the cartilage, possibly leading to perforation (1). The mucoperichondrial and mucoperiosteal flaps have no inherent elasticity, but they can be expanded, over time, without apparent loss of function (15).

Blood supply to the nasal mucosa is derived primarily superiorly and posteriorly from the ethmoid and sphenopalatine arteries. The anterior supply is provided by the greater palatine artery, after it traverses the incisive canal, and by nasal branches of the superior labial artery. The vascular supply is interconnected by abundant anastomoses (1,3). Nasal mucosal flaps are generally planned to preserve either one or both of these sources of blood supply. Bipedicled flaps preserve blood supply from both sources. Unipedicled flaps preserve blood supply only from one source but allow a greater degree of arc rotation.

Oral cavity mucosa consists of nonkeratinized, stratified, squamous epithelium that can secrete mucus but has no ciliary function. Thus, a buccal mucosal flap, while providing closure, will not preserve regional mucociliary function. The FAMM flap, which is pedicled on the facial artery, consists of buccal mucosa, submucosa, a small amount of buccinator muscle, and the deeper plane of the orbicularis oris muscle (16). Extranasal mucosal flaps are mentioned only briefly here; a more extensive discussion may be found in our original publications.

FLAP DESIGN AND DIMENSIONS

Closure of perforations with intranasal mucosal flaps hinges on the premise that residual, uninvolved, nasal mucosa, although inelastic, may be mobilized with relaxing incisions that do not compromise major vascular supply. Fewer incisions are preferred, but not at the expense of adequate mobilization of mucosa.

At the minimum, an anterior-to-posterior directed incision is required in the region of the inferior meatus that allows the advancement of thicker, more robust mucoperiosteum from the nasal floor and lateral wall in a medial and superior direction. If mucosal advancement is still not adequate, a caudad-to-cephalad superior incision may be placed near the junction of the septum and upper lateral cartilages, allowing advancement of a septal flap in a medial and inferior direction. A transverse incision connecting the former two incisions may be made, to create a unipedicled flap, thus increasing the arc of rotation. The incision is placed at the level of the posterior nasal spine and across the anterior nasal sill (12).

The size and location of the perforation dictate the degree of surgical exposure required. The amount of available mucosa for approximating edges of perforation varies inversely with the size of perforation (3). Therefore, larger perforations require greater exposure, in order to mobilize a sufficiently large flap. Posterior perforations are difficult to access with an endonasal approach. Thus, although endonasal approaches, with or without alotomy, are adequate for small, anterior perforations, large and posterior perforations generally require the exposure provided by external rhinoplasty and midface degloving. The senior author uses an extended external rhinoplasty approach, with or without a midface degloving, employing the standard transcolumellar, full transfixion, bilateral intercartilaginous, and gingivobuccal incisions (13).

If the amount of uninvolved nasal mucosa is not adequate to allow tension-free perforation closure, tissue expansion is a means of flap lengthening that preserves nasal histology and, therefore, physiology (Fig. 1). A gain of 5 cm is expected from a 1-cm × 3-cm tissue expander (PMT Accuspan Corp., Chanhassen, MN), described in the senior author's previous study. Expansion is a multistage process, requiring a period of at least 6 weeks (15).

More successful outcomes are associated with a multilayered closure involving grafts of connective tissue interposed between the left and right repaired mucoperichondrium. The interposition grafts help prevent incisional breakdown and reperforation, by serving as templates for overlying mucosal-tissue migration and vascularization and by providing a barrier between the healing flaps. Possible grafting materials include uninvolved septal cartilage, ethmoid bone, auricular cartilage, temporalis fascia, mastoid perichondrium, and human acellular dermal graft (Alloderm, LifeCell Corp., The Woodlands, TX). The advantage of Alloderm is the elimination of donor-site morbidity (2).

Inferior turbinate flaps involve the inferior half of the turbinate, pedicled anteriorly, which may include part of the bone. The flap is rotated anteriorly and adjusted to fill the perforation. The contralateral side may be left to heal by secondary intention, or bilateral turbinate flaps may be used. The pedicle is taken down after 3 weeks (7).

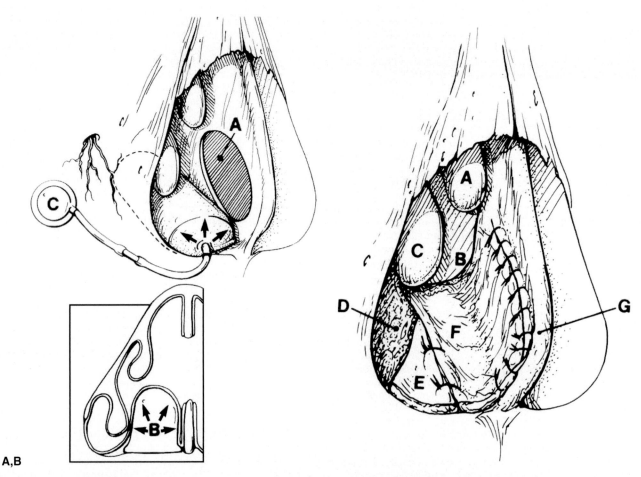

FIG. 1. A: A. 1-cm × 3-cm tissue expander is inserted into a submucoperiosteal pocket on the nasal floor. A, Nasal septal perforation. B, Long-term expanded nasal-floor mucosa (arrows). C, Peripheral port implanted onto the maxillary fossa. B: Completion of flap elevation rotation and repair of perforation. A, Middle turbinate. B, Posterior naris. C, Inferior turbinate infractured. D, Raw surface area left by flap rotation. E, Full-thickness skin graft on floor of nose. F, Rotated flap. G, Anterior septal angle.

OPERATIVE TECHNIQUE

Preoperative intensive nasal care and hygiene are recommended. The latter may include antibiotic use, frequent saline irrigation, and lubrication with emollients. Once proper hygiene is established, chronic inflammation may be stabilized with a topical nasal steroid spray.

The senior author has developed a graduated approach to septal perforation repair with mucoperichondrial/periosteal advancement flaps (12). For anterior perforations less than 0.5 cm, an endonasal approach is used (Fig. 2), to develop opposing bipedicled flaps. For perforations 0.5 to 2 cm, an external rhinoplasty approach is used (Fig. 3), to develop bilateral, posteriorly based, unipedicled flaps. For perforations larger than 2 cm, the closure is undertaken in two stages. The first involves placing an intranasal tissue expander for 6 weeks, and the second involves an external rhinoplasty approach, with midface degloving, to develop bilateral, posteriorly based, unipedicled flaps.

The nose is prepared with sponges or pledgets soaked with a topical decongestant, such as phenylephrine or oxymetazoline. The nasal and paranasal soft tissues are injected with standard lidocaine (Xylocaine)/epinephrine preparations.

For the external rhinoplasty approach, a transcolumellar incision is first made at the base of the columella and dissected inferiorly under the feet of the medial crura and posteriorly to the caudal septum. Bilateral intercartilaginous incisions are made and connected to a full transfixion incision that spans over the septal angle and through the membranous septum. The columellar and medial crural flaps are elevated superiorly, thus exposing the caudal septum.

For midface degloving, a complete gingivobuccal sulcus incision is made, with cautery, between the right and left upper first molars. The osseocartilaginous nose is then degloved over the upper lateral cartilage and nasal bones. The dissection is carried posteriorly and laterally over the nasal bones down onto the maxilla. The intranasal incisions are then connected

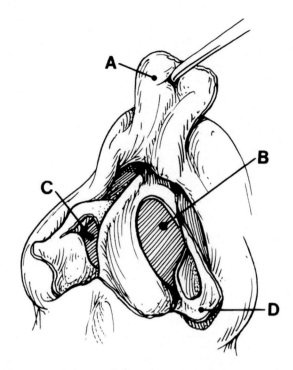

FIG. 3. Extended external rhinoplasty approach. Exposure of nasal septal perforation using the extended external rhinoplasty approach. *A*, Columella flap retracted. *B*, Cartilaginous perforation. *C*, Mucosal perforation. *D*, Mucosa elevated and reflected laterally.

sharply to the gingivobuccal incision, between the pyriform apertures across the anterior nasal spine. The face of the maxilla is then stripped with a periosteal elevator, identifying the edges of the pyriform aperture and the infraorbital nerves. This dissection is connected with the nasal degloving dissection. The tip structures and upper lip are retracted superiorly, and the last remaining bridge of tissue lateral to the pyriform aperture and upper lateral cartilages is divided with cutting cautery. The midface is now degloved, isolating the nasal fossae at the level of the pyriform aperture, nasal valve, and anterior septal angle. The nasal tip, upper lip, and midfacial soft tissues are retracted superiorly and secured with half-inch Penrose drains.

Once the appropriate exposure is established, the rim of the perforation is debrided. The mucoperichondrial flaps are elevated bilaterally along the remainder of the septum, which, if deviated, is removed or straightened. The flap is elevated superiorly to the junction of the septum and upper lateral cartilage, anteriorly to the anterior septal angle, and inferiorly to the maxillary crest. A transverse mucosal incision may be made from the posterior nasal spine across the anterior nasal sill, up onto the lateral pyriform aperture, to the level of the insertion of the inferior turbinate.

The mucoperiosteum of the nasal floor and inferior meatus is elevated laterally to the insertion of the inferior turbinate, medially to the maxillary crest (where the decussating fibers are carefully incised), and posteriorly to the junction of the hard and soft palates. The inferior turbinate is fractured medially, allowing a full-thickness incision to be made through the inferior meatal mucosa just below the insertion of the turbinate. A back cut is made at the posterior portion of this incision toward the nasal floor, allowing full medialization of this posteriorly based mucoperiosteal flap.

Now, the intranasal mucosa is mobile from the upper lateral cartilages down to the maxillary crest, across the nasal floor, and up to the inferior turbinate. The flap is rotated medially across the floor and up the septum, until the inferior and superior edges of the perforation meet. These two

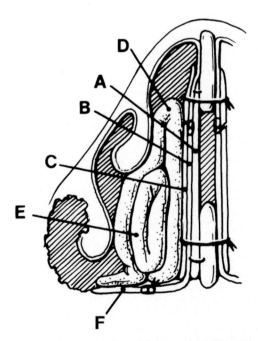

FIG. 2. Completed repair with nasal floor mucosal flaps. Closure of perforation and nasal packing. *A*, Alloderm dermograft. *B*, Rotated nasal-floor mucosal flaps. *C*, Thin silicone sheeting secured to nasal mucosal flaps. *D*, Surgical sponge (Telfa) dressing. *E*, Surgical sponge (Merocel). *F*, Skin graft covering donor site.

mucosal edges are closed with interrupted 5–0 Vicryl suture from posterior to anterior. If excess tension remains, a relaxing incision is made near the septum–upper lateral cartilage junction, allowing inferior displacement of the superior flap.

The senior author's interposition graft of choice is AlloDerm. This is secured between the two nasal mucosal flaps to the septal cartilage with 5–0 Vicryl suture, superior to the perforation, and allowed to drape over and totally cover the perforation on one side of the septal cartilage. The repaired mucoperichondrial flaps are placed into position, and the denuded nasal floor is covered with a full-thickness postauricular skin graft to prevent vestibular stenosis. This graft is secured in place to the nasal sill and medialized mucosal flap with interrupted 5–0 Vicryl suture.

For external rhinoplasty, the intercartilaginous and transfixion incisions are then closed with 4–0 chromic suture, and the columellar incision is closed with 6–0 Prolene suture. When necessary, the medial crural feet are resuspended from the caudal septum with a 4–0 chromic mattress suture. For midface degloving, the intraoral incision is closed with a running 3–0 chromic suture.

Bilateral silicone sheeting is fixated external to the mucosal flaps with 4–0 nylon suture. Finally, a Telfa pad, wrapped over a Merocel sponge, is placed as packing and intranasal support. The packing and external splints are removed on the seventh postoperative day, while the silicone splint is maintained in position until the fourth to sixth postoperative week.

For those defects that require tissue expansion, the previously mentioned procedure is preceded by placement of tissue expanders under a mucoperiosteal pocket in the bilateral nasal floors. The mucosa of the anterior nasal sill is incised and carried laterally up onto the pyriform aperture. The nasal floor and inferior meatal mucoperiosteum are elevated, and a 1-cm × 3-cm tissue expander is inset into the nasal floor pocket. Elevation of medial maxillary soft tissue is accomplished through a mucosal incision at the inferior pyriform aperture. The peripheral port of the expander is placed onto the maxilla and connected to the expander. Care is taken to prevent bending or kinking of the tubing. Approximately 0.2 mL of sterile saline dyed with methylene blue is instilled into the peripheral port, to slightly inflate the expander. The mucosal incision is closed with interrupted 4–0 chromic suture; nasal packing is not used.

Two weeks postoperatively, small aliquots (0.5 to 1.0 mL) of sterile saline are injected into the peripheral port through an intraoral approach. A transcutaneous injection into the peripheral port may be performed, but this usually requires a preinjection, infraorbital nerve block with local anesthesia. Expansion is performed on a weekly basis and typically requires 6 to 8 weeks to reach a total expander volume of 4 to 7 mL. Once the desired amount of mucosal expansion is achieved, the repair is performed, as previously described, after a midface degloving approach and removal of the tissue expanders.

Caudal perforations of a moderate size are amenable to an inferior turbinate flap (7). After the nose is prepared, a full-thickness incision is started from the posteromedial margin of the turbinate and extended anteriorly. The incision is ended prior to the turbinate's insertion into the lateral wall, thus preserving the anterior blood supply. In cross-section, the U-shaped flap contains mucosa and submucosa from both the medial and lateral surfaces of the turbinate and possibly turbinate bone within. The flap is rotated medially and anteriorly on itself. The distal segment is opened and fit to fill the perforation, such that the submucosal surface faces medially and the mucosal surface faces the nasal airway. It is sutured with 4–0 plain gut suture to the septal rim. The donor site is typically left to heal by secondary intention. The contralateral side of the perforation may also be left to heal by secondary

intention, or bilateral inferior turbinate flaps may be created. The pedicle is taken down in 3 weeks.

CLINICAL RESULTS

Results over the past 30 years by the author and others (6,9,12,17) have shown good to excellent closure of defects utilizing a variety of approaches, from the smallest to the largest and more complex approaches. Reports vary from 75% to 100% of closure over all techniques.

Causes for reperforation include perioperative infection, closure under tension, lack of intervening connective tissue, and presence of persistent inflammatory or neoplastic disease (2). Complications specific to the inferior turbinate flap include the development of synechiae and nasal stenosis (7). Complications associated with tissue expansion include infection, expander exposure, implant failure, ischemia of expanded mucosa, seroma formation, and widening of donor scars (15).

SUMMARY

Advancement of mucoperichondrial/periosteal flaps, with placement of connective tissue interpositional grafts, can lead to a successful and functional repair of septal perforations. The appropriate approach for a particular perforation allows adequate mucosa to be mobilized for a tension-free closure. Tissue expansion facilitates lengthening of nasal mucosa, thus avoiding the use of extranasal tissues. Alternative methods, such as inferior turbinate flaps or oral mucosal flaps, may be useful in particular situations.

References

1. Fairbanks DN. Closure of nasal septal perforations. *Arch Otolaryngol* 1980;106:509.
2. Kridel RW. Septal perforation repair. *Otolaryngol Clin North Am* 1999;32:695.
3. Gollom J. Perforation of the nasal septum. The reverse flap technique. *Arch Otolaryngol* 1968;88:518.
4. Karlan MS, Ossoff R, Christu P. Reconstruction for large septal perforations. *Arch Otolaryngol* 1982;108:433.
5. Belmont JR. An approach to large nasoseptal perforations and attendant deformity. *Arch Otolaryngol* 1985;111:450.
6. Vuyk HD, Versluis RJ. The inferior turbinate flap for closure of septal perforations. *Clin Otolaryngol Allied Sci* 1988;13:53.
7. Friedman M, Ibrahim H, Ramakrishnan V. Inferior turbinate flap for repair of nasal septal perforation. *Laryngoscope* 2003;113:1425.
8. Tipton JB. Closure of large septal perforations with a labial-buccal flap. *Plast Reconstr Surg* 1970;46:514.
9. Heller JB, Gabbay JS, Trussler A, et al. Repair of large nasal septal perforations using facial artery musculomucosal (FAMM) flap. *Ann Plast Surg* 2005;55:456.
10. Hier MP, Yoskovitch A, Panje WR. Endoscopic repair of a nasal septal perforation. *J Otolaryngol* 31:323, 2002.
11. Kridel RW, Appling WD, Wright WK. Septal perforation closure utilizing the external septorhinoplasty approach. *Arch Otolaryngol Head Neck Surg* 1986;112:168.
12. Romo T 3rd, Foster CA, Korovin GS, Sachs ME. Repair of nasal septal perforation utilizing the midface degloving technique. *Arch Otolaryngol Head Neck Surg* 1988;114:739.
13. Romo T 3rd Sclafani AP, Falk AN, Toffel PH. A graduated approach to the repair of nasal septal perforations. *Plast Reconst Surg* 1999;103:66.
14. Karlan MS, Ossoff RH, Sisson GA. A compendium of intranasal flaps. *Laryngoscope* 1982;92(7 Pt 1):774.
15. Romo T 3rd, Jablonski RD, Shapiro AL, McCormick SA. Long-term nasal mucosal tissue expansion use in repair of large nasoseptal perforations. *Arch Otolaryngol Head Neck Surg* 1995;121:327.
16. Pribaz J, Stephens W, Crespo L, Gifford G. A new intraoral flap: facial artery musculomucosal (FAMM) flap. *Plast Reconstr Surg* 1992;90:421.
17. Pedroza F, Patrocinio LG, Arevalo O. A review of 25-year experience of nasal septal perforation repair. *Arch Facial Plast Surg* 2007;9:12.

CHAPTER 80 ■ EAVE SKIN FLAP FOR HELICAL RECONSTRUCTION

M. L. LEWIN*

The helix is the most prominent part of the external ear, visible when viewing the face from the front and even more conspicuous in profile. The most frequent deformity of the helix occurs in facial burns. Because of its prominence and its thin skin and cartilage, the helix is often destroyed, leaving the auricle with a flat, scarred, jagged rim (Figs. 1A and 2A). Other helical deformities are due to lacerations, excision of tumors, or harvesting of large composite grafts (1).

INDICATIONS

If the helical defect is small, it is best repaired by a chondrocutaneous flap, but if the defect is larger than 2.5 cm, this procedure will reduce the size of the auricle. Several procedures are recommended for reconstruction of the helix. Some may require multiple stages, may leave conspicuous scars, or are applicable only to small helical losses.

The eave skin flap was devised primarily for isolated defects of the helix (2). It can be used to reconstruct the entire helix or a portion of it (3) in a two-stage procedure that can be performed with the patient under local anesthesia without hospitalization. It uses the postauricular and mastoid skin, which is a good match for the skin of the ear. The flap donor-site scar or skin graft is concealed behind the ear.

In assembling the cartilaginous framework in total ear reconstruction provision is made for the helix. A vertical strip of cartilage extends above the horizontal plane of the scapha; however, the skin flap that covers the cartilaginous framework frequently effaces the prehelical sulcus so that the helical outline is lost. An eave flap can restore the sharp delineation of the helix. The eave flap is not advised when the ear framework is of alloplastic material.

FLAP DESIGN AND DIMENSIONS

The procedure is based on the observation that a skin flap that is dissected free and held at both ends will curl until it sponta-

neously tubes itself. This curling is caused by the contracture of the denuded undersurface of the flap. If half the width of the flap is inserted into the tissue and the other half is unattached, the latter will curl until its undersurface becomes completely epithelialized.

OPERATIVE TECHNIQUE

The defective margin of the auricle is denuded by excision of the marginal scar (Fig. 1B). If a portion of the helix remains on either end of the defect, it is incised for a few millimeters.

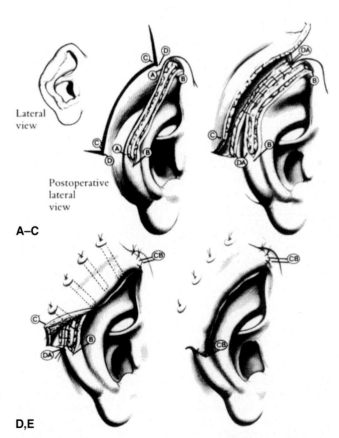

Lateral view

Postoperative lateral view

A–C

D,E

FIG. 1. Diagram of procedure (see text). **A:** Preoperative appearance. **B:** Helical defect denuded by excision of marginal scar. The mastoid flap is incised. **C:** Formation of postauricular skin tunnel. **D:** Mastoid flap overlapping helical defect like an eave. **E:** Postoperative appearance. (From Lewin, ref. 2, with permission.)

* Deceased.

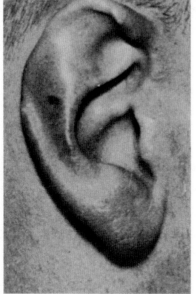 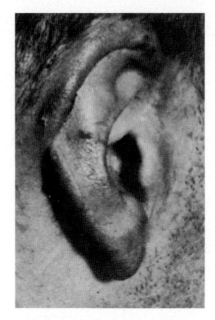 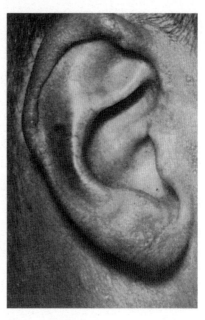

A–C

FIG. 2. A: Loss of helix due to burn. **B:** Eave flap after first stage. Overlap is tapered so that it flattens at the inferior pole. **C:** Final appearance. Soft curvature and delicate outline of the helix. Smooth junction at both ends. (From Lewin, ref. 2, with permission).

Later, the tips of the flap will be inserted into these cuts to obtain a tongue-in-groove junction.

By pressing the auricle against the mastoid, the length of the flap is outlined, and an incision is made a few millimeters posteriorly. At both ends of this incision, perpendicular divergent incisions are made, thus widening the flap as it extends posteriorly (Fig. 1B). The upper incision is about 2.5 cm long, and the lower is considerably shorter. The latter can be dispensed with if the lower pole of the flap extends below the middle of the auricle where the helix is flat. These incisions outline the mastoid skin flap.

The anterior margin of the postauricular incision (Fig. 1B, DD) is approximated to the posterior edge of the denuded helical defect (Fig. 1B, AA), which forms a skin-lined tunnel and also bends the auricle backward, holding it in close approximation to the mastoid (Fig. 1C). The suturing is done with fine catgut or Dexon, knotted on the skin surface inside the tunnel.

The incised mastoid skin flap is undermined for a distance of about 3 cm. Its anterior free margin (Fig. 1B, CC) then can easily overlap the margin of the auricle (Fig. 1D). The overlapping must be free of any tension, or the flap will retract and flatten during the healing period. The upper and lower corners of the flap are sutured into the open incisions along the margin of the defect.

The anterior margin of the mastoid skin flap—the eave flap—overlaps the scaphal surface for a distance of 3 to 6 mm (Fig. 1D, C–CB). More overlap is allowed in the upper portion to obtain the effect of tapering off. Three or four double-armed nylon sutures are inserted into the anterior lip of the helical defect (Fig. 1D, B–CB) and passed through the flap. They then are tied over bolsters about 2.5 cm posterior to the free margin of the flap (Fig. 1E). The sutures control the amount of overlapping.

Packing is inserted into the postauricular skin tunnel and underneath the overlap. Within 3 weeks, the undersurface of the overlap is epithelialized, and there is a noticeable curling of the anterior border of the flap (Fig. 2B).

The second stage is usually carried out 3 weeks later. The necessary width of the flap is estimated, and the flap is cut free from the mastoid. The skin-lined tunnel is incised, allowing the pinna to return to its normal position. The posterior border of the flap then is trimmed as needed and sutured to the remaining skin on the medial surface of the auricle (Fig. 1B, AA). With the flap widening at its base, the divergent suture lines facilitate a smooth junction with the edges of the defect. The mastoid defect can be closed by advancing scalp skin, although a skin graft is usually used.

This procedure can be modified according to the requirements of each patient. If the helical defect is wide and a longer flap is needed, the mastoid flap can be made longer by dispensing with the skin tunnel and using all the skin on the medial surface of the auricle so that the entire auricle adheres to the skull.

CLINICAL RESULTS

The curling effect of the thin mastoid or auricular skin gives an excellent simulation of the normal helix (Fig. 2C). If the helical flap includes scalp skin or a skin graft, however, the result is usually less satisfactory because the reconstructed helix is thicker, bulkier, and curls irregularly.

SUMMARY

The eave skin flap can be used to recreate the helical rim by taking advantage of the natural tendency of the free edge of a flap to curl.

References

1. Lewin ML. Reconstruction of the helix. *Arch Otolaryngol* 1948;47:802.
2. Lewin ML. Formation of the helix with a postauricular flap. *Plast Reconstr Surg* 1950;5:432.
3. Argamaso RV, Lewin ML. Repair of partial ear loss with local composite flap. *Plast Reconstr Surg* 1968;42:437.

CHAPTER 81 ■ RETROAURICULAR TUBED SKIN FLAP TO THE HELICAL RIM

D. N. STEFFANOFF

The retroauricular tubed skin flap has proved an excellent choice for reconstruction of the auricle because of its color and texture match, rich blood supply, and proximity to the deformity (see also Chap. 85).

INDICATIONS

Problems of auricular reconstruction involve restoring cartilaginous support, supplying soft-tissue coverage of similar color and texture, and positioning the auricle at the proper angle to the side of the head (1–5). The retroauricular tubed skin flap allows the surgeon to meet all these requirements for a satisfactory cosmetic reconstruction of a partially mutilated auricle (6).

ANATOMY

The retroauricular skin and subcutaneous tissue are supplied by the postauricular artery, which is a branch of the external carotid artery. The anterior and lateral auricular skin is supplied by branches of the temporal artery.

OPERATIVE TECHNIQUE

The first patient benefiting from this surgical approach presented with a loss of 60% of the helical rim and 40% of the chonchal-anthelical skin and cartilaginous support as a result of a human bite (Fig. 1). The following steps illustrate the initial reconstruction:

1. Forming the retroauricular tubed skin flap, which in this patient measured 68 mm long and 16 mm wide (Figs. 1B and 1C). The postauricular artery is included in the flap.
2. Delaying the incision through half the circumference of the cephalic end of the flap.
3. Transferring the cephalic end of the tubed flap to the cephalic portion of the helical rim (Fig. 1D).
4. Delaying the incision through half the circumference of the caudal end of the tubed flap and delaying the incision and undermining of the mastoid skin, where a cartilage graft will be placed, partially to reconstruct the concha and anthelix.
5. Transferring the caudal end of the tubed skin flap to the caudal end of the deformity, near the earlobe.
6. Burying the carved cadaver cartilaginous support to simulate the lost portion of the concha and anthelix (Fig. 1E). This cartilage was stored in absolute ethyl alcohol, but it was placed in saline for 30 minutes prior to its use.
7. Incising behind the cartilage graft to permit the external ear to be elevated to the proper angle with the side of the head. Soft tissue is maintained with the cartilage to accept a 0.016-in. split-thickness skin graft from the medial upper arm (Fig. 1F).

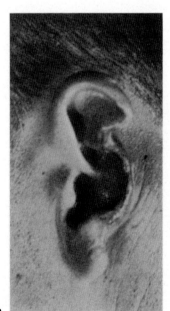

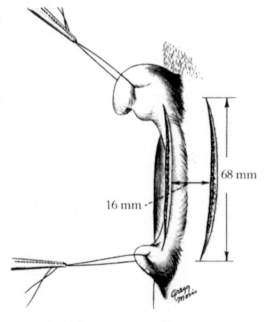

A,B

FIG. 1. **A:** Human bite deformity with 60% loss of helical rim and 40% loss of the chonchal-anthelical skin and cartilaginous support. **B:** Incisions for the bipedicle retroauricular flap. *(Continued)*

227

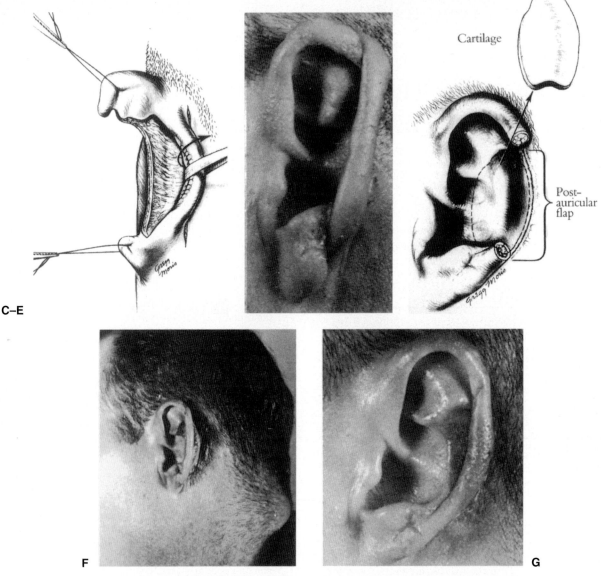

C–E

F   G

FIG. 1. *Continued.* **C:** Tubed skin flap partly retracted, revealing denuded donor site, which was closed by direct suture of wound edges. **D:** Retroauricular tubed skin flap sutured to the cephalic portion of the helical rim. **E:** Postauricular flap of mastoid skin and the underlying cartilaginous graft for reconstruction of the partially deficient concha and anthelix. **F:** The postauricular flap with underlying cartilage graft and split-thickness skin graft placed on the back side of the cartilage and the flap donor site. **G:** Closeup of auricular reconstruction.

8. The tubed flap is incised longitudinally along its original suture line and sutured to the incised margin of the postauricular flap using a plaster cast model of the opposite ear for comparison.

The completed reconstruction is shown in Fig. 1G.

SUMMARY

The retroauricular tubed skin flap can be used to reconstruct large defects of the helical rim of the external ear.

References

1. Ford JF. A method of plastic reconstruction of the auricle: preliminary report. *Plast Reconstr Surg* 1946;1:332.
2. Fomon S. *The surgery of injury and plastic repair.* Baltimore: Williams & Wilkins, 1939.
3. Maliniac JW. Reconstruction for partial loss of ear. *Plast Reconstr Surg* 1946;1:124.
4. Barsky AJ. *Plastic surgery.* Philadelphia: W. B. Saunders, 1938.
5. O'Connor GB. Establishment of cartilage depots for military and civil use (editorial). *Am J Surg* 1942;58:313.
6. Steffanoff, DN. Auriculomastoid tube pedicle for otoplasty. *Plast Reconstr Surg* 1948;3:352.

CHAPTER 82 ■ CHONDROCUTANEOUS ADVANCEMENT FLAP TO THE HELICAL RIM

N. H. ANTIA

EDITORIAL COMMENT

This is an excellent procedure for restoring substantial defects of up to 3 cm of the helix of the ear. It gives predictably good results. Its only drawback is the lowering of the height of the ear. A good portion of the scar line is not as obvious as noted in the postoperative photographs, when the incision is placed within the helical sulcus (see diagrams).

Many acquired defects of the ear involve small segments of the helical margin, usually less than a quarter of the circumference of the ear. Such defects commonly result from the excision of tumors such as basal cell carcinoma or burns. Although small, the defect is very noticeable, especially in men. The chondrocutaneous advancement flap is a relatively simple and safe single-staged operative procedure that provides an almost normal contour to the ear (1,2).

INDICATIONS

Several techniques have been described for the correction of helical defects, such as postauricular, cervical, or mastoid flaps or composite grafts. To correct such a defect and produce a good cosmetic result is difficult because of the intricate nature of the chondrocutaneous sandwich that gives the delicate configuration to the auricle.

The chondrocutaneous advancement flap recreates the normal delicate contours of the ear that are difficult to achieve by any other procedure. There is also no donor defect.

FLAP DESIGN AND DIMENSIONS

The principle underlying this procedure is that of advancement of the adjacent intact helical margin as a chondrocutaneous flap based on a wide postauricular skin pedicle. The ear lobule, which can be quite variable in size, is also advanced upward with this procedure.

If the defect is large, involving 3 to 4 cm of the helix, a double chondrocutaneous advancement of the helix can be performed by including the intact cephalic segment of the helix as a second flap (Fig. 1). It is important to extend the triangular tail of this flap right into the depth of the concha so that even after advancement the pleasing question mark shape of the helix is preserved. When such a large defect is closed by this technique (as shown in Fig. 2), it is often necessary to reduce the size of the contralateral ear to provide earlobe symmetry.

OPERATIVE TECHNIQUE

The technique of the operation is shown diagrammatically in Fig. 3, and the result is shown in Fig. 4. In this case, the scarred margins of the defect were pared to recreate the original defect, and reconstruction was undertaken as a secondary procedure.

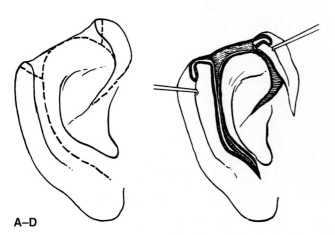
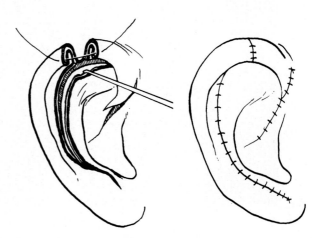

A–D

FIG. 1. A–D: Diagrammatic representation of double chondrocutaneous advancement flaps for reconstruction of a large (3 to 4 cm) helical defect. (From Antia and Buch, ref. 1, with permission.)

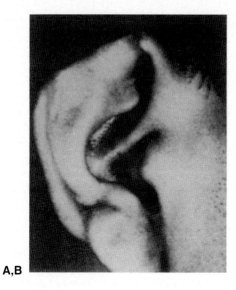
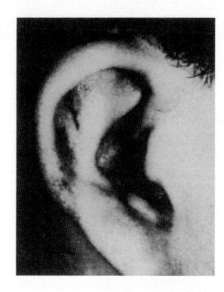

A,B

FIG. 2. A: Preoperative appearance of a large superior helical defect. B: Postoperative result. The size of the contralateral ear was reduced to produce symmetry. (From Antia and Buch, ref. 1, with permission.)

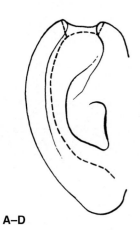
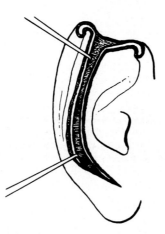
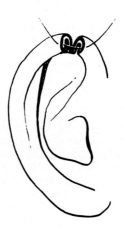
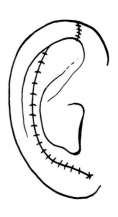

A–D

FIG. 3. A–D: Diagrammatic representation of a chondrocutaneous advancement flap from the caudal portion of the helix for reconstruction of a small (1 to 2 cm) helical defect. (From Antia and Buch, ref. 2, with permission.)

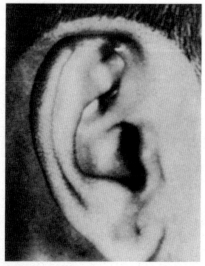
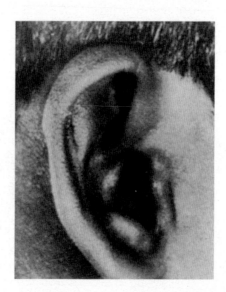

A,B

FIG. 4. A: Preoperative appearance of a small helical defect. B: Postoperative result. Note how the lobule has been pulled upward and the circumference of the ear has decreased. (From Antia and Buch, ref. 2, with permission.)

The skin on the lateral surface of the ear and the underlying cartilage are incised along the line of the anthelix between the helix and the anthelix, and the incision is extended into the soft tissue of the lobule (Fig. 3A). This is followed by careful dissection of the postauricular skin from the posterior surface of the concha and from the mastoid (Fig. 3B).

This dissection is especially difficult in the region of the groove between the mastoid and the ear, where there are dense, fibrous adhesions. Care must be taken to preserve the blood supply to the flap by keeping as close to the cartilage and bone as possible. The chondrocutaneous sandwich, on a wide and highly vascular pedicle, can now be advanced to close the defect. It is necessary only to obtain accurate apposition of the skin (Fig. 3D), since the cartilage can be held in place by a well-molded dressing.

SUMMARY

The chondrocutaneous advancement flap is a simple, safe, one-stage procedure that gives excellent results for correction of partial losses of the helix of the ear.

References

1. Antia NH, Buch VI. Chondrocutaneous advancement flap for the marginal defect of the ear. *Plast Reconstr Surg* 1967;39:472.
2. Antia NH. Repair of segmental defects of the auricle in mechanical trauma. In: Tanzer R, Edgerton M, eds., *Symposium on Reconstructive Surgery of the Auricle*. St. Louis: Mosby, 1974;218–220.

CHAPTER 83 ■ ANTEGRADE TRIANGULAR COMPOSITE EAR FLAP FOR HELIX-SCAPHA DEFECTS OF THE EAR

R. V. ARGAMASO AND C. A. RHEE

EDITORIAL COMMENT

This is an outstanding method of ear reconstruction; it extends Antia's procedure for the lateral ear defect. The result is an ear that appears almost normal but is slightly smaller than on the unopetated side.

The antegrade triangular chondrocutaneous flap is useful for single-stage reconstruction of defects measuring less than 2.0 cm that involve the helix scaphal region of the upper ear (1–3).

INDICATIONS

The antegrade triangular composite ear flap is a simple method that can be used to correct defects or deformities of 2.0 cm or less in the helix or scaphal region of the upper segment of the ear (Fig. 1). This technique offers the advantages of a single-stage procedure and obviates the need for the additional use of cartilage and skin grafts. A disadvantage is that, depending on the extent of the defect, the overall size of the ear is reduced.

ANATOMY

The auricle or pinna has a somewhat oval shape; the upper half is usually wider and gradually tapers bluntly toward the lobe. At the helical rim, the tail of the rim and antitragus, the skin can be separated easily from the underlying cartilage. Therefore, it is possible to skeletonize the entire lower portion of the ear and to advance the skin mantle superiorly. The blood supply of this flap is based in the skin pedicle of the lower pole of the ear.

FLAP DESIGN AND DIMENSIONS

A skin marking for the incision is drawn on the lateral side, along the most anterior rim of the defect, and arching downward toward the fold between the helix and anthelix just above the ear lobe. A second marking is drawn along the margin of the upper stump of the helix.

OPERATIVE TECHNIQUE

The incision is made through and through the lateral skin, cartilage, and skin of the medial ear, creating a triangular chondrocutaneous flap (Fig. 2). At the inferior end of the incision, the skin is elevated from the medial and lateral sides of the concha (Figs. 3 and 4). The tail of the helix is cut and detached from the main cartilaginous portion of the ear. The blood supply of the composite flap is now based on its inferior skin pedicle. Detachment of the cartilage facilitates advancement of the tail of the helix and antegrade advancement and rotation of the triangular composite flap over the defect. An incision then is made at the upper stump to open up a triangular space for accepting the apex of the chondrocutaneous flap.

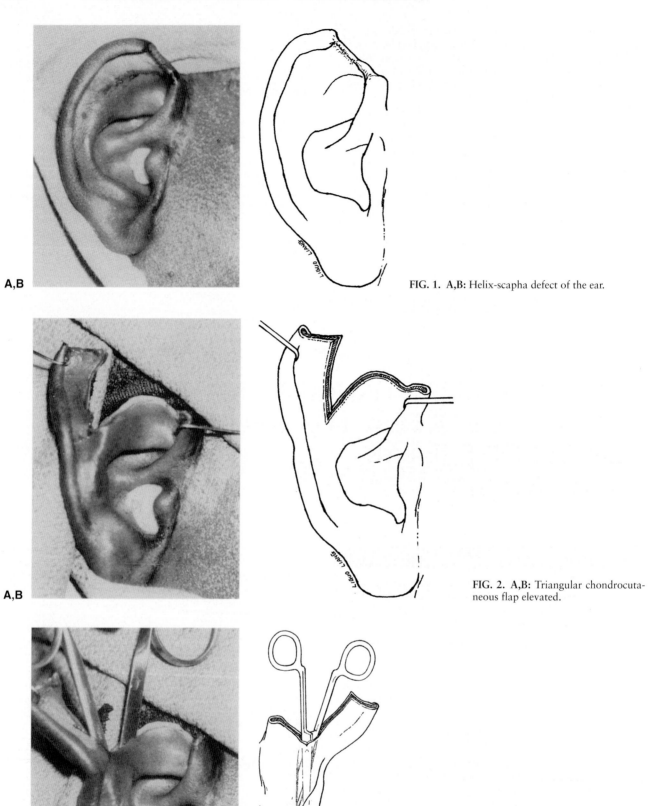

FIG. 1. A,B: Helix-scapha defect of the ear.

FIG. 2. A,B: Triangular chondrocutaneous flap elevated.

FIG. 3. A,B: Skin elevated from medial concha.

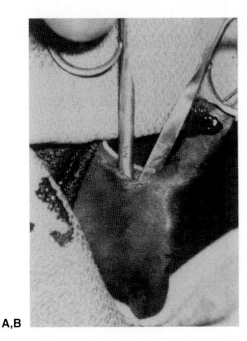

A,B

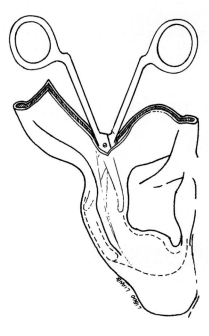

FIG. 4. **A,B:** Skin elevated from lateral ear.

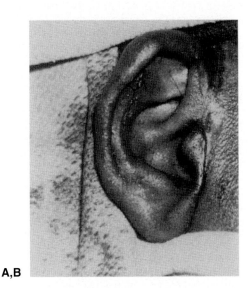

A,B

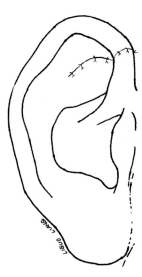

FIG. 5. **A,B:** End result after antegrade advancement and rotation of triangular composite flap.

Closure is accomplished in layers and includes the approximation of cartilage to cartilage, with particular attention to the helical margins. This maneuver brings the helical rims together and recreates the scaphoid fossa (Fig. 5).

SUMMARY

An antegrade triangular chondrocutaneous flap can be used in one stage for reconstructing defects of less than 2.0 cm that involve the helix scaphal region of the upper ear.

References

1. Argamaso RV, Lewin M. Parial deformities of the ear. In: Hinderer UT, od. *Plastic Surgery,* vol. 1, Amsterdam: Elsevier, 1992; 249–255.
2. Argamaso RV. Ear flaps. *Ear Nose Throat* 1972;51:310.
3. Argamaso RV, Lewin ML. Repair of partial ear loss with local composite flaps. *Plast Reconstr Surg* 1968;42:437.

CHAPTER 84 ■ FLAP CORRECTION FOR CRYPTOTIA

R. V. ARGAMASO

A retroauricular retrograde skin flap can be used to correct a congenital, bilateral, ear deformity. The procedure places scar lines in areas that reduce scar visibility and also circumvents the need for skin grafts.

INDICATIONS

The term *cryptotia* is applied to a congenital anomaly of the ear characterized by the disappearance of the superior pole from view; the pole telescopes and hides beneath the scalp. When the invaginated upper pole is retracted out from under the scalp, the helix usually appears intact; however, the scapha may have some deformity associated with a rather sharply folded superior antihelical crus. A third crus may be present. After retraction is released, the upper pole returns into the scalp pocket.

Elevation of the upper pole of the ear from the side of the head is indicated for aesthetic reasons and also offers convenience and support for eye glasses or hearing aids. Many methods of releasing the upper pole have been described (1–6). Elevation from the side of the head creates a skin defect of the scalp and on the medial aspect of the ear. This open area requires coverage with adjacent scalp flaps, skin grafts, or a combination of these. The resultant scalp scars are readily seen but may be hidden if the hair is kept long.

The retrograde medial-ear skin flap is a random flap that is useful for the correction of cryptotia (7) as well as for defects of the lower pole of the ear (8). Scar lines are placed in areas which limit scar visibility, and the need for skin grafts is circumvented.

ANATOMY

The primary blood supply to the medial skin of the ear comes from the posterior auricular artery. Its branches freely anastomose with those vessels on the lateral surface of the ear coming from branches of the superficial temporal artery. The rich network of anastomosing vessels, arranged randomly at the periphery of the ear, safely permits elevation of skin flaps on the medial side, based virtually from any direction.

FLAP DESIGN AND DIMENSIONS

The extent of the skin incision is outlined, with the upper pole retracted from its pocketed position in the scalp. Starting at about the level of the earlobe, the incision follows along the auricular cephalic sulcus on the mastoid side and continues superiorly, arching anteriorly, and terminating at the helical crus, where a Z-plasty is also outlined (Fig. 1A–C). At the inferior extremity of this skin marking, a small back-cut is marked and extends toward the earlobe, which will allow further rotation of the medial-ear skin flap. Thus, the flap encompasses nearly the entire medial skin of the ear based on a broad pedicle along the helical margin.

OPERATIVE TECHNIQUE

The incision is made along the predetermined skin marking. The segment of ear cartilage buried beneath the scalp is liberated from its soft-tissue moorings by transecting its attachments to the periosteum of the temporal bone. When detachment is complete, the upper pole of the ear stays out of the scalp and assumes its normal projection. The skin flap then is elevated in a retrograde manner from the perichondrium toward the helical rim. The communicating branches through the cartilage (perforators) are identified and electrocoagulated. Electrocoagulation of bleeders on the flap side should be minimized or avoided. Dissection toward the helix is done carefully, as close to the perichondrium as possible, to avoid interruption of the intercommunicating vessels crossing over the helix from the lateral side of the ear.

The retrograde skin flap then is rotated superiorly. Additional superior advancement of the flap is gained by a back-cut. The medial ear skin thus stretched and expanded toward the upper pole becomes sufficient to resurface the medial side of the exteriorized segment of the ear. A small dog-ear that develops inferiorly is trimmed. The small triangular skin flap, based anteriorly at the region of the helical crus, is transposed in Z-plasty fashion to recreate and maintain a deep auricular cephalic sulcus. The flaps finally are inset using fine sutures of 5–0 or 6–0 nylon (Fig. 1D–F). A conforming dressing is applied with mild compression.

CLINICAL RESULTS

In the retrograde flap, edema is to be expected during the early postoperative stage. This edema gradually subsides within a period of days or a few weeks. The scar lines are found in inconspicuous areas along the postauricular sulcus, and the hairline is not disturbed (Fig. 2).

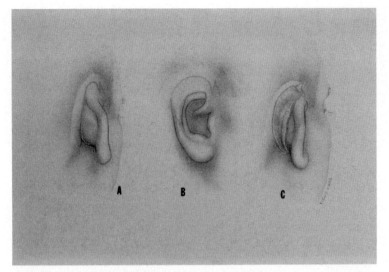

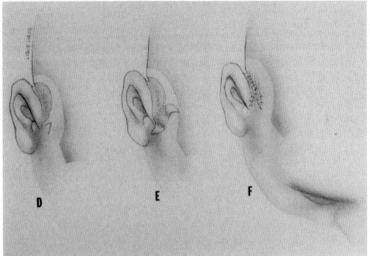

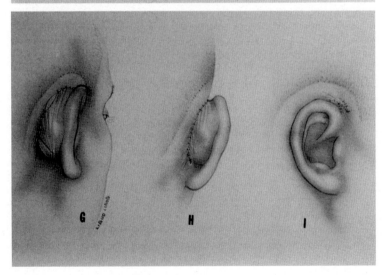

FIG. 1. A–C: Artist's rendition showing outline of skin incision on mastoid skin along the retroauricular sulcus, terminating anteriorly as a Z. Note back-cut toward the earlobe. **D–F:** Upper pole is released and triangular flaps are interposed. **G–I:** Retrograde flap is rotated and set in place.

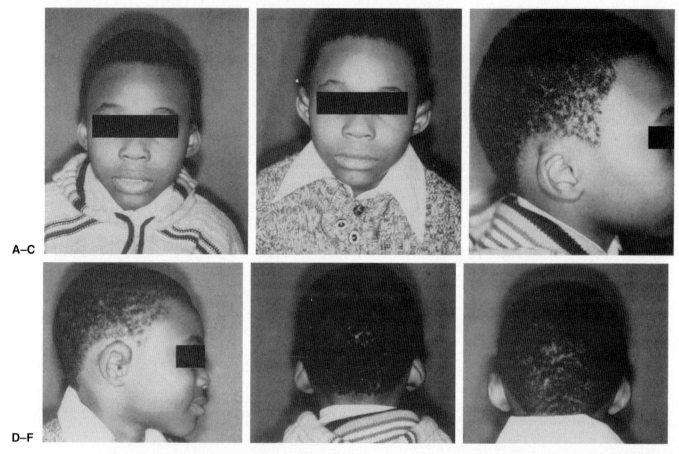

A–C

D–F

FIG. 2. **A:** Preoperative frontal view. **B:** Postoperative frontal view. **C:** Preoperative lateral view. **D:** Postoperative lateral view. **E:** Preoperative back view. **F:** Postoperative back view.

SUMMARY

The retroauricular retrograde skin flap is useful for the correction of cryptotia. Placement of the scar lines along the retroauricular groove minimizes their exposure from casual frontal, lateral, or back views.

References

1. Burian F. Correction of pocketed auricle. In: *The plastic surgery atlas*, vol. 2. London: Butterworth, 1967;470.
2. Cowan RJ. Cryptotia. *Plast Reconstr Surg* 1969;27:209.
3. Fukuda O. Otoplasty of cryptotia. *Jpn J Plast Reconstr Surg* 1968;11:L117.
4. Pollack WJ. Technique for correction of cryptotia: Case report. *Plast Reconstr Surg* 1969;44:501.
5. Washio H. Cryptotia: pathology and repair. *Plast Reconstr Surg* 1973;52:648.
6. Wesser DR. Repair of a cryptotic ear with a trifoil flap. *Plast Reconstr Surg* 1972;50:192.
7. Argamaso RV. Cryptotia: its surgical correction. *Ann Plast Surg* 1979;2:109.
8. Argamaso RV. Techniques for the reconstruction of the earlobe. *Philippine J Surg Spec* 1979;35:31.

CHAPTER 85 ■ RETROAURICULAR BIPEDICLE SKIN FLAP FOR PARTIAL EAR RECONSTRUCTION

S. ZENTENO ALANIS

Partial losses of the auricle often give the misleading impression that the defect is smaller than it is in reality.

INDICATIONS

When the defect is in the posterior margin of the ear, a large bipedicle flap of posterior ear skin is recommended (see Chapter 81). These tissues are thin, well vascularized, pliable, and of the same color as the rest of the ear.

If the defect is in the superior portion of the external ear, a cartilage graft may be required for support. If the defect is in the inferior portion of the ear, there is no need for cartilage because the force of gravity does not alter the shape obtained with a skin flap (1–18).

ANATOMY

The bipedicle flap from the retroauriculomastoid area has a superior pedicle located next to the helix insertion and an inferior pedicle behind the earlobe (Fig. 1). The postauricular artery is included in the flap.

FLAP DESIGN AND DIMENSIONS

This flap is about 2 cm wide and 5 cm long. The anterior line of the flap is drawn on the posterior ear surface, leaving a portion of skin about 2 mm wide between this line and the edge of the defect. The posterior line of the flap will be parallel to the anterior line and located next to the retroauricular hairline (Figs. 1 and 2B). The transverse measurement must be more than double the width of the defect.

OPERATIVE TECHNIQUE

The bipedicle skin flap is raised and folded longitudinally on itself. The anterior edge of the flap is sutured to the anterior edge of the ear defect. The posterior edge of the flap is sutured to the 2-mm skin bridge left behind when the anterior edge of the flap is incised. The skin graft that will cover the flap donor area then is sutured to the posterior edge of the same skin bridge (Fig. 2C).

In the case of major loss of the posterior margin of the ear, a cartilage segment taken from the ipsilateral concha as a composite flap or a cartilage graft taken from the contralateral ear will be required to maintain the shape of the ear (Fig. 3C).

The second stage is performed 3 to 4 weeks later. Both pedicles are divided so that an extra portion of skin is included to provide helical continuity.

SUMMARY

The retroauricular bipedicle flap is used for large defects of the posterior margin of the external ear.

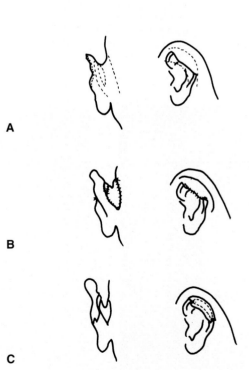

FIG. 1. A: Posteroanterior and lateral views of the flap design. **B:** Mobilization of the flap to cover the posterosuperior marginal defect. The flap donor area has been skin grafted. **C:** Final result after transposing the flap pedicles. A cartilage graft has been inserted to support the helical rim.

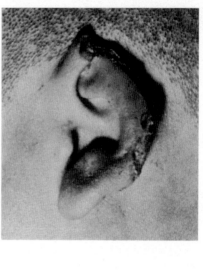

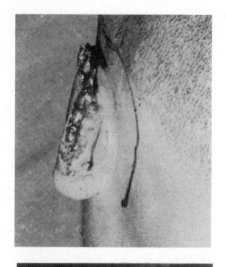

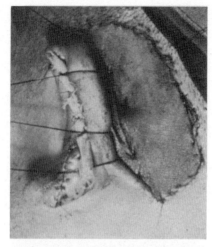

A–

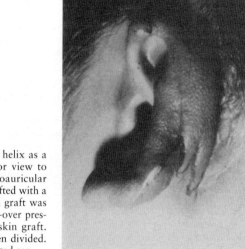

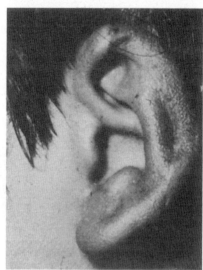

D,E

FIG. 2. A: Loss of a portion of the helix as a result of a human bite. **B:** Posterior view to demonstrate the outline of the retroauricular bipedicle skin flap. **C:** The flap was lifted with a segment of conchal cartilage. A skin graft was sutured to the flap donor area. A tie-over pressure dressing will be used for the skin graft. **D:** The pedicles of the flap have been divided. **E:** Final appearance of the reconstructed ear.

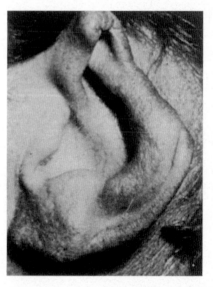

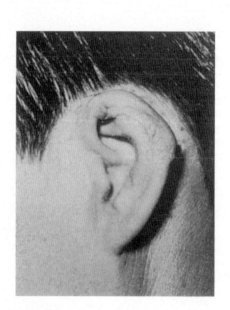

A,B

FIG. 3. A: Defect of half of the helical rim, superior crus of the anthelix, and triangular fossa as a result of trauma. **B:** After transposition of the skin-flap pedicles. *(Continued)*

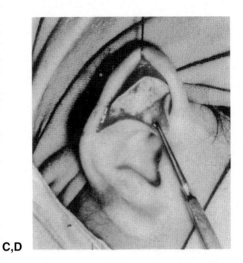
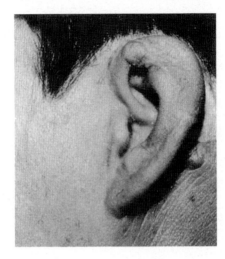

C,D

FIG. 3. *Continued.* **C:** *A cartilage graft was taken from the contralateral ear.* **D:** *Final appearance of the reconstructed ear.*

References

1. Maliniac JW. Reconstruction for partial loss of the ear: case reports. *Plast Reconstr Surg* 1946;1:124.
2. Stefanoff DN. Auriculomastoid tube pedicle for otoplasty. *Plast Reconstr Surg* 1948;3:352.
3. Lewin ML. Formation of the helix with a postauricular flap. *Plast Reconstr Surg* 1950;5:432.
4. Cronin TD. One-stage reconstruction of the helix: two improved methods. *Plast Reconstr Surg* 1952;9:547.
5. Spina VA. A simpler method of partial reconstruction of the external ear. *Plast Reconstr Surg* 1954;13:488.
6. Gillies, HD, Millard, DR. *The principles and art of plastic surgery.* Boston: Little, Brown, 1957. P. 312.
7. Converse, JM. Reconstruction of the auricle. Part II. *Plast Reconstr Surg* 1958;22:230.
8. Luna, C. Partial auricular plastic surgery. *Rev Lat Am Cirug Plast* 1961;5:28.
9. Navabi, A. One-stage reconstruction of a partial defect of the auricle. *Plast Reconstr Surg* 1964;33:77.
10. Pigossi, N. Repair of partial losses of the external ear. *Rev Lat Am Cirug Plast* 1965;9:35.
11. Steffensen, WH. A method of total ear reconstruction. *Plast Reconstr Surg* 1965;36:97.
12. Cosman B, Crikelair G. The composed tube pedicle in ear reconstruction. *Plast Reconstr Surg* 1966;37:517.
13. Millard DR. The chondrocutaneous flap in partial auricular repair. *Plast Reconstr Surg* 1966;27:523.
14. Zenteno Alanis S. Reconstruccíon de pabellon auricular. *Rev Anales Soc Otorinolaringol* 1968.
15. Zenteno Alanis S. Creación de la Clínica de 1° y 2° Arcos Branquiales. *Rev Lat Am Cirug Plast* 1970;14:65.
16. Orticochea M. Reconstruction of partial loss of the auricle. *Plast Reconstr Surg* 1971;47:220.
17. Zenteno Alanis S. Severe problems in total ear reconstruction. In: *Transactions of the 5th International Congress of Plastic and Reconstructive Surgery.* Melbourne, Australia: Butterworth, 1971.
18. Zenteno Alanis S. Reconstruccíon de Pérdidas Parciales del Pabellón Auricular. *Trib Med Mex* 1975;29:A3.

CHAPTER 86 ■ CHONDROCUTANEOUS CONCHAL FLAP TO THE UPPER THIRD OF THE EAR

J. E. DAVIS

Loss of the upper third of the ear can be repaired in one stage with a chondrocutaneous flap raised from the concha.

INDICATIONS

This type of reconstruction is indicated in deformities resulting from trauma and after surgical ablation, but in congenital microtia the concha is too small to provide donor tissue (1–12).

ANATOMY

The very narrow pedicle is at the helix radicis. The blood supply is of the random-pattern type, and the pedicle itself consists of three layers: skin, cartilage, and skin.

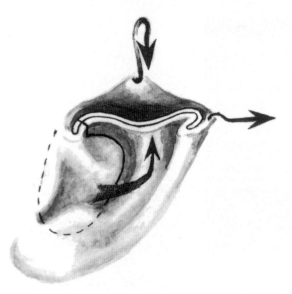

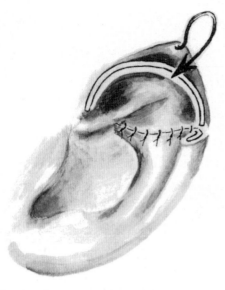

FIG. 1. The solid and dotted lines outline the chondrocutaneous conchal flap, which will be rotated upward on its narrow pedicle. The postauricular skin is dissected from the auricular cartilage at the margins of the upper ear defect.

FIG. 2. The chondrocutaneous conchal flap has been rotated to reconstruct the upper third of the external ear. A mastoid skin flap covers the exposed cartilage.

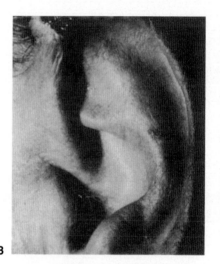

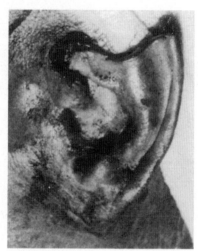

A,B

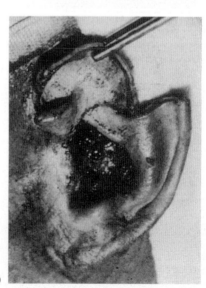

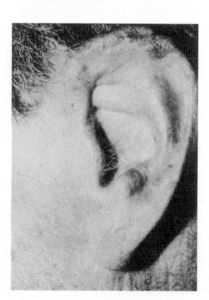

C,D

FIG. 3. A: Ulcerated skin cancer of superior helix of the left external ear. **B:** Operative photograph after excision of the skin cancer. **C:** The chondrocutaneous flap is rotated into position. **D:** Postoperative appearance. (From Davis, ref. 10, with permission.)

FLAP DESIGN AND DIMENSIONS

The flap is unique because it can be mobilized on a very small pedicle as a result of the abundant blood supply at this point.

OPERATIVE TECHNIQUE

An incision is made (Fig. 1) through the skin and conchal cartilage. The incision commences just behind the radix, falls below the inferior crus, runs along the anthelical insertion at the conchal floor, and continues forward at the lower cavum conchae until reaching the posterior border of the external auditory meatus. It comes up vertically inside the tragus to the anterior border of the helix radicis at the sulcus auricularis superior.

Then the dissection proceeds under the posterior conchal perichondrium. The chondrocutaneous flap is raised with hooks until it remains attached by a pedicle of only about 8 mm at the radix helicis.

The flap is now rotated upward into position to form the ear dome (Figs. 2 and 3C). The position is held by the elasticity of the cartilage as the flap tends to return to its original position, and one cartilage border presses gently against the other. These borders are trimmed until they coapt exactly. There is no need to suture the cartilages together because the position is maintained adequately with skin sutures. A mastoid skin flap can be raised to cover the border and posterior surface of this upper dome. The raw surface on the conchal floor is grafted with full-thickness contralateral retroauricular skin.

CLINICAL RESULTS

The resulting aesthetic appearance of the ear is not perfect because the radix helicis pedicle is prominent in the area normally occupied by the fossa triangularis depression (Fig. 3D).

However, most of my patients were satisfied, and only one wished to have a secondary procedure to form the fossa triangularis.

SUMMARY

A chondrocutaneous conchal flap can be used to reconstruct the upper third of the ear.

References

1. Adams WM. Construction of the upper half of the auricle utilizing composite conchal cartilage graft with perichondrium attached on both sides. *Plast Reconstr Surg* 1955;16:88.
2. Crikelair GF. A method of partial ear reconstruction for avulsion of the upper portion of the ear. *Plast Reconstr Surg* 1956;17:438.
3. Antia NH, Buch VI. Chondrocutaneous advancement flap for the marginal defects of the ear. *Plast Reconstr Surg* 1967;39:472.
4. Argamaso RV, Lewin ML. Repair of partial ear loss with local composite flap. *Plast Reconstr Surg* 1968;42:437.
5. Nagel F. Reconstruction of partial auricular loss. *Plast Reconstr Surg* 1972;49:340.
6. Davis JE. On auricular reconstruction. *Internatl Microform J Aesthet Plast Surg Otoplasty* 1972:1.
7. Davis JE. Discussion. In: RC Tanzer, MT Edgerton, eds. *Symposium on reconstruction of the auricle.* St. Louis: Mosby, 1974;247.
8. Davis JE. Auricle Reconstruction. In: MN Saad, P Lichtvelt, eds. *Reviews of plastic surgery.* Amsterdam: Excerpta Medica, 1974;129.
9. Lewin ML, Argamaso RV. Repair of major defects of the auricle in mechanical trauma. In: Tanzer RC, Edgerton MT, eds. *Symposium on reconstruction of the auricle.* St. Louis: Mosby, 1974;221.
10. Davis JE. Acquired deformities of the auricle. In: Converse JM, ed. *plastic and reconstructive surgery,* 2d ed. Philadelphia: WB Saunders, 1977;1755.
11. Converse JM. Acquired deformities of the ear. In: Converse JM, ed. *Plastic and reconstructive surgery,* 2d ed. Philadelphia: WB Saunders, 1977;1724.
12. Brent B. Reconstruction of traumatic ear deformities. In: Furnas DW, ed. *Clinics in plastic surgery: deformities of the external ear.* Philadelphia: WB Saunders, 1978;441.

CHAPTER 87 ■ RETROGRADE AURICULAR FLAP FOR PARTIAL EAR RECONSTRUCTION

H. W. LUEDERS

The retrograde auricular flap is useful for reconstruction and enlargement of an ear that has been burned, avulsed, or injured in such a manner that the upper part of the scapha or fossa triangularis has been lost, leaving a residual mass of skin and cartilage close to the concha (1).

ANATOMY

The posterior surface of the ear is supplied principally by terminal branches of the auricular artery from the postauric-ular artery. Care must be taken not to injure this artery in its location along the postauricular groove when dissecting over the mastoid.

FLAP DESIGN AND DIMENSIONS

The postauricular skin is used as the base to carry the composite skin and cartilage to the new enlarged position of the ear rim. The flap base extends from the anterior scalp to the mastoid.

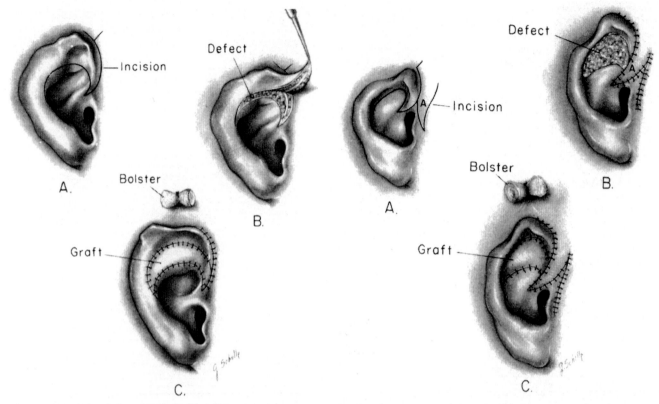

FIG. 1. A–C: Case 1. The patient was 34 years old when both ears were burned in May 1959, the right more severely. Surgery of the ear was performed in 1960. Preoperative ear height was right ear 5.0 cm and left ear 6.2 cm. A pedicle suspension suture was fixed to a bolster. (From Lueders, ref. 1, with permission.)

FIG. 3. A–C: Case 2. The patient was 43 years old when burned in February 1962. Surgery of the ear was performed in September 1962. Preoperative ear height was right ear 5.0 cm and left ear 6.5 cm. Postoperative height of the right ear was 6.5 cm. *Note:* The defect represents the pedicle of postauricular skin advanced off the concha. (From Lueders, ref. 1, with permission.)

OPERATIVE TECHNIQUE

The anterior skin and cartilage are incised on the remaining ear mass, starting at the onset of the helix anteriorly and curving to the temple (Figs. 1 and 2). The other inferior incision starts at the helix anteriorly and proceeds across the ear cartilage toward the opposite helical rim, creating a triangular flap anteriorly up to the limit of the temple. It is through the inferior incision that the dissection is carefully taken just to the postauricular skin, and the skin and subcutaneous tissue are dissected off the remaining concha onto the mastoid groove

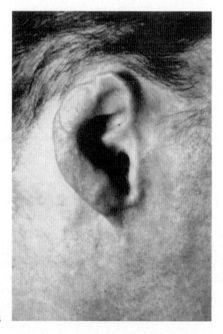
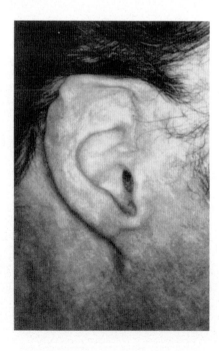

A,B

FIG. 2. Case 1. **A:** Preoperative appearance. **B:** Postoperative appearance. Increase in height of right ear was 1.5 cm. (From Lueders, ref. 1, with permission.)

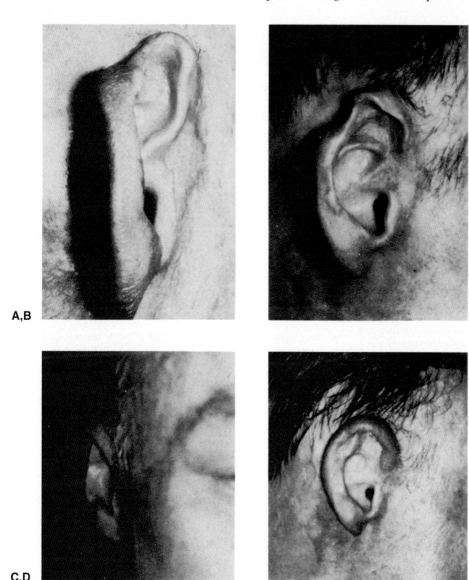

A,B

C,D

FIG. 4. Case 2: **A:** Preoperative view showing loss of the postauricular groove. **B:** Postoperative view. Increase in height of the right ear was 1.5 cm. Axis of ear is anterior: **C:** Anterior view of reconstructed ear. **D:** Lateral postoperative view with completed neck tubed pedicle. (From Lueders, ref. 1, with permission.)

and off the mastoid and temple. To mobilize this flap and give it freedom to move upward and backward, an incision is made transversely in the temple skin.

The skin defect may be so large anteriorly that it is advantageous to elevate a preauricular superiorly based flap to fill in the defect (Fig. 3). This has the advantage of wedging the upper limb in place. The defect created by the advancing helix is covered with a full-thickness skin graft or a thick, split, nonperforated skin graft. The graft is placed in the exposed subcutaneous fat of the postauricular skin composite flap. The graft is sutured in and immobilized by a tie-over dressing over nonadherent gauze. A subcutaneous suture placed from the scalp to the flap and back to the point of origin and tied over a bolster may help support the flap in its new position. The rest of the ear is splinted with saline-moistened gauze and a bulky dressing.

CLINICAL RESULTS

On completion of the dissection, the tip of the flap may be blue. Carefully placed dressings that avoid undue pressure

have prevented skin losses. Long-term follow-up demonstrates no loss of position or problems. The technique allows the formation of a framework of cartilage in the ear rim in the first stage, to which additional tubed pedicles can be attached to shape the ear further (Fig. 4). To avoid creating an ear that appears vertical or whose axis is forward, the initial temple incision should be curved back toward the mastoid. On the average, a 1.5-cm increase in the vertical height of the ear can be anticipated by the initial flap procedure.

SUMMARY

A retrograde auricular flap can be used to reconstruct partial ear losses that involve the upper part of the ear.

Reference

1. Lueders HW. One-stage enlargement of the burned ear. *Plast Reconstr Surg* 1966;37:512.

CHAPTER 88 ■ SUBCUTANEOUS PEDICLE FLAP FOR RECONSTRUCTION OF THE ANTERIOR SURFACE OF THE EXTERNAL EAR

J. K. MASSON

EDITORIAL COMMENT

This is an easy and reliable technique to reconstruct full-thickness defects on the lateral surface of the ear using postauricular skin. When planning the flap, one should, make sure that the subcutaneous vascular pedicle lies at or close to the center of the defect.

After excision of benign or malignant lesions from the helix and conchal regions of the external ear, the defect, if small, can be sutured directly. More often, however, it may be of such size or in such a location that a free graft or a local flap is needed for satisfactory repair. A simple skin flap on a subcutaneous pedicle from the uninvolved postauricular surface of the ear and the adjacent mastoid area has been useful in repairing a number of defects that involve the anterior skin surface and the underlying cartilage (1).

INDICATIONS

The main advantage offered by the subcutaneous pedicle flap is its ease of application. The flap provides an ideal color match and does not require the special dressing techniques that are necessary for immobilization of a free graft.

The flap is not limited to the concha, as Figures 1 and 2 might suggest, but in fact can be used in the triangular and scaphoid fossa areas. The flap has been used to cover a large part of the external canal and can be used even for some defects involving the helical rim. In one extreme case, a large flap was used to provide coverage for the entire anterior surface of the ear out to the helical rim, which had been avulsed in an automobile accident.

ANATOMY

The fairly rich blood supply to the external ear arises from the external carotid artery by way of the superficial temporal artery in front and from the posterior auricular artery behind. The venous drainage enters the superficial temporal vein in front and the external jugular vein below.

From the medial aspect of the ear and the posterior aspect of the auditory meatus, the lymphatic vessels collect in the mastoid glands at the mastoid tip. The efferent lymphatic trunks enter the deep cervical chain near the origin of the sternocleidomastoid muscle. The lymphatic vessels of the external

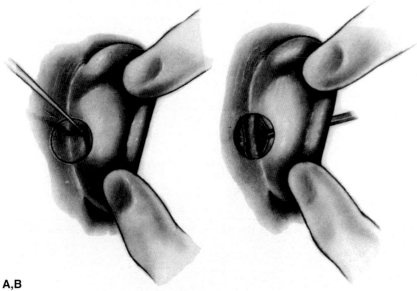

A,B

FIG. 1. **A:** Postauricular subcutaneous pedicle flap showing incision extending through ear. **B:** Flap is rolled or pulled through to the anterior surface. *(Continued)*

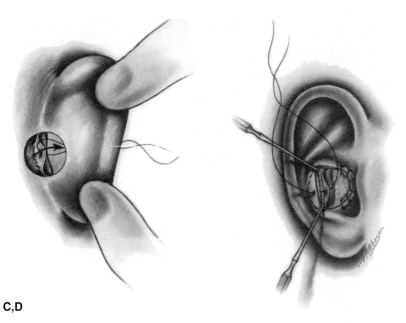

C,D

FIG. 1. *Continued.* **C,D:** Flap is brought forward and sutured in place. (From Masson, ref. 1, with permission.)

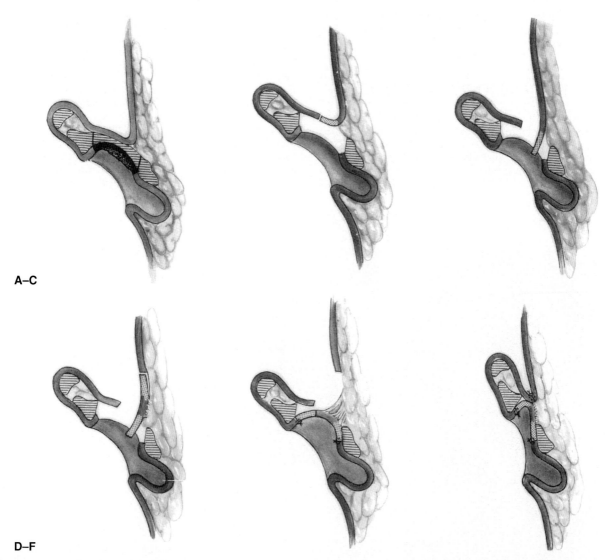

A–C

D–F

FIG. 2. Cross section through ear at level of external auditory canal. **A:** Lesion in concha. **B:** Remainder of flap incised and undermined. **C–E:** Flap pulled through and sutured to anterior surface of the ear. **F:** Flap sutured into place and the donor site closed primarily. (From Masson, ref. 1, with permission.)

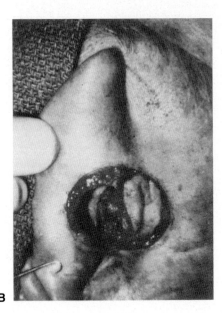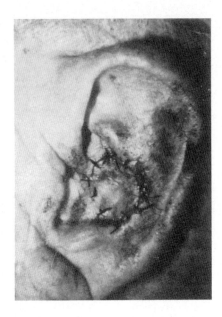

A,B

FIG. 3. **A:** Postauricular flap mobilized on a subcutaneous pedicle after excision of a basal cell carcinoma of the anterior surface of the concha. Note the opening through to the anterior surface. **B:** Flap fits the defect with ear pushed back to the head.

ear drain to the anterior or preauricular glands and, to some extent, to the glands about the parotid and eventually into the deep cervical chain.

FLAP DESIGN AND DIMENSIONS

After excision of the lesion from the anterior (lateral) surface of the ear, including the cartilage immediately beneath the tumor, a flap about the same size as the skin defect is marked out on the postauricular skin, overlapping the palpable margin of the surgical defect, and extending onto the cephaloauricular sulcus and mastoid area (see Figs. 1 and 2).

OPERATIVE TECHNIQUE

This roughly circular flap is incised around its borders, coming through on one border into the defect on the anterior surface of the pinna. The margins of this skin and subcutaneous flap are undermined quite generously, preserving a pedicle of subcutaneous tissue roughly in the center of the island-like postauricular flap.

Now, with the ear pushed back, the flap is apparent through the perforating defect in the external ear. With a hook or tissue forceps, the flap margins are brought through the defect to the anterior surface of the ear and secured with interrupted skin sutures about the entire periphery of the flap. This closes the operative defect on the lateral surface (Figs. 3 and 4).

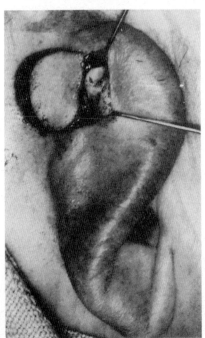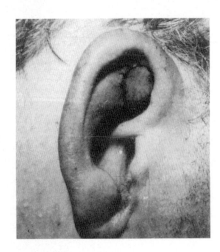

A,B

FIG. 4. **A:** Postauricular subcutaneous pedicle flap for closure of a defect in the upper part of the anterior ear. **B:** Flap in the triangular fossa 3 days after operation.

The donor area of the flap behind the ear then is closed directly. Only a light protective dressing is necessary over the ear for the first postoperative day.

CLINICAL RESULTS

In no case has there been any circulatory disturbance or unsatisfactory healing, although these possibilities must be considered and theoretically could happen. The final appearance after healing is complete has been excellent.

SUMMARY

The subcutaneous pedicle flap is a simple, reliable method of closing defects on the anterior surface of the external ear.

Reference

1. Masson IK. A simple island flap for reconstruction of concha-helix defects. *Br J Plast Surg* 1972;25:399.

CHAPTER 89 ■ RETROAURICULAR DERMAL PEDICLED SKIN FLAP TO THE EAR

A. J. RENARD

Techniques described to correct defects of the external ear usually fall into two categories. The first includes circumference-reducing procedures with the necessary removal of normal tissue and a resulting small ear (1–4). The second includes various techniques designed to maintain the size of the ear by interposition of a flap or graft or both (5–9). The use of a retroauricular flap for reconstruction of the auricle through an opening in the cartilage is well known. The flap described in Chapter 88 uses this technique; however, it is based on a rather nonmobile subcutaneous pedicle (10).

ANATOMY

This is usually a random-pattern skin flap (11,12). It is not uncommon to find a direct cutaneous artery at its base (Fig. 1). When this is the case, this retroauricular flap is an axial-pattern flap, receiving its blood supply in a retrograde fashion by the anastomosis between the superficial temporal artery and the retroauricular artery (Fig. 2).

FLAP DESIGN AND DIMENSIONS

The retroauricular dermal pedicled skin flap is designed as an ellipse (instead of a triangle) with its long axis oriented slightly obliquely, downward, and forward (Fig. 3). This orientation is important because as the donor defect is closed, the base of the flap is in a position that avoids distortion and undue tension on its dermal pedicle (Fig. 4). The base of the flap is deepithelialized over a length of about 1.5 to 2 cm.

The greatest width usually measures approximately 2 to 3 cm (Fig. 3A).

OPERATIVE TECHNIQUE

Once the flap is elevated, it can be used in two ways. It can be carried directly to a helical defect for peripherally located lesions (Figs. 5 and 6), or it can be tunneled through an opening made in the cartilaginous framework for use on the lateral surface of the ear (Figs. 7 and 8). This hiatus should be made wide enough to avoid constriction of the pedicle. The dermal deepithelialized surface of the pedicle always remains in apposition to the deep dermis of the overlying retroauricular skin (see Fig. 4). The distal portion of the flap is then trimmed to fit the contour of the defect (Figs. 5C and 7C). The retroauricular donor site can be closed with a minimum of tension.

CLINICAL RESULTS

In a small series of patients seen by the author, all the flaps have survived, the suture line of the flap donor site healed well, and aesthetic results have been quite satisfactory.

SUMMARY

The retroauricular flap based on a dermal pedicle provides coverage for ear defects in one stage without the need to sacrifice healthy tissue. It can be used for peripherally as well as centrally located lesions.

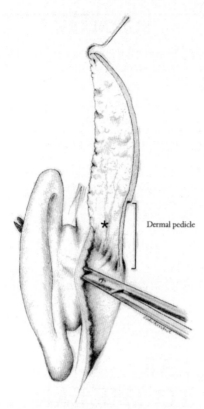

FIG. 1. The skin behind the concha is undermined to allow passage of the flap. The *asterisk* indicates the presence of a small direct cutaneous artery occasionally found in the base of the flap.

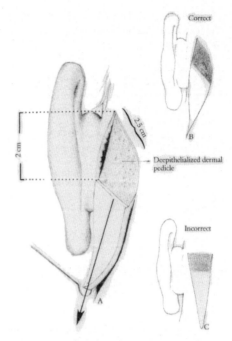

A–C

FIG. 3. A–C: The flap is designed as an ellipse with its axis oriented downward and slightly forward. The base of the flap is deepithelialized over a length of about 2 cm.

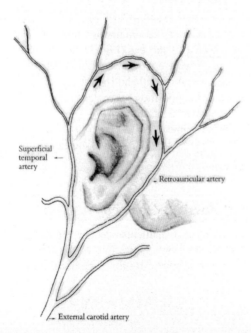

FIG. 2. Blood supply around the ear. There is an anastomosis between the superficial temporal artery and the retroauricular artery. When the retroauricular flap is elevated with its dermal pedicle based superiorly, the blood supply is maintained in a retrograde fashion by the anastomosis between the two arteries.

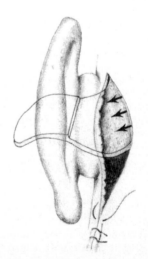

FIG. 4. The flap is tunneled under the skin to be delivered centrally or peripherally. The base of the flap is in a position that avoids distortion at the time of closure of the defect.

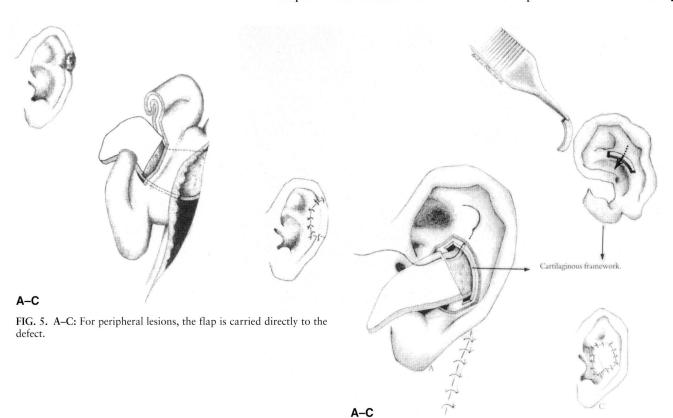

A–C

FIG. 5. A–C: For peripheral lesions, the flap is carried directly to the defect.

A–C

FIG. 7. A–C: For centrally located lesions, the flap is brought through the cartilaginous framework after removing a strip of cartilage. The hiatus in the cartilaginous framework should be made wide enough to avoid constriction of the pedicle.

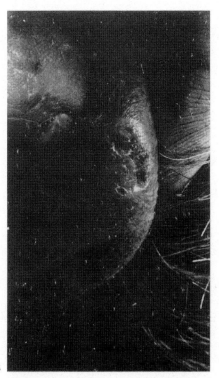

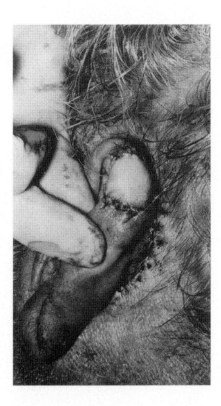

A,B

FIG. 6. A: A 63-year-old white man with a squamous cell carcinoma of his left ear located at the superior helix. **B:** The lesion was removed and the defect was closed with a retroauricular flap elevated on a deepithelialized dermal pedicle and carried directly to the defect behind the cartilaginous framework. (From Renard, ref. 11, with permission.)

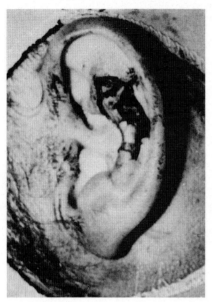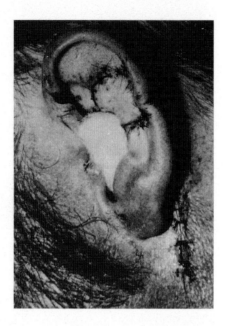

A,B

FIG. 8. A: A 28-year-old white man with a crush-avulsion injury of the skin and cartilage of the concha, anthelix, and scapha of his left ear. **B:** The retroauricular flap based on its dermal pedicle was brought through the cartilaginous framework to the lateral surface of the ear. (From Renard, ref. 11, with permission.)

References

1. Crikelair GF. A method of partial ear reconstruction for avulsion of the upper portion of the ear. *Plast Reconstr Surg* 1956;17:438.
2. Antia NH, Buch VI. Chondrocutaneous advancement flap for marginal defect of the ear. *Plast Reconstr Surg* 1967;39:472.
3. Tanzer RC, Belluci RJ, Converse JM, Brent B. Deformities of the auricle. In: Converse JM, ed., *Reconstructive plastic surgery*. Philadelphia: WB Saunders, 1977; Chap. 35.
4. Songcharoen S, Smith RA, Jabaley M. Deformities of the external ear: tumors of the external ear and reconstruction of defects. *Clin Plast Surg* 1978;5:447.
5. Pegram M, Peterson R. Repair of partial defect of the ear. *Plast Reconstr Surg* 1956;18:305.
6. Kazanjian VH. Surgical treatment of congenital deformities of the ears. *Am J Surg* 1958;95:185.
7. Owens N. An effective method for closing defects of the external auditory canal. *Plast Reconstr Surg* 1959;23:381.
8. Gingrass RP, Pickrell KL. Techniques for closure of conchal and external auditory canal defects. *Plast Reconstr Surg* 1968;41:568.
9. Nagel F. Reconstruction of a partial auricular loss: case report. *Plast Reconstr Surg* 1972;49:340.
10. Masson JK. A simple island flap for reconstruction of concha-helix defects. *Br J Plast Surg* 1972;25:399.
11. Renard A. Postauricular flap based on a dermal pedicle for ear reconstruction. *Plast Reconstr Surg* 1981;68:159.
12. Tanzer RC. Postauricular flap based on a dermal pedicle for reconstruction (Discussion). *Plast Reconstr Surg* 1981;68:165.

CHAPTER 90 ■ AURICULAR, PREAURICULAR, AND POSTAURICULAR SKIN FLAPS TO THE EXTERNAL AUDITORY CANAL

W. B. MACOMBER* AND J. D. NOONAN

Stenosis of the external auditory canal is an infrequent but serious consequence of congenital malformation, auricular trauma, or surgical extirpation. Even relatively minor scarring can cause marked functional and physical impairment. Not only is there a possibility of hearing deficit, but there is also the probability of chronic inflammation and infection.

* Deceased.

INDICATIONS

The use of skin grafts may provide a temporary solution; however, late results have shown that the ongoing process of wound contraction invariably produces further reduction in the lumenal diameter. To rectify this problem, a variety of local flaps can be used to break up the concentric scarring (1–4).

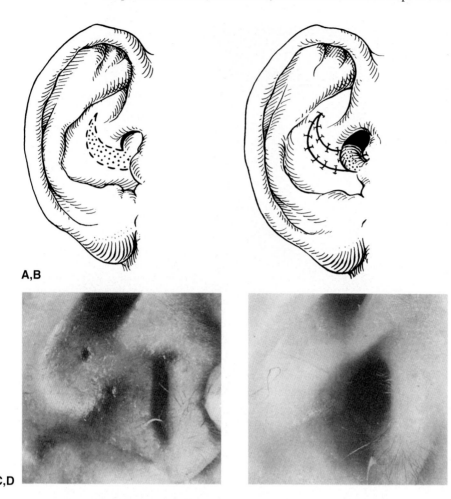

A,B

C,D

FIG. 1. A: Outline of the conchal skin flap. B: Conchal skin flap in place with skin graft applied to the donor site. C: Preoperative stenosis of the auditory canal. D: Postoperative result following meatus reconstruction with a conchal skin flap. (From Macomber, ref. 4, with permission.)

ANATOMY

The vascularity of these flaps is based on the rich dermal network that exists in this region arising from both the preauricular and postauricular vessels.

OPERATIVE TECHNIQUE

Conchal Skin Flap

This is an excellent choice, provided the auricular tissue has not been damaged by antecedent trauma. Based either inferi-orly (Fig. 1) or superiorly, the entire conchal skin and subcutaneous tissue can be elevated and transposed across the meatus of the external auditory canal. Care must be taken not to denude the conchal cartilage of its perichondrium, and a relatively wide base ensures flap viability. The flap donor site is usually closed with a skin graft.

Preauricular Flap

The preauricular flap (Fig. 2) is based inferiorly to minimize the arc of rotation; however, care must be taken, particularly in men, to avoid pulling the sideburn immediately adjacent to or onto the ear itself at the time of closure of the flap donor

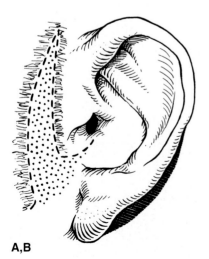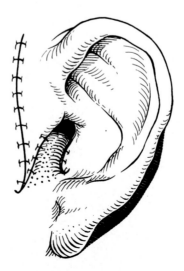

A,B

FIG. 2. A: Outline of the preauricular skin flap. B: Preauricular skin flap in place. *(Continued)*

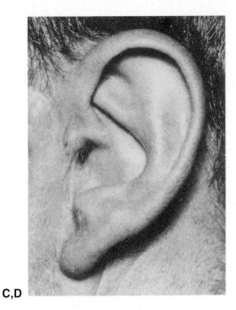
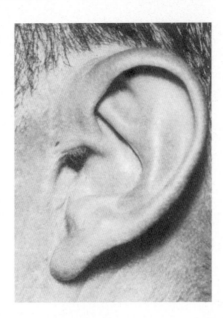

C,D

FIG. 2. *Continued.* **C:** Preoperative stenosis of the auditory canal. **D:** Postoperative result following release of the meatal stenosis with a preauricular skin flap. (From Macomber, ref. 4, with permission.)

site. To avoid this untoward result, the postauricular flap is quite a satisfactory alternative.

Postauricular Flap

This flap is outlined in the retroauricular area over the mastoid prominence immediately adjacent to the postauricular sulcus. The flap usually measures 3 to 4 cm long and at least 1 cm wide. The base is located below the level of the external auditory canal, separated only by the conchal portion of the ear. The flap then is elevated just above the periosteum and tunneled through the concha, with the small portion of the flap within the tunnel being deepithelialized.

On completion of any of these operations, a Xeroform- or mineral oil-soaked gauze packing is placed into the newly formed canal and left there for 7 to 10 days. This dressing is repeated once or twice until adequate wound healing is appreciated. At this point, a soft rubber tube or ear plug of appropriate size is introduced into the external auditory canal and maintained there until the scar has softened satisfactorily. The plug is removed periodically and the canal is irrigated to avoid buildup of cerumen.

CLINICAL RESULTS

The resulting orifice is quite patulous, and the untoward effect of subsequent stenosis is averted.

SUMMARY

Auricular, preauricular, and postauricular flaps, compared to skin grafts, provide a more permanent solution for stenosis of the external auditory meatus.

References

1. Owens N. An effective method for closing defects of the external auditory canal. *Plast Reconstr Surg* 1959;23:381.
2. Renard A. Postauricular flap based on dermal pedicle for ear reconstruction. *Plast Reconstr Surg* 1981;68:159.
3. Songcharoen S, Smith RA, Jabaley M. Tumors of the external ear and reconstruction of defects. *Clin Plast Surg* 1978;5:447.
4. Macomber WB. Reconstruction of the traumatically stenosed external auditory canal. *Plast Reconstr Surg* 1958;22:168.

CHAPTER 91 ■ SKIN FLAP TO THE TORN EARLOBE

A. M. PARDUE

The earliest known reference to a flap concerned the repair of cleft earlobes (1). Cleft earlobe deformity may be congenital or acquired (2–4). Acquired cleft earlobe may be complete or incomplete (3,5).

INDICATIONS

Repair of congenital cleft earlobe consists of excising the skin of the opposing surfaces of the cleft and approximating the two sides with or without a small Z-plasty within the suture line as it curves around the earlobe (1,3,6). Acquired cleft of the earlobe is usually due to a tear through the lobe by a sudden pull on an earring or by prolonged pull of a heavy earring.

Here we are primarily concerned with a repair of a complete or incomplete cleft of the earlobe with preservation of an earring opening that is correctly positioned. If the cleft is incomplete, the bridging tissue should be excised, creating a complete cleft, to avoid bulging of the bridging tissue (3).

ANATOMY

The repair of a cleft earlobe with preservation of the earring opening consists of raising a small transposition flap whose blood supply is derived from the ample vascularity of the earlobe and the rich plexus of vessels in the skin and subdermal areas (5).

FLAP DESIGN AND DIMENSIONS

The flap is based superiorly to one side of the upper end of the cleft. The width of the flap is the width of the inner surface of the cleft near its superior end. The flap is approximately 3 mm long and 1 mm thick.

OPERATIVE TECHNIQUE

The procedure starts with outlining the flap and the area to be excised (Fig. 1A). The margins of the cleft are excised, and a

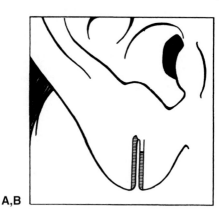
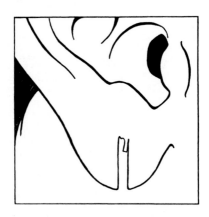
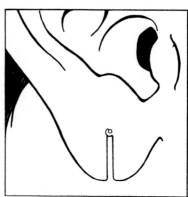
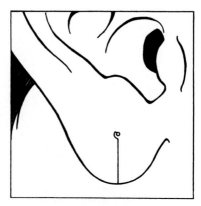

A,B

C,D

FIG. 1. **A:** The shaded areas show the opposing surfaces of the cleft to be excised. **B:** The skin has been excised, and the backcut for the transposition flap is shown. **C:** The small flap is transposed to the opposite side and sutured. **D:** The cleft is closed in a straight line.

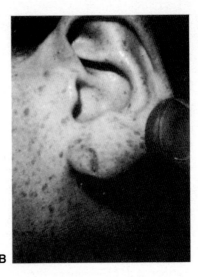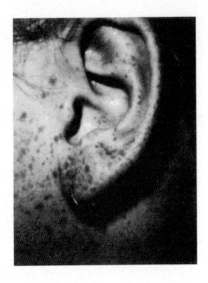

A,B

FIG. 2. **A:** Preoperative view showing an incomplete cleft. **B:** Postoperative view showing the repaired cleft with the loop of clear nylon passing through the perforation.

small flap is raised on one side at the upper end of the cleft (Fig. 1B). The distal edge of the flap is sutured to the opposite side so that the suture line is not at the dependent area of the perforation (Fig. 1C). The raw surfaces of the cleft are approximated with two to three sutures of 5–0 Vicryl, and the skin margins are closed with 6–0 Prolene (Fig. 1D). A Z-plasty may be used to interrupt the suture line on the curve of the earlobe. A single loop of 4–0 clear nylon suture is left within the perforation for 4 to 6 weeks and then is replaced with an earring. The technique is simple and is readily done with the patient under local anesthesia (Fig. 2).

A different technique (7) using a posterior transposition flap has been reported, but the design of this flap requires excising more normal skin from one side of the cleft, with possible distortion of the flap as it is transposed and twisted into the perforation canal.

CLINICAL RESULTS

Results with this technique have been uniformly good for both complete and incomplete clefts. There have been no reports of failures of the flap. The patient should be instructed not to wear heavy earrings again or ones that might be snagged easily, thereby retearing the earlobe.

SUMMARY

A skin flap can be designed from the margin of a torn earlobe to correct the deformity and at the same time provide a skin-lined canal for a new earring opening.

References

1. McDowell F. Sushruta's ancient earlobe and rhinoplastic operations in India (Editorial comment on classic reprint). *Plast Reconstr Surg* 1969; 43:517.
2. Yamada A. The evaluation of the cleft earlobe. *Jpn J Plast Reconstr Surg* 1976;19:171.
3. Boo-Chai K. The cleft earlobe. *Plast Reconstr Surg* 1961;28:681.
4. Dibbell DG. Split earlobe deformities. *Plast Reconstr Surg* 1970;45:77.
5. Pardue AM. Repair of torn earlobe with preservation of the perforation for an earring. *Plast Reconstr Surg* 1973;51:472.
6. Hamilton R, LaRossa D. Method for repair of cleft earlobes. *Plast Reconstr Surg* 1975;55:99.
7. Buchan NG. The cleft earlobe: A method of repair with preservation of the earring canal. *Br J Plast Surg* 1975;28:296.

CHAPTER 92 ■ REPAIR OF THE CLEFT EARLOBE WITH AN ADVANCEMENT FLAP AND TWO UNILATERAL Z-PLASTIES

B. STRAUCH AND M. KEYES-FORD*

EDITORIAL COMMENT

This is an excellent technique to avoid secondary notching and indentation of a traumatic laceration of the lobule of the ear. The combination of a sliding advancement flap with Z-plasties gives a rounded appearance to the earlobe and lengthens the surgical scar.

Many flaps have been described for repair of the cleft earlobe (1–8). Our preferred technique uses an advancement flap with two unilateral Z-plasties.

INDICATIONS

This procedure allows repair of the cleft, and retention of the normal curve of the earlobe, as well as preventing late notching.

ANATOMY

The transposed flaps created by the advancement flap and Z-plasties are supplied by a rich plexus of perforators from both the superficial temporal and posterior auricular arteries, which are branches of the external carotid. Venous drainage is from the accompanying veins (9).

FLAP DESIGN AND DIMENSIONS

The procedure is designed so that an advancement flap from the posterior limb of the cleft provides the rounded contour of the lower edge of the lobule. Two unequal, unilateral Z-plasties are transposed in a superior direction. An incision on the posterior limb of the cleft bisects this limb, using the lower third as the advancement flap (A–B), and the upper two thirds (B-C-E') becomes the lower unilateral Z-plasty. An incision (D–C') on the anterior limb of the cleft creates the second unilateral Z-plasty (see Fig. 1, D–C'). The inferior border of the anterior limb of the cleft is deepithelialized to accept the advancement flap (see Fig. 1, B'–A').

* Deceased.

OPERATIVE TECHNIQUE

First, markings similar to those in Fig. 1 are made on the anterior and posterior limbs. The healed edges of the cleft are excised. The lower edge of the anterior limb is excised to the subcutaneous level (Fig. 2, B'–A'). The incision at the lower edge of the posterior limb is incised to create an advancement flap that corresponds to the length of the deepithelialized portion of the anterior limb (see Fig. 2, A–B). The two unilateral Z-plasties are created by making incisions into the anterior and posterior limbs, as previously mentioned (see Fig. 2, E'–C–B, C'–D–E').

All flaps are transposed by starting with the lower advancement flap (A–A'). Flap E–C–B is transposed into the defect D–C' created in the anterior limb of the cleft. Flap C'–D–E is transposed into the defect E'–D' created in the posterior limb. If point E is in excess, it may bulge and should be trimmed or, alternatively, a relaxing incision can be made in the apex of the cleft to allow point E to lie flat (Fig. 3). The lateral surface suture line of the earlobe is sutured with 6–0 nylon, the medial surface with 5–0 nylon.

CLINICAL RESULTS

Good results using this technique can be obtained with complete as well as incomplete cleft earlobes. (Incomplete clefts should be converted into complete ones.) Once the incisions have healed, a rounded contour at the lower rim of the earlobe is formed, without notching. Patients can have the ear pierced in approximately 6 months or when the suture line has softened. They are discouraged from wearing heavy, hanging earrings that can recreate the same deformity.

SUMMARY

An advancement flap and two unilateral Z-plasties provide a simple solution for the repair of the cleft earlobe, by creating a smooth, round contour at the lower edge and by preventing recurrent notching.

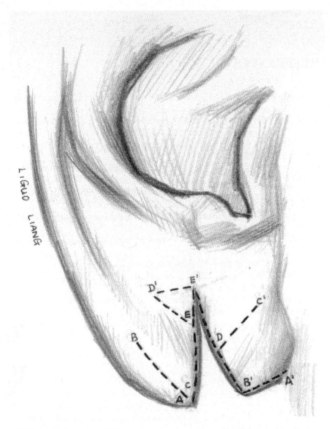

FIG. 1. Diagram of plan of proposed flaps. (From Strauch, Keyes-Ford, ref. 8, with permission.)

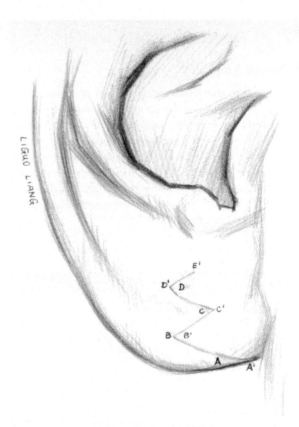

FIG. 3. Diagram of flap transpositions. (From Strauch, Keyes-Ford, ref. 8, with permission.)

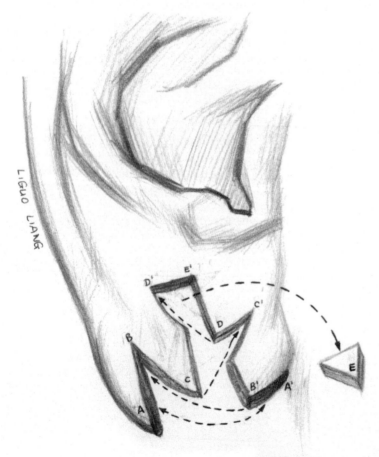

FIG. 2. Diagram of flap incisions. (From Strauch, Keyes-Ford, ref. 8, with permission.)

References

1. Argamaso RV. The lap joint principle in the repair of cleft earlobe. *Br J Plast Surg* 1978;31:337.
2. Buchan BG. The cleft earlobe: A method of repair with preservation of the earring canal. *Br J Plast Surg* 1975;28:296.
3. Hamilton R, Donato L. Method for repair of cleft earlobes. *Plast Reconstr Surg* 1975;55:99.
4. Khoo Boo-Chai MD. The cleft earlobe. *Plast Reconstr Surg* 1961;28:681.
5. Pardue AM. Repair of the torn earlobe with preservation of the perforation for an earring. *Plast Reconstr Surg* 1973;51:475.
6. Dibbell DG. Split earlobe deformities. *Plast Reconstr Surg* 1970;45:77.
7. McLaren L. Cleft earlobes: A hazard of wearing earrings. *Br J Plast Surg* 1954;7:102.
8. Strauch B, Keyes-Ford M. Repair of the cleft earlobe with an advancement flap and two unilateral z-plasties. *Plast Reconstr Surg* 1997;99:1074.
9. Cormack GC, Laberty BG. *The arterial anatomy of skin flaps.* Edinburgh: Churchill Livingstone, 1986;116–121.

CHAPTER 93 ■ ROLL-UNDER (OR FOLD-UNDER) FLAP FOR RELEASE OF EARLOBE CONTRACTURES

J. R. LEWIS, JR.*

EDITORIAL COMMENT

As pointed out by the author, this technique is also applicable to secondary face lifts where there has been a downward pull and distortion of the earlobe.

The roll-under (or fold-under) flap for rounding of a contracted earlobe has been very useful in this author's experience, particularly in secondary face-lifts. When the original face-lift has been performed and it pulls down on the earlobe, a tight, tapered lobe often follows. It is unsightly and makes difficult a secondary meloplasty without an obvious scar below the lobe. Some lobes are naturally tapered, and these can be rounded as well, both to simplify wearing earrings and to hide the scar at the junction of lobe to cheek.

INDICATIONS

The procedure is probably used in one patient of four in whom the author performs a meloplasty, either to avoid tapering the borderline lobe or to correct a lobe that is already tapered or contracted. Obviously, the need for performing this as a secondary procedure will be decreased greatly by care in the original surgery to give adequate support to the anterior and posterior flaps at a higher level, so that no pull is carried to the earlobe itself.

ANATOMY

The circulation comes from small branches of the superficial temporal artery to the anterior aspect of the ear and from the posterior auricular vessels that supply the superficial aspects of the ear and the earlobe. There should be no problems with circulation if the flap is not overly and unnecessarily thinned.

FLAP DESIGN AND DIMENSIONS

The roll-under flap is a relatively broad-based flap, with the length of the flap generally no longer than its width. The flap has a thick base because it is not thinned except in its terminal end for fitting into the V resection (Fig. 1).

The incision is outlined by a skin pencil at the time of meloplasty, or the correction may be of an earlobe alone. It is necessary to carry the incision upward in front of the ear to about the tragus and posterior to the ear for about the same distance to slide the skin anteriorly and posteriorly upward to avoid additional pull on the lobe once the rounding has been accomplished (see Fig. 1).

Generally, it is not difficult to correct this during a meloplasty or as an earlobe correction alone because the tissue along the jawline usually will give enough for adequate correction, even when it has been pulled tightly or has been scarred by the previous surgery. In such cases, however, the flap may be outlined more posteriorly. With overly tight closure and overzealous skin resection, the earlobe is usually pulled not only downward but anteriorly. Correction of the positioning and of the rounding of the lobe is therefore accomplished simultaneously.

* Deceased.

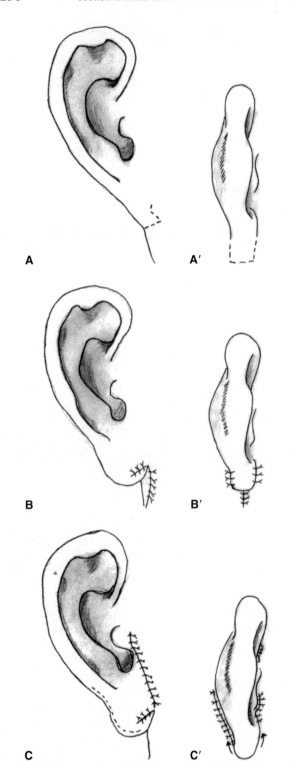

OPERATIVE TECHNIQUE

A number of methods for correcting this problem have been devised, but for about 25 years, the author has used the following simple technique. A small skin flap based on the lobe is outlined along the jawline below the earlobe and rolled (or folded) up under the lobe to separate the lobe from the cheek. The jawline defect is small and is corrected by simply pulling the cheek upward in front of the ear and upward and backward behind the ear as in a face-lift procedure. Deep support of the cheek tissue is carried upward anteriorly to the temporal scalp and to the deep fascia of the cheeks in front of the ear, and posterior to the ear it is carried to the mastoid fascia and the occipital scalp. Thus, there is no residual pull on the earlobe.

CLINICAL RESULTS

The success rate of correction of earlobe deformities by this simple method has been high. Because of the give in the tissues over a period of months or years following the meloplasty, adequate support is generally achieved posteriorly and anteriorly, and the lobe is adequately rounded to allow for this. On occasion, the earlobe may be left a little too redundant, but this is considered in planning the procedure.

When the lobe is naturally too redundant already, a similar procedure may be used to reduce the length or width of the lobe by additional vertical resections within the lobe and horizontal resection of the lobe itself rather than by creating the skin flap below the lobe. Reduction of the earlobe is beyond the scope of this chapter, but it may be carried out along with the rounding and correction of contractures.

SUMMARY

The roll-under (or fold-under) flap has proved quite effective over the years for rounding of a contracted earlobe.

◄ FIG. 1. **A,A′**: Outline of flap, rectangular in shape, below and slightly behind the ear and based on the lobe itself. **B,B′**: Roll-under (or fold-under) of the flap medially and upward to round the earlobe. In isolated lobe reconstruction, the donor defect may be closed as a simple linear closure below the earlobe and slightly behind the angle of the jaw. **C,C′**: Use of the roll-under flap to round the earlobe along with a meloplasty. Note that the incision was carried upward in front of the ear and upward behind the ear, bringing the cheek and neck tissues upward to close the defect against the newly rounded lobe rather than closing a donor defect below the lobe. Obviously, the incisions would extend farther superiorly with the usual meloplasty.

CHAPTER 94. Lateral Neck Skin Flap for Earlobe Reconstruction

S. Zenteno Alanis

www.encyclopediaofflaps.com

CHAPTER 95 ■ TEMPOROPARIETAL FASCIAL FLAP TO THE EAR

S. OHMORI*

In employing Cronin's technique using a silicone frame in the repair of microtia (1), I found that the mastoid needed to be excavated to house the concha (created by a silicone prosthesis). The overlying flap must be created in such a way that no tension is produced. I used the method on 87 patients, and follow-up study showed that although a fairly deep concha could be created by this method, minor fistulas developed in 25 sites in the area where the L-shaped incision was made (Fig. 1). These fistulas led to infection, which necessitated removal of the silicone frame in nine of 87 reconstructed ears. The incidence of removal was considerable enough to make one hesitate to adopt the silicone frame (2–4). The temporoparietal fascial flap can resolve this problem.

INDICATIONS

The temporoparietal fascia is brought to the conchal part of the silicone frame and anchored to the surrounding skin. The concha is made deeply concave, and the helix becomes clearly visible. The fascia then is skin-grafted. Because there is no tension over the frame, fistula formation is less likely. The fascia is thin, has an excellent blood supply, and leaves no functional donor defect.

ANATOMY

See Chapter 6.

FLAP DESIGN AND DIMENSIONS

Preoperatively, the course of the superficial temporal artery is marked on the temporal skin using palpation or the Doppler probe (Fig. 2A). During the operation, a T-shape is drawn, following the marked course of the artery (Fig. 2B). A line of 5.5 to 6.0 cm in length is drawn at a distance of 7.5 to 8.0 cm from the hairline.

OPERATIVE TECHNIQUE

The first stage of microtia reconstruction is the switch back of the lobule. This is followed in 3 months by inlay grafting as a second stage (see Fig. 2).

Dacron mesh is bonded to the rim of the silicone frame using artificial thread and then sterilized. Saline solution is injected subcutaneously into the operative area. (Epinephrine should never be used.) An L-shaped skin incision then is made, followed by skin dissection, first with a scalpel and then with scissors, in the direction of the hairline. Hemostasis should be meticulous.

The soft tissue of the mastoid area, including part of the parotid gland, is excised by electrocautery to the depth of the mastoid periosteum in such a way that the conchal part of the silicone frame is easily housed. At the same time, a subcutaneous tunnel is excavated at the anterior aspect of the auricle. The ear lobule then is made into two skin flaps so that the tail of the frame can be accommodated. The adequacy of the dissection is checked by inserting a frame without a Dacron mesh into the sterilized area. A silicone tube (3 mm in outer diameter with multiple holes) is inserted into the dissected area so that suctioning can be performed easily.

A T-shaped incision is made (Fig. 2B), and the scalp skin is separated from the underlying temporoparietal muscle, making sure that hair follicles are not unnecessarily destroyed. Care should be taken that the vasae temporales superficiales are not damaged. When the dissection is completed, the fascia

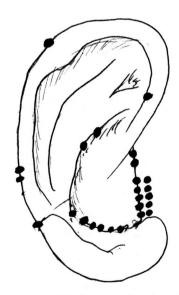

FIG. 1. Minor exposure of the frame was found mostly along the L-shaped incision scar, proving that there is a shortage of skin in the flap that covers the frame. The *dots* show the sites that have been exposed in the past. (From Ohmori, Matsumoto, ref. 2, with permission.)

* Deceased.

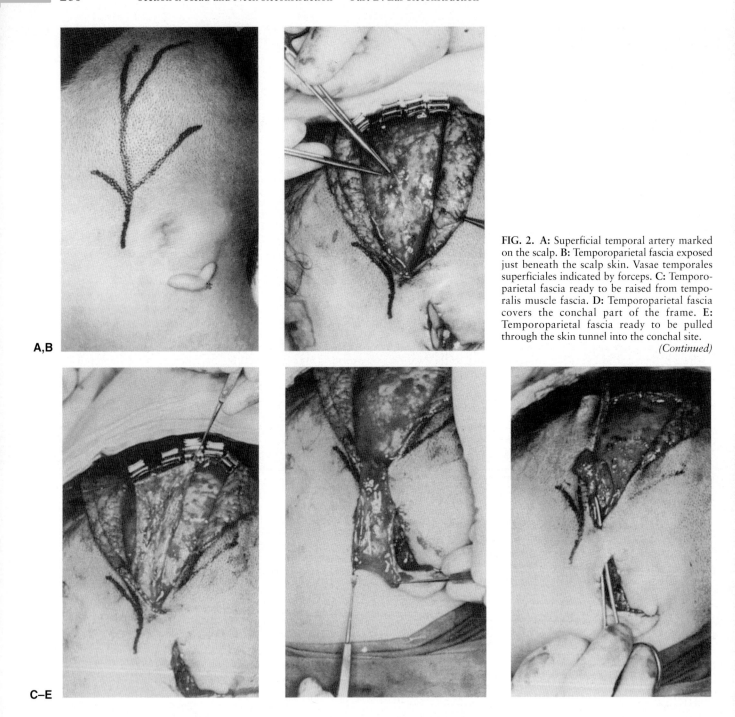

A,B

C–E

FIG. 2. A: Superficial temporal artery marked on the scalp. **B:** Temporoparietal fascia exposed just beneath the scalp skin. Vasae temporales superficiales indicated by forceps. **C:** Temporoparietal fascia ready to be raised from temporalis muscle fascia. **D:** Temporoparietal fascia covers the conchal part of the frame. **E:** Temporoparietal fascia ready to be pulled through the skin tunnel into the conchal site.

(Continued)

is separated from the underlying lamina temporalis and brought to the conchal site through the subcutaneous tunnel (Fig. 2D and E) previously created at the site of the anterior part of the auricle. The prepared silicone frame is inserted into the excavated area, and a suction tube is applied at the site of the anthelix (Fig. 2F).

The fascia is anchored to the surrounding skin. When suction is applied, the shapes of the concha, helix, and anthelix become visible. Also apparent is the shortage of skin necessary for covering the silicone frame. The end of the skin flap is trimmed to a clean edge, which is sewn onto the underlying frame, making all convolutions clear.

A 4 × 5-cm full-thickness skin graft taken from the inguinal region is placed over the temporoparietal fascia and sutured to the surrounding skin (Fig. 2G). This may result in an excess of skin at some points, but the concavity of the concha remains clearly visible. Wet cotton wool is packed into this concavity, followed by dry gauze on top of the cotton, to make a tie-over dressing. Pressure is exerted by applying an ample amount of wet cotton wool packed into the other convolutions.

A third-stage procedure, skin grafting to raise the reconstructed auricle off the skull, can be performed 3 months after the second-stage procedure of inlay grafting.

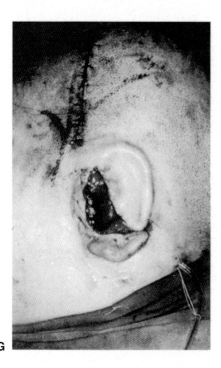
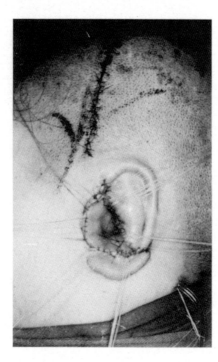

FIG. 2. *Continued.* **F:** After the temporoparietal fascia is anchored to the surrounding conchal skin, suction is applied to clarify conchal depth. **G:** Full-thickness skin is grafted onto the fascia. Good conchal shape is apparent.

F,G

CLINICAL RESULTS

In the period between September of 1974 and June of 1981, this refined technique was used on 147 patients (150 ears) with typical microtia (Fig. 3). Two silicone frames had to be removed, one because of fistula from the parotid gland and the other because of sudden edema of unknown origin in the reconstructed ear. The remaining 144 patients (147 ears) did not need frame removal, which I believe is an outstanding outcome.

I contacted approximately 66% of these patients; about 20% were not contacted; and about 14% did not respond. These two latter groups are considered to be retaining their frames uneventfully as untoward results generally seem to motivate patient contact.

Concerning the attitudes of my patients and their parents after 2 or more years postoperatively, (a) they cease to pay particular attention to preventing exposure of the reconstructed ear to trauma, (b) exposure to temperatures down to −1 or −2°C causes no trouble, and (c) the patients tend to have long hair, indicating that they are still aware that their ears have been reconstructed.

Further disadvantages of the procedure are that the size and position of the reconstructed ear are not always the same as those of the normal ear. This is due to the fact that there is only one type of prosthesis.

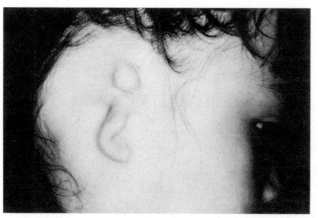
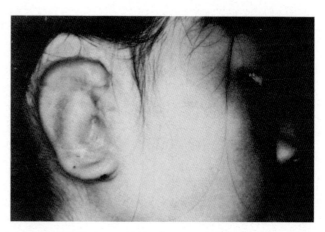

A,B

FIG. 3. **A:** Preoperative view of a patient with congenital microtia. **B:** Postoperative result using a temporoparietal fascial flap over a silicone frame. The fascia was covered with a full-thickness skin graft taken from the inguinal region.

SUMMARY

In what I believe is an improved technique, the temporoparietal fascia is brought to the conchal part of the silicone frame and anchored to the surrounding skin using extensive suction. Skin shortage is solved by skin grafting, which prevents fistula formation. The method allows uniform reconstruction of the auricle. There are few instances of removal of the silicone frame in follow-up 2 to 7 years postoperatively.

References

1. Cronin TD. Use of a Silastic frame for total and subtotal reconstruction of the external ear: Preliminary report. *Plast Reconstr Surg* 1966;37:399.
2. Ohmori S, Matsumoto K. Follow-up study on reconstruction of microtia with a silicone frame. *Plast Reconstr Surg* 1974;53:555.
3. Ohmori S. Reconstruction of microtia using the Silastic frame. *Clin Plast Surg* 1978;5:379.
4. Ohmori S, Nakai H, Takada H. A refined approach to ear reconstruction with Silastic frames in major degrees of microtia. *Br J Plast Surg* 1979;32:267.

CHAPTER 96 ■ V–Y ADVANCEMENT SKIN FLAPS

E. G. ZOOK AND R. C. RUSSELL

These flaps have an excellent blood supply from subcutaneous tissue and are ideal for use on the face (1–7). They are superior to rotation flaps (which leave dog-ears), skin grafts (which are depressed and shiny), and primary closure (where tension is present).

INDICATIONS

Excision of facial lesions frequently leaves a circular or elliptical defect. If the skin is loose and can be approximated without deformity of the surrounding tissue, that is the treatment of choice. The use of a V–Y advancement flap eliminates secondary procedures to revise dog-ears that occur with rotation flaps.

In our patients, the most common of the V–Y flaps are the nasal dorsal flap to cover defects on the nasal dorsum or ala and nasolabial flaps to cover defects of the ala or alar base. The flaps also have been found to be excellent to close defects of the nasal tip and eyelid. They have been used in numerous areas on the face (Fig. 1).

We found that large defects of the lower eyelid skin can be closed with a V–Y flap from the cheek without ectropion. V–Y glabellar advancement flaps are excellent for closure of wounds of the medial canthal area. V–Y flaps are also excellent for closure of forehead defects, where the flap can be advanced in the transverse wrinkle lines of the forehead. We found this flap to be especially good in the area of the sideburn in men, where one flap can be brought up from the beard area and another down from the temple area, which reconstructs the sideburn (Fig. 3).

FLAP DESIGN AND DIMENSIONS

After adequate excision and clear frozen-section margins on malignancies, closure by simple approximation is evaluated. If significant distortion of the surrounding tissues results, a V–Y flap is designed to close the defect. When possible, the line of advancement of the flap is designed parallel to the skin tension lines. If there is a significant difference in the diameters of the defect, the flap is designed to have the shortest advancement. The flap is designed 1½ to 2 times the length of the diameter of the defect in the direction of the closure. Flaps from the nasolabial fold in older persons with lax skin can be moved 3 to 4 cm onto the side of the nose, and nasal dorsal flaps can be moved 2 cm to cover tip or alar defects.

OPERATIVE TECHNIQUE

After marking the flap, incisions are made completely through the skin. Vigorous skin hook traction on the

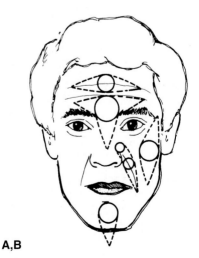
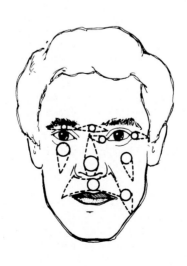

A,B

FIG. 1. **A,B:** Some of the defects and flaps used to close them are shown. (From Zook, ref. 7, with permission.)

263

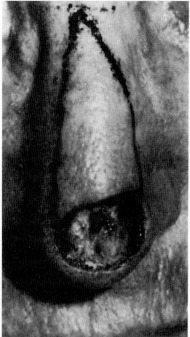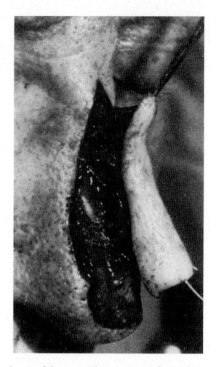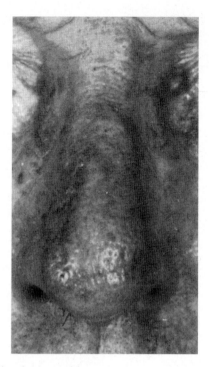

A–C

FIG. 2. **A:** 1- × 1.5-cm defect on the tip of the nose. The superior V flap is designed so that most of the incisions fall beyond the crest of the nose. **B:** The V flap on the dorsum of the nose has been mobilized with loupe magnification and freeing of bands that prevent motion. Several of the remaining vessels can be seen to feed the flap. **C:** The nose 6 months later with little scar, no depression, and uniform skin quality of the nose tip. (From Zook, ref. 7, with permission.)

opposite sides of the incision is used to stretch the soft tissue and free the flap (Fig. 2B). Blunt scissor dissection is carried out, if necessary, identifying and cutting bands that inhibit the advancement of the flap, in the direction necessary to close the defect.

The V tip of the flap is the most frequent area of tightness and must be released. If extensive freeing is necessary, it is done with loupe magnification until the flap moves easily into the defect. If adequate advancement cannot be obtained without significant tension on the flap, a second flap is designed and advanced from the opposite side. In the area of the nose and surrounding tissue, the flap will survive on only a few small arteries and veins and can be dissected using loupe magnification.

The flap is sutured into place with subcuticular sutures at the advancing edge and at the base of the Y. It is important in certain closure areas, such as the lower eyelid, that the Y be closed tightly to hold the flap up in place and prevent ectropion (Fig. 3).

CLINICAL RESULTS

We have used more than 150 V–Y flaps over 5 years for defects secondary to excision of skin malignancies and benign lesions (skin grafts placed where malignancies have previously been excised, large nevi, and others). The flaps have been used equally in men and women. Eighty percent of defects were closed with a single flap, and the remainder were closed with either two or three V–Y advancement flaps. The only complications have been loss of the edge of a flap from too much tension (not enough freeing), loss of one of the pair

of V–Y flaps over the nasal ala, and lack of hair growth after a V–Y scalp flap.

Of the 150-plus V–Y flaps we have used, none has required revision. In many areas, such as the dorsum and tip of the nose, the advancement of local skin is the nearest possible color match and avoids the depression that one gets with a skin graft (see Fig. 2). Early in our use of V–Y flaps, we used a flap from the nasal dorsum and one from the columella to close nasal tip defects. As we have become more familiar with and braver in mobilizing the dorsal nasal skin, we have closed such defects with only a single dorsally based flap. This dorsal nasal flap is designed wide enough to place the scars lateral to the nasal dorsum, so that they are least visible (Fig. 2A).

Over the nasal ala, the skin is tightly adhered to the cartilage; so it is not safe to advance a small local V–Y flap. In this case, we advance a V–Y flap from the lax skin of the dorsum of the nose to close the defect. The blood supply of the scalp is primarily transverse rather than vertical, and therefore use of the V–Y flap is not advisable.

We have used V–Y flap closure on the trunk and upper extremity with good results also. It must be pointed out, however, that the blood supply is not as good and more frequently two flaps have to be advanced, each to close half the defect.

SUMMARY

V–Y advancement flaps are particularly useful for defects of the face, especially because secondary revision is very rarely necessary.

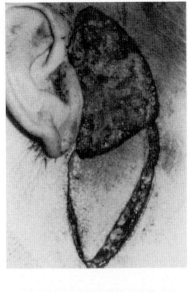
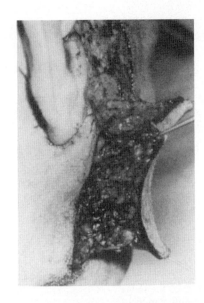

A,B

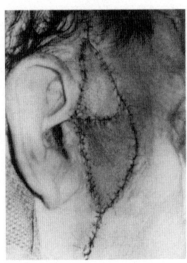
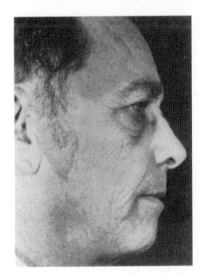

C,D

FIG. 3. **A:** A man with a recurrent basal cell carcinoma in the preauricular area involving most of the right sideburn. After excision and free margins, the defect is seen. The V–Y flap is designed inferiorly in beard-bearing skin and one superiorly in the temple area. **B:** Inferior flap is mobilized vigorously. The vessels in the flap pedicle can be seen. **C:** Lower pedicle is raised; the upper is brought distally and closed. **D:** Patient 1 year postoperatively with his sideburn preserved and minimal scarring.

References

1. Esser FJS. Island flaps. *NY State J Med* 1917;106:264.
2. Kubacek V. Transposition of flaps on the face on a subcutaneous pedicle. *Acta Chir Plast* 1965;2:108.
3. Barron JN, Emmett AJJ. Subcutaneous pedicle flaps. *Br J Plast Surg* 1965;18:51.
4. Trevaskis AE, Rempel J, Okuneki W, et al. Sliding subcutaneous pedicle flaps to close a circular defect. *Plast Reconstr Surg* 1970;46:155.
5. DuFourmental C, Tallat SM. The kite-flap. In: *Transactions of the fifth international congress of plastic and reconstructive surgery.* Melbourne: Butterworth, 1971;1223.
6. Argamaso RV. V–Y–S plasty for closure of a round defect. *Plast Reconstr Surg* 1974;53:99.
7. Zook EG. V–Y advancement flap for facial defects. *Plast Reconstr Surg* 1980;65:786.

CHAPTER 97 ■ TRIANGULAR AND HATCHET SUBCUTANEOUS PEDICLE SKIN FLAPS

A. J. J. EMMETT

It is the natural elasticity of skin that enables defects to be closed, and it has been usual to fit the long axis of the defect into the lines of minimal tension (1). Where a rounded defect is to be closed, the shape of the defect may be tapered into the line of closure by adding a triangle at either end of the rounded defect to produce a tapered elliptical shape. These triangles of tissue then are discarded. As the size of this round defect becomes larger, the size of the triangle to be discarded also increases, to the point where these triangles themselves may be used as a flap and slid into the original round defect with a V–Y closure of the base from which they have come (2–10).

INDICATIONS

Various triangular flaps are a safe and interesting way to close medium-sized defects in the 1.5- to 3-cm range in all areas of the body. They have been used on the back, foot, hand, face, and chest. They are a versatile design, with a great bulk of pedicle relative to the size of the flap, providing great flap viability. The single triangular flap has an advantage for closure of rounded defects when one side of the defect is closed by a natural boundary. The double-triangular subcutaneous pedicle skin flap has been used for forehead defects above the eyebrow, eyebrow defects, and some hairy scalp defects. I have

used the hatchet flap for repair of the chin, eyelid, cheek, and lower lip.

ANATOMY

The pedicle is the subcutaneous tissue that lies beneath triangular flaps, and this can then be extended as deep as necessary. It is all the better if muscle lying beneath is included. The flap is based on a random arterial blood supply, but occasionally, it can be based over a direct nutrient artery.

FLAP DESIGN AND DIMENSIONS

These flaps are all rather free form and have a degree of adjustability; so the surgeon is not rigidly committed to the original cutout flap pattern and can vary the fit of the flap as the operation progresses.

A general principle of these flaps is that the defect is narrowed in around the pedicle. The tail of the flap is closed in a V–Y fashion so that as the donor site is closed, it pushes the tapered tail of the flap forward toward the recipient site. The line of the triangular flap is that of the line of minimal tension closure (Figs. 1 and 2).

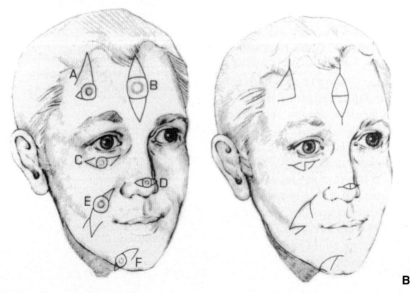

FIG. 1. A,B: Various forms and modifications of double triangular flaps, single triangular flaps, and hatchet flaps. (From Emmett, ref. 10, with permission.)

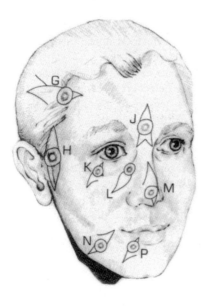
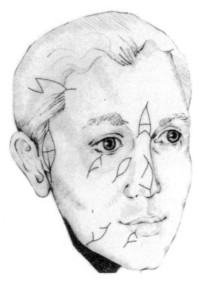

FIG. 2. A,B: Various forms and modifications of double triangular flaps, single triangular flaps, and hatchet flaps. (From Emmett, ref. 10, with permission.)

A,B

OPERATIVE TECHNIQUE

Double Triangular Subcutaneous Pedicle Skin Flap

In a procedure to close a defect in the central forehead (see Fig. 1B), the flaps are incised down into the subcutaneous tissue, tapering outward. The principle is that the pedicle should be dissected downward sufficiently deeply and laterally so that the triangular flap will move freely into the defect. At times, this may be down to deep fascia and muscle.

The two triangular defects then are sutured together, and the defect is closed in a V–Y fashion behind each flap. Thus, the tension of the closure lies in the wound on either side, and the flap itself has minimal tension (11).

On the face, I close the dermis with interrupted sutures to produce an even contour before inserting the skin stitches. A variant with a fishtail or W flap at the lower end to fit the crease lines of the glabella is shown in Fig. 2J. Double triangular flaps in the preauricular region and on the nasal bridge are also illustrated (Figs. 1D and 2H). Closure of a forehead defect above the eyebrow, with preservation of the underlying nerves, is illustrated in Fig. 3.

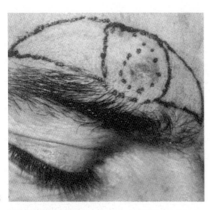
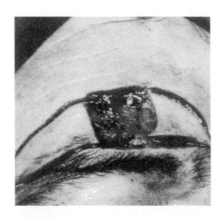

A,B

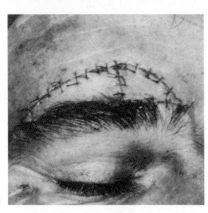
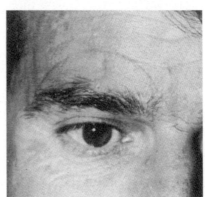

C,D

FIG. 3. A–D: Closure of a forehead defect above the eyebrow. The underlying nerves were preserved. Eyebrow defects and some hair-bearing scalp defects can be closed this way.

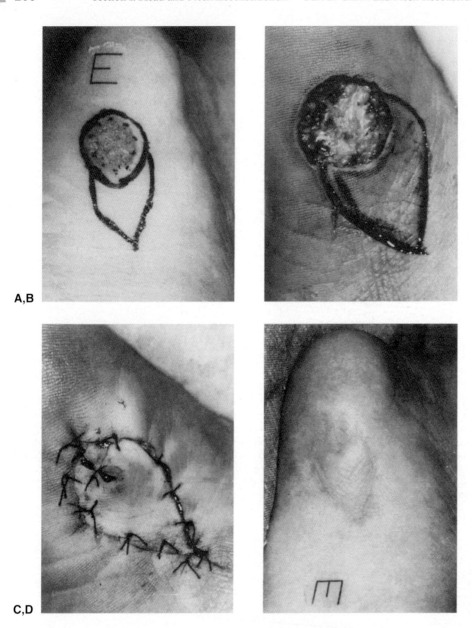

A,B

C,D

FIG. 4. A–D: Variant of the single triangular flap in which the horns of the flap end are brought together to make a secondary advancement using the two extra triangles that sometimes are discarded. This case shows that the indications for these flaps are not limited to the face.

Another variant of this flap, the V–Y–S flap, keeps partial skin pedicles that interrupt the pattern of circumferential scar (Fig. 1C).

Single Triangular Flap

In a procedure using this flap for repair of an inner canthal area defect (Fig. 2L), one corner of the leading edge is slid forward so that the end result is a tapered contour. This may better fit the scar line to the crease lines.

In another variant (Fig. 4A), the horns of the flap end are brought together to make a secondary advancement using the two extra triangles that sometimes are discarded. By using this method, the flap need not advance so far, and shallower dissection is sufficient, preserving skin sensation more adequately.

Hatchet Flap

In areas of loose tissue, the subcutaneous attachment may be left even to the flap tip. In areas of greater fixity, the flap can be mobilized further and a smaller subcutaneous pedicle left. Illustrations are provided for the use of the hatchet flap in repairing the chin (Fig. 1F), eyelid (Fig. 2K), cheek (Fig. 2N), and lower lip (Fig. 2P). In these procedures, the tail of the flap closes in V–Y fashion as the flap slips forward into the defect.

Where the hatchet flap is in more rigid skin, folding of the pedicle in V–Y fashion and shortening and insetting of the trailing edge, pedicle side, may be difficult. In these circumstances, a secondary V flap helps close the base (Figs. 1E and 2G). In a case of excision of a skin lesion of the cheek (Fig. 5A), a hatchet flap is mobilized.

CLINICAL RESULTS

I have used various triangular flaps extensively over the last 20 years. The dissection around the pedicle of the flap can be as deep as is permitted by the anatomy of the region, and in the central area of the face, inclusion of the facial muscles is an advantage. Division of facial muscles is not a problem, since I have repeatedly seen direct reinnervation of divided muscles in this area.

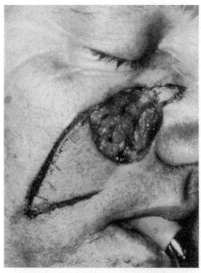
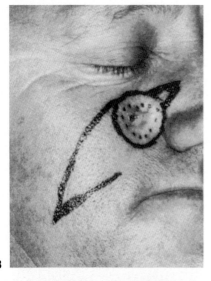

A,B

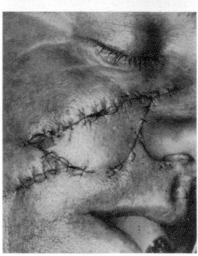
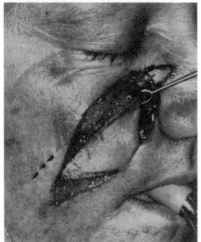

C–E

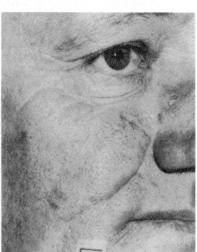

FIG. 5. **A–E:** As the flap is drawn into the defect, the tail tends to kick out (**C**) over the area, and a secondary triangular flap is raised just enough to fill the defect. It need not go right up to the angle of the base. The front of the flap is sutured with buried dermal sutures before the tail of the flap is fitted with the secondary triangular flap.

SUMMARY

Double triangular flaps, single triangular flaps, and the hatchet flap are all extremely useful for closure of defects about the face.

References

1. Cox HT. The cleavage lines of the skin. *Br J Surg* 1941;29:234.
2. Kutler W. A new method for fingertip amputation. *JAMA* 1947;133:29.
3. Kubacek V. Transposition of flaps on the face on a subcutaneous pedicle. *Acta Chir Plast* 1960;2:108.
4. Barron JN, Emmett AJJ. Subcutaneous pedicle flaps. *Br J Plast Surg* 1965;18:51.
5. Fischl RA. A flap for nasolabial defects, or "save the dog-ear." *Br J Plast Surg* 1969;22:351.
6. Atasoy E, Ioakimidis E, Kasdan M, et al. Reconstruction of the amputated fingertip with a triangular volar flap. *J Bone Joint Surg* 1970;52:921.
7. Trevaskis AE, Rempel J, Okenski W, et al. Sliding subcutaneous pedicle flaps to close a circular defect. *Plast Reconstr Surg* 1970;46:155.
8. DuFourmentel C, Tallat SM. The kite-flap. In: *Transactions of the fifth international congress of plastic and reconstructive surgery*. Melbourne: Butterworth, 1971;1223.
9. Argamaso RV. V–Y–S plasty for closure of a round defect. *Plast Reconstr Surg* 1974;53:99.
10. Emmett AJJ. The closure of defects by using adjacent triangular flaps with subcutaneous pedicles. *Plast Reconstr Surg* 1977;59:45.
11. Esser FJS. Island flaps. *N Y Med J* 1917;106:264.

CHAPTER 98 ■ TRANSPOSITION CHEEK SKIN FLAPS: RHOMBIC FLAP AND VARIATIONS

J. P. GUNTER AND R. W. SHEFFIELD

EDITORIAL COMMENT

The editors commend this flap to you. The detailed explanation of the base geometry unravels the mysteries of the rhombic flap.

Because of the different sizes and shapes of defects, the conditions, availability, and extensibility of surrounding skin, and the proximity of different anatomic structures, there is no single transposition flap to reconstruct all cheek defects. The rhombic flap is frequently used for reconstructing small to moderate-sized cheek defects. Although is not applicable in all cases, an understanding of its basic principles is often helpful in the plan and design of other transposition flaps.

INDICATIONS

The rhombic flap, described by Limberg (1), is the one we use most for reconstructing cheek defects. It has a precise geometric design, and knowledge of its principles helps to understand flap transfer and to plan and execute other transposition flaps.

ANATOMY

Axial-pattern (arterial) flaps are seldom used for reconstructing cheek defects. Random-pattern (cutaneous) flaps are the rule, as there is little concern about their viability because of the favorable blood supply to the cheek skin. Random-pattern flaps of the cheeks are raised at a level that preserves the subdermal vascular plexus, which requires that a layer of the subcutaneous tissue remain on the flap.

The skin of the cheek is richly vascular. Perfusion is mainly through the facial artery, which courses superiorly and medially from the inferior border of the mandible to the nasofacial groove. Other arteries supplying the cheek skin are the transverse facial artery (a branch of the superficial temporal), the buccal branch of the maxillary artery, the infraorbital artery (one of the terminal branches of the maxillary artery), and the zygomatic branch of the lacrimal artery (a branch of the ophthalmic artery).

All the arteries supplying the cheek have corresponding veins that accompany them. The facial vein is the chief vein of the cheek. It lies posterior to the facial artery and follows the course of the artery. It communicates with the ophthalmic vein, which empties into the cavernous sinus, and with the infraorbital and deep facial veins, which communicate with the cavernous sinus through the pterygoid plexus. It drains into the internal jugular vein in the upper neck (2–4).

FLAP DESIGN AND DIMENSIONS

Transposition skin flaps use tissue adjacent to the defect but from a different plane to effect closure. Such flaps are designed adjacent to the defect so that they share a portion or all of one side of the defect. Although flap shapes may vary, all can be thought of as having two sides, a distal end and a base. If excision of a lesion can be designed in the shape of a rhombus, with adequate margins that do not excessively sacrifice normal tissue, the rhombus is marked around the lesion with two sides parallel to the lines of maximum extensibility of the skin (LME), when possible.

The rhombic flap is designed to reconstruct a 60-degree rhombic defect (1,5–10) (ADEF in Fig. 1). In such a defect, the length of all the sides and the short diagonal are equal (i.e., two equilateral triangles with a common base). The distal end of the flap (D'C') is a continuation of the short diagonal of the defect (FD) and of equal length. The side of the flap next to the defect (AD') is also a side of the defect (AD). The side of the flap farthest from the defect (BC') is parallel to the near side (AD') and equal in length. All sides of the defect and the flap are equal in length.

Four potential donor sites then are mentally pictured (Fig. 2), and the site with the most available skin is determined by manual pinching, pushing, and pulling of the skin in these areas. (This is also helpful in assessing the effect donor-site closure will have on surrounding anatomic structures.) The rhombic flap then is drawn in the most favorable area and mentally transposed, checking the direction of the vectors of tension (VOT) and looking for possible problems.

When possible, the flap should be planned so that the short diagonal of the flap donor site (DB) is in the same direction as the lines of maximum extensibility (Fig. 3). This facilitates closure of the donor site by taking advantage of the extensibility of the skin in that direction. We accomplish this by designing the rhombic defect so that two parallel sides are in the same direction as the lines of maximum extensibility. Of the four rhombic flaps possible, two will have their short diagonals in the direction of the lines of maximum extensibility (Fig. 4). One of these flaps should be chosen for reconstruction, if there are no contraindications.

The near corner of the flap base is adjacent to the defect. The far corner is the width of the base away from the defect and serves as the pivot point during transfer of the flap. In the description of the classic transposition flap, the pivot point is assumed to be stationary. This requires that the flap be longer

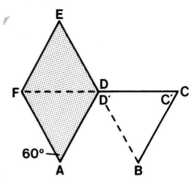

FIG. 1. Sixty-degree rhombic defect with adjacent rhombic flap. All sides of the defect and flap and the short diagonals are equal in length.

than the defect in order to reach the distal end of the defect when it is transferred (11–13). In the type of transposition flaps we commonly use, however, the pivot point is advanced toward the defect as the flap is transposed. This facilitates primary closure of the donor site and obviates additional length requirement.

When the shape of a lesion is predetermined and it is not practical to convert it to a rhombus, the elements of design of the rhombic flap are often useful in devising other transposition flaps for closure (Fig. 5). This is particularly true for circular, oval, and teardrop-shaped defects. A rhombus is drawn around the defect, and the most favorable donor site is determined by using the same method already described for reconstruction of a rhombic defect. A rhombic flap is drawn in that area. Inside the outline, a flap with dimensions and shape similar to the defect is drawn, filling the rhombic flap outline in the same manner that the defect fills its surrounding rhombus (Fig. 5B). The flap then is visually transposed into the defect, assessing the areas that will be under tension and the direction of the vectors of tension. If an area under tension is near a mobile anatomic structure and the vector of tension points toward that structure, it will probably be distorted if that flap is used. In such cases, another flap should be considered.

OPERATIVE TECHNIQUE

After the flap has been designed and it appears that there are no contraindications to its use, minor alterations for improving the reconstruction are considered. It may be possible to make the defect smaller by undermining and advancing the edges without distorting any anatomic landmarks. If so, the flap can be planned smaller, facilitating closure of the donor site. As long as the donor site can be closed without undue tension, it is best to keep the flap large, because this will result in less tension on the flap edges when they are sutured into the defect.

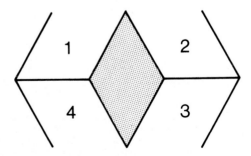

FIG. 2. Possible rhombic flap donor sites. There are four theoretical donor sites for every 60-degree rhombic defect.

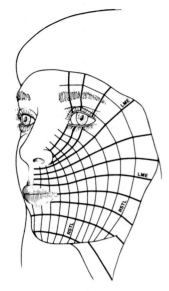

FIG. 3. Lines of maximum extensibility (LME). (From Borges, ref. 15, with permission.) These lines run perpendicular to the relaxed skin tension lines (RSTL). The skin is most extensible in the direction of the lines of maximum extensibility.

The key to successful transfer of the rhombic flap is primary closure of the donor site. As the flap is transposed to the defect, the edges of the donor site are approximated by advancing the pivot point of the flap (B) toward the corner, at the junction of the short diagonals of the defect and donor site (D in Fig. 6). Closure occurs in one of two ways (Fig. 7). The optimal procedure is for the pivot point of the flap (B) to move to a point D at the junction of the short diagonals of the flap donor site and defect. When this occurs, there is no distortion of the defect or flap. The sides of the flap can be approximated to the corresponding sides of the defect without tension. The only area of tension will be along the donor-site closure, with the greatest amount at the end where point B is approximated to point D. This will result in a vector of tension that is parallel to side DE.

In many situations it is impossible to move point B the entire distance to point D. In such cases, point D must move toward point B to effect donor-site closure. When this occurs, it results in a distortion of the defect. Side DE must either

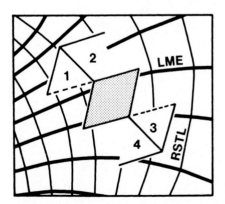

FIG. 4. Choosing the correct rhombic flap. The rhombic defect should be designed so that two sides are as close to parallel to the lines of maximum extensibility (LME) as possible. This will result in the short diagonals of two of the donor sites being nearly parallel to the lines (donor sites 1 and 3). One of these donor sites should be used, when possible, to facilitate primary closure of the donor site.

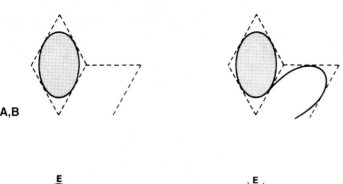

A,B

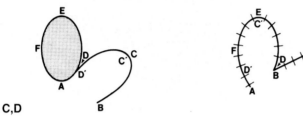

C,D

FIG. 5. Reconstruction of an oval defect using rhombic flap principles. **A:** Rhombus drawn to encompass defect, with rhombic flap outlined. **B:** Oval flap drawn to fill the outlined rhombic flap in the same manner that defect fills the rhombus. **C:** Final design of the flap. **D:** Flap transposed with primary closure of the donor site.

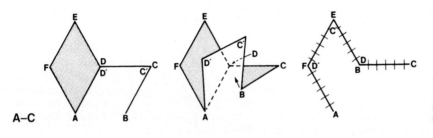

A–C

FIG. 6. **A–C:** Transfer of flap. As the flap is transferred, point *B* (pivot point of the flap) is moved toward point *D*, resulting in primary closure of the donor site.

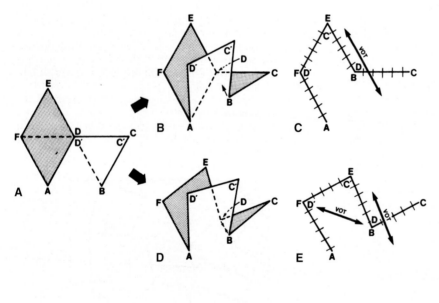

FIG. 7. Effects of donor-site closure. **A:** Point *D* remains stationary as point *B* moves toward *D* to accomplish closure of the donor site. **B:** This results in a vector of tension (VOT) parallel to side *ED* without distortion of the flap or defect. **C:** Points *D* and *B* move toward each other for donor-site closure. **D:** This results in a widening of the defect and the short diagonal of the flap (*D'B*), with an additional VOT in the direction of the short diagonal (**E**).

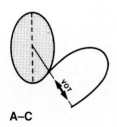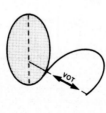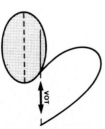

A–C

FIG. 8. Changing direction of the vector of tension (VOT) of the donor-site closure by altering the length of far side of the flap. **A:** Direction of vector after closure of donor site in routine design of flap. **B:** Vector of tension becomes more perpendicular to long axis of defect if far side is shortened. This creates a tendency for the defect to widen as the flap is transferred and the donor site closed. **C:** Lengthening of far side results in less tendency for widening of defect, since closure of donor site will result in downward pull on side of defect.

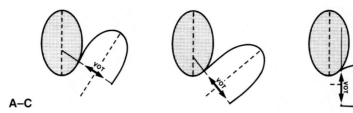

A–C

FIG. 9. Effect of changing relationships of long axes of defect and donor site on the direction of the vector of tension (VOT) of donor-site closure. **A:** The more nearly parallel the axes, the more nearly perpendicular the vector of tension of closure of the donor site is to the long axis of the defect. This creates a greater tendency for widening of the defect as the donor site is closed. **B:** As the axes become more perpendicular, the direction of the vector of tension changes toward the same direction as the long axis of the defect. **C:** When long axes of defect and donor site are perpendicular, the direction of the vector of tension of the donor-site closure is parallel to the long axis of defect, creating a downward pull on side of defect without a tendency for widening of the defect as the donor site is closed.

elongate, or point *E* must move in the same direction and for the same distance as point *D*. If side *DE* elongates, side *BC'* of the flap also must elongate in order to approximate *DE*.

As point *D* moves toward point *B*, the short diagonal of the defect (*FD*) is elongated, resulting in a widening of the defect. When this happens, the short diagonal of the flap *BD'* also must elongate to fill the defect. This, in effect, requires a widening of the flap. If the skin of the flap is extensible, this may not cause any problems, but if the skin is not extensible, an area of tension will be created where point *D'* is approximated to point *F*. The resulting vector of tension will be in the direction of the short diagonal of the defect (*FD*).

The farther point *D* has to move to meet point *B* and the less the extensibility of the flap, the greater will be the tension at closure site *D'F*. As this tension increases, flap survival is jeopardized. A way to relieve this tension is to undermine the skin adjacent to side *AFE*. This will allow point *F* to move toward point *D*, lessening the length requirement of *BD'*. If there are anatomic structures in the proximity of point *F*, however, they may be distorted as the area moves.

If the direction of the vector of tension created by closure of the donor site is not ideal, it can be changed somewhat by extending or shortening the far side of the flap (Fig. 8). By extending the far side, the vector of tension will rotate in a direction more parallel to the long axis of the defect (Fig. 8C).

The more parallel the vector of tension is to the long axis of the defect, the less tendency there is for the defect to widen as the donor site is closed. As the length of the far side increases, that corner of the base of the flap moves farther from the point at which it has to be approximated for donor-site closure. The farther apart these points are, the greater the tension created by their approximation. If this distance grows too large, it may prevent primary closure of the donor site. Varying the distance of the far side of the flap will cause discrepancies in the length of the opposing sides of the flap and defect that must be sutured together. If this discrepancy is not too great, the elastic characteristics of the skin will compensate.

Another way to change the direction of the vector of tension created by donor site closure is to change the direction of the longitudinal axis of the flap in relation to the longitudinal axis of the defect (Fig. 9). As the axis of the flap rotates away from the defect, the vector of tension of the donor-site closure rotates in the same direction. The more nearly parallel the direction of the longitudinal axis of the defect and donor site, the more tendency there is for the defect to increase in width as the donor site is closed. If the longitudinal axis of the donor site is perpendicular to that of the defect, closure of the donor site will result in a downward pull on the proximal side of the defect without a tendency for widening the defect (14,15). This will result in less tension on the flap edges after closure (Figs. 10 and 11).

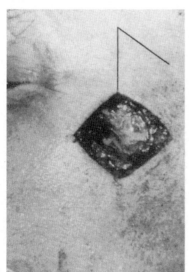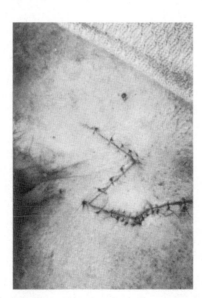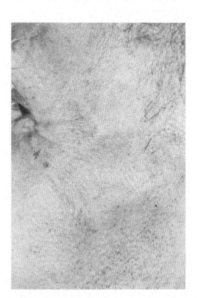

A–C

FIG. 10. A: Closure of a rhombic defect with a rhombic flap. The rhombic defect has two sides parallel to the lines of maximum extensibility. The donor site is favorable with the short diagonal running in the direction of the lines of maximum extensibility. **B:** The flap transferred and closed under little tension. **C:** Final result 1 year later. (From Gunter et al., ref. 8, with permission.)

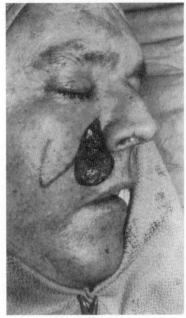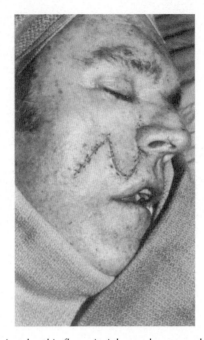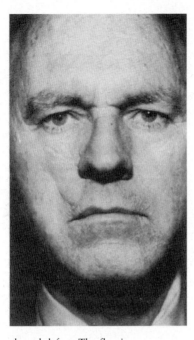

A–C

FIG. 11. **A:** Flap designed using rhombic flap principles to close a teardrop-shaped defect. The flap is designed so that the vectors of tension are directed between the upper lip and the base of the nose. **B:** The flap sutured into place with little tension on the base of the nose or the upper lip. **C:** The final result 2 years later.

SUMMARY

Although the rhombic flap is not applicable in all cases, an understanding of these principles is often helpful in the plan and design of other transposition flaps.

References

1. Limberg AA. Design of local flaps. In: Gibson T, ed. *Modern trends of plastic surgery.* London: Butterworth, 1966;38–61.
2. Warwick R, Williams P, eds. *Gray's anatomy,* 35th ed. Philadelphia: WB Saunders, 1973;626–630.
3. Hollinshead WN, ed. *Anatomy for surgeons,* vol. 1: *The head and neck,* 2d ed. New York: Hoeber, 1968;341–346.
4. Woodburne RT. *Essentials of human anatomy,* 3d ed. New York: Oxford University Press, 1965;219–222.
5. Becker FF. Rhomboid flap in facial reconstruction. *Arch Otolaryngol* 1979;105:569.
6. Borges AF. The rhombic flap. *Plast Reconstr Surg* 1981;67:458.
7. Brobyn TJ. Facial resurfacing with the Limberg flap. *Clin Plast Surg* 1976;3:481.
8. Gunler JP, Carder HM, Fee WE. Rhomboid flap. *Arch Otolaryngol* 1977;103:206.
9. Jervis W, Salyer KE, Busquets MAV, Atkins RW. Further applications of the Limberg and Dufourmentel flaps. *Plast Reconstr Surg* 1974;54:335.
10. Lister GD, Gibson T. Closure of rhomboid skin defects: the flaps of Limberg and Dufourmentel. *Br J Plast Surg* 1972;25:300.
11. Converse JM, ed. *Reconstructive plastic surgery,* Vol. 1: *General principles,* 2d ed. Philadelphia: WB Saunders, 1977;202–207.
12. Grabb WC, Myers MB, eds. *Skin flaps.* Boston: Little, Brown, 1975;111–131.
13. McGregor IA, ed. *Fundamental techniques of plastic surgery,* 6th ed. London: Churchill-Livingstone, 1975;119–129.
14. Schrudde J, Petrovici V. The use of slide-swing plasty in closing skin defects: A clinical study based on 1308 cases. *Plast Reconstr Surg* 1981;67:467.
15. Borges AF, ed. *Elective incisions and scar revision.* Boston: Little, Brown, 1973;1–15.

CHAPTER 99 ■ RHOMBIC AND RHOMBOID *SCHWENKLAPPEN*-PLASTY

E. ROGGENDORF

EDITORIAL COMMENT

The reader will find this chapter difficult to assimilate. The mathematics are correct and helpful in the planning of flaps; however, one should realize that the skin is an elastic tissue, but with varying degrees of elasticity, depending on anatomic location and age of the patient.

The term *Schwenklappen* comes from the German *schwenken*, meaning "to move, swing, or turn about." Whereas a transposition flap rotates only about a pivot point, a *Schwenklappen* flap not only rotates about a pivot point, but the reserve skin adjacent to the base slides in the direction of the rotation as the flap donor site is closed (1–4). (Note that a rhombus, e.g., a Limberg flap, is an equilateral parallelogram, with all four sides equal, whereas a rhomboid is an oblong parallelogram, with only opposite sides and angles equal.)

INDICATIONS

Rhombic and rhomboid *Schwenklappen*-plasties can be applied in any region of the body if blood supply, skin reserves, and the need for flap delay are taken into account. One of their advantages is that the optimal use of existing skin reserves can easily be calculated. These flaps are especially suited for skin defects in the face and on the neck because of the good blood supply found in these areas. In other regions, flap design and flap delay also can favor their application.

Skin defects should be closed under minimum tension by making use of available skin reserves. This includes mobilization of defect margins for diminishing the size of the primary defect, extension of the flap itself (pure advancement or extension flaps), extension of the surrounding skin of the donor area (pure *Schwenklappen*-plasties), and no extension of skin at all (pure transposition flaps). Figures 4 to 7 illustrate the ease with which *Schwenklappen*-plasties may be performed in various combinations with other techniques for covering skin defects when skin reserves are minimal.

FLAP DESIGN AND DIMENSIONS

Planimetric *Schwenklappen*-Plasties

Planimetric *Schwenklappen*-plasties are flaps that involve only two dimensions of the skin; stereometric *Schwenklappen*-plasties use three dimensions, creating curved surfaces.

For these flaps, the shapes of rhombi (Limberg, Fig. 1A) and rhomboids (Roggendorf, Fig. 1B) provide skin-saving incisions, since Burow's triangles are included in the flap design. Primary closure of the donor area is a prerequisite for *Schwenklappen*-plasties. As the donor area is closed, the flap base is rotated; as a result, the flap transfer is effected. Tension is thus shifted into the suture line of the flap donor area. With exact planning, therefore, the flap itself can be transferred into the defect without any tension.

The skin reserve r must be equal to or greater than the required skin extension s. Planning of planimetric *Schwenklappen*-plasties is simplest if small circular defects are to be covered by rhombic flaps with angles between 60 and 70 degrees. Whatever the direction of extension, the skin extension vector s can be planned in line with the maximum skin reserve vector r_{max} without any difficulty (Fig. 2).

In oblong skin defects, the skin reserve will lie mostly in the direction of the long axis of the primary defect, and here too rhomboids with angles α of 60 to 75 degrees are best (Fig. 3A). These rhomboids can be constructed easily using the angle α plus the width and length of the defect.

If skin reserve is smaller than required skin extension (that is, $r < s$), the maximum skin reserve vector r_{max} should be determined and the skin extension vector s planned in that direction.

The mutual dependence between *Schwenkungs*-angle α and the direction of skin extension s (Fig. 3A) makes it possible to calculate the ideal angle α for planimetric *Schwenklappen*-plasties by using the formula $\alpha = 2\,(90 + \delta)/3$ (Fig. 3B). This formula can be applied in rhomboid as well as rhombic planimetric *Schwenklappen*-plasties.

Stereometric *Schwenklappen*-Plasties

As has been pointed out, the direction of the skin extension vector s depends on the transfer angle α in planimetric *Schwenklappen*-plasties (Fig. 3A). This leads to a limited applicability of planimetric *Schwenklappen*-plasties in difficult reconstructions; however, when a stereometric *Schwenklappen*-plasty with additional transposition is used, better results are obtained (Fig. 4C).

The stereometric *Schwenklappen*-plasty is modeled from a foldlike elevation surrounding the flap base (Fig. 8A and B). In this case, the skin extension vector s is brought in line with the maximal skin reserve vector r_{max} (Fig. 9). When the smallest skin extension vector s_{min} is chosen, maximal skin reserve will result (Fig. 9A).

If the *Schwenklappen*, after its transfer by rotation of the flap and its base (i.e., *Schwenkung*, Fig. 8B), is additionally transposed (further rotation of the flap, Fig. 8C), stereometric unevenness in the flap surface may result. The elevation in the area surrounding the flap base (Fig. 9C) will level out by itself or can be excised or retransferred later.

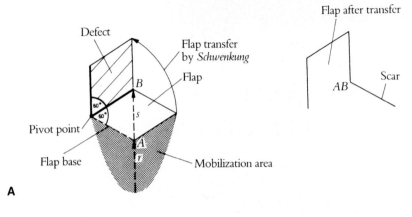

A

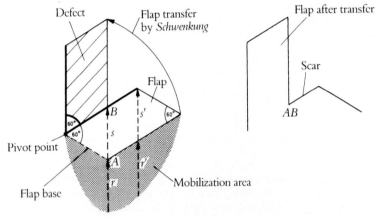

B

FIG. 1. A,B: *Schwenklappen*-plasty with *Schwenkungs*-angle α of 60 degrees. Rhombic (**A**) and rhomboid (**B**) designs, the latter covering nearly twice the extent of the former, although the same skin reserve vector r is used. s, skin extension vector; r, skin reserve vector.

To plan a transposed stereometric *Schwenklappen*-plasty to make full use of all available skin reserve, first outline the defect (Fig. 9A). Then calculate the maximum skin reserve vector r_{max} in the direction of C_1 (Fig. 9A). The width of the defect is marked with the minimum skin extension vector s_{min}, determining the preferred donor site. The flap length is determined using an overlong flap design that includes Burow's triangle (Fig. 9B and C). The combined stereometric *Schwenklappen*-plasty can be carried out if r is greater than s.

A combination of stereometric *Schwenklappen*-plasty with additional transposition has the advantages of ease in calculating dimensions, permits optimal utilization of maximum skin reserve, allows extensive choice of donor site, and leaves no permanent skin reserve in the area surrounding the flap base. When closure of the primary defect does not require all the skin in a planned flap, the flap can be adjusted to any shape; however, until the final decision (Fig. 7), the whole of the flap skin is available for defect closure.

Compared with planimetric *Schwenklappen*-plasties, the transposed stereometric *Schwenklappen* needs a somewhat greater length because of the additional transposition. The additional length required in elderly patients or for regions other than the head and neck may be provided by flap delay for 8 to 10 days, using parallel incisions in the long sides of the flap with undermining, and/or inclusion of direct cutaneous vessels.

CLINICAL RESULTS

In my experience with more than 75 *Schwenklappen*-plasties, minor marginal tip necroses developed in a few aged patients but without major consequences. In all patients, the incision lines calculated preoperatively were quite adequate, and no additional incisions were required (Figs. 5 and 6).

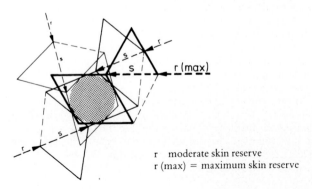

r   moderate skin reserve
r (max) = maximum skin reserve

FIG. 2. If the donor site can be freely selected, the skin extension vectors of rhombic *Schwenklappen*-plasties can easily be brought in line with the maximum skin reserve r_{max}.

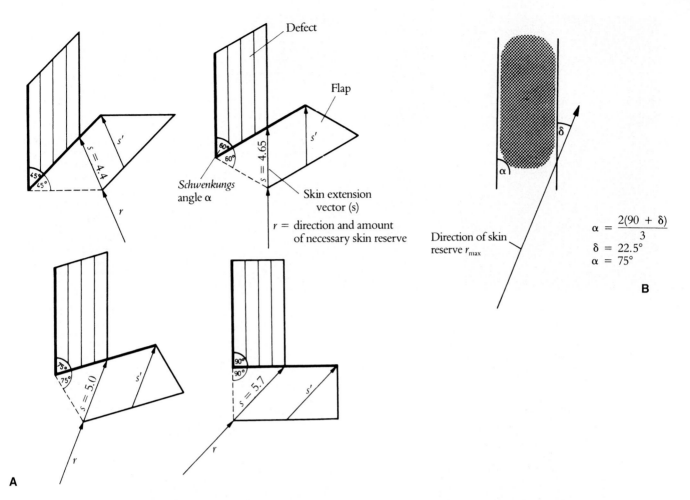

FIG. 3. Interrelationship of the direction of skin reserve, *Schwenkungs*-angle α, and donor site for both rhomboid and rhombic *Schwenklappen*-plasties. **A:** Direction and size of the skin extension vector *s* as a function of the *Schwenkungs*-angle α. Note the increase in length of skin extension vector *s* from angle α = 0 to 90 degrees. If angle α = 60 degrees, the tension lines run parallel to the margin of the primary defect. If angle α is smaller, the tension lines run across the primary defect and could broaden it eventually. If the angle is larger, the tension lines do not touch the primary defect but, under certain circumstances, could tighten it. Not only is the skin extension vector *s* determined by the planimetric *Schwenkungs*-angle α but so also are the donor site and flap shape. **B:** Calculation of the ideal *Schwenkungs*-angle α that brings skin extension vector *s* in line with the maximum skin reserve r_{max}. Applicable for both rhomboid and rhombic *Schwenklappen*-plasties.

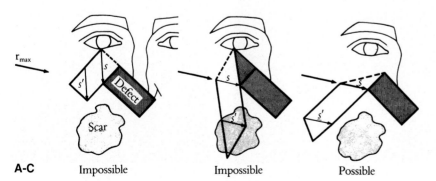

A–C   Impossible   Impossible   Possible

FIG. 4. Adjustment of the *Schwenklappen*-plasty to the maximum skin reserve. Defect, possible flap donor site, and maximum skin reserve are determined by the needs of the case. **A:** Planimetric *Schwenklappen*-plasty with angle α = 90 degrees, taking into account the defect and flap donor site, but not the direction of the maximum skin reserve r_{max}. Skin extension vector *s* shows that realization is not possible. **B:** Planimetric *Schwenklappen*-plasty with the angle α = 40 degrees. Skin extension vector *s* and maximum skin reserve r_{max} lie in the same direction, but raising the flap is not possible. **C:** Skin extension vector *s* lies in the direction of maximum skin reserve r_{max}. No interference with the lower eyelid or the scarred area. (From Roggendorf, ref. 4, with permission.)

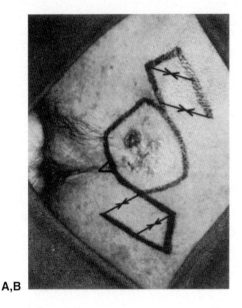

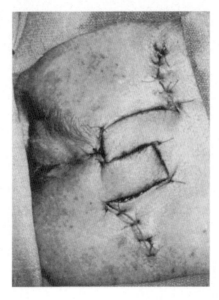

FIG. 5. A: Closure of oversized rhombic defects by a rhomboid two-flap plasty if coverage by rhombic flaps is insufficient. A recurrent basal cell carcinoma with reduced skin reserve due to previous tumor excision. Defect closure is achieved with two planimetric *Schwenklappen*-plasties, additional flap transposition, and small diminution of the defect. The skin extension vectors relate to the maximum skin reserve next to the primary defect. **B:** Note that tension occurs only at the donor site and that there is no tension in the flap itself.

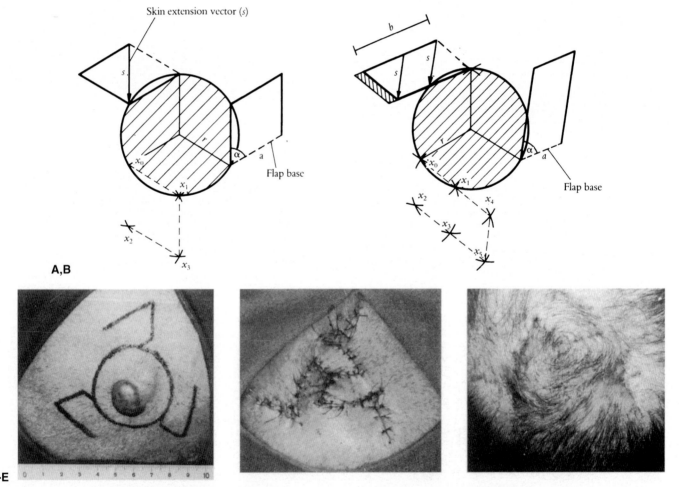

FIG. 6. Closure of circular defects by rhombic and rhomboid three-flap plasties. **A:** Planning and construction of a rhombic three-flap plasty using a pair of compasses, with the distance between the two branches being $a = s =$ radius progressing from x_0 to x_3. **B:** Planning and construction of the rhomboid three-flap plasty in the same manner, but $a = r = 0.75$ radius only, progressing from x_0 to x_5; $b = 2a - 10\%$. With the rhomboid three-flap plasty, 77% more defect area can be covered than with rhombic flaps if the skin reserve vectors are the same. **C:** Tumor of the scalp; diameter of the skin defect was 4.5 cm. **D:** After defect closure by rhomboid three-flap plasty. **E:** Same area 5 weeks later.

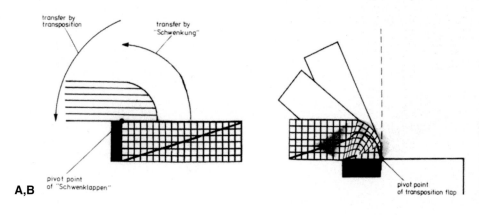

FIG. 7. Maximum skin rotation obtained by combining two techniques: planimetric *Schwenklappen*-plasty and transposition flap. **A:** Note pivot point of *Schwenkung*. **B:** Note pivot point of transposition. With an increasing transposition angle, flap length available for covering the defect is reduced.

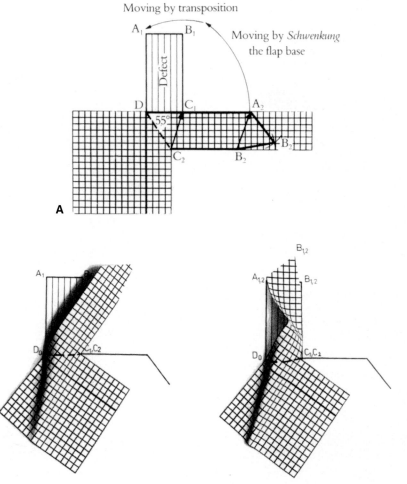

FIG. 8. Stereometric local flap composed of a stereometric *Schwenklappen* and a transposition flap. **A:** Calculating the stereometric flap by choosing the flap base DC_2 and angle $\alpha = 55$ degrees. **B:** After stereometric transfer of the flap base, $\alpha = 55$ degrees. **C:** Stereometric flap model after stereometric transfer of the flap base and transposition of the flap itself. (From Roggendorf, ref. 4, with permission.)

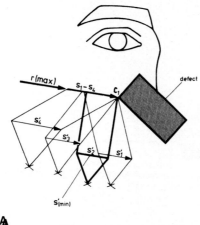

s_2 = Skin extension vector s(min)
   = Optimum utilization of
     maximum skin reserve r(max)

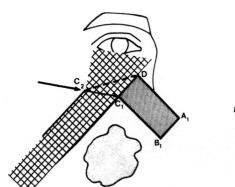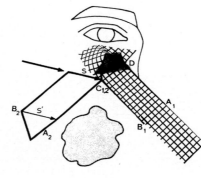

FIG. 9. Planning transposed stereometric *Schwenklappen*-plasty to make full use of available skin reserve. **A:** Maximum skin reserve vector r_{max} in direction of C_1 is defined. Marking the defect width either with minimum skin extension vector s_{min} or at a preferred donor site. In the first case, the utilization of maximum skin reserve is optimal. In the second case, length of skin extension vector s is increasing and flap shape is changing. **B:** Using an overlong flap model with the flap base C_2D. **C:** Stereometric flap transfer by convergence of $C_2 \rightarrow C_1$. Fitting the flap model into the stereometric elevation of the flap base. Marking the flap model at A_1 and B_1. Copying the marked outlines onto the donor site in order to fix A_2 and B_2. Raising Burow's triangle from s.

SUMMARY

Schwenklappen-plasties, which involve both transposition of the flap and rotation of the flap base, can be used to close many defects of the face. These flaps also can be extended by using a flap that creates a curved surface at the flap base.

References

1. Borges AF. Choosing the correct Limberg flap. *Plast Reconstr Surg* 1978;62:542.
2. Limberg AA. *Planimetrie und Stereometrie der Hautplastik.* Jena: Fischer Verlag, 1967.
3. Lister GD, Gibson T. Closure of rhomboid skin defects: the flap of Limberg and DuFourmentel. *Br J Plast Surg* 1972;25:300.
4. Roggendorf E. The oblong parallelogram-shaped *Schwenklappen*-plasty. *Plast Reconstr Surg* 1980;65:635.

CHAPTER 100 ■ RHOMBOID-TO-W FLAP

H. BECKER

The rhomboid-to-W flap eliminates many of the problems associated with other flaps (1–3). The rhomboid defect is converted into a W-shaped scar, which is easier to conceal in the natural crease lines. It is possible to borrow tissue from all four directions, thereby causing minimal distortion of tissue with no dog-ear formation. A scar that has a W shape is also less likely to develop trapdoor scarring (Fig. 1)

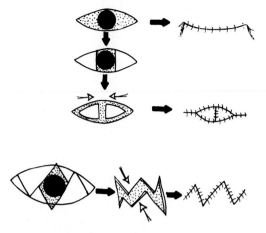

FIG. 1. When a circular lesion is excised, the adjacent triangles are normally discarded to avoid dog-ear formation. This tissue can normally be salvaged and advanced as sliding subcutaneous pedicle flaps. However, the resultant scar is not very desirable, and trapdoor scarring is common. With the rhomboid-to-W technique, the tissue of the adjacent triangles is used. By transposing this tissue into the defect, a W-shaped closure is achieved. (From Becker, ref. 3, with permission.)

INDICATIONS

The rhomboid-to-W technique has been used most successfully for the closure of facial defects. The W-shaped scar is easily concealed, and other problems associated with local flaps are largely overcome. This technique also has been used successfully on the dorsum of the hand, on the digits, and for the closure of small decubitus ulcers.

FLAP DESIGN AND DIMENSIONS

In planning the rhomboid-to-W flap, the axis of the W should follow the crease lines. The availability of skin is assessed in all directions, and the flap is planned according to the amount of tissue to be borrowed in each direction.

OPERATIVE TECHNIQUE

The lesion is excised as close to a rhomboid as possible. Reciprocal flaps are raised on each side (Fig. 2). The rhomboid-to-W technique involves a combination of Z-plasty lengthening and V–Y advancement in four different directions. It is noted that by transposing flaps *A* and *B* and *C* and *D*, the Z-plasty transposition effect is used on either side of the rhomboid. Further tissue borrowing is achieved by

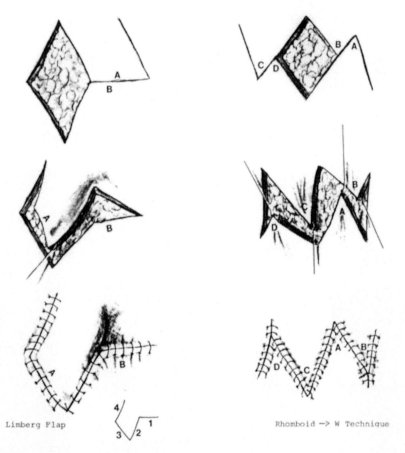

FIG. 2. Difference between the Limberg flap and the rhomboid-to-W technique. Note the large dog-ear formation with the Limberg flap and tissue borrowing from one direction only. With the rhomboid-to-W technique, there is no dog-ear formation and tissue is borrowed in all four directions.

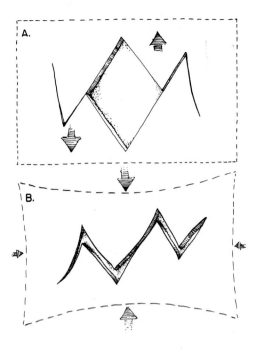

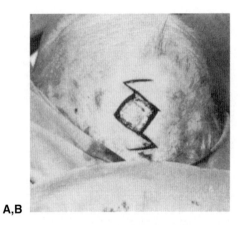

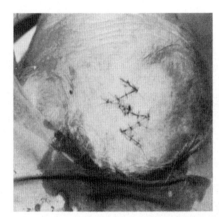

FIG. 3. A,B: Note that tissue is borrowed from all directions for closure of the defect. (From Becker, ref. 3, with permission.)

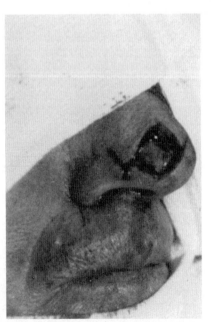

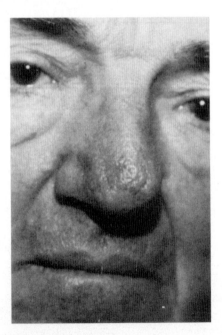

A,B

FIG. 4. A: Lesion excised from scalp, showing outline of flaps. **B:** After transposition of flaps, closure is achieved. (From Becker, ref. 3, with permission.)

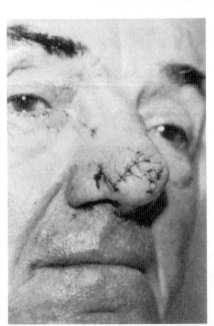

A–C

FIG. 5. A: Patient with lesion on tip of nose excised, showing rhomboid defect. **B:** Closure after rhomboid-to-W technique. **C:** Final result.

advancing flap *A* to the apex of the rhomboid and flap *C* to the opposite of the apex of the rhomboid.

Thus tissue is borrowed from all directions (Fig. 3). By altering the size of flaps *A* and *C*, the amount of tissue borrowing from either direction can be preplanned. The shorter flaps *A* and *C* are made, the greater is the V–Y advancement effect. By extending flaps *A* and *C* to the apices of the rhomboid, minimal V–Y advancement is used and greater tissue borrowing is achieved by the bilateral Z-plasty transposition effect.

Once flaps *A* and *C* are sutured to each other, the donor defects are closed by flaps *B* and *D* (Figs. 4 and 5). If flaps *B* and *D* do not close the defects completely, they can be closed as a V–Y and, in some cases, even left open to heal spontaneously, or rarely, they can be skin-grafted.

SUMMARY

The rhomboid-to-W technique has several advantages over standard techniques, especially for closure of defects of the face and hands.

References

1. Becker H. The rhomboid-to-W technique for excision of some skin lesions and closure. *Plast Reconstr Surg* 1979;64:444.
2. Becker H. The use of a new flap in the management of facial lesions. *Plast Surg Forum* 1979;II:198.
3. Becker H. Rhomboid-to-W flap. *Ann Plast Surg* 1983;11:125.

CHAPTER 101 ■ DOUBLE-Z RHOMBOID PLASTY FOR RECONSTRUCTION OF FACIAL WOUNDS

F. N. GAHHOS

EDITORIAL COMMENT

This is a good alternative procedure, particularly for defects in which there is no mobility for correction with a single rhomboid flap. The use of two flaps gives a more satisfactory result without creating secondary deformities.

The double-Z rhomboid plasty, a technique of four transposition pedicle flaps, is characterized by borrowing the required tissue from two nonadjacent, opposite sides of the defect (1). When used in the face, where primary closure or reconstruction with direct tissue advancement is not feasible, the technique will avoid displacement or distortion of mobile anatomic landmarks (2). The flaps can be developed as strictly cutaneous, fasciocutaneous, or myocutaneous.

INDICATIONS

There are four main indications for the use of the double-Z rhomboid plasty in the face and neck: (a) when there is tissue availability in only two opposite directions, where closure by advancement flaps is not possible; (b) for prevention of the displacement of tissue landmarks such as lips, eyebrows, and nose; (c) for reconstruction of defects of two different tissue

types, such as skin and mucosa or skin and hair-bearing skin; and (d) in the presence of wrinkles, to support the requirements of placing most scars in that direction. Proper orientation, planning, and rotation of the flap axis and placement of mobile landmarks along relaxed skin tension lines, as well as minimizing the need for advancement of the transposed flaps, will provide excellent cosmetic results.

ANATOMY

The double-Z rhomboid plasty is a technique involving multiple transposition pedicle flaps. The underlying muscle fascia or muscle can be incorporated into the flaps in areas of compromised circulation. As with other cutaneous flaps in the face, the axial skin blood supply can be disregarded. The design is simple, and the orientation is based on relaxed skin tension lines.

FLAP DESIGN AND DIMENSIONS

The first consideration in design is the optimal orientation of the rhombus containing the lesion, which is marked along with an appropriate margin of normal skin. A standard rhombic defect has a long and short axis; the double-Z rhomboid plasty borrows from each side of the long axis. Determining the optimal orientation is perhaps the most

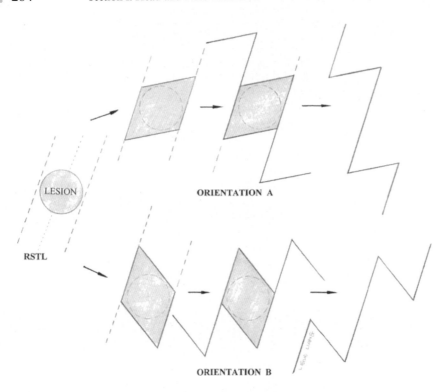

ORIENTATION A

LESION

RSTL

ORIENTATION B

FIG. 1. Technique of determining optimal orientation of the double-Z rhomboid plasty in relation to relaxed skin tension lines (RSTL). Two orientations of the excisional rhombus are possible (see text for description). In both orientations, three of the five suture-line segments will parallel the RSTL.

difficult aspect, and adequate time should be taken to design the flaps correctly. The relaxed skin tension line is determined, which can be done by pinching the skin between the thumb and index finger in the area of the lesion to determine the direction of maximum tissue availability. Two lines are drawn along the edges of the planned skin defect, which must be parallel to the relaxed skin tension lines (Fig. 1). There are two possible orientations that will result in both minimal closure tension and maximal cosmesis. The surgeon will choose the design that least distorts adjacent anatomic landmarks.

The desired direction of the final incisions may also aid in the choice of orientation. Regardless of the orientation used, the major incision and two of the minor incisions will end up parallel to the relaxed skin tension lines and to each other. The remaining two incisions will vary in direction, depending on the chosen rhombic orientation.

Frequently, when reconstructing defects in the face, tissue may be available in all directions; in such cases, the relaxed skin tension lines can be ignored. The rhombus can be oriented to avoid displacement of tissue landmarks. In cases where the excisional defect contains more than one tissue type, the rhombus can be oriented so that one of the long pedicle flaps contains tissues similar to those resected.

After determining orientation, designing the flap is relatively simpler (Fig. 2). The excisional defect is a standard 60/120 degree rhombus, and all four sides are the same length. Four flaps (A, B, C, and D) are designed in the form of Z-plasties. Flaps A and D have long pedicles and are used to reconstruct the excisional defect; their short sides are equal in length to the sides of the rhombus, and their long sides are equal to twice that length. Flaps B and C have short pedicles and are used to reconstruct the long flap (A, D) donor-site defects. Both sides of these two short-pedicled

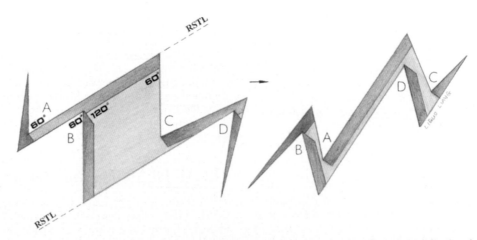

FIG. 2. Multiple pedicle flap design of the double-Z rhomboid plasty technique. The length of all sides of the rhombus and each limb of the Z-plasty flaps are equal. Closure of the rhombic excisional defect is accomplished by transposition of the four pedicle flaps: A with B and C with D.

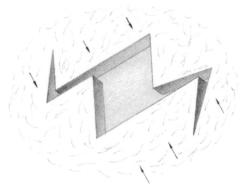

FIG. 3. Wide undermining (*stippled area*) is required for optimal cosmetic results. *Arrows* show direction of tissue advancement.

flaps are equal in length to the sides of the rhombus; all four flap corners are 60 degrees. Establishing the correct 60-degree angle for each of the four Z-plasty flaps requires no angle measurements because the backcuts are made parallel to two of the sides of the rhombic defect. Closure of the rhombic excisional defect is accomplished by elevation and transposition of all four flaps (Fig. 2).

OPERATIVE TECHNIQUE

Once orientation of the double-Z plasty and limb design have been completed, execution of the technique requires only basic surgical skills. The rhombic-shaped tissue containing the lesion is excised to the indicated depth; the underlying muscle fascia can be included in the specimen, when indicated, as with melanomas. The four pedicle flaps can be elevated as cutaneous, fasciocutaneous, or myocutaneous flaps by including underlying muscle fascia or muscle. Incisions must be made perpendicular throughout the flap thickness in order not to compromise blood flow to the four flap tips. Incisions can be made at an angle when preservation of hair follicles

is desirable. Adequate undermining of the area (Fig. 3) is imperative to prevent dog-ear formation. Also, adequate wide undermining will reduce tension along the central long segment of the incision, thus improving circulation. Following creation of the four flaps, adequate undermining, and hemostasis, the flaps are transposed (see Fig. 2). Closure of the four short incisions is easier and should be performed first. This leaves the long central segment, which is usually closed under moderate tension.

Thin cutaneous flaps can be approximated in a single layer using nondissolvable skin sutures. Thicker flaps containing subcutaneous tissue, fascia, or muscle can be closed in layers, using dissolvable sutures for the deep layers. Cutaneous flaps under great tension also may benefit from a layered closure, which facilitates early removal of skin sutures.

Use of drains in the face is rarely required; however, elevation of the flaps and undermining at the level of the superficial muscle fascia are more likely to result in postoperative seromas. In these cases, as well as where excessive bleeding is encountered, use of drains may be indicated. As with all flaps, use of tight dressings should be avoided. With thin cutaneous flaps showing signs of vascular distress, use of an ointment or cream may prevent drying and facilitate survival as a composite graft. Use of 60-degree angles throughout the double-Z rhomboid plasty minimizes dog-ear formation; the tested technique of subcutaneous fat removal at the corners will avoid the occurrence of dogears altogether.

CLINICAL RESULTS

Experience with 197 double-Z rhomboid plasties over a 10-year period has shown that skin grafting seems a much faster procedure at the nasal tip and alar margin, with equally good results; use of the plasty procedure also results in a slightly depressed scar at this site. Among other perceived disadvantages of the double-Z rhomboid plasty are that it is a lengthy procedure compared with skin grafting or the rhomboid flap. Recurrence of tumor along the edges of rhombic excision will result in multiple local recurrences. Also, there is a possibly higher incidence of flap-tip necrosis compared with advancement, rotation, and rhomboid flaps.

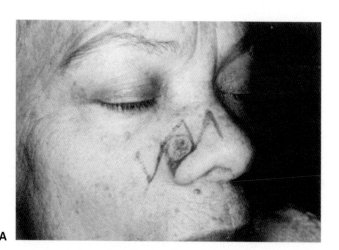
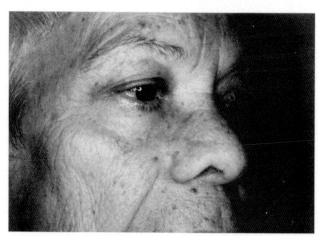

A   B

FIG. 4. An 82-year-old woman with a large basal-cell carcinoma of the nose. **A:** The excisional rhombus was oriented in such a direction that the alar rim and inner canthus location would not change with reconstruction **B:** Results 1 year following surgery, showing no alar rim displacement (*right*). (From Gahhos, Cuono, ref. 2, with permission.)

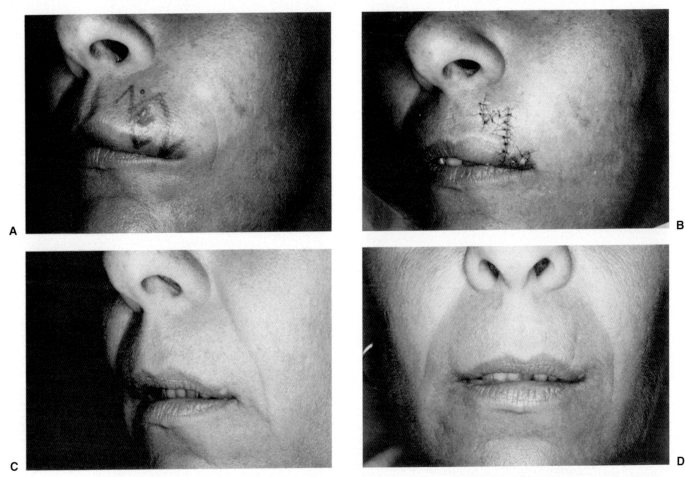

FIG. 5. Basal-cell carcinoma of the upper lip in a 49-year-old patient. A,B: Immediate reconstruction of
the rhombic defect with the double-Z rhomboid technique. The tissue to be excised contains upper-lip
skin, vermilion border, and mucosa. The rhombus is oriented in such a way that the superiorly based
lateral-pedicle flap contains equivalent amounts of skin, vermilion, and mucosa. C,D: Appearance
15 months after surgery shows reasonable upper-lip symmetry and an uninterrupted vermilion border.
(From Gahhos, Cuono, ref. 2, with permission.)

SUMMARY

Where primary closure is not possible and displacement of
adjacent mobile landmark structures needs to be avoided, the
double-Z rhomboid plasty is the technique of choice in the
reconstruction of difficult facial skin defects.

References

1. Cuono CB. Double-Z plasty repair of large and small defects: the double-Z
   rhomboid. *Plast Reconstr Surg* 1983;71:658.
2. Gahhos FN, Cuono CB. Double-Z rhombic technique for reconstruction of
   facial wounds. *Plast Reconstr Surg* 1990;85:869.
3. Katoh H, Nakajima T, Yoshimura Y. The double-Z rhomboid plasty: an
   improvement in design. *Plast Reconstr Surg* 1984;74:817.

CHAPTER 102 ■ SUBCUTANEOUS PEDICLE FLAPS

J. N. BARRON* AND M. N. SAAD

The use of subcutaneous pedicle flaps in the repair of cheek and neck defects is governed by the same basic principles laid out in Chapter 44 on the use of these flaps for the repair of nasal defects (1–3).

INDICATIONS

Skin and lining defects of the cheek can be repaired by mobilizing an appropriate island of skin from adjacent redundant areas of the cheek (Figs. 1 and 2). The nasolabial fold is an ideal abundant source of tissue for the repair of adjacent skin defects (4,5). It has a robust blood supply and provides an excellent texture and color match. Circular defects of the cheek also can be repaired by using two sliding subcutaneous pedicle flaps (6) (Fig. 3). Skin defects of the neck can be repaired by suitably designed subcutaneous pedicle flaps, although other techniques, such as free skin grafts or standard flaps, are usually preferred.

It should be noted that subcutaneous pedicle flaps should not be used to repair circular defects less than 2 cm in diameter, especially in the lax region of the cheek, because peripheral scar contraction can cause mushrooming of the flap.

ANATOMY

It has been suggested that flaps used for the repair of lower cheek defects should be based inferiorly on the branches of the facial artery, while flaps for the repair of upper cheek defects should be based laterally on the transverse facial artery (7).

*Deceased.

FLAP DESIGN AND DIMENSIONS

The design, geometry, and pivot point at the base of the pedicle must be arranged so that there is no longitudinal tension on the transplanted pedicle. Whenever possible, the pedicle should contain an axial vascular system, such as the terminal branch of the facial artery. Otherwise, one should ensure that the subcutaneous pedicle contains sufficient vascular elements to sustain the viability of the flap. It is advantageous to include the platysma in the pedicle when a subcutaneous pedicle flap is taken from the neck. (This no longer constitutes a subcutaneous pedicle flap but is a musculocutaneous flap based on the platysma; see Chapter 122.)

Whether the subcutaneous pedicle is based inferiorly or laterally, the actual geometry of the skin flap is planned in V-Y fashion, thus siting the scars in the lines of facial expression.

For the repair of lining defects of the cheek, an adjacent skin flap based on the subcutaneous tissues at the edges of the defect may be turned in and sutured to the mucosal defect (2) (Fig. 4). In female patients, the flaps should be based on the mandibular or submandibular region, while in male patients, the hairless malar region is preferred (2).

OPERATIVE TECHNIQUE

The operative technique of raising and insetting a subcutaneous pedicle flap has been fully described in Chapter 44. Atraumatic technique and thorough hemostasis are essential, and if necessary, suction drainage should be provided.

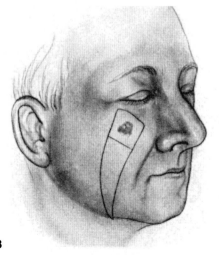
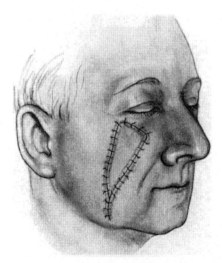

A,B

FIG. 1. A,B: The design of the V-Y cheek advancement flap based on a subcutaneous pedicle.

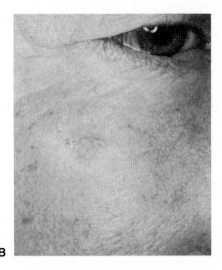
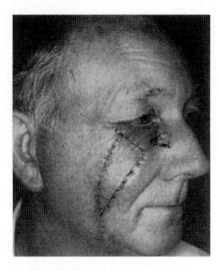

A,B

FIG. 2. A,B: Basal cell carcinoma of the cheek excised and repaired by a V-Y subcutaneous pedicle flap. Note the tulle gras bolster anchoring the deep-ithelialized medial corner of the flap, thus relieving the tension on the flap and minimizing the risk of ectropion.

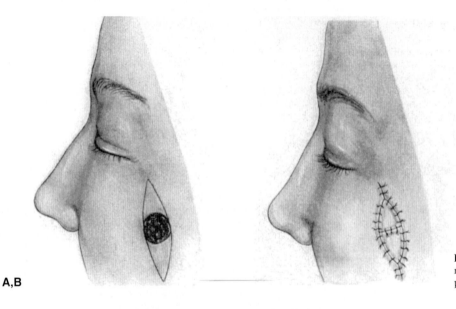

A,B

FIG. 3. A,B: Closure of elliptical defects repaired by two V-Y sliding subcutaneous pedicle flaps.

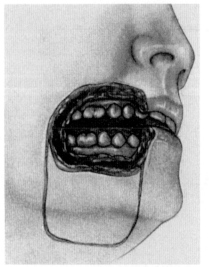
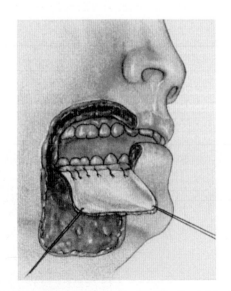
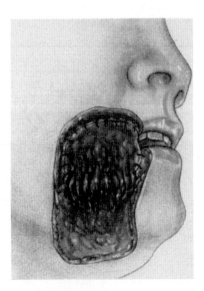

A–C

FIG. 4. A: Technique for the repair of cheek lining defects (2). The flap is based on a subcutaneous pedicle at the inferior margin of the defect. **B:** Proximal upper edge of the flap sutured to the inferior edge of the mucosal defect. **C:** Flap turned up and fully inset into the mucosal defect.

Instead of discarding the pointed corners of cheek flaps to fit the defect, it is advantageous to deepithelialize them and use them as subcutaneous anchorage points. This relieves the tension on the flap proper and eliminates the risk of ectropion (Fig. 2).

SUMMARY

Subcutaneous pedicle flaps can be used in many instances for repair of cheek, neck, or intraoral defects.

References

1. Barron JN, Emmett AJJ. The subcutaneous pedicle flaps. *Br J Plast Surg* 1965;18:51.
2. Chongchet V. Subcutaneous pedicle flaps for reconstruction of the lining of the lip and cheek. *Br J Plast Surg* 1977;30:38.
3. Spira M, Gerow FJ, Hardy SB. Subcutaneous pedicle flaps on the face. *Br J Plast Surg* 1974;27:258.
4. Herbert DC, De Geus J. Nasolabial subcutaneous pedicle flaps. *Br J Plast Surg* 1975;28:90.
5. Grate MR Jr, Hicks JN. Nasolabial subcutaneous pedicle flap. *South Med J* 1973;66:1234.
6. Herbert DC, Harrison RG. Nasolabial subcutaneous pedicle flaps. *Br J Plast Surg* 1975;28:85.
7. Trevaskis AE, Rempel J, Okunski W, Rea M. Sliding subcutaneous pedicle flaps to close a circular defect. *Plast Reconstr Surg* 1970;46:155.

CHAPTER 103 ■ NASOLABIAL SKIN FLAPS TO THE CHEEK

H. OHTSUKA

EDITORIAL COMMENT

In treating defects of the face, the possibility of primary closure and even the use of split- or full-thickness skin grafts should be considered first. The cases illustrated demonstrate a good alternative when the simpler techniques will not suffice.

The nasolabial flap has long been used for coverage or reconstruction of the nose and its neighboring regions (Fig. 1). The flap can be either inferiorly or medially based (1–4).

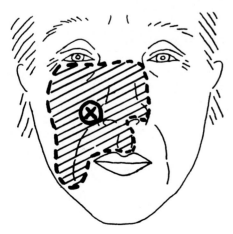

FIG. 1. Range of coverage of a medially based nasolabial skin flap. *X* is at the site of the medial pedicle. (From Ohtsuka et al., ref. 4, with permission.)

ANATOMY

The facial artery and its main branches lie deep and run close to the oral and mucous membranes (Fig. 3A). In contrast, the alar branch of the facial artery has a rich anastomosis with other arteries and supplies the overlying skin and subcutaneous tissue (Fig. 2C). Based on these facts, the nasolabial flap may be elevated as an axial-pattern flap centering around the alar base, even if the main artery itself is not actually contained in the flap.

FLAP DESIGN AND DIMENSIONS

The flap is limited in size to about 3 × 10 cm from the standpoint of donor-site closure. The lower part of the flap usually contains some hair in male patients.

OPERATIVE TECHNIQUE

This elliptical flap is designed along the nasolabial fold. The pedicle of the flap is usually located near the alar base (like a mushroom), although it can be based near the mandibular end (Fig. 2B–D). The medially based flap can be raised from the mandibular margin to the alar base. Some parts of the zygomaticus major and other cutaneous muscles may be included in the flap. The flap can be transposed to cover the lower eyelid, cheek, nose, and upper lip (see Fig. 1).

CLINICAL RESULTS

The nasolabial flap was used for coverage or reconstruction of the nose, lip, and cheek in 29 patients with satisfactory results. Among them were seven reconstructions of the ala, seven of

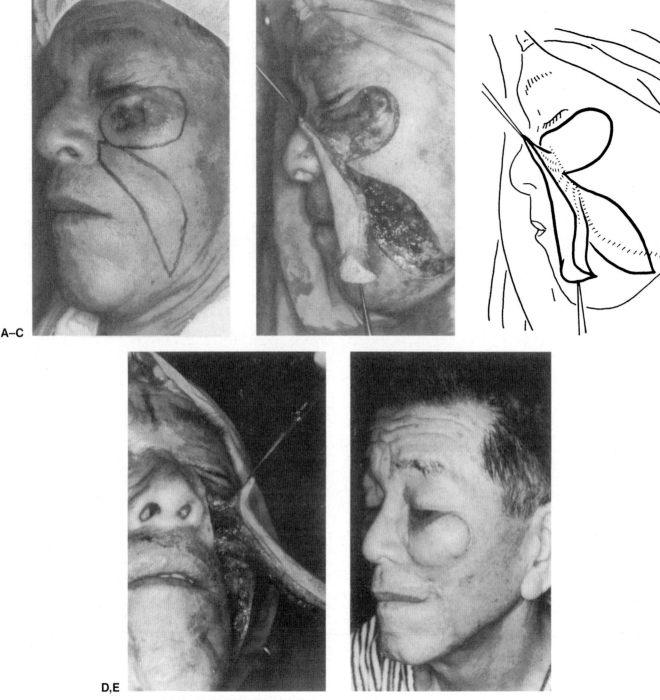

FIG. 2. A: A 78-year-old man with a basal cell carcinoma on the left upper cheek. Preoperative planning of the nasolabial skin flap. **B:** The basal cell carcinoma was excised, and a 3 × 8-cm left nasolabial skin flap with a mushroom-shaped pedicle is being raised adjacent to the nasal ala. **C:** The relationship between the nasolabial flap and the facial artery is illustrated. (The labial arteries are omitted.) **D:** Medial view of the raised flap and its pedicle. **E:** Appearance 3 weeks postoperatively.

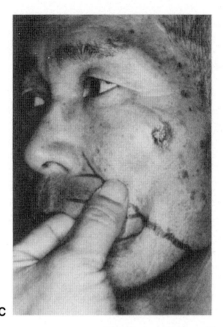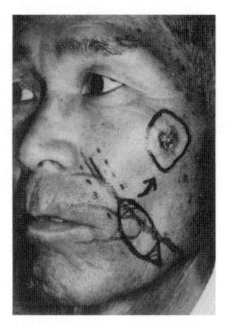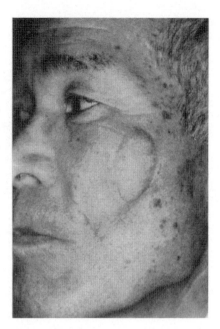

A–C

FIG. 3. **A:** A 63-year-old man with a basal cell carcinoma on the upper lateral cheek treated by using subcutaneous nasolabial flap. The route of the facial artery has been identified by palpation and marked on the skin. **B:** Region to be excised and the flap are marked. **C:** Appearance 3 months postoperatively.

the cheeks, four of the upper lips, two of the nasal dorsum, one of the columella, four improvements of nasal stenosis, and four others. The flap was designed with its base medially in 26 patients and inferiorly in three patients. No significant complications occurred. Occasionally, minor revisions were performed. Color and texture match of nasolabial flaps was far superior to that of split-thickness or full-thickness skin grafts.

SUMMARY

The nasolabial flap, especially when based medially, is a good flap for cheek defects.

References

1. Barron JN, Emmett AJ. The subcutaneous pedicle flap. *Br J Plast Surg* 1965;18:51.
2. Herbert DC, Harrison RG. Nasolabial subcutaneous pedicle flaps: I. Observations on their blood supply. *Br J Plast Surg* 1975;28:85.
3. Herbert DC, DeGeus J. Nasolabial subcutaneous pedicle flaps: II. Clinical experience. *Br J Plast Surg* 1964;28:63.
4. Ohtsuka H, Shioya N, Asano T. Clinical experience with the nasolabial flap. *Ann Plast Surg* 1981;6:207.

CHAPTER 104 ■ BILATERALLY PEDICLED V-Y ADVANCEMENT FLAP

L. PONTES AND M. RIBEIRO

EDITORIAL COMMENT

A modification of the V-Y flap that allows greater mobility of the flap.

The bilaterally pedicled V-Y advancement flap, based on two lateral subcutaneous pedicles and subtotally freed from its underlying bed on the superficial muscular aponeurotic system (SMAS), is a versatile, cosmetically elegant flap, with a reliable blood supply.

INDICATIONS

Traditional V-Y advancement flaps for reconstruction of soft tissue have been widely used for decades (1–3). Several

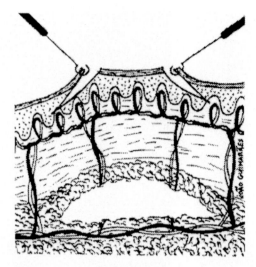

FIG. 1. The blood supply to the skin island is based on the subdermal plexus flow through subcutaneous bilateral bridges. In contrast to the traditional V-Y flap, the central subdermal base is cut from its bed on the superficial musculoaponeurotic system, so that the skin island can be advanced more freely, based only on its bilateral pedicles, to cover a further defect.

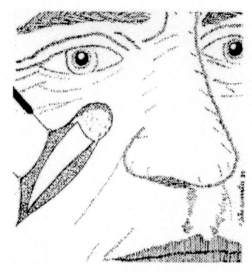

FIG. 3. The incisions of the lateral segments of the flap are made by beveling outward just until the subdermal plane, continuing the dissection in this plane by undermining both cheek flaps.

subsequent modifications have been proposed to maximize its advancement, fundamentally by ameliorating its undermining (4) or by the addition of an extended flap segment (5,6). The laxity of the underlying subcutaneous tissue and its attachments to the fascia determine the degree of advancement in traditional V-Y flaps. When a thin subcutaneous layer is present, this movement is restricted and results in tension on the flap. The subcutaneous bilateral bridges of the flap we present allow for more extensive advancement and coverage of the defect.

ANATOMY

The advancement principle of this flap is based on the subdermal plexus flow to the skin island via subcutaneous bilateral bridges (7) (Fig. 1). It differs from traditional V-Y advancement flaps in that it does not rely on the classic sub-

cutaneous central "vertical" pedicle, so that the flap can be advanced more freely to cover a more extensive defect, based only on its bilateral pedicles.

FLAP DESIGN AND DIMENSIONS

The V-Y flap is designed on the skin, taking account of the fact that the ratio of flap length to defect diameter must range between 2:1 and 3:1 (Fig. 2). However, this is not necessarily pertinent if the blood supply of the flap is not totally random. The lateral portions of the flap are positioned, whenever possible, to consider the aesthetic units and subunits of the face, the presence of skin folds and preexisting scars, the quality of the neighboring skin (including the effects of irradiation), the maximum extensibility lines and rest tension lines, and the overall facial appearance.

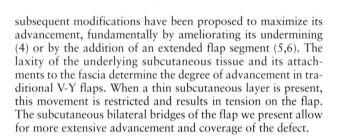

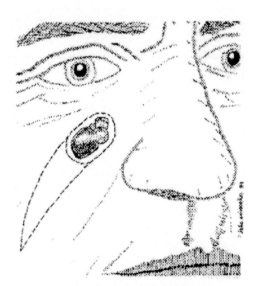

FIG. 2. With Bonney blue, the V-Y flap is planned on the skin, taking into account that the flap length to defect diameter ratio must range between 2:1 and 3:1. However, this does not necessarily always need to be the case if the blood supply of the flap is not totally random.

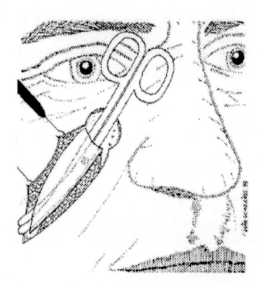

FIG. 4. Elevation of the central part of the flap from its bed on the superficial musculoaponeurotic system, extending its dissection with scissors laterally under the cheek flaps, to create and to free the inferior aspect of the pedicles.

OPERATIVE TECHNIQUE

The incisions of the lateral portions of the flap are made by beveling outward just up to the subdermal plane, continuing the dissection in this plane by undermining both cheek flaps (Fig. 3). Often, when a higher blood perfusion of the subcutaneous tissue is presumed, due to unilateral anatomic proximity of a major artery, just one pedicle at that side can be taken. The next step is to dissect and elevate the whole central segment of the flap from its bed on the SMAS, extending the dissection with scissors laterally under the cheek flaps, to create and to free the inferior aspect of the pedicles (Fig. 4). At this point, the tip of the V is freed, and with the help of a skin hook, the top of the flap is extended. Very cautious blunt dissection is performed on the lateral pedicles until the flap covers the defect without tension. Although this technique is also possible in younger patients, it is in older ones that the tissue moves more freely. The skin is closed with nylon 4-0 stitches, creating a classic "Y" pattern (Fig. 5).

CLINICAL RESULTS

The bilaterally pedicled V-Y advancement flap, based on the two subcutaneous pedicles that vascularize the skin island via subdermal plexus lateral bridges, was used in 959 soft-tissue reconstructions all over the face after oncologic resections. Three hundred ninety-eight (41.5%) were located on the cheek, 328 (34.2%) were periorbital, 165 (17.2%) were buccomandibular, and 68 (7.1%) were paranasal. All 959 flaps survived, except in 11 cases (1.15%) in which complete necrosis occurred in patients who had previous local irradiation. In 29 patients (3.02%), local infection occurred, which resolved by conservative means. The flaps healed without further problems, with a very low frequency of congestion or edema, and a good cosmetic result was consistently obtained. No major revisions were required, except in cases of local recurrence.

SUMMARY

The bilaterally pedicled V-Y advancement flap, with its subcutaneous bilateral bridges, reliable blood supply, and versatility,

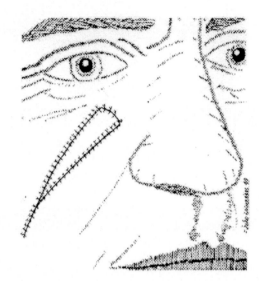

FIG. 5. Skin closure with nylon 4-0 sutures, creating a classic Y pattern.

adds to the armamentarium of traditional V-Y advancement flaps, allows for coverage of more extensive defects, and produces good cosmetic results.

References

1. Bairon JN, Emmet AJ. Subcutaneous pedicle flap. *Br J Plast Surg* 1965;18:51.
2. Zook EG, Van Beek AL Russell RC. V-Y advancement flap for facial defects. *Plast Reconstr Surg* 1980;65:786.
3. Peled I, Kaplan H, Wexler MR. Lower eyelid reconstruction by V-Y advancement cheek flap. *Ann Plast Surg* 1980;5:321.
4. Chan ST. A technique of undermining a V-Y subcutaneous island flap to maximize advancement. *Br J Plast Surg* 1988;41:62.
5. Pribaz JJ, Chester CH, Barral DT. The extended V-Y flap. *Plast Reconstr Surg* 1992;90:275.
6. Terashi H, Kurata S, Hashimoto H. Extended V-Y flap: reports and reconsideration. *Ann Plast Surg* 1997;38:147.
7. Pontes L, Ribeiro M, Vrancks JJ, Guiniarães J. The new bilaterally pedicled V-Y advancement flap for face reconstruction. *Plast Reconstr Surg* 2002;109:1870.

CHAPTER 105 ■ FOREHEAD SKIN FLAPS

J. S. P. WILSON AND N. M. BREACH

The forehead flap provides the largest area of donor skin with matching color and texture to facial skin (Fig. 1). It is one of the safest cutaneous flaps available in reconstructive surgery (1,2).

INDICATIONS

A forehead flap is long enough to reach any part of the ipsilateral face and will provide cover to the carotid artery in the upper neck. It also can be used to reconstruct the cervical esophagus, provided that it is passed under the malar region and that the body of the mandible is removed. The elderly patient is not confined to bed with a limitation of neck movements with the use of a forehead flap.

Skin taken from other regions for facial reconstruction does not provide a good color and texture match and does not supply the deep support necessary, as in the reconstruction of a nose. The difference in color and texture is difficult to disguise.

ANATOMY

A knowledge of the arterial pattern of this flap and its variations is essential to enable the full use of the forehead skin in reconstructive surgery (3). The lateral forehead is supplied by the zygomatic and anterior branches of the superficial temporal artery. The main artery arises as a terminal branch of the external carotid artery. It comes to lie in a superficial plane just anterior to the tragus of the ear (4). Proximal to this, it lies deep in the parotid gland, which prevents its further mobilization.

The superficial temporal artery ascends superficial to the zygomatic arch and soon divides into the anterior superficial temporal branch (ASTB), which passes upward and medially into an ascending posterior superficial branch that passes vertically to supply the scalp.

Cadaver studies revealed that in 80% of cases the zygomatic branch arises from the trunk of the superficial temporal artery, and in the remaining 20% of cases, it arises from the anterior branch (Fig. 2) (5,6). It also has been found that the point of origin of the zygomatic artery was 60% above the zygomatic process, 32% over the zygomatic process, and 2% below the level of the zygomatic process (7). Failure to include a large zygomatic branch may be the reason for reported cases of failure. The ASTB sends perforating branches through the frontalis muscle that is included in the flap to supply the skin. The flap should therefore be regarded as a musculocutaneous flap.

Centrally, the forehead is supplied bilaterally by the supratrochlear artery, which becomes superficial 1 cm medial to the inner canthus, and the supraorbital artery, which is palpable at the junction of the lateral two thirds of the rounded supraorbital ridge with the sharp medial one third. Both vessels are branches of the ophthalmic artery and then pass vertically upward to the scalp.

Micropaque injections of the superficial temporal artery (STA) in cadaver specimens show the rich anastomotic plexus between these vessels (Fig. 3). The blood supply to the

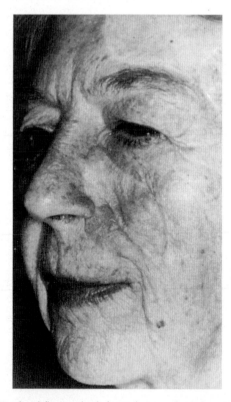

FIG. 1. Forehead flap to cheek for melanoma showing restoration of contour.

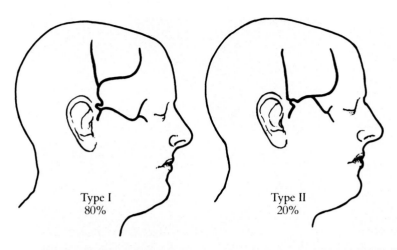

FIG. 2. Variations in terminal branching of the superficial temporal artery (6).

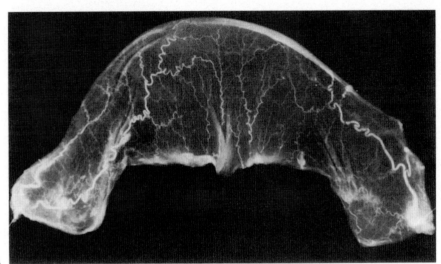

Hairline

Anastomotic network

Anterior branch of superficial temporal artery

Supra-orbital artery

Supratrochlear artery

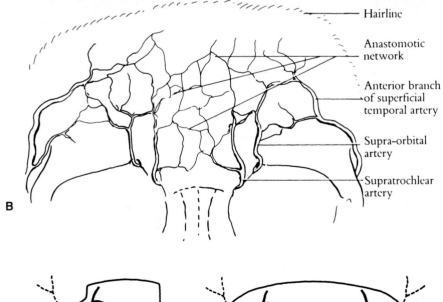

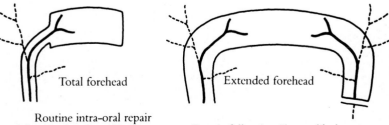

Total forehead

Routine intra-oral repair following hemimandibulectomy

Extended forehead

Repair following ⅔ mandibulectomy

FIG. 3. A: Injection of Micropaque in the extended forehead showing contralateral anastomoses. **B:** Diagram of anastomoses following injection studies. **C:** Vascular supply of the total forehead: (*left*) total forehead, and (*right*) extended forehead flap, the contralateral superficial temporal vessels having retrograde flow to the level of the malar bone.

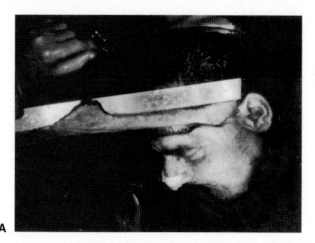
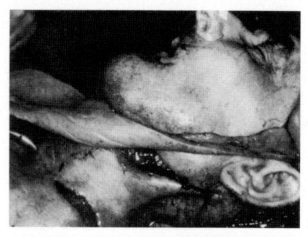

FIG. 4. A,B: Clinical example of extended forehead flap showing that it can reach to the cervical region. (From Narayanan, ref. 17, with permission.)

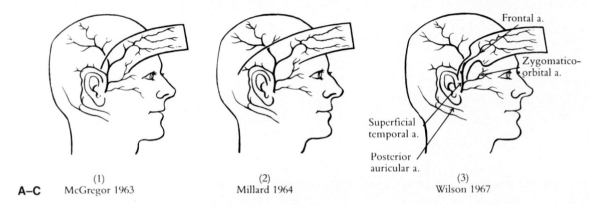

(1)
McGregor 1963

(2)
Millard 1964

(3)
Wilson 1967

Frontal a.

Zygomatico-orbital a.

Superficial temporal a.

Posterior auricular a.

A–C

FIG. 5. A–C: Variations of pedicle of forehead flap (5,9,10,20).

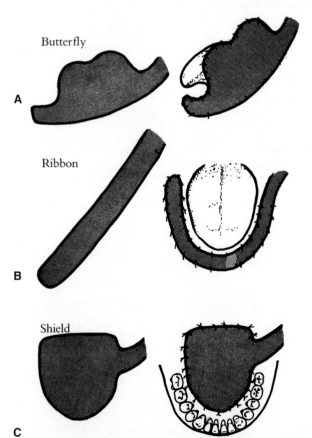

Butterfly

A

Ribbon

B

Shield

C

FIG. 6. Outline of types of forehead flaps for intraoral use. **A:** The butterfly shape is used to repair defects of the posterior tongue to allow mobility, the other wing closing the defect in the cheek. The distal extension provides cover and seal, being supported by the cut end of the mandible. **B:** The narrow flap repairs central and alveolar defects. **C:** The repair following total glossectomy should be in the form of a shield.

forehead is therefore basically four interconnecting vascular territories or angiotomes.

FLAP DESIGN AND DIMENSIONS

If Micropaque is injected into one ASTB, the dye flows across the forehead into the supraorbital and supratrochlear angiotome and hence to the contralateral STA, in which the flow is reversed (Fig. 3A). This allows the creation of an extended flap passing from one malar bone to the contralateral malar bone (Fig. 3C). The flap is 25 cm long in an average adult and can be carried safely on a pedicle no wider than 2 cm at its base. It is obvious that this pedicle, based just anterior to the tragus containing the STA, is highly mobile (8) (Fig. 3C). This flap, provided that the STA and its small accompanying veins are intact, is perfectly safe in clinical practice (Fig. 4).

The course of the STA must be identified and marked on the forehead. The pedicle of the flap must be of sufficient length to transpose the flap without tension. The maximum mobility of the flap is achieved by using a narrow 2-cm pedicle, including the STA. If the STA has been previously sacrificed, a broad-based McGregor flap will be required, which should be delayed (9). If there is any doubt as to the viability of the flap, a flap that includes the postauricular vessel or a posteriorly based flap can be used, but this reduces flap mobility (10,11) (Fig. 5).

Intraoral Reconstruction (12)

The flap should be of a correct size to repair an intraoral defect. Too much tissue provides excessive bulk that impedes swallowing, and too little leads to secondary deformities and oral disability. There are three basic shapes. The butterfly can

repair defects of the posterior tongue to allow mobility, the other wing closing the defect in the cheek. The distal extension provides cover and seal, being supported by the cut end of the mandible. The narrow flap repairs central and alveolar defects. The repair following total glossectomy should be in the form of a shield (Fig. 6).

Neck Reconstruction

The dependability of the vascular supply of the forehead flap is such that it can be used to cover an exposed carotid artery in the neck (13). The extended forehead flap can be cut long enough to reconstruct the cervical esophagus safely, provided that the resection of the tumor had required sacrifice of the hemimandible (Fig. 7).

OPERATIVE TECHNIQUE

The STA lies superficial to the epicranial aponeurosis and thus is easily identified when the flap is raised on its narrow pedicle. As the flap is raised, care must be taken not to lift the periosteum from the frontal bone, and coagulation diathermy should be minimal. If either of these points is not observed, delayed healing of the applied skin graft will result.

Small defects can be repaired by a flap taken high in the forehead, the pedicle donor site being closed by direct suture and a small graft applied to the flap donor site (Fig. 8). This donor site can easily be disguised by a change of hairstyle in the female patient.

The most satisfactory cosmetic result is achieved when the whole forehead is raised as a cosmetic unit by beveling the margins of the flap to 45 degrees (Fig. 9). The marginal step deformity is thus kept to a minimum. The line of the upper

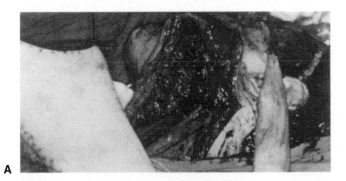

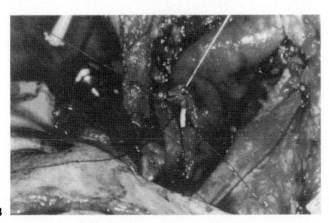

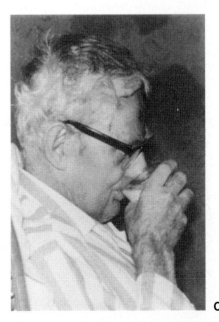

FIG. 7. A: Flap raised. B: Flap used to reconstruct the esophagus. C: Postoperative result at 1 month.

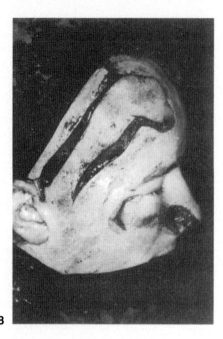
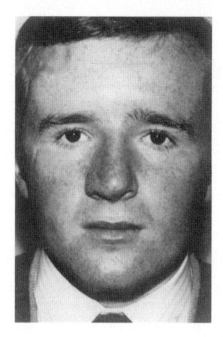

A,B

FIG. 8. **A:** High forehead flap. **B:** Post-operative photograph showing reconstruction of the right side of the nose.

incision should be just below the hairline and the lower incision just above the eyebrows. In the midline, it is carried down onto the glabellar region of the nose. The temporal hairline should be preserved, if possible.

The forehead should be repaired with a sheet of skin taken by a dermatome, applied immediately, and sutured into place with a tie-over foam dressing or as an exposed graft at 48 hours. The upper edge of the graft is disguised in the bald patient by a wig.

Intraoral Reconstruction

When the flap is used for intraoral reconstruction, it may be introduced through a transverse skin incision 1.5 cm below the zygomatic arch (9). Blunt dissection avoids injury to the branches of the facial nerve and the parotid duct. A tun-

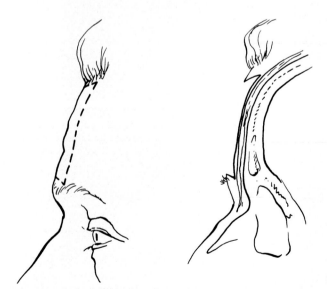

FIG. 9. The beveling of the skin by removal of two triangles of deep tissue to restore contour to the forehead.

nel of adequate size is therefore created to the edge of the intraoral defect. In central arch defects using a narrow pedicle flap, the side of the tunnel can be at the nasolabial groove (Fig. 10).

A technique that increases the versatility of the flap is its introduction into the oral cavity deep to the zygomatic arch (5) (Fig. 11). The coronoid process of the mandible is divided and passed upward, with its temporal insertion under the zygoma to 4 cm above the arch. The segment of muscle then is excised to provide an adequate tunnel. Only on rare occasions is it necessary to divide the zygoma or to remove a segment to provide a larger tunnel to avoid compression of the narrow pedicle. This technique has the advantage of positioning the temporary fistula above the level of the floor of the mouth, thereby establishing an immediate salivary seal.

Additional tissue may be gained for closure of soft-palate defects by using the severed end of the pedicle. This can be performed at 14 days if no complication has occurred (14).

Variations in the Flap Pedicle

Shaved Pedicle

Immediate one-stage reconstruction can be performed by deepithelializing the pedicle. The pedicle then can be permanently buried in the tunnel under the skin (15). This technique avoids a second operation in the elderly, poor-risk patient but may result in some additional bulk or eventually the occasional development of epithelial cysts.

Island Flap

A true island flap may be used to fill a defect. The course of the ASTB is carefully defined, and an incision is made 1 cm medial to this. The skin then is elevated to expose the vessel. A 1-cm pedicle of vessels and subcutaneous tissue of sufficient length to carry the flap to the defect without tension then is carefully elevated. A subcutaneous tunnel between the base of the pedicle and the edge of the defect is created by blunt dis-

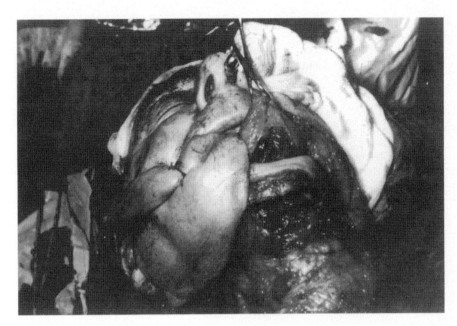

FIG. 10. Introduction of flap through the nasolabial groove.

section, and the island flap is passed through the tunnel and sutured into the defect.

If the flap blanches, it should be returned to the forehead for 10 minutes to relieve the vessel spasm that is often caused by excessive stretching of vessels not supported by a skin pedicle. Particular attention should be paid to obtaining complete hemostasis because hematoma in the tunnel will lead rapidly to necrosis of the flap.

Modifications of the Flap

Various modifications of the forehead flap are usually necessary to provide full-thickness repairs.

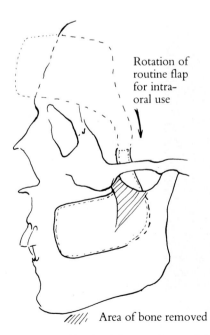

Rotation of routine flap for intra-oral use

///// Area of bone removed

FIG. 11. Transposition of forehead flap into the mouth by means of a submalar approach.

Lined Flap

Two weeks before the flap is required, it is lined by a split-thickness skin graft mounted on a stent mold that is inserted by means of an incision in the hairline into a pocket under the forehead flap. Thus, preliminary grafting of the forehead is achieved, and a lined flap is produced for the repair of full-thickness defects of the face.

Split Flap

The forehead flap may be split to provide lining and cover to two separate cosmetic units. The position of the vessels is studied on the undersurface of the flap, and the flap is divided into two parts, each containing a branch of the ASTB. This is well illustrated in a patient requiring reconstruction of upper and lower lips with the adjacent tissues in the nasolabial region. The two flaps are folded axially to provide lining and cover to the lip (Fig. 12).

Axial Fold

This is the safest method of folding, since it is carried out in the axis of the vessels. It is most useful when the defect involves a free margin, such as in the full-thickness reconstruction of a lip (Fig. 13). If a vermilion border is required, the appropriate area of the fold can be deepithelialized and a tongue flap sutured to the raw area. If the mucosa is intact, this can be sutured to the free margin of the lip and the flap then provides a base to the piriform opening to provide support for the simultaneous reconstruction of the nose.

Contraaxial Fold

This flap provides both lining and cover, but folding the flap through 180 degrees causes an acute angulation of the vessels. On occasion, it is possible to deepithelialize the fold and obtain an immediate 90% inset; however, if the flap is first folded and delayed (Fig. 14), the technique is usually free of complications. Alternatively, the fold can be inset later, after leaving a temporary fistula. The flap then can be safely inset at 14 days.

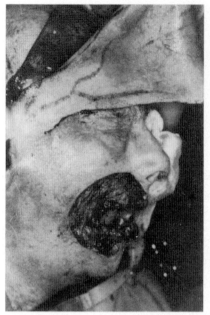
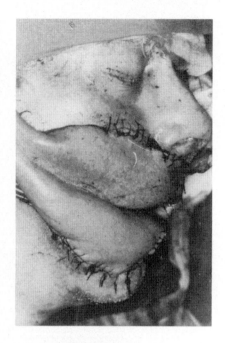

A,B

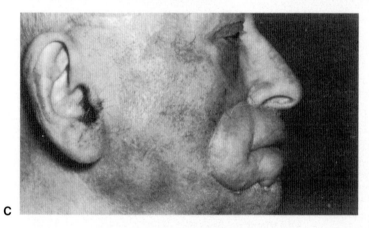

C

FIG. 12. **A:** Defect of lip following resection of a tumor. Vessels seen on undersurface of the flap are marked prior to splitting the flap. **B:** Flap split and folded to provide lining and cover and a commissure of the mouth. **C:** Early postoperative result.

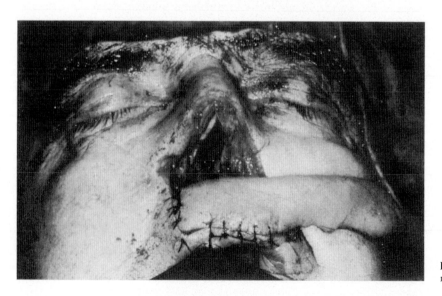

FIG. 13. Forehead flap with axial fold to reconstruct full thickness of upper lip.

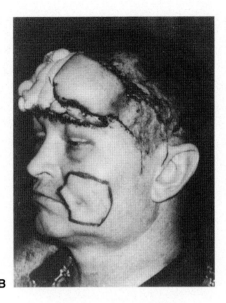

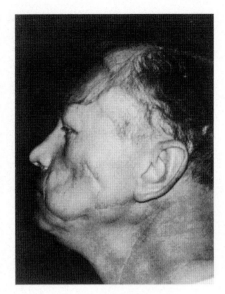

A,B

FIG. 14. **A:** Delayed contraaxial folding of the flap. **B:** Early postoperative result for full-thickness defect of the cheek following excision of a tumor.

Innervated Flap

If innervation is desirable in the flap, as in the case of reconstruction of the nose following ulceration resulting from trigeminal anesthesia, a contralateral central flap including the supratrochlear nerve in its shaved pedicle may be passed by means of a subcutaneous tunnel to provide a repair with normal sensation (16).

Centrally Based Forehead Flaps

See Chapters 52 to 54.

Combined Centrally and Laterally Based Forehead Flaps

If two separate cosmetic units require simultaneous reconstruction, a synchronous narrow-pedicle lateral flap and a central flap may be used. The lateral flap based on the ASTB provides skin to the cheek and lip, which gives an adequate soft-tissue platform for reconstruction of the nose by a central forehead flap based on the supratrochlear artery. An area on the cheek flap is deepithelialized to provide a base for reconstruction of the nose. This technique clearly defines the nose from the cheek, giving a superior cosmetic result.

In the elderly patient in whom a one-stage full-thickness reconstruction is required, a central flap and a lateral island flap may be used (Fig. 15). The central flap provides lining to the nose, and the lateral flap provides the skin cover.

Bipolar Scalp and Forehead Flaps

The use of both terminal branches of the external carotid artery in full-thickness reconstructions has been suggested (17). The ASTB is used to provide a lining flap for intraoral reconstruction, and a scalp flap based on the posterior

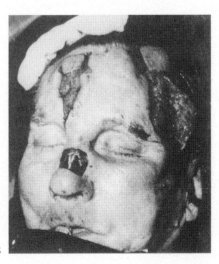

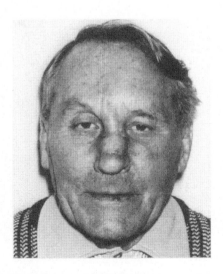

A,B

FIG. 15. **A:** Central and lateral island forehead flaps for full-thickness nasal defect, the central flap for lining and the lateral flap for cover, passing subcutaneously to the defect. **B:** Early postoperative result.

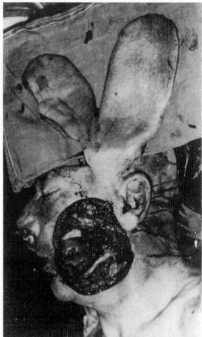
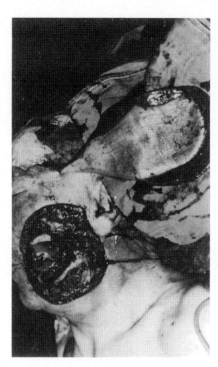
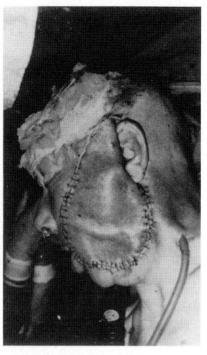

A–C

FIG. 16. Bipolar forehead and scalp flap for reconstruction of a full-thickness defect of the cheek. **A:** Defect with the flaps raised on the anterior and posterior branches of the superficial temporal artery. **B:** Flaps folded on each other to show the smaller flap internally to provide valvular seal. **C:** Flap sutured into position.

superficial temporal branch (PSTB) is used to repair the skin defect in the male patient (Fig. 16).

Transposition of Forehead on a Narrow Scalp Pedicle

Despite findings that there is decreased vascularity in the region of the vertex of the skull (18), the rich vascular anastomosis between the PSTB and the ASTB allows the construc-

tion of a narrow-pedicle flap containing the ipsilateral PSTB to be extended across the scalp to the contralateral forehead, anastomosing with the contralateral ASTB and allowing reversed flow in the artery. This technique (Fig. 17) allows the safer transfer of skin from one temple to the denuded bone of the other temple.

Investigations into the vascular supply to the skin of the forehead and clinical trials lead to the conclusion that provided there is a proper artery arising from one of the major perforators included in the narrow pedicle, the lengths of the

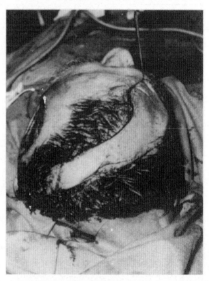
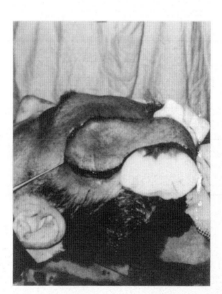
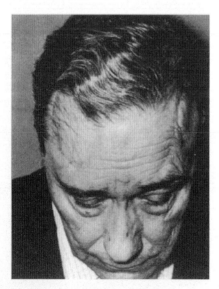

A–C

FIG. 17. A: Flap based on the posterior branch of the superficial temporal artery from the contralateral receding hairline. **B:** Flap transposed into position. **C:** Early postoperative result.

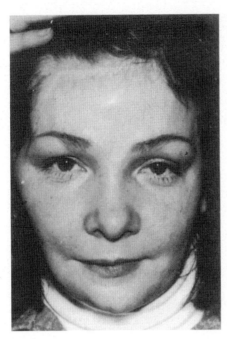

FIG. 18. Postoperative appearance of total forehead graft at 3 months.

pedicle and the flap are dependent solely on the strength of the vascular links between the adjacent vascular territories, called *angiotomes* (19).

CLINICAL RESULTS

The main contraindication to the use of the forehead flap is the resultant smooth forehead with a lack of expression (Fig. 18);

however, it is possible to disguise this deformity with a change of hairstyle.

Another disadvantage of the forehead flap is its relative lack of elasticity that results in a degree of trismus when it is used for the repair of full-thickness cheek defects. This may be partially overcome by a well-placed Z-plasty in the region of the oral commissure after primary healing has occurred. A further significant problem that results when the flap is used for full-thickness defects of the cheek is the apparent loss of bulk of the cheek as a result of the relative lack of subcutaneous fat of the forehead skin (20).

Our series consists of 513 vascularly based narrow-pedicle flaps. The broad-based flaps are excluded because they are usually required only if the superficial temporal system has previously been damaged.

One narrow-pedicle forehead flap in an elderly patient was too thick to allow its safe transposition into the mouth; it was returned to the donor area without loss, and a deltopectoral repair was performed.

There was a marginal loss in 17 patients that was easily corrected by secondary advancement of the flap. There was a partial loss in 10 patients that was treated by the secondary use of the pedicle or a local flap. Ten flaps failed to survive. Four of these were true island flaps, and the cause was probably damage to the vessel or tension on the transported fascial pedicle. It must therefore be concluded that this procedure demands the most careful surgical technique (Figs. 19–21).

In one patient, a prosthetic nose was substituted when further reconstruction was refused. In the other cases, flaps were introduced from another region.

SUMMARY

The forehead flap can be used in a variety of ways to cover cheek, neck, and intraoral defects. Nasal reconstruction and centrally based forehead flaps are discussed further in other chapters.

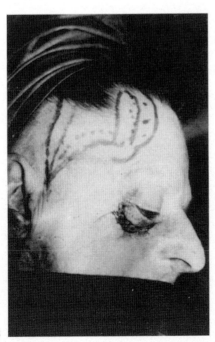
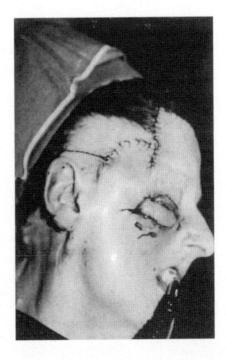

A,B

FIG. 19. A: Island forehead flap designed for reconstructing lower eyelid. B: Flap sutured into position.

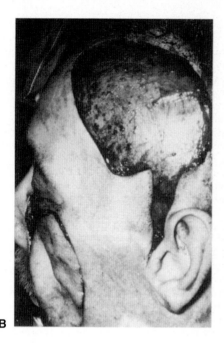
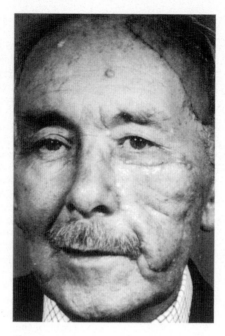

A,B

FIG. 20. A: Large island flap transposed from the forehead of a patient with a receding hairline. B: Early postoperative result.

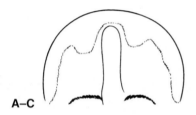
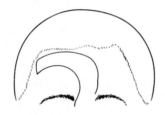
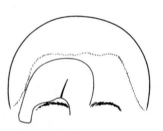

A–C

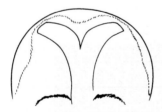
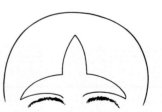

D,E

FIG. 21. Diagram illustrating the various forms of forehead flaps (see Chapters 52–54). A: Extended central forehead flap. B: L-shaped flap. C: Extended flap to malar region. D: Bipolar flap. E: Tripolar flap.

References

1. Gillies HD. *Plastic surgery of the face.* Oxford, England: Oxford Medical Publications: Henry, Frowde, Hodder and Stoughton, 1920.
2. Conway H, Stark RB, Kavanagh JD. Variations of the temporal flap. *Plast Reconstr Surg* 1952;9:140.
3. Esser JFS. *Biological or artery flaps of the face.* London: Royal Society of Medicine, 1931.
4. Manchot C. *Die Hautarterien des Menschlichen Corpers.* Leipzig, 1889.
5. Wilson JSP. The application of the two-centimetre pedicle flap in plastic surgery *Br J Plast Surg* 1967;20:278.
6. Richbourg B, Mitz V, Lassau JP. Artère temporale superficielle. Etude anatomique et dèductions pratiques. *Ann Chir Plast* 1975;2:197.
7. Stock AL, Collins HP, Davidson T. Anatomy of the superficial temporal artery. *Head Neck Surg* 1980;2:466.
8. Wilson JSP. Major flaps in the reconstruction of defects of the head and neck: cancer of the head and neck. In: *Proceedings of the International Symposium, Montreaux, Switzerland, April 2–4, 1975* (Series 365). Amsterdam: Excerpta Medica, 1976.
9. McGregor, IA. The temporal flap in intraoral cancer: its use in repairing the postexcisional defect. *Br J Plast Surg* 1963;16:4.
10. Millard DR. Immediate reconstruction of the lower jaw. *Plast Reconstr Surg* 1964;35:60.
11. Hamaker RC, Conley J. Modified nondelayed forehead flaps. *Arch Otolaryngol* 1975;101:189.
12. Lee ES, Wilson JSP. Carcinoma involving the lower alveolus: An appraisal of past results and an account of current management. *Br J Surg* 1973;60.
13. Smalley JJ, Cunningham MD. Forehead flap rotation to protect the carotid artery. *Plast Reconstr Surg* 1972;49:96.
14. Chambers RG, Edwards SC. Palatal reconstruction utilizing retrieved forehead flap. *J Surg Oncol* 1975;7:191.

15. Kemahan DA, Littlewood AHM. Experience in the use of arterial flaps about the face. *Plast Reconstr Surg* 1961;28:207.
16. McLean NR, Watson ACH. Reconstruction of a defect of the ala nasi following trigeminal anaesthesia with an innervated forehead flap. *Br J Plast Surg* 1982;35:201.
17. Narayanan MS. Immediate reconstruction with bipolar scalp flap after excisions of huge cheek cancers. *Plast Reconstr Surg* 1970;46:548.
18. Corso PF. Variations of the arterial, venous and capillary circulation of the soft tissues of the head by decades as demonstrated by the methyl methacry-

late injection technique and their application to the construction of flaps and pedicles. *Plast Reconstr Surg* 1961;27:160.
19. Behan FC, Wilson JSP. The principle of the angiotome: a system of linked axial-pattern flaps. In: *Transactions of the sixth international congress of plastic and reconstructive surgeons.* Paris: Masson, 1975.
20. McGregor IA, Reid WH. The use of the temporal flap in the primary repair of full-thickness defects of the cheek. *Plast Reconstr Surg* 1966;38:1.

CHAPTER 106 ■ BILOBAR AND TRILOBAR FOREHEAD AND SCALP FLAPS

M. NARAYANAN

Immediate reconstruction of head and neck defects resulting from excisions of huge cancers is a unique procedure in plastic surgery. The principles of immediate reconstruction after excision of oropharyngeal cancers are well documented (1–3).

Wide variations are reported in the geographic incidence of squamous cell carcinoma of the mouth. Although it is as low as 2% of all cancers in Western countries, it offers a formidable problem in South India, accounting for 39.52% of all cancers in males and 18.80% of all cancers in females. Management becomes even more difficult because 86% of these patients report in the late stages of their disease; consequently, conventional radiotherapy cannot cure the primary growth more than 50% (4).

In patients with residual primary growth, the threat to life can be treated only operatively. If the tumor and the draining lymph nodes can be excised and the face reconstructed, solutions to the problems of offensive odor, trismus, pain, and drooling can be offered. Fortunately, distant metastasis occurs in only 1% of patients. The predominant concern of the surgeon is cancer clearance, however mutilating the excision may be. Not less important, though, are reconstruction and rehabilitation of the patient. The surgeon is encouraged to perform a wider excision if a versatile flap that can effectively reconstruct large postexcisional defects is available.

INDICATIONS

In the flaps described below, irradiation is still possible postoperatively because the blood supply to the flaps is quite good. In males, a beard can be grown to help conceal facial asymmetry.

The anatomic locations of postexcisional facial and neck defects are shown in Fig. 1. Treatment of the primary tumor, including neck dissection, was previously described by the author (5).

FLAP DESIGN AND DIMENSIONS

Bilobar Flap

The superficial temporal artery divides into a frontal and an equally large parietal (posterior) branch. The frontal branch is the one used for the forehead flap, and it can be used to reconstruct the intraoral mucosa. The scalp, supplied by the parietal branch, can be used for external skin coverage (see also Chapter 107).

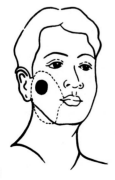
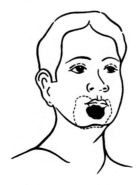
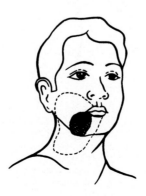

A–C

FIG. 1. Anatomic distribution of cheek cancers. *Dotted lines* indicate the extent of possible postexcisional defects in huge facial cancers. The probable carcinogen is chewing tobacco in the buccolabial sulci. **A:** Retromolar. **B:** Anterior. **C:** Intermediate.

OPERATIVE TECHNIQUE

Bilobar Flap

The branches of the superficial temporal artery are identified by palpation or with a Doppler device. The lines of incision start as with the standard forehead flap, but at a point about 5 cm above the bifurcation of the anterior and posterior branches of the temporal artery, the incision deviates posteriorly to enclose a wide parietal scalp flap that has the exact dimensions of the skin defect. The flaps can be measured accurately by cutting out patterns of the mucosal and skin defects on sterile gauze. The frontalis muscle and the parietal scalp flap are raised at this same loose areolar tissue level.

The single bilobar flap narrows to a small pedicle 2.5 cm wide just above the zygomatic arch (6). The whole flap is everted and turned down (Fig. 2B). The forehead flap at this stage fits snugly into the mucosal defect, where it is sutured. The parietal scalp flap then is folded forward across the face to fit exactly into the skin defect of the cheek, chin, and lips (Figs. 2C and 3). It is sutured there except for the fold at the posterior border. To cover the raw area of the forehead, a split-thickness skin graft from the clavicular area is applied. The scalp defect is covered with a split-thickness skin graft from the trunk.

A fistula will present at the folded portion of the flap just in front of the ear. This fistula drains the pterygoid fossa and the submandibular area. Saliva may leak through, but this is not a great disadvantage because the patient is tube fed for the first 2 weeks. The flap pedicle is returned after a convenient interval.

Island Bilobar Flap (7)

Where it is possible to isolate the superficial temporal vascular pedicle without injury, the fistula can be avoided. This is done by raising a rectangular scalp flap of skin only overlying the branching of the superficial temporal artery and above (Fig. 4A). When this is done, the superficial temporal vessels soon come into view. The vessels, surrounded by dense fibrous tissue, are preserved to form the vascular pedicle. Often it is not safe or easy to isolate the vessels completely. In such cases, the skin alone is undermined at the upper end of the carrier pedicle for a suitable distance.

The rectangular scalp flap overlying the pedicle of the island flap then is cut off and discarded. The superficial temporal vessels and surrounding fibrous tissue are retracted posteriorly, and a vertical incision is made in the zygomatic skin bridge (Fig. 4B). The edges of this are turned back, and the incision is deepened and spread, taking care to avoid injury to

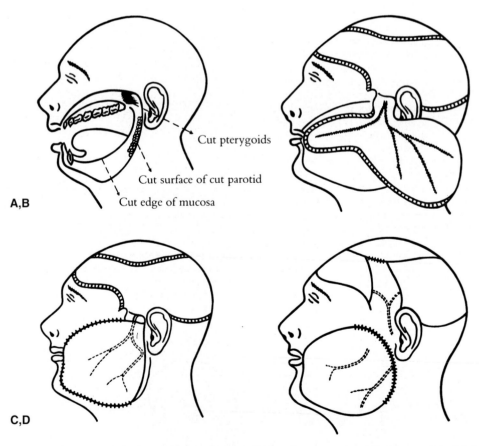

Cut pterygoids

Cut surface of cut parotid

Cut edge of mucosa

A,B

C,D

FIG. 2. **A:** Defect of cheek and upper neck at completion of tumor excision. **B:** Scheme of the bilobar forehead skin and scalp flap based on the frontal and parietal branches of the superficial temporal artery. The forehead portion is used to restore cheek lining to the defect. **C:** Scheme of folding over the scalp portion of the flap to provide skin coverage. Note that the fold posteriorly is not divided or set into place at this operation, so a fistula is present. The scalp defect is skin-grafted. **D:** Several weeks later, the fold in the flap is divided. The inner edge is used to close the lining, and the outer edge is used to close the skin surface. (From Narayanan, ref. 5, with permission.)

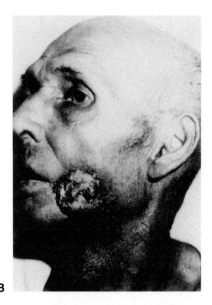
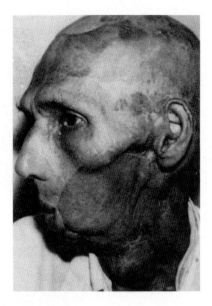

FIG. 3. A: A retromolar growth perforating the cheek. B: Postoperative result 3 years later.

A,B

the facial nerve branches to the eyelids. As soon as a suitable trough is prepared, the fibrous tissue-vascular pedicle is placed within it (Fig. 4B). The skin flaps over the zygomatic arch are brought together, and the forehead and parietal scalp flaps are sutured in place. This island-flap technique has the advantage of further reducing morbidity and hospital stay.

Trilobar Flap

Where the skin loss is below and posterior to the ear, this area cannot be covered by the bilobar forehead and scalp flap. A trilobar flap is designed consisting of the usual forehead and parietal flap with an added vertical flap from the frontal area of scalp on the end of the forehead flap. This whole flap is turned down so that the transverse portion of the forehead flap covers the mucosal defect. When the scalp flap is folded forward, the portion of flap from the frontal scalp (the third lobe) everts posteriorly to cover the defect on the surface of the neck. The parietal scalp covers the cheek (Fig. 5).

Every effort should be made to improve the cosmetic appearance of the forehead. Methods include the use of total forehead flaps (8) and use of a supraclavicular skin graft (9).

CLINICAL RESULTS

Hemorrhage from the flaps and excised area has been noticed only in association with partial tracheal obstruction and was largely relieved when the airway was cleared. There were only two partial necroses of the forehead flap in a series of 132 patients. There has been no delay in wound healing. When the scalp flap is larger than the size of the defect, contractures occur and produce secondary trismus. Blowing exercises should be encouraged in such patients.

The method cannot be employed in those rare patients in whom the tumor involves the superficial temporal artery. Growth of hair on a female's face is a disability, and an epilation dose of irradiation is advised. A narrow forehead flap may not provide full mucosal cover in some patients.

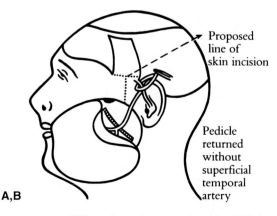
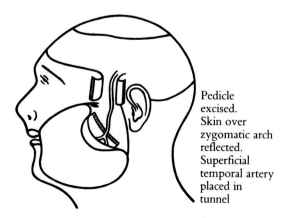

A,B

FIG. 4. Operative steps of an island bilobar flap. A: The superficial temporal artery and surrounding fibrous tissue are isolated as a pedicle in the first stage. B: Final position of the island carrier pedicle and the flaps before suturing. (From Narayanan, ref. 5, with permission.)

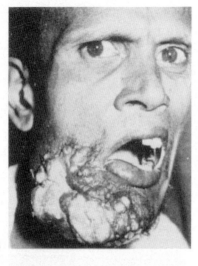
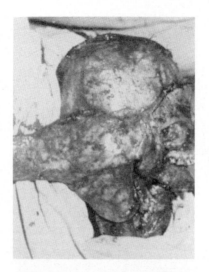

A,B

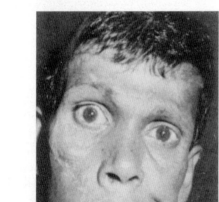
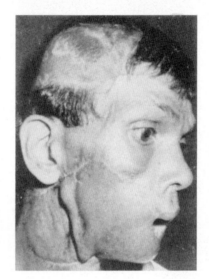

C,D

FIG. 5. **A:** Huge fungating carcinoma of the intermediate area of the cheek. **B:** Trilobar flap raised and everted. The parietal scalp flap extends to the left. Note the third lobe directed inferiorly in lower part of the photograph. This lobe is the vertical extension into the frontal scalp on the end of the forehead flap. **C, D:** Final result 3 years later. Note the area behind and below the ear that has been reconstructed with the third "lobe" of the flap. Notice also the donor defect.

SUMMARY

Bilobar forehead and scalp flaps can be used to cover both the mucosal and skin surfaces in cheek defects. A third lobe can be added to cover the neck area if necessary.

References

1. Conley J. Crippled oral cavity. *Plast Reconstr Surg* 1962;30:469.
2. Edgerton MT, DePrez JD. Reconstruction of the oral cavity in treatment of cancer. *Plast Reconstr Surg* 1957;19:89.
3. Millard DR Jr. Forehead flap in immediate repair of head, face and jaw. *Am J Surg* 1964;108:508.
4. Krishnamurthy O, Shanta V. In: *Proceedings of the 11th international congress of radiology and combined therapy in oral cancer.*
5. Narayanan M. Immediate reconstruction with bipolar scalp flap after excision of huge cheek cancers. *Plast Reconstr Surg* 1970;46:548.
6. Wilson JSP. The application of two-centimetre pedicle flaps in plastic surgery. *Br J Plast Surg* 1967;20:278.
7. Narayanan M. New variation of cheek reconstruction. *Plast Reconstr Surg* 1971;48:3.
8. Hoopes JE, Edgerton MT. Immediate forehead flap repair in resection of oropharyngeal cancer. *Am J Surg* 1966;112:527.
9. Edgerton MT, Hansen FC. Matching facial contour with split-thickness graft from adjacent areas. *Plast Reconstr Surg* 1960;25:455.

CHAPTER 107 ■ SUPERFICIAL TEMPORAL ARTERY FOREHEAD AND SCALP FLAPS

I. K. DHAWAN

The first flap to use the superficial temporal artery specifically included the forehead skin supplied by the frontal branch (1). Subsequently, flaps using both branches of the superficial temporal artery were described (2–4).

The scalp is vascular and richly supplied by branches of the superficial temporal artery. Defects on the scalp can be camouflaged easily, and scalp skin is a large reservoir situated away from radiated areas in the neck and face.

INDICATIONS

I have used these flaps for the repair of extensive defects in the cheek after excisions for cancer. Flaps can be designed to fit the particular defect. In two patients in whom the external carotid artery had to be ligated, a bilobar flap was successfully used after a delay.

ANATOMY

The external carotid artery divides into its two terminal branches behind the neck of the mandible. The branches are the superficial temporal and the internal maxillary arteries. The former pierces the deep fascia under cover of the parotid gland and then ascends over the zygomatic arch. It enters the scalp in a plane superficial to the aponeurosis of the

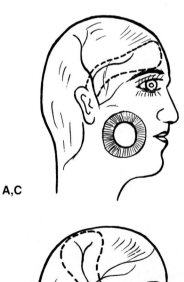

A,C

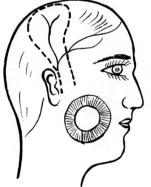

B,D

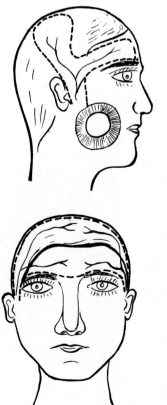

FIG. 1. Flaps based on the superficial temporal artery may be designed in various ways. Either only the forehead (**A**) or the parietal scalp (**B**) or both the forehead and parietal scalp (bilobar flap) (**C**) may be used. Also, the forehead and hairy scalp based on the superficial temporal artery of both sides may be carried down as a visor flap (**D**).

309

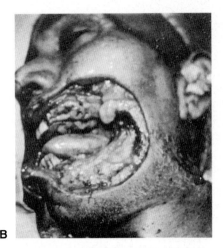
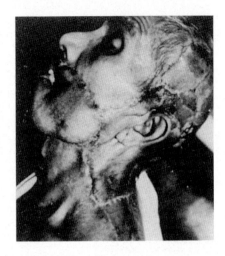

A,B

FIG. 2. A: Defect after excision of cheek cancer. B: Postoperative appearance with a parietal scalp flap replacing cheek skin. A posterior cervical skin flap provided the lining for the cheek.

occipitofrontalis muscle. At a variable distance above the zygomatic arch, it divides into a frontal branch going to the forehead and a posterior branch supplying the temporal and parietal regions. The artery and its branches are easily palpated. The accompanying veins are often prominent and mark the course of the artery.

FLAP DESIGN AND DIMENSIONS

The variety of flaps based on the superficial temporal artery may be classified as follows (Fig. 1): (a) flaps using one branch of the artery (i.e., frontal [forehead] or parietal [scalp]); (b) flaps using both branches of the superficial temporal artery (i.e., the bilobar forehead skin and scalp flaps); and (c) flaps using the frontal branch of both superficial temporal arteries to carry large areas of the forehead and scalp to cover the face (i.e., the visor flap) (see Fig. 3).

During excision of a facial tumor, care must be exercised to prevent damage to the external carotid artery if it is not involved in the tumor. It is especially vulnerable near its bifurcation into its terminal branches, where the internal maxillary artery should be carefully ligated to preserve the superficial temporal artery. Preoperatively, the superficial temporal artery and its branches are carefully marked out on the skin by palpation. The nonhairy frontal flap forms the lining of a cheek defect, and the hairy parietal flap forms the skin cover of a cheek defect in a male patient (Fig. 2).

OPERATIVE TECHNIQUE

The requisite length of the carrier segment of the flap is marked, depending on the distance of the defect from the base of the pedicle. The required dimensions of the flaps for lining and cover are marked on the forehead and parietal scalp. The flaps are raised in the loose areolar plane between the pericranium and the frontalis muscle—the galea aponeurotica. Great care is taken not to damage the superficial temporal artery near the ear. If the entire forehead is needed for repair and must be carried on a single pedicle, one delay 7 to 10 days earlier improves flap survival. The flaps also may be carried as island flaps on a subcutaneous vascular pedicle (Fig. 3).

CLINICAL RESULTS

The forehead in dark-skinned people is not a suitable donor site because of the cosmetic defect that results. The scalp is not a suitable donor site for females because the cover provided by it is hairy. Partial flap loss has been seen in one forehead and one scalp flap.

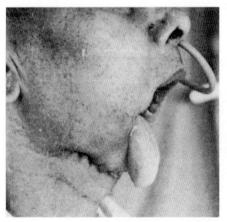
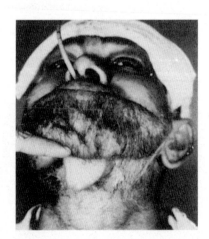
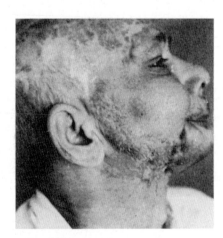

A–C

FIG. 3. A: Appearance after the excision of a lower lip cancer involving the mandible. B: The visor flap brought down to reconstruct the lower lip and chin. C: Postoperative appearance with the visor flap shaved of hair. (From Dhawan, Aggarwal, ref. 3, with permission.)

SUMMARY

Scalp flaps are ideally suited to repair large defects in the face after excisions for cancers of the cheek, alveolus, floor of the mouth, and tongue. Both lining and cover can be provided, and very large defects may be repaired. However, if the external carotid artery is compromised during excision, then the flaps lose their main blood supply and are in danger of being lost.

References

1. McGregor IA. The temporal flap in intraoral cancer: its use in repairing the postexcisional defect. *Br J Plast Surg* 1963;16:318.
2. Narayanan M. Immediate reconstruction with bipolar scalp flap after excision of huge cheek cancers. *Plast Reconstr Surg* 1970;46:548.
3. Dhawan IK, Aggarwal SB. The use of scalp flaps following resection of oral cancer. *Aust N Z J Surg* 1972;41:363.
4. Zembacos J. Bipolar scalp flaps. In: *Transactions of the sixth international congress of plastic and reconstructive surgeons*. Paris: Masson, 1976;392.

CHAPTER 108 ■ GALEAL FLAPS

J. M. PSILLAKIS, J. AVELAR, AND J. PERSSONELLI

EDITORIAL COMMENT

This flap is based on the same principle as the temporoparietal fascial flap. Galea can be included when a thicker flap is desired. In ear reconstruction, the thinner fascial flap by itself is preferable.

Aponeurotic galeal flaps can be used for the correction of various facial deformities. They can be used not only for bulk but also to support skin and bone grafts through their increased vascularity.

INDICATIONS

Reconstruction of the Auricular Framework (1,2)

See Chapter 95.

Cancer Surgery of the Head and Neck

Tumors of the orbital and frontal regions sometimes necessitate resection of soft tissue, including periosteum. A galeal flap with the superficial temporal artery as its pedicle can be rotated for coverage of the bone and as a vascular bed for a skin graft.

Hemifacial Atrophy

Patients with hemifacial atrophy have very thin skin and a poor blood supply. Management sometimes calls for segmental osteotomies of the maxilla and mandible with bone grafts.

The galeal flap introduced subcutaneously ensures a successful surgical outcome because of increased volume of skin coverage and improvement in vascularity (Fig. 4).

Treacher Collins Syndrome

The cleft and hypoplasia of the orbital framework require a bone graft. The lack of soft tissue necessitates Z-plasties, skin grafts, or flaps. The galeal flap over the bone graft makes an increase in the thickness of soft tissue possible; consequently, a smoother bone contour can be achieved.

Other Deformities (3)

The aponeurotic flap is also useful in patients with sequelae of facial fractures as well as in those with hemicraniofacial microsomia (4). Again, the flap also may be used as coverage for bone grafts.

ANATOMY

The cranial galea aponeurotica is the tendinous aponeurosis that connects the frontal and occipital muscles. Originating laterally in the anterior and superior auricular muscles, it loses its aponeurotic character and continues with the temporal fascia up to the zygomatic arch. It adheres to the skin of the scalp by means of a firm, thick layer of fibroadipose tissue, forming the superficial fascia of the scalp. Its adherence to the periosteum by means of loose cellular tissue confers mobility to the scalp. Together with the temporal fascia, the galea forms the substrate for the superficial network of vessels and nerves that irrigate the scalp (5).

Branches of the occipital, superficial temporal, and posterior auricular vessels are the possible pedicles for galeal flaps (Fig. 1). These vessels anastomose, forming a real vascular

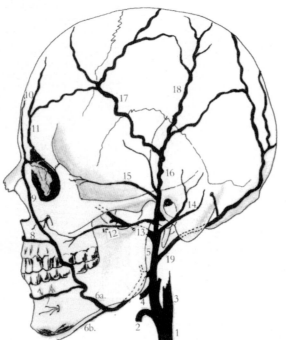

1. common carotid artery
2. superior thyroid artery
3. internal carotid artery
4. lingual artery
5. external carotid artery
6a. facial artery
6b. submental artery
7. inferior labial artery
8. superior labial artery
9. angular artery
10. medial supraorbital artery
11. lateral supraorbital artery
12. transverse facial artery
13. maxillary artery
14. posterior auricular artery
15. zygomatico-orbital artery
16. superficial temporal artery
17. frontal branch superficial temporal artery
18. parietal branch superficial temporal artery
19. occipital artery

FIG. 1. Blood vessels that form the pedicles of galeal flaps.

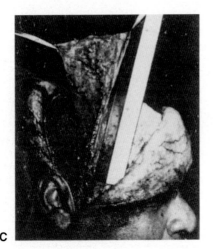
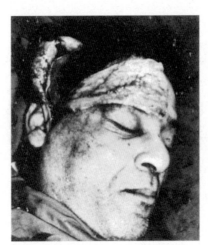
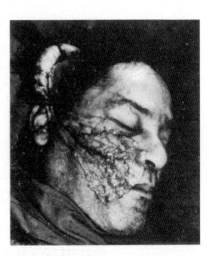

A–C

FIG. 2. A: Racquet-shaped galeal flap. B,C: Arc of rotation.

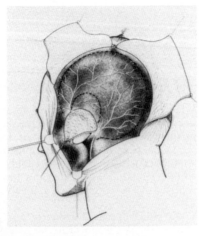
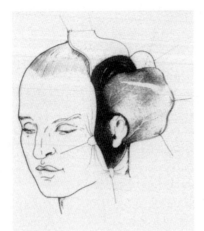
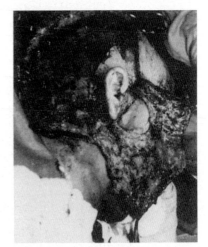

A–C

FIG. 3. A–C: Bipedicled galeal flap based on both the superficial temporal and posterior auricular arteries.

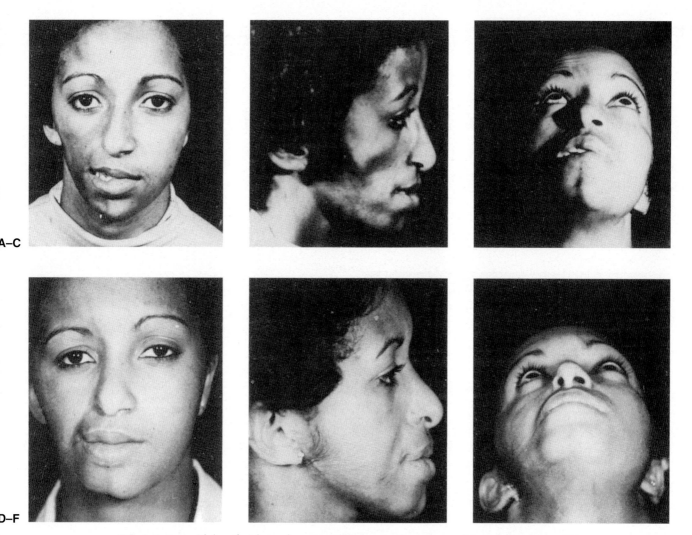

A–C

D–F

FIG. 4. Patient with hemifacial atrophy managed by segmental osteotomy of the maxilla and mandible and a bipedicled galeal flap. **A–C:** Preoperative appearance. **D–F:** Postoperative appearance.

network. Thus, the anterior occipital artery anastomoses with its contralateral counterpart and with the parietal branch of the superficial temporal artery, the posterior auricular artery anastomoses with the parietal branch of the superficial temporal artery, the parietal and frontal branches of the superficial temporal artery anastomose with their contralateral counterparts.

FLAP DESIGN AND DIMENSIONS

Various shapes of galeal flaps are possible, including different lengths of a racquet-shaped flap with one of the vascular pedicles as its base (Fig. 2) or a bipedicle flap on the superficial temporal and posterior auricular vessels (Figs. 3 and 4). The size of the flaps, starting from the insertion on the zygomatic arch to the midline of the cranium, varies from 15 to 17.5 cm.

SUMMARY

Galeal flaps can be used to reconstruct various areas of the face, providing increased vascularity to support skin and bone grafts.

References

1. Fox JW, Edgerton MT. The fan flap, an adjunct to ear reconstruction. *Plast Reconstr Surg* 1976;58:663.
2. Avelar J. Total reconstruction of the auricle in one stage. *Rev Bras Cir* 1977; 67:139.
3. Holmes AO, Marshall KA. Uses of the temporalis muscle flap in blanking out orbits. *Plast Reconstr Surg* 1979;63:336.
4. Avelar J, Psillakis JM. The use of galea flaps in craniofacial deformities. *Ann Plast Surg* 1981;6:464.
5. Perssonelli J. The anatomy of the vascularization of aponeurotic galeal flaps. Presented at the Annual Meeting of the Brazilian Society of Plastic Surgery, São Paulo, Brazil, 1980.

CHAPTER 109 ■ POSTAURICULAR AND RETROAURICULAR SCALPING FLAP (THE PARAS FLAP)

A. D. DIAS AND P. CHHAJLANI

EDITORIAL COMMENT

This would not be the editors' first choice for donor tissue material, although the flap will survive on the axial blood supply.

The skin behind the ear and in the retroauricular region, although restricted in area, can be raised as an axial pattern flap with wide maneuverability. It provides a good skin match for the face without leaving any defect on the front of the face (1–6).

INDICATIONS

This axial-pattern scalp flap with a random extension is an alternative choice for covering facial defects. The flap is easy to dissect and raise without prior delay. It can reach nearly the whole face and down to the hyoid bone on the contralateral side. The donor site is not visible from the front and, in profile, the skin-grafted area is covered by hair. The absence of any visible donor-site defect and an excellent color match are worth the possibility of a certain amount of morbidity in the postoperative period.

ANATOMY

There is a cross-communication between the frontal branches of the superficial temporal arteries, with the artery dividing into two branches: frontal and parietal. The frontal branch divides into two parts, one supplying the forehead and the other the hair-bearing scalp of the frontoparietal region. The forehead branch communicates with the ipsilateral frontal and bilateral supraorbital and trochlear vessels.

The main vessel of the flap is the posterior branch supplying the hair-bearing scalp. This is a constant vessel of about 1 mm in diameter running across the flap and beyond the midline up to the glabrous skin but not entering it. The postauricular and retroauricular scalping flap (PARAS) flap has a profuse circulation, primarily from the contralateral superficial temporal vessels, boosted by the postauricular and occipital vessels, the frontal branch of the ipsilateral superficial temporal vessels, and the bilateral supratrochlear and supraorbital vessels (Fig. 1).

FLAP DESIGN AND DIMENSIONS

The flap is designed for a transverse incision at the level of the lower limit of the concha, going across postauricular and retroauricular skin and ascending anteriorly upward just behind the helical margin of the ear (see Fig. 1A). Posteriorly, the transverse incision goes into the hair-bearing scalp for 1.5 to 2 cm and then ascends, running parallel to the anterior incision in a slightly expanding fashion. The flap is elevated just superficial to the perichondrium of the ear and in the loose areolar plane of the scalp. Flap-delineating ascending incisions are extended transversely across the scalp. A posterior incision extends across one parietal eminence and ends just after crossing the opposite one; the anterior incision stops at the midline. Forehead skin and flap base are undermined (7), leading to descent and rotation of the flap and providing an additional 4 to 5 cm.

The postauricular and retroauricular skin can be considered to be a random pattern extension of an axial pattern flap (8). It is advisable that a 1:1 ratio be maintained. With its ample circulation, it seems justifiable to transfer the flap in single stages, keeping the random pattern extension limited to the 1:1 ratio. The postauricular (mastoid region) and retroauricular (posterior surface of the pinna) areas provide, on average, 20 to 25 cm of skin. The width of the flap is at least 10 cm in the sagittal plane. The reach of the flap extends down to the hyoid bone in the neck on the contralateral side.

Even in cases where only hairless skin is required, some of the hair-bearing scalp from the mastoid region is included to give uniform width to the flap; it is returned in a second stage.

OPERATIVE TECHNIQUE

The donor site is examined and the superficial temporal vessels palpated. The hair is trimmed and shampooed 2 days before the operation. With the patient under general anesthesia, the flap is marked out using a pattern made preoperatively. Saline-adrenaline 1:150,000 is infiltrated and the flap is raised. The width of the flap increases gradually as the base is approached, taking care to prevent narrowing at the top of the ear.

The anterior incision runs within 1.5 to 2 cm of the hairline in a normally hirsute scalp and goes up to the midline. The posterior incision runs over the ipsilateral parietal eminence and gradually deviates posteriorly to run behind the contralateral parietal eminence, just beyond which it stops. The forehead and base are undermined, bringing the flap down by 4 to 5 cm. The length of the incisions ultimately will depend on the area of the face to be covered.

Glabrous skin is sutured over the defect, and the donor raw area behind the ear is covered with a split-thickness skin graft. The rest of the raw area on the skull is covered with either amniotic membrane or a split-thickness skin graft. The raw area in the bridge segment partly folds on itself, and

314

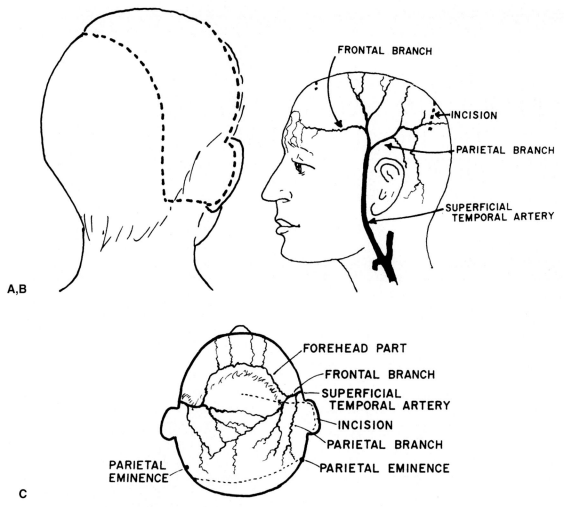

FIG. 1. A: Schematic delineation of the flap on the ipsilateral side. **B:** Vascular pattern on the contralateral side (base). **C:** Relationship of the flap incision to the vascular network. The forehead branch (ipsilateral) escapes the incision and anastomosis with the contralateral forehead branch and both the supraorbital and trochlear branches bilaterally. (From Dias, Chhajlani, ref. 6, with permission.)

the remainder is suitably dressed. Three weeks later, the flap is divided and the bridge segment returned to the donor-site area.

CLINICAL RESULTS

There have been circulatory problems in the distal few millimeters of the flap, but they have not compromised the end result; there is enough laxity in the flap to excise the problem margin, if necessary, and resuture without any significant defect. Rather than delay the flap, it might be preferable to keep its distal margin a few millimeters more proximal.

Dissection of the skin on the back of the ear may result in venous damage. This skin is very thin and floppy and may suffer venous thrombosis as a result of kinking. It might be preferable to include the perichondrium of the back of the ear in the flap, to increase its stiffness, and also to protect the venous circulation during dissection. Problems of skin grafting the donor area will arise; if small strips of cartilage are removed at short intervals, skin grafts could take. It is also suggested that the temporal fascia should be included while the flap is being harvested to protect the scalp circulation, as there is no galea aponeurotica in this area.

SUMMARY

Postauricular and retroauricular skin flaps have withstood the test of time with respect to color match, and the skin texture is quite good. This flap can be a useful addition to the various other flaps used for facial reconstruction.

References

1. Crickelair GF. A method of partial ear reconstruction for avulsion of the upper portion of the ear. *Plast Reconstr Surg* 1956;17:438.
2. Washio H. Retroauricular temporal flap. *Plast Reconstr Surg* 1969;43:162.
3. Orticochea M. A new method for total reconstruction of the nose: the ears as donor areas. *Br J Plast Surg* 1971;26:150.
4. Nahai P, Hurteau J, Vasconez LO. Replantation of an entire scalp and ear by microvascular anastomosis of only one artery and one vein. *Br J Plast Surg* 1978;31:339.
5. Galvao MSL. A post-auricular flap based on the contralateral superficial temporal vessels. *Plast Reconstr Surg* 1981;68:891.
6. Dias AD, Chhajlani P. The post- and retro-auricular scalping flap (the PARAS flap). *Br J Plast Surg* 1987;40:360.
7. Converse JM. Clinical application of the scalping flap in reconstruction of the nose. *Plast Reconstr Surg* 1969;43:247.
8. Smith PG, McGregor IA. The vascular basis of axial pattern flaps. *Br J Plast Surg* 1973;26:150.

CHAPTER 110 ■ LATERAL CHEEK AND POSTERIOR AURICULAR TRANSPOSITION FLAP

R. O. DINGMAN* AND G. H. DERMAN

The posterior auricular transposition skin flap provides an excellent donor source to close soft-tissue defects in the buccal and parotid-masseteric areas. Even large areas can be reconstructed by this flap alone or with additional transposition, advancement, or bilobed flaps (1–4) (Figs. 1 and 2).

INDICATIONS

Primary closure of defects or local flap reconstruction is complicated by the proximity of important anatomic structures that are fixed or easily distorted when tension is applied. Important among these are the facial nerve, ears, lips, eyelids, nose, and hairline. Exact or close matches of skin color, texture, and contour are prime considerations because of the highly visible location of these areas and the concern regarding an optimal aesthetic result.

ANATOMY

The posterior auricular transposition flap is composed of non–hair-bearing skin and a thin layer of subcutaneous tissue overlying the superficial cervical fascia covering the sternocleidomastoid, occipitalis, and posterior auricular muscles anteriorly as well as the superior portions of the splenius capitis, semispinalis capitis, and trapezius muscles further posteriorly. The platysma muscle is present sometimes at the extreme anterior portion of the flap base. This muscle is not included in the flap but is left in place to protect the cervical and mandibular branches of the facial nerve.

This flap is richly vascularized, with its major blood supply entering the dermal-subdermal plexus from the base of the flap in the neck and originating from the superior thyroid branch of the external carotid artery (5). Muscular perforators supply the flap after piercing through the sternocleidomastoid muscle. Branches of the sternocleidomastoid artery as well as direct superficial skin branches from the superior thyroid artery also supply the flap.

Venous drainage is by means of a plexus of small branches feeding the posterior auricular and external jugular system. Sensory nerve supply is from branches of the greater auricular (C2–3) and lesser occipital (C2) nerves entering at the base of

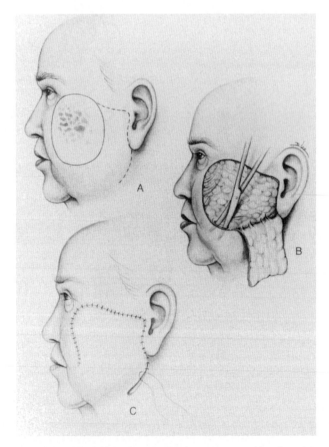

FIG. 1. A–C: This older patient with a large amount of lax skin of the cheeks had malignant degeneration of a deeply pigmented lesion of the left face. The diagnosis was malignant melanoma. The lesion was excised with moderately wide margins and closed by development of a large cheek-neck flap advanced and rotated into the defect. If the single flap is not adequate for closure of the defect, it can easily be combined with a postauricular transposition flap (see Fig. 3).

---

* Deceased.

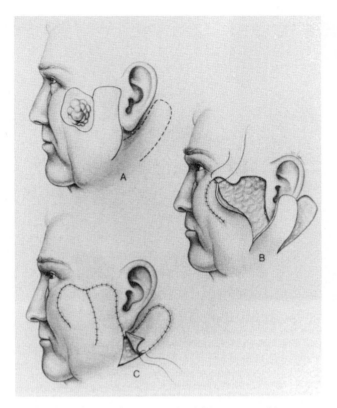

FIG. 2. A–C: Planning for closure of a defect anticipated by excision of a benign lesion of the lateral face. The combination of a preauricular and a postauricular flap provides a generous amount of tissue of the desired skin for facial repair. The donor site is repaired with a split-thickness skin graft.

the flap. Preservation of these branches should retain flap sensibility; however, patients should be cautioned regarding the possibility of sensibility loss about the ear.

FLAP DESIGN AND DIMENSIONS

The flap is designed using a rotation template such as a cloth towel. The longest flap we elevated was 10 cm, and we have used this as our size limit. The base of the flap should be designed along the path of the sternocleidomastoid muscle obliquely across the neck. The sides of the flap are cut parallel to the muscle belly, with an extra width of skin approximately 1 cm on either side, anterior or posterior, included if necessary. Tissue expansion similar to that used in ear reconstruction can also be used to increase the size of the flap and to aid in donor site closure.

OPERATIVE TECHNIQUE

The incision is carried down to the plane just above the superficial fascia overlying the posterior auricular musculature, and the flap is developed in the subcutaneous plane, similar to a neck lift. Care is taken to avoid injury to the cervical and mandibular branches of the facial nerve by dissecting superficial to the platysma muscle and designing the flap so that it lies posterior to the angle of the mandible. Careful dissection will prevent injury to the greater auricular nerve, the external jugular vein, and the spinal accessory nerve. These structures should all be kept deep to the level of elevation of the flap.

Once the flap has been elevated and transposed into position, the donor defect can be closed primarily, skin-grafted, or

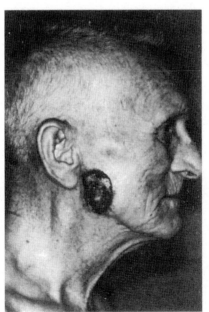
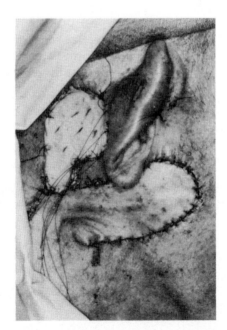
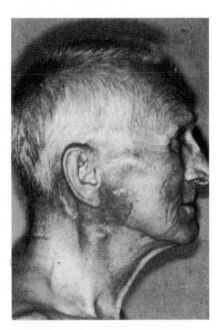

A–C

FIG. 3. A: A healthy 77-year-old man 24 hours after removal of a squamous intraepidermal carcinoma of 5 months' duration over the angle of the right mandible. This had been removed one day earlier by Mohs' surgical treatment with microscopically clear margins. B: A postauricular pedicle flap was developed and rotated into the defect over the masseteric-parotid area. The donor site was dressed with a full-thickness skin graft. The ear is temporarily held forward with a nylon suture. C: The postoperative course was uneventful. At 3 months, the flap is well healed. There is a small dog-ear at the anteroinferior turning point of the flap. This should flatten out without further surgical care.

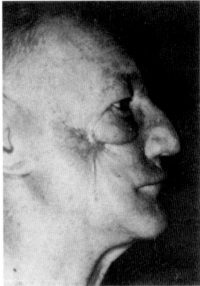
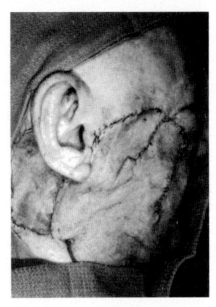
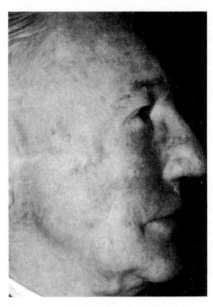

A–C

FIG. 4. A: A 65-year-old man with scar lesion of the right cheek following spontaneous closure of a large defect incident to Mohs' chemosurgery. Note ectropion of the right lower lid and lymphedema due to interruption of lymphatics to the right lower lid. B: View at termination of surgery showing flap from the right preauricular region advanced to the right lower lid and right postauricular flap advanced into the preauricular area. C: Ten years postoperatively.

closed by local rotation or advancement of a second flap. The bilobed flap technique also can be used to close defects further anterior on the face. A dog-ear of excess tissue may be present at the anterior rotation point. If it does not resolve spontaneously (as most do), revision at a later date may be necessary (Figs. 3 and 4).

CLINICAL RESULTS

The posterior auricular flap was used to close defects in the buccal and parotid-masseteric regions of several patients. One patient required a bilobed flap for coverage further anteriorly. The only complication encountered was a superficial skin slough at the distal end of the flap, and this subsequently healed completely. Patient satisfaction was high, with no functional deficits noted, except for a mild transient sensory loss in the occipital and posterior auricular region.

SUMMARY

The lateral cheek and posterior auricular flaps provide one of the better cosmetic alternatives for reconstructing cheek defects. With the use of tissue expansion the range and versatility of the flap may also be augmented.

References

1. Converse JM. Defect of cheek closed by preauricular and postauricular flaps. In: Converse JM, ed. *Reconstructive plastic surgery*, 2d ed. Philadelphia: WB Saunders, 1977;1582–1583.
2. Esser JFS. *Die Rotation der Wang*. Leipzig: Vogel Verlag, 1918.
3. Zimany A. The bilobed flap. *Plast Reconstr Surg* 1953;11:424.
4. DeCholonky T. The repair of extensive soft-tissue defects of the cheek. *Plast Reconstr Surg* 1955;16:288.
5. Clemente CD. *Anatomy: a regional atlas of the human body*, 2d ed. Baltimore: Urban & Schwarzenberg, 1981; Fig. 510.

CHAPTER 111 ■ SLIDE-SWING SKIN FLAP

J. SCHRUDDE AND V. PETROVICI

The slide-swing skin flap combines the principle of transposition with skin sliding. It can be used to close large, round defects with a flap that is smaller than the original defect (1).

In the literature, it is stated that larger defects cannot be closed by means of simple transposition flaps; multiple flaps must be used. According to our method, larger defects may be closed without any variation of the line of incision. In the case of Limberg and his followers, a generally rounded defect must be turned into a geometric figure, which inevitably results in the further excision of healthy skin. The flap must be cut exactly to the same size as the defect. Our three types of flaps allow the line of incision to be adjusted to the shape of the defect, and the flap is not only swung but slid into place.

INDICATIONS

Coverage of a round or oval defect is always difficult if the wound is large in relation to its surroundings. Among the many procedures possible, a local pedicle flap is most advantageous because it matches skin color and texture and has the potential for preserving sensibility. The slide-swing skin flap permits closure of a wound using flaps that are small in comparison to the defect. The flap is swung over as usual, with the base of the flap following in the same direction. Concurrently, the skin surrounding the defect is slid. The principle involves exploiting the displacement of the skin necessary to close the secondary defect while reducing the original defect as a result.

The slide-swing plasty may be employed on almost all parts of the body. The size of the flap is dependent on the elasticity of the skin. This is greatest in the region of the trunk, especially in the area of the flank, and in the back, abdomen, and buttocks. Skin reserves decrease in the distal regions of the limbs and are reduced on the scalp. The possibilities of closing a defect are dictated by its size and location.

The main indications for the slide-swing plasty are the defects that remain after removing tumors (see Fig. 3), skin dysplasias, or scars that result from injuries. To avoid distortion of facial structures in the case of larger defects, undermining of the skin and subcutaneous tissue should be undertaken mainly in the direction of the peripheral parts of the face. The slide-swing flap may be used even in places where other methods are doomed to failure. For example, the slide-swing plasty can be used on the nose and in other less elastic skin areas where pure transposition flaps require skin grafting.

FLAP DESIGN AND DIMENSIONS

A more thorough analysis of the slide-swing skin flap reveals that it is in part founded on the principles of the triangular exchange plasty (Z-plasty), the exact trigonometric rules for which were laid down by Limberg (2). The slide-swing plasty is partly a combination of two asymmetrical figures with a common median incision, also known as the *basic incision*. In contrast to the exchange plasty and to other methods further developed by Limberg in which all incisions were straight, all lines of incision in slide-swing flaps take the form of arcs that are partly stretched, with one exception (i.e., the initial section of the median incision that forms the bottom angle of the defect).

The additional mobilization of the skin around the defect as a part of the technique leads to a reduction in the size of the defect. Exploiting the extent of skin reserves, the flap can be cut smaller than the defect. This has the effect of reducing the size of the defect as well as the resultant scars. Unlike conventional transposition flaps and those of Limberg, incisions in our flap types are never made parallel. Instead, the flap narrows to a point. In addition, the sides of the flap are not cut to the same length, thus increasing the size of the flap base. Three basic types of flaps have been developed (Fig. 1).

Type 1

This technique is used to close a round defect. The flap can be laid out at any point on the round defect. The excision of the defect is arranged so that a right angle is formed at the base of the flap. The resulting movement of the skin reduces the size of the formerly round defect so that the shape of the closed defect corresponds more or less to that of the flap.

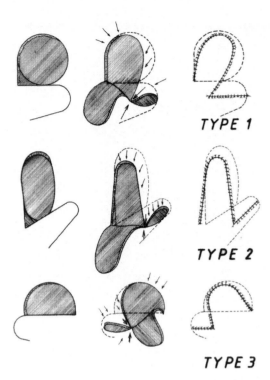

FIG. 1. The three types of slide-swing skin plasty. (From Schrudde, Petrovici, ref. 1, with permission.)

Type 2

The same principle is involved when using an oblong flap to close a defect. Here care must be taken to ensure that when closing the secondary defect the movement of the skin leads to a reduction in the length of the defect. This technique is significant for the blood supply because the width is in inverse proportion to the length. Therefore, the pole of the incision made at the flap base, removed from the defect, is placed vertically under the slip of skin to be slid into the place created by the formation of the flap and the edge of the defect.

Type 3

This technique allows the use of a straight stretch of an otherwise round defect edge when forming the flap. The actual flap is kept quite small as a result of skin sliding to close the secondary defect and of further sliding of the skin surrounding the defect. Relative to the size of the area operated on, there are few scars. Depending on the site of the defect, a type 2 flap is sometimes converted into a type 3 flap to improve blood supply.

Mobilization of both the rounded flap and the three-cornered flap to close the secondary defect calls for elasticity of the surrounding skin. The slide-swing plasty combines the principle of transposition flaps with that of skin sliding. The triangular flap with which the secondary defect is closed is extremely mobile. By sliding it in the direction of the secondary defect, some of the circumference is drawn with it, thus reducing the size of the defect. The secondary defect extends only marginally into healthy surrounding tissue, and less scar formation is the welcome result. In the case of a Z-plasty, the triangular skin flaps are separated from their underlying tissue down to their bases. When using the slide-swing flap, the skin surrounding the defect is also mobilized, resulting in skin movement in all directions. The special recommendation of this method is that all the skin reserves around the defect are exploited.

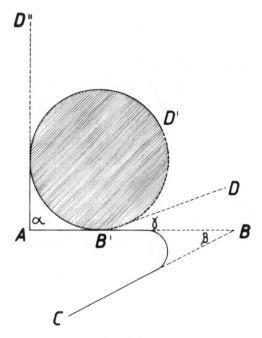

FIG. 2. Geometric principles of slide-swing plasty with exchange of asymmetrical triangles. (From Schrudde, Petrovici, ref. 1, with permission.)

Head and Neck Area

In the head and neck area, the more caudal the defect, the easier it is to use the method because of the elasticity of the skin. When properly planned, the technique permits optimal restoration of the contours of the head and neck. The slide-swing plasty produces especially good results in early treatment of a facial injury. The injury is thoroughly cleaned, and its irregular edges are excised slightly to give it a more or less round shape. A slide-swing plasty then is outlined in accordance with the position and extent of the defect. A type 3 flap, with the advantages already mentioned, is best.

OPERATIVE TECHNIQUE

In the case of type 1 slide-swing flaps, two skin flaps and the underlying tissue are mobilized and swung into place (Figs. 2 and 3). First, there is the round flap with sides to meet at an acute angle (β), if one imagines them extended. On the opposite side, on the median incision AB, there is a right angle (α). The flap $AB'C$ is used to close the defect. Second, the flap employed in closing the secondary defect is situated between the defect and the transposition flap at an acute angle (γ). The median line $B'B$ between the angles (β) and (γ) is part of the basic incision AB, which belongs to the figure $D'ABC$.

Swinging the flap into the defect is the equivalent of an asymmetric exchange plasty ($D'ABC$), with the basic incision AB and the differing side angles (α) and (β). The flap $AB'C$ is thereby rounded off to fit the defect, resulting in better blood supply. Along with the transposition of the flap, angle γ is moved into the place of angle β; angle γ is increased, following the movement to C that results from straightening the line $D'B'$, increasing the blood supply.

CLINICAL RESULTS

The slide-swing flap has proved to be of great practical use. This plasty was used in more than 1,600 patients between 1962 and 1982 at the Department of Plastic Surgery at the University of Cologne. Primary healing was achieved in almost every patient. Delayed healing as a result of necrosis of the distal portions of the flap usually was the consequence of poor design in the ratio of length and width, as well as impaired circulation postoperatively because of pressure. We never observed total flap loss. In case of partial necrosis, another slide-swing plasty or free skin transplant should be tried. If granulation tissue cannot be removed completely, as is often the case in bedsores, fistulas may result. Hematomas under

A–C

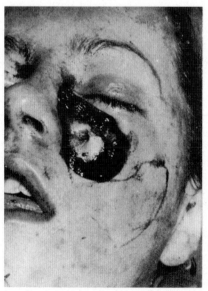
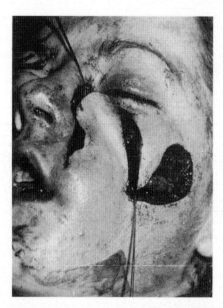
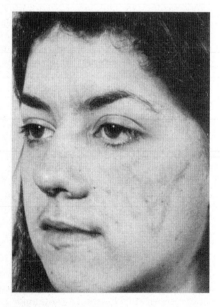

FIG. 3. A: Rhabdomyosarcoma on left cheek removed, leaving a defect of 8 × 5 cm. A type 2 slide-swing plasty is drawn. **B:** Transposition of the flap. **C:** After 5 years, no signs of relapse or metastases of the tumor.

large flaps are not unusual and should be removed completely as soon as possible.

SUMMARY

The slide-swing flap combines the principle of transposition with skin sliding. This permits the closure of large, round defects with flaps that are smaller than the original defect.

References

1. Schrudde J, Petrovici V. The use of slide-swing plasty in closing skin defects: a clinical study based on 1308 cases. *Plast Reconstr Surg* 1981; 67:467.
2. Limberg AA. Design of local flaps. In: Gibson T, ed., *Modern trends of plastic surgery*. London: Butterworth, 1966;38–61.

CHAPTER 112 ■ CERVICAL SKIN FLAPS TO THE CHEEK

V. Y. BAKAMJIAN

See Chapters 118 and 120. The same cervical skin flaps as are described for intraoral lining can be used to cover external cheek defects (Figs. 1 and 2).

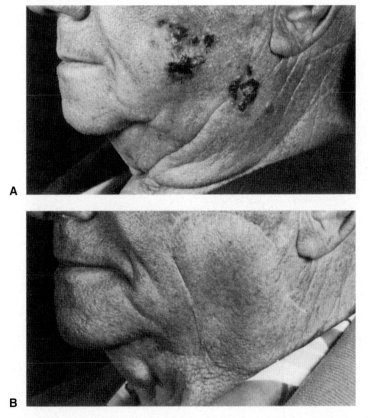

FIG. 1. Transverse cervical skin flap to the cheek in a male patient. **A:** Multicentric pigmented basal cell carcinoma. **B:** Result after wide resection and repair.

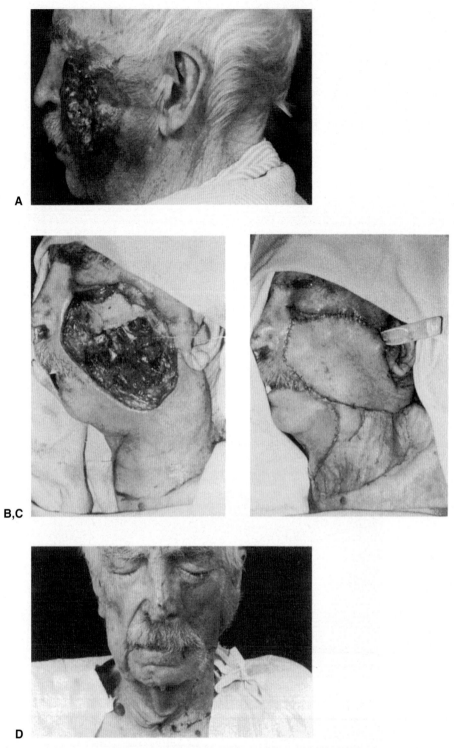

FIG. 2. Oblique cervical skin flap to the cheek in a 90-year-old patient. **A:** Neglected squamous cell carcinoma. **B:** Defect after wide resection with outline of the flap. **C:** The repair with the donor site covered with a split-thickness skin graft. **D:** The final result.

CHAPTER 113 ■ TRANSPOSITION NECK-TO-CHEEK SKIN FLAPS

C. C. COLEMAN, JR., AND M. J. TAVIS*

The need for an abundance of relaxed tissue lying within the operative field has prompted the use of a posteriorly based neck flap to cover cheek defects.

INDICATIONS

The posteriorly based flap, when raised, affords a broad exposure for formal neck dissection and also provides tissue for defects in the cheek and mandibular regions. The posteriorly based neck flap can be used for various defects, including cancers of the parotid, radionecrosis with persistent cancer invading the mandible, and skin malignancy involving the jaw and mouth.

ANATOMY

The neck skin has been used as a pedicle-flap donor site by numerous workers (1–4). Most of the reports deal with neck flaps that are based inferiorly and are migrated in a clockwise direction (5–9), primarily by stretching the posterolateral neck skin. Such flaps will successfully close sizable cheek defects, but their blood supply is greatly jeopardized by an associated radical neck dissection. The division of the deep fascia requires that all three branches of the supraclavicular plexus of arteries, veins, and nerves be ligated.

Studies have shown that the blood flow in the cervical skin comes from a lateral direction (10). The posteriorly based flap is not compromised by an associated radical neck dissection because muscular branches of the vertebral, occipital, and superior thyroid arteries are not affected by the dissection. Although the posteriorly based cervical skin flap includes the platysma muscle, the blood supply is random in nature.

FLAP DESIGN AND DIMENSIONS

With the patient supine, the neck is extended and the head is rotated in the opposite direction, thus placing the deep cervical fascia under maximal tension and thereby facilitating ele-

vation of the flap. The flap is based on the anterior border of the trapezius muscle. It is outlined roughly parallel to the mandible over as far as the midline of the neck as a well-rounded structure. The lower border of the flap parallels the clavicle. The degree of rotation depends on the angle. The lower incision follows over the posteroinferior trapezius (Fig. 1A).

OPERATIVE TECHNIQUE

Following surgical delineation of the cheek resection, the neck flap is elevated down to the deep cervical fascia and reflected posteriorly. The extirpative procedure then is carried out through this ample exposure. When the composite resection is completed, the adjustment in the lower incision will provide easy relaxed closure of the face with the rotation neck flap (Fig. 1B). Although there are some reports (4–9) to the contrary, we believe that closure of the neck defect always requires a split-thickness skin graft (Fig. 1C) or, in some cases, a rotation chest flap (also based posteriorly) (Figs. 2–4).

CLINICAL RESULTS

In no patient has there been any tissue loss in these flaps, and the associated grafts on the donor site have been successful in every patient. Because of the position and size of the neck defect in rounded, laterally based flaps, a skin graft or additional chest rotation flap is always necessary.

Another disadvantage of these flaps is that they are so thin that contour problems are frequently present, particularly when segments of the facial skeleton are removed in the resection. In such instances, the bulky pectoralis major island musculocutaneous flap is more desirable.

All neck flaps produce rotation redundancies that necessitate secondary minor surgical procedures. At least one segment of the facial scar (medial) and the medial edge of the skin graft or second rotation flap will require Z-plasty release.

SUMMARY

Posteriorly based neck flaps are helpful, time-proven adjuncts to extirpative surgery of the face and jaws.

---

* Deceased.

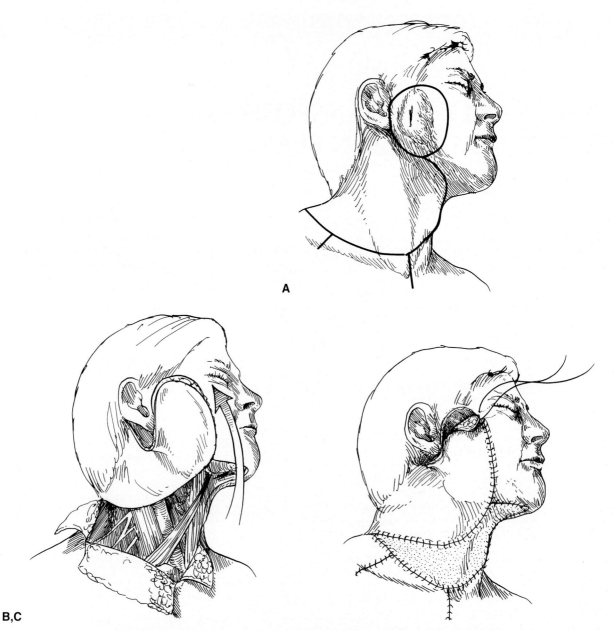

FIG. 1. A: Drawing of large round rotation flap extending to or slightly beyond the midline of the neck. As the inferior part of the incision is carried over the trapezius, the degree of cephalad extension will determine the amount of rotation. **B:** The donor wound in the neck gives ample room for radical neck dissection. Occasionally, two divergent radial incisions in the lower part of the neck skin are necessary in order to gain access to the insertion of the sternocleidomastoid muscle and internal jugular vein. **C:** Closure of the neck is accomplished with a split-thickness skin graft.

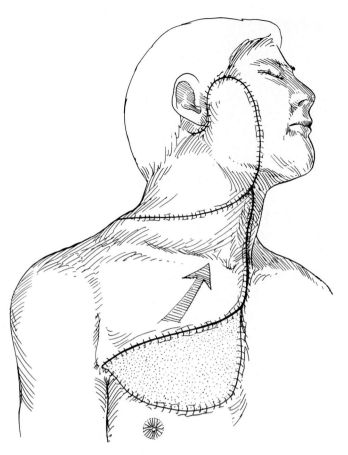

FIG. 2.   In some patients, a second rotation flap in the upper lateral chest is used to close the neck wound. This obviates placing a skin graft over the carotid axis and transfers skin-graft coverage to a less vital area.

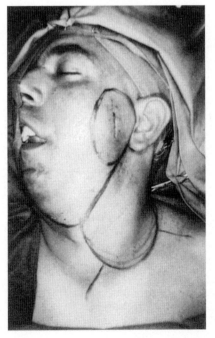
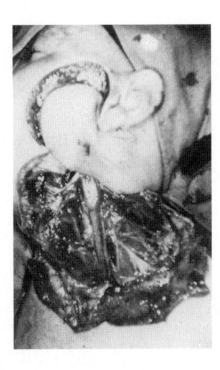

A,B

FIG. 3. **A:** Composite resection of cheek and parotid outlined. Injudicious open biopsy of tumor necessitated the cheek resection. **B:** The exposure of the neck structures affords ample room for radical neck dissection. Note blood stain on central portion of flap.

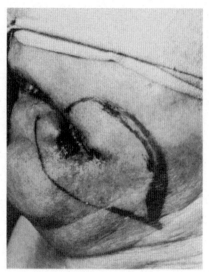
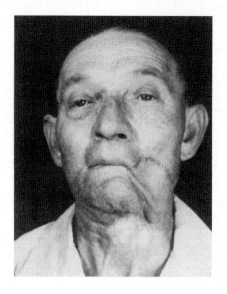

A,B

FIG. 4. **A:** Deeply infiltrating basal cell carcinoma extending through full thickness of cheek and oral commissure. The tumor extended along the gingivobuccal sulcus at the level of the jaw. An anteriorly based tongue flap was used for lining. **B:** Rotation neck flap transferred as cover for the operative defect. A split-thickness skin graft was needed for closure of the defect.

References

1. Hadjistomaff B. Restoration of the cheek by using the skin of the jaw-neck region. *Plast Reconstr Surg* 1947;2:127.
2. Hoffman G. Full-thickness resection of the cheek with one-stage reconstruction. *Am Surg* 1968;34:68.
3. Conley J. *Regional flaps of the head and neck*. Philadelphia: WB Saunders, 1976;176–187.
4. Kaplan I, Goldwyn RM. The versatility of the laterally based cervicofacial flap. *Plast Reconstr Surg* 1978;61:390.
5. Smith F. Flaps utilized in facial and cervical reconstruction. *Plast Reconstr Surg* 1951;7:415.
6. Stark RE, Kaplan J. Rotation flaps, neck to cheek. *Plast Reconstr Surg* 1972;50:230.
7. Crow ML, Crow J. Resurfacing large cheek defects with rotation flaps from the neck. *Plast Reconstr Surg* 1976;58:196.
8. Juri J, Juri C. Advancement and rotation of large cervicofacial flaps for cheek reconstruction. *Plast Reconstr Surg* 1979;64:692.
9. Coleman CC. Flaps for floor of the mouth and cheek reconstruction. In: Grabb WC, Myers MB, eds., *Skin flaps*. Boston: Little, Brown, 1975; 337–350.
10. Freeland AP, Rogers J. The vascular supply of the cervical skin with reference to incision planning. *Laryngoscope* 1975;85:714.

CHAPTER 114 ■ CERVICAL ROTATION SKIN FLAP FOR RECONSTRUCTION OF THE CHEEK

R. B. STARK

The cervical rotation flap, well vascularized by branches of the external carotid artery, offers a nearly ideal means of surfacing the aesthetic unit of the cheek (1–5).

INDICATIONS

Cervical flaps have been used to resurface the cheek when dermatoses have been removed (i.e., epitheliomas, hemangiomas, radiodermatitis, superficial melanoma, blue nevus of Ota, and

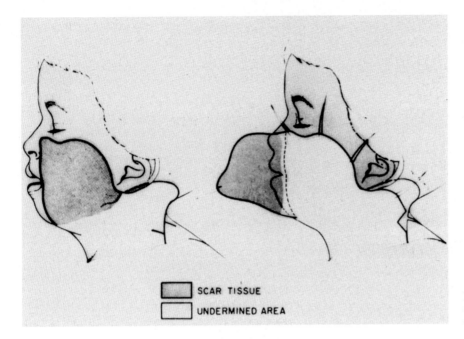

SCAR TISSUE

UNDERMINED AREA

FIG. 1. The area of scar tissue (*shaded*) is excised, and the cervical flap is undermined completely and rotated to cover the defect.

noma) and for oral-cutaneous fistulas and scarring from burns and lupus erythematosus.

FLAP DESIGN AND DIMENSIONS

The size of the flap is dependent on the surface area of the neck. In the average-sized adult, the rotation flap, which resembles an acute angle more than it does a hemicircle, may measure 10 cm on each of its two sides (along the body of the mandible and along the hairline of the neck).

OPERATIVE TECHNIQUE

With rotation superiorly and medially, the side adjacent to the mandibular body shifts to the nasolabial line and side wall of the nose. The side next to the hairline is elongated by a generous back cut into the base of the flap (parallel to the clavicle). The flap then shifts up to the infraorbital rim, the zygomatic arch, and along the posterior hairline. The back-cut incision opens as a V when rotation of the flap begins and is virtually a straight line when it reaches its final position. A cut a few centimeters proximally on the opposite side of the wound produces a Z that facilitates wound closure at this point.

As a general principle, the flap should be raised before the lesion is removed to determine adequacy of cover and vascularity (Fig. 1). The flap consists of full-thickness skin and subcutaneous tissue whose thickness is that of a rhytidectomy flap.

In the postoperative period, tension on the flap can be minimized by positioning. The head is turned toward the flap, and the ipsilateral shoulder is hunched, with that arm placed across the chest, the hand resting on the opposite shoulder. This arm-chest relationship is maintained by a padded elastic bandage of Velpeau design. A head cap of the operating room type is joined to the Velpeau by adhesive bands.

CLINICAL RESULTS

In a series of 27 patients, there was one incident of a postoperative hematoma when the flap replaced a hemangioma, necessitating evacuation and resuture. In three instances, the distal end of the flap failed to survive. The remaining flap was later rerotated successfully.

SUMMARY

The cervical rotation skin flap is ideal for reconstructing cheek defects.

References

1. Gonzalez-Ulloa M, Castillo A, Stevens E, et al. Preliminary study of total restoration of facial skin. *Plast Reconstr Surg* 1954;13:151.
2. Stark RB. The pantographic expansion principle as applied to the advancement flap. *Plast Reconstr Surg* 1955;15:222.
3. Stark RB. *Plastic surgery.* New York: Hoeber, 1962;106,146.
4. Stark RB, Kaplan M. Rotation flaps neck to cheek. *Plast Reconstr Surg* 1972;50:230.
5. Stark RB. Resurfacing the face. *Clin Plast Surg* 1975;2:577.

CHAPTER 115 ■ CERVICOFACIAL SKIN FLAP TO THE CHEEK

R. M. GOLDWYN

The cervicofacial flap involves the lower cheek and upper neck. It is based laterally not medially, as is usually described (1).

INDICATIONS

The cervicofacial flap is particularly suitable for patients who are middle-aged or older because of the laxity of the cervical skin that allows a primary closure of the donor area. It has been used without difficulty in younger patients; however, a skin graft may be required in the neck to prevent excessive pulling on the lower lid. The flap can be used, with or without lining, for closure of a cheek defect that also requires a radical neck dissection because the opening on the neck can be approximated without resorting to a distant flap. In my experience, this flap has its greatest usefulness for closure of cheek defects ranging from 4 × 4 cm to 6 × 7 cm.

ANATOMY

Although random, the cervicofacial skin flap is richly supplied, primarily by the external maxillary artery and vein and their branches. It is not necessary to include the platysma for blood supply.

FLAP DESIGN AND DIMENSIONS

No flap delaying procedure is required. The skin portion of this laterally based flap usually measures 9.5 cm wide at its base and 12 cm long.

OPERATIVE TECHNIQUE

Flap dissection on the cheek usually follows or parallels the nasolabial fold and then goes across the mandible down to the midcervical region or lower, where dissection is maintained superficial to the platysma muscle to avoid injury to the mandibular branch of the facial nerve. In the midneck, the flap is cut transversely to a point over the sternocleidomastoid muscle and then superiorly and posteriorly to the earlobe or mastoid area.

If the flap is rotated into the lower eyelid, it is advisable to anchor it to the deep tissues of the orbit and the nose to avoid ectropion from its weight. Similarly, the excision should be carried laterally beyond and above the outer canthus onto the temporal region, where the flap also can be fastened to provide a supportive sling under the lower lid.

Closure of the donor area in the neck can be accomplished usually by beginning posteriorly and laterally and going medially, ending with a Y. If necessary, a split-thickness skin graft can be taken from an inconspicuous donor area and used in the neck to decrease tension on the flap, thereby lessening the possibility of ectropion. A few months later, the skin graft can be excised on an outpatient basis under local anesthesia.

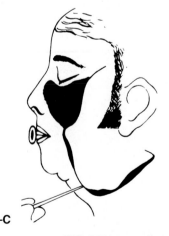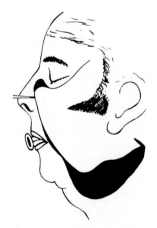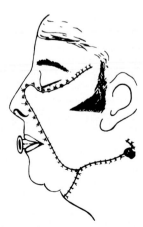

A–C

FIG. 1. Diagram of patient at time of operation. **A:** After excision of tumor and development of the cervicofacial flap. **B:** Rotation of flap. **C:** Closure.

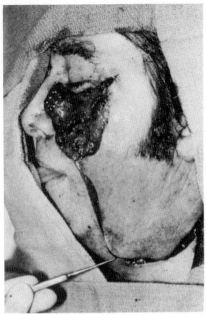
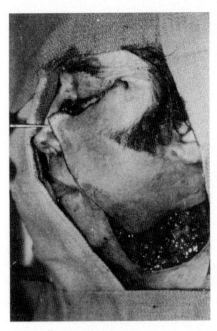
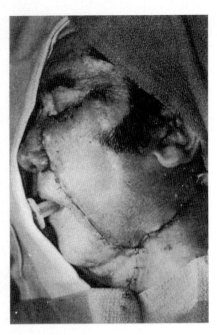

A–C

FIG. 2. A 46-year-old man with sclerosing basal cell carcinoma of 2 years' duration. **A:** After excision of tumor and development of the cervicofacial flap. **B:** Flap rotated. **C:** Primary closure of recipient and donor sites. (From Kaplan, Goldwyn, ref. 1, with permission.)

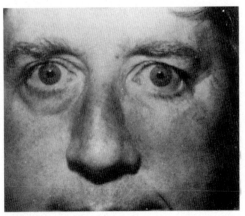
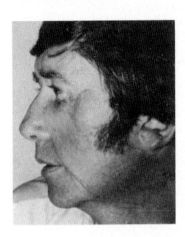

A,B

FIG. 3. **A,B:** Appearance 3 years postoperatively. (From Kaplan, Goldwyn, ref. 1, with permission.)

At completion of the operation, a Penrose drain can be placed inferiorly and posteriorly, extending upward for the length of the flap. It is removed in 36 to 48 hours. If the patient's head is kept slightly flexed postoperatively, the flap will be subjected to less pull (Figs. 1–3).

In 6 months, this discomfort disappeared. Two patients for whom a skin graft was used for closure of the donor site later had their graft excised and a Z-plasty used to avoid a straight-line hypertrophic scar under the neck. No patient has reported any functional deficit from the use of the flap.

CLINICAL RESULTS

If the flap is contemplated in male patients, they should be warned that their beard line will be slightly higher than normal. This discrepancy has not caused any complaints in my patients. In none of the 17 patients for whom this flap has been used within the past 4 years has there been a problem with necrosis, infection, or failure to achieve adequate closure of the defect and donor site. One patient had the sensation of "pulling" of his lower lid but no evidence of actual ectropion.

SUMMARY

The cervicofacial flap is a useful, well-tolerated flap for closing cheek defects with or without an associated radical neck dissection.

Reference

1. Kaplan I, Goldwyn RM. The versatility of the laterally based cervicofacial flap for cheek repairs. *Plast Reconstr Surg* 1978;61:390.

CHAPTER 116. Cervicopectoral Skin Flap to the Cheek *D. W. Becker, Jr*
www.encyclopediaofflaps.com

CHAPTER 117 ■ KITE FLAP IN FACIAL RECONSTRUCTIVE SURGERY

J.-L. DUCOURS, P. POIZAC, D. RICHARD, J. AFTIMOS,
J. UNANUE, B. MARAUD, A. WANGERMEZ,
C. ORRETEGUY, AND C. AUGUSTIN

EDITORIAL COMMENT

This is a nice design modification of the subcutaneous advancement flap that will cover a circular defect with good cosmetic results.

The kite flap is a triangular cutaneous advancement flap with a subcutaneous pedicle. Vascularization is ensured by a segmental arterial network made up of vertical ascending branches that guarantee considerable security. The flap is relatively easy to transfer and yields excellent cosmetic results (1,2).

INDICATIONS

Use of this flap is mainly in reconstructive facial surgery for repair of defects following excision of cutaneous tumors (3), preferentially in the cheek and in the suborbital and glabellar regions. Because the flap depends on linear sliding rather than rotation, distortion is reduced in adjacent areas, and the initial loss of substance in the defect can be distributed around the flap and along the V–Y closure. For extensive orbital tumors (4), external canthus loss near the eyelid edge (5), or scar ectropion requiring skin grafting (6), solutions other than the kite flap are necessary. This applies also to defects of the chin or upper lip.

ANATOMY

The area of the subcutaneous pedicle is not well defined, and its extent is greater than mere projection from the cutaneous plane would indicate. Mobilization of the cutaneous triangle of the kite flap requires a considerable amount of adjacent subcutaneous tissue. This increases flap vascularization and ensures greater ease of transfer. The pedicle is usually fatty but sometimes can be muscular, particularly in the suborbital region when pedicled on the orbicularis oculi muscle.

According to the arterial classification proposed by Kunert (7), the kite flap is a segmental flap based on ascending vessels from an axial network comprising longitudinal vessels that make the flap quite reliable (see Fig. 3). Venous return is modeled on the arterial network.

FLAP DESIGN AND DIMENSIONS

The flap is designed after tumor excision (Figs. 1 and 2), when the margins of healthy tissue can be determined. To ensure optimal advancement, the subcutaneous tissue must be sufficiently thick and loose to allow efficient flap transfer. A line is drawn from the center of the defect and parallel to minimal lines of tension on the skin. The tip of this triangular-shaped flap is positioned on the initial vertical incision line (Fig. 3). Flap length is generally equal to 2.5 times its width. The kite-flap variation proposed by Ichiro (8), although reducing the length of the necessary incision and allowing the scar to be

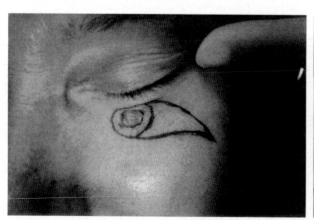
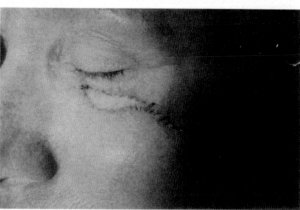

FIG. 1. Basal-cell carcinoma of the median suborbital region. **A:** Flap design and excision limits. **B:** Flap in place.

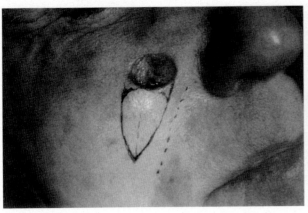
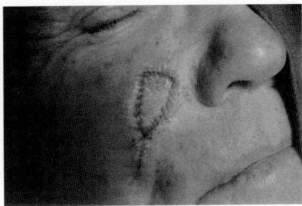

A   B

FIG. 2. After excision of nasogenian basal-cell carcinoma. **A:** Drawing of the flap. **B:** Immediate result.

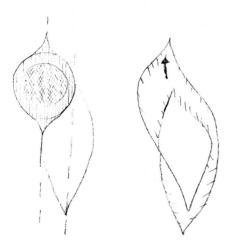

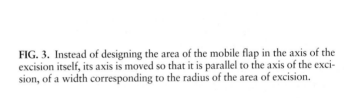

FIG. 3. Instead of designing the area of the mobile flap in the axis of the excision itself, its axis is moved so that it is parallel to the axis of the excision, of a width corresponding to the radius of the area of excision.

inserted in a fold slightly outside the area of flap excision, nevertheless appears to create local distortion of the subcutaneous tissue.

OPERATIVE TECHNIQUE

The incision reaches the fatty subcutaneous plane. It is advisable to undermine widely around the flap in the same plane, especially at the flap tip, to ensure ease of transfer. Traction with Gillies' hooks enables noting the areas where additional tissue removal is necessary.

When the upper part of the flap can be easily inset into the defect without tension, the first subcutaneous stitch is placed at the middle of the flap base and then at both ends, corresponding to an acute angle that matches the shape of the defect. Subcutaneous stitches then are placed from the base to the tip of the flap. These are important in avoiding the "cushion" effect that some detractors of this flap have criticized (9).

Closure of the donor site is carried out in a simple V–Y fashion. It is often necessary to position the closure to avoid a cutaneous dog-ear. A corner stitch is placed at the junction of the V–Y flap closure, and overstitching with Prolene ensures optimal apposition of the cutaneous edges.

CLINICAL RESULTS

The kite flap has been used in areas where slackness and thickness of subcutaneous tissue allow optimal advancement. In the suborbital region, it has been used for external and median

defects, with care taken not to turn out the lower eyelid. In the nasogenian region, we have repaired defects not extending into the nasal or orbital regions, and the flap has also been used in the glabellar region for defects between the eyebrows. The kite flap should not be used for reconstructing defects of the chin or upper lip.

SUMMARY

Because this flap allows cutaneous transfer by linear sliding, without rotation or distortion, it can yield excellent cosmetic results.

References

1. Dufourmentel C. Le lambeau cerf-volant: Le lambeau insulaire de glissement avec plastie en VY. *Ann Chir Plast* 1970;15:344.
2. Marchac D. *Chirurgie des baso de la face*, Geneva: Medicate Hygiene, 1986.
3. Ducours JL, Richard D, Aftimos J, et al. Le lambeau "cerf-volant" dans la reconstruction après exérèse de carcinome baso-cellulaires de la face. *Rev Stomatol Chir Maxillofac* 1989;90:345.
4. Mustardé JC. The use of flaps in the orbital region. *Plast Reconstr Surg* 1970;45:146.
5. Converse JM. *Reconstructive plastic surgery*, vol. II. Philadelphia: WB Saunders, 1964;676.
6. Grignon JL. L'ectropion de la paupière inférieure post-traumatique et après chirurgie correctrice. *Ann Chir Plast* 1971;16:127.
7. Kunert P. Structure and construction: the system of skin flaps. *Ann Plast Surg* 1991;27:509.
8. Ono I, Gunji H, Sato M, Kaneko F. Use of the oblique island flap in excision of small facial tumors. *Plast Reconstr Surg* 1993;91:1245.
9. Lejour M, De Mey A, Andry G. Revue de 52 lambeaux de glissement en llot de la joue. *Ann Chir Plast* 1982;27:20.

CHAPTER 118 ■ POSTERIOR CERVICAL FLAPS

I. K. DHAWAN AND N. C. MADAN

The skin from the back of the neck has not been used often for facial reconstruction. Its use as a random flap raised in vascular areas of the scalp on the neck has been described for the repair of pharyngeal fistulas (1) and for other head and neck defects (2). We have described a posterior cervical flap for facial defects (3).

INDICATIONS

We have used this flap in the repair of cheek and lip defects after excisional surgery for tumors and trauma (see Figs. 2 and 3). It can provide either lining or cover or both for a full-thickness defect.

ANATOMY

The flap depends on the occipital artery for its nutrition, and its base is formed by a horizontal line joining the mastoid process to the midline posteriorly. The flap extends vertically downward to the nape of the neck, up to the D2–3 spinous process (Fig. 1). For better reach, the trunk of the occipital artery may be divided and the flap extended into the temporal region, where it depends for its blood supply on the posterior branch of the superficial temporal artery and its anastomosis with the occipital artery (see Fig. 3).

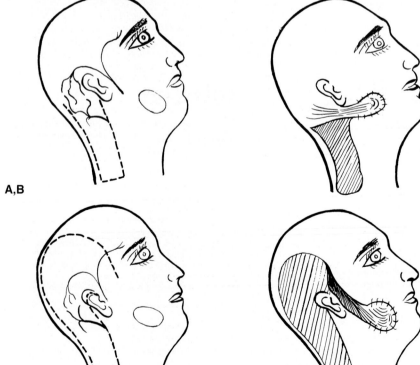

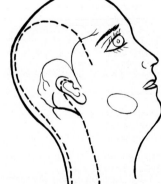

A,B

C,D

FIG. 1. **A,B:** The flap may have its base between the mastoid and occiput and is then served by the occipital artery. **B–D:** When an extra length is required for a longer reach, however, it may be extended into the temporal region, where it is served by the posterior branch of the superficial temporal artery and its anastomosis with the occipital artery. (From Dhawan et al., ref. 3, with permission.)

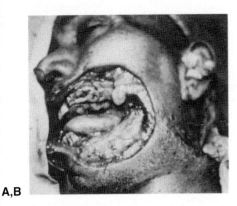
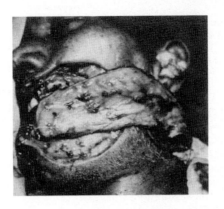

A,B

FIG. 2. A: The defect after excision of cheek mucosa cancer B: The posterior cervical flap in place for lining. Cover was provided by a scalp flap. (From Dhawan et al., ref. 3, with permission.)

The occipital artery runs on the superior oblique muscle and enters the superficial fascia of the scalp at the junction of the medial and intermediate thirds of the superior nuchal line, passing either through the trapezius or between the trapezius and the sternocleidomastoid. At this point, its pulsations are palpable. Its terminal branches anastomose freely with the superficial temporal artery, and a descending branch has been described arising from it.

FLAP DESIGN AND DIMENSIONS

Such a flap in an adult is usually about 8 cm wide and 20 cm long. It is unlikely to survive when the external carotid artery has been ligated during excisional surgery of the face. The flap needs to be raised in a lateral position, which involves either a change of position after excisional surgery or carrying out the excisional surgery in a lateral position, which is a bit awkward. The base of the flap is on the superior nuchal line, and the incisions extend vertically down to the D2–3 level. Such a flap can be rotated through 90 degrees with its pivot point at the medial end of the base and will reach to provide hairless

lining or cover for cheek defects. The flap leaves no frontal defect and can provide a large amount of skin.

OPERATIVE TECHNIQUE

The occipital artery is marked preoperatively at the superior nuchal line as it enters the superficial fascia of the scalp. The posterior branch of the superficial temporal artery is also marked. The flap is raised with the patient in the lateral position. The incisions extend through the deep fascia, the flap is raised with the deep fascia up to the nuchal line, and great care is taken to preserve the occipital artery. Because the deep fascia is closely applied to the muscle, raising the flap necessarily involves cutting through the muscle.

When a longer length of carrier segment is required, however, such as when the flap needs to be turned in for lining also, the trunk of the occipital artery may be ligated deep to the trapezius insertion and very close to the periosteum. The flap is then extended to the temporal region on a pedicle that includes the posterior branch of the superficial temporal artery. The pedicle is raised in a plane between the periosteum and the

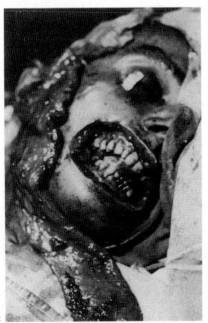
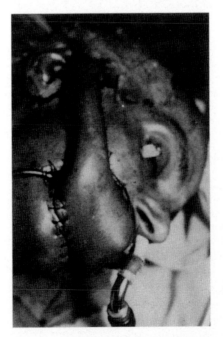
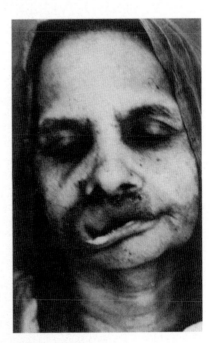

A–C

FIG. 3. A: A large squamous cell cancer of the lip. The defect left after excision and the posterior cervical flap raised and extended into the temporal region. B: The appearance after the flap is inserted. C: The final result. (From Dhawan et al., ref. 3, with permission.)

aponeurosis. The flap then derives its blood supply from the posterior branch of the superficial temporal artery and its free anastomosis with the occipital artery. When using this flap for lining and cover, it should preferably be folded axially unless the amount of lining required is small (Figs. 2 and 3).

CLINICAL RESULTS

We have used the posterior cervical flap based on the occipital artery in 16 patients to provide lining (13 patients), cover (two patients), and for both functions (one patient) in large orocutaneous fistulas left after excision of cheek cancer. Among these 16 patients, one flap was lost, and an additional flap was required. There was partial marginal loss in another three patients, but these did not require new flaps. In the remaining 12 patients (75%), there was no loss and the flaps functioned well.

Extension of the posterior cervical flap into the temporal region to the territory of the posterior branch of the superficial temporal artery was used in another 12 patients. With these, there was no loss in seven patients (about 60%). There was a partial loss in two patients (16%), requiring additional flaps. In 10 of the 12 patients, the flap was used to provide lin-

ing and cover in large orocutaneous fistulas left after excision of cheek cancer. In another two patients, it was used to provide total repair of upper lip loss following an injury. Flap loss can be reduced when providing both lining and cover by folding the flap axially rather than contraaxially. In addition, the mouth should be kept open, because a closed mouth is likely to compress the flap at the fold.

SUMMARY

A posterior cervical flap can be used for both lining and cover in the reconstruction of cheek defects.

References

1. Zovickian A. Pharyngeal fistulae, repair and prevention, using mastoid occiput based shoulder flaps. *Plast Reconstr Surg* 1957;19:355.
2. Chretien PB, Ketcham AS, Hage RC, Gretner HR. Extended shoulder flap and its use in reconstruction of the defects of head and neck. *Am J Surg* 1969;18:752.
3. Dhawan IK, Madan NC, Mehta, SN. Posterior cervical flaps for the repair of defects of the face. In: *Transactions of the sixth international congress of plastic and reconstructive surgeons*. Paris: Masson, 1976;387.

CHAPTER 119 ■ SUBMENTAL ADVANCEMENT SKIN FLAP TO THE CHIN

J. W. SNOW

Occasionally, one is presented with the problem of resurfacing the skin over the chin, a situation usually secondary to a skin defect created by excision of cancerous or precancerous tissue.

FLAP DESIGN AND DIMENSIONS

A submental advancement flap whose superior margin is the mental sulcus can be used for resurfacing the chin. Excision of most of the anatomic unit of the chin is marked out (Fig. 1A). As much skin and deeper tissue as necessary is removed for complete tumor excision. The fat pad will be carried with the submental skin to help carry the blood supply.

OPERATIVE TECHNIQUE

Fig. 1B shows the outline of the submental flap. The submental keyhole-like flap was elevated to the junction with the neck. The lateral triangles produced by the configuration of the flap (Fig. 1C) were sutured together to advance the submental flap.

The neck then was slightly flexed and the flap advanced to the mental sulcus. Subcuticular sutures were used at the base of the flap to advance it distally and to release pressure at the distal suture line (Fig. 1D).

CLINICAL RESULTS

The wound healed per primam in the patient illustrated. The multicentric basal cell carcinoma was completely excised. With healing, full neck extension was obtained gradually, and the patient's cosmetic results were satisfactory (Fig. 1E). It has now been 6 years since her surgery; there has been no evidence of recurrence, and her surgical reconstruction is generally not noticeable.

SUMMARY

A submental skin flap can be advanced to reconstruct chin defects.

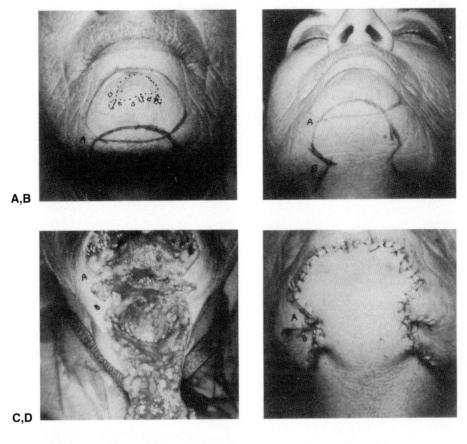

A,B

C,D

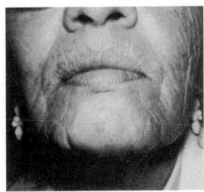

E

FIG. 1. **A:** In the midportion of the chin was what appeared to be a 3 × 1.5-cm basal cell carcinoma with adjacent atrophic skin and suspicious additional small lesions as seen in multicentric basal cell carcinoma. Notice the outline of area to be resected and the dotted outline of the position of tumor that did not show well on the photograph. **B:** Outline of keyhole-shaped submental flap. **C:** Tumor excised and flap elevated back to the neck, leaving the submental fat pad attached to the flap. Note triangles *A* and *B*. **D:** Triangles *A* and *B* sutured together and subcuticular stitches and flexion of the neck allow advancement of the flap to resurface the chin. **E:** Appearance 6 months postoperatively.

CHAPTER 120 ■ BIPEDICLE SUBMENTAL SKIN FLAP

V. Y. BAKAMJIAN

INDICATIONS

The same cervical skin flaps that were described for intraoral lining (see Chapter 184) are easily applied for both the external and internal coverage of facial defects (1). Cervical skin flaps also provide distinctly cosmetic advantages—those of matching color, texture, and degree of hairiness with facial skin.

FLAP DESIGN AND DIMENSIONS

Two mirror-image flaps of a transverse or slightly oblique projection meeting across the midline form a particularly safe

bipedicle variant that may be very useful for chin and lip area applications. The central segment of the bipedicle flap is applied to the area of reconstruction; the pedicles are tubed as carriers on each side.

OPERATIVE TECHNIQUE

Depending on its width, the cervical donor wound is closed either by direct approximation of the edges or with a skin graft. At the time of division, the pedicles are returned to replace all or most of the skin-graft covering on the donor wound (Figs. 1 and 2).

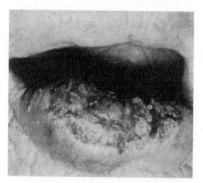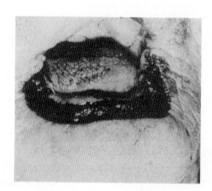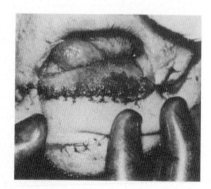

A–C

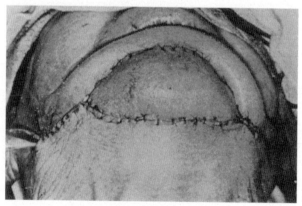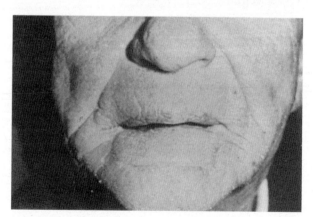

D,E

FIG. 1. Bipedicle submental skin flap to lower lip. A: Squamous cell carcinoma. B: Lower lip total resection. C: Skin flap supplying outer layer and lingual flap providing inner layer and vermilion for the new lip. D: Submental closure of the donor wound. E: Final result. (From Bakamjian, ref. 1, with permission.)

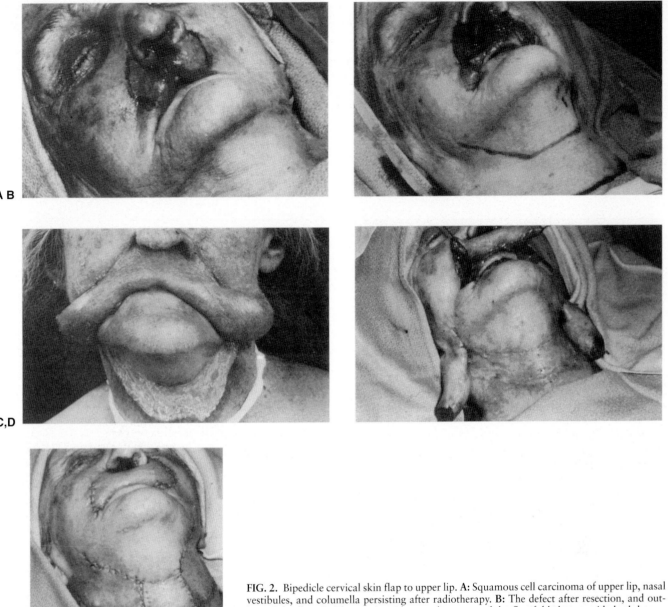

FIG. 2. Bipedicle cervical skin flap to upper lip. **A:** Squamous cell carcinoma of upper lip, nasal vestibules, and columella persisting after radiotherapy. **B:** The defect after resection, and outline of the flap. **C:** The repair, with central segment of the flap folded to provide both layers, and skin graft for the donor wound. **D:** Division of pedicles. **E:** Pedicles returned to replace most of the skin graft on the neck. (From Bakamjian, ref. 1, with permission.)

SUMMARY

Bipedicle submental cervical skin flaps can be used to cover full thickness lip and other facial defects.

Reference

1. Bakamjian VY. The reconstructive use of flaps in cancer surgery of the head and neck. In: Saad MN, Lichtveld P, eds. *Reviews in plastic surgery: general plastic and reconstructive surgery.* Amsterdam: Excerpta Medica, 1974.

CHAPTER 121 ■ SUBMENTAL ISLAND SKIN FLAP

D. MARTIN, P. PELISSIER, AND J. BAUDET

The submental island flap is presented as another cervical flap (1,2) that provides a reliable technique for soft-tissue coverage of the face and also overcomes some inherent disadvantages of random (3,4), superiorly based platysmal muscular or myocutaneous (5–8), and supraclavicular neurovascular flaps (9) (e.g., limited mobility, unacceptable donor-site scars, unpredictable outcomes).

INDICATIONS

This flap has a long (up to 8 cm), reliable pedicle, and cutaneous dimensions can reach up to 7 × 16 cm. It can be used as a cutaneous, musculofascial (cervicofascial and platysma), or osteocutaneous flap. It has an excellent skin color match and a wide arc of rotation, and it can extend over the whole face except for part of the forehead and the whole oral cavity (9). The donor-site scar, concealed under the mandibular arch, is quite acceptable.

ANATOMY

The submental artery (SMA) is a constant branch arising 5 to 6.5 cm from the origin of the facial artery (1,10,11) (Fig. 1). The SMA runs in a groove on the medial aspect of the submandibular gland and is bound medially by the mylohyoid muscle and above by the mandibular border. It ends at the level of the anterior belly of the digastric muscle and may give off a branch to the sublingual gland or one to the lower lip. The skin territories measure 4 × 5 cm to 15 × 7 cm, but possible dimensions of the skin flap are much larger because of the rich subcutaneous and subdermal anastomoses between the two submental arteries.

There is a constant submental vein draining into the facial vein and at least one anastomosing vein between facial and external jugular veins. In some cases, the submental vein may be used for venous drainage of the flap.

FLAP DESIGN AND DIMENSIONS

The upper limit of the flap is along the mandibular arch in the submental region, from the ipsilateral angle to a contralateral point across the midline (Fig. 2). The extent of the flap depends on the width of the cutaneous paddle at the midline. If cervical and submental skin has enough laxity, a 7 × 16-cm flap is possible. A pedicle flap may reach any part of the oral cavity or the lower two thirds of the side of the face and a part of the forehead. A free flap, using good-caliber vessels in the pedicle, including facial artery and veins, and is extremely reliable. It is also possible to use a distal or composite pedicle, taking a segment of the internal basilar margin (Fig. 3).

For a distally based flap with a slightly greater arc of rotation than the proximally based flap, the position of the mandibular branch of the facial nerve, which is the pivotal point for flap rotation, may be a restricting factor in dissection of the pedicle. An osteocutaneous flap can be raised along with a segment of the rim of the mandible, supplied by small periosteal vessels (Fig. 4). Inner cortex is preferable to preserve a smooth mandibular contour. Care should be taken not to injure the inferior alveolar nerve. This flap may be useful in

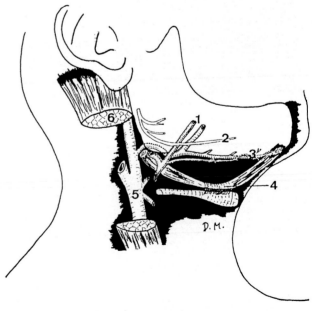

FIG. 1. Diagram of the anatomy: *1*, facial vessels; *2*, mandibular branch of facial nerve; *3*, submental artery and vein; *4*, digastric muscle; *5*, common carotid artery; *6*, sternocleidomastoid muscle. (From Martin et al., ref. 1, with permission.)

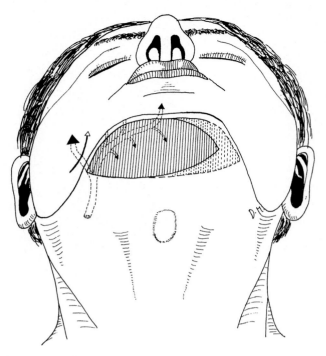

FIG. 2. Outlining of the flap. (From Martin et al., ref. 2, with permission.)

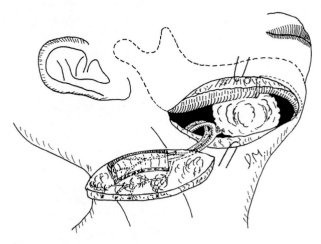

FIG. 4. Compound osteocutaneous flap. (From Martin et al., ref. 1, with permission.)

reconstruction of segmental contralateral mandibular defects or those of the malar region. It is also possible to harvest just the subcutaneous fascia along with the platysma and adipose tissue to correct soft-tissue defects due to trauma or as a result of Romberg's disease (Fig. 5).

OPERATIVE TECHNIQUE

The flap is marked with the patient in the supine position and the head extended (see Fig. 2). The inferior limit (possible width) is outlined by an index finger-thumb pinch test to assess primary closure. An incision is made at the lower margin of the flap. Undermining is continued superiorly, keeping

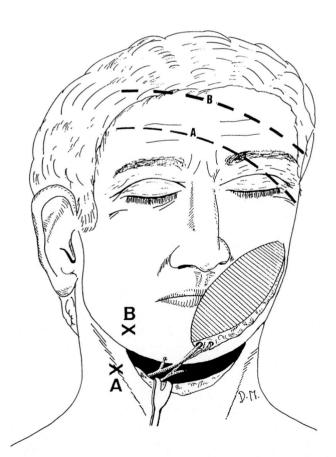

FIG. 3. Arc of rotation of the flap. A: Proximally based. B: Distally based. (From Martin et al., ref. 2, with permission.)

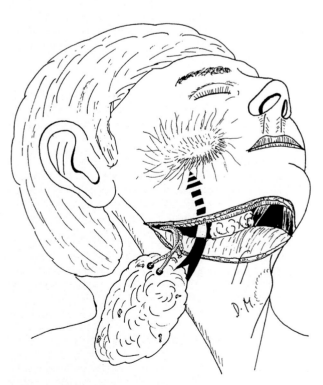

FIG. 5. Fascioplatysmal flap. (From Martin et al., ref. 1, with permission.)

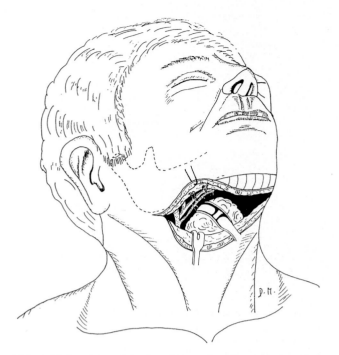

FIG. 6. Undermining of the flap close to the submandibular gland. (From Martin et al., ref. 2, with permission.)

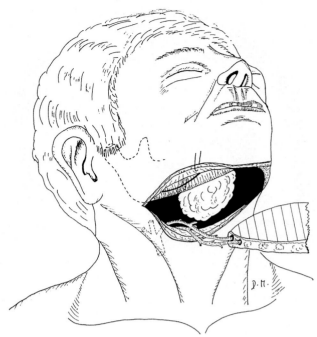

FIG. 7. Raising the flap from distal to proximal. (From Martin et al., ref. 2, with permission.)

the subcutaneous adipose tissue with the flap and dissecting close to the submandibular gland and mylohyoid and digastric muscles (Fig. 6).

An incision then is made at the upper extent of the flap along the mandibular margin, and the flap is raised beginning at the distal tip and including the platysma and adipose tissue layers; gentle traction eases dissection. Dissection is carried down to the origin of the facial artery (Fig. 7), and the facial vein also is identified. When raising the flap, it is important to begin the dissection by the exposure of the submandibular gland. This gland will be thoroughly undermined until it remains attached only by its inferior aspect. Care should be taken during the dissection to ligate the very short vessels coming from the facial and submental pedicles.

When one needs a very wide arc of rotation for the flap, for instance, to reach the forehead, the facial vein is too short. In such a situation, it is possible to use the constant anastomosing vein between the facial and external jugular vein as the drainage of the flap by dividing the facial vein. We have used this reliable procedure six times in our 19 submental flaps. We have described it as a Y-V lengthening of a vein. It avoids the need for a microsurgical anastomosis when transferring a submental flap as far as the forehead.

Closure of the donor area is accomplished by some undermining, restricted to cervical skin only. The skin is sutured to the hyoid bone to create a well-defined cervicomental angle. Flexion of the neck to facilitate closure should be avoided because it causes subsequent hypertrophic scars.

CLINICAL RESULTS

In a series of 19 patients, only one complication was encountered: A hematoma at the recipient site was evacuated with an uneventful final outcome. The blood supply is robust, the vascular pedicle is constant, and the dissection is not difficult, with care taken to avoid injury to the mandibular branch of

the facial nerve. There are a few limitations to its use, including thickness of the flap and hairy skin in males.

SUMMARY

When considering orofacial or similar reconstructions, the submental flap is recommended for excellent color match, for overcoming the disadvantages of other local flaps, and for its versatility of design as a composite flap.

References

1. Martin D, Baudet J, Mondie JM, Peri G. A propos du lambeau cutané sous mental en îlot: protocole opératoire. Perspectives d'utilisation. *Ann Chir Plast* 1990;35:480.
2. Martin D, Pascal JF, Baudet J, et al. The submental island flap: a new donor site. Anatomy and clinical applications as a free or pedicled flap. *Plast Reconstr Surg* 1993;92:867.
3. Jellouli M, Soussaline M, Richard JM, Luboinski B. Choix des méthodes de reconstruction de la joue après exérèse carcinologique au vu d'une étude retrospective de 32 cas sur 8 ans de 1980 à 1987, a l'Institut Gustave Roussy. *Ann Otolaryngol Chir Cervicofac (Paris)* 1990;107:265.
4. Mazzola RF, Oldini C, Sambataro G. Use of the submandibular flap to close pharyngostomes and other defects of the lower anterior neck region. *Plast Reconstr Surg* 1979;64:340.
5. Coleman JJ, III, Nahai F, Mathes SJ. Platysma musculocutaneous flap: Clinical and anatomic considerations in head and neck reconstruction. *Am J Surg* 1982;144:477.
6. Fan HW, Jean-Gilles B, Die A. Cervical island skin flap repair of oral and pharyngeal defects in the composite operation for cancer. *Am J Surg* 1969;118:759.
7. Futrell JW, Johns ME, Edgerton MT, et al. Platysma myocutaneous flap for intraoral reconstruction. *Am J Surg* 1978;136:504.
8. Hurwitz DJ, Rabson JA, Futrell JW. The anatomic basis for platysma skin flap. *Plast Reconstr Surg* 1983;72:302,22.
9. Baudet J, Martin D, Ferreira R, et al. The supraclavicular neurovascular free flap: anatomy and clinical application. In: G. Brunelli, ed., *Textbook of Microsurgery*. Paris: Masson, 1988.
10. Salmon M. *Les arteres de la peau*. Paris: Masson, 1936.
11. Whetzel TP, Mathes SJ. Arterial anatomy of the face: an analysis of vascular territories and perforating cutaneous vessels. *Plast Reconstr Surg* 1992; 89:591.

CHAPTER 122 ■ PLATYSMAL FLAPS FOR CHEEK AND INTRAORAL RECONSTRUCTION

J. N. BARRON,* M. N. SAAD, AND L. O. VASCONEZ

A turnover platysma muscle flap based superiorly and including an island of skin in its distal third is admirably suited for resurfacing the intraoral mucosa following excision of buccal mucosal tumors and cicatricial release of caustic burn scars as well as for resurfacing the oral surface of the lower lip and creating a deeper sulcus. It has the added attraction of providing sensitive skin to the buccal mucosa as well as to the lower lip (1).

INDICATIONS

Clinical experience has demonstrated that defects in the buccal mucosa should be resurfaced with flap tissue, avoiding the use of skin grafts, which usually contract and produce trismus. The platysma is admirable for this purpose because it provides a flap that is quite thin and has skin devoid of hair. As a turnover flap pivoting along the mandible, it is introduced intraorally through a small tunnel. Although the flap has been used for extraoral coverage, to accomplish this, an additional twist must be added that may compromise the blood supply.

ANATOMY

The platysma is a well-defined, thin muscular sheet in males, but it can be hypoplastic, especially in females. It consists of paired muscles that are obliquely oriented and flat and that phylogenetically represent the remnants of the panniculus carnosus (2).

The platysma extends from above the mandible to below the clavicle, and its cephalad and caudad edges insert into the skin. The blood supply to the muscle comes most often from the submental branch of the facial artery superiorly, and a smaller vessel is noted that is a branch of the superficial cervical artery inferiorly. The skin overlying the platysma derives its sensory supply from the cutaneous branches of the cervical plexus. Its medial and lateral borders are easily identified from the strap muscles and the trapezius muscle, respectively.

FLAP DESIGN AND DIMENSIONS

A skin-flap island is designed in the form of an ellipse on the lateral aspect of the neck and above the clavicle. Because the blood supply to the flap is from the submental branches of the facial artery, one should be careful in the dissection along the medial edge and also should avoid elevating the flap beyond the lower border of the mandible. It is safer to make a back-cut on the posterior edge along the trapezius muscle. The flap usually reaches the highest point of the intraoral buccal mucosa and also will reach and serve quite well to recreate the commissure of the mouth, both on the inner lining and outer layer.

OPERATIVE TECHNIQUE

Vertical and lateral extensions are made through the skin, and the superior skin flap is dissected above the mandible superficial to the platysma muscle. The inferior skin flap is also dissected to just below the clavicle.

The muscle is divided at least 1 cm below the lower edge of the skin island and is freed up along its medial extent from the strap muscles in a relatively avascular plane. The muscle is also freed up laterally from the anterior edge of the trapezius muscle, but care must be used to avoid an injury to the eleventh cranial nerve. The muscle and the skin island are freed up to the level of the mandible, where the mandibular branch of the facial nerve is identified and preserved intact. At this point, the intraoral defect has been marked out or created and a tunnel is opened bluntly to allow for passage of the flap. Once this is done, the flap is inset with fine sutures. Back-cutting on the posterior edge along the trapezius muscle and careful dissection along the medial flap edge, as well as avoiding flap elevation beyond the lower mandibular border, will prevent disturbing the blood supply from the submental branches of the facial artery.

The neck incision then is resutured with fine nylon. Small defects usually close primarily. A temporary Penrose drain may be left in place (Figs. 1 and 2).

---

* Deceased.

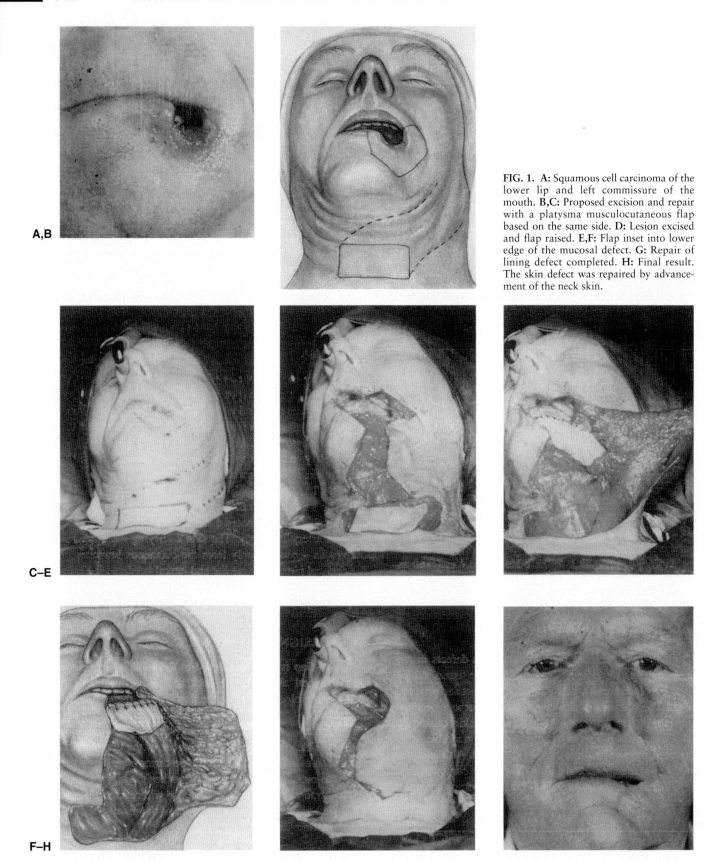

FIG. 1. A: Squamous cell carcinoma of the lower lip and left commissure of the mouth. **B,C:** Proposed excision and repair with a platysma musculocutaneous flap based on the same side. **D:** Lesion excised and flap raised. **E,F:** Flap inset into lower edge of the mucosal defect. **G:** Repair of lining defect completed. **H:** Final result. The skin defect was repaired by advancement of the neck skin.

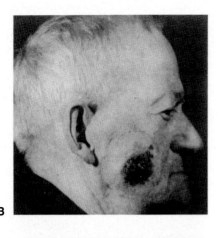
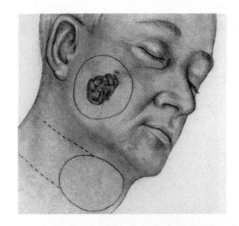
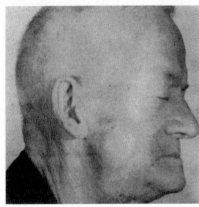
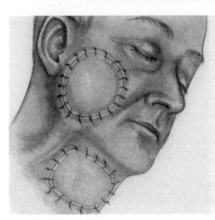

FIG. 2. A: Malignant melanoma of the cheek. **B:** Planned repair with a platysma musculocutaneous flap. **C,D:** Flap in situ. The neck defect was too large for direct suture, and a skin graft was applied.

Precautions

Injury to the eleventh nerve is potentially disastrous, particularly as one dissects and frees up the posterior edge of the platysma muscle. An injury to the mandibular as well as the cervical branches of the facial nerve is also possible.

In patients with thin platysma muscles, it is quite easy to "buttonhole" the muscle and thus to jeopardize the blood supply. Obviously, the procedure is not possible in patients who have undergone neck dissections and is not advised on irradiated necks.

CLINICAL RESULTS

Considerable safety has been reported in using the musculocutaneous unit for the resurfacing of intraoral defects, with relatively minor complications and no significant deficits other than the occasional loss of the eleventh nerve and some asymmetry of the lower lip.

SUMMARY

The platysma muscle with an island of skin provides an elegant way to resurface intraoral defects.

References

1. Coleman J, Jurkiewicz MJ, Nahai F, Mathes SJ. The platysma musculocutaneous flap: experiences with 24 cases. *Plast Reconstr Surg* 1983; 72:315.
2. Hurwitz DJ, Rabson JA, Futrell JW. The anatomic bases for the platysma skin flap. *Plast Reconstr Surg* 1983;72:302.

CHAPTER 123 ■ NAPE OF THE NECK FLAP

T. D. R. BRIANT AND V. V. STRELZOW

In 1842, Mutter first described his "autoplasty technique," using a superiorly based posterolateral neck flap from the shoulder and deltoid region to correct a cicatricial burn contracture of the anterior neck (1). Since then, several variously named, constructed, and applied shoulder neck flaps have been suggested (2–9).

INDICATIONS

The nape of neck flap has been used to cover a wide variety of defects. In the neck, these include closure of pharyngocutaneous fistulas, replacement of soft tissue lost through excision or slough, pharyngolaryngeal reconstruction, release of contractures, and provision of protective coverage for the great vessels.

Uses on the face or scalp include replacement of excised facial or scalp skin (see Fig. 5), repair of through-and-through cheek defects, closure of orocutaneous fistulas (see Fig. 4), and coverage along an exposed mandible. Repair of the lower face and mandibular margin is often beyond the range of the forehead flap and somewhat awkward for the deltopectoral flap.

Intraoral applications include palate reconstruction, floor of mouth repair, coverage of lateral oropharyngeal wall defects, and lateral commissure reconstruction. This flap is a particularly useful alternative to the forehead flap in repair of palatal defects, both because of its proximity and also because its bulk provides a very appropriate thickness to the reconstructed palate (see Fig. 3).

The advantages of the flap include its high reliability, ease of construction, and constant anatomic basis. The bulk and generous amount of usable flap area are sufficient for large, full-thickness defect replacement with or without the use of other flaps. The donor site is usually beyond neck radiation fields, thus allowing the flap to be used even in heavily irradiated necks. Cosmetically, the texture and color match are good and the donor-site defect, after skin grafting, is acceptable. This compares with the forehead flap and anterior chest wall flap, which usually result in a much more obvious cosmetic deformity, especially in women.

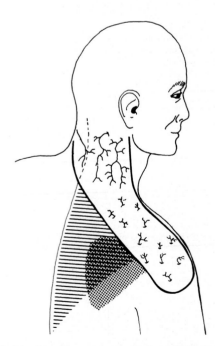

FIG. 1. The blood supply to the nape of the neck flap is mainly random via perforating vessels. An axial supply to the proximal flap is disputed. (From Briant et al., ref. 11, with permission.)

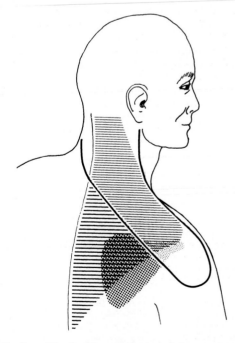

FIG. 2. Outline of the flap. Posteriorly, its inferior margin crosses the midline to ensure optimal blood supply, and anteriorly, its margin continues along the trapezius muscle edge. (From Briant et al., ref. 11, with permission.)

344

ANATOMY

The blood supply of the nape of the neck flap usually has been described as being based on main branches of the posterior auricular and occipital arteries, implying it to be primarily an arterialized flap in its proximal half, with random supply by means of perforating vessels in its distal half. No significant branches, however, have been found running longitudinally within this flap (10,11). There is strong evidence that the nape of the neck flap has a random vascular supply by means of perforating vessels (Fig. 1). Should the flap be used in its musculocutaneous form, the trapezius musculocutaneous flap, the descending branch of the occipital artery, running deep to the trapezius muscle, then is included in the proximal part of the flap (see Chapter 130).

FLAP DESIGN AND DIMENSIONS

After routine assessment of defect size, need for lining, and distance from the flap turning point, the nape of neck flap is measured and outlined on the patient (Fig. 2). The anterior margin descends from the region of the mastoid tip along the leading edge of the trapezius muscle for the desired length. The posterior margin begins 2 to 3 cm across the midoccipital line and curves down the neck to become approximately horizontal over the scapular spine. The outline is roughly rectangular, approximately 10 to 12 cm wide at its base, with a length approaching 30 to 35 cm. The flap often tapers gently as it continues farther down onto the shoulder.

OPERATIVE TECHNIQUE

If only a short flap is required (i.e., one not extending beyond the midclavicular point) delay of the flap is unnecessary (7–9); however, we believe that if a longer flap is required or if the distal tip of the flap requires split-thickness skin graft lining, the flap should be delayed for 3 weeks (Fig. 3A). This is accomplished by elevating the distal half to two thirds of the flap along with the fascia of the underlying muscles and then resuturing it to its bed. Should the flap be used in its musculocutaneous form (by dividing the trapezius muscle and leaving the proximal portion of the trapezius muscle in continuity with the proximal third to half of the flap), the flap need not be delayed unless it is extended well over the shoulder.

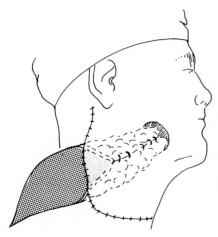
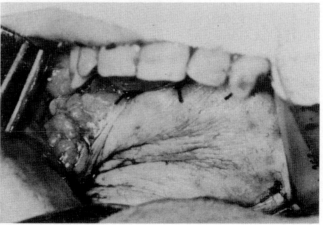
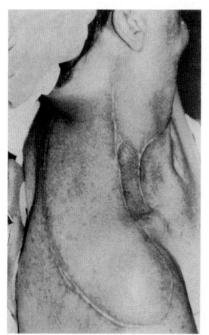
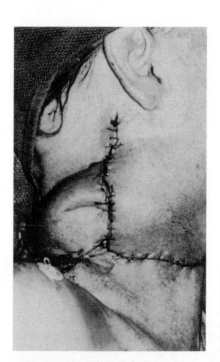

A,B

C,D

FIG. 3. A: Delayed right nape of the neck flap in a patient with adenoid cystic carcinoma of the oropharynx and palate. B,C: The flap has been inwardly tubed and passed into the palatal region under previous neck flap. D: The flap inset into the palatal defect. (From Briant et al., ref. 11, with permission.)

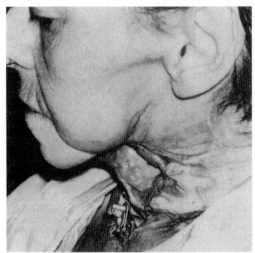
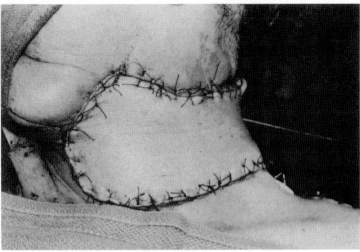

A,B

FIG. 4. **A:** A 63-year-old woman with a left base of tongue carcinoma previously unsuccessfully treated with cryotherapy and radiotherapy who underwent a left composite resection complicated by an orocutaneous fistula. **B:** A left nape of the neck flap was used for closure of the fistula. (From Briant et al., ref. 11, with permission.)

After transferring the flap, the bared shoulder area is covered with a split-thickness skin graft. Tubing the proximal flap with skin rolled inward (Fig. 3B,C) or outward is often expedient where the flap is transposed over or transferred beneath intact skin en route to its final destination. It is better to insert the whole pedicle when possible, by removing any poor-quality skin that it may cross, to provide better tissue cover and resultant cosmetic effect (Fig. 4). After 3 weeks, the final detachment of the distal portion of the flap is undertaken, and the remaining unused pedicle is returned to the donor site (Fig. 5).

CLINICAL RESULTS

Of 13 patients, in only one, a hemiplegic with severe premature arteriosclerotic vessel disease, was full-thickness loss of the distal 1.5 cm of the flap noted (the flap was delayed). The resultant defect healed uneventfully by secondary intention. In such cases, or in patients who appear significantly undernourished or debilitated, or if previous radiation fields overlap the lower lateral neck, a second delay may be contemplated.

It should be noted that commonly after elevation of the flap the distal few centimeters may appear mottled and may stay so for several days. Rarely, some epithelial sloughing is seen in association with this discoloration. These events appear to be independent of the patency of the external carotid artery system.

Disadvantages of the flap include delay procedures that we believe necessary to ensure reliability of long flaps and that can mean that head and neck reconstructive procedures may become three- or four-stage operations. Certain midline defects, especially high on the face, or those extending vertically in the neck region are either not accessible or may require bilateral flap closure.

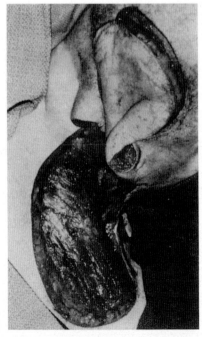
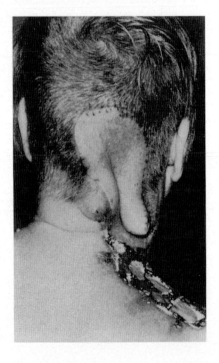

A,B

FIG. 5. **A:** A 59-year-old woman with a squamous cell carcinoma of the occiput previously unsuccessfully treated with local surgery and radiotherapy. **B:** After a radical full-thickness excision including occipital bone, a right nape of neck flap was placed over dura. The donor defect was covered with split-thickness skin grafts. (From Briant et al., ref. 11, with permission.)

SUMMARY

The nape of neck flap is a superiorly based posterolateral neck flap that can be used to cover defects of the neck, face, scalp, and intraoral region.

References

1. Mutter TD. Case of deformity from burns relieved by operation. *Am J Med Sci* 1842;4:66.
2. Owens N. A compound neck pedicle designed for the repair of massive facial defects: formation, development and application. *Plast Reconstr Surg* 1955;15:369.
3. Zovickian A. Pharyngeal fistulas: repair and prevention using mastoid-occipital based shoulder flaps. *Plast Reconstr Surg* 1957;19:355.
4. Kirschbaum S. Mentosternal contracture: preferred treatment by acromial flap. *Plast Reconstr Surg* 1958;21:131.
5. Corso PF, Gerold FP, Frazell EL. Rapid closure of large salivary fistulae by an accelerated shoulder flap technique. *Am J Surg* 1963;106:691.
6. Chretien PB, Ketcham AS, Hoy RC, Gertren HR. Extended shoulder flap and its use in reconstruction of defects of head and neck. *Am J Surg* 1969;188:752.
7. Conley J. The use of regional flaps in head and neck surgery. *Ann Otol* 1960;69:1223.
8. Tardy MD. Regional flaps, principles and application. *Otolaryngol Clin North Am* 1972;5:551.
9. Shumrick DA. Reconstructive flaps in head and neck surgery. *Otolaryngol Clin North Am* 1969;2:685.
10. Scheim MD, Kahane JC, Myers EN. Blood supply to nape of neck flap: Implications from a fetal anatomic study. *Ann Otol* 1977;86:329.
11. Briant TDR, Strelzow VV, Bird RJ. Nape of neck flap. *J Otolaryngol* 1980;9:35.

CHAPTER 124 ■ DELTOPECTORAL SKIN FLAP

V. Y. BAKAMJIAN

EDITORIAL COMMENT

This landmark chapter should be studied with considerable care and detail. The deltopectoral flap preceded the pectoralis major flap in head and neck reconstruction, and although it is not as reliable as the latter for intraoral resurfacing or in postradiation patients, the versatility and reach of the deltopectoral flap are admirable. Safety is ensured by preservation of the second perforating branch of the internal mammary artery and by flap design and subfascial elevation, as emphasized by the author.

Developed in the early 1960s, the deltopectoral flap was the first axial-pattern skin flap derived from an outside area for direct reconstructive applications in regions of the head and neck (1–10).

INDICATIONS

With optimal flap reach occurring in stockier patients with broad shoulders and short necks, the flap may serve at almost any head and neck level below the ipsilateral eyebrow (Fig. 6) or below midlevel of the contralateral face, if necessary (Fig. 7).

The deltopectoral flap can be used for either external cover or intraoral lining or both simultaneously. It also can be combined with another deltopectoral flap or a pectoralis major musculocutaneous flap (11–15).

ANATOMY

Two contiguous but separate axially vascularized zones are distinguishable in the area of the flap (Fig. 2), with or without a random narrow zone at the far end (16). Intercostal perforating branches from the internal mammary artery arborize outward in the pectoral zone; a cutaneous vessel from the thoracoacromial artery does the same in the deltoid zone; and a few musculocutaneous short twigs from the subscapular and circumflex humeral vessels pierce into the random distal zone. When the flap is elevated, however, its survival will depend entirely on the flow of blood in the branches from the internal mammary to the pectoral zone passing by means of rich dermal and subdermal plexus connections into the axially oriented vasculature of the deltoid zone and beyond. Clinical experience has amply demonstrated that the blood supply of internal mammary origin suffices for full survival of the flap, without delay, in 85% to 90% of patients.

FLAP DESIGN AND DIMENSIONS

Based parasternally over the three or four upper intercostal spaces, the flap extends horizontally to the anterior aspect of the shoulder, where its curvilinear distal margin may reach to

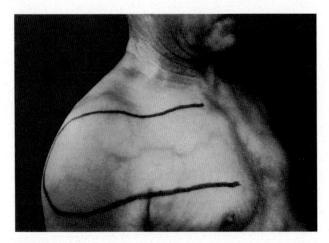

FIG. 1. Outline of a typical deltopectoral flap. Infrared photograph showing the axiality of venous return.

the anterolateral, midlateral, or even posterolateral contour line of the deltoid region, depending on specific case requirements (Fig. 1). It then can carry a generous portion of deltoid skin, not damaged by prior radiotherapy or compromised by incisions used in resecting head and neck cancer, on the end of a pedicle of pectoral skin.

The actual reach of the raised flap is longer than would be surmised from its outlined dimensions when the patient's arm lies by his or her side. This can be explained by the considerable elongation that characteristically occurs along the lower border of the flap as it is raised in cephalad rotation. The phenomenon is due to the better than average stretching ability of skin in the vicinity of the axillary fold—essential for the full range of abduction and elevation of the arm (Fig. 5). Consequently, the pivot point for rotation of the flap shifts from the lower to the upper medial corner of its base. Tilting the patient's head toward the base of the flap also helps determine proper flap dimensions.

OPERATIVE TECHNIQUE

Should the poor general health of a patient—anemia, advanced arteriosclerosis, diabetes, or lupus—give cause for concern, a simple delay some 7 to 10 days before using the flap may be a wise choice.

In the case of a flap of conventional size, incising its outline and limited undermining into the triangle of the infraclavicular fossa to divide the cutaneous branch of the thoracoacromial artery should suffice (Fig. 3A). In effect, this will amount to cutting nearly all flow into and out of the area of the flap, except that which enters and leaves by means of the vessels of the base. For a delay with equivalent effect in a longer and larger flap than is conventional, however, additional undermining of the narrow random zone of its far end will be needed (Fig. 3B).

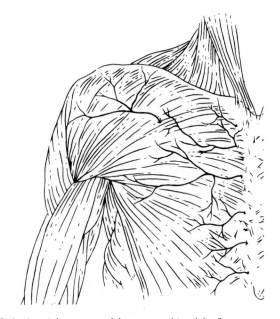

FIG. 2. Arterial anatomy of donor area skin of the flap.

From tip to base, the flap is raised with knife dissection along the subfascial plane, stopping at intervals to test its reach into the area of the recipient defect without tension. Excessive dissection toward the feeding vessels of the flap base is avoided in this manner. Also, one may be pleasantly surprised to find that a longer than conventional-sized flap may reach its destination without having to divide the cutaneous branch of the thoracoacromial artery. This vessel may be found at a more proximal point than just at the medial side of

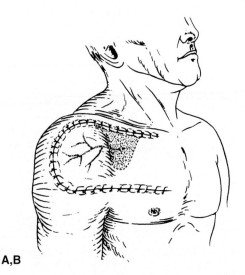
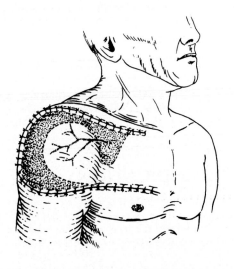

A,B

FIG. 3. A,B: Modes of delay.

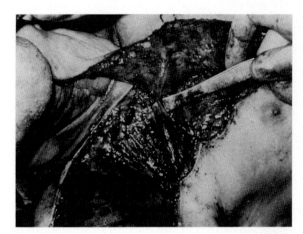

FIG. 4. The cutaneous branch of the thoracoacromial artery seen here emerging from muscle into skin at a more proximal point than its usual one just at the medial side of the deltopectoral groove, thereby permitting its preservation in the use of an extended flap.

the deltopectoral groove, where it usually emerges from muscle to enter the skin (Fig. 4).

A *rotation transfer* of the open flap can resurface the entire adjacent side or front of the neck (Fig. 8). This greatly simplifies the decision in a radical neck dissection to sacrifice cervical skin infiltrated with advanced cancer or severely damaged by prior radiation.

A *subcutaneous transfer* through the dissected neck with the flap pedicle deepithelialized, simulating an island flap, may be used for covering a high cervical and parotid area defect (Fig. 9). This technique eliminates the need for division of the pedicle in a second stage and may bring welcome protection to the dissected neck as well as contour augmentation.

Bridging over the neck, with the pedicle tubed and with an intervening span of intact cervical skin from the donor area, is a more commonly employed method for transfer to locations on the head (Fig. 10). Additionally, splitting the flap end (Fig. 11), folding it to provide two layers (Fig. 12), and deepithelializing the folded edge, if necessary (Fig. 13), are auxiliary maneuvers that may be used under special circumstances.

The bridging over the neck technique is employable also for intraoral defects, but with a two-directional instead of the one-directional method of tubing the pedicle (Fig. 14). As in the case of cervical flaps, entry is made through a portal high

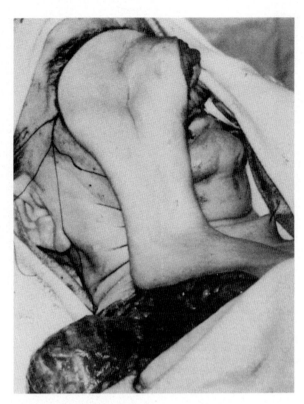

FIG. 6. Ipsilateral high reach of the flap.

in the neck, usually created at the time of resecting intraoral cancer. The distal portion of the flap is dressed into the defect, after which the intermediate short segment within the portal of entry is entubed (skin side facing inward), and the remainder is tubed in ordinary fashion (skin facing outward). The entry, when a segment of mandible has not been resected, is

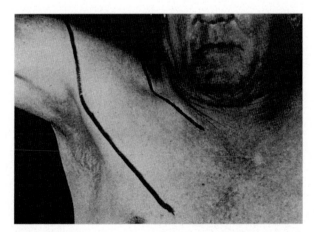

FIG. 5. The reserve of stretching along the inferior border of the deltopectoral flap, demonstrated by abduction of the arm.

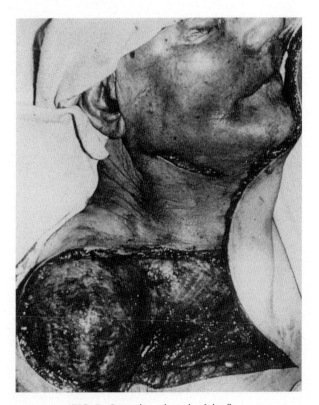

FIG. 7. Contralateral reach of the flap.

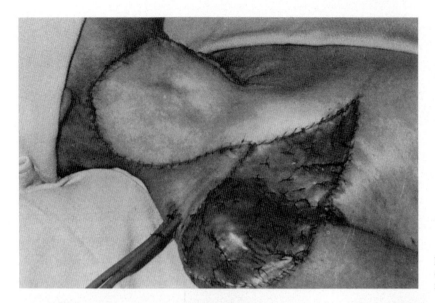

FIG. 8. Rotation transfer of the open flap to cover one side of the neck denuded of its skin in radical neck dissection.

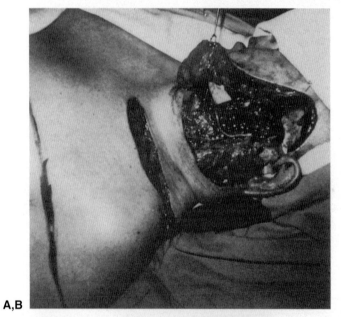

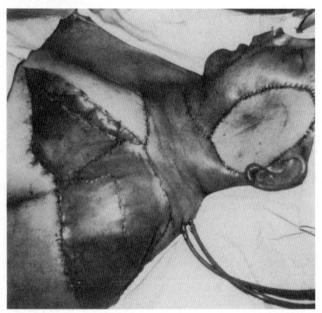

A,B

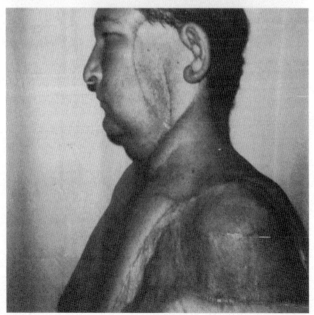

C

FIG. 9. Subcutaneous transfer of the flap with deepithelialized pedicle. **A:** Defect resulting from radical parotidectomy, mandibulectomy, and radical neck dissection for advanced recurrent cancer. **B:** The repair. **C:** The result.

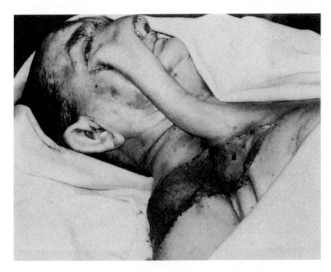

FIG. 10. Transfer to orbitonasal skin defect with tubing of the pedicle.

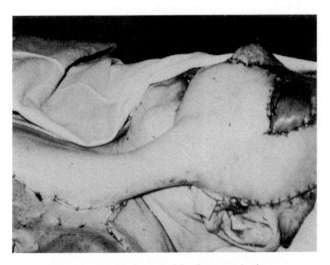

FIG. 11. Split in the end of the flap over the face.

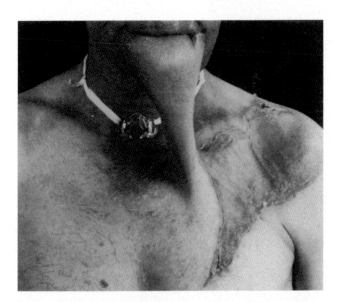

FIG. 12. Folded end of the flap to provide two layers for a total lower lip reconstruction.

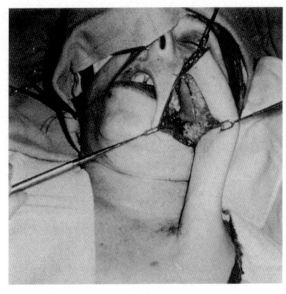

FIG. 13. Deepithelialization of folded edge of flap in closing a through-and-through defect in the cheek.

deep for defects of the floor of the mouth, tongue, or oropharynx (Fig. 15) and superficial to it for defects of the cheek and maxillary area (Fig. 16). Needless to say, this reversal in direction from the skin-inward to the skin-outward type of tubing demands meticulous care to avoid a possible strangulation of the blood supply to its distal end.

Whether it is tubed in one or two directions, the pedicle is always available for secondary use by upward waltzing if there is a need for additional tissue to improve on, or to complete, the reconstruction (Fig. 16).

Finally, there are varied and numerous possibilities of using the flap simultaneously with its twin from the opposite side (Fig. 17), with a temporal forehead flap from the same side (12) or with the pectoralis major musculocutaneous flap from the same side (Fig. 18).

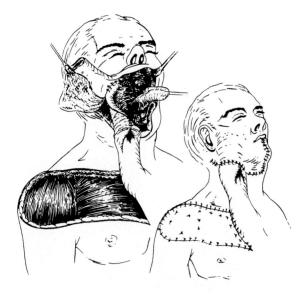

FIG. 14. The two-directional method of tubing the pedicle as seen in transfer to the oropharynx in a patient in whom a segment of the mandible had to be sacrificed.

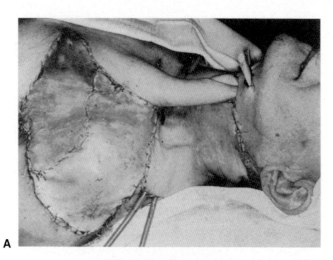

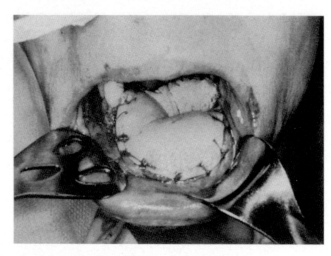

A

B

FIG. 15. Two-directional tubing of the pedicle in passage on deep side of mandible into the oral cavity.
A: External view. B: Intraoral view.

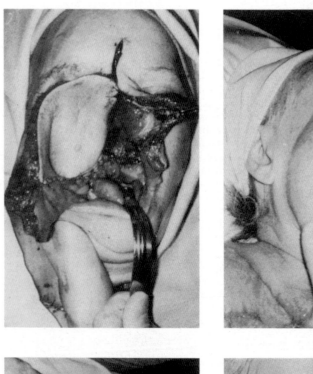

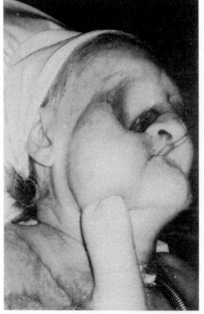

A,B

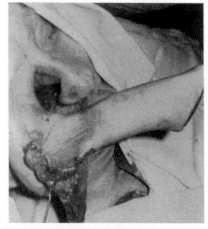

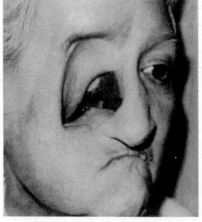

C,D

FIG. 16. Two-directional tubing of pedicle in passage superficial to the mandible into a defect of radical orbitomaxillary resection. A: Flap in the defect. B: Appearance after healing. C: Waltzing the pedicle. Tubed pedicle divided from its base on the chest and ready for use in restoring the palatal defect. D: The end result.

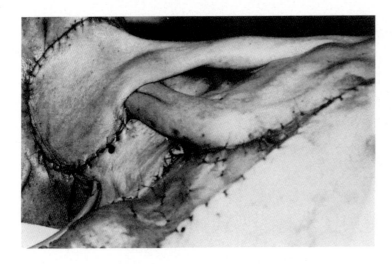

FIG. 17. Deltopectoral twin flaps.

CLINICAL RESULTS

Of the first 53 flaps I used in the early period of flap development at the Roswell Park Memorial Institute, 41 were completely successful. Of the remaining 12 flaps, seven suffered minor losses of no particular consequence, each progressing to a satisfactory outcome either with healing by secondary intention or with a minor readjustment when dividing the pedicle in a second stage. Only five flaps sustained more than a minimal loss, ranging up to a distal third of the flap. Two such losses were caused by the hanging weight of the pedicle against the hard edge of a mandibular rib graft over which the flap had been wrapped. Another occurred in a diabetic and arteriosclerotic patient in whom hematoma formation and infection caused the loss in a "trial" delay that consisted of undermining the entire area of the flap. It is interesting to note that in none of the patients did the amount of loss prevent the completion of an intended reconstruction, which involved the use of additional stages with the remaining portion of the flap.

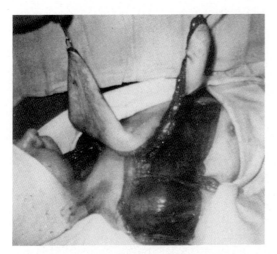

FIG. 18. Deltopectoral and pectoralis major musculocutaneous flaps simultaneously raised from the same side.

SUMMARY

The deltopectoral flap is a well-established technique for reconstruction of head and neck defects.

References

1. Bakamjian VY. A two-stage method for pharyngoesophageal reconstruction with a primary pectoral skin flap. *Plast Reconstr Surg* 1965;36:173.
2. Bakamjian VY, Cuff NK, Bales HW. Versatility of the deltopectoral flap in reconstructions following head and neck cancer surgery. In: *Transactions of the fourth international congress of plastic and reconstructive surgeons, 1967:* Amsterdam: Excerpta Medica, 1969;808–815.
3. Bakamjian VY. The reconstructive use of flaps in cancer surgery of the head and neck. In: Saad MN, Lichtveld P, eds. *Reviews in plastic surgery: general plastic and reconstructive surgery.* Amsterdam: Excerpta Medica, 1974.
4. Bakamjian VY, Cervino L, Miller S, Henz VR. The concept of cure and palliation by surgery in advanced cancer of the head and neck. *Am J Surg* 1973;126:482.
5. Bakamjian VY, Long M, Rigg B. Experience with the medially based deltopectoral flap in reconstructive surgery of the head and neck. *Br J Plast Surg* 1971;24:174.
6. Bakamjian VY. The deltopectoral flap. In: Grabb WC, Myers MB, eds. *Skin flaps.* Boston: Little, Brown, 1975.
7. Bakamjian VY, Poole M. Maxillofacial and palatal reconstructions with the deltopectoral flap. *Br J Plast Surg* 1977;30:17.
8. Bakamjian VY, Dhooge PL. The contralateral deltopectoral flap in repeat resections for recurrent cancer of the head and neck. *Chir Plast (Ber.)* 1979;4:243.
9. Bakamjian VY, Ciano M. The reconstructive role in cancer surgery of the head and neck. *Ann Chir Plast* 1982;27:133.
10. McGregor IA, Jackson IT. The extended role of the deltopectoral flap. *Br J Plast Surg* 1970;23:173.
11. McGregor IA, Reid WH. Simultaneous temporal and deltopectoral flaps for full-thickness defects of the cheek. *Plast Reconstr Surg* 1970;45:326.
12. Krizek TJ, Robson MC. Split flap in head and neck reconstruction. *Am J Surg* 1973;126:488.
13. Leonard AG. Reconstruction of the chest wall using a deepithelialized "turn over" deltopectoral flap. *Br J Plast Surg* 1980;33:187.
14. Konno A, Towaga K, Izuka K. Primary reconstruction after total or extended total maxillectomy for maxillary cancer. *Plast Reconstr Surg* 1981;67:440.
15. McGregor IA, Morgan RG. Axial and random pattern flaps. *Br J Plast Surg* 1973;26:202.
16. Daniel RK, Cunningham DM, Taylor GI. The deltopectoral flap: an anatomical and hemodynamic approach. *Plast Reconstr Surg* 1975; 55:275.

CHAPTER 125 ■ DELTOPECTORAL SKIN FLAP AS A FREE SKIN FLAP USING THE INTERNAL MAMMARY VESSELS, REVISITED: FURTHER REFINEMENT IN FLAP DESIGN, FABRICATION, AND CLINICAL USAGE

K. SASAKI, M. NOZAKI, T. HONDA, K. MORIOKA, Y. KIKUCHI, AND T. HUANG

EDITORIAL COMMENT

This chapter shows how anatomic analysis can be used to make a previously difficult free flap anastomosis more reliable.

The deltopectoral skin flap described by Bakamjian (1) in 1965 is an axial flap; therefore, it can be harvested as a free skin flap for distant transfer by means of a microsurgical technique (2,3). This skin flap was useful for facial resurfacing because of excellent color and texture match. Shortness of the vascular pedicle and smallness of the vessel caliber, on the other hand, render flap revascularization technically difficult. The method is further plagued by problems attributable to bulkiness of the skin flap and morbidities associated with donor-site deformity. These problems have been ameliorated by extending the pedicle to the internal mammary vessel and defatting the flap.

INDICATIONS

Between 1985 and 1998 at our hospital, a total of 27 patients underwent reconstruction of head and neck deformities due to various causes, using a free deltopectoral skin flap. There were 14 men and 13 women. The youngest patient was 11 years old, and the oldest was 66 years of age; the average age of this group was 36 years. Twelve patients had burn deformities of the face. A large facial hemangioma was seen in seven individuals. The flap was often used to reconstruct defects consequential to cancer extirpation. The indications and the number of patients with head and neck deformities managed with a free deltopectoral flap were as follows: burn contracture, $n = 12$; hemangioma, $n = 7$; malignant tumors, $n = 4$; pigmented nevus, $n = 1$; neurofibroma, $n = 1$; epidermal nevus, $n = 1$; and silicone granuloma, $n = 1$. Although the flap was sufficient to cover any defect around the face and the neck, it was never used to reconstruct the upper eyelid deformity. Resurfacing of the facial defect, however, did not follow the concept of facial aesthetic units. The distribution of the 31 recipient sites was as follows: frontal scalp forehead, $n = 5$; orbital area, $n = 1$; nose, $n = 1$; cheek, $n = 13$; mouth, $n = 2$; and chin/neck, $n = 9$. For three patients, the defect involved more than one area of the face.

ANATOMY

The lateral edge of the flap is bound by a line drawn 2 to 3 cm beyond the deltopectoral sulcus, alias Mohrenheim's fossa. The boundary is especially important in individuals for whom a concomitant defatting/thinning of the skin flap is contemplated at the time of initial flap harvesting. The medial boundary of the flap is located usually at the sternal edge on the same side. The medial boundary of the flap can be expanded by 3 to 4 cm beyond the ipsilateral parasternal line, especially where a segment of the internal mammary vessel is included in fabricating a vascular pedicle.

Length and size of the vessel can vary depending on the location of the flap marked over the upper chest and the distance from the parasternal line. Diameter of the arterial pedicle can be increased from 0.9 to 2.9 mm by incorporating a segment of the internal mammary artery. Similarly, elongation of the vascular pedicle can be achieved by removing the skin and the soft tissues surrounding the vessels at the medial edge of the flap (Fig. 1).

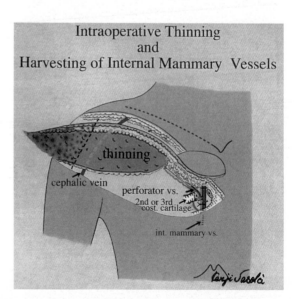

FIG. 1. Demonstrating the continuation of the medial vessel into the internal mammary vessel. Use of the latter vessel makes the final anastomosis easier and safer.

FLAP DESIGN

The extent of the tissue defect around the recipient site is measured, and the area is traced with a piece of paper. The pattern of defect is transferred onto the deltopectoral area over the second and third intercostal spaces. The course of intercostal vessels supplying the area is traced and marked using a Doppler device.

OPERATIVE TECHNIQUE

Dissection of the flap is best started from the lateral edge. The incision is carried down to the muscular layer. The dissection is continued to include the fascial layer of the pectoralis major muscle and the deltoid muscle, making the fascia a part of the flap. As dissection is continued medially, care is taken not to injure the anterior perforating branches of the internal mammary vessel. The vessels usually emerge through the pectoralis major muscle at the second and third intercostal spaces, one finger width lateral to the sternal border. The origin of the pectoralis major muscle may be divided and retracted laterally to facilitate dissection of the anterior perforating branches of the internal mammary vessel and to expose the costal cartilage at a point 1.5 to 2 cm from the sternal border. A small segment of the costal cartilage is removed with a rongeur to expose the internal mammary vessel/anterior perforating vessel junction. The cartilage is removed carefully to avoid injuring the vessels that are positioned closely against the inner surface of the cartilage. The sternal and the anterior intercostal branches are ligated to include a segment of the internal mammary vessel in fabricating the vascular pedicle (Fig. 2).

The anterior perforator of the internal mammary artery assumes the course paralleling the long axis of the skin flap. It extends toward the deltopectoral sulcus, that is, Mohrenheim's fossa, once it comes through the muscle and enters the skin. In the pectoral area, several vertical rami branch off this artery to form the subdermal vascular network. The vascular network in the distal end of this flap is expanded by anastomosis between the anterior perforating artery and the cutaneous branches of

the thoracoacromial artery and the deltoid musculocutaneous arteries (3–5). That is to say, a skin flap 7 to 10 mm thick can be fabricated safely without the need for subcutaneous fatty tissues to maintain vascular supplies to the skin flap.

The soft-tissue defect resulting from costal cartilage resection is obliterated by suturing the previously detached pectoralis major muscle bundle to the cartilage. In instances in which a complete closure of the wound per primum is not feasible, would distort the nipple areola configuration, or both, a V-to-Y skin flap advancement technique of wound closure is used. This approach is especially useful in closing the central defect where the primary closure would otherwise distort the surrounding structures, for example, nipples and chest configuration.

To close a wound, a triangular skin marking with its base adjacent to the wound length is made in the caudal or the lateral section of the chest wall. The length of the flap is determined by the extent of skin laxity surrounding the triangular skin flap. The triangular island skin flap is advanced cephalad or medialward to compensate for the tissue defect. The V-shaped donor defect is closed primarily into a Y shape—hence, a V-to-Y skin flap advancement wound closure. Flap revascularization is accomplished by coapting the graft vessels with the facial artery/vein or the superficial temporal artery/vein under magnification.

CLINICAL RESULTS

The length of follow-up in this group of patients varied between 14 years and 2 months, and 13 months, with an average of 5 years and 4 months.

The size of nutrient vessels was quite variable. As expected, the caliber of anterior perforating artery and vein was small. Of seven flaps with the anterior perforators as the nutrient vessels, the arterial size varied between 0.6 and 1.2 mm, with an average size of 0.9 mm. The vein was similarly quite small. The venous caliber varied between 1.5 and 3.2 mm, with an average size of 2.3 mm. The length of vascular pedicle was inconsistent. The longest one was 4.8 cm, and the shortest one was 1.8 cm, with an average length of 3.5 cm. Vascular anastomosis was, as expected, technically difficult. Thrombosis occurred at the anastomotic site in three instances. The secondary intervention saved two flaps. That is, we encountered a complete flap necrosis in one individual in this group of patients.

In 20 flaps in which a segment of the internal mammary vessel was included in vascular pedicle fabrication, the caliber of the artery and vein was noticeably larger. The arterial size varied between 1.4 and 3.0 mm, with an average size of 2.1 mm. The internal mammary vein was noted to vary between 2.0 and 3.8 mm. The average venous size was 2.9 mm. The shortest vascular pedicle with a segment of internal mammary vessel included was 3.5 cm, and the longest one was 7.1 cm. Although necrosis of the flap was not seen in this group of patients, we encountered venous thrombosis in one patient due to torsion of the vascular pedicle at the anastomotic site. However, a revisional procedure prevented flap necrosis.

Concomitant thinning of the skin flap at the time of initial surgery was carried out in only 15 patients. However, secondary thinning of the flap was deemed necessary in two of these patients because of bulkiness of the flap noted in the area of vascular pedicle attachment. In contrast, debulking procedures were needed in 6 of 10 flaps that had not had the primary intraoperative thinning. On the other hand, we had encountered partial necrosis of the flap around the tip in four individuals who had intraoperative thinning procedures. Derangement of subdermal vascular supplies attributable to defatting was thought to be the cause.

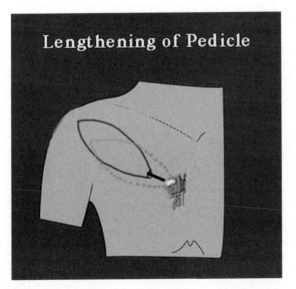

FIG. 2. The medial pectoralis vessels are dissected through the second and third intercostal spaces. A small segment of cartilage is excised and the vessel traced to the internal mammary vessel.

The V-to-Y flap advancement technique of closing the flap donor site defect was used in eight patients. The appearance of the wound was judged to be cosmetically satisfactory. The appearance of the donor site in patients who had undergone a conventional method of skin grafting, in contrast, was unsightly.

SUMMARY

Between 1985 and 1998, a total of 27 patients underwent head and neck reconstruction using a deltopectoral skin flap, alias dictus a Bakamjian flap, fabricated as a free flap and transferred by means of a microsurgical technique. We have instituted several technical refinements in flap fabrication. A segment of the internal mammary artery and vein was incorporated in the fabrication of the flap's vascular pedicle. A more than twofold increase in the vessel size and the vascular pedicle length rendered flap revascularization technically easier. The frequency of secondary flap debulking was similarly drastically reduced by incorporating the maneuver of thinning of the skin flap before transfer. Furthermore, the use of V-to-Y technique of wound closure simplified the closure of the flap donor defect. The outcome was considered to be much better than that with the conventional technique of primary closure with concomitant skin grafting.

References

1. Bakamjian VY. A two-stage method of pharyngoesophageal reconstruction with a primary pectoral skin flap. *Plast Reconstr Surg* 1965;36:173.
2. Harii K, Ohmori K, Ohmori S. Free deltopectoral skin flap. *Br J Plast Surg* 1974;27:231.
3. Taylor GI, Daniel RK. The anatomy of several free flap donor sites. *Plast Reconstr Surg* 1975;56:243.
4. Daniel RK, Cunningham DM, Taylor GI. The deltopectoral flap: an anatomical and hemodynamic approach. *Plast Reconstr Surg* 1975; 55:275.
5. Palmer JH, Taylor GI. The vascular territories of the anterior chest wall. *Br J Plast Surg* 1986;39:287.

CHAPTER 126 ■ DELTOSCAPULAR SKIN FLAP

C. J. SMITH

The deltoscapular flap, perceived by several independent observers as a mirror image of the Bakamjian deltopectoral flap (1), has been used for reconstruction of a posterior neck and back defect (2), an occipital defect (3), and defects of the lateral and anterolateral neck (4).

INDICATIONS

This flap is useful as an adjunct to the head and neck surgeon's armamentarium, but because of its anatomic position, it does not equal the deltopectoral flap in versatility. In addition, the thickness of the skin of the back limits the mobility of the flap and prohibits tubing of the proximal portion.

The primary advantages of this flap are (a) the location of its base inferior to the posterior neck skin, which commonly receives radiation in cases of head and neck cancer and which constitutes the base of the classic shoulder flap (5); (b) its arc of rotation, which extends to difficult-to-reach occipital and posterior neck wounds; and (c) its use as an additional source of tissue when other methods have failed or are not feasible (3,4). The flap can be used simultaneously with or subsequent to the use of an ipsilateral deltopectoral flap by designing the superior limb to superimpose the distal limb of the deltopectoral flap.

ANATOMY

The blood supply is from the perforating branches of the posterior intercostal arteries (2–4) and, if not elevated extensively from the trapezius muscle, also from musculocutaneous branches of the descending branch of the transverse cervical artery (2,4). It has not been unequivocally demonstrated clinically or in the laboratory that this mirror image of the deltopectoral flap is a true axial flap capable of transposition without delay.

FLAP DESIGN AND DIMENSIONS

The dimensions of this flap are essentially the same as those of the deltopectoral flap, beginning adjacent to the midline of the back, spanning three to four intercostal spaces from the first thoracic vertebra, and extending laterally across the back onto the posterolateral shoulder (Fig. 1). The pivot point is at the most medial aspect of the inferior limb incision, which can be slightly back-cut to increase the reach of the flap. The arc extends to the occipital scalp, the auricular region, and the lateral or anterolateral neck.

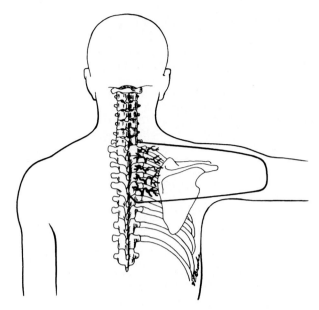

FIG. 1. Outline of deltoscapular flap with arm elevated in anatomic position. Undermining extends only to lateral border of neck for transfer to anterolateral side of neck. Inferior incision can be back-cut for greater reach. (From Smith, ref. 4, with permission.)

The deltoscapular flap is designed to avoid the occipital and nuchal region of patients who have received extensive radiation to the head and neck. The superior aspect of the limb is placed at the level of the spine of the seventh cervical or first thoracic vertebra and is extended laterally onto the deltoid region and upper extremity (Fig. 1). When a deltopec-

toral flap has been used previously, the superior part of the limb curves gently downward onto the upper extremity to join the distal incision of the deltopectoral flap (see Fig. 2).

As recommended for the shoulder flap (6), the proposed incision lines must be marked preoperatively on the skin while the patient is sitting because of the distortion of the skin relative to the bony landmarks when the patient is in a lateral decubitus position.

OPERATIVE TECHNIQUE

The inferior incision is always started as far medial as the fourth or fifth thoracic vertebral spine and may even be back-cut, if necessary, to improve mobility of the flap. The flap is gradually tapered while distally incorporating the thinner, more pliable skin of the deltoid region and upper extremity. Undermining usually need not be carried farther medial than the lateral aspect of the neck. It is hypothesized that this permits incorporation of anastomotic branches of the dorsal scapular artery in addition to the posterior perforating arteries.

Undermining is more difficult than with the deltopectoral flap because of the rigidity of the skin of the back and the tight adherence of the deep fascia to the muscles. As the undermining proceeds from inferior to superior, care must be taken not to undermine deep to the deltoid muscle. By limiting the undermining to a vertical line that extends from the lateral margin of the neck, the flap may extend well onto the posterior aspect of the upper extremity. Thus, the length and pliability necessary to reach the anterolateral side of the neck are obtained without excessive tension (Fig. 2).

By delaying the flap in multiple stages and limiting medial undermining to a vertical line at the lateral border of the neck, a length comparable with the deltopectoral flap may be

A–C

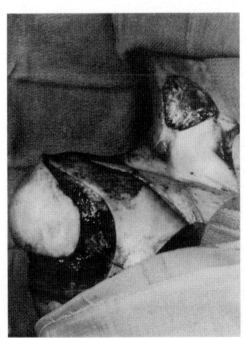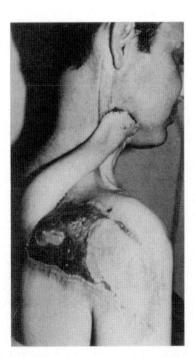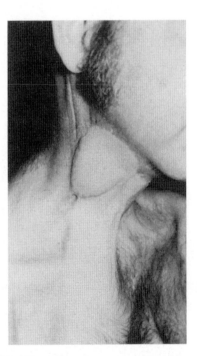

FIG. 2. A: Pharyngocutaneous fistula was prepared by excision of excess surrounding skin and rotation of local flap as internal lining. Delayed deltoscapular flap extends well onto upper third of upper extremity just prior to transfer. B: Distally tubed deltoscapular flap at 2 weeks is shown healing well without necrosis. Initial drainage beneath flap was promptly controlled by pressure dressings for 7 days. C: Transferred segment of deltoscapular flap heals to right deltopectoral flap anteriorly. (From Smith, ref. 4, with permission.)

obtained. In the initial stage, superior and inferior incisions are made, which are followed in 10 to 14 days by undermining. Ten to 14 days later, the distal end is incised. The flap may be transferred in 2 to 3 days, when viability is ascertained (Fig. 2). As suggested for the shoulder flap (7), undermining the distal end in long flaps as a separate procedure may be wise and is recommended. Because of the unknown qualities of this flap and the circumstances in which it was used (after necrosis of a deltopectoral flap), meticulous, although perhaps excessive, care and delay have been the rule.

CLINICAL RESULTS

The disadvantages of this flap are awkward postoperative positioning of the patient, inflexibility of the proximal pedicle of thick back skin that reduces the length of the arc of rotation, and an apparent (but unestablished) necessity for delay. The flap has been used successfully without delay (2), but was simply transposed as a broadly based, obliquely designed flap with a large dog-ear to an adjacent defect on the back and inferior posterior neck. On the other hand, it has been recommended that a delay be performed for flaps that are to be interpolated to more distant defects (3,4).

SUMMARY

The deltoscapular flap is geometrically a mirror image of the deltopectoral flap and is based on perforating cutaneous branches of the posterior intercostal arteries. Its use has been limited to major reconstructive problems of the head and neck when more conventional methods have not been applicable. Application has been limited by the development of reliable musculocutaneous and free flaps, but it remains a useful alternative flap for unusual circumstances.

References

1. Bakamjian VY. A two-stage method for pharyngoesophageal reconstruction with a primary pectoral skin flap. *Plast Reconstr Surg* 1965;36:122.
2. Doldan FG, Shatkin S. The deltoscapular flap. *Plast Reconstr Surg* 1975;55:708.
3. Harashina T, Nakajima T, Maruyama Y. Deltovertebral flap to cover a large scalp defect. *Plast Reconstr Surg* 1977;59:851.
4. Smith CJ. The deltoscapular flap. *Arch Otolaryngol* 1978;104:390.
5. Mutter TD. Cases of deformity from burns, relieved by operation. *Am J Med Sci* 1842;4:66.
6. Zovickian A. Pharyngeal fistulas, repair and prevention, using mastoid-occiput based shoulder flaps. *Plast Reconstr Surg* 1957;19:355.
7. Chretien PB, Ketcham AS, Hage RC, Gretner HR. Extended shoulder flap and its use in reconstruction of the defects of head and neck. *Am J Surg* 1969;118:752.

CHAPTER 127 ■ DORSAL SCAPULAR ISLAND FLAP

C. ANGRIGIANI

The dorsal scapular island flap is raised from the back and can be transferred as an island vascular flap to the anterior part of the thorax, the face, or the cranial vault without disruption of trapezius muscle function; therefore, there is no morbidity of shoulder joint motion (1). The flap is irrigated by the cutaneous branch of the superficial branch of the dorsal scapular artery, which is consistently present (2) (Fig. 1). It can be elevated with vascularized bone (the medial border of the scapula).

INDICATIONS

The procedure is indicated for resurfacing of the neck, the face, or the anterior thorax whenever a microsurgical free-tissue transfer is not indicated or cannot be carried out. It is also indicated for mandibular reconstruction as a salvage procedure when free vascularized bone graft cannot be performed.

ANATOMY

The dorsal scapular artery originates from the posterior scapular artery as a deep branch or as a direct branch of the subclavian artery (3,4). It runs posteriorly and almost horizontally, deep or through the branches of the brachial plexus. The artery then courses under the trapezius, the omohyoid, and levator scapulae muscles on top of the rib cage. During its course, it gives off branches to these muscles. At the medial angle of the scapula, the dorsal scapular artery gives off a superficial branch that pierces the rhomboid muscle and runs under the deep surface of the lower part of the trapezius; it then gives off one or two cutaneous branches that pierce this muscle and reach the skin.

The anatomic course of this artery must be differentiated from the superficial branch of the posterior scapular artery,

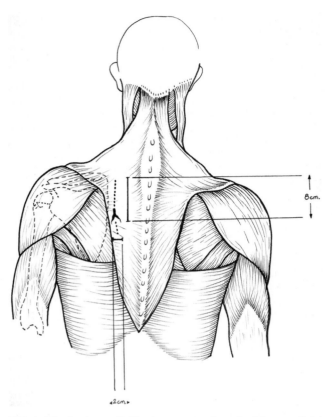

FIG. 1. The flap is supplied by the cutaneous branch of the superficial branch of the dorsal scapular artery. This is a consistent vessel.

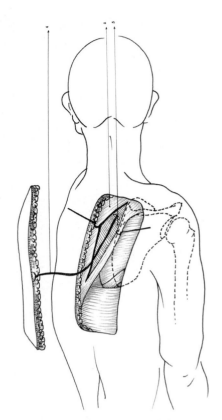

FIG. 2. The dorsal scapular flap vascular pedicle pierces two muscles before reaching the skin: the rhomboideus and the trapezius.

which is the main pedicle of the trapezius muscle (5). The dorsal scapular artery runs deep to the levator scapular and the omohyoid muscle; it is not related to the trapezius main pedicle. This is not a conventional lower trapezius flap, which is irrigated by the descending branch of the superficial branch of the posterior scapular artery. The traditional lower trapezius flap disrupts the main vascular pedicle of the trapezius muscle and impairs its function.

The dorsal scapular flap utilizes a double perforator, as the pedicle pierces two muscles before reaching the skin: the rhomboideus and the trapezius (Fig. 2).

The main trunk of the dorsal scapular artery divides into two branches when it reaches the angle of the scapula: the superficial (which irrigates the dorsal scapular flap) and the deep branch (which irrigates the medial border of the scapular bone).

FLAP DESIGN AND DIMENSIONS

The skin projection of the medial border of the scapula, the superomedial angle of the scapula, and the tip of the scapula are marked with the patient in a standing position and the arms at the sides of the body; the spinous processes of the vertebrae are also marked. A line is drawn between the spine of the scapula and the spinous process of the tenth thoracic vertebra, which indicates approximately the lateral border of the trapezius muscle. A point is marked 2 cm medial to the lateral border of the trapezius muscle at the level of the middle of the scapula. This point represents the emergence of the cutaneous perforator through the trapezius muscle, and it must be included in the flap design. A 20-cm-long skin paddle oriented in any direction can be safely designed.

OPERATIVE TECHNIQUE

The patient is placed in a prone decubitus position. The procedure is prepared with the skin infiltrated with 1% lidocaine (Xylocaine) along the flap margins already marked. The skin is incised, and dissection is performed above the deep fascia. The lateral border of the trapezius muscle is identified and retracted superiorly, in order to observe its deep surface, where the superficial branch of the dorsal scapular artery is easily seen. The skin island is dissected, and the perforator is now observed on the surface of the muscle; it is then dissected free from the muscle. The vascular pedicle is liberated from the muscle belly, and dissection continues up to the point where the pedicle pierces the rhomboideus muscle; the pedicle is dissected in depth through this muscle, and the main trunk of the dorsal scapular artery is exposed. The deep branch to the scapular bone is ligated and sectioned, unless a bone segment is included in the flap.

A long retractor is placed, pulling up the trapezius, the omohyoid, and the levator scapula muscles and creating a tunnel. The muscle branches to these muscles are coagulated and sectioned. A cannula is passed through this tunnel up to the supraclavicular skin, which is incised. The flap is passed to the anterior incision. The donor site of the back is closed, and the patient is turned to a dorsal decubitus position. The flap is inset into the anterior thorax, the face, or the neck (Fig. 3).

CLINICAL RESULTS

The DSAP flap was used in 42 cases in our clinical series (25 female and 17 male patients). Patient ages ranged from 9 to 65

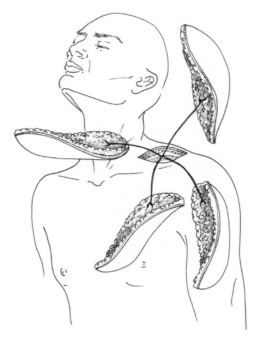

FIG. 3. After transposing the flap anteriorly, the arc of rotation allows for inset into the anterior thorax, the face, or the neck.

years. The flap was used as a single skin and subcutaneous tissue flap in 36 cases. In seven cases, it was utilized as compound soft tissue and vascularized bone (using the medial part of the scapula bone); four of these cases were mandibular reconstructions, one case was a clavicle pseudoarthrosis, and a sixth case was a superior maxillary reconstruction.

The skin flaps were used for anterior chest-wall resurfacing after release of burn scar contraction in 6 cases, for neck resurfacing (partial or total) in 18 cases, for cranial-vault reconstruction in 4 cases, and for cheek reconstruction in 8 cases.

There were three complete flap losses and four partial tissue losses suffered at the distal part, which eventually healed. The complete failures were related to technical errors during flap elevation in two cases; in one case, the flap could not be carried out as planned due to absence of the skin branch of the dorsal scapular artery. The direct cutaneous branch of the great intercostal (third space) was used as the vascular pedicle of the skin island, which was transferred as a free flap.

SUMMARY

The dorsal scapular flap represents an additional way to transfer an island flap from the medial part of the back (corresponding to the area of the traditional lower trapezius musculocutaneous flap) to the anterior thoracic wall, the neck, the face, or the cranial vault.

References

1. Angrigiani C, Grilli D, Karanas YL, Longaker M. The dorsal scapular island flap: an alternative for head, neck, and chest reconstruction. *Plast Reconstr Surg* 2003;111:67.
2. Weiglein AH, Hass F, Pierer G, et al. Anatomic basis of the lower trapezius musculocutaneous flap. *Surg Radiol Anat* 1996;18:257.
3. Huelke DF. A study of the transverse cervical and dorsal scapular arteries. *Anat Rec* 1958;103:233.
4. Daseler EH, Anson BJ. Surgical anatomy of the subclavian artery and its branches. *Surg Gynecol Obstet* 1959;108:149.
5. Salmon M. *Les artères des muscles du tronc.* Paris: Masson, 1933.

CHAPTER 128. Tubed Abdominal and Chest Skin Flaps *M. F. Stranc and W. E. Stranc*
www.encyclopediaofflaps.com

CHAPTER 129 ■ LATISSIMUS DORSI MUSCULOCUTANEOUS FLAP TO THE HEAD, NECK, CHEEK, AND SCALP

W. Y. HOFFMAN, R. M. BARTON, AND L. O. VASCONEZ

The latissimus dorsi muscle, with its long vascular pedicle, can be converted to a flap of considerable length that, combined with the substantial bulk and reliable vascular supply of the muscle, makes this muscle ideal for major head and neck reconstruction. Moreover, the length and diameter of the primary vascular supply allow the fashioning of an excellent free flap.

INDICATIONS

The latissimus dorsi has proved especially useful in resurfacing defects of the cheek and lateral scalp. Although most of the neck can be reached for coverage by the latissimus dorsi, the pectoralis major is generally preferred for neck and intraoral reconstruction. The latissimus dorsi is used in these areas when a great deal of bulk or skin or both are needed (1–7).

For reestablishing oropharyngeal continuity, the musculocutaneous flap has been used with the skin portion placed inward and with skin grafts placed on the exposed muscle surface (8). The split flap, with two musculocutaneous units, has been applied to reconstruction of the pharynx while simultaneously providing outer skin coverage (9,10).

The free latissimus dorsi flap was first described for coverage of a chronically infected scalp after multiple skin grafts had failed (11). Since that time, the free latissimus dorsi has been used as a muscle alone with skin graft cover (12,13), as a musculocutaneous flap both for scalp and other head and neck defects (14,15), and as an osteomusculocutaneous composite transfer to achieve internal and external wound closure and to restore mandibular continuity (16). Whenever possible, however, the long vascular pedicle of the muscle should lead to consideration of a pedicled flap rather than a free flap.

ANATOMY

The latissimus dorsi muscle originates from the lower thoracolumbar vertebrae, the thoracolumbar fascia, the lumbar and sacral vertebrae, and the posterior iliac crest. It inserts into the intertubercular groove of the humerus, serving to adduct, extend, and internally rotate the arm and to lift and stabilize the pelvis in walking (2,17).

The blood supply to the muscle comes primarily from the thoracodorsal artery, with secondary contributions from perforating branches of the lower posterior intercostal arteries. The thoracodorsal artery, arising at a bifurcation with the circumflex scapular artery, is a terminal branch of the subscapular artery that enters the muscle on the deep surface 8 to 10 cm from the axillary artery and 2 cm from its free anterior edge. There is a constant branch to the serratus anterior muscle. The diameter of the most proximal part of the thoracodorsal artery averages 1.5 to 3.0 mm, making it an excellent vessel for microvascular anastomosis.

At the point of entry into the muscle, the thoracodorsal artery splits into a lateral branch that is parallel to and 2 cm from the anterior border of the muscle and a medial branch that runs obliquely near the upper border of the muscle. This anatomic formation constitutes the basis for the "split" flap with two musculocutaneous units on a single pedicle and has been found in 85% to 95% of cadavers studied (9,10,18).

The secondary blood supply, originating in the intercostal vessels that also nourish the ribs, is important in head and neck reconstruction and forms the basis for the osteomusculocutaneous flap that carries viable rib with the muscle based only on the thoracodorsal vessels (16,19,20).

Musculocutaneous perforators are widely distributed over the entire muscle surface and supply the overlying skin. Inclusion of the thoracolumbar fascia will provide blood to skin down to the iliac crest if the proximal musculocutaneous perforators are also preserved. This "extended," or musculofascial, flap is not completely reliable, and some authors recommend delaying this flap by ligating the posterior perforating vessels (3,5,7,21).

FLAP DESIGN AND DIMENSIONS

Planning backward from the expected defect ensures that the skin island is placed sufficiently inferior on the muscle (Fig. 1). Small island flaps may be excluded from any direct musculocutaneous perforators and may not survive. Using a Doppler probe to locate perforators has been reported, but this is difficult to perform accurately. The largest flap reported is 20 × 30 cm. The donor defect may be closed primarily if the skin island is smaller than 8 to 10 cm.

OPERATIVE TECHNIQUE

Muscle and Musculocutaneous Flap

An incision is made just beyond the free edge of the muscle to expose the vascular pedicle. The incision is carried posteriorly to join the incised skin island, which is sutured to the muscle fascia early in the procedure to avoid shearing any musculocutaneous perforators. The pedicle can be dissected up to the axillary vessels, dividing the circumflex scapular vessels if necessary. The nerve also may be divided to cause later atrophy of the muscle that will create better contour. The muscle is dissected superficial to the serratus anterior and the scapula. If a transfer of vascularized rib is planned, the perforators to that rib are preserved; otherwise, all the posterior vessels are divided.

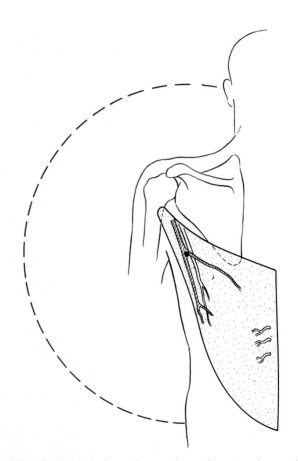

FIG. 1. This diagram shows the partial arc of rotation that can be extended with a distal fascial portion of the flap. The arterial configuration and the secondary pedicles are shown.

After detaching the origin of the muscle, the flap is tunneled with the attached skin island *under* the pectoralis major muscle and *over* the clavicle. If necessary, the base of the muscle and pedicle are thinned to prevent pressure on the vessels, and the muscle then is brought either subcutaneously or over the neck skin to the cheek or scalp, fitting nicely into the defect left after removal of the sternocleidomastoid muscle in radical neck dissections.

Free-flap Technique

The technique for a free flap is similar to that of a muscle flap, except that the insertion of the muscle is divided as well. The dissection under the muscle is best done in a retrograde fashion to identify the vascular supply as early as possible. The donor vessels are divided close to the axillary vessels only after the recipient defect and vessels have been prepared. For head and neck reconstruction, the superficial temporal and the fascial vessels are used most frequently as the recipient vessels.

CLINICAL RESULTS

One of the main problems with the latissimus dorsi for head and neck reconstruction is its location and the difficulty in positioning the patient for simultaneous resection and flap elevation. This can be overcome by lateral decubitus positioning for lateral lesions or by closing most of the posterior wound before beginning resection.

The functional deficit is minimal, except in certain athletic endeavors (swimming, climbing) and in patients who have some pelvic or hip instability.

Temporary brachial plexus palsy has been reported in up to 10% of patients, because of manipulation and hyperextension or abduction of the arm during the operation. The flap itself is extremely reliable. Any tissue loss is usually caused by compression of the pedicle or technical difficulty with a microvascular anastomosis (22).

SUMMARY

With a pivot point in the axilla, the latissimus dorsi muscle and musculocutaneous flap can reach not only the anterior or posterior neck but also the chin, cheek, and lateral scalp.

Other areas that are not within reach can be closed with a free flap.

References

1. Quillen CG, Shearin JC, Georgiade NG. Use of the latissimus dorsi myocutaneous island flap for reconstruction in the head and neck area. *Plast Reconstr Surg* 1978;62:113.
2. Mathes SJ, Nahai F. *Clinical atlas of muscle and musculocutaneous flaps.* St. Louis: Mosby, 1979;369–392.
3. Quillen CG. Latissimus dorsi myocutaneous flaps in head and neck reconstruction. *Plast Reconstr Surg* 1979;63:664.
4. Krishna BV, Green MF. Extended role of latissimus dorsi myocutaneous flap in reconstruction of the neck. *Br J Plast Surg* 1980;33:233.
5. Maxwell GP, Leonard LG, Manson PN, Hoopes JE. Craniofacial coverage using the latissimus dorsi myocutaneous flap. *Ann Plast Surg* 1980;4:410.
6. Morris RL, Given KS, McCabe JS. Repair of head and neck defects with the latissimus dorsi myocutaneous flap. *Am Surg* 1981;47:167.
7. Barton FE, Spicer TE, Byrd HS. Head and neck reconstruction with the latissimus dorsi myocutaneous flap: anatomic observations and report of 60 cases. *Plast Reconstr Surg* 1983;71:199.
8. Watson JS, Lendrum J. One-stage pharyngeal reconstruction using a compound latissimus dorsi island flap. *Br J Plast Surg* 1981;34:87.
9. Tobin GR, Spratt JS, Bland KI, Weiner LJ. One-stage pharyngoesophageal and oral mucocutaneous reconstruction with two segments of one musculocutaneous flap. *Am J Surg* 1982;144:489.
10. Tobin GR, Moberg AW, Dubou RH, et al. The split latissimus dorsi myocutaneous flap. *Ann Plast Surg* 1981;7:272.
11. Maxwell GP, Stueber K, Hoopes JE. A free latissimus dorsi myocutaneous flap. *Plast Reconstr Surg* 1978;62:462.
12. Mathes SJ, Vasconez LO, Rosenblum ML. Management of the difficult scalp and intracranial wound. *Clin Plast Surg* 1981;8:327.
13. Alpert BS, Buncke HJ, Mathes SJ. Surgical treatment of the totally avulsed scalp. *Clin Plast Surg* 1982;9:145.
14. Maxwell GP. Experience with 13 latissimus dorsi myocutaneous free flaps. *Plast Reconstr Surg* 1979;64:1.
15. Maxwell GP. Musculocutaneous free flaps. *Clin Plast Surg* 1980;7:111.
16. Schmidt DR, Robson MC. One-stage composite reconstruction using the latissimus dorsi myo-osteocutaneous free flap. *Am J Surg* 1982;144:470.
17. Bartlett SP, May JW, Jr., Yaremchuk MJ. The latissimus dorsi muscle: a fresh cadaver study of the primary neurovascular pedicle. *Plast Reconstr Surg* 1981;67:631.
18. Tobin GR, Schusterman MA, Peterson GH, et al. The intramuscular neurovascular anatomy of the latissimus dorsi muscle: the basis for splitting the flap. *Plast Reconstr Surg* 1981;67:637.
19. Schlenker JD, Indresano AT, Raine T, et al. A new flap in the dog containing a vascularized rib graft and the latissimus dorsi myocutaneous flap. *J Surg Res* 1980;29:172.
20. Schlenker JD, Robson MC, Parsons RW. Methods and results of reconstruction with free flaps following resection of squamous cell carcinoma of the head and neck. *Ann Plast Surg* 1981;6:362.
21. Bostwick J, Nahai F, Wallace JG, Vasconez LO. Sixty latissimus dorsi flaps. *Plast Reconstr Surg* 1979;63:31.
22. Vasconez LO, McCraw JB, Hall EJ. Complications of musculocutaneous flaps. *Clin Plast Surg* 1980;7:123.

CHAPTER 130 ■ TRAPEZIUS MUSCLE AND MUSCULOCUTANEOUS FLAPS

K. F. HAGAN AND S. J. MATHES

The trapezius muscle is the basis for muscle and musculocutaneous flaps that are of great usefulness in reconstructing defects of the head and neck and of the upper back (1–12). Its location makes it frequently the flap of choice for defects of the occipital, parotid, and cervical spine areas. In addition, it may be used for intraoral and anterior neck coverage. The posterior trapezius musculocutaneous flap should be considered the flap of choice for defects of the lateral face, posterior scalp and neck, and the upper third of the posterior trunk.

ANATOMY

Muscle Function

The muscle may be functionally separated into three parts (Fig. 1). The upper occipital and cervical part acts to elevate the shoulder, holding it in normal postural position by slight, continuous, tonic contraction. This action is not shared with other muscles (although the levator scapulae exerts an upward pull on the scapula, it does not have the same effect on the shoulder girdle), and hence denervation of the trapezius or functional loss of its upper fibers will result in the shoulder-drop deformity (13,14).

The medial fibers, originating from the upper thoracic region, pull the scapula backward toward the midline and act to square the shoulders. This function is shared with the rhomboid muscles.

The inferior fibers from the lower thoracic region act in concert with the upper fibers to rotate the scapula, assisting in abduction of the arm above the horizontal plane; however, loss of function of lower fibers alone usually has minimal effect on arm abduction because the serratus anterior is a more powerful rotator of the scapula than the trapezius. Therefore, selective loss of the middle and inferior fibers has no significant clinical sequelae (see Fig. 1).

The trapezius is a broad, flat, triangular-shaped muscle that, when combined with its contralateral mate, forms a trapezium (see Fig. 1). It originates medially from the external occipital protuberance, the medial part of the superior nuchal line of the occipital bone, the ligamentum nuchae, and the spinous processes of the seventh cervical and all the thoracic vertebrae. The superior portion of the muscle that originates from the occipital and upper thoracic areas inserts into the posterior aspect of the lateral third of the clavicle (Figs. 1 and 2). The middle portion, originating from the lower cervical and upper thoracic areas, inserts onto the acromion and the superior spine of the scapula. The inferior fibers, originating from the lower thoracic vertebrae, insert into the base of the spine of

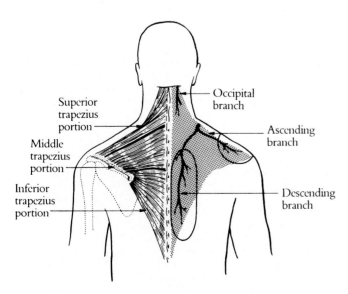

FIG. 1. Trapezius anatomy. The relationship of the three functional portions of the trapezius muscle to the vascular supply to the trapezius is demonstrated. The location of the anterior and posterior skin islands is shown.

363

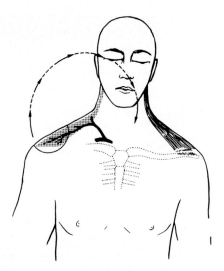

FIG. 2. Trapezius muscle, anterior view. The anterior portion is inserted into the clavicle. The anterior skin island flap, based on the anterior branch of the transverse cervical artery, is illustrated with its arc of rotation.

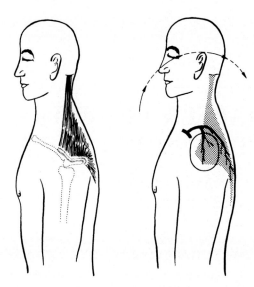

FIG. 3. Lateral view. Both anterior and posterior branches of the transverse cervical artery are illustrated. The arc of rotation is demonstrated.

the scapula. The muscle overlies the splenius capitis, levator scapulae, supraspinatus, rhomboidus minor and major, and the upper medial portion of the latissimus dorsi muscle.

The vascular supply consists of a dominant pedicle and several minor pedicles (Figs. 1–3B). The dominant blood supply originates from the transverse cervical artery and vein, a branch of the subclavian artery or thyrocervical trunk and associated veins. This vascular pedicle courses between the sternocleidomastoid and the scalenus muscles, crosses the anterior margin of the trapezius, and enters the deep surface of the muscle at the base of the neck. It then divides into ascending and descending branches that are the basis for the separate superior and inferior musculocutaneous flaps. The descending branch courses along the deep surface of the muscle, between the spine and the scapulae, supplying musculocutaneous perforators to the overlying skin. The ascending branch, which may occasionally arise as a separate branch from the thyrocervical trunk, courses laterally on the deep surface of the superior portion of the muscle, giving perforating vessels to the overlying skin just posterior to the clavicle. The average length of this dominant pedicle is 4 cm, with an average diameter of 1.8 mm.

Several minor pedicles also supply this muscle. The largest of these is a branch of the occipital artery (which arises from the external carotid). It supplies the superomedial portion of the muscle (see Fig. 1). This branch is the basis for McCraw's technique for augmenting the Mutter flap with the upper portion of the trapezius (9). It is approximately 3 cm long and 1 mm in diameter.

The remaining minor pedicles consist of perforating branches of the posterior intercostal arteries and veins that enter the muscle along the midline adjacent to the cervical and thoracic vertebral bodies. These are 1 to 2 cm in length and 0.5 mm in diameter.

A musculocutaneous flap based on these vessels alone has not been described, but these vessels have been used as the vascular basis for a medially based turnover muscle flap for coverage of the cervicothoracic spine, similar to the medially based pectoralis major flap used for sternal wound coverage (see Chapter 342).

The nerve supply to the trapezius consists of the spinal accessory nerve (cranial nerve XI) that enters the deep surface

of the muscle about 5 cm above the clavicle and direct branches of the ventral rami of the third and fourth cervical nerves. The accessory nerve is the primary motor nerve, and it must be preserved if the muscle is to remain functional. Cervical nerves III and IV provide sensory (proprioceptive) fibers. The cutaneous sensory nerves to the skin overlying the trapezius consist of the branches of the cervical nerves anteriorly and the intercostal nerves posteriorly. Because these nerves must be cut during flap elevation, a neurosensory flap is not possible unless these sensory nerves are connected to preserved sensory nerves at the flap recipient site.

The entire cutaneous territory of the trapezius measures 34 × 28 cm, which includes several centimeters superiorly and inferiorly beyond the muscle fibers. The cutaneous perforators are located throughout the muscle surface, but the largest and most consistent occur along the medial aspect 2 to 3 cm from the midline. For clinical purposes, the entire muscular unit is almost never used.

FLAP DESIGN AND DIMENSIONS

Clinically useful flaps consist of two anterior flaps based on either the ascending branch of the transverse cervical artery or on the occipital perforating branch with a skin paddle located laterally over the shoulder (see Figs. 1–3) and a posterior flap based on the descending branch of the dominant artery with a vertical skin island located between the spine and the scapula (Figs. 1 and 5).

Anterior Transverse Flap

The arc of rotation of the flap will reach the temporal area (see Figs. 2 and 3) and across to the midline floor of the mouth and neck when mobilized as an island on the transverse cervical vessels. Even as a pedicle flap, it will easily reach into the hypopharynx and laryngeal areas (11,14). An osteocutaneous flap for mandibular reconstruction may be elevated by preserving the insertion of the trapezius to the acromion and spine of the scapula and removing the entire acromion and scapular spine en bloc with the muscle (9).

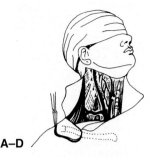
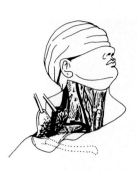
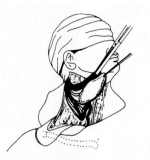
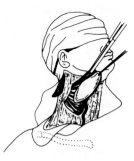

A–D

FIG. 4. Dissection of anterior transverse flap. **A:** Skin incision is made along the anterior border of trapezius. The trapezius muscle is exposed along with the transverse cervical vessels. Skin incision is made over skin paddle. **B:** Dissection is performed in a subfascial plane over the acromion, dissecting beneath the trapezius muscle. The posterior descending branch of the transverse cervical artery is ligated. **C:** The skin island is now elevated along with the intact superior portion of trapezius muscle. **D:** The fibers of origin of the superior trapezius muscle may be completely divided, maintaining only the continuity of the vascular pedicle, if a wider arc of rotation is desired.

Posterior Vertical Flap

The posterior trapezius musculocutaneous flap was developed in an attempt to avoid the loss of function of the superior fibers and thus to maintain proper shoulder position (13) (see Fig. 5). This musculocutaneous flap is based on the middle and inferior portion of the trapezius muscle. The posterior muscle is supplied by the descending branch of the transverse cervical vessels. The skin island is located between the scapula and the spine; skin island dimensions may be up to 25 × 8 cm, extending as much as 5 cm below the inferior border of the scapula. It may be raised as a musculocutaneous flap with skin continuity maintained for defects of the upper thoracic verte-brae (Fig. 7). For defects of the lateral face, neck, and shoul-der, a skin island is preferred (Figs. 1, 5, and 8). The arc of rotation of this flap will extend to the shoulder, upper third of the posterior scalp, and lateral neck (Figs. 5 and 6). The skin island will easily reach the anterior floor of the mouth and anterior midline of the neck.

Variations

When bulk alone is needed in the lateral neck, as in parotidec-tomy defects or hemifacial microsomia patients, the posterior muscle alone may be transferred to the neck, although the resulting bulk at the base of the neck may require delayed revi-sion. Other flaps, such as the sternocleidomastoid or platysma, are often preferred for smaller defects.

The trapezius can be used as a free flap. However, the accessibility and functional expendability of other flaps, such as the latissimus dorsi muscle, make the trapezius a poor choice for transfer.

OPERATIVE TECHNIQUE

Anterior Transverse Flap

The flap may be raised as a pedicle from 6 to 10 cm wide and 8 to 30 cm long. This is raised from lateral to medial, similar to the cervicohumeral flap (see Chapter 131), raising the distal skin in a subfascial plane until the midportion of the trapezius muscle is reached. At this point, the muscle is transected and raised with the flap, severing the dominant pedicle from the

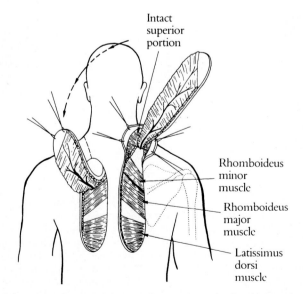

Intact superior portion

Rhomboideus minor muscle

Rhomboideus major muscle

Latissimus dorsi muscle

FIG. 5. Posterior vertical flap. Flap is raised, exposing the latissimus dorsi and rhomboid muscles. Note descending branch of the trans-verse cervical vessel supplying the overlying trapezius muscle. Superior portion of muscle is left intact to prevent shoulder drop. Arc of rotation is shown for the right side flap.

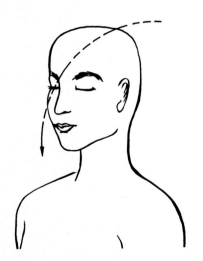

FIG. 6. Anterior arc of rotation for posterior vertical trapezius mus-culocutaneous flap.

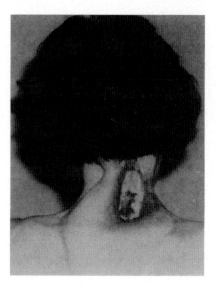

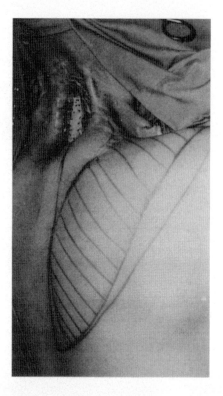

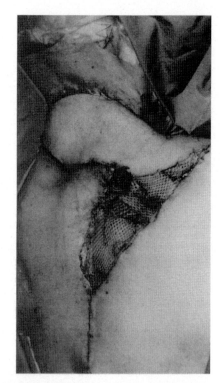

A–C

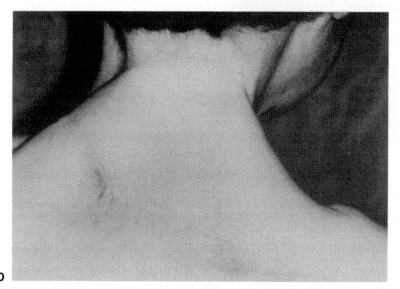

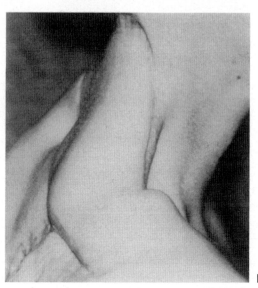

D

E

FIG. 7. Posterior vertical trapezius musculocutaneous flap for posterior neck coverage. A: Osteoradionecrosis of cervical vertebral column following failure of local flap coverage. B: Design of posterior trapezius flap with skin intact. C: Flap is rotated to provide coverage of the cervical defect. Skin graft is required to cover the upper portion of the defect. D: Healed flap, anterior view. E: Healed flap, lateral view. (From Mathes, Nahai, ref. 13, with permission.)

attached portion of muscle that is supplied only by the occipital perforating branches. The skin over the lateral third of the clavicle on this flap is unreliable, and a delay may be helpful.

A more reliable and versatile flap consists of the entire upper portion of the trapezius muscle based on the dominant anterior ascending branch of the pedicle, the transverse cervical artery (Figs. 1–4). This flap is raised as a skin island, with the skin paddle centered over the acromion, extending several centimeters in all directions as needed. The flap may be raised from lateral to medial, but the preferred method is medial to lateral (9), especially because this step is frequently done in conjunction with a neck dissection.

The skin island is designed and marked, and a skin incision is made from the medial portion of the island to the upper neck, paralleling the anterior border of the muscle (Fig. 4A). Dissection is carried deep to the anterior border, identifying and preserving the transverse cervical vessel (Fig. 4B). The superior fibers of the muscle are then removed from their insertions into the lateral third of the clavicle, the acromion, and the upper portion of the spine of the scapula. The dissection is carried beneath the distal random portion of the skin island in a subfascial plane. The upper portion of the muscle itself may be left intact, attached to its origin as a muscle pedicle (Fig. 4C), or it may be divided, resulting in a skin and mus-

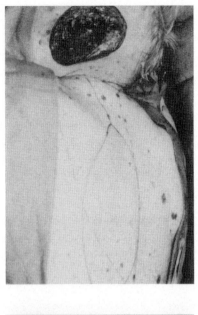
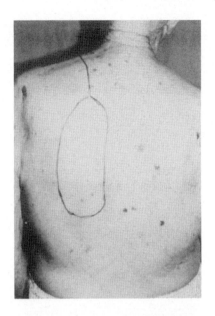

A,B

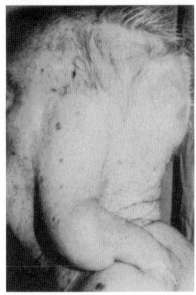
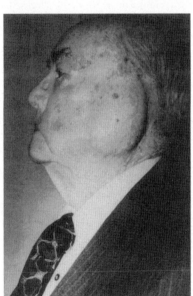

C,D

FIG. 8. Posterior vertical trapezius island musculocutaneous flap for lateral face coverage. **A:** Defect following removal of squamous cell carcinoma of the ear, parotid, and zygoma. **B:** Design of skin island of vertical trapezius. **C:** Healed flap. Note that skin grafts cover exposed inferior muscle fibers. **D:** Final result following division of muscle flap at base of neck. (From Mathes Nahai, ref. 12, with permission.)

cle island supported only by the ascending branch of the transverse cervical vessels (Fig. 4D). In the latter case, the accessory nerves to the remaining muscle may be preserved if the muscle is transected distal to the site of entrance of the nerve.

The donor area usually will require a skin graft. Only the smallest skin island will allow primary closure in this area.

Posterior Vertical Flap

This flap is best raised from inferior to superior (distal to proximal). Flap elevation begins by dissecting the extended portion of the skin flap off the upper fibers of the latissimus dorsi (see Fig. 5). When the inferior border of the trapezius is identified, it is elevated with the flap, dividing its vertebral origin. At the level of the scapula, care must be taken to avoid raising the rhomboid muscles with the flap, which would lead beneath the scapula. The descending branch of the vascular supply will be visualized on the undersurface. The muscle is divided at the lateral edge of the skin paddle, taking care to

preserve the uppermost fibers between the skull and clavicle, which are responsible for shoulder elevation.

The donor defect usually may be closed primarily. Nevertheless, muscle bulk at the base of this flap is often aesthetically objectionable (see Fig. 8C); therefore, debulking or division of this muscle pedicle is frequently necessary. This is done after a delay of 3 to 4 weeks in healthy recipient beds and 6 to 8 weeks in irradiated wounds.

CLINICAL RESULTS

The primary disadvantage of the anterior trapezius flap is the potential shoulder-drop deformity and the continuity of the donor-site defect with the neck wound of a radical neck dissection.

Complications may arise from errors in planning or technique. The most common planning error in raising trapezius flaps relates to their blood supply. The dominant pedicle, the transverse cervical artery, is frequently divided during head and neck procedures or is damaged by local radiation treatment to the neck area. If doubt exists as to the integrity of this vessel, an arteriogram should be obtained. If an anterior trapezius flap is based on the occipital perforating branches (augmented Mutter flap), the skin portion is less reliable and flap delay may be necessary for extension beyond the lateral third of the clavicle.

Technical errors most often occur when elevating the posterior flap. Care must be taken to avoid dissection beneath the rhomboid muscles. In addition, the spinal accessory nerve to the upper portion of the muscle must be preserved. Constrictive dressings around the neck must be avoided.

SUMMARY

Trapezius muscle and musculocutaneous flaps are extremely useful for reconstructing defects of the head and neck, upper posterior thorax, and anterior neck.

References

1. Mutter TD. Case of deformity from burns, relieved by operation. *Am J Med Sci* 1842;4:66.
2. Zovickian A. Pharyngeal fistulas: repair and prevention using mastoid occiput based shoulder flaps. *Plast Reconstr Surg* 1957;19:355.
3. Chretien PB, Ketcham AS, Hoye RC, Gertren HR. Extended shoulder flap and its use in reconstruction of defect of the head and neck. *Am J Surg* 1972;118:752.
4. Robson MC. The undelayed Mutter flap in head and neck reconstruction. *Am J Surg* 1976;132:472.
5. McCraw J, Dibbell D, Carraway J. Experimental definition of independent myocutaneous vascular territories. *Plast Reconstr Surg* 1977;60:212.
6. McCraw J, Dibbell D, Carraway J. Clinical definition of independent myocutaneous vascular territories. *Plast Reconstr Surg* 1977;60:341.
7. Demurgasso F. Reconstruction con colgajo osteo cutaneo trapecial en reseccion mandibulares segmentarias por cancer de cabeza y cuello. Presented at the Premio Anual, Sociedad Argentina de Patologia de Cabeza y Cuello, Buenos Aires, 1977.
8. Demurgasso F, Piazza M. Trapezius myocutaneous flap in reconstructive surgery of head and neck cancer: an original technique. *Am J Surg* 1979;138:533.
9. McCraw JB, Magee WP, Jr., Kalwaic H. Uses of the trapezius and sternocleidomastoid myocutaneous flap in head and neck surgery. *Plast Reconstr Surg* 1979;63:49.
10. Bertolti JA. Trapezius musculocutaneous island flap in the repair of major head and neck cancer. *Plast Reconstr Surg* 1980;65:16.
11. Mathes SJ, Vasconez LO. Head, neck and truncal reconstruction with the myocutaneous flap: anatomical and clinical considerations. In: *Transactions of the Seventh International congress of Plastic and Reconstructive Surgeons, 1979.* São Paulo, Brazil: Cartgraf, 1980;178–182.
12. Mathes SJ, Nahai F. Muscle flap transposition with functional preservation: technical and clinical considerations. *Plast Reconstr Surg* 1980;66:242.
13. Mathes SJ, Nahai F. *Clinical atlas of muscle and musculocutaneous flaps.* St. Louis: Mosby, 1979.
14. Mathes SJ, Nahai F. *Clinical applications for muscle and musculocutaneous flaps.* St. Louis: Mosby, 1982.

CHAPTER 131 ■ CERVICOHUMERAL FLAP

E. A. LUCE

The musculocutaneous "revolution" in reconstructive surgery has allowed refinement of the principle of primary reconstruction of head and neck defects following extirpative cancer surgery. The cervicohumeral flap was designed as an extension of the trapezius flap for reconstruction in the midface, oral cavity, neck, and anterior chest.

INDICATIONS

At present, I limit the use of the cervicohumeral (and trapezius) flap to coverage of anterior cervical defects or to situations where other alternatives are not available (see Fig. 5). In most head and neck cancer patients, I prefer the modified pectoralis major island flap (1,2) as the "workhorse" in head and neck coverage.

ANATOMY

The cervicohumeral flap is based on the posterior shoulder and supraclavicular region, extends across the acromioclavicular joint, and continues down the lateral aspect of the arm (Fig. 1). The axis of rotation, and presumably the blood sup-

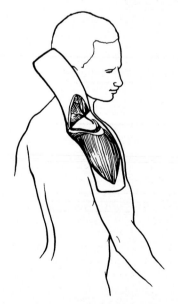

FIG. 1. Dominant and minor blood supplies to the trapezius and cervicohumeral flap.

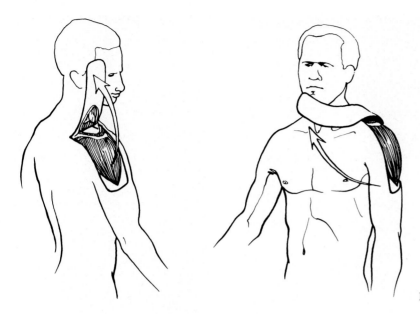

FIG. 2. Arc of rotation of the flap.

ply, is the trapezius muscle (3,4). The dominant vascular pedicle to the trapezius is the transverse cervical artery, although branches (probably minor in significance) are contributed by the occipital artery proximally, the superficial cervical artery in the midportion of the muscle, and branches of the suprascapular in the distal portion (3).

Beyond the distal insertion of the trapezius, the skin over the deltoid on the lateral proximal arm is supplied by the posterior circumflex humeral artery. This skin, when included with the trapezius musculocutaneous unit and with sacrifice of the posterior circumflex humeral artery, is random in blood supply. The skin distal to the insertion of the deltoid probably is derived from the lateral head of the triceps and the biceps-triceps intermuscular septum (5).

FLAP DESIGN AND DIMENSIONS

The cervicohumeral flap has been described as reliable when raised undelayed with a length-width ratio of 3:1. The flap has

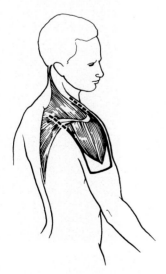

FIG. 3. Limits of the cervicohumeral flap.

been centered over the acromioclavicular joint and extended down the anterolateral arm. On occasion, the flap has been extended to a distance of 30 cm, although not with consistent success.

The wide arc of rotation of the flap (Fig. 2) has permitted reconstruction of a wide variety of defects in the past, including the oral cavity, midface and cheek, temple, and neck (Fig. 4); however, the flap has not been as consistent and reliable as initially anticipated (5) (Fig. 3).

OPERATIVE TECHNIQUE

My standard procedure has been to perform a preliminary delay 10 days prior to definitive rotation of the cervicohumeral flap. This initial delay consists of parallel incisions of the distal 10 to 12 cm of the flap with subfascial undermining of the included skin. This delay ligates the posterior circumflex humeral artery. Definitive rotation of the flap requires mobilization proximally to the acromioclavicular joint, including detachment of the trapezius muscle from the spine of the scapula. The arm donor site has been skin grafted in every case (Figs. 4 and 5).

Clearly, if an associated radical neck dissection is necessary, care must be taken to identify the transverse cervical artery at the base of the neck. In my experience, the course of this artery varies from patient to patient, and at times I have identified the artery as high as 5 or 6 cm superior to the clavicle.

CLINICAL RESULTS

I reviewed my experience over a 16-month period with use of the cervicohumeral flap for coverage of head and neck defects and compared the results to the standard flap in use at that time, the deltopectoral flap. The location of the lesion, the nature and extent of the resection, the use of radiotherapy, the length of the flap, and outcome were tabulated. A comparison was made between the cervicohumeral and the deltopectoral flap when used for similar reconstructive needs.

The cervicohumeral flap was used in 15 patients during the 16-month period for reconstruction of head and neck defects following cancer resection in patients aged 32 to 91 years. All flaps had prior delay. Ten of the 15 patients had radical neck

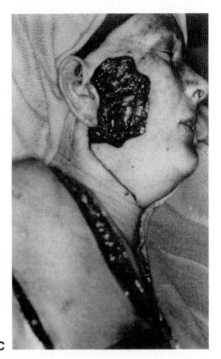
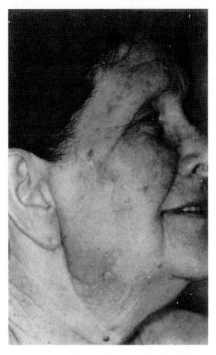
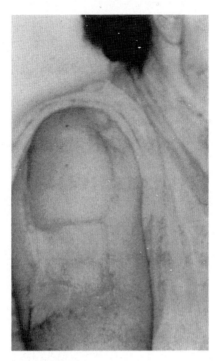

A–C

FIG. 4. **A:** Level IV malignant melanoma of the cheek diagnosed by excisional biopsy. Wide skin excision, superficial parotidectomy, upper neck dissection. A cervicohumeral flap was mobilized on the right shoulder. **B:** Patient 6 months postoperatively. **C:** Donor site on upper arm and shoulder.

dissections, and two patients had previous radiotherapy. Necrosis of the cervicohumeral flap occurred in six patients (40%). Three major sloughs required alternative methods of coverage, and three tip sloughs had wound disruption that required advancement reinsertion of the flap. Age of the patient, location of lesion, or associated radical neck dissection did not influence flap survival.

During the same time period, 10 deltopectoral flaps were used for similar reconstruction, and flap necrosis occurred in two patients.

The determining factor in survival of the cervicohumeral flap was the length of the flap. Extension of the cervico-

humeral flap beyond the distal insertion of the deltoid at the middle or proximal third of the humerus was associated with a high probability of flap necrosis despite prior delays. Experience has indicated that proximal mobilization of the trapezius muscle is preferable to distal skin extension (Fig. 3).

SUMMARY

The cervicohumeral skin flap can be used to reconstruct various head and neck defects; however, the flap should not be extended beyond the insertion of the deltoid.

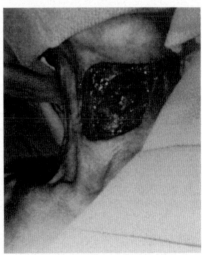
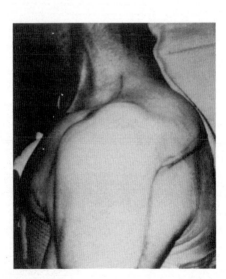
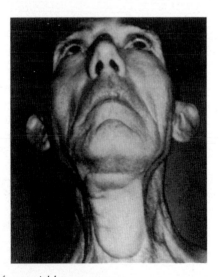

A–C

FIG. 5. **A:** Chondroradionecrosis of the larynx with skin ulceration. Defect after partial laryngectomy and wide excision of ulcer and surrounding damaged skin. **B:** Outline of cervicohumeral flap that extends to the insertion of the deltoid only. **C:** Result several weeks following retrieval of flap.

References

1. Ariyan S. The pectoralis major myocutaneous flap. *Plast Reconstr Surg* 1979;63:73.
2. Luce EA, Gottlieb SE. Versatility of a pectoralis major flap in head and neck reconstruction. Movie presented at the Annual Meetings of the American Society of Plastic and Reconstructive Surgeons, New Orleans, La., October 1980, and the Society of Head and Neck Surgery, Marco Island, Fla., April 1982.
3. Mathes SJ, Vasconez LO. The cervical humeral flap. *Plast Reconstr Surg* 1978;61:7.
4. McCraw JB, Magee WP, Kalwaich H. Uses of the trapezius and sternocleidomastoid myocutaneous flaps in head and neck reconstruction. *Plast Reconstr Surg* 1979;63:49.
5. Blevins PK, Luce EA. Limitations of the cervical humeral flap in head and neck reconstruction. *Plast Reconstr Surg* 1980;66:220.

CHAPTER 132 ■ PECTORALIS MAJOR MUSCLE AND MUSCULOCUTANEOUS FLAPS

S. ARIYAN

EDITORIAL COMMENT

This is one of the most significant musculocutaneous flaps for head and neck reconstruction. It is extremely versatile and has a hardy blood supply. The aesthetic appearance of the donor scar can be minimized by using the parasternal paddle, allowing for a curving midline scar with a transverse extension. This scar in women is almost completely hidden by the overlying breast.

The pectoralis major muscle and musculocutaneous flaps are reliable flaps that can be used for various head and neck defects (1–11).

INDICATIONS

The pectoralis major musculocutaneous flap can be used to reconstruct the oropharynx or the defect left after orbital exenteration or temporal bone resection as well as for mandibular reconstruction. (See Chapter 212 for reconstruction of the esophagus and Chapter 388 for chest wall reconstruction.)

Oropharynx (1–6)

In most cases, tumors of the floor of the mouth or lateral tongue can be reconstructed by other flaps, such as the sternocleidomastoid, platysma, nasolabial, or tongue flaps. If the surgical wound is larger than these flaps can cover, however, more tissue can be provided with the pectoralis major musculocutaneous flap, with either a single skin paddle, two skin paddles in tandem (Fig. 5), or two split-skin paddles side by side (Fig. 6). Previously, reconstructions of the tongue and piriform sinus with forehead flaps or deltopectoral flaps did not provide sufficient bulk. These cutaneous flaps are relatively thin flaps, and reconstructions using them often led to a "funnel" that directed fluids toward the laryngeal airway, frequently leading to aspiration of fluids.

Resection of the lateral floor of the mouth, alveolar ridge, posterior half of the tongue, and piriform sinus requires sufficient skin and bulk for reconstruction. This can be achieved with a pectoralis major musculocutaneous flap in one stage. The bulk provided by this flap appears to be sufficient to avoid aspirations, either by directing fluids past the airway or by diverting fluids to the contralateral normal piriform sinus, as a result of fullness on the operated side.

Orbital Exenteration

The wound resulting from an orbital exenteration has been reconstructed by a variety of flaps, including forehead flaps (12) and temporalis muscle flaps (13–16). The pectoralis major musculocutaneous flap is particularly useful for reconstruction in this area because it provides bulk and well-vascularized tissue to fill the cavity, to seal cerebrospinal fluid (CSF) leaks, and to provide greater protection against bacterial invasion (1–3).

Temporal Bone Resection

Resections of malignant tumors of the external auditory canal and mastoid can cause significant disability because of the proximity of the disease to the brain, the major dural sinuses, the carotid artery, and the cranial nerves, or because of the surgical treatment necessary to control the malignancy. Adequate tumor resection often has been compromised because of the complexity of the surgery as well as the difficulty of the reconstruction. In addition, these wounds often have been complicated by CSF leaks and bacterial contamination.

Because these cancers are otherwise uniformly fatal, treatment should consist of a radical en bloc resection of the tumor and temporal bone, together with a full course of postoperative radiation therapy (17,18). Although these wounds have been covered with rotation scalp flaps and deltopectoral flaps, the pectoralis major musculocutaneous flap is ideal for these reconstructions because it provides sufficient bulk and soft tissue to cover the dura and seal it against CSF leaks and it provides a rich vascularity to permit uncomplicated healing despite bacterial contamination of the wounds (19).

Mandibular Reconstruction

Bone grafts often fail to reconstruct a mandibular segment because of the poor vascularity in the recipient bed resulting from radiation fibrosis or dermal scarring from previous surgical procedures or injuries.

Because I was able to demonstrate that rib grafts would survive on their periosteal blood supply, I then employed the pectoralis major musculocutaneous flap, incorporating a segment of underlying rib to reconstruct a jaw (9). Although this extended pectoralis major flap may be used for reconstruction of segmental resections of the mandible, it does not appear to be suitable for reconstruction of the entire mandible.

ANATOMY

Although the thoracoacromial artery had been previously described in the literature as running along the undersurface of the pectoralis minor muscle, fresh cadaver dissections confirmed the consistent presence of this vessel along the undersurface of the pectoralis major muscle, with a branch from this vessel to the pectoralis minor. There are additional arteries to the pectoralis major, namely, the lateral thoracic artery to the lateral and inferior portions of the muscle, the superior thoracic artery to the clavicular portion, and the intercostal perforators from the internal mammary artery, providing some supply to the sternal portion of the muscle (2,20–22).

Nevertheless, the dominant blood supply is the thoracoacromial artery, a branch of the subclavian, which traverses laterally from the midportion of the clavicle for about 4 cm until it reaches the "axis" from the acromion to the xiphoid, where it then turns and runs along this line (Fig. 1). The thoracoacromial artery is accompanied along its course by its corresponding vein (or two veins) and by one of the motor nerves to the pectoralis major muscle, the lateral pectoral nerve (lateral anterior thoracic nerve) (2).

The pectoralis major muscle could be classified, along with the latissimus dorsi muscle, as a type V muscle—a single dominant vascular pedicle close to the insertion with additional segmental pedicles (22). Flat muscles (such as the pectoralis major, latissimus dorsi, and trapezius) have a dominant vascular pedicle traveling along the undersurface of the muscle. These muscles may be split such that only a portion of the muscle need be elevated with its underlying vessels to provide a reliable muscular pedicle to transport portions of overlying skin.

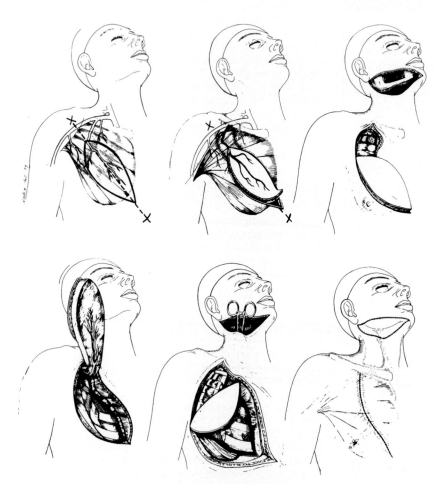

FIG. 1. The various stages in outlining the pedicle, identifying the axial vessels within the subpectoral fascia, dissecting the skin paddle with a narrow pedicle of only a portion of the muscle, freeing the neurovascular "island" pedicle, and transporting the flap to the recipient site.

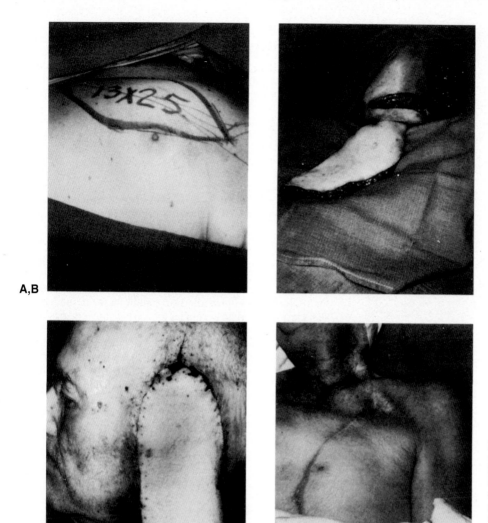

A,B

C,D

FIG. 2. **A–C:** A large (13 × 25 cm) paddle of skin was used to cover a large wound following a temporal bone resection. The skin paddle extended beyond the pectoralis major muscle by 8 cm and included the anterior rectus fascia. **D:** The donor defect was closed primarily with generous elevation and advancement of the chest skin and subcutaneous tissue. The donor site seen at 1 year.

FLAP DESIGN AND DIMENSIONS

Prior to outlining the skin paddle, the vascular axis must be drawn across the chest from the tip of the shoulder to the xiphoid (Fig. 1). The thoracoacromial artery and vein exit at a right angle from the midportion of the clavicle until they reach this axis, at which point they proceed inferomedially along this line. The paddle of skin (or two paddles), in a size and shape to fit the surgical defect, then can be outlined at the appropriate location on this vascular axis to provide the length to the muscle pedicle necessary to reach the defect. If additional skin is desired, or if additional length is necessary for the pedicle to reach a cranial defect, the paddle may be extended farther beyond the pectoralis major muscle. In these cases, the underlying rectus fascia must be elevated with the pectoralis major muscle.

Use of the pectoralis major musculocutaneous flap may pose some problems on the chests of female patients. In my experience, most of my female patients have been older, and their breasts have been atrophic and ptotic and lie laterally when the patient is supine (Fig. 3). The skin paddle may therefore be outlined on the medial aspect of the breast skin over the thin parasternal area, where little breast tissue is incorpo-

rated in the skin paddle (4). The skin is then easily advanced to close the donor defect.

In the younger patient who has fuller breasts, thinner inframammary skin is used on the muscle pedicle to prevent distortion of the breast (5). After the inframammary skin incision is made, the breast is completely elevated off the pectoralis major muscle, as in an augmentation mammaplasty (Fig. 4).

OPERATIVE TECHNIQUE

Donor Site

Skin Paddle

There are any number of ways to proceed with the dissection whereby the vascular pedicle is identified early to avoid any damage to it during the dissection. The method used most often is to incise along the inferolateral portion of the skin paddle first. The dermis of the skin paddle is sutured to the muscle fascia with several interrupted sutures along the entire skin paddle as the dissection proceeds around the paddle.

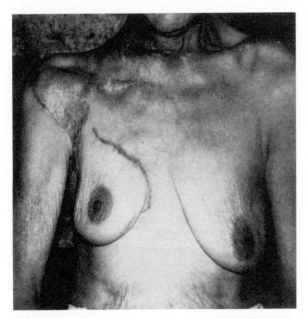

FIG. 3. The pectoralis major flap may be outlined medial to a ptotic and atrophic breast in the older patient. This may be done reliably even after a previous harvesting of a deltopectoral flap. (From Ariyan, ref. 4, with permission.)

Once the skin is incised along the inferolateral border of the outline, the muscle fibers are split to enter the subpectoral space. Care must be taken to enter the space deep to the subpectoral fascia; when the muscle is dissected from this subpectoral fascia, the vascular pedicle in this fascia is separated from the muscle. To do this safely, the dissection is carried sharply to the ribs before the loose areolar space can be identified. Once this space is entered, the pectoralis major muscle may be readily elevated with finger dissection. A large retractor is now placed to elevate the pectoralis major muscle to identify the thoracoacromial vessels in this fascia. With the vascular pedicle clearly identified, the remainder of the dissection of the flap may be done with relative ease. The location of the vessels, relative to the dissection site, is frequently checked to avoid inadvertent damage to the blood supply.

Muscle Pedicle

After the skin paddle has been dissected fully, the size of the muscle pedicle must be determined to complete the dissection. This pedicle of muscle may be as wide or as narrow as desired, for it merely transports the skin paddle with the underlying vasculature. If the sternocleidomastoid muscle has been removed in a neck dissection, the muscle pedicle of the pectoralis major flap is dissected as wide as the contralateral sternocleidomastoid appears in that patient so that it may serve to replace the missing sternocleidomastoid (2) and to restore contour and symmetry to the neck. It is rarely necessary to dissect the entire pectoralis major muscle.

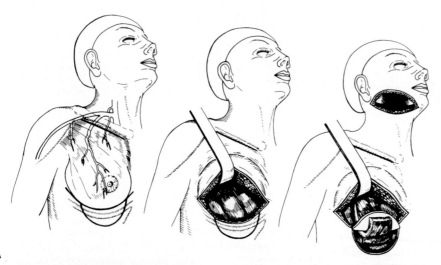

A

FIG. 4. A: In the younger woman, the skin paddle may be taken from the inframammary area after the breast is completely elevated off the muscle and returned again. B–D: Clinical example. (Periareolar depigmentation is vitiligo.) (From Ariyan, Cuono, ref. 5, with permission.)

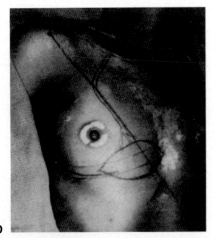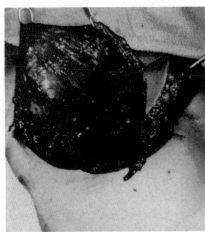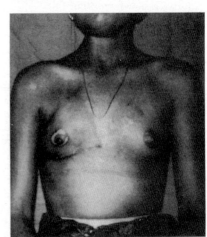

B–D

The muscle pedicle is dissected on each side parallel to the vascular pedicle directly up to the clavicle. This flap is then freed of all its attachments to the clavicle by resecting approximately 4 to 6 cm of the infraclavicular portion of the muscle, which is left attached only by its neurovascular pedicle as an "island" flap (2,3). These vessels should not be skeletonized during the dissection; they should be left with their adventitial and fascial attachments intact to prevent spasm or traction damage during the postoperative period.

When the flap is brought up to the neck, the portion of the pedicle that rests over the clavicle is then only the thin neurovascular bundle, with the muscle stump lying above the clavicle. In this manner, an unsightly bulge of muscle overlying the clavicle is avoided. Additional length may be provided to the pedicle by transecting the lateral pectoral nerve that tethers the vascular pedicle at this point. If muscle bulk is important (as in the replacement of a resected sternocleidomastoid), the nerve may be left intact to allow for less atrophy. Otherwise, it is best to transect the nerve for additional pedicle length and to allow for muscle atrophy and less bulk with the passage of time.

Chest Skin

Although the skin above the outlined skin paddle on the chest may be incised to lay open the pectoralis major muscle for facilitation of dissection of the muscle pedicle, and although this may make the first few cases easier for the surgeon, it is not necessary. In previous reports of this flap (2,3), the illustrated cases demonstrated the flap tunneled under the skin of the deltopectoral region to avoid marring this skin area.

Some surgeons have advocated the use of a deltopectoral flap for outer covering of the muscle pedicle of the pectoralis major musculocutaneous flap. I have not found this necessary, for I frequently tunnel this muscle pedicle under the neck skin. Nevertheless, this concept has led some authors to incorporate an ipsilateral deltopectoral flap with a pectoralis major flap as a single "bilobed" flap (23). Others have suggested elevating a deltopectoral flap to facilitate the dissection of a pectoralis major flap and then replacing the deltopectoral flap back on the shoulder (24). This would provide ready access to the muscle for dissection without marring the chest skin if it should be needed in the future. I have found this unnecessary,

for the skin of the deltopectoral area may be elevated as a bipedicle flap that can be retracted for ready access for muscle dissection.

Closure of Donor Site

Although some surgeons have covered the chest donor site with skin grafts, I have found this totally unnecessary. The chest skin is dissected laterally for advancement and closure of the defect. If the flap is dissected as a cutaneous flap without incorporating the pectoralis major muscle, the flap may be dissected as far posteriorly as the posterior axillary line if necessary. This can provide generous advancement, and I have been able to close each of my donor sites without skin grafts—even donor sites for cutaneous paddles as large as 13 × 25 cm (Fig. 2).

Recipient Site

Orbital Exenteration

Following resection of the tumor and the globe, the wound is evaluated for the depth and volume that needs to be filled (Fig. 7). A pectoralis major musculocutaneous flap is planned with the width equivalent to the defect that needs to be reconstructed and the length sufficient to fill the orbital cavity with soft tissue. The flap is elevated with chest skin intact over the entire length of the flap.

This flap is not tunneled under the neck or facial skin because an unacceptable cosmetic deformity would result. It is brought up to the wound over the neck and face, with its pedicle exposed on one side. The skin is removed from the distal 4 to 6 cm, the exposed muscle and soft tissues are used to fill the orbital cavity, and the margins of the skin of the flap are sutured to the skin edges of the orbit. The undersurface of the flap pedicle may be protected against infection by the application of topical antibacterial cream (such as silver sulfadiazine) and covered with petrolatum gauze.

The flap may be divided and inset at about 2 weeks. The remainder of the flap pedicle may be discarded because the donor site is usually healed by this time. It should be noted that if the lateral pectoral nerve has not been cut during the

A–C

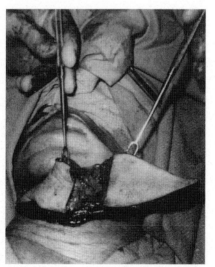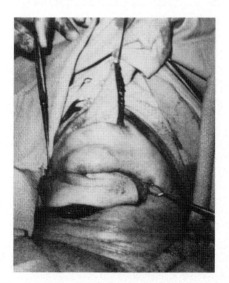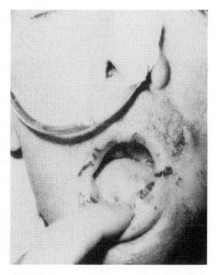

FIG. 5. **A:** Double skin paddles in tandem to resurface a through-and-through defect. **B:** The proximal paddle is used for the chin, and the distal paddle is used for the floor of the mouth. **C:** The distal paddle at 2 weeks.

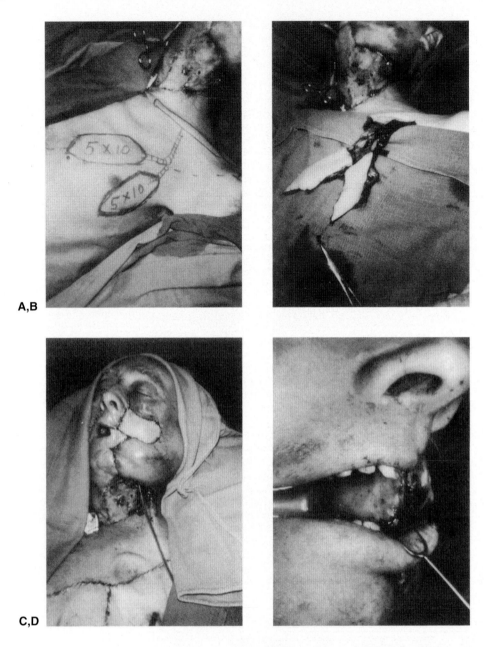

A,B

C,D

FIG. 6. A: A split pectoralis major muscle with two side-by-side skin paddles. **B,C:** These were used to line and resurface a through-and-through defect of the cheek. **D:** The lining at 3 weeks.

first procedure, a local anesthetic should be given around the neurovascular bundle as well; otherwise, the patient will feel a deep, dull pain as the neurovascular bundle is clamped.

Temporal Bone Resection

Following resection of the tumor and the temporal bone, the size and extent of the defect are determined and a paddle of skin of appropriate size is outlined over the vascular axis of the pectoralis major muscle. This flap can be tunneled under the neck skin on its narrow muscle pedicle to reach the cranial resection and cover the wound in one stage. This musculocutaneous flap can tolerate a full course of radiation therapy without complications in the postoperative period.

Mandibular Reconstruction (7–11)

In patients in whom I employed the pectoralis major musculocutaneous flap incorporating a segment of underlying rib to reconstruct a jaw (9), the body and symphysis of the mandible were reconstructed with the attached rib while the floor of the

mouth and chin were reconstructed with the overlying double-paddle musculocutaneous flap (Fig. 8). The viability of this rib was confirmed through the use of flourochrome markers (9).

However, for reconstruction of the entire mandible, the paddle of skin that is needed would require a long segment of bone along its longitudinal axis. To accomplish this would require elevating the entire pectoralis major muscle to transport such a paddle of skin and bone, and this would be much too bulky. Under these circumstances, I prefer to reconstruct the jaw with free bone grafts in the traditional manner and to cover it with a pectoralis major musculocutaneous flap so that the bone graft is sandwiched within a well-vascularized muscle.

CLINICAL RESULTS

The pectoralis major musculocutaneous flap has been a very reliable and successful flap in my early experience of 40 consecutive patients (six patients had esophageal reconstruc-

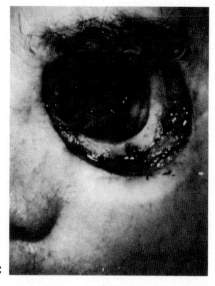
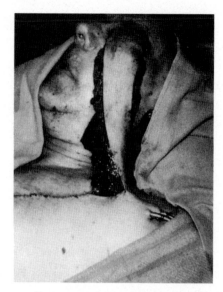
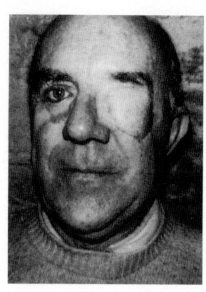

A–C

FIG. 7. A: An extensive squamous cell carcinoma that invaded the globe and orbital contents was widely resected. B: The cavity was filled with the soft tissue of the distal portion of a pectoralis major flap. C: The appearance of the patient at 6 months. (From Ariyan, ref. 4, with permission.)

tions). In half these patients, the size of the skin paddle exceeded 150 cm², with the largest paddle recorded at 13 × 25 cm for a temporal bone resection (see Fig. 2). All the donor sites were closed primarily and healed without complication. In eight patients, the flap was elevated with double paddles, either in tandem or split side by side (see Figs. 5 and 6).

There were nine complications in eight patients. There were three cases of separation of the skin paddle along a portion of the suture line; however, in each instance, the muscle did not separate and the wound healed without additional surgical treatment. An orocutaneous fistula developed in three patients, two of whom had oropharyngeal reconstruction with the tip of the skin paddle in the piriform sinus; there was only one orocutaneous fistula in the six reconstructions of the esophagus (all of which had a full course of preoperative radiation therapy). Each of these three fistulas closed within 2 weeks without requiring additional surgery.

There were three cases of partial loss of the skin paddle, one for a jaw reconstruction, one for an orbital reconstruc-tion, and one in a double paddle. Two were debrided and allowed to close by secondary contraction, while a third required surgical debridement and secondary closure of the wound. There was no case of total loss of a pectoralis major flap.

The patients in this series did not have any evidence of dis-ability from a partial loss of the pectoralis major muscle, whether the lateral pectoral nerves were cut or left intact. In two patients, both pectoralis major muscles were used for reconstructions, and these patients had no disability. All six patients with esophageal reconstructions are able to eat regu-lar or mechanically soft diets without difficulty in swallowing.

SUMMARY

The pectoralis major musculocutaneous flap is very reliable for head and neck reconstruction. There are few complica-tions and little or no disability from the loss of muscle.

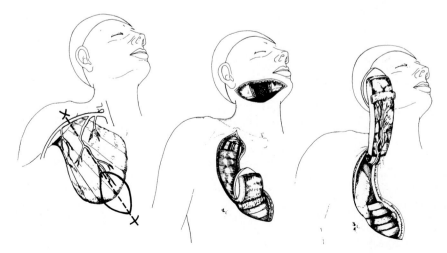

FIG. 8. Artist's depiction of pectoralis major flap elevated with underlying segment of rib. Note that the skin paddle is used for oral lining and the rib is used to bridge the mandibular resection.

References

1. Ariyan S, Krizek TJ. Reconstruction after resection of head and neck cancer. CINE Clinics. Clinical Congress of the American College of Surgeons, Dallas, Texas, October 1977.
2. Ariyan S. The pectoralis major myocutaneous flap: a versatile flap for reconstruction in the head and neck. *Plast Reconstr Surg* 1979;63:73.
3. Ariyan S. Further experiences with the pectoralis major myocutaneous flap for the immediate repair of defects from excisions of head and neck cancer. *Plast Reconstr Surg* 1979;64:605.
4. Ariyan S. Pectoralis major, sternomastoid, and other musculocutaneous flaps for head and neck construction. *Clin Plast Surg* 1980;7:89.
5. Ariyan S, Cuono CB. Myocutaneous flaps for head and neck reconstruction. *Head Neck Surg* 1980;2:321.
6. Sharzer LA, Kalisman M, Silver CE, Strauch B. The parasternal paddle: a modification of the pectoralis major myocutaneous flap. *Plast Reconstr Surg* 1981;67:753.
7. Brown RG, Fleming WH, Jurkiewicz MJ. An island flap of the pectoralis major muscle. *Br J Plast Surg* 1977;30:161.
8. Arnold PG, Pairolero PC. Chondrosarcoma of the manubrium: resection and reconstruction with pectoralis major muscle. *Mayo Clin Proc* 1978;53:54.
9. Cuono CB, Ariyan S. Immediate reconstruction of a composite mandibular defect with a regional osteomusculocutaneous flap. *Plast Reconstr Surg* 1980;65:477.
10. Bell MSG, Barron PT. The rib-pectoralis major osteomusculocutaneous flap. *Ann Plast Surg* 1981;6:347.
11. Green MF, Gibson JR, Bryson JR, Thomson E. A one-stage correction of mandibular defects using a split sternum pectoralis major osteomusculocutaneous transfer. *Br J Plast Surg* 1981;34:11.
12. Thomson HG. Reconstruction of the orbit after radical exenteration. *Plast Reconstr Surg* 1970;45:119.
13. Murray JE, Matson DD, Habal MB, et al. Regional cranio-orbital resection for recurrent tumor with delayed reconstruction. *Surg Gynecol Obstet* 1972;134:437.
14. Bakamijian VY, Souther SG. Use of temporal muscle for reconstruction after orbitomaxillary resections for cancer. *Plast Reconstr Surg* 1975;56:171.
15. Sypert GW, Habal MB. Combined cranio-orbital surgery for extensive malignant neoplasms of the orbit. *Neurosurgery* 1978;2:8.
16. Holmes AD, Marshall KA. Uses of the temporalis muscle flap in blanking out orbits. *Plast Reconstr Surg* 1979;63:336.
17. Parsons H, Lewis JS. Subtotal resection of the temporal bone for cancer of the ear. *Cancer* 1954;7:995.
18. Ward GE, Loch WE, Lawrence W. Radical operation for carcinoma of the external auditory canal and middle ear. *Am J Surg* 1951;82:169.
19. Ariyan S, Sasaki CT, Spencer D. Radical en bloc resection of the temporal bone. *Am J Surg* 1981;142:443.
20. Manktelow RT, McKee NJ, Vettese T. An anatomic study of the pectoralis major muscle as related to functioning free-muscle transplantation. *Plast Reconstr Surg* 1980;65:610.
21. Freeman JL, Walker EP, Wilson JSP, Shaw HJ. The vascular anatomy of the pectoralis major myocutaneous flap. *Br J Plast Surg* 1981;34:3.
22. Mathes SJ, Nahai F. Classification of the vascular anatomy of muscles: experimental and clinical correlation. *Plast Reconstr Surg* 1981;67:177.
23. Meyer R, Kelly TP, Failat ASA. Single bilobed flap for use in head and neck reconstruction. *Ann Plast Surg* 1981;6:203.
24. Donegan JO, Whiteley J, Gluckman JL, Shumrick DA. Improved method of harvesting the pectoralis major myocutaneous flap. *Am J Otolaryngol* 1981;2:223.

CHAPTER 133 ■ FREE GROIN FLAP RECONSTRUCTION OF SEVERE BURN NECK CONTRACTURE

K. HARII

Reconstruction of a severe burn scar contracture of the neck occasionally requires skin-flap coverage to prevent recurrence, of the contracture or to reestablish chin prominence. Conventional flaps such as the deltopectoral, acromiopectoral, and shoulder flap are available for this purpose, but a free skin flap from the groin region is an alternative because it can provide sufficient skin for coverage of the total anterior neck surface in one operation (1–3). The donor scar in the grout can be easily concealed.

ANATOMY

There are dual arterial supplies to the groin flap that consist of the superficial circumflex iliac artery (SCIA) and the superficial epigastric artery (SEA). Both arteries form complex vascular patterns in nourishing the groin flap. In a typical case, the separate SCIA and SEA originate directly from the femoral artery, but on some occasions, their points of origin vary from the profunda femoris, the deep circumflex iliac artery and so on. In 16% of cadaver dissections, either or both the SCIA and the SEA emerged from arteries other than the femoral artery (1,4).

In 30% to 50% of cases, the SCIA and SEA together form a single common trunk at their origin, but they are of separate origin in the remainder of cases. The SCIA is constant, with a reliable anatomic course, but the SEA occasionally is deficient. Both arteries form a closed vascular network in nourishing the groin skin, and a free groin flap can therefore be isolated with a pedicle of either of the arteries or the common trunk.

There are two venous drainage systems in the groin. The dominant venous system is usually composed of the superficial cutaneous veins involving the superficial circumflex iliac vein and the superficial epigastric vein. In more than 60% of cases, both veins form a common trunk and flow into the saphenous bulb after crossing over the femoral artery. When both veins are duplicated or branch farther out, the dominant venous flow usually is maintained by the superficial circumflex iliac vein. The deep veins, such as the venae comitantes of the two arteries, are additional drainage systems in the groin and can, in some cases in which the superficial veins do not develop well, be reliable drainage veins.

FLAP DESIGN AND DIMENSIONS

The femoral artery, the inguinal ligament, and the anterosuperior iliac spine are first marked as definite anatomic landmarks. The base of the flap should be placed over the femoral artery. The center of the flap is positioned a little higher than the axial line, which is drawn from a point on the femoral artery about 3 cm below the inguinal ligament to the anterosuperior iliac spine, because the base of the flap can include the origins of both the SCIA and the SEA (Fig. 1).

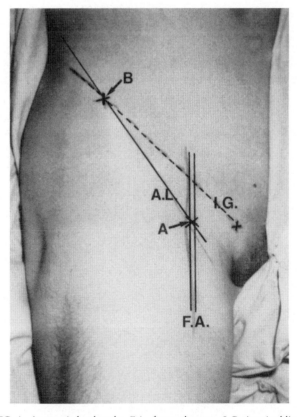

FIG. 1. Anatomic landmarks: *F.A.*, femoral artery; *I.G.*, inguinal ligament; *A.L.*, axial line; *arrow A*, point on femoral artery 3 cm below the inguinal ligament; *arrow B*, the anterosuperior iliac spine. (From Harii, ref. 3, with permission.)

OPERATIVE TECHNIQUE

All the scar tissue causing the neck contracture is completely excised. If the anterior cervical muscles are affected by the contracture, they also are excised to minimize recurrence of the contracture. It is important to create a deep groove along the chin-neck angle, because an obtuse angle may give a poor aesthetic result.

During preparation of the recipient site, exposure of a suitable artery and vein is required. The facial artery and vein at the mandibular angle are generally preferred, but if the facial vessels are not available, the superficial cervical, lingual, or other vessels are used.

Following preparation of the recipient site, a groin flap of the required size is isolated. The flap then is elevated from the lateral margin toward the femoral artery. At the lateral border of the sartorius muscle, a terminal cutaneous branch of the SCIA is clearly observed piercing the sartorius fascia to the skin. To secure a blood supply in the distal part of the flap, the branch should be included in the flap with a piece of the sartorius fascia. The dissection then proceeds toward the medial border of the sartorius muscle, and here the root of the SCIA should be identified (2).

After dissection of the medial border of the sartorius fascia, the flap is further elevated toward the femoral artery, tracing the root of the SCIA. On reaching the lateral wall of the femoral artery, the SCIA is usually observed originating from the femoral artery itself or one of the major branches. The SEA also is dissected after the root of the SCIA has been exposed. The venae comitantes of the two arteries should be preserved.

The base of the flap finally is incised to dissect the superficial cutaneous veins. The flap is thus elevated as an island flap with the nutrient vessels composed of the SCIA, the SEA (or the common trunk of both arteries), the venae comitantes of the two arteries, and the superficial cutaneous veins; however, one artery and one vein that appear optimal for microvascular anastomoses are finally selected.

The isolated groin flap is then transferred to the recipient defect and fixed with several marginal sutures. Microvascular anastomoses between flap and recipient vessels then are performed. After observation of good vascular return to the flap, both the donor and recipient sites are closed. The skin defect in the groin is approximated as directly as possible, but a skin graft may be required (Fig. 2).

CLINICAL RESULTS

The main drawbacks of the free groin flap are the complex vascular anatomy of the groin and the short and small stalk of the pedicle vessels, which sometimes make the operation difficult.

SUMMARY

A free groin flap is an alternative for release of neck scar contractures when standard flaps are not available.

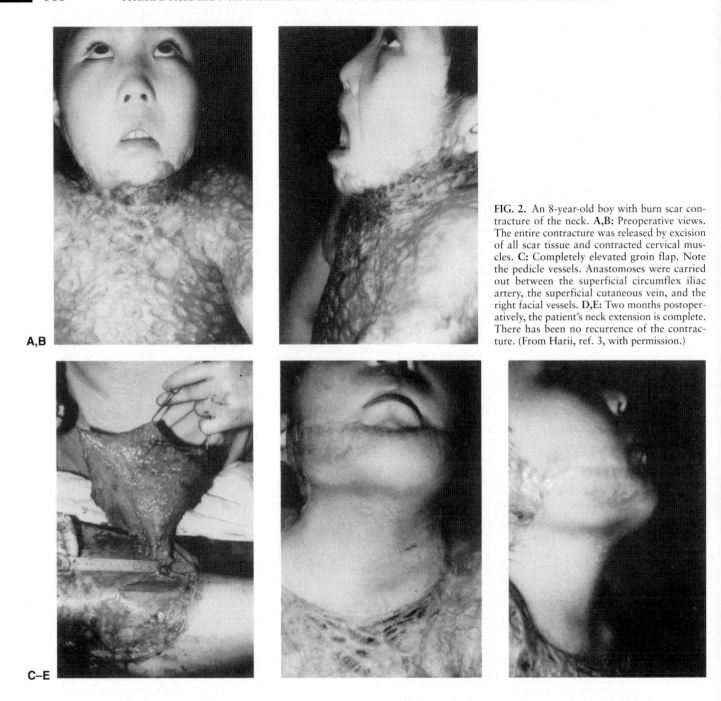

A,B

C–E

FIG. 2. An 8-year-old boy with burn scar contracture of the neck. **A,B:** Preoperative views. The entire contracture was released by excision of all scar tissue and contracted cervical muscles. **C:** Completely elevated groin flap. Note the pedicle vessels. Anastomoses were carried out between the superficial circumflex iliac artery, the superficial cutaneous vein, and the right facial vessels. **D,E:** Two months postoperatively, the patient's neck extension is complete. There has been no recurrence of the contracture. (From Harii, ref. 3, with permission.)

References

1. Harii K, Ohmori K, Torii S, Sekiguchi J. Microvascular free skin flap transfer. *Clin Plast Surg* 1978;5:239.

2. Harii K. Microvascular transfer of free skin flaps. In: Wilson JSP, ed. *Operative surgery,* 3d ed. London: Butterworth, 1981;83.
3. Harii K. Microvascular free tissue transfers. *World J Surg* 1979;3:29.
4. Taylor GI, Daniel RK. Anatomy of several free-flap donor sites. *Plast Reconstr Surg* 1975;56:243.

CHAPTER 134 ■ LATERAL INTERCOSTAL MICROVASCULAR FLAP FOR RELEASE OF NECK SCAR

H. A. BADRAN

This is a sizable neurovascular skin flap from the anterolateral abdomen, based on the lateral cutaneous branch of any one of the lower three posterior intercostal vessels or the subcostal artery. It can have varying forms and a wide spectrum of applications, including use for posttraumatic scarring of the face, neck, and extremities, to correct facial contour deformities, and in breast and penile reconstruction (Fig. 3).

INDICATIONS

Lateral intercostal flaps share indications with other upper-quadrant flaps (1–8) but without the need for delay or the inclusion of intercostal or abdominal musculature. The flaps are innervated by the lateral cutaneous nerve, which contains between two and four fascicles for total flap supply. A vascularized rib segment may be incorporated for an osteocutaneous flap (9), and the flap may be deepithelialized (10).

Other advantages of the flap include its large size (up to 25 × 20 cm), its long pedicle (8–15 cm), easy anastomosis of relatively large-diameter intercostal vessels (1.5–2.0 mm), and relative thinness. There is a choice between several pedicles, and the flap can be defatted and beveled without compromising its vascularity; primary tailoring minimizes the need for future revisions. The donor defect is closed directly, even in larger flaps, because of the redundancy of the abdominal skin.

ANATOMY

For purposes of description, the posterior intercostal artery, which is a branch of the thoracic aorta, can be divided into four segments: vertebral, costal groove, intermuscular, and rectus sheath segments (7). The vertebral segment gives off a nutrient branch to the rib, a spinal branch, and a collateral branch. In the intermuscular segment, the artery gives off mainly muscular and intermuscular branches. In the rectus sheath segment, the vessel terminates by anastomosing with the epigastric system. In the costal groove segment, the vessel gives off the following branches.

The *lateral cutaneous branch* arises near the anterior end of the costal groove and is accompanied by a vein of similar diameter lying above and a nerve below. The lateral cutaneous bundle courses obliquely in the intercostal space deep to the internal and external intercostal muscles and under cover of the slip of origin of the external oblique. It leaves the intercostal space at the anterior border of this slip and emerges to the subcutaneous tissue lying on the superior slip, 1 to 2 cm in front of the anterior border of the latissimus dorsi muscle. At this point, the artery has an internal diameter of 0.5 to 1.0 mm.

The bundle courses for a short distance superficial to the muscle fascia, to which it is firmly attached, before dividing into a smaller posterior and a larger anterior branch. Early

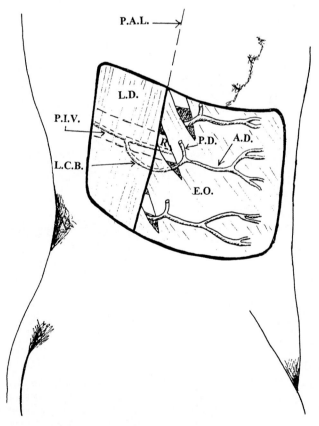

FIG. 1. Diagram of surface anatomy of the flap. *P.A.L.,* posterior axillary line; *L.D.,* latissimus dorsi; *P.I.V.,* posterior intercostal vessels; *R,* rib; *L.C.B.,* lateral cutaneous branch; *P.D.,* posterior division; *A.D.,* anterior division; *E.O.,* external oblique.

division of the lateral cutaneous bundle may occur in 40% of cases. In these instances, the posterior division exits in the normal position described for the lateral cutaneous bundle. On the other hand, the anterior division continues deeply between the slips of the external oblique to emerge several centimeters anterior to the point of emergence of the posterior division. Injury of this anterior division in the depth of the intercostal space, or mistaking it for the anterior continuation of the pos-

terior intercostal bundle, could lead to flap loss. In 5% of cases, the two divisions of the lateral cutaneous branch arise separately from the posterior intercostal artery.

Periosteal branches arise directly or from the muscular branches of the vessel. These branches supply the anterior and posterior periosteum and are located well protected within its layers. These vessels can support a vascularized rib segment without the need for an endosteal supply (9).

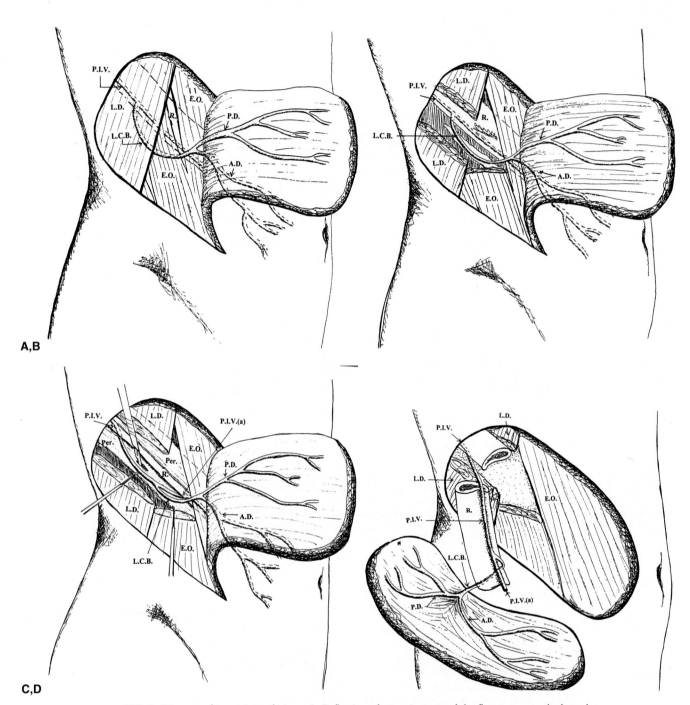

FIG. 2. Diagram of operative technique. **A:** Reflection of posterior part of the flap to expose the lateral cutaneous branch between the slips of origin of the external oblique. **B:** The branch is traced back into the intercostal space. The slip of origin of the external oblique is detached, the latissimus dorsi is cut, and the intercostal muscles are divided. **C:** Delivery of the posterior intercostal bundle out of the subcostal groove. The periosteum (*Per.*) is incised at the lower border of the rib and again at the roof of the groove, to facilitate the delivery. **D:** Diagram of osteocutaneous flap. The posterior intercostal bundle is left in place in the subcostal groove of the harvested rib segment and is dissected out only for the desired pedicle length from the portion of the rib posterior to that segment.

Musculocutaneous branches usually anastomose with the musculocutaneous branches of the thoracodorsal system before emerging to the subcutaneous tissues. This is a hemodynamic basis for inclusion of ribs and latissimus dorsi muscle together in one vascularized unit.

FLAP DESIGN AND DIMENSIONS

The flap is outlined within the skin territory supplied by the artery with the patient standing. The point of pedicle exit into the subcutaneous plane can be roughly marked at the intersection of the anterior border of the latissimus dorsi and the lower border of the rib, corresponding to the bundle selected, usually the tenth or eleventh.

With the chosen pedicle lying in the center, the skin territory of the flap can extend to incorporate four intercostal spaces in the vertical dimension, and from the lateral border of the rectus abdominis anteriorly to the lateral border of the sacrospinalis posteriorly. The posterior border of the flap should lie at least 5 cm behind the posterior axillary line to ensure that the lateral cutaneous branch of the lower three posterior intercostal arteries and the subcostal artery are included in the flap (Fig. 1).

OPERATIVE TECHNIQUE

The part of the flap posterior to the pedicle is elevated first with the muscle fascia to protect the vessels (Fig. 2A). Once the lateral cutaneous branch is identified, it is traced back to its origin from the posterior intercostal artery in the intercostal space. The slip of origin of the external oblique from the same rib is detached, and the latissimus dorsi and inter-

costal muscles are divided (Fig. 2B). For the desired pedicle length, the bundle then is dissected out from the subcostal groove in a posterior direction. To do this, the periosteum is incised on the lower border of the rib and is reflected down (Fig. 2C). It is again incised in the area of the roof of the costal groove. In this way, the delivery of the intercostal bundle is facilitated by pulling the incised edge of the periosteum down.

This step is better done under loupe magnification and can be time consuming. Care should be taken to identify and coagulate the periosteal branches arising directly from the vessels to the periosteum of the undersurface of the groove; their injury could lead to troublesome bleeding. Dissection between the point of exit of the branch from the mother vessels to its emergence in the subcutaneous level should be done with utmost care because of the possibility of branching anomalies.

Anteriorly, the posterior intercostal bundle is dissected to just beyond the lateral cutaneous branch, ligated, and cut. The lateral cutaneous nerve can be stripped from the main nerve for the desired length. Dissection then proceeds carefully to free the lateral cutaneous bundle from the fascia on the slip of origin of the external oblique on which it lies. This step is also better done under loupe magnification. The rest of the flap borders then are incised down to and including the muscle fascia. The flap is quickly elevated and its circulation tested before the pedicle is clamped.

In cases of osteocutaneous flaps, raising the skin portion of the flap is initially done in the usual fashion. The lateral intercostal branch then is traced into the intercostal space as usual, but the posterior intercostal bundle is not dissected out and is kept in the costal groove. The rib is harvested based on the periosteal blood supply given by the artery while inside the groove. At the posterior end of the harvested rib segment, the posterior intercostal vessels are dissected out of the groove and traced for the desired length (Fig. 2D).

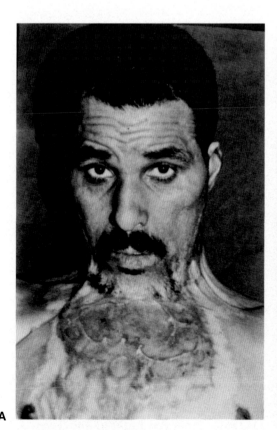
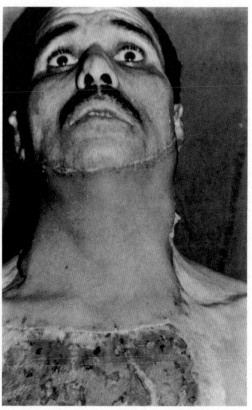

A   B

FIG. 3. Severe post-burn contracture of the neck. **A:** Preoperative view. **B:** Postoperative view showing the large dimensions of the flap.

SUMMARY

The varying forms possible in using the lateral intercostal flap and its advantageous properties make it useful in a wide variety of applications.

References

1. Badran HA, El-Helaly M, Safe I. The lateral intercostal neurovascular free flap. *Plast Reconstr Surg* 1984;73:17.
2. Esser JFS. *Biological or artery flaps of the face.* Monaco: Institut Esser de Chirurgie Structive, 1931.
3. Dibbel DG. Use of long island flaps to bring sensation to the sacral area in young paraplegics. *Plast Reconstr Surg* 1974;54:200.
4. Daniel RK, Terzis JK, Cunningham DM. Sensory skin flaps for coverage of pressure sores in paraplegic patients: a preliminary report. *Plast Reconstr Surg* 1976;58:317.
5. Daniel RK, Kerrigan CI, Gard DA. The great potential of the intercostal flap for torso reconstruction. *Plast Reconstr Surg* 1978;61:653.
6. Little JW, Fontana DJ, McCulloch DT. The upper quadrant flap. *Plast Reconstr Surg* 1981;68:175.
7. Kerrigan CL, Daniel RK. The intercostal flap: anatomical and hemodynamic approach. *Ann Plast Surg* 1979;2:411.
8. Drever JM. Total breast reconstruction with either of two abdominal flaps. *Plast Reconstr Surg* 1977;59:185.
9. Badran HA, Safe I, El Fayoumy S. Simplified technique for isolating vascularized rib periosteal grafts. *Plast Reconstr Surg* 1990;86:1208.
10. Badran HA, Yousef MK, Shaker A. Management of facial contour deformities with deepithelialized lateral intercostal free flaps. *Ann Plast Surg* 1996;37:94.

CHAPTER 135 ■ MICROVASCULAR FREE TRANSFER OF A DEEPITHELIALIZED GROIN FLAP TO THE CHEEK

L. A. SHARZER

Soft-tissue augmentation with autogenous dermis and fat is a well-known and well-accepted technique. Composite dermal fat segments may be transferred as grafts (nonvascularized) (1–4), as pedicle flaps (vascularized) (5–7), or as free flaps (microvascular) (8–12). Nonvascularized grafts undergo 40% to 50% resorption and must therefore be overcorrected at the time of transfer. Even then, resorption is unpredictable and the ultimate outcome uncertain. Because flaps retain their circulation, the volume transferred is the volume that remains, barring excessive generalized weight gain or weight loss. Free flaps, in general, allow greater leeway in flap design and donor-site choice than pedicle flaps, and this is true for deepithelialized free flaps as well.

INDICATIONS

The most common indications for deepithelialized free-flap transfer are Romberg's hemifacial atrophy, congenital or acquired hemifacial microsomia, and contour defects related to trauma or cancer surgery.

ANATOMY

The deepithelialized groin flap based on the superficial circumflex iliac vessels is particularly well suited to contour reconstructions and has been my flap of choice.

FLAP DESIGN AND DIMENSIONS

The flap should be designed to the exact recipient-site requirements (Figs. 1 and 2). The flap outline will often be quite irregular, as there may be projections into the temporal, malar, or mental regions. Recipient vessels are planned in advance, so they can be oriented on the flap template. In general, it is best to use vessels in the neck such as the facial artery and vein or other branches of the external carotid artery. In this way, if the planned-for vessels are found to be unsuitable, the vascular pedicle will be located where it can be anastomosed (with a vein graft, if necessary) to another neck vessel.

The flap template then is transferred to the groin area, where the flap outline is marked. The flap pedicle is oriented toward the takeoff of the superficial circumflex iliac artery, and the long axis of the flap lies along the course of the artery two fingerbreadths below the inguinal ligament. It is helpful to tattoo key points of the flap to aid in orientation after the flap is elevated.

OPERATIVE TECHNIQUE

Donor Site

The flap is elevated as a standard free groin flap. My preferred technique is a lateral to medial elevation after preliminary identification of the superficial circumflex iliac artery and vein through an incision over the femoral artery. It is best not to

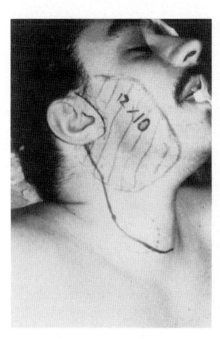

FIG. 1. Soft-tissue defect outlined on the cheek.

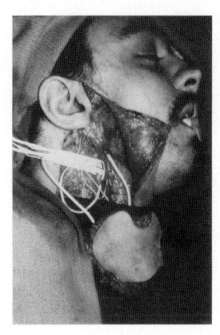

FIG. 3. Dissected flap has been transferred to the face. (*White vessel loops* mark the external carotid artery and its branches.)

deepithelialize any portion of the flap until it has been revascularized at the recipient site. The donor site is always closed primarily. It is often necessary to excise dog-ears at both medial and lateral ends of the defect because of the irregularity of flap design.

Recipient Site

A preauricular incision is made and extended into the submandibular area if necessary. A cheek flap is elevated, as for a face-lift. If the proposed recipient vessels are in the neck, epinephrine may be infiltrated in the cheek area to aid in hemostasis. Epinephrine should not be used anywhere near the recipient vessels. The recipient vessels are identified and marked with vessel loops, but they are not divided until the

flap has been transferred. Care must be taken to avoid injury to the marginal mandibular branch of the facial nerve.

After completion of donor- and recipient-site dissections and observation of the flap for adequacy of circulation, the flap is transferred to the face and held in place with a few sutures while the vascular anastomoses are carried out. I prefer to perform the arterial anastomosis first because this decreases ischemia time and allows a longer period of observation of the arterial anastomosis.

Once the flap has been revascularized, it is oriented in its new position. Key sutures are placed in the dermis of the flap and brought out through the facial skin to be tied later over a bolster. The cheek flap then is placed without tension over the free flap to determine how much of the free flap may be deepithelialized (Figs. 3 and 4). Often, the added bulk of the soft tissue from the flap makes the facial skin inadequate, and a

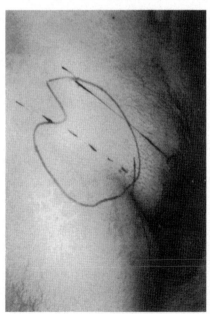

FIG. 2. Pattern of required flap transferred to the groin. (*Solid line* is at the inguinal ligament; *broken line* is along the course of superficial circumflex iliac artery.)

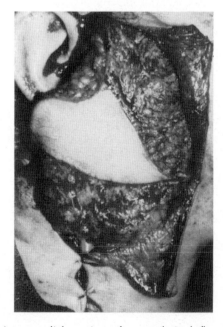

FIG. 4. Anteromedial portion of revascularized flap has been deepithelialized.

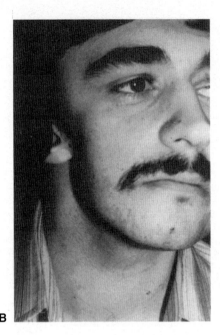
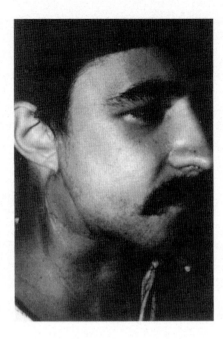

FIG. 5. A: Preoperative appearance of acquired hemifacial microsomia. **B:** Postoperative appearance following flap transfer.

A,B

portion of free-flap skin must be left intact. Even if it is not necessary to leave a portion of flap skin intact, it is desirable to leave at least a small patch to serve as a monitor of circulation during the postoperative period. This can later be removed, leaving a linear scar. A tight closure of facial skin over the free flap should be avoided. The dermis should be anchored to facial fascia or periosteum of the zygoma to avoid "drooping" later on. Deepithelialization is then carried out and the wound is closed over suction drains (Fig. 5).

CLINICAL RESULTS

Complications that may arise from any free groin flap transfer, such as vascular thrombosis, are possible with this procedure. Two complications, in particular, must be anticipated. The recipient vascular anatomy is frequently anomalous in congenital cases, and it is important to identify the common carotid and the carotid bifurcation before dividing any vessels. The internal and external carotid arteries may be small and confused with branches of the facial or superior thyroid arteries. The other complication is sagging of the flap if it is not well anchored to fascia or periosteum.

SUMMARY

Deepithelialized groin flaps are a safe, reliable operation for autogenous soft-tissue augmentation of the cheek.

References

1. Thompson N. The subcutaneous dermis graft: a clinical and histological study in man. *Plast Reconstr Surg* 1960;26:1.
2. Leaf N, Zarem HA. Correction of contour defects of the face with dermal and dermal fat grafts. *Arch Surg* 1972;105:715.
3. Sawhney CP, Banerjee TN, Chakravarti RN. Behavior of dermal fat transplants. *Br J Plast Surg* 1969;22:169.
4. Scheussler WW, Steffans DN. Dermal grafts for correction of facial defects. *Plast Reconstr Surg* 1949;4:341.
5. Converse JM, Betson RJ. A twenty-year follow-up of a patient with hemifacial atrophy treated by a buried de-epithelialized flap. *Plast Reconstr Surg* 1971;48:2.
6. Dey DL. Hemifacial atrophy: repair with a buried flap. *Aust N Z J Surg* 1974;44:379.
7. Neumann CG. The use of large buried pedicle flaps of dermis and fat. *Plast Reconstr Surg* 1953;11:315.
8. Fujino T, Tanino R, Sugimoto C. Microvascular transfer of a free deltopectoral dermal fat flap. *Plast Reconstr Surg* 1975;55:428.
9. Harashina T, Nakajima T, Yoshimora Y. A free groin flap reconstruction in progressive facial hemiatrophy. *Br J Plast Surg* 1977;30:14.
10. Wells JH, Edgerton MT. Correction of severe hemifacial atrophy with a free dermis-fat flap from the lower abdomen. *Plast Reconstr Surg* 1977;59:223.
11. O'Brien BM, Russell RC, Morrison WA, Sully L. Buried microvascular free flaps for reconstruction of soft-tissue defects. *Plast Reconstr Surg* 1981;68:712.
12. Shintomi Y, Ohura T, Honda K, Iida K. The reconstruction of progressive facial hemiatrophy by free vascularized dermis fat flaps. *Br J Plast Surg* 1981;34:398.

CHAPTER 136 ■ MICROVASCULAR TRANSFER OF A SCAPULAR/PARASCAPULAR FLAP TO THE CHEEK

T. BENACQUISTA AND B. STRAUCH

EDITORIAL COMMENT

The use of scapular/parascapular flaps in this area is quite effective, not only for the correction of cheek skin deformities but also for the augmentation of subcutaneous tissue, especially in patients with Romberg's disease or hemifacial microsomia.

The use of scapular and parascapular microvascular free flaps in cheek reconstruction is gaining more popularity (1,2). These fasciocutaneous flaps have great versatility, allowing for good contour in many types of cheek defect and in cases of facial asymmetry. The flaps also have been used in the lower extremity and hand.

INDICATIONS

When used as fasciocutaneous flaps, these free-tissue transfers can fill in large cheek defects after trauma or tumor ablation. When deepithelialized, the flaps can be used in the correction of facial asymmetry. Advantages in these cases include reliability, appropriate bulk for the cheek, and lack of atrophy; the latter characteristic is not found in muscle flaps (1,2). The color match of scapular and parascapular flaps may be troublesome when they are used with skin to fill in cheek defects, but the excellent contour that can be achieved may outweigh this shortcoming.

These free flaps not only provide sufficient bulk for cheek defects but have a quite constant and reliable pedicle, with a long pedicle length (7–8 cm) and wide-caliber vessels (2–3 mm). If bone is required in the reconstruction, the flap can be taken with the lateral border of the scapula. About 10 to 14 cm of bone can be harvested, depending on the amount required by the individual patient (3).

The major disadvantage is patient positioning during flap harvesting and closure of the donor site. Dissection of the vascular pedicle can be tedious because of the numerous muscular and bony branches that must be divided. Also, the donor site does not have a cutaneous sensory nerve, and there is no possibility for a sensate flap.

ANATOMY

The cutaneous flaps are supplied by the circumflex scapular artery, which emerges from the scapular artery about 4 cm from its origin from the axillary artery (4). The circumflex scapular artery emerges from the triangular fossa on the back at the edge of the lateral border of the scapula. This space is formed by the long head of the triceps and the teres major and minor muscles (5) (Fig. 1). The artery then terminates into two fasciocutaneous branches, one oriented transversely (scapular flap [6]) and one oriented vertically (parascapular flap [7]).

Before dividing into terminal branches, the circumflex scapular artery gives off several branches to the lateral border of the scapula in its superior portion. These branches supply the periosteum of the lateral border of the scapula and the attached muscles, thus allowing bone to be harvested with the flap.

FLAP DESIGN AND DIMENSIONS

Because of the orientation of the fasciocutaneous branches, the flaps can be designed as an ellipse, either horizontally

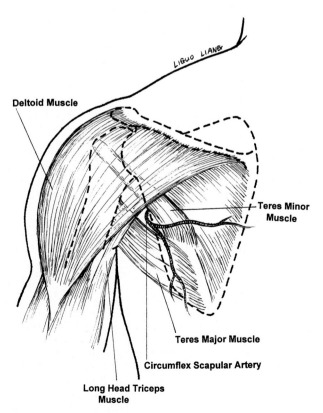

FIG. 1. Vascular anatomy of the scapular region.

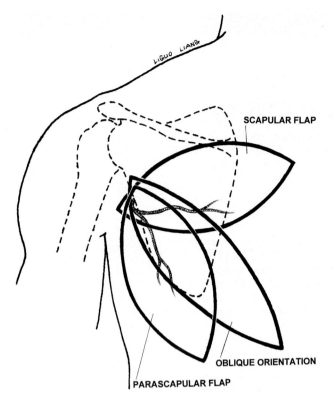

FIG. 2. Dorsal aspect of the scapular area with schematic outlining of the various technical possibilities: scapular or parascapular flaps, oblique orientation or in combination.

(scapular flap) or vertically (parascapular flap). More commonly, the flap is designed in an oblique configuration between these two orientations to allow easier primary skin closure of the back and a better cosmetic result (Fig. 2).

Depending on the laxity of the skin, up to 10 cm of skin width can be harvested and closed primarily. Much larger widths can be harvested with a good blood supply; however, the resultant defect must be skin grafted, or preoperative skin expansion must be planned. The length that can be harvested depends on the patient's size and can be up to 30 cm. Combinations of cutaneous flaps are possible for larger defects. Even the latissimus dorsi muscle, with or without a cutaneous paddle, may be harvested on the thoracodorsal pedicle if more bulk is necessary; this is rare for defects limited to the cheek. A combination of the two cutaneous territories as two separate paddles can be useful in through-and-through defects to provide both external skin coverage and inner-mouth lining.

OPERATIVE TECHNIQUE

The patient is placed in a lateral decubitus position with the side of the cheek defect facing upward using the ipsilateral back for the harvest site, which allows a two-team approach to the procedure, although the work space may be somewhat cramped. The team at the head will prepare the cheek to receive the flap and will dissect out the recipient vessels. In cases of facial asymmetry due to hemifacial microsomia or Romberg's disease, a skin flap is raised via a preauricular incision on the affected side to the extent of the deficiency to accommodate a deepithelialized scapular or parascapular flap.

The incision can be extended into the neck if the facial artery and vein or other neck vessels are to be used as recipient

vessels, or it can be limited to the preauricular region with a better cosmetic result if the superficial temporal artery and vein are used as recipient vessels (8). Because the superficial temporal vein is quite fragile, this may not always be possible.

If there is an ablative portion to the procedure, the patient is usually placed first in a supine position, as most head and neck surgeons are not amenable to operating with the patient in a lateral decubitus position. In this case, once the ablation is completed, the vessels in the neck are prepared for the anastomoses, and the patient then is turned onto the side. After the flap has been harvested, it is best to detach it, put it aside, and close the donor defect. This should be done as expediently as possible because the flap is ischemic during this period. The wound then is dressed, and the patient can return to a supine position without reprepping and draping.

The location of the triangular fossa is palpated just lateral to the scapula. If it is not palpable, it can be located using the following measurements. The triangle is located at distance $D_1 = (D - 1)/2$, where D is the distance between the middle part of the spine and the tip of the scapula (7) (Fig. 3).

As mentioned, the flap is usually oriented in an oblique direction from the shoulder toward the middle of the back. Dissection starts at the distal end of the flap, and a fasciocutaneous flap is raised off the underlying muscle fascia. With an oblique orientation, this is usually the latissimus dorsi muscle. Fascial extensions can be harvested to fill in subtle deficiencies in cases of facial asymmetry (1).

As the dissection is carried proximally, the borders of the omotricipital space are identified, the teres major first laterally and the teres minor medially. Once these are identified, the

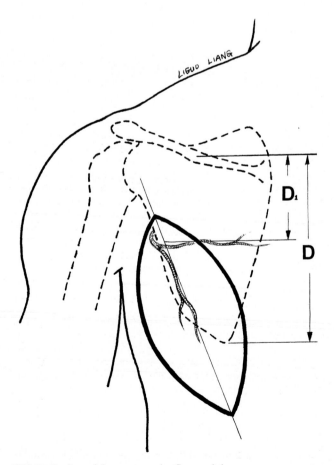

FIG. 3. Outline of the parascapular flap, and the measurement procedure (D, D_1) to determine the emergence of the pedicle, as shown.

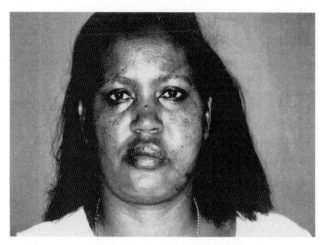

FIG. 4. Clinical case. A 35-year-old woman with a history of an enlarging left-cheek mass, which was adherent to the skin but without invasion of buccal mucosa. Pathology showed dermatofibrosarcoma protuberans.

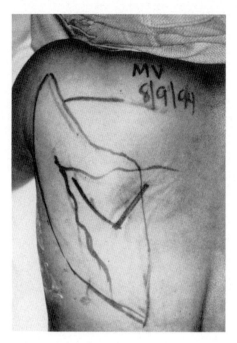

FIG. 6. Markings drawn for a very large parascapular flap in an oblique orientation shaped to fit the defect.

pedicle is usually visible. At this point, the upper incision can be made and the long head of the triceps will be seen. The pedicle is traced back into the triangle toward the cirumflex scapular artery or to the scapular artery, depending on the length of pedicle required. The dissection should be carried out as bloodlessly as possible because blood staining the tissues in this area makes for a frustrating experience, especially when dissecting the periosteal branches.

Once the flap is transferred to the face and revascularized, it is sculpted to fit the defect. Preoperative fabrication of a facial moulage may help to obtain better results (2). The flap should be anchored to bone whenever possible to prevent descent over time, especially when very large flaps are being used. If flap deepithelialization is required and the flap is to be placed under a facial skin flap, a lateral skin paddle may be constructed for postoperative monitoring (Figs. 4–8).

CLINICAL RESULTS

All series reporting the use of scapular/parascapular free flaps in head and neck reconstruction are quite favorable. Some authors state that this is their first choice for reconstruction of major defects in this area (1–3,8–10). In a series of 28 patients, Upton et al. reported little less than half requiring

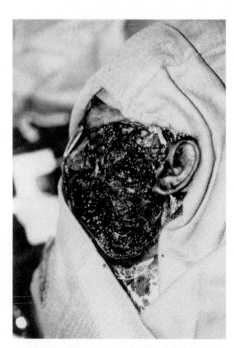

FIG. 5. Defect of the entire left cheek after tumor resection.

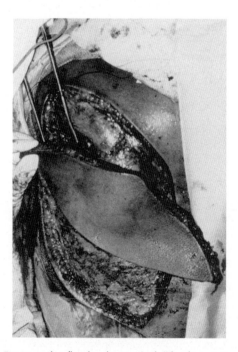

FIG. 7. Parascapular flap has been raised. The donor site required skin grafting to close the defect.

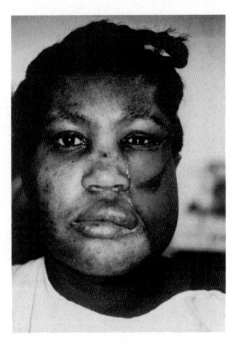

FIG. 8. Postoperative appearance at 6 months.

SUMMARY

Scapular/parascapular flaps are excellent for cheek reconstruction and may be the best choice for this purpose. The flaps are vigorous and have constant vascular anatomy, good pedicle length, and large vessel caliber. Although there is no long-term atrophy, patients may require flap revision to achieve the best results.

References

1. Siebert JW, Anson G, Longaker MT. Microsurgical correction of facial asymmetry in 60 consecutive cases. *Plast Reconstr Surg* 1996;97:354.
2. Upton J, Albin RE, Mulliken JB, Murray JE. The use of scapular and parascapular flaps for cheek reconstruction. *Plast Reconstr Surg* 1992; 90:959.
3. Swartz WM, Banis JC, Newton D, et al. The osteocutaneous scapular flap for mandibular and maxillary reconstruction. *Plast Reconstr Surg* 1986;77:530.
4. Strauch B, Yu HL. *Atlas of microvascular surgery: anatomy and operative approaches.* New York: Thieme Medical Publishers, 1993.
5. dos Santos LF. The vascular anatomy and dissection of the free scapular flap. *Plast Reconstr Surg* 1984;73:599.
6. Barwick WJ, Goddkind DJ, Serafin D. The free scapular flap. *Plast Reconstr Surg* 1982;69:779.
7. Nassif TM, Vidal L, Bovet JL, Baudet J. The parascapular flap: a new cutaneous microsurgical free flap. *Plast Reconstr Surg* 1982;69:591.
8. Longaaker MT, Siebert JW. Microvascular free-flap correction of severe hemifacial atrophy. *Plast Reconstr Surg* 1995;96:800.
9. Chandrasekhar B, Lorant JA, Terz JJ. Parascapular free flaps for head and neck reconstruction. *Am J Surg* 1990;116:160.
10. Sullivan MJ, Carroll WR, Baker SR. The cutaneous scapular free flap in head and neck reconstruction. *Arch Otolaryngol Head Neck Surg* 1990; 116:600.

secondary procedures to achieve better contour (2). Another series of 57 patients reported excellent contour using the flap with fascial extensions (1), with revisions performed in about a third of patients and no significant sagging or atrophy reported over time.

CHAPTER 137 ■ MICROVASCULAR FREE TRANSFER OF OMENTUM TO THE CHEEK

S. K. DAS AND M. A. LESAVOY

EDITORIAL COMMENT

The major problem of free omentum to the face for contour restoration is the late sagging of the omentum. For this reason, other procedures are being used, such as those described in preceding chapters, especially deepithelialized skin flaps.

The search for ideal tissue to reconstruct contour deformity in the face still goes on. Various autogenous and synthetic materials have been tried.

INDICATIONS

Omentum is one of the satisfactory alternatives for reconstruction of contour defects produced by facial atrophy (Romberg's disease) (1–4); hemifacial microsomia (5,6), or trauma. Correction of the underlying bony defect is necessary first, followed by soft-tissue reconstruction.

ANATOMY

The size of the omentum is not a problem, and it has been shown that omentum is almost always present, with an average length of 25 cm and an average width of 33 cm. Omental size can be predicted from the sex, height, and weight of the patient (7,8). Only in rare cases of total lipodystrophy is omental fat, as well as mesenteric fat, totally absent (9).

The structure and vascular anatomy of the omentum make it suitable for use in facial reconstruction (3,8). The fatty structure gives it pliability and softness, and the distribution of omental vessels helps divide the omentum into vascular units. The right gastroepiploic vascular pedicle length ranges from 9 to 12 cm, and the size of the vessels ranges from 1.5 to 3 mm for artery and 2.5 to 3.5 mm for vein. The length of the pedicle permits the selection of donor vessels far away from the recipient site and allows for minimal size discrepancy with recipient vessels, such as the facial, superior thyroid, and superficial temporal vessels.

The unique vasculature of the omentum, in the form of parallel vessels ranging between two and eight in number running distally from the gastroepiploic arch, allows the omentum to be split into units with an artery and vein surrounded by a segment of omentum. Thus, one can augment a specific portion of the face by placing strips of omentum one upon the other.

FLAP DESIGN AND DIMENSIONS

A clever technique has been devised (3) using the unique vasculature of omentum in an attempt to counter the gravitational sag of omental transfer over time and the accumulation of bulk along the dependent mandibular margin. The face is divided into three sections (Fig. 1): a frontotemporal area above the line drawn from the tragus to the lateral canthus of the eye, a zygomaticomaxillary area above a line drawn from the tragus to the lateral commissure of the mouth, and a mandibular area above a line drawn from the lobule of the ear along the inferior border of the mandible.

Usually, the base of the omentum with the gastroepiploic arch is placed vertically and along the preauricular area and the omentum is spread as a fan anteriorly and medially.

OPERATIVE TECHNIQUE

The most common recipient vessels are the facial, because of easy access and corresponding vessel size. The superficial tem-

poral artery is an excellent alternative, but one should be aware that in some cases of hemifacial atrophy the superficial temporal vessels can be atrophic or hypoplastic.

The face is explored through a preauricular face-lift type of incision, with extension below the mandibular area. The skin flap is raised as in a face-lift, but the attachment of the skin to deeper tissue (dermis to premuscular fascia) along the three lines mentioned above is kept intact. The recipient vessels, the facial or the superficial temporal vessels, are exposed and the anastomoses are performed.

The distal omentum is split into several tongues or peninsulas and is placed in the already dissected pockets as required to correct the deformity. Usually, a slight overcorrection is recommended. Pull-out bolster sutures (Fig. 2C) are placed through the distal end of the tongues of omentum over forehead, supraorbital area, zygomaticofrontal area, nasolabial area, and mandibular area. The skin flap is closed, and a drain is placed over the most dependent part (postauricular).

CLINICAL RESULTS

In most cases, reoperation and revision of excess omentum are necessary. The reason for this is generally overaugmentation, with the expectation of resorption; however, because this flap is vascularized immediately, the amount of resorption is less than one would expect. Other possible complications related to this procedure occur from harvesting the omentum through a laparotomy.

The success rate with this flap for facial reconstruction has been high, and surgeons using the procedure are consistently satisfied. The difficulty with late gravitational sagging over the mandibular area has been minimized through the modifications described.

SUMMARY

The omentum, through microvascular transfer, has provided a good flap for reconstructing contour deformities of the face.

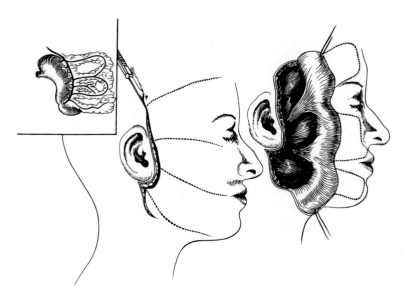

FIG. 1. Three compartments of the face divided by three lines (see text). (From Upton et al., ref. 3, with permission.)

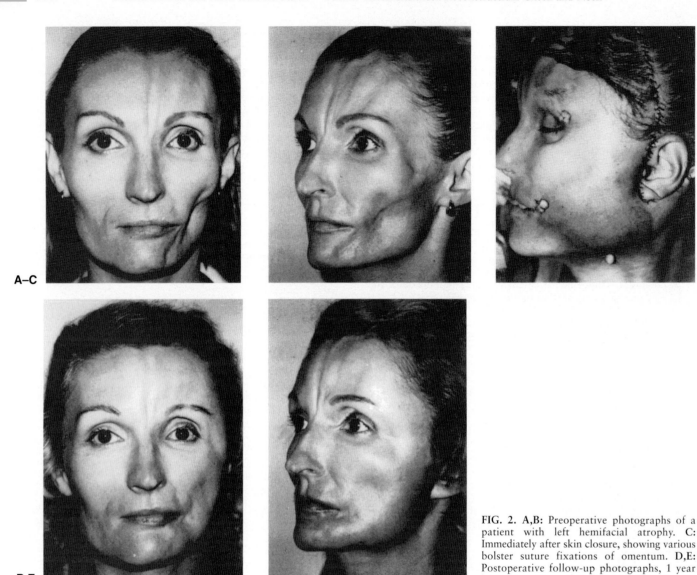

A–C

D,E

FIG. 2. **A,B:** Preoperative photographs of a patient with left hemifacial atrophy. **C:** Immediately after skin closure, showing various bolster suture fixations of omentum. **D,E:** Postoperative follow-up photographs, 1 year later. (From Das, ref. 8, with permission.)

References

1. Harii K. Free omental transfer. In: *Transactions of the Sixth International Congress of Plastic and Reconstructive Surgery.* Paris: Masson, 1976;61.
2. Harii K. Clinical application of free omental flap transfer. *Clin Plast Surg* 1978;5:273.
3. Upton J, Mulliken JB, Hick PD, Murray JE. Restoration of facial contour using free vascularized omental transfer. *Plast Reconstr Surg* 1980;66:560.
4. Zuo SL. Reconstruction of facial atrophy defect by transplantation of free great omentum: case report (Author's translation). *Chung Hua Kou Chiang Ko Tsa Chih* 1981;16:14.
5. Rheiner P, Montandon D. Correction d'une hemiatrophic faciale par transfert libre de l'épiploon. *Helv Chir Acta* 1980;47:141.
6. Wallace JG, Schneider WJ, Brown RG, Nahai FM. Reconstruction of hemifacial atrophy with a free flap of omentum. *Br J Plast Surg* 1979;32:15.
7. Das SK. The size of the human omentum and methods of lengthening it for transplantation. *Br J Plast Surg* 1976;29:70.
8. Das SK. Use of the omentum in reconstructive surgery. In: Barron J, Saad M, eds. *Manual of operative plastic and reconstructive surgery.* Edinburgh: Churchill-Livingstone, 1980.
9. Personal communication with Dr. M. Jurkiewicz, 1988.

CHAPTER 138 ■ FREE DELTOID FLAP

J. D. FRANKLIN AND R. D. GOLDSTEIN

For details of anatomy, flap design and dimensions, operative technique, and clinical results, see Chapter 308. This chapter shows one indication for the flap—coverage of a defect in the cheek (Fig. 1).

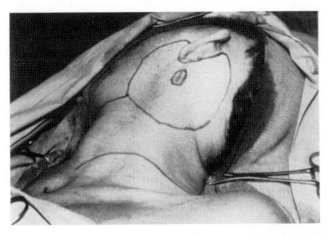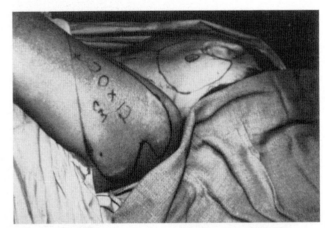

A,B

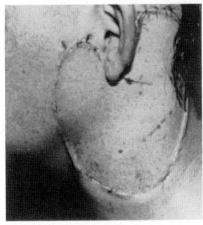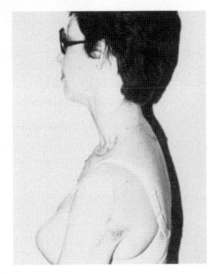

FIG. 1. **A:** A 36-year-old woman prior to wide excision for a neck dissection for nodular level IV 1.2mm thick melanoma. **B:** The donor site for the flap is 20 × 12 cm at its greatest dimensions. **C:** Early postoperative appearance. **D:** Result, 1 year later. Note that the donor site was closed primarily, because the flap was taken more down on the shoulder on the inferior portion of the arm, rather than on the shoulder.

C,D

CHAPTER 139 ■ SCAPULAR AND PARASCAPULAR FLAPS

J. BAUDET, T. NASSIF, J. L. BOVET, AND B. PANCONI

For details of anatomy, flap design and dimensions, operative technique, and clinical results, see Chapter 309. This chapter illustrates the use of the parascapular flap for release of a scar contracture in the neck (Fig. 1).

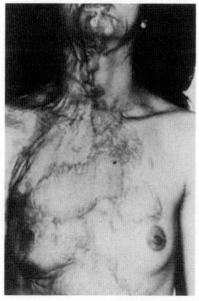
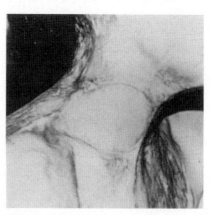

FIG. 1. A: Sequelae of burn with contracture of the right side of the neck. B: Satisfactory release of skin contracture after transfer of a parascapular flap. Z-plasties are planned for the anterior part. (Clinical case courtesy of Dr. J. Fissette et al., Department of Maxillofacial Surgery and Plastic Surgery, and Professor A. Castermans, Hopital de Baviere, Liege, Belgium.)

CHAPTER 140 ■ THORACODORSAL ARTERY PERFORATOR (TDAP) FLAP

C. ANGRIGIANI

This flap was originally described in 1995 as a method for diminishing the volume of the conventional latissimus dorsi myocutaneous flap (1). Various methods had been previously described to split the muscle, either longitudinally or transversely, to diminish flap bulk (2,3). The same area of skin and subcutaneous tissue island can be harvested without the muscle, using the perforator-flap technique.

The thoracodorsal artery perforator (TDAP) flap is another example of the independence of the skin paddle from the underlying muscle from the standpoint of irrigation.

INDICATIONS

The TDAP, as well as its predecessor, the latissimus dorsi musculocutaneous flap, can be used as an island or as a free transferred flap. It is indicated when a thin, large flap with a long vascular pedicle is necessary. It is used as an island for resurfacing of axillary, shoulder, or ipsilateral breast, or anterior thorax, lesions.

As a free flap, it is indicated whenever a large area of skin and subcutaneous tissue is necessary, and a long and large vascular pedicle is preferred (for example, for large ankle and lower-leg lesions or cranial lesions when the anastomoses are performed to the neck vessels).

As the skin island can be designed in any direction, the TDAP flap is a very convenient way to harvest skin from the lateral thoracic wall and the inframammary area; this is an excellent donor area, with low morbidity and acceptable aesthetic results, and is easy to close directly.

ANATOMY

The vascular anatomy of this flap has been studied extensively. The thoracodorsal artery originates from the subscapular artery. It runs under the deep surface of the latissimus dorsi, where it bifurcates into two main branches: horizontal and vertical (or descending) branches. Both branches give off cutaneous branches, which pierce the muscle and distribute in the subcutaneous tissue; the larger ones arise from the descending branch at 6 to 8 cm inferior to the axillary crease and 1 to 2 cm posterior to the anterior border of the muscle (Fig. 1). This main cutaneous artery frequently surrounds the anterior border of the muscle or pierces it through a few anterior fibers. In summary, the thoracodorsal artery consistently gives off several cutaneous branches through the muscle, although the first one may be attached to the anterior border (Fig. 2).

FLAP DESIGN AND DIMENSIONS

The flap is designed with the patient in a standing position. The arm is abducted 90 degrees. An assistant holds the elbow, and the patient is asked to adduct the arm against opposition. The anterior border of the latissimus dorsi is clearly observed and is marked. A point is marked over this line at 7 cm below the axillary crease. A 2-cm radial circumference centered at this point is marked. This is the approximate location of the proximal cutaneous branch of the thoracodorsal artery. A Doppler probe is applied, and the vessel is precisely located.

From this point, a 25-cm-long ellipse skin paddle is designed with the longitudinal axis placed in any direction. The cutaneous vessel that irrigates the flap does not need to be in the center. Usually, the flap is designed in an oblique anterior position for better donor-area closure. No relation exists between the flap design and the limits of the underlying muscle: the flap may be designed almost completely beyond the anterior border of the muscle.

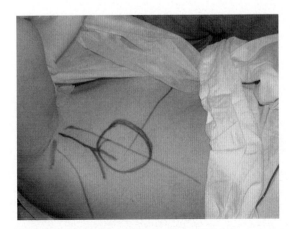

FIG. 1. The thoracodorsal artery runs under the deep surface of the latissimus dorsi muscle, where it bifurcates into two main branches: horizontal and descending branches. Both branches give off cutaneous branches that pierce the muscle. The larger ones come off the descending branch at 6 to 8 cm inferior to the axillary crease and 1 to 2 cm to the border of the muscle.

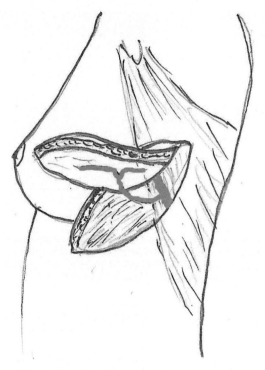

FIG. 2. Anatomy of the course of cutaneous vessels.

OPERATIVE TECHNIQUE

The patient is positioned in a lateral decubitus position with the arm in 90-degree abduction and 90-degree elbow flexion. Once the operative field is prepared, the dermis is infiltrated with lidocaine (Xylocaine) 1% with epinephrine where the skin will be incised. The skin incision starts at the inferior border of the flap. The anterior border of the latissimus dorsi is exposed, and dissection continues superiorly above the deep fascia with optical magnification. The cutaneous vessels are identified, and careful dissection is performed between the muscle fibers to the main pedicle, which is completely exposed. The muscle branches are coagulated or clipped and sectioned. The muscle nerve is preserved.

The cutaneous perforator can be easily dissected from the muscle fibers because it is surrounded by fatty tissue. It is not advisable to perform this procedure as a muscle-sparing technique, because a greater risk of damaging the vessels exists.

CLINICAL RESULTS

Seventy-five patients were operated on by using TDAP flaps (42 male and 33 female patients). Patient ages ranged from 2 to 78 years. Thirty-five cases used islands and 40 used free flaps. In 26 cases, the muscle was used as an independent unit. The island flaps were used mainly for burn scar–contracture release at the mammary or axillary area, or for shoulder resurfacing after tumor resection. The free flaps were used for cranial-vault coverage and knee, ankle, and elbow coverage.

Five flaps were lost. In three cases, the skin island was lost, and the muscle was eventually used as a free muscle flap and skin grafted. In two cases, the flap was lost after having been transferred, because of technical problems at the anastomosis. In three cases, the perforator was not found or was destroyed during flap elevation. Considering that in more than 50 specimen dissections done in injected cadavers, the cutaneous branches of the thoracodorsal artery were consistently found, we believe that technical error was the main factor for flap loss.

SUMMARY

The thoracodorsal perforator flap is very reliable; the cutaneous branches of the thoracodorsal are a constant finding (the skin paddle of the traditional latissimus dorsi musculocutaneous flap is consistently irrigated by these branches). The flap allows a better "handling" of the skin island and the underlying muscle.

References

1. Angrigiani C, Grilli D, Sebert J. Latissimus dorsi musculocutaneous flap without muscle. *Plast Reconstr Surg* 1995;96:1608.
2. Godina M. The tailored latissimus dorsi free flap. *Plast Reconstr Surg* 1987;80:304.
3. Hayashi A, Maruyama Y. The "reduced" latissimus dorsi musculocutaneous flap. *Plast Reconstr Surg* 1989;84:290.

CHAPTER 141 ■ FREE ANTEROLATERAL THIGH FLAPS FOR RECONSTRUCTION OF HEAD AND NECK DEFECTS

I. KOSHIMA

EDITORIAL COMMENT

This chapter describes another source of tissue for your reconstructive efforts in the head and neck area. The solution is especially attractive, inasmuch as it does not require changing the position of the patient.

The anterolateral thigh flap is based on the septocutaneous or muscle perforators of the lateral descending branch of the lateral circumflex femoral system. It is useful for reconstruction of defects in the head and neck and in the extremities.

INDICATIONS

This flap is suitable for coverage of defects in the head and neck regions, such as the oral floor with or without tongue and hypopharyngeal defects, and also the cervical esophagus with the anterior cervical wall (1). It is also suitable for reconstruction of scalp defects. Even in infected cranial full-thickness defects involving the dura, one-stage reconstruction is possible using an anterolateral thigh fasciocutaneous flap because the dural defect can be replaced with the vascularized fascia lata. The fasciocutaneous flap is also suitable for the repair of large, full-thickness defects of the lip. Instead of the oral orbicular muscle, the vascularized tensor fascia lata can be used to suspend the lower or upper lip. In obese patients, the flap can be made thinner with primary defatting (1).

The main advantage is that, with the use of the vascular system of this flap, massive complex defects in the head and neck can be easily reconstructed in one stage with combined "chimeric" flaps with the same vascular source. The flap can be combined with other flaps or tissue (chimeric combined flap), such as the paraumbilical flap (rectus abdominis musculocutaneous flap), vascularized iliac bone or fibula, rectus femoris muscle, or sartorius muscle (2). In addition, this flap can be connected with other adjacent flaps ("mosaic" flaps), such as the connected anterolateral thigh-groin flap and/or anterolateral thigh-medial thigh flap (3).

ANATOMY

The lateral circumflex femoral system is composed of three main branches: the *ascending branch,* which passes through the intermuscular space between the sartorius and vastus lateralis muscles and terminates in the outer cortex of the iliac bone; the *transverse branch,* which terminates in the tensor fasciae latae muscle; and the *(lateral) descending branch,* which runs downward through the intermuscular space between the rectus femoris and the vastus lateralis muscles and finally terminates in the vastus muscle near the knee joint. The perforator of the anterolateral thigh flap usually is derived from the transverse branch or the descending branch, and the proximal perforator is situated around the proximal third of the thigh through the lateral longitudinal line of the thigh. Usually, a few cutaneous perforators are found passing through the intermuscular septum or the vastus lateralis muscle. Even in cases with no septocutaneous perforators, there are cutaneous perforators penetrating the vastus lateralis muscle (1–5,7,8) (Fig. 1).

FLAP DESIGN AND DIMENSIONS

The anterolateral thigh flap commands a skin territory of up to 600 cm^2 (30 × 20 cm), almost the same area as the tensor fasciae latae musculocutaneous flap. The upper border of the skin territory is the line through the iliac crest, and the lower border is the level of the lateral femoral condyle. The posterolateral skin territory is a longitudinal line drawn from the greater trochanter distally to the fibular head. The anteromedial margin of the skin territory is a line placed through the midportion of the rectus femoris muscle.

The skin, lateral femoral cutaneous nerve, fascia lata, rectus femoris muscle, and vastus lateralis muscle are elevated as a unit based on the skin perforator. The main pedicle perforator is located at the proximal third of the longitudinal line through the intermuscular space between the rectus femoris and vastus lateralis muscles. Other small perforators are located in the middle third of the lateral aspect of the thigh. Clinically, preoperative stereoangiograms or simple angiograms and Doppler audiometry are essential to determine the locations of the perforators and vascular variations of the lateral circumflex femoral system; however, using the Doppler is sometimes unreliable in cases in which the descending branch runs downward near the lateral skin surface of the thigh because the sound of the descending branch is enhanced rather than the perforators.

The skin territory can be extended with the use of connected (supercharged or mosaic) flaps (6). An upper extension is possible with the combined anterolateral thigh flap-groin flap, -vascularized iliac bone graft, -rectus abdominis musculocutaneous flap, or -latissimus dorsi musculocutaneous flap. A medial extension can be made with the combined anterolateral thigh flap-medial thigh flap-saphenous flap. A posterior extension is also possible with the anterolateral thigh flap-posterior thigh flap (Fig. 2).

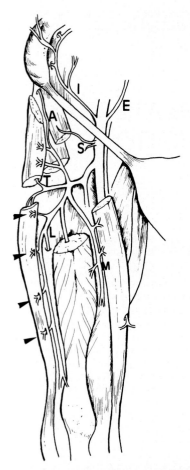

FIG. 1. Diagram of the surgical anatomy of the anterolateral thigh. The lateral circumflex femoral system is composed of the ascending branch (*A*), the transverse branch (*T*), the lateral descending branch (*L*), and the medial descending branch (*M*). Perforators (*arrowheads*) of the anterolateral thigh flap usually are derived from the lateral descending branch (or directly from the transverse branch). (From Koshima et al., ref. 1, with permission.)

OPERATIVE TECHNIQUE

With the patient in the supine position, flap elevation is begun simultaneously with tumor resection or recipient-bed preparation in the head and neck region; the donor area is relatively distant compared with other flaps, and early recipient-site preparation reduces operating time.

The first incision is made through the longitudinal line at the middle of the anterior aspect of the thigh (the middle on the rectus femoris muscle). Lateral skin is elevated subfascially through the incision with a pair of retractors, and the septocutaneous or musculocutaneous artery can be seen (Fig. 3). The septocutaneous artery comes through the intermuscular septum between the rectus femoris and vastus lateralis muscles. The musculocutaneous artery penetrates the vastus lateralis muscle. If the pedicle perforator is absent in the lateral septum (extremely rare), it is often located at the medial intermuscular septum between the rectus femoris and sartorius muscles. It often emerges at the juncture of the rectus femoris, sartorius, and vastus medialis muscles in the midthigh.

Before raising the skin flap, with transection of several muscle branches and retraction of the rectus femoris muscle medially, the pedicle is dissected and traced proximally, from the descending or transverse branch up to the division of the

rectus femoris muscular branch. If possible, the rectus muscle branch is preserved to maintain muscle vascularization. The branch of the femoral nerve running parallel to or across this vascular system must be separated carefully. Usually, the operating time required for tumor resection is longer than that for dissection of the flap pedicle vessels.

When tumor resection is completed, the skin flap is outlined to include the perforator in the anterolateral thigh region. After an incision through the outline, the flap is elevated from the distal portion, as the amount of bleeding from this portion is small. When a fasciocutaneous flap is required, the flap is raised subfascially. In obese patients, a thin anterolateral thigh flap can be created by removal of a considerable amount of fatty tissue. Regarding the creation of a thin flap: After the island flap pedicled by only one perforator is raised over the fascia, the flap can be made thinner by excising the subcutaneous fatty tissue with scissors (Fig. 4). Because the subdermal plexus of the capillary vessels is preserved, the peripheral region of the flap can be as thin as necessary, and only a thin layer of superficial fat (approximately 5 mm thick) is retained to protect the subdermal plexus. Resection of the

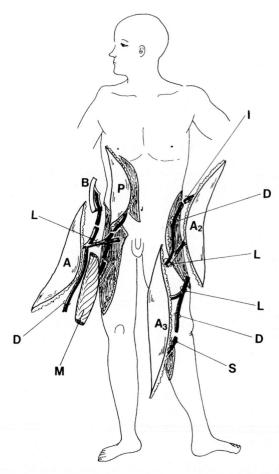

FIG. 2. Schema of flap design and dimensions. The lateral half of the thigh usually can provide a single dominant perforator for the anterolateral thigh flap. The flap can be combined with other adjacent flaps or tissues with the same vascular source (chimeric combined flaps). The flap territory can be extended superiorly or inferiorly by using connected "mosaic" or supercharged flaps. *A*, anterolateral thigh flap; *B*, iliac bone graft; *M*, rectus femoris muscle; *P*, paraumbilical flap; *L*, lateral circumflex femoral system (*LCFS*); *D*, descending branch of *LCFS*; *A₂*, connected anterolateral thigh-groin flap; *I*, superficial circumflex iliac vessels; *A₃*, connected anterolateral thigh-saphenous flap; *S*, saphenous vessels.

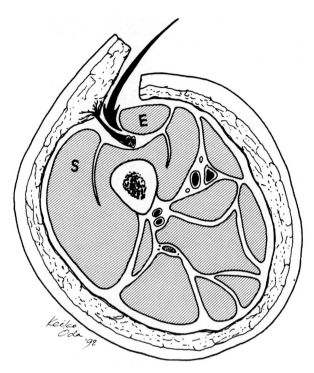

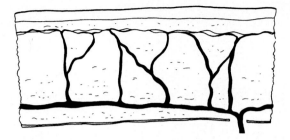

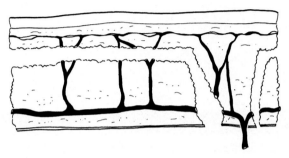

FIG. 3. Cross-sectional schema of flap elevation (right thigh). The septocutaneous perforator (sometimes penetrating the vastus lateralis muscle) can be seen through the first incision, which is made through the longitudinal line at the middle of the anterior aspect of the thigh. *E*, rectus femoris muscle; *S*, vastus lateralis muscle. (From Koshima et al., ref. 1, with permission.)

FIG. 4. Diagram of method for obtaining a thin anterolateral thigh flap. With preservation of the subdermal plexus, a thin flap can be obtained primarily by removing a considerable amount of fatty tissue. (From Koshima et al., ref. 1, with permission.)

fatty tissue about 2 cm around the perforator is impossible because of potential damage to the pedicle perforator. Relatively large flaps (up to 30 cm long and 20 cm wide usually can survive with only a single perforator.

The donor site is closed primarily or, if too large for direct closure it is covered with a mesh skin graft. Even with a split-thickness skin graft on the bare muscle, there is no deficit in walking.

CLINICAL RESULTS

Regarding complications, sensory disturbance in the distal portion of the flap is the result of sacrificing the lateral femoral cutaneous nerve. In cases with a small perforator less than 0.8 mm in caliber, the skin territory is limited to a maximum of 20 × 10 cm. Use of the rectus femoris muscle with this flap results in little functional deficit. In some patients, the rectus femoris muscle has a single vascular source with no collateral routes; therefore, when the muscle is preserved in the donor leg, the feeding artery also should be preserved.

SUMMARY

The anterolateral thigh flap ideally can reconstruct defects in the head and neck regions and, when combined or connected with other flaps from the same vascular source, is especially useful for complicated facial defects.

References

1. Koshima I, Fukuda H, Yamamoto H, et al. Free anterolateral thigh flaps for reconstruction of head and neck defects. *Plast Reconstr Surg* 1993;92:421.
2. Koshima I, Yamamoto H, Hosoda M, et al. Free combined composite flaps using the lateral circumflex femoral system for repair of massive defects of the head and neck regions: an introduction to the chimeric flap principle. *Plast Reconstr Surg* 1993;92:411.
3. Koshima I, Yamamoto H, Moriguchi T, Orita Y. Extended anterior thigh flaps for repair of massive cervical defects involving pharyngoesophagus and skin: an introduction to the "mosaic" flap principle. *Ann Plast Surg* 1994;32:321.
4. Song YG, Chen GZ, Song YL. The free thigh flap: a new concept based on the septocutaneous artery. *Br J Plast Surg* 1984;37:149.
5. Koshima I, Fukuda H, Utsonomiya R, Soeda S. The anterolateral thigh flap: variations in its vascular pedicle. *Br J Plast Surg* 1988;42:260.
6. Koshima I. Reply (see ref. 3). *Ann Plast Surg* 1994;33:462.
7. Xu DC, Zhong S, Kong J, et al. Applied anatomy of the anterolateral femoral flap. *Plast Reconstr Surg* 1988;82:305.
8. Zhou G, Qiao, Q, Chen GY, et al. Clinical experience and surgical anatomy of 32 free anterolateral thigh flap transplantations. *Br J Plast Surg* 1991;44:91.

CHAPTER 142 ■ MICROVASCULAR TRANSFER OF ANTEROLATERAL THIGH FLAPS FOR RECONSTRUCTION OF HEAD AND NECK DEFECTS

R. S. ALI AND F.-C. WEI

EDITORIAL COMMENT

The ALT flap has become a workhorse flap because of its donor site, which is easily covered by clothing, and its flap tissue pliability. The reader must be aware of the variability of the blood supply.

The anterolateral thigh (ALT) flap was first described as a free cutaneous flap from the anterolateral aspect of the thigh, based on a septocutaneous perforator. In fact, the majority of ALT flaps are based on musculocutaneous perforators. As surgical techniques to dissect musculocutaneous perforators have developed, the ALT flap has been at the forefront of the "perforator flaps." Rapid assimilation of the ALT flap into multidisciplinary head and neck practices attests to its versatility, based on characteristics such as: (a) a large cutaneous surface area; (b) multiplicity of tissue components that can be included in the flap (skin, fat, fascia, muscle, nerve, tendon); (c) freedom with which the tissue components can be separated on individual musculocutaneous perforators or septocutaneous vessels; (d) a long, wide-caliber pedicle; and (e) minimal donor morbidity.

INDICATIONS

General

The ALT flap, first described by Song et al. (1), is an ideal soft-tissue flap and is used in the reconstruction of many soft-tissue defects, including those following tumor resection, lower-limb trauma, or congenital deficiency.

Head and Neck

Indications for ALT flap use in head and neck surgery include the following: external face resurfacing, intraoral mucosal lining, soft-tissue volume replacement, palate and maxillary reconstruction, filling of dead space/sinus/cavity, reconstruction of the floor of the mouth, reconstruction of the tongue, reconstruction of the pharyngoesophagus, and scalp and skull-base reconstruction.

Buccal Mucosa

The cutaneous or fasciocutaneous ALT flap is a moderately thin, pliable flap that is ideal for resurfacing intraoral defects (Fig. 1). The long pedicle allows suitable inset of the ALT flap intraorally, with tunneling of the pedicle, to allow comfortable microvascular anastomosis to facial or cervical recipient vessels. The greater surface area of the ALT flap, compared with the radial forearm flap, along with versatility in tissue design due to the often multiple perforators supplying the skin paddle, permits the resurfacing of larger defects, multiplanar defects (2), and bilateral defects (3).

An ALT flap with more than one tissue paddle, based on widely separated perforators, is invaluable in the reconstruction of intraoral defects located in nearby but different sites or on different axial planes (2) (Fig. 2). More recently, the double-paddled ALT flap has evolved into harvesting two separate ALT flaps from one thigh, based on a single source vessel (3). This offers infinite degrees of freedom when positioning the flaps but requires the preparation of additional recipient vessels and additional microvascular anastomoses (Fig. 3).

Tongue Reconstruction

A thin fasciocutaneous or cutaneous ALT flap is ideal for reconstructing the partial glossectomy defect. The large cutaneous paddle permits resurfacing of an extensive surface area, and the relatively pliable flap can be molded to the three-dimensional contours of the tongue (Fig. 4).

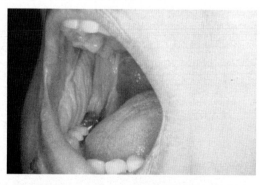

FIG. 1. Thin fasciocutaneous anterolateral thigh (ALT) flap, to resurface extensive defect of right buccal mucosa. Note large surface area and excellent contour of flap.

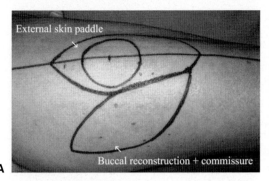
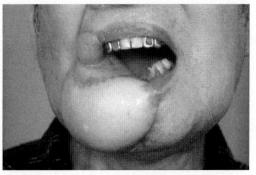

FIG. 2. ALT flap with multiple Doppler-detected perforator signals. **A:** Two eccentrically aligned skin paddles are marked, based on widely separate perforators. The flap is raised on a single pedicle and requires only a single anastomosis. **B:** Flap design allows more exact inset into the multiplanar defect involving the right commissure and buccal mucosa, as well as the right lower lip.

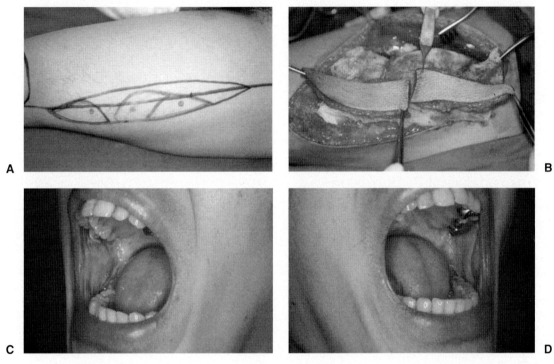

FIG. 3. Widely separated perforators permit planning of a large fasciocutaneous ALT flap (**A**), which is then divided between the perforators and raised as two separate ALT flaps (**B**). **C,D:** Bilateral intraoral defects may be reconstructed with two separate flaps harvested from a single thigh.

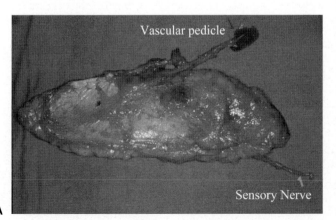
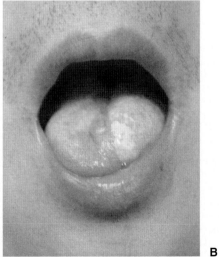

FIG. 4. A: ALT fasciocutaneous flap raised, with an additional length of sensory nerve proximally (anterior branch of lateral femoral cutaneous nerve of thigh). **B:** The large surface-area, pliable flap is used to reconstruct the mobile, three-dimensional tongue, following partial glossectomy. Sensory reinnervation may facilitate more rapid return of protective sensation.

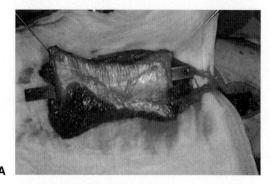
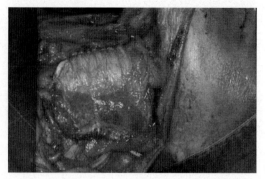

FIG. 5. **A:** Wide musculocutaneous ALT flap, raised and tubed, to form a neo-pharyngoesophagus in situ. **B:** Skin paddle faces inward, and harvesting an additional width of fascia, to over-sew the suture line, ensures a watertight, three-layer closure. Muscle component adds extra vascularity to the flap bed and additional coverage of exposed cervical structures.

Total glossectomy requires reconstruction with a flap of large cutaneous surface area and sufficient soft-tissue volume; the musculocutaneous ALT flap is excellent for reconstructing such defects. Incorporation of vascularized nerve in the ALT flap (anterior branch of the lateral femoral cutaneous nerve) confers the additional option of sensory reinnervation (4).

Pharyngoesophageal Reconstruction

A rapidly developing indication for use of the ALT flap is in pharyngoesophageal reconstruction. A wide fasciocutaneous or musculocutaneous ALT flap is raised with supplementary vascularized fascia and tubed to form a wide-bore, relatively rigid cylinder. The fascial layer augments the water-tight closure requisite to preparing the neo-pharyngoesophagus. The ALT flap can be raised simultaneously with tumor resection and recipient-site preparation; furthermore, the neo-pharyngoesophagus may be tubed and prepared with the flap still in situ on the thigh (Fig. 5). The free ALT flap can withstand extended ischemia time, compared with the free jejunal flap. There is growing evidence that postoperative complications are reduced by using the ALT flap, with concomitant superior functional outcome (5,6).

Maxillary and Palatal Defects

Maxillary tumor resection often results in complex three-dimensional defects requiring multiple skin paddles, in addition to soft-tissue volume replacement and/or the need to separate compartments or pack sinuses/dead spaces. The ALT flap harvested with additional vascularized fascia and/or muscle is ideal for reconstructing such multidimensional defects alone or in combination with a bone flap (Fig. 6).

Through-and-Through Cheek Defects

A musculocutaneous ALT flap incorporating a portion of vastus lateralis provides excellent approximation of the bulk required to reconstruct a full-thickness cheek defect. The musculocutaneous ALT flap may be used to provide tissue bulk and external skin cover only. If the commissure is involved, the ALT flap may be folded around the commissure, to provide soft-tissue bulk and intraoral and extraoral skin cover (Fig. 7). If the commissure is not involved, an area of the ALT flap may be deepithelialized, and the flap "posted" into the oral cavity to provide intraoral coverage. Alternatively, a mul-

tiple-paddled ALT flap may be designed, which can be divided between widely separated perforators, and the separated tissue paddles inset to provide both intraoral and extraoral coverage (2).

Mandibular Defects

Oromandibular resections, resulting in significant volume loss, require a large bulky flap for adequate soft-tissue reconstruction. It has become established practice to reconstruct major oromandibular defects with a combination of two flaps: a bone/internal lining flap and a soft-tissue/external skin flap (7,8). The ALT musculocutaneous flap has been extensively used in conjunction with the fibula osteoseptocutaneous (OSC) flap (Fig. 8). Both flaps can be harvested from the same lower limb, simultaneously with recipient-site preparation, in a multidisciplinary two-team approach. In recurrent or complex cases with limited local recipient vessels, the ALT perforator flap may be raised with a length of distal vessel, for use as a flow-through flap (9) or to "piggy back" a distal flap.

Face and Scalp Resurfacing/Craniofacial

Large malformations, tumors, or traumatic defects of the face and scalp may warrant major resurfacing and necessitate a pliable and robust flap with a large surface area (Fig. 9). Scalp and dura defects necessitate inclusion of vascularized fascia, which can be used to reconstruct the dura with a water-tight

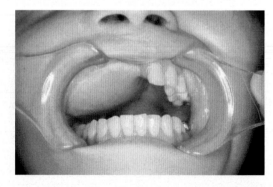

FIG. 6. Musculocutaneous ALT flap for reconstruction of the right palate, following excision of a maxillary tumor. Subsequent bony reconstruction with a free fibula flap was followed by the insertion of osseointegrated teeth.

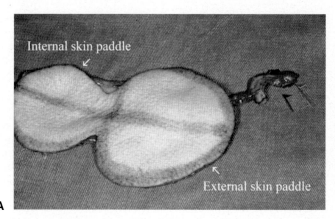
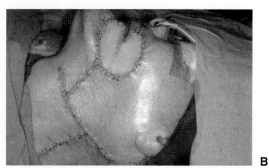

FIG. 7. **A:** Fasciocutaneous ALT flap designed with a large external skin paddle and a smaller skin paddle for reconstruction of the buccal mucosa. **B:** The flap is inset by folding around the full-thickness defect, to provide internal and external skin coverage and to create a new oral commissure.

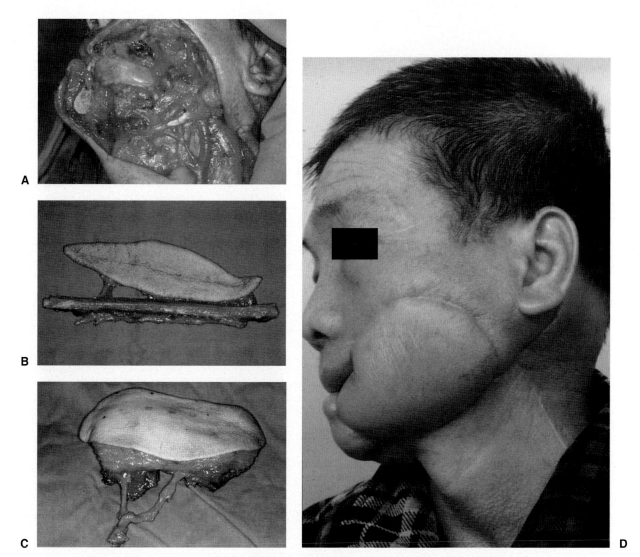

FIG. 8. **A:** Full-thickness oromandibular defect with segmental mandibulectomy and neck dissection. **B:** Fibula-osteoseptocutaneous (OSC) flap used to reconstruct the bony defect and internal oral lining. **C:** Large-surface-area, bulky musculocutaneous flap raised to reconstruct full-thickness soft-tissue defect and to provide well-vascularized coverage of the underlying bone flap and metal work. **D:** Combined fibula-OSC and ALT flaps inset. ALT flap provides sufficient soft-tissue bulk and large-surface-area skin paddle and is pliable enough to fold over to form a neo-commissure.

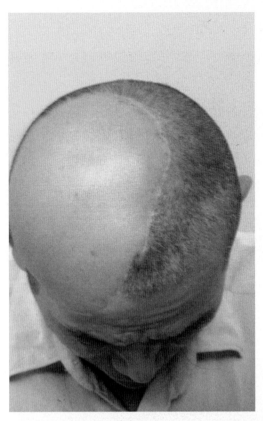

FIG. 9. Large fasciocutaneous ALT flap, inset following resection of an ulcerative incision, with exposed skull. Flap is thin, pliable, and large enough to provide scalp reconstruction.

seal, in conjunction with a large cutaneous component for resurfacing work.

Skull Base

A musculocutaneous or cutaneous ALT flap is ideal for use in this vital area, and can be tailored to fill any dead space and to provide a large surface area of robust skin. The fascial component of a fasciocutaneous ALT flap may also be used and is especially suitable if the dead space is narrow.

ANATOMY

The area of the anterolateral thigh supplied by the lateral circumflex femoral artery (LCFA) extends from the iliac crest to the lateral femoral condyle and from the medial border of the rectus femoris to the posterior midline. A line joining the anterior superior iliac spine (ASIS) to the superolateral margin of the patella indicates the longitudinal axis of the anterolateral thigh flap, and approximates the intermuscular septum between the vastus lateralis and rectus femoris (Fig. 10).

The LCFA usually arises from the profunda femoris but may also arise from the main femoral artery. The LCFA trifurcates into ascending, transverse, and descending branches and supplies much of the skin and underlying musculature of the anterolateral thigh, including the tensor fasciae latae and quadriceps femoris muscle mass, comprising the vastus lateralis, v. intermedius, v. medialis, and rectus femoris.

The vascular pedicle of the ALT flap is usually the descending branch (75% of cases), which is also the largest and longest of the LCFA branches. In a significant minority of cases, however, the ALT musculocutaneous perforators may arise from the transverse branch (25% of cases). The descending branch has a length of 8 to 12 cm and runs in the intermuscular septum between the vastus lateralis and rectus femoris. The pedicle of the ALT flap is therefore readily located, of significant length, has an arterial diameter of 2.1 ± 0.1 mm, and is typically accompanied by two venae comitantes (d = 1.8−2.3 ± 0.1 mm) (10).

Perforating arteries from the descending branch of the LCFA localize to the middle third of the anterolateral thigh. A 3-cm circle radius bisecting the longitudinal axis of the anterolateral thigh flap contains the majority (92%) of Doppler-audible perforators, most (87%) of which lie just lateral to the longitudinal axis (10) (Fig. 10). On average, two to four perforating arteries supply the cutaneous territory of the ALT flap (11). In general, the blood supply to the ALT flap is via musculocutaneous perforators traversing through the vastus lateralis (59.2%–84%), giving rise to the ALT musculocutaneous perforator flap. The remaining (16%–40.8%) flaps are supplied by septocutaneous vessels that pass directly through the intermuscular septum, to give rise to a septocutaneous flap. Rarely are there no suitable perforators on which to base an ALT flap (12,13). In such cases, the skin paddle may be raised with the underlying vastus lateralis muscle as a carrier, flap design can be altered to that of a medial thigh or tensor fasciae latae flap, or the contralateral thigh can be explored.

The ratio of musculocutaneous perforators to septocutaneous vessels varies considerably and varies with the location of the skin paddle. Septocutaneous vessels are more prevalent in the proximal thigh, whereas musculocutaneous perforators predominate in more distally located skin flaps. The distinction between septocutaneous vessel and musculocutaneous perforator is worth making, because the "true" perforator flap relies on intricate dissection of the musculocutaneous perforator through the underlying musculature and is the hallmark of "perforator flap surgery" (14). The septocutaneous ALT flap, raised on shorter, more direct vessels penetrating the intramuscular septum, presents a more rapid and straightforward dissection.

Variability in the vascular pedicle of the ALT flap and the differential ratio of musculocutaneous perforators to septocutaneous vessels are well-recognized characteristics of the ALT flap. Perforator-flap harvest relies on retrograde dissection; therefore, providing that the surgeon is aware of potential vascular variations, there is seldom any contraindication to raising an ALT flap.

Sensory innervation of the anterolateral thigh is via the lateral femoral cutaneous nerve of the thigh (L2–L3), which enters the proximal thigh deep to the inguinal ligament and passes over the sartorius proximally, to pierce the deep fascia 7 to 10 cm inferomedial to the ASIS. The sensory nerve then divides into anterior and posterior branches; the larger anterior branch passes downward along the longitudinal axis of the anterolateral thigh to supply the ALT cutaneous-flap territory. Motor innervation of the quadriceps musculature is via the femoral nerve (L2–L4). The motor nerve to the vastus lateralis (VL) travels superolaterally with the vascular pedicle and is preserved whenever possible.

FLAP DESIGN AND DIMENSIONS

The ALT flap is marked with the patient supine on the operating table. The readily palpable bony landmarks—the ASIS and the superolateral margin of the patella—are identified. A line connecting the ASIS to the superolateral patella is drawn and bisected with a 3-cm circle radius. A 5- to 8-MHz handheld Doppler probe is used to audibly identify cutaneous perforators, which are localized to the lateral half of the marked cir-

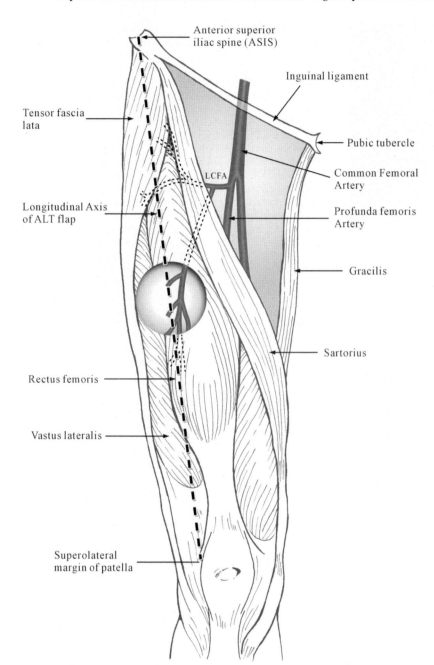

Anterior superior
iliac spine (ASIS)

Inguinal ligament

Tensor fascia
lata

LCFA

Pubic tubercle

Common Femoral
Artery

Longitudinal Axis
of ALT flap

Profunda femoris
Artery

Gracilis

Sartorius

Rectus femoris

Vastus lateralis

Superolateral
margin of patella

FIG. 10. Diagrammatic representation of ALT flap, demonstrating bony landmarks [anterior superior iliac spine (ASIS), patella], longitudinal axis of flap, location of ALT-flap perforators, and relationship to underlying musculature.

cle. If Doppler volume and probe pressure are kept constant, louder signals generally correspond to greater flow; therefore, more dominant perforators can be identified and designated with a larger marking.

A longitudinally orientated skin paddle is designed around the marked perforator(s). A skin paddle of 8 to 10 cm in width lends itself to direct closure (depending on skin laxity), whereas wider skin paddles will require alternate closure techniques such as skin grafting. Longer ALT flaps (20–25 cm) are increasingly preferred because they facilitate longer proximal pedicle dissection, without compromising donor-site closure or cosmesis. The flap may be designed more distally or extended laterally, as required, providing it includes the selected perforator(s). If multiple skin paddles are to be harvested from one thigh, each skin paddle is designed around widely separated, suitable perforators.

OPERATIVE TECHNIQUE

The patient is positioned supine and the whole lower limb circumferentially sterilized and draped. A sandbag placed under the ipsilateral hip, or tethering the ipsilateral foot to the contralateral side, will keep the limb internally rotated slightly and presents better access to the lateral aspect of the thigh.

Under loupe magnification, an initial exploratory incision is performed along the medial side of the planned flap. The ALT flap may be raised in a suprafascial or subfascial plane, depending on which tissue components are required and the desired thickness of the ALT flap. The cutaneous or fasciocutaneous tissue paddle is elevated sufficiently, to allow visual confirmation of the presence, position, and size of the perforators. Modification of ALT flap design may be conducted at

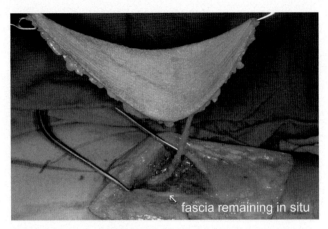

FIG. 11. Very thin ALT flap can be raised in a suprafascial plane, consisting of only skin, dermis, and minimal subcutaneous fat. Fascia is incised, to allow dissection of the perforator, but is repaired following flap harvest, resulting in negligible functional donor morbidity.

this stage, depending on perforator attributes. Once suitable perforators have been visualized, the flap is elevated by retrograde dissection of the selected perforator(s) to the source vessel in the intermuscular septum. A small cuff of fascia may be retained around the entry point of the perforator complex into the cutaneous paddle, to protect against damage or twisting of the perforator vessel.

Meticulous intramuscular dissection is the sine qua non of "perforator flap surgery" and mandates scrupulous hemostasis. Musculocutaneous perforators are dissected by initially "deroofing" or exposing the vessel, by incising the muscle fibers above the perforator. The perforator is then dissected free of the muscle tissue on either side, and, finally, the underside of the perforator is freed. Multiple side branches to the adjacent muscle are encountered and necessitate careful ligation, using hemoclips or coagulation with bipolar diathermy.

Perforator dissection continues proximally until the required length of pedicle is achieved. If the cutaneous flap to be raised is supplied by more than one perforator and the motor nerve to the vastus lateralis runs between the perforators and is unable to be preserved, it is incised near its entry point into muscle and repaired directly, under microscope magnification.

A fasciocutaneous ALT flap is raised in the relatively avascular subfascial plane and allows full exposure of the intermuscular septum and easy visualization of the perforators. Flap harvest is technically straightforward and results in a flap that includes the rich vascular network of the deep fascia. The cutaneous ALT flap is raised in the suprafascial plane and permits harvest of the thinnest possible flap, containing only skin and subcutaneous tissue (Fig. 11).

If an even thinner cutaneous flap is required, the ALT perforator flap may be thinned primarily, before ligation of the pedicle. Thinning to a uniform thickness of 3 to 5 mm can be performed safely under microscope guidance, as long as a small area of tissue (radius: 2–4 cm) surrounding the perforator is preserved (15). Thinning prior to vascular ligation permits monitoring of flap viability and allows precise hemostasis.

The ALT musculocutaneous flap is dissected anterograde, the flap pedicle is identified in the intermuscular septum, and the vastus lateralis is split along its longitudinal axis, to ensure inclusion of the vascular pedicle. Musculocutaneous ALT flap harvest may include as much or as little muscle as required by the dimensions of the defect.

Perforators supplying the skin overlying the muscle may be visualized prior to flap harvest, and the cutaneous and muscle components can each be tailored to the requirements of the defect (Fig. 12A). Alternatively, the muscle and skin components can be raised en bloc, and skin viability ensured by including the perforator Doppler signals heard at the beginning of the procedure (Fig. 12B).

Incorporating the anterior branch of the lateral femoral cutaneous nerve proximally raises the potential to develop a sensate ALT flap. Such reinnervation by coaptation of the sensory nerve to the recipient nerve(s) allows protective sensation to be achieved more rapidly. Additional fascia lata can be rolled to form a tendonlike structure that can function as a static sling in adjuvant procedures associated with facial resurfacing.

A longer ALT flap may be raised, and the extra length deepithelialized and buried, to minimize contour deformities or fill dead space (Fig. 13). This has proved valuable following cervical lymph-node dissection and serves to protect vital structures in the neck from potential radiotherapy effects (16). A deepithelialized ALT flap is also suitable for correcting contour deformities, such as hemifacial microsomia (17).

Direct closure of the thigh is possible for defects of less than 8 to 10 cm in width and is generally performed in two

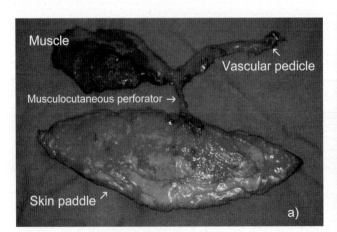
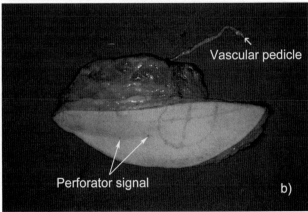

FIG. 12. A: Musculocutaneous ALT flap, in which the skin component has been separated on an individual perforator. In this way, the flap can be tailored to an individual defect, and the muscle component used as a soft-tissue filler, to separate compartments or to provide extra bulk where required. **B:** Musculocutaneous ALT flap, in which the muscle is raised en bloc with the skin paddle, making sure to include the perforator signals marked on the flap.

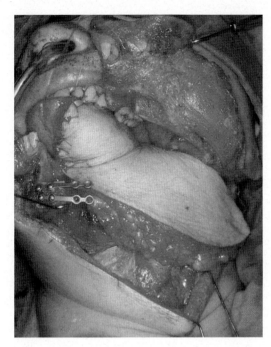

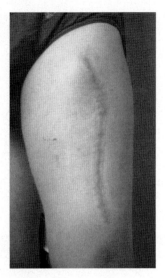

FIG. 14. ALT-flap donor site can usually be closed directly for flaps of less than 8 to 10 cm width. There are rarely any functional sequelae, and the majority of patients express satisfaction with the discrete, easily hidden donor site.

FIG. 13. Thick fasciocutaneous ALT flap inset into a left partial glossectomy defect. The remaining flap is deepithelialized and positioned under the facial and cervical skin flaps, to minimize any contour defect, following cervical lymph-node dissection. The additional tissue also serves to protect underlying vascular and neural structures from the potentially harmful effects of radiotherapy. Deepithelialization may be performed before or after microanastomosis.

layers (Fig. 14). Drainage is not required, and the patient is mobilized on postoperative day 1. Harvesting of a suprafascial flap entails additional closure of the remaining deep fascia. Musculocutaneous flap harvest often allows easier closure of the relatively "debulked" thigh. If a wide flap has been harvested that precludes direct closure of the thigh, a split-thickness skin graft is applied to the muscle or fascial bed of the residual defect.

CLINICAL RESULTS

The ALT flap has become our workhorse soft-tissue flap for head and neck reconstruction. Since 1999, between 200 and 300 ALT flaps have been used for head and neck reconstruction each year.

SUMMARY

The ALT flap has demonstrated primacy in microvascular head and neck reconstruction, whether used as a cutaneous/fasciocutaneous flap for resurfacing, or as a musculocutaneous flap for complex maxillary and oromandibular defects or total tongue reconstruction. The flap has rapidly established a dominant role in pharyngoesophageal reconstruction, due to its ease of handling and improved functional outcome. Microvascular transfer of an ALT flap results in a discrete donor site, with minimal reported functional or aesthetic morbidity.

Favorable anatomic characteristics of the flap include a large cutaneous surface area and reliable distribution of perforators. Recent advances in surgical technique and instrumentation have encouraged the development of the double-paddle ALT flap and harvesting of multiple ALT flaps from a single thigh. This allows bilateral pathologies to be treated simultaneously and has extended the reach of the reconstructive sur-

geon to premalignant progressive conditions, such as oral submucosal fibrosis.

References

1. Song YG, Chen GZ, Song YL. The free thigh flap: a new free flap concept based on the septocutaneous artery. *Br J Plast Surg* 1984;37:149.
2. Lin YT, Lin CH, Wei FC. More degrees of freedom by using chimeric concept in the applications of anterolateral thigh flap. *J Plast Reconstr Aesthet Surg* 2006;59:622.
3. Chou EK, Ulusal B, Ulusal A, et al. Using the descending branch of the lateral femoral circumflex vessel as a source of two independent flaps. *Plast Reconstr Surg* 2006;117:2059.
4. Yu P. Reinnervated anterolateral thigh flap for tongue reconstruction. *Head Neck* 2004;26:1038.
5. Yu P, Lewin JS, Reece JP, Robb GL. Comparison of clinical and functional outcomes and hospital costs following pharyngoesophageal reconstruction with the anterolateral thigh free flap versus the jejunal flap. *Plast Reconstr Surg* 2006;117:968.
6. Yu P, Robb GL. Pharyngoesophageal reconstruction with the anterolateral thigh flap: a clinical and functional outcomes study. *Plast Reconstr Surg* 2005;116:1845.
7. Koshima I, Fukuda H, Soeda S. Free combined anterolateral thigh flap and vascularized iliac bone graft with double vascular pedicle. *J Reconstr Microsurg* 1989;5:55.
8. Wei FC, Celik N, Chen HC, et al. Combined anterolateral thigh flap and vascularized fibula osteoseptocutaneous flap in reconstruction of extensive composite mandibular defects. *Plast Reconstr Surg* 2002;109:45.
9. Koshima I, Hosoda S, Inagawa K, et al. Free combined anterolateral thigh flap and vascularized fibula for wide, through-and-through oromandibular defects. *J Reconstr Microsurg* 1998;14:529.
10. Xu DC, Zhong SZ, Kong JM, et al. Applied anatomy of the anterolateral femoral flap. *Plast Reconstr Surg* 1988;82:305.
11. Kawai K, Imanishi N, Nakajima H, et al. Vascular anatomy of the anterolateral thigh flap. *Plast Reconstr Surg* 2004;114:1108.
12. Kimata Y, Uchiyama K, Ebihara S, et al. Anatomic variations and technical problems of the anterolateral thigh flap: a report of 74 cases. *Plast Reconstr Surg* 1998;102:1517.
13. Wei FC, et al. Have we found an ideal soft-tissue flap? An experience with 672 anterolateral thigh flaps. *Plast Reconstr Surg* 2002;109:2219, discussion: 2227.
14. Wei FC, Celik N. Perforator flap entity. *Clin Plast Surg* 2003;30:325.
15. Kimura N, Satoh K. Consideration of a thin flap as an entity and clinical applications of the thin anterolateral thigh flap. *Plast Reconstr Surg* 1996;97:985.
16. Ao M, Uno K, Maeta M, et al. De-epithelialised anterior (anterolateral and anteromedial) thigh flaps for dead space filling and contour correction in head and neck reconstruction. *Br J Plast Surg* 1999;52:261.
17. Ji Y, Li T, Shamburger S, et al. Microsurgical anterolateral thigh fasciocutaneous flap for facial contour correction in patients with hemifacial microsomia. *Microsurgery* 2002;22:34.

CHAPTER 143 ■ MUSCLE VASCULARIZED PEDICLE FLAP AND BONE

Y. SHINTOMI, K. NOHIRA, Y. YAMAMOTO, AND L. O. VASCONEZ

EDITORIAL COMMENT

This procedure may open up new possibilities in coverage of difficult defects. However, as pointed out so aptly by Buncke (2), other methods should be considered that are reliable and involve a single stage.

The introduction of free-tissue transfer and refinements of microvascular techniques have made it possible to reconstruct difficult defects expeditiously; however, available flap donor sites are often limited by local vascular anatomy. This chapter presents a unique technique of allowing the custom design of free flaps that fit the tissue requirements of specific defects. The muscle vascularized pedicle (MVP) flap, which is actually a secondarily vascularized flap, is developed by implanting a vascular bundle surrounded by a small cuff of muscle into a selected donor site (1). With extension of the concept of the MVP flap, any tissue, such as bone, tendon, and nerve, can be revascularized and applied as a source of free tissue transfer (1–3).

INDICATIONS

When thin flaps are needed for head and neck and upper and lower extremity reconstruction, a free skin flap can be pro-

vided that has a thickness of 1 cm or less. The donor site can be chosen so that it provides skin of good color, texture, and volume in facial reconstruction. The donor site also can be chosen not only so that it provides bone of specific contour in maxillary or mandibular reconstruction but also so that it results in as little morbidity as possible.

ANATOMY

Any muscle vascular pedicle can be used. Especially desirable muscles are those that have large, long vascular pedicles providing easy microvascular anastomosis in free tissue transfer, such as the latissimus dorsi and serratus anterior muscle with the thoracodorsal vessels and the rectus abdominis muscle with the inferior epigastric vessels.

FLAP DESIGN AND DIMENSIONS

The cuff of muscle needed to revascularize the custom tissue should be approximately 10% to 20% of the size of the flap. The skin of the lateral thoracic, medial arm, and anterior chest are typically good donor-site choices for facial reconstruction. They are successfully revascularized by implantation of a small cuff of the latissimus dorsi or serratus anterior muscle with the thoracodorsal pedicle. The iliac bone is a typically

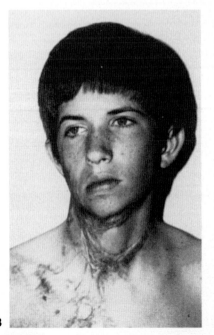
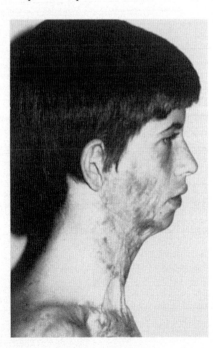

A,B

FIG. 1. **A,B:** A 15-year-old boy who sustained multiple flame burns 2 years previously. The preoperative frontal and lateral appearance of the burn scar. Note the significant right-sided burn scar contracture, which is pulling the right side of the mouth downward and preventing adequate neck extension.

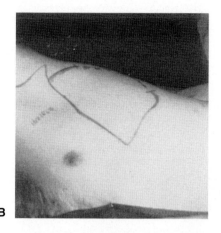
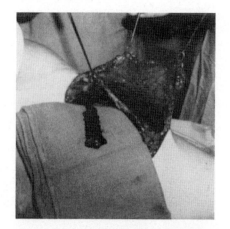

A,B

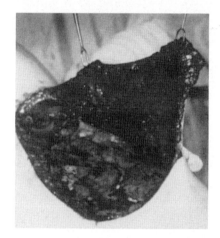
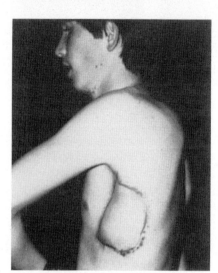

C,D

FIG. 2. **A:** The patient in the lateral decubitus position with the skin over the right lateral chest wall marked in an exact pattern to cover the planned defect. The initial incision will be through the anteromedial portion of this outline. **B:** The skin flap elevated at the level of appropriate thickness. The bulks of the latissimus dorsi muscle and the small sheath of muscle surrounding the thoracodorsal vessels. **C:** The positioning of the small muscle sheath to the undersurface of the skin flap. Note that a thin silicone sheet has already been placed over the underlying remaining subcutaneous tissue and latissimus dorsi muscle. **D:** The planned skin flap several days following the delay procedure, at which a complete division of all remaining skin attachments to the flap was done. Approximately 1 week later, this newly vascularized skin flap underwent free-tissue transfer to resurface the neck burn scar defect.

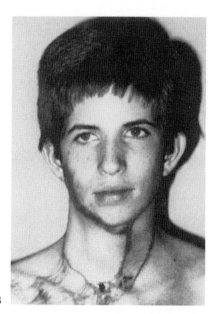
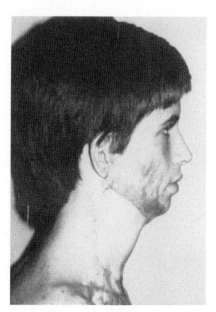

A,B

FIG. 3. **A,B:** Anterior and lateral views approximately 1 month following transfer of the flap. Although the edges of the wounds have not yet completely settled, note the good color and texture match. Also note the correction of the contracting forces on the right corner of the mouth.

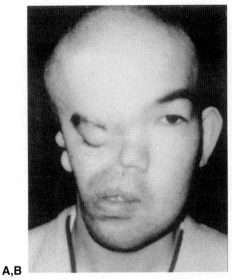
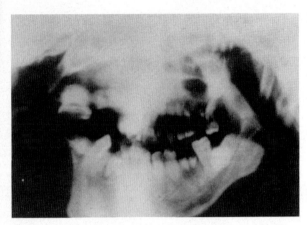

A,B

FIG. 4. A, B: A 27-year-old man with defect of the right mandible following cancer resection. Mandibular reconstruction with a free muscle vascularized pedicle iliac bone was scheduled.

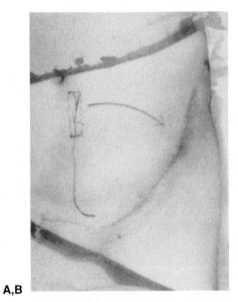
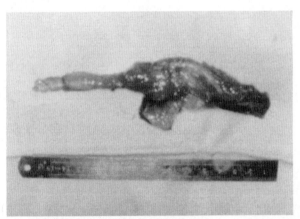

A,B

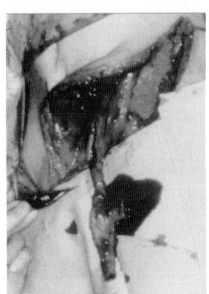
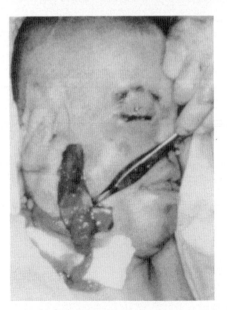

C,D

FIG. 5. A: The left inferior epigastric vascular pedicle surrounded by a small cuff of the rectus abdominis muscle was designed with the patient in the supine position. B: After a total of 4 weeks from the first surgery, with one surgical delay procedure to the iliac bone, the revascularized iliac bone was elevated. Good bleeding was noticed from the incised margin of the revascularized iliac bone. C: View of the muscle vascularized pedicle bone based on the left inferior epigastric vessels after isolation. D: The revascularized iliac bone was transferred to the defect. Microvascular anastomosis with the right facial artery and vein was performed.

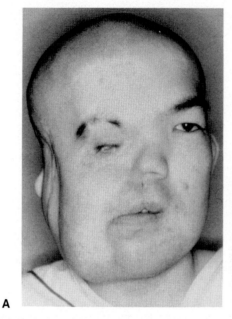

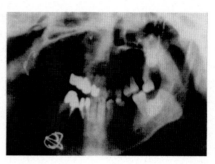

A   **B**

FIG. 6. **A:** Anterior view approximately 6 months after transfer of the bone. **B:** Postoperative radiograph showing a good bony synthesis of the reconstructed mandible.

good donor site choice for maxillary or mandibular reconstruction. It can be successfully revascularized by implantation of a small cuff of the rectus abdominis muscle with the inferior epigastric pedicle.

OPERATIVE TECHNIQUE

The procedure involves three stages. In the first stage, a pattern of the required flap is designed on the selected donor site. The flap is undermined with the appropriate thickness, including the subdermal plexus. The selected vascular bundle, surrounded by a small cuff of muscle, is dissected and implanted into the undersurface of the flap. A thin silicone sheet occasionally is placed under the implanted vascular pedicle to avoid neovascularization from the bed. When bone is to be revascularized, the surface of the donor bone that is to be attached with the selected vascular bundle and a small cuff of muscle is rasped to the cancellous bone layer to provide rapid, reliable revascularization from the implanted pedicle. Two weeks later, a surgical delay procedure is performed by cir-

cumferentially incising the skin flap or bone on its remaining borders. From 1 to 3 weeks later, in the third stage, the revascularized tissue then can be transferred as a conventional free flap to the recipient site (Figs. 1–6).

SUMMARY

A custom-designed secondarily vascularized flap, which can include bone, can be developed by implanting a vascular pedicle surrounded by a small cuff of muscle into a selected donor site.

References

1. Shintomi Y, Ohura T. The use of muscle vascularized pedicle flaps. *Plast Reconstr Surg* 1982;70:725.
2. Buncke HJ. The use of muscle vascularized pedicle flaps (discussion). *Plast Reconstr Surg* 1982;70:735.
3. Shintomi Y, Nohira K, Yamamoto Y, et al. MVP (muscle vascularized pedicle) Flap and Bone. Panel Discussion, Yokohama: IPRAS, 1995.

CHAPTER 144 ■ PRINCIPLES OF PREFABRICATED FLAPS

J. BAUDET AND D. MARTIN

Flap prefabrication may be considered a generic description referring to the remodeling, reshaping, or rebuilding of pedicled or free flaps, in effect, a tailored or customized flap. Using the concept of prefabrication, the area of the potential flap can be enlarged, a more reliable vascularity can be achieved, and the availability of donor materials can be maximized before transfer of the flap.

INDICATIONS

Because the use of prefabrication involves a wide variety of complementary or associated surgical techniques, perhaps the only common denominator is the ability to extend the indications and potentials of pedicled or free flaps in several donor and recipient body areas. Techniques can include the use of delay as a preliminary stage for a free flap, thus increasing the survival area by enlargement of the choke vessels that link vascular territories (1,2). Flap preexpansion can enhance the available area of a flap, contribute to better vascularity and safety, and allow easier primary closure at the donor site (3–6). Induced neovascularization or preliminary vascular induction can expand the possibilities of tissue use by delaying or staging transfer until dependable vascularization is achieved (7–24). Combinations using several elements of prefabrication make it possible to reconstruct several anatomic and aesthetic units in sequential procedures done at a single donor site with the addition of free or pedicled flaps (25–27).

OPERATIVE TECHNIQUE

Induced Neovascularized Flap

Orticochea (13) was the first to use this principle for reconstruction of the nose. He transferred the superficial temporal vessels to the retroauricular conchal area, which then was used in a second stage as a pedicled composite flap. Subsequently, Erol (14) developed the conversion of a thick split-thickness skin graft as a secondary vascularized flap. The temporopari-etal branch or the frontal branch of the superficial temporal vessels was used in nine patients to prepare vascular pedicled flaps, which then were transferred at least 3 weeks later for reconstruction of the infraorbital, zygomatic, or buccal regions as well as for nose and ear reconstruction.

Shen (16) reconstructed the helix of the ear after implanting the superficial temporal artery and vein into a long, thin tube on the neck. The average time between the two operations was 4.5 weeks. He also was the first to transfer a prefabricated flap with preliminary vascular induction successfully (17). In a first stage, the descending branch of the lateral femoral circumflex artery was implanted beneath the skin territory of the lateral aspect of the thigh. Six weeks later, a 2.6 × 16-cm flap was transferred and revascularized in the neck for treatment of a severe burn contracture. According to the same principle, a skin territory can be neovascularized by the free transfer of an arteriovenous pedicle and its surrounding fascia or a muscle cuff done as a first stage (18,19).

Prefabricated Composite Flap

A total nose reconstruction was prefabricated on the forearm, with incorporation of the radius in the flap as vascularized bone. In a first stage, the nose was adequately shaped and 1 month later was transferred to the recipient site, including part of the vascularized radius for support of the nasal spine and reconstruction of the columella. The eyebrows and upper and lower eyelids were reconstructed in the same patient by a unipedicled galea and scalp flap plus skin graft (Figs. 1–7).

Reconstruction of Several Anatomic and Aesthetic Units by Prefabrication

A complex reconstruction was carried out in which the first set of microsurgical transfers included an inguinal flap to the cheek and an osteocutaneous transfer from the dorsum of the foot, including the second metatarsal, to reconstruct the nose (Figs. 8 and 9). The eyebrow, both eyelids, orbital cavity, and lips were prefabricated in situ on the radial artery of the forearm (Figs. 10–13). The whole prefabricated construct finally was successfully transferred, with the deepithelialized zone of the transfer buried under the free inguinal flap previously used to reconstruct the cheek. Preserved bovine cartilage was used to support the lower eyelid, and a split palmaris longus muscle was inserted into the lips for better contour and definition.

Text continued on page 416.

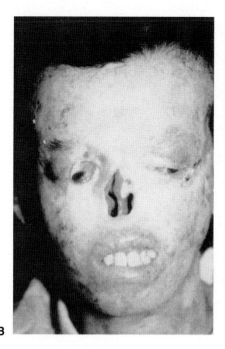
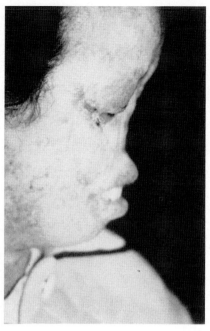

A,B

FIG. 1. A,B: Xeroderma pigmentosum of the face in a young female with a history of numerous destructive basal cell carcinomas and superficial malignant melanomas. Nose, upper and lower eyelids, and both eyebrows require reconstruction. (From Baudet, ref. 27, with permission.)

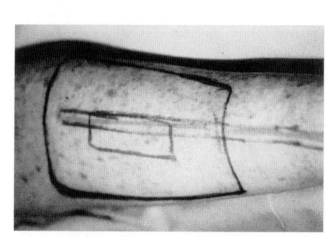

FIG. 2. Marking of cutaneous territory of the left forearm centered on the radial artery designed for prefabrication of the nose. Rectangle at right center corresponds to the territory of the radius that will be incorporated in the flap as vascularized bone to ensure support of the nose. (From Baudet, ref. 27, with permission.)

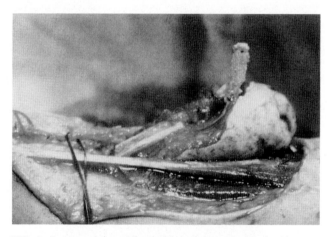

FIG. 4. One month later. The prefabricated nose is raised with a segment of radius divided into two segments: one for the support of the nasal bridge, the other for reconstruction of the columella. (From Baudet, ref. 27, with permission.)

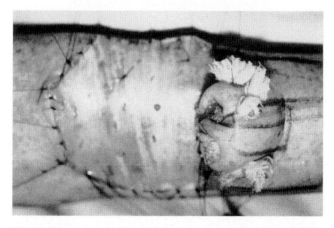

FIG. 3. Illustration of the prefabrication; the nose has been modeled and the donor site grafted. (From Baudet, ref. 27, with permission.)

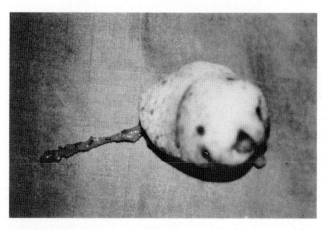

FIG. 5. Appearance of the prefabricated nose before revascularization. (From Baudet, ref. 27, with permission.)

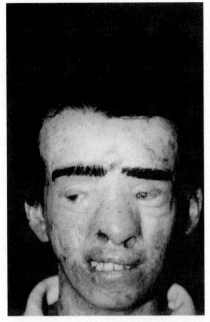
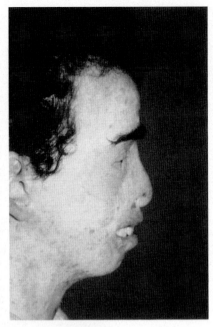

A,B

FIG. 6. A, B: Final result. Note the excellent texture and projection of the recreated nose. Eyebrows and upper and lower eyelids were reconstructed by a unipedicled galea and scalp flap plus skin graft. (From Baudet, ref. 27, with permission.)

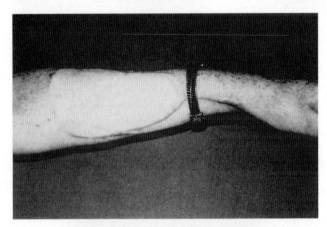

FIG. 7. Sequelae at the grafted donor site. (From Baudet, ref. 27, with permission.)

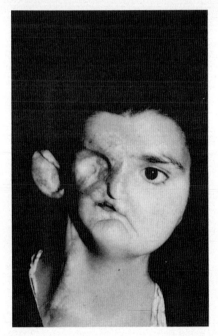

FIG. 8. Patient after childhood radiotherapy for an immature angioma. (From Baudet, ref. 27, with permission.)

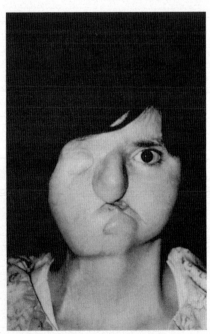

FIG. 9. Appearance after the first two microsurgical transfers, an inguinal flap to the cheek and osteocutaneous transfer from the dorsum of the foot for nose reconstruction. (From Baudet, ref. 27, with permission.)

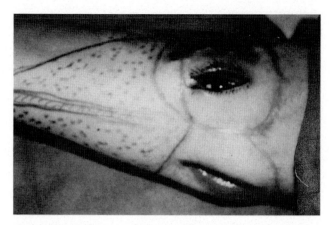

FIG. 10. Prefabrication on the radial artery of the foream. *Above:* An orbital cavity with an ocular prosthesis already in place; reconstruction of the eyebrow by end-to-side scalp transfer on the radial artery. *Below:* Creation of upper and lower lips. (From Baudet, ref. 27, with permission.)

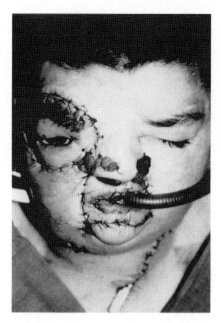

FIG. 12. Immediate postoperative appearance. (From Baudet, ref. 27, with permission.)

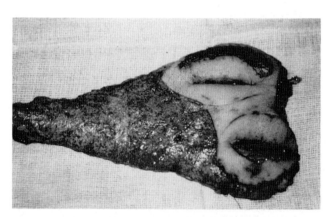

FIG. 11. Appearance of the free transfer after pedicle separation. The deepithelialized zone is buried under the free inguinal flap previously used to reconstruct the cheek. (From Baudet, ref. 27, with permission.)

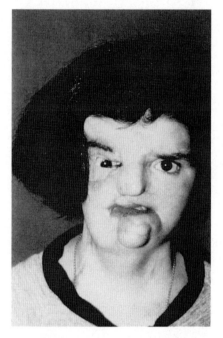

FIG. 13. Final appearance of this complex reconstruction with four microsurgical transfers, including a prefabricated free flap. (From Baudet, ref. 27, with permission.)

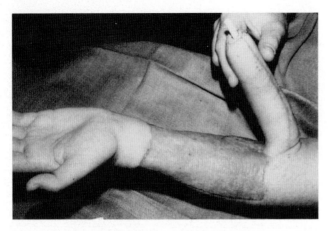

FIG. 14. Prefabricated penis on forearm of a female transexual patient. Appearance at 1 month. (From Baudet, ref. 27, with permission.)

Another complex reconstruction involved prefabrication of the penis on the forearm. The unit was transferred 1 month later after excellent healing of the neourethra and good tolerance of the prosthesis had been demonstrated (Figs. 14 and 15).

CLINICAL RESULTS

Preexpansion of flaps is associated with a significant rate of complications (hematoma, seroma, infection, superficial or full-thickness skin necrosis). Partial thrombosis of the main vascular axis and its branches can occur in induced neovascularization. When using delay techniques or induced neovascularized expansion, it is advisable to use silicone sheets or interpositional skin grafting to prevent neoconnections of the flap to the donor site or adhesions of the vascular carrier to the recipient bed and subsequent tedious and hazardous dissection at the time of flap transfer.

It is imperative to emphasize that all prefabrication procedures, whether used singly or in combination, must be planned meticulously. The surgeon must have not only a wide

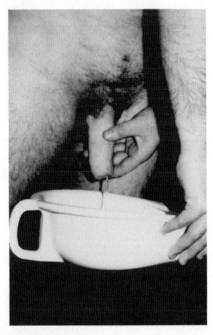

FIG. 15. Postoperative view; satisfactory cosmetic result and adequate micturition. (From Baudet, ref. 27, with permission.)

anatomic knowledge of tissue behavior and vascularity but also must exhibit technical expertise.

SUMMARY

Indications for prefabrication of any sort must be evaluated carefully. Such procedures should be undertaken only when these techniques are the most suitable, or possibly the only, solution. Nevertheless, when carefully planned and executed, customized or prefabricated flaps currently may be the most ambitious and exciting advance in reconstructive plastic surgery.

References

1. Callegari PR, Taylor GI, Caddy C, Minabe T. An anatomic review of the delay phenomenon. I. Experimental studies. *Plast Reconstr Surg* 1992; 89:397.
2. Taylor GI, Corlett R, Caddy C, Zelt RG. An anatomic review of the delay phenomenon. II. Clinical applications. *Plast Reconstr Surg* 1992;89:408.
3. Shenaq JM. Pretransfer expansion of a sensate lateral arm free flap. *Ann Plast Surg* 1987;19:558.
4. Leighton WD, Russel RC, Fellar AM, et al. Experimental pretransfer expansion of a free flap donor site. II. Physiology, histology, and clinical correlation. *Plast Reconstr Surg* 1988;82:76.
5. Masser MR. The preexpanded radial free flap. *Plast Reconstr Surg* 1990; 86:295.
6. Vergote T, Revol M, Servant JM, Banzet P. Lambeaux musculocutanés de grand dorsal expanses micro anastomosés. *Ann Chir Plast Esthet* 1993;38:323.
7. Dickerson RC, Duthies RB. The division of arterial blood flow to bone. *J Bone Joint Surg Am.* 1963;45A:356.
8. Woodhouse CF. The transplantation of patent arteries to bone. *J Int Coll Surg* 1963;39:437.
9. Hirase Y, Valauri FA, Buncke HJ. Neovascularized bone, muscle and myo osseous free flap: an experimental model. *Plast Reconstr Surg* 1988;4:209.
10. Duarte A, Valauri FA, Buncke HE Creating a free muscle flap by neovascularization: an experimental investigation. *J Reconstr Microsurg* 1987;4:15.
11. Hirase Y, Valauri FA, Buncke HJ. Neovascularized free cutaneous cartilage flap transfer with microsurgical anastomosis: an experimental study in the rabbit. *Ann Plast Surg* 1988;21:342.
12. Hirase Y, Valauri FA, Buncke HJ. Neovascularized free fat flaps: an experimental model. *J Reconstr Microsurg* 1988;4:197.
13. Orticochea M. A new method for total reconstruction of the nose: The ears as donor area. *Br J Plast Surg* 1971;24:225.
14. Erol OO. The transformation of a free skin graft into a vascularized pedicled graft. *Plast Reconstr Surg* 1976;58:470.
15. Erol OO, Spira M. Development and utilization of a composite island flap employing omentum: experimental investigation. *Plast Reconstr Surg* 1980; 65:405.
16. Shen TY. Vascular implantation into skin flap: experimental study and clinical application. A preliminary report. *Plast Reconstr Surg* 1981;68:404.
17. Shen TY. Microvascular transplantation of a prefabricated thigh flap. *Plast Reconstr Surg* 1982;69:568.
18. Khouri RK, Upton J, Shaw WW. Principles of flap prefabrication. *Clin Plast Surg* 1992;4:763.
19. Khouri RK, Upton J, Shaw WW. Prefabrication of composite free flaps through staged microvascular transfer: an experimental and clinical study. *Plast Reconstr Surg* 1991;87:108.
20. Falco NA, Pribaz JJ, Eriksson E. Vascularization of skin following implantation of an arteriovenous pedicle: implications in flap prefabrication. *Microsurgery* 1992;13:249.
21. Pribaz JJ, Maitz PKM, Fine NA. Flap prefabrication using the "vascular crane" principle: an experimental study and clinical application. *Br J Plast Surg* 1994;47:250.
22. Maitz PKM, Pribaz JJ, Hergrueter CA. Manipulating the prefabricated flap: an experimental study examining flap viability. *Microsurgery* 1994; 15:624.
23. Maitz PKM, Pribaz JJ, Duffy FJ, Hergrueter CA. The value of the delay phenomenon in flap prefabrication: an experimental study in rabbits. *Br J Plast Surg* 1994;47:149.
24. Khouri RF. Panel discussion on the "prefabricated flap." Presented at the 11th Congress of the International Confederation of Plastic, Reconstructive and Aesthetic Surgery. Yokohama, Japan, April 16–21, 1995.
25. Baudet J, River D, Martin D, Boileau R. Prefabricated free flap transfer. In: Swartz WM, Banis J., eds. *Head and neck microsurgery.* Baltimore: Williams & Wilkins, 1992.
26. Brent B, Byrd HS. Secondary ear reconstruction with cartilage graft covered by axial random and free flaps of temporoparietal fascia. *Plast Reconstr Surg* 1983;72:141.
27. Baudet J. Prefabrication of facial flaps. In: Rose E., ed. *Aesthetic facial restoration.* Philadelphia: Lippincott-Raven, 1998.

CHAPTER 145 ■ PREFABRICATED INDUCED EXPANDED (PIE) SUPRACLAVICULAR FLAP

R. K. KHOURI AND P. PELISSIER

Prefabrication of flaps opens interesting, new possibilities (1–5). The prefabricated induced expanded (PIE) supraclavicular flap involves the staged transfer of expanded supraclavicular skin, with a fascial flap used as a carrier (7,8). The PIE supraclavicular flap is ideally suited for nasal reconstruction, when a forehead flap option is not available or when a forehead scar is not desirable.

INDICATIONS

Facial defects are best reconstructed with facial tissue. When this option is not available, the next best tissue match is supraclavicular skin, which has no practical vascular pedicle that would allow its transfer as a thin flap. The PIE flap is an ideal alternative for reconstruction of facial units using tissue that best matches facial tissue. Total cheek, forehead, nasal, and even hemifacial reconstructions are possible with a single PIE flap. With judicious design, the flap can be made large enough to reconstruct major facial defects that extend to the contralateral side well beyond the midline.

ANATOMY

When available, the temporoparietal fascia is the preferred carrier. (For details of flap dissection, see Chapters 58 and 95 on temporoparietal fascia flaps.) If the temporoparietal fascia is not available, the next best alternative is the radial forearm fascial free flap. (See Chapters 198 and 200 for details of flap anatomy.) Any other fascial flap with a long vascular pedicle is suitable as a carrier.

Although expanded tissue can be transferred only to adjacent sites with traditional skin expansion, the presence of a long vascular pedicle in the carrier placed over the expander makes it possible to transfer the expanded tissue as an island flap to distant sites. Furthermore, the angiogenic effect of the expander capsule improves the neovascularization between the fascia carrier and the expanded skin.

A temporoparietal fascia flap is transferred to a subcutaneous pocket in the ipsilateral supraclavicular fossa, and a skin expander is simultaneously placed under both the fascia flap and the elevated supraclavicular skin, thereby precluding the need for microsurgical expertise and eliminating the potential complications associated with microvascular anastomoses. The PIE flap is a two-staged transfer.

FLAP DESIGN AND DIMENSIONS

The fascia flap can be either a distant microvascular free flap or a pedicled temporoparietal fascial flap. The fascia is tacked under the supraclavicular skin, and a skin expander is placed under both fascia and skin. After adequate expansion, the fascia is incorporated within the capsule of the expander, and the composite capsulofasciocutaneous flap can be transferred based on the vascular pedicle of the fascia flap.

OPERATIVE TECHNIQUE

In the first stage, an extended superficial temporoparietal fascia flap is dissected (Fig. 1). To reach the supraclavicular fossa, flap dissection must extend cephalically nearly up to the vertex. The vascular pedicle will need to be dissected inside the

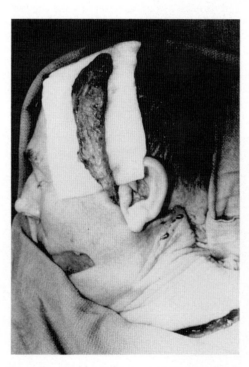

FIG. 1. Temporoparietal fascia flap is raised. The superficial temporal vessels are dissected inside the parotid gland down to the main trunk of the facial nerve.

417

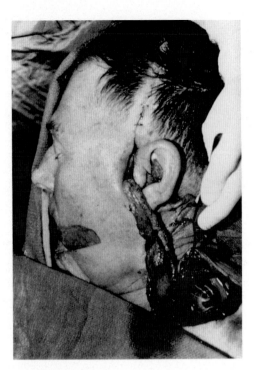

FIG. 2. A thin subcutaneous pocket is made in the supraclavicular area using a preauricular incision extended to the mastoid hairline. To dissect the pocket fully and help with insertion of the fascia and the expander, a counterincision is made at the level of the acromion. The temporoparietal fascia flap has been turned down, and the expanders are visible inside the supraclavicular pocket.

parotid gland down to the level of the main trunk of the facial nerve. A thin subcutaneous pocket is dissected in the supraclavicular area. Superficial undermining of the skin is achieved through a rhytidectomy-type incision extended to the mastoid hairline and through a counterincision on the superior aspect of the shoulder (Fig. 2). The fascia flap then is transferred inside the supraclavicular pocket and temporarily tacked to the skin with retention sutures. An expander is placed under both the fascia flap and the supraclavicular skin. It is important to sandwich the vascular pedicle between Silastic sheets along its entire length to facilitate its dissection in the second stage.

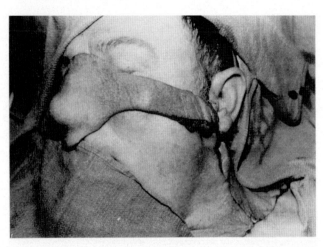

FIG. 4. At the second stage, the prefabricated induced expanded (PIE) flap has been dissected and transferred to the nose. The expanders are removed, and the donor site is closed primarily. Displacement of the anterior Silastic sheet made it impossible to separate the vascular pedicle safely from the overlying cervical skin; the latter had to be included in the pedicle and resected at a later stage.

The expander is gradually inflated starting 10 days later. During the course of the inflation, it is possible to trace the course of the temporal artery under the supraclavicular skin with Doppler examination. It is preferable to expand slowly and to gather enough well-expanded skin; this interim period typically may last 2 to 3 months (Fig. 3).

In a second operative stage, after adequate expansion is achieved, the PIE supraclavicular flap is raised as an island flap pedicled on the fascia vessels. The vascular pedicle that was sandwiched between Silastic sheets is readily available and allows flap transfer to the facial defect. With adequate planning, the donor site can be closed primarily (Fig. 4). If required, the pedicle component can be resected at a later date (Fig. 5).

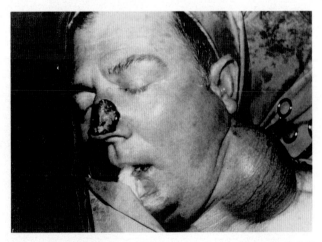

FIG. 3. Before the second stage, the supraclavicular skin is well expanded and the temporal artery can be subjected to Doppler evaluation over the expander.

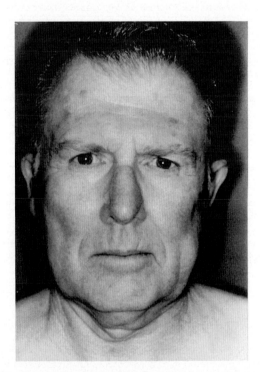

FIG. 5. Frontal view 6 months after the nasal reconstruction.

CLINICAL RESULTS

Despite a limited degree of overlap between the fascia carrier and the skin paddle, the potent angiogenic effect of the expander is such that we have not observed any marginal skin flap necrosis. In our experience, as little as a one to four ratio of overlap between the fascia carrier and the expander allows adequate perfusion of the skin overlying the entire expander capsule.

Complications may relate to temporoparietal fascia flap elevation or to extrusion of the expander. Displacement of the Silastic sheets may render the secondary dissection of the pedicle very tedious.

In ten cases, we had only one venous thrombosis in a microvascular free flap; that flap was salvaged by timely reexploration. We also experienced two expander exposures, necessitating premature transfer of the PIE flap. In both these cases, the reconstruction was salvaged at the expense of a larger donor-site defect.

SUMMARY

The PIE flap allows safe pedicle transfer of an expanded thin supraclavicular skin flap to any facial unit. It uses the principle of carrier-mediated staged transfer, in which the carrier is a fascia flap. If that fascia flap is a pedicled temporoparietal flap, no microsurgical anastomoses are needed.

References

1. Khouri RK, Upton J, Shaw WW. Principles of flap prefabrication. *Clin Plast Surg* 1992;19:763.
2. Khouri RK, Upton J, Shaw WW. Prefabrication of composite free flaps through staged microvascular transfer: an experimental and clinical study. *Plast Reconstr Surg* 1991;87:108.
3. Yao ST. Vascular implantation into skin flap: experimental study and clinical application. A preliminary report. *Plast Reconstr Surg* 1981;68:404.
4. Bricout N, Arrouvel C, Banset P. Résultats préliminaires d'une étude éxperimentale sur les lambeaux "à pédicule vasculaire axial induit." *Ann Chir Plast Esthet* 1984;29:376.
5. Hirase Y, Valauri FA, Buncke HJ, Newlin LY. Customized prefabricated neovascularized free flaps. *Microsurgery* 1987;8:218.
6. Khouri RK, Ozbek MR, Hruza GJ, Young VL. Facial reconstruction with prefabricated induced expanded (PIE) supraclavicular skin flaps. *Plast Reconstr Surg* 1995;95:1007.
7. Olenius M, Dalsgaard CJ, Wilkman M. Mitotic activity in expanded human skin. *Plast Reconstr Surg* 1988;81:30.
8. Bengtson BP, Ringler SL, George ER, et al. Capsular tissue: a new local flap. *Plast Reconstr Surg* 1993;91:1073.

CHAPTER 146 ■ PARTIAL FACE TRANSPLANT

B. DEVAUCHELLE

Extended soft-tissue defects of the face are very difficult to reconstruct, especially when multiple anatomic units like the nose, lips, and chin are missing simultaneously. Under such circumstances, several conventional autologous tissue transfers are necessary to restore the form and, if possible, the function, of each of the missing parts of the damaged face. The idea was raised that in such cases, a one-stage reconstruction of the central and lower face could be achieved by microsurgical transfer of a full-thickness composite tissue allograft harvested on the cephalic extremity of a brain-dead donor with similar morphologic characteristics.

INDICATIONS

Previous procedures, which often required several secondary corrections, usually led to poor cosmetic and functional outcomes. The original face of the reconstructed patient had an unattractive appearance with many scars and several mismatching skin paddles, all of them remaining mostly immobile and devoid of any future expressive mobility.

The partial face transplant is a full-thickness composite soft-tissue allograft, including all anatomic components of the nose-lips-chin triangle, harvested down to their skeletal bone support (Fig. 1). The transplant is sensate and aims at restoring all complex motor functions devoted to orality—competent feeding, intelligible speech, and restoration of the aesthetic appearance of the central and lower face, with no donor-site morbidity. Furthermore, it allows a one-stage high-quality restoration of an acceptable aesthetic appearance of the central and lower face. Although the ultimate goal of the procedure is certainly not to reach an exact restitution of the recipient's previous facial identity, the new face, which is finally created with the contribution of the graft, restores a real morphologic individuality to the facial image. A lifelong immunosuppressive treatment remains, at present, a drawback, but is a mandatory medical requirement to obtain the durable benefit of all the surgical advantages.

ANATOMY

The graft is supplied by the right and left facial arteries and veins that, during their ascending course to the medial canthi, give rise to a large number of medial and lateral collateral vessels running into the subcutaneous and submuscular planes. Lateral branches (long and short facial collaterals) are directed to the cheeks, and medial branches distribute to the submental area (submental vessels), to the lips (upper and lower labial vessels), and to the nose. All of these collaterals are richly connected with each other and with branches from adjacent angiosomes. Major right-left anastomoses crossing the midline exist between the labial, submental, and nasolobar arteries and veins. Thanks to these numerous functional connecting vascular channels, the graft may be revascularized on a single vascular pedicle.

Sensitive nerves to the graft arise from the infraorbital (V2) and mental (V3) nerves on both sides. These nerves leave the corresponding bone foramina on the maxilla and the mandible, and then enter the soft tissues of the mid and lower face; they then quickly divide into small rami distributed to the skin. Due to this early spread in the small terminal rami, the main stem of the maxillary (V2) and inferior alveolar (V3) nerves need to be exposed by an endo-osseous dissection, in order to obtain, after deep subperiosteal elevation of the graft, large proximal nerve stumps suitable for reliable microsurgical anastomoses.

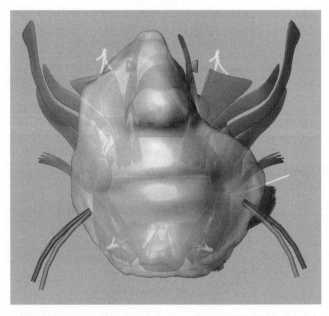

FIG. 1. Schematic anatomic drawing of the nose-lips-chin allograft. Preoperative virtual three-dimensional model of the first partial human face allograft.

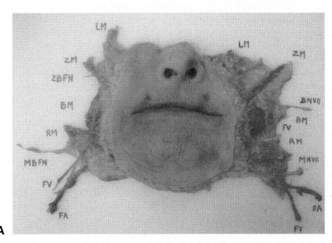
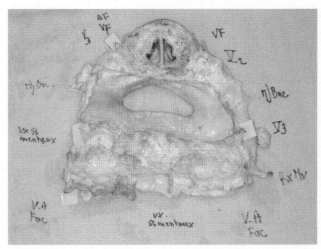

FIG. 2. Anatomic specimen of a partial face transplant. The dissected allograft, shown from its outer (**A**) and inner (**B**) aspects, is elevated on both facial vascular pedicles containing all the muscles of orofacial expression with their intact motor-nerve supply, V2 and V3 sensitive nerves, the whole nasal pyramid, and a large patch of anterior oral mucosa.

Motor nerves to the graft originate from the terminal zygomatic, buccal, and mandibular branches of the facial nerves, which arise from the parotid area, run laterally above the masseteric fascia, then reach [deep to the superficial muscular aponeurotic system (SMAS) layer] the levator and depressor muscles of the lips. Depending on the extent of the graft, they need to be dissected separately at their exit from the parotid gland or, otherwise, inside the gland or more proximally on the cervico- and temporofacial trunks of the facial nerves.

FLAP DESIGN AND DIMENSIONS

The partial central and lower face allograft is a full-thickness composite tissue transfer, which includes the exact amount of skin necessary to close the recipient's cutaneous defect, the underlying subcutaneous fat, the four sensitive nerves to these integuments, all perioral muscles with their intact segmental motor nerve supply, the missing cartilage of the nose, the inner lining of both nasal vestibules, and a large patch of anterior and lateral oral mucosa (Fig. 2). If necessary, the graft may be enlarged laterally by including the cheeks, with the corresponding buccinator muscles, buccal nerves, and the anterior portion of Bichat's fat pads.

A brain-dead donor is selected according to strong morphologic and immunologic criteria. Ideally, the anatomic requirements include a similar range of age (within the same decade), the same color and texture of skin, and a comparable overall body habitus. The donor and the recipient should also share the same blood group and have several (as many as possible) positive human leukocyte antigen (HLA) cross-match tests.

OPERATIVE TECHNIQUE

Graft Harvesting

The face transplant is elevated on both right and left facial vessels exposed on the basilar border of the mandible. The contour of the skin flap is designed very precisely, following a sterile, rigid pattern, previously fabricated on the recipient, in order to match exactly the dimensions and shape of the defect to be repaired. After the circumferential skin incision, a deep subcutaneous dissection is made laterally on both sides of the graft, in order to expose the proximal heads of the levator and zygo-

matic muscles superiorly, and the risorius and platysma muscle sheets inferiorly. Below the lower border of the mandible, the latter is incised in order to expose the facial artery, the facial vein, and the mandibular branch of the facial nerve, which usually crosses the pedicle at that point. Buccal and zygomatic branches are then identified on the outer surface of the masseteric fascia and of Bichat's fat pad. Stensen's parotid duct is ligated and not included in the composite tissue transfer.

Along the infraorbital segment of the skin incision, the orbicularis oculi muscle is divided between its preseptal and preorbital parts. The lower orbital septum is then transected in order to expose and to cut the maxillary nerve in the proximal portion of the infraorbital groove. Thereafter, the upper part of the graft is elevated from the maxilla through a subperiosteal plane dissection, allowing inclusion inside the medial part of the transfer of the intact periosteal attachments of all levator muscles to the upper lip, which are inserted on the anterior surface of the bone. When the proximal heads of the zygomatic and levator anguli oris muscles are cut more laterally, they are tagged individually on small silicone markers, in order to identify them and to prevent their retraction inside the graft fatty tissue. On the dorsum of the nose, the integuments are elevated from the nasal bones under the deep surface of the nasalis muscle. Then, the lateral nasal cartilages are incised along their bone attachments, and the whole nasal pyramid is separated from the bony piriform aperture with a simple, sharp blade, descending the frontal section of the nasal septum and of the mucosae of both nasal cavities.

Along the inferior skin incision line, the depressor muscles to the lower lip are freed from their mandibular insertions. Then, the mental foramina are exposed through a subperiosteal approach, and a small cortical bone window is drilled on the lateral side of each of them, in order to expose and transect the main stem of the inferior alveolar nerve inside the distal part of the mandibular canal. The transplant elevation finally ends with a sharp breakdown of the oral mucosa, occurring centrally along the upper and lower vestibular sulci close to the gingiva and laterally on the cheek inner lining in front of the opening of the parotid duct. At the end of the harvesting procedure, the graft remains pedicled on both right and left facial blood vessels, which are dissected from the submandibular gland and traced proximally down to the large neck vessels, in order to obtain the longest and most extensive donor blood vessels for revascularizing the transplant. If a lower suprahyoid skin extension is included in the graft design, care is taken

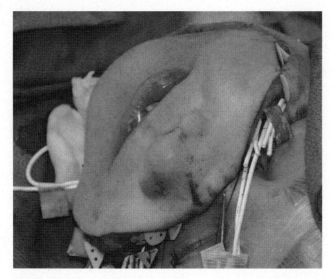

FIG. 3. Early revascularization of the first partial face transplant. Facial artery anastomosis on the right side of the graft, 30 seconds after clamp release. Note the uniform recovery of normal skin perfusion on the nearly whole allograft surface.

during this dissection not to damage the thin submental blood vessels that are responsible for the supply of that area.

After harvest, the facial graft is irrigated with 500 mL of ILG-1 organ preservation solution at 4°C, and then placed in double plastic bags and in a standard icebox. After multiorgan procurement, the donor's nose-lips-chin triangle is cautiously reconstructed, using a custom-made, carved, and colored silicone mask inside a plaster cast molded on the face before any incision and at the very beginning of the procedure.

Recipient Allograft

The recipient's face is prepared to receive the graft after a tracheotomy is performed. An extended facial dissection is then performed in order to obtain regular, healthy skin edges around the soft-tissue defect, to remove deep scar tissue, and to isolate each anatomic structure to be joined to those dissected and individually tagged on the graft. Superficial muscle dissection attempts to individualize all remaining stumps of the elevator and depressor muscle bellies and the segmental motor branches of the facial nerves. Deeply, terminal sensitive branches of the maxillary and mandibular nerves are exposed at the origin of their supraperiosteal course and prepared for further microsurgical anastomoses at the point at which they leave the infraorbital or mental foramina. Blood vessels selected to revascularize the transplant are usually the right and left facial vessels carefully exposed in the submandibular area or in the neck.

After a complementary microsurgical preparation performed on a bed of iced sponges, the graft is transferred to the recipient's face and secured along one edge of the skin defect by several temporary stitches. Revascularization is then carried out by anastomosing donor and recipient facial vessels on one side of the transplant (Fig. 3). When the clamps are released, the whole composite allograft rapidly recovers a normal color and volume. Due to the right-left vascular anastomoses running mostly in the labial networks, active bleeding is also quickly observed on the free end of the contralateral vessels. Further repair includes, sequentially, the circumferential closure of the oral vestibule; the clockwise suture of mental and infraorbital sensitive nerves that start from the responsible facial pedicle; and, finally, the anastomoses of the contralateral facial artery and vein.

Facial mimic muscles are sutured in layers, with an attempt to join them individually whenever possible. If not possible, an approximation is made by joining together the buccinator mass deeply and vectorial groups of levator muscles superficially. On the lower edge of the transplant, the depressor muscles of the lower lip are reinserted on the periosteum of the mandibular border. To reanimate the face, several motor-nerve coaptions are conducted in a termino-terminal or termino-lateral fashion, depending on the location of injuries on the available facial nerve branches. Final inset of the transplant then includes the ascending repair of both nasal vestibules, the upper periosteal suspension of the deep graft layer on the recipient facial skeleton, the lower closure of the nasal SMAS layer, and, finally, subcutaneous and skin suture. Silkworm guts are used to drain the subcutaneous space by capillarity, and the wounds are lightly dressed with short sterile skin closure strips (Steri-Strips) only. Silicone drains are inserted in both nasal fossae to maintain their permeability and to ensure hemostasis. The whole graft is left uncovered for postoperative monitoring.

CLINICAL RESULTS

The first partial face transplantation was carried out in Amiens, France, on November 27, 2005, to reconstruct the central and lower face of a 38-year-old woman who had suffered, 6 months previously, a severe dog bite that amputated her distal nose, both lips, chin, and adjacent parts of the cheeks (Fig. 4). The donor's face was harvested and transplanted according to the previously described technique, and a standard immunosuppressive treatment was instituted to prevent graft rejection. The initial postoperative course was uneventful. No surgical complication occurred, wound healing was rapid, and immunosuppression well tolerated. Nevertheless, the patient developed, at week 3 (W3) and month 7 (M7), two moderate rejection episodes that were easily controlled by increasing corticosteroid doses. Immediate anatomic integration and psychologic acceptance of the face transplant were excellent.

From this inaugural experience, it was determined that, functionally, the patient was able to eat and drink almost normally at the end of the first postoperative week. Rehabilitation training was started at day 1, repeated twice a day, and tried to create, very early, an intimate functional sensory relationship between the sensate autologous tongue and the "dead" deep surface of the lips on the graft. Facial static and dynamic exercises were mainly focused on the restoration of lip suspension and mouth occlusion.

Sensation of the graft recovered quite rapidly and was probably favored by the positive neurotrophic effects of the immunosuppressive drugs. Assessed by the progression of the Tinel sign and by repeated heat-cold and Semmes-Weinstein testing, sensitive recovery began around the infraorbital and mental areas at the end of M1 and occurred more quickly for epicritic than for discriminative sensitivity. Later, the reinnervated area reached the lateral part of the lips at M2 and thereafter involved the whole surface of the transplant at M4. The oral mucosa of the graft also became sensate over the same interval of time, since at the end of M2, routine mucosal biopsies performed for immunologic monitoring needed to be done under local anesthesia.

Motor recovery was slower but became progressively more effective. Dynamic motions were first observed on the upper lip and arose from transmission of contractions generated in the healthy proximal stumps of the repaired levator and zygomatic muscles (M3). Thereafter, real autonomous contractions of the transplanted muscle bellies, causing natural skin wrinkling, became obvious from M4 on. Of course, these phenomena occurred as results of a complex random biological process, which probably involved both intramuscular neurotization taking place in the areas of muscle repair and intraneural axonal regeneration spreading through the motor-nerve coaptation

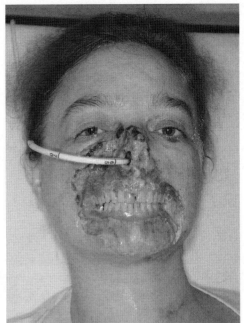
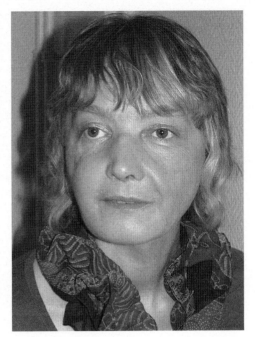

A,B

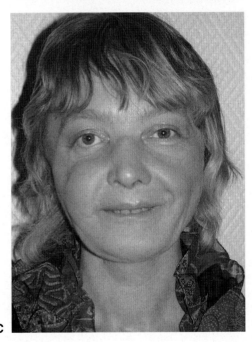

C

FIG. 4. Anatomic and functional results of the first partial facial composite tissue allograft. After a dog-bite trauma, the patient completely lacked the distal nose, both lips, and chin (**A**). One year after transplantation, she has recovered her static rest face image (**B**) and also a dynamic, perfectly symmetric smile (**C**).

sites. A paralytic sagging of the lower lip remained present until W20, and hypertonic and hypotonic areas may have also coexisted temporarily inside the face graft. Nevertheless, complete active, then passive, lip occlusions were achieved at M6 and M8, respectively, and a perfect symmetric smile was restored at M10. Over the same period, other relevant facial expressive motions involving the antagonistic depressor muscles, as in fear, pain, and hesitation, also recovered progressively.

The partial face transplant is fully sensate and contains, in exact anatomic position, all the functional muscle vectors responsible for delicate lip movements involved in feeding, speech, and facial expression. After revascularization, the allograft immediately recovers its form, volume, and contour, therefore allowing a one-stage reconstruction of several neighboring anatomic units within a severely damaged face, with highly natural curves, nearly inconspicuous transitions between autologous and heterologous tissue, and no additional scars to the surrounding skin. There is no donor-site morbidity in the

recipient body and, thanks to the rapid sensitive nerve recovery, the neurologic reintegration of the transplant into the brain cortex seems to favor a relatively rapid psychologic acceptance of the new face inside the body scheme.

Technically, face transplant is a long and serious procedure requiring two teams of experienced microsurgeons able to carry out, simultaneously and in perfect time planning, operations on the brain-dead donor and on the recipient patient. For the recipient, facial reconstruction would obviously be delayed until a compatible and adequate donor becomes available. Additionally, after successful surgery, a lifelong immunosuppressive treatment is mandatory, to prevent allograft rejection until a hypothetic state of tolerance is achieved. Well-known side effects of the drugs commonly used for this purpose include, in addition to potential negative alterations of renal and hepatic functions, an increased risk of viral, microbial, and fungal infections; of skin cancer (×15); and of lymphoma (1%). At the present time, the lifelong results of a facial transplant cannot be predicted; in cases of early or late failures (acute or chronic rejections), the transplantectomy site would then need to be reconstructed secondarily by another graft or by conventional autologous tissue transfer.

SUMMARY

Although the ultimate goal of the procedure is certainly not to reach exact restitution of the recipient's facial identity, the new face that is recreated with the contribution of the graft restores a real morphologic individuality.

References

1. Devauchelle B, Badet L, Lengelé B, et al. First human face allograft: early report. *Lancet* 2006;15:368.
2. Monaco AP, Maki T, Hale D, et al. The enigma of tolerance and chimerism: variable role of T cells and chimerism in induction of tolerance with bone marrow. *Transplant Proc* 2001;33:3837.
3. Dakpe S. Image d'une transplantée faciale: à propos de l'intégration neurologique d'une allotransplantation du triangle nez-lèvres-menton. Thèse pour le doctoral en medicine No. 71, Oct. 2006. Université de Picardie, France.
4. Giraux P, Sirigu A, Schneider F, Dubernard JM. Cortical reorganization in motor cortex after hand graft of both hands. *Nat Neurosci* 2001;4:691.
5. Dubernard JM, Lengelé B, Morelon E, et al. First human face transplantation at 18 months' follow-up. *N Engl J Med* 2007;357:2451.

CHAPTER 147 ■ FACIAL TRANSPLANTATION—THE ANATOMIC BASIS

M. SIEMIONOW, G. AGAOGLU, AND S. UNAL

EDITORIAL COMMENT

The editors know of only a few partial face transplantations that have been done up to now. Nonetheless, anyone who is interested in facial transplantation will be well served by studying the descriptive anatomy of the donor and the recipient dissections as outlined in this chapter. Without clinical experience, it is likely that some of the indications outlined in the chapter may be modified with clinical experience.

Lifelong immunosuppression therapy, due to serious side effects, is the main obstacle to routine use of composite tissue allografts. When the subject is a candidate for face transplantation, there are ethical, social, and psychologic issues to be considered. In addition, the technical aspects of face transplantation have to be outlined. To mimic the clinical scenario of a facial transplantation procedure, we have performed a mock facial transplantation by harvesting a total facial-scalp flap from donor cadavers and transferring the flap to recipient cadavers.

INDICATIONS

Since the first successful hand allograft transplantation in France in 1998 (1), composite tissue allograft transplantation has opened a new era in the field of reconstructive surgery. However, the final cosmetic and functional outcomes of currently available reconstructive procedures for severe soft-tissue defects of the face are not optimal. Face transplantation is a promising alternative to the conventional reconstructive procedures. Successful partial face transplantation cases have been reported in France and in China (2–4). We have designed a cadaveric facial allograft transplantation model (5,6) to support application of facial allografts, as a new treatment option for reconstruction of facial defects in patients with severe facial deformities due to burn, trauma, and cancer ablation.

ANATOMY

In donor cadavers, a full facial-scalp flap was elevated to include the entire facial skin and the scalp. The flap also incorporated the superficial muscular aponeurotic system (SMAS) of the face; the parotid gland; the inferior and superior tarsal plates; and the great auricular, facial, supraorbital, infraorbital, and mental nerves. This composite facial-scalp flap is based bilaterally on the external carotid arteries, including superficial temporal and facial arteries, and on the external jugular and facial veins.

FLAP DESIGN AND DIMENSIONS

The flap was designed to include the entire facial skin and the scalp, including both ears, based on the external carotid arteries and external jugular and facial veins. The mean horizontal-vertical dimensions for the total facial-scalp flaps were 57 × 30 cm, and the mean surface area was 1,192 cm². The mean horizontal and vertical dimensions for facial flaps without scalp were 33 × 28 cm, and the mean surface area was 675 cm².

OPERATIVE TECHNIQUE

Mock Facial Transplantation: Technique of Donor Facial-Scalp Flap Harvesting

A midline vertical incision from mentum to suprasternal notch was performed to the depth of the platysmal layer (Fig. 1A). From the lower end of the vertical incision, horizontal incisions were extended bilaterally, to be met posteriorly in the neck midline at the scalp hairline. With the cadaver in the left lateral position, the incision was extended vertically in the midline to the vertex of the scalp.

In the subplatysmal plane, the flaps were elevated from medial to lateral and caudal to cranial, exposing the strap muscles at the midline and the sternocleidomastoid muscle (SCM) more laterally. The caudal portions of the external jugular veins (EJVs) were found bilaterally underneath the platysmal layer, ligated, transected, and incorporated into the skin-platysmal flap. The great auricular nerves were both identified on the lateral edges of the SCM and incorporated into the flap.

The scalp-flap dissection was performed in the subgaleal plane, with the cadaver turned to the left lateral and right lateral positions. The supraorbital rims were reached, and the supraorbital nerves were traced down to their exit from the supraorbital foramen and transected. Then, the external ear canals were reached and transected to incorporate the ears within the flap.

In the neck, the SCM was cut close to its clavicular and sternal insertions, and the carotid sheath underneath was exposed. The omohyoid muscle was cut at its tendinous junction, to better expose the caudal portion of the carotid sheath. The carotid sheath was incised and the carotid artery, along with the internal jugular vein, was dissected cranially to reach the carotid bifurcation. After the bifurcation of the common carotid to internal and external carotid arteries, the external carotid artery was transected, to become the arterial pedicle of the flap.

At this point, the attachments of the stylohyoid and digastric muscles on the hyoid bone were cut, to get a better exposure of the underlying structures. The ascending pharyngeal, the superior thyroid, and the lingual arteries were ligated close to their branching from the external carotid, and the dissection was further carried cranially. The hypoglossal nerve was also exposed and transected. The facial artery, branching from the anteromedial side of the external carotid artery, was carefully dissected in a cranial direction as it entered the submandibular gland. The artery was traced and separated from the gland with a tedious dissection, and the gland was not incorporated in the platysmal skin flap (Fig. 1B).

Then, the second venous pedicle of the flap, the facial vein, was also isolated from the surrounding soft tissue and the submandibular gland. After dissection of the vein toward its entrance to the internal jugular vein, it was ligated and transected, leaving sufficient pedicle to become the second venous pedicle of the flap. After the mandibular border was reached at the midline, the dissection was continued cranially underneath the SMAS, to reach the lips. The vermilion of the lips was incorporated within the flap, as the sub-SMAS dissection was deepened to incise the gingivobuccal mucosa. Through intraoral incision, the mental nerves were exposed, traced, and incorporated within the flap.

After keeping the facial artery intact, the external carotid artery was further traced cranially behind the ramus of the mandible as it continued deep to the parotid gland. The gland was incorporated within the flap. Before becoming the superficial temporal artery, the external carotid gives off the occipital, the maxillary, the transverse facial, and the middle temporal branches, each of which was ligated and transected sequentially.

In the cheek flap dissections continued in a sub-SMAS plane, a fashion similar to a face-lift dissection was used. Intraoral incision was circumferentially carried onto the upper gingivobuccal sulcus, and the soft tissues were sharply incised. Through the upper gingivobuccal incision, in the subperiosteal plane, the infraorbital nerve was explored, traced, and included in the flap.

On both sides, the upper and lower palpebral fornix conjunctival incisions were performed in a circumferential manner just at the tarsal margins and joined with the sub-SMAS flap dissection plane, in order to incorporate the upper and lower lids within the flap. At the midline, the nasal soft tissue was elevated, leaving the osseocartilaginous framework behind, and the elevation of the total facial-scalp flap was completed (Fig. 1C and D).

Technique of Recipient Facial Skin Harvesting as a "Monoblock" Full-Thickness Skin Graft

Incisions were made in a fashion similar to that described previously. The entire skin of the neck, face, and scalp was incised and elevated as a "monoblock" full-thickness skin graft in a plane above the platysma, SMAS, and galea, respectively (Fig. 2A and B). The great auricular nerve was identified at the posterior border of the SCM muscle, dissected from the surrounding tissue, and the maximal access to the nerve was preserved. Through the upper and lower gingivobuccal incisions, the vermilion of the upper and lower lips was excised with the entire facial skin. At the infraorbital and mental regions, both the infraorbital and mental nerves were explored and dissected from their surrounding tissue, respectively, until an adequate length of the nerves was achieved for future coaptation. The upper and lower circumferential conjunctival incisions were performed at the tarsal margins and were joined with the facial skin dissection plane, incorporating the upper and lower lids. At the supraorbital rims, the supraorbital nerves were explored and traced down to the supraorbital foramen, until adequate length was obtained.

Next, the arterial and venous pedicles were dissected and prepared for the future anastomoses. External jugular veins were bilaterally explored under the platysma and were prepared to serve as one of the recipient venous pedicles. SCM muscle was retracted laterally, and the carotid sheath was reached and incised. The external carotid artery was dissected, separated from the internal carotid artery, and prepared as the recipient's arterial pedicle. The facial vein was identified at its entrance into the internal jugular vein and dissected to obtain adequate length to serve as the second venous pedicle in the recipient.

Technique of Donor Facial-Scalp Flap Transplantation into Recipient Facial-Scalp

The inset of the donor flap began with markings of the regions at which the donor facial-scalp flap would be anchored against gravity. These anchoring sites included the mandibular and zygomatic ligament regions, preauricular area, mastoid fascia, temporalis fascia, and frontal bone. The harvested facial-scalp flap was transferred from the donor to the recipient site, and the sequence of flap inset was as follows. First, the supraorbital, infraorbital, and mental nerves of the facial flap were approximated to their respective nerves in the recipient. Next, the flap was sutured to the marked regions at the level of the mandibular and zygomatic ligaments bilaterally (Fig. 3A). This was followed by anchoring the flap into the preauricular regions, to the mastoid fascia behind the ears, and to the temporalis fascia at the temporal region (Fig. 3B). At the frontal region, the flap was fixed to the frontal bone

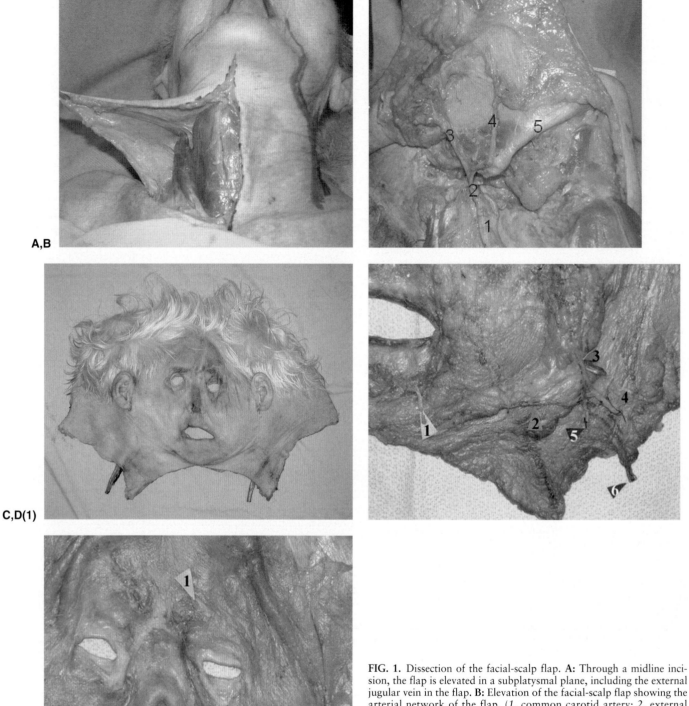

A,B

C,D(1)

D(2)

FIG. 1. Dissection of the facial-scalp flap. **A:** Through a midline incision, the flap is elevated in a subplatysmal plane, including the external jugular vein in the flap. **B:** Elevation of the facial-scalp flap showing the arterial network of the flap. (*1*, common carotid artery; *2*, external carotid artery: *3*, superficial temporal artery: *4*, facial artery: *5*, lower border of mandible.) **C:** Harvested total facial-scalp flap. **D1:** Inverted surface of the harvested total facial-scalp flap showing sensory nerves, and arterial and venous pedicles. (*1*, mental nerve; *2*, facial artery; *3*, superficial temporal artery; *4*, external carotid artery; *5*, facial vein; *6*, external jugular vein. **D2:** (*left*). *1*, supraorbital nerve; *2*, infraorbital nerve (*right*).

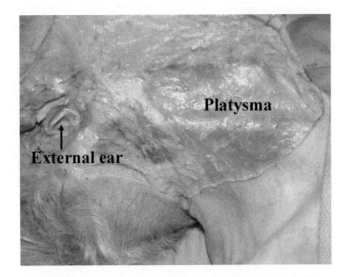
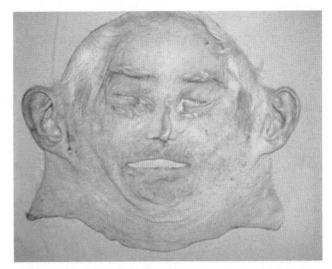
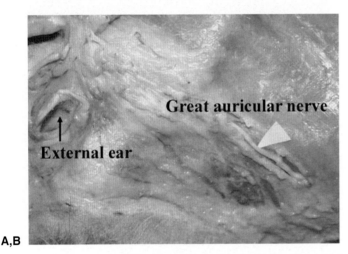
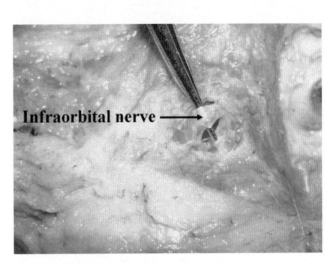

A,B

FIG. 2. **A:** Elevation of the facial skin of the recipient cadaver above the superficial muscular aponeurotic system (SMAS)–platysmal plane as "monoblock" skin graft. In the neck, the skin is elevated above the platysmal plane (**B**, *above*). The total facial-scalp skin in the recipient cadaver harvested as a "monoblock" full-thickness skin graft (*right, above*).

with 4–0 Prolene sutures passed through the cortical bone tunnels created by the electric drill (Fig. 3C).

Next, the upper and lower gingivobuccal and conjunctival incisions were closed. The vascular pedicles, consisting of the external carotid arteries and facial veins, were approximated to their respective recipient vessels (Fig. 3D). The great auricular nerves and the external jugular veins of the facial flap were approximated to their respective nerves and vessels in the recipient for future nerve coaptation and vascular anastomoses. There was no attempt to perform vessel or nerve repair, because vessels are collapsed in cadavers and lack elasticity and turgor, and nerves easily become dried during flap harvesting. Finally, the skin incisions were closed, and the inset of the flap was completed.

EXPERIMENTAL RESULTS

Mock Facial Transplantation

In our cadaver studies, in the donor cadavers, the mean harvesting time of the total facial-scalp flap was 235.62 minutes. The mean length of the supraorbital, infraorbital, men-

tal, and great auricular nerves was 1.5, 2.46, 3.02, and 6.11 cm, respectively. The mean length of the external carotid artery, facial, and external jugular veins was 5, 3.15, and 5.78 cm, respectively. In the recipient cadavers, the mean harvesting time of facial skin as a "monoblock," full-thickness graft was 47.5 minutes (Table 1). The mean time for the preparation of the arterial and venous pedicles and sensory nerves for the future anastomoses and coaptation was 30 minutes. The mean time for the facial flap anchoring was 22.5 minutes. The total mean time of mock facial transplantation without vessels and nerve repair was 320 minutes (Table 2). The sequence of the mock facial transplantation is presented in Table 3.

So far, two partial face transplantations have been performed, the first one in France and the second one in China. The first patient was a woman, aged 38 years, who had suffered amputation of the central and lower face, including nose, upper and lower lips, chin, and adjacent parts of the cheeks (2). The transplantation procedure consisted of bilateral facial arteries and vein anastomoses, mucosal repair of the oral and nasal vestibules, bilateral coaptation of the infraorbital and mental nerves, joining of mimic muscles with motor nerve suture on the mandibular branch of the left facial nerve, and skin closure.

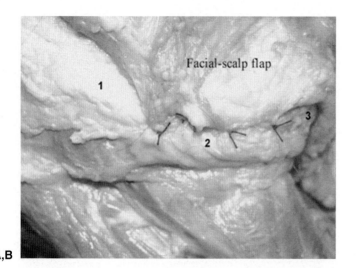

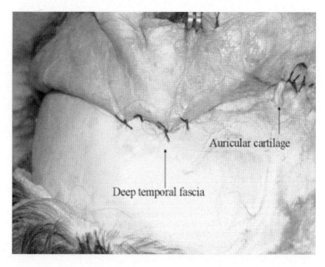

A,B

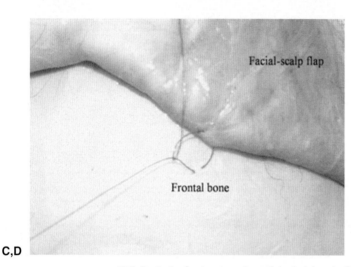

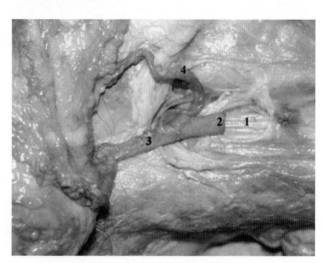

C,D

FIG. 3. **A:** Anchoring procedure of the facial-scalp flap in the recipient cadaver. Fixation to the mandibular ligament region (*left, above*). (*1*, platysma; *2*, mandibular border; *3*, mentum). **B:** Facial flap fixation to the temporalis fascia region and suturing of the auricular cartilages of the external ears. **C:** Flap anchoring to the frontal bone by the suture passing through the tunnel created in the cortical bone (*left, below*). **D:** The vascular pedicles of the donor facial flap are approximated to their respective vessels in the recipient for future vascular anastomoses. (*1*, recipient's external carotid artery; *2*, donor's external carotid artery: *3*, donor's superficial temporal artery; *4*, donor's facial artery).

TABLE 1

SUMMARY OF THE HARVESTING TIME AND VASCULAR PEDICLE AND NERVE LENGTH IN THE DONOR CADAVERS

Cadaver no.	Facial flap harvesting time in the donor (min)	Facial skin graft harvesting, time in the recipient (min)	External carotid artery pedicle length (cm)	Facial vein pedicle length (cm)	External jugular vein pedicle length (cm)	Supraorbital nerve length (cm)	Infraorbital nerve length (cm)	Mental nerve length (cm)	Great auricular nerve length (cm)
1	250	—	5.1	2.8	5.8	1.7	2.4	3.2	6.4
2	280	—	4.8	3.3	6.7	1.5	2.2	3.6	6.1
3	220	—	5.6	3.5	6	1.3	2.5	3.1	5.7
4	240	—	4.9	3.2	5.2	1.4	2.4	2.9	6.3
5	235	—	4.5	3.6	5.3	1.4	2.1	2.5	6.4
6	220	—	5.1	3.2	6.2	1.7	2.8	2.8	5.9
7	210	—	5.2	2.7	5.7	1.6	2.5	3	5.4
8	230	—	4.8	2.9	5.4	1.4	2.8	3.1	6.7
Mean	235.62 ± 21.94	47.5 ± 3.53	5.0 ± 0.32	3.15 ± 0.32	5.78 ± 0.5	1.50 ± 0.15	2.46 ± 0.25	3.02 ± 0.31	6.11 ± 0.42

TABLE 2

TOTAL MEAN TIME NEEDED FOR PREPARATION OF THE RECIPIENT'S DEFECT AND INSET OF THE DONOR FACIAL FLAP TO THE RECIPIENT CADAVERS

Surgical procedure	Cadaver no. 1	Cadaver no. 2	Mean time
Facial skin graft harvesting in the recipient (min)	50	45	47.5 ± 3.53
Preparation of the arterial and venous pedicles and nerves for anastomoses and repair (min)	30	30	30 ± 0
Inset of the donor facial flap into the recipient (min)	25	20	22.5 ± 3.53
Facial flap harvesting time from the donor cadavers (min)	210	230	220 ± 14.14
Total time for mock facial transplantation (min)	315	325	320 ± 7.07

The initial postoperative course of the first clinical case was reported to be uneventful. No surgical complications occurred. Anatomic and psychologic integration and recovery of sensation were excellent. The 4-month outcome revealed the feasibility of the procedure and was considered successful, with respect to appearance, sensibility, and acceptance by the patient. The clinicopathologic findings from the skin and oral mucosa of the patient during the first 8 months were also reported (3). The patient developed clinical rejection episodes at days 20 and 214 postgraft, which disappeared after increasing the dose of immunosuppressants. Pathologic changes suggestive of rejection were more severe in the oral mucosa than in the facial skin. Close clinicopathologic monitoring of the facial skin and oral mucosa was considered the most reliable way to detect rejection in the setting of human facial tissue allotransplantation.

TABLE 3

MOCK FACIAL TRANSPLANTATION PROCEDURE

Sequence of Procedures

1 Transfer of the donor facial flap into the recipient's facial defect
2 Coaptation of the supraorbital, infraorbital, and mental nerves
3 Anchoring of the flap at the region of the mandibular and zygomatic ligaments
4 Anchoring of the flap to the preauricular region, mastoid fascia, and temporal fascia
5 Anchoring of the flap to the frontal bones
6 Closure of the upper and lower gingivobuccal incisions
7 Closure of the upper and lower conjunctival incisions
8 Anastomoses of the external carotid arteries between the donor and recipient
9 Anastomoses of the facial veins between the donor and recipient
10 Coaptation of the great auricular nerves
11 Anastomoses of the external jugular veins between the donor and recipient
12 Closure of the skin incisions

The second partial face transplantation, according to media reports, was performed in a Chinese hunter, aged 30 years, who was disfigured after being attacked by a bear (4). In this case, the defect included nose, upper lip, and cheek. The hospital reported: "The operation is considered successful and the patient is in good condition." However, currently, there is no more information available on this patient's follow-up. The long-term results of the reported cases of partial facial transplantations will be critical, to assess the future applications of partial or total face transplantation.

SUMMARY

Total facial-scalp flaps from donor cadavers were harvested and transferred to recipient cadavers. In the donors, the time of facial-scalp flap harvesting was measured, as well as the length of the arterial and venous pedicles and sensory nerves, which were included in the facial flaps. In the recipients, the time of facial skin harvest as a "monoblock," full-thickness graft was measured, as were the anchoring regions for the inset of the donor flaps and the time sequences for the vascular pedicle anastomoses and nerve coaptations (7).

References

1. Dubernard JM, Owen E, Herzberg G, et al. Human hand allograft: report on first 6 months. *Lancet* 1999;353:1315.
2. Devauchelle B, Bodet L, Lengete B, et al. First human face allograft: early report. *Lancet* 2006;368:203.
3. Kanitakis J, Badet L, Petruzzo P, et al. Clinicopathologic monitoring of the skin and oral mucosa of the first human face allograft: report on the first eight months. *Transplantation* 2006;82:1610.
4. http://news.bbc.co.uk/2/hi/asia-pacific/4910372.stm
5. Siemionow M, Unal S, Agaoglu G, et al. What are alternative sources for total facial defect coverage? A cadaver study in preparation for facial allograft transplantation in humans—part I. *Plast Reconstr Surg* 2006;117:864.
6. Siemionow M, Agaoglu G, Unal S. Mock facial transplantation: a cadaver study in preparation for facial allograft transplantation in humans—part II. *Plast Reconstr Surg* 2006;117:876.
7. Siemionow M, Agaoglu G. The issue of facial "appearance and identity transfer" after mock transplantation: a cadaver study in preparation for facial allograft transplantation in humans. *J Reconstr Microsurg* 2006;22:329.

CHAPTER 148 ■ NASOLABIAL DERMAL FLAPS FOR SUSPENSION IN LOWER FACIAL PALSY

M. R. WEXLER AND I. J. PELED

The variety of possible procedures to correct facial palsy is enormous (1). The best results are with those that restore normal dynamic forces by cross-face reinnervation (2) or bridging nerve grafts to the missing facial nerve and autogenous muscle (3).

INDICATIONS

Patients are often interested in a simpler procedure and reject the idea of an operation on the normal side of the face or elsewhere on the body. We offer our patients a variety of procedures, and our experience is based on those who objected to more sophisticated techniques.

For several years, we have used dermal nasolabial flaps for suspension to improve lower facial palsy (4,5). The advantages of this method are its simplicity, the use of tissue otherwise discarded, and the creation of a fibrotic cheek that improves speech. The nasolabial fold is simulated by the new scar. Correction of lower eyelid ectropion can be achieved at the same time, although the results are only average. Elevation of redundant ala nasi can be achieved as well. If the results are not satisfactory, further procedures can be performed.

FLAP DESIGN AND DIMENSIONS

A fusiform area is marked along the nasolabial fold of the affected side (Figs. 1 and 2B) from the upper pole of the ala nasi to the border of the mandible. The average size of the flap is 9 cm long and 3 cm wide. The rich blood supply of the

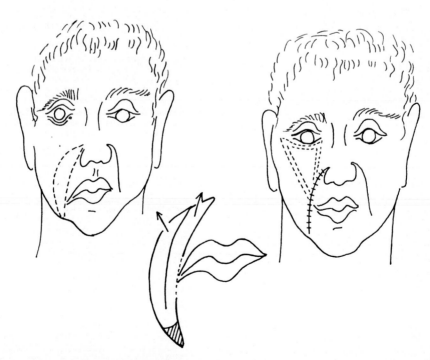

FIG. 1. Schematic drawing of the procedure. Note that the lateral flap is elongated in the lower part. (From Wexler et al., ref. 5, with permission.)

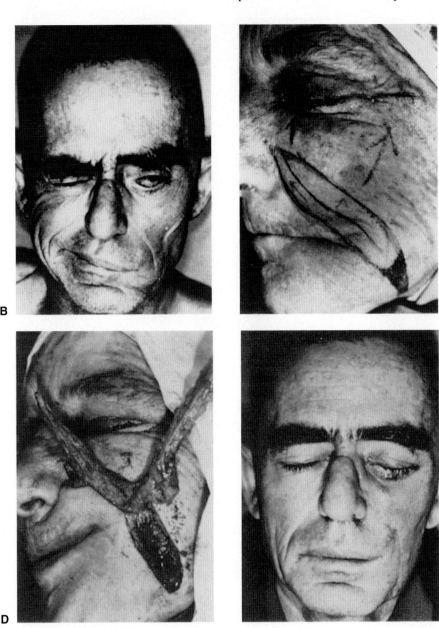

A,B

C,D

FIG. 2. **A:** A 51-year-old man before surgery. **B:** Outline of the flap. **C:** The deepithelialized dermal suspension flaps before being tunneled. **D:** Same patient 2 years after surgery. (From Wexler et al., ref. 5, with permission.)

nasolabial area allows the raising of quite long flaps that are narrowly based at the corner of the mouth.

OPERATIVE TECHNIQUE

The skin is very superficially incised around the marked fusiform area, which is carefully deepithelialized. The circumference of the deepithelialized area then is incised to the subcutaneous tissue except for the area adjacent to the corner of the mouth, the base of the flap. It then is incised in its middle (Fig. 1), thus creating two dermal flaps attached to the corner of the mouth. One is short, about 4 cm long, and the second is longer, about 10 cm, and about 1 to 2 cm wide.

The cheek is undermined from the corner of the mouth to the corner of the orbit over the zygoma and the zygomaticofrontal process. A 3-cm incision is made in this region parallel to the senile creases (crow's feet). A tunnel is created from this incision toward the medial canthal tendon along the lower eyelid. The long flap is passed through the cheek tunnel, thus pulling the corner of the mouth obliquely upward (Fig. 2). Two

separate 3–0 nylon sutures are woven into the dermis flap and pulled with it from the corner of the mouth to the zygoma. Then 4–0 nylon sutures are used to anchor the dermis flap to the periosteum in that location.

If ectropion of the lower eyelid is present as well, the end of the flap is rotated medially and passed through the lower eyelid tunnel, anchoring it lower to the medial canthal tendon and then pulling it laterally to attach it to the periosteum of the lateral orbital wall on the zygomaticofrontal process. The short flap is pulled upward and sutured to the periosteum of the inferior orbital margin.

CLINICAL RESULTS

Improvement was noted in all patients, especially after our addition of 3–0 nylon suspension sutures to the dermis flap (Figs. 2 and 3). Since then, we have noticed that there is no recurrence of drooping of the corner of the mouth, and our initial overcorrection is now done more conservatively. We have not observed flap necrosis with subsequent drop of the oral commissure.

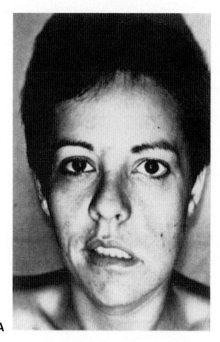
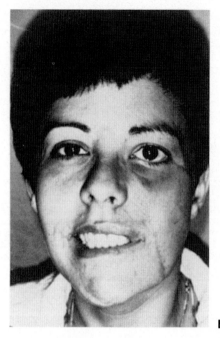

FIG. 3. A: A 28-year-old woman before surgery. **B:** Same patient 1 year after surgery. The lateral flap was not rotated to the medial canthal region. (From Wexler et al., ref. 5, with permission.)

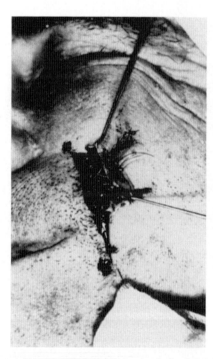

FIG. 4. A complication of pilonidal cyst formation in a male patient that had to be excised. (From Wexler et al., ref. 5, with permission.)

This procedure is not suitable for hairy patients, in whom pilonidal cysts may appear and in whom long-term infection may persist for 1 to 6 months postoperatively (Fig. 4). The technique does not restore animation to the face, but it does improve the obvious deformity.

SUMMARY

Dermal nasolabial flaps can be used to improve the appearance of patients who have facial paralysis. Such flaps are good for patients who are not suitable for more extensive nerve-grafting procedures.

References

1. Freeman BS. Facial palsy. In: Converse JM, ed., *Reconstructive plastic surgery*, 2d ed. Philadelphia: WB Saunders, 1977;1774–1867.
2. Anderl H. Reconstruction of the face through cross-face nerve transplantation in facial paralysis. In: Converse JM, ed., *Reconstructive plastic surgery*, 2d ed. Philadelphia: WB Saunders, 1977;1848–1864.
3. Thompson N. Autogenous muscle grafts in the reconstruction of the paralyzed face. In: Converse JM, ed., *Reconstructive plastic surgery*, 2d ed. Philadelphia: WB Saunders, 1977;1841–1848.
4. Pitanguy I, Cavalcanti MA, Caland M, Guevara E. Steps for the diagnosis and treatment of peripheric facial palsy. *Rev Bras Cir* 1976;66:63.
5. Wexler MR, Kaplan H, Peled I, Rousso M. Nasolabial dermal flaps for lower facial palsy improvement. In: Bernstein L, ed., *Transactions of the Third International Symposium of Plastic and Reconstructive Surgery of the Head and Neck*, Vol. 2. New York: Grune & Stratton, 1981;108.

CHAPTER 149 ■ MICRONEUROVASCULAR FREE GRACILIS MUSCLE TRANSFER FOR FACIAL REANIMATION

K. HARII AND H. ASATO

The free gracilis muscle transfer with microneurovascular anastomoses is currently a worthwhile and reliable procedure, especially in the successful reconstruction of a paralyzed face.

INDICATIONS

Since our clinical introduction of the free gracilis muscle transfer with microneurovascular anastomoses in 1976 (1), this procedure has provided many advantages for successful facial reanimation in long-standing or established facial paralysis. This procedure is indicated for a complete paralysis without regard to etiology. It can also be used for incomplete or partial paralysis.

The motor nerve of the gracilis muscle can be sutured to either the ipsilateral facial nerve or the stump of a previously performed cross-facial nerve graft (2). On some occasions, a branch of the hypoglossal nerve can be used.

ANATOMY

The gracilis muscle is the most superficially located muscle in the thigh adductor group. It arises from the medial margin of the lower half of the pubic arch and inserts into the medial surface of the upper end of the tibia. It forms a flat and narrow muscle belly.

The dominant nutrient vessels of the gracilis muscle originate from either the profunda femoris or the medial circumflex femoral vessels and enter the muscle from its upper third. Although there are a few additional small nutrient vessels ramifying directly from the femoral vessels to the distal portion of the muscle, the dominant nutrient vessels alone can nourish the entire muscle belly (Fig. 1A).

The motor nerve of the gracilis muscle is derived from the anterior branch of the obturator nerve with the sensory nerve to the thigh, which separates from the motor nerve at the gracilis hilus and finally terminates at the skin of the inner medial thigh. The motor nerve of the gracilis muscle is accompanied by the dominant nutrient vessels and can easily be identified between the adductor longus and brevis muscles (Fig. 1B).

OPERATIVE TECHNIQUE

Isolation of the Muscle

An incision approximately 10 cm long is placed along the posterior border of the adductor muscle. After separation of the fascia over the adductor longus and gracilis muscles, the dominant nutrient pedicle of the gracilis is normally identified between the adductor longus and brevis muscles. Blunt careful finger dissection around the muscles can easily expose the pedicle vessels and nerve without injury.

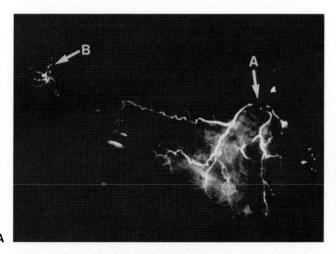
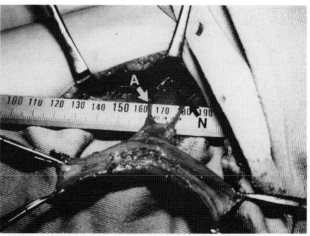

A   B

FIG. 1. **A:** Vascular supply to the gracilis muscle. *Arrow A*, dominant nutrient vessels. *Arrow B*, small additional nutrient vessels. **B:** Elevated gracilis muscle. *Arrow A*, pedicle vessels. *Arrow N*, motor nerve.

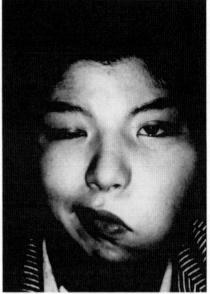
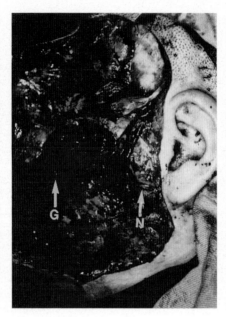
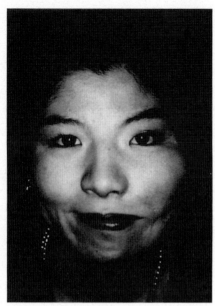

A–C

FIG. 2. **A:** A 25-year-old woman with complete paralysis of the left lower face after multiple ablative procedures for a large lymphangioma of the left cheek. Preoperative view. **B:** A gracilis muscle transplanted beneath the undermined cheek skin, with suturing of its motor nerve to a stump of the facial nerve severed in the previous ablative surgery. *Arrow G,* Gracilis muscle; *A,* site of vessel anastomoses; *N,* site of nerve suture **C:** One-and-a-half years postoperatively. Good contraction of the transplanted muscle upon smiling is obtained.

Following exposure of the pedicle vessels and the accompanying motor nerve, the distal part of the muscle is bluntly dissected. The pedicle vessels and nerve should be extensively dissected toward their origin to obtain as long and large a pedicle as possible. Finally, a muscle belly of the required size is harvested. A proximate linear cutter (Ethicon Co.) is useful to cut the muscle belly. It can simultaneously achieve hemostasis and creation of a rigid muscle stump by its staplers. This facilitates a secure fixation of the muscle stump to the subcutaneous tissues of the face upon transplantation.

One-Stage Reconstruction

In cases of facial paralysis such as those following excision of buccal or parotid tumors (including a facial nerve or a major portion of the mimetic muscles), the transected facial nerve stump is usually available as a motor source in the recipient paralyzed cheek. An acquired contraction of the transferred muscle, innervated with the ipsilateral facial nerve, can be quite natural.

Through a preauricular incision in the affected cheek, a cheek flap is raised, and suitable vessels and the facial nerve stump are exposed first. Usually, either the superficial temporal artery and vein or the facial artery and vein are available for the recipient vessels. The facial nerve stump is simultaneously exposed at its transected site. It is further dissected proximally to obtain a healthy stump. The facial nerve canal in the temporal bone can be opened to acquire a suitable nerve stump.

The cheek then is widely undermined to accept the subsequent muscle transfer. Subcutaneous soft tissue over the zygoma should be partly excised to avoid bulkiness after fixing the muscle in this region.

Simultaneously with the preparation of the recipient cheek, the gracilis muscle is harvested by a second operating team. The harvested muscle is finally transferred to the recipient

cheek, and the neurovascular anastomoses are performed under an operating microscope. After revascularization and neurorrhaphy of the muscle, the two ends of the muscle are fixed to the zygoma and the nasolabial region under proper tension (Fig. 2).

Two-Stage Operation

In many cases with long-standing paralysis, the facial nerve stump is not available in the paralyzed cheek (3). A new facial nerve stump, created by a cross-facial nerve graft from the intact facial nerve branch, has great potential for reinnervation of the transferred muscle, thereby obtaining a natural or near-natural facial animation.

The operative procedure is performed in two stages. In the first stage, through a 2-cm vertical incision at the anterior margin of the parotid gland, as many buccal and zygomatic branches as possible are exposed after their emergence from the anterior border of the parotid gland. A long sural nerve graft approximately 20 cm long and harvested by the second team is placed subcutaneously from the intact cheek to the affected cheek. Endoscopic harvest of the sural nerve can leave a minimal scar.

Usually, the sural nerve graft is reversed. The distal stump of the nerve graft, placed close to the exposed facial nerve branches at the intact cheek, is sutured to selected funiculi in the facial nerve branches. The proximal stump is passed through either the upper lip or the chin and anchored subcutaneously close to the suitable vessels expected to be used as recipient vessels in the second-stage operation.

In the second stage, about 8 to 10 months after the first-stage operation or 1 to 2 months after a Tinel's sign has advanced to the grafted nerve stump in the affected cheek, a cheek flap is elevated, and the cross-facial nerve stump and the recipient vessels are exposed. The gracilis muscle then is transferred with microneurovascular anastomoses (Fig. 3).

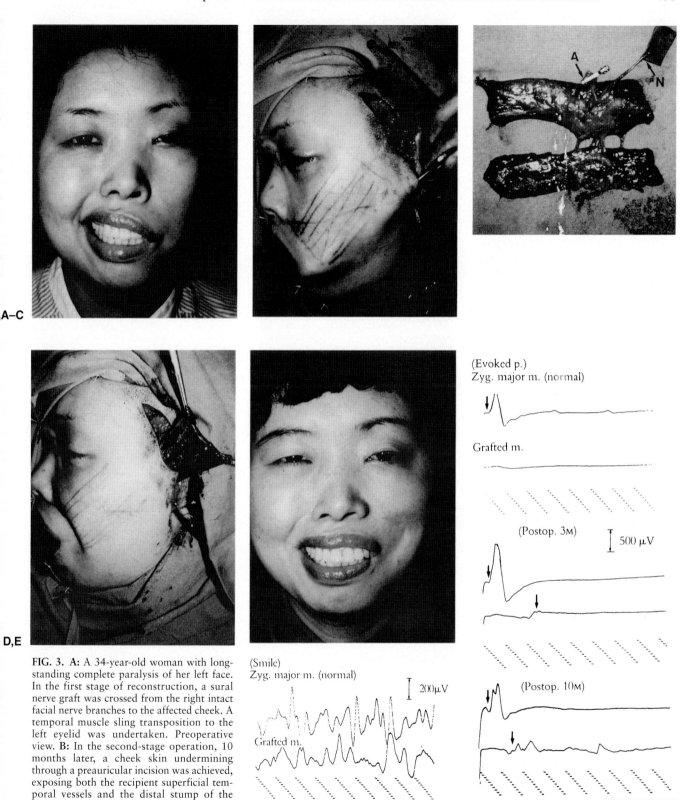

FIG. 3. A: A 34-year-old woman with long-standing complete paralysis of her left face. In the first stage of reconstruction, a sural nerve graft was crossed from the right intact facial nerve branches to the affected cheek. A temporal muscle sling transposition to the left eyelid was undertaken. Preoperative view. **B:** In the second-stage operation, 10 months later, a cheek skin undermining through a preauricular incision was achieved, exposing both the recipient superficial temporal vessels and the distal stump of the cross-facial sural nerve graft. **C:** Gracilis muscle segment. *A,* dominant nutrient vessels; *N,* motor nerve. **D:** Gracilis muscle set in place; note creation of nasolabial fold. Microneurovascular anastomoses were performed. **E:** Two-year postoperative view upon smiling, which corresponds well to contralateral facial animation. **F:** Electromyogram showing good action potentials at postoperative follow-up 15 months later. **G:** Low evoked potentials on stimulation to the contralateral facial nerve trunk were recorded from the transplanted muscle at the 10th postoperative month. Evoked potentials then became higher and the distal latency shortened when muscle neurotization became complete.

SUMMARY

The paralyzed face can be reanimated successfully with a free gracilis muscle graft. Microneurovascular anastomoses can be performed to the recipient vessels and the nerve, which is either the ipsilateral facial nerve, if available, or the stump of a previously performed cross-facial nerve graft. Innervation to the grafted muscle will usually occur between 8 to 10 months postoperatively. The muscle contractile power will then increase and on average, reach its maximum at two years postoperatively.

References

1. Harii K, Ohmori K, Torii S. Free gracilis muscle transplantation with microneurovascular anastomoses for the treatment of facial paralysis. *Plast Reconstr Surg* 1976;57:133–143.
2. Harii K. Microneurovascular free muscle transplantation. In: Rubin LR, ed. *The paralyzed face*. St. Louis: Mosby-Year Book, 1991.
3. Harii K. Refined microneurovascular free muscle transplantation for reanimation of paralyzed face. *Microsurgery* 1988;9:169–176.

CHAPTER 150 ■ MICROVASCULAR FREE TRANSFER OF A PARTIAL GRACILIS MUSCLE TO THE FACE

R. M. ZUKER

EDITORIAL COMMENT

This is an elegant modification of the use of the free gracilis muscle for restoration of the paralyzed face. It allows a sufficient amount of muscle to be transferred to the face and avoids some of the bulkiness that was associated with the transfer of the entire muscle.

The use of a portion of the gracilis muscle is particularly well suited for facial reanimation. The desired length of muscle can be harvested with a percentage of muscle circumference as long as great care is taken to maintain the integrity of the pedicle (1,2). Excess bulk can be avoided (3), and a reliable, innervated flap of the required dimensions can be obtained.

INDICATIONS

Indications for facial reanimation using innervated muscle flaps relate to the extent of the paralysis, the age of the patient, and the patient's needs and desires. A significant degree of facial paralysis, with inability to elevate the commissure and upper lip, warrants consideration for reconstruction. Although possible in older age groups, I believe that reinnervation of a transferred muscle, particularly through cross-face nerve grafts, begins to lose its effectiveness in the sixth and seventh decades of life. Some patients require a rapid, static, alteration and would not benefit from the time-consuming cross-face nerve graft/free muscle transfer. Other patients may be quite well adjusted to their condition and not wish to

undergo any surgical reconstruction. Thus, it is crucial to present what is possible and what is not possible to the patient. Elevation of the commissure and upper lip is usually an attainable goal (4). The direction of movement can be adjusted to match the normal side; however, perfect symmetry is never achieved. This procedure addresses only elevation of the commissure and upper lip and does not reconstruct the multitude of other fine movements of the face associated with smiling.

There are three situations that can be addressed by muscle transfer in facial paralysis, depending on the availability of a motor nerve (5). If the stump of the ipsilateral facial nerve is available, as may follow tumor excision, this stump can be used directly to innervate the transferred gracilis. The second situation is a unilateral facial paralysis where there is no ipsilateral facial nerve; for example, a case following acoustic neuroma surgery where the seventh nerve is nonfunctional at the intracranial level. In this case, a portion of nerve activity from the normal side can be transferred across the face through a cross-face nerve graft. This involves a preauricular incision with dissection of the normal nerve. The specific branches that go to the zygomatics major and minor are identified, and a portion of these can be taken for anastomosis to the nerve graft. The sural nerve graft is tunneled across the face through incisions in the nasal floor and preauricular region; after nerve repair on the normal side, it is banked in the preauricular area of the paralyzed side. One year later, this banked stump of the sural nerve can be used to innervate the transferred partial gracilis.

A third situation is when there is no facial nerve available bilaterally, as occurs in congenital conditions such as Mobius syndrome and also occasionally in patients with bilateral acoustic neuromata. In this situation, a partial gracilis transfer can be used to provide elevation of the commissure and upper lip, but it must be innervated by a regional motor nerve. Available motor nerves include the fifth, the eleventh, and the twelfth. I have found the motor branch to the masseter (V) to be extremely useful in this situation.

The advantages of the partial gracilis are numerous. The neurovascular pedicle is reliable and the flap can be easily harvested. The partial gracilis can be specifically designed and sculpted to meet specific requirements for variability of length and width. The bulkiness of the transfer is minimized by using only a partial segment of the muscle. Finally, there is virtually no donor-site morbidity except for the scar in the upper medial portion of the thigh and minimal early postoperative discomfort.

ANATOMY

The basic anatomy of the gracilis muscle is adequately described elsewhere in this volume (see Chapter 329). The muscle is identified and isolated, and the neurovascular pedicle is carefully dissected. The muscle remains on its vascular pedicle until it has been fully prepared and is ready for transfer, as described subsequently.

FLAP DESIGN AND DIMENSIONS

The required length of muscle then is assessed. The muscle will originate from the zygomatic arch and temporal fascia and will insert into preplaced sutures that have been sited carefully to replicate the activity on the normal side. Generally, four such sutures are used. One is into the lower lip, the second is into the modiolus, the third is into the more lateral portion of the upper lip, and the fourth is into the midportion of the upper lip. These four sutures are securely anchored; they will be used to maintain insertion of the muscle flap into place.

The functional length of the muscle is measured from the modiolus to the most lateral portion of the zygomatic arch. The obliquity of the muscle can be adjusted by altering the position of the origin to match the normal side. To provide sufficient muscle tissue for suturing, 1-cm length is added at each end. Thus, if the functional length required is 9 cm, 11 cm of muscle would be harvested.

The volume of the muscle is assessed in the thigh; usually, about 40% to 50% of the circumference of the muscle is sufficient. This volume is determined by the size of the gracilis in the thigh, the location of the neurovascular pedicle, and the innervation pattern, as will be described.

OPERATIVE TECHNIQUE

With a nasotracheal tube in the contralateral side, the involved side is prepared and the operative field extended to include the entire mouth, chin, and neck region. The ipsilateral thigh is generally used, and the limb is prepared to at least below the knee and draped free. The facial dissection begins with a preauricular incision and a submandibular extension. The cheek is elevated above the level of the submuscular aponeurotic system (SMAS). Appropriate anchoring sutures are placed into the lower lip, modiolus, and upper lip, as described above. The site of origin of the muscle is prepared on the zygomatic arch and temporal fascia. The recipient vessels then are dissected free; these are usually the facial artery and vein. They are traced upward, divided, and then reflected posteriorly, where they will lie in an excellent position for anastomosis to the vessels of the gracilis. Last, the motor nerve that will power the muscle is found.

If there is an ipsilateral branch of the facial nerve, a standard facial nerve dissection is necessary. If innervation is to be by a cross-facial nerve graft, the graft generally is found quite easily and traced a sufficient distance to be reflected downward to provide for a tensionless nerve repair. If the motor nerve to the masseter is to be used, it is found on the undersurface of the masseter muscle. The masseter is reflected downward from the zygomatic arch and the nerve coursing transversely and then entering the deep surface of the masseter is found. It is traced into the muscle, divided, and reflected upward so that it lies at the level of the zygomatic arch and provides ease in repair.

The muscle is dissected simultaneously. A segment of muscle is freed circumferentially, and the neurovascular pedicle is dissected fully. The single artery and paired veins are dissected back to their origin so that the longest possible pedicle is obtained. The nerve is also dissected proximally as it courses upward and anteriorly, bisecting the 90-degree angle of muscle and the vascular pedicle. Depending on the length of nerve required, it can be traced all the way to the inguinal ligament. Then it is divided proximally and reflected downward so that each of its fascicles can be evaluated and stimulated individually. The muscle itself is freed circumferentially above and below the pedicle so that the required length can be removed easily. In general, the pedicle should lie at about the midportion of the selected segment of muscle so that adequate vascularity is assured on both ends. The width is assessed, and the segment of muscle that will be harvested is determined. Usually, 40% to 50% of the muscle circumference is required, as this provides a healthy strip of about 2 cm in width without excessive bulk.

A nerve stimulator is used to stimulate each of the fascicles at the site of division. The muscle is observed for segmental contraction so that if only a single fascicle is available for innervation, the appropriate fascicle in the motor nerve to the gracilis can be determined.

The location of the pedicle relative to the entire muscle in an anterior/posterior plane then is assessed. Usually, the anterior 40% of the muscle can be taken, preserving the vascular pedicle. Evaluation of the muscle includes determination of the natural cleavage plane. This plane is dissected, with division of the nerves and vessels going to the more inferior portion, which will not be used. During this segment of the dissection, great care must be taken not to damage the main pedicle.

The required length of muscle is separated from the posterior segment, which will be left behind. The required length is measured with the hip in abduction and the knee in extension. In this way, the segment of muscle that will be taken is in a stretched position. If 11 cm is required, then 5.5 cm is taken on either side of the pedicle (Fig. 1). The muscle then is divided on either end and thus remains attached only by its vascular pedicle.

After the muscle segment has been isolated and divided, the end that will insert into the commissure and lips is prepared. A small central wedge of about 0.5 cm of muscle tissue is removed from this end, and the outer components are sutured together with mattress sutures and carried out along the free edge of the muscle. They will function as anchors or the insertion sutures that have been placed in the lower lip, modiolus, and upper lip.

Muscle preparation is now complete and, after the circulatory status has been assured, the muscle can be removed and transferred (Fig. 2). The vascular pedicle of the partial gracilis is divided and the donor site closed in layers. The muscle is transferred to the face, where the insertion sutures are placed just proximal to the anchorage mattress sutures that were previously inserted. The muscle then is drawn beneath the cheek flap toward the mouth, and the sutures are tied sequentially.

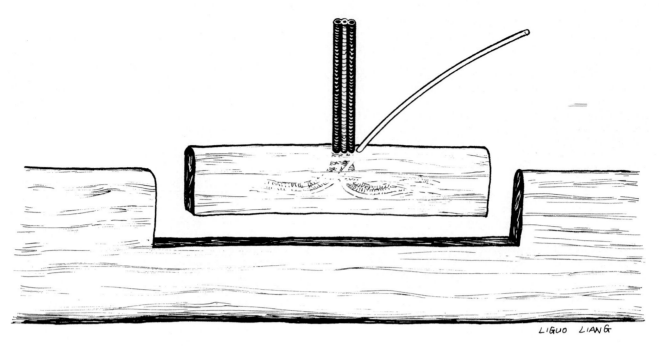

FIG. 1. Schematic diagram of a selected segment of gracilis muscle.

The muscle is stretched to its normal resting length and then tacked to its site of origin with mattress sutures. Tension is such that it just barely pulls on the modiolus. Measurements will show that this is the maximal resting extended length. The muscle is anchored securely to the zygomatic arch and temporal fascia. It is spread over the fascia to avoid any excessive bulk in this region.

Then the microvascular repairs are carried out. First, the larger vena comitans of the partial gracilis is sutured to the facial vein end-to-end. The artery to the partial gracilis then is anastomosed to the facial artery, again in an end-to-end fashion. Once the circulation has been reestablished, the nerve repair is carried out (Fig. 3). This is a crucial part of the procedure and must be done with extreme precision. The stump of the facial nerve, the cross-facial nerve graft, or the motor nerve to the masseter is sutured to the motor nerve of the gracilis. This repair is done without tension under high magnification, with appropriate fascicles accurately aligned. The wound then is closed in layers, with a Penrose drain below the earlobe. No suction drains are used.

The muscle begins to function about 2 to 3 months after the transfer if a direct nerve repair has been carried out. If a cross-facial nerve graft has been used, reinnervation is somewhat slower and may not occur until 4 to 5 months. Once reinnervation begins however, simple exercises are used to increase excursion of the muscle and to achieve symmetry. In bilateral cases, the second side is done 3 to 6 months after the first side.

CLINICAL RESULTS

Results of the procedure have been quite satisfactory. The degree of excursion produced by the gracilis seems to be adequate, especially in cases where direct nerve repairs are carried out. In congenital facial paralysis, there is often some activity

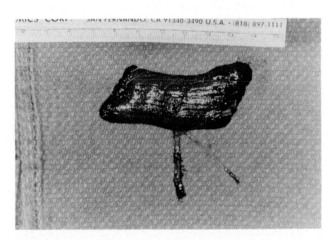

FIG. 2. Partial gracilis muscle prepared and ready for insertion into face.

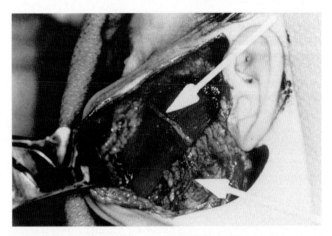

FIG. 3. Partial gracilis muscle in the face with microvascular and microneural repairs.

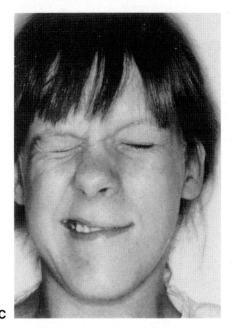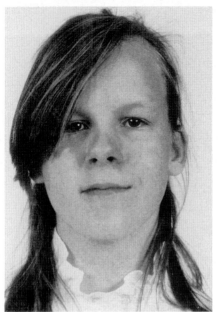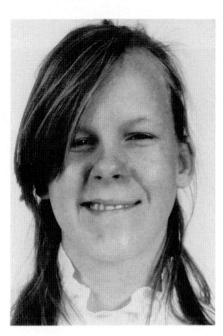

A–C

FIG. 4. Unilateral congenital facial paralysis. **A:** Preoperative: smiling. **B:** Postoperative: at rest. **C:** Postoperative: smiling. (From Zuker, ref. 5, with permission.)

around the eye or in the paranasal region. The main deficit appears to be in elevation of the corner of the mouth and upper lip. In this situation, a cross-facial nerve graft, followed by a partial gracilis transfer, provides an acceptable reconstruction (Fig. 4). I have also been pleased with the results of the reconstruction that can be achieved in bilateral conditions, such as Mobius syndrome.

This procedure allows one to tailor the size of the muscle to the dimensions required, thus avoiding excessive bulk. It also allows the surgeon to place the muscle in the exact location that will produce the required movement. Thus, the muscle can be placed to provide symmetrical motion with the normal side. In unilateral cases, the appropriate nerve (seventh nerve) can be used to innervate the muscle, thus achieving synchronous and spontaneous activity.

SUMMARY

The gracilis muscle can be sculpted to provide the exact length required with minimal bulk. It has been successfully used in facial reanimation for congenital or acquired conditions, whether unilateral or bilateral. Appropriate positioning of the muscle is possible, and adequate excursion can be achieved. By using only a portion of the muscle, the problem of excess bulk is avoided.

References

1. Manktelow RT, Zuker RM. Muscle transplantation by fascicular territory. *Plast Reconstr Surg* 1984;73:751.
2. Manktelow RT. *Microvascular reconstruction: anatomy, applications and surgical techniques. Facial paralysis reconstruction.* Heidelberg: Springer Verlag, 1986;128.
3. Zuker RM. Facial reanimation: Cross-face nerve grafting and muscle transplantation. In: Cohen M, ed. *Mastery of plastic and reconstructive surgery. Facial reanimation, cross face nerve grafting and muscle transplantation;* Vol. 1, Boston: Little, Brown, 1994. Chap. 58.
4. Harii K, Ohmori K, Torii S. Free gracilis muscle transplantation with microvascular anastomoses for the treatment of facial paralysis. *Plast Reconstr Surg* 1976;57:133.
5. Zuker RM. Facial paralysis in children. *Clin Plast Surg* 1990;17:95.
6. Zuker RM, Manktelow RT. A smile for the Mobius syndrome patient. *Ann Plast Surg* 1989;22:188.

CHAPTER 151 ■ MICRONEUROVASCULAR FREE TRANSFER OF THE SERRATUS ANTERIOR MUSCLE

J. C. GROTTING

The serratus anterior muscle is a small, thin muscle that can be used as a free vascularized transfer for cover or function, especially in the hand, foot, and face (1–3). It has a predictable anatomic configuration and blood supply. As long as its upper portion is kept intact, the use of the lower one to three slips in reconstruction has little, if any, effect on normal function.

INDICATIONS

The serratus anterior muscle has been most useful in situations where a small, relatively thin, and potentially functional muscle is needed. As a free transfer, one or two slips are ideal for use in the hand or foot (4). The segmental organization allows careful axial division between slips for placement of portions of the muscle into various locations within a wound. Reanimation in facial paralysis requires three slips. In most cases, a cross-facial nerve graft is performed as a first stage. When axonal growth has advanced across the face, the lower three slips of the serratus can be inserted for functional replacement of the paralyzed muscle units (Fig. 5). With the muscle turned over, the neurovascular repairs are protected and only a short pedicle is required.

ANATOMY

The serratus anterior muscle is a broad, flat muscle that forms the medial wall of the axilla. Its dual blood supply and unique organization into separate slips that originate from each of the first nine ribs make it ideal for segmental transfer of only the lower three to four slips, thereby preserving muscle function (Fig. 1). The lateral thoracic artery vascularizes the upper four or five slips, whereas the lower portion is consistently supplied by a large branch of the thoracodorsal artery. This vessel enters the serratus in its posterior third and gives off segmental branches to each of the lower five slips (Fig. 2), each branch accompanied by a corresponding vein and a twig of the long thoracic nerve. The most inferior three slips are particularly suitable for use as a free muscle transfer and will have a long pedicle if the serratus branch is dissected back to include the subscapular-thoracodorsal axis (Fig. 3).

The serratus anterior stabilizes the scapula by its broad insertion along the medial and inferior border. It is innervated by the long thoracic nerve that arises from C5, C6, and C7 and travels inferiorly along the serratus fascia, joining with the serratus branch of the thoracodorsal artery at about the level of the sixth slip (Fig. 2). Loss of the long thoracic nerve will cause winging of the scapula, a complication that

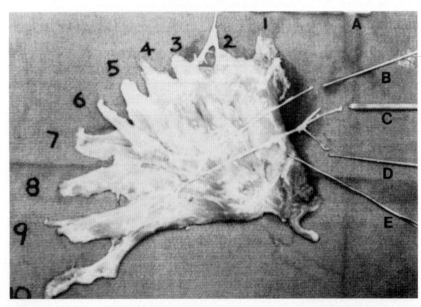

FIG. 1. A cadaver dissection of the serratus anterior muscle illustrates its organization into separate slips. (In this case, ten are present; usually only nine are found.)

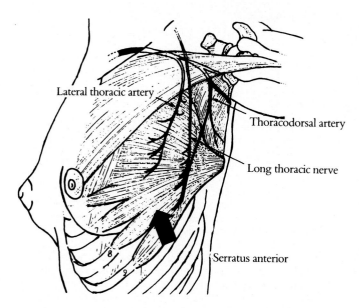

Lateral thoracic artery

Thoracodorsal artery

Long thoracic nerve

Serratus anterior

FIG. 2. The upper five slips of the serratus anterior receive their blood supply from the lateral thoracic artery. The lower three to four slips are consistently supplied by a large branch of the thoracodorsal artery. The long thoracic nerve lies on the serratus fascia anterior to this large branch.

can be avoided by separating the discrete fascicles of the long thoracic nerve to only the lower three slips. The proximal serratus innervation must be preserved to maintain the muscle as a functional unit. With magnification, the long thoracic nerve can be split into fascicular groups to the level of the axillary vein, but this tedious exercise probably puts the proximal nerve at unnecessary risk of injury. Therefore, it is better to use a shorter nerve segment and to interpose a nerve graft at the recipient site if a long nerve pedicle is needed. Removal of the lowest three slips of the serratus will not result in winging of the scapula as long as the proximal muscle retains its innervation.

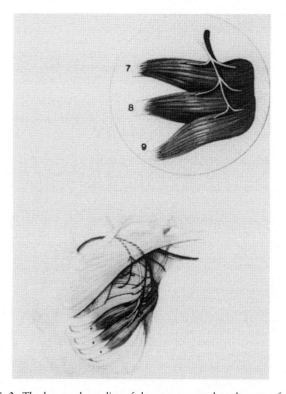

FIG. 3. The lowest three slips of the serratus can be taken as a free, potentially functional muscle flap without producing winging of the scapula. The segmental nature of the blood supply and innervation to each slip is illustrated.

Because the blood supply to the lower portion of the serratus anterior arises from the subscapular-thoracodorsal axis, a long vascular pedicle can be obtained by dividing the thoracodorsal branch to the latissimus dorsi and continuing the dissection superiorly, taking the subscapular artery off at its origin from the third portion of the subclavian artery. A 15-cm pedicle can be obtained by this technique, but if a long pedicle is not needed, the serratus branch from the thoracodorsal artery is usually large enough for a technically straightforward microvascular anastomosis, thereby preserving the major blood supply to the latissimus dorsi.

Although the proximal serratus anterior has a broad insertion along the medial border of the scapula, the seventh, eighth, and ninth slips tend to merge and overlap each other, inserting at the inferior pole by means of a short tendinous attachment. The latissimus dorsi must be raised off the lower pole of the scapula to facilitate this portion of the dissection.

OPERATIVE TECHNIQUE

The serratus anterior is most easily dissected with the patient in either the full-lateral or half-lateral position. The tip of the scapula must be accessible and the arm prepped free, as in the latissimus dissection. The incision is planned 3 to 4 cm anterior to the posterior axillary fold formed by the latissimus muscle. I have found it useful to curve the incision anteriorly over the eighth rib to allow access to the origin of the muscle (Fig. 4). The incision is deepened to the deep fascia, and the anterior edge of the latissimus is identified.

Dissection of the posterior skin flap off the anterior latissimus fold to below the ninth rib will help identify the important landmarks. The latissimus and serratus muscles are easily separated superiorly because the serratus muscle passes deep to the latissimus. Inferiorly, however, the fibers of the two muscles interdigitate and must be separated sharply. As the latissimus is dissected from the underlying serratus, the thoracodorsal artery and vein soon will come into view. The branch to the lower slips of the serratus anterior then can be identified and must be carefully protected.

The long thoracic nerve is always located anterior to the serratus branch and runs over the surface of the muscle, joining the artery and vein at about the sixth slip. The dissection of these structures should be left until after the entire outer surface of the lowest slips have been exposed. The long thoracic nerve can be densely adherent to the serratus fascia.

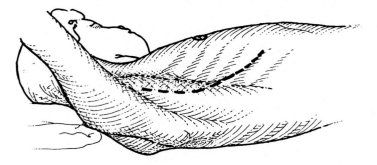

FIG. 4. The incision is planned just anterior to the latissimus dorsi fold and is extended forward along the eighth rib. This allows access for both the origin and insertion of the serratus anterior muscle.

The fascia below the ninth slip is sharply incised, mobilizing the inferior border of the serratus from its origin along the ribs to the scapular tip. The plane between the chest wall and the serratus is avascular and can be developed easily with the gloved hand. From the undersurface of the serratus, the slips can be palpated and the true division between them identified. Using a hand behind the muscle as a guide, the fascia between the sixth and seventh slips can be incised, staying well in front of the neurovascular pedicle. Posterior to the neurovascular pedicle, the division between slips is less distinct and must be sharply divided.

If the serratus is being used for function, the length of the muscle should be measured and markers placed every 5 cm before dividing the origin and insertion. This allows careful reapproximation of the resting length after transfer, an important consideration in restoring its ability to perform work.

The neurovascular pedicle is isolated next. If the lowest three serratus slips are to be used, the small branches that enter slips 5 and 6 must be carefully divided between fine ligatures to gain pedicle length. If these tiny branches are overlooked, accidental avulsion and injury to the main vessels may be precipitated. The branches from the long thoracic nerve to the upper serratus slips must be separated from the fascicles continuing into the flap if neural repair is anticipated. Otherwise, the nerve may be divided distal to its last branch to the sixth slip. Intraneural dissection can be accomplished quite far proximally if performed with care under loupe magnification. A 3- to 5-cm nerve pedicle is usually all that is necessary when using the serratus for facial reanimation. If a long nerve pedicle is required, an interpositional nerve graft will place the proximal long thoracic nerve at less risk of inadvertent division. The vascular pedicle can be extended to 15 cm by continuing the dissection to the level of the axillary vein. The origin and insertion of the serratus are divided sharply. Intercostal perforators that are encountered must be ligated. The lowest slip often interdigitates with the fibers of the external oblique muscle. The insertions of the lowest three slips seem to wrap around the tip of the scapula and attach to it by a very short tendon that also will bleed when divided. When the muscle is to be used as a free transfer, it should be allowed to perfuse on its dissected pedicle for 10 to 20 minutes before division and transfer.

Because the perforating intercostal vessels communicate with the serratus branch from the thoracodorsal system, the serratus muscle may support an osseous component consisting of the underlying one or two ribs (see Chapter 207). The muscle also can be taken with a skin island.

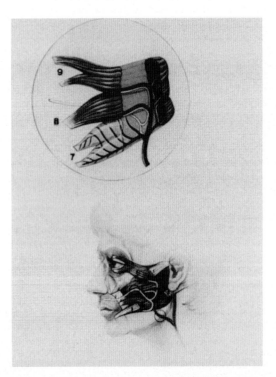

FIG. 5. The serratus can be used for reanimation in facial paralysis. The muscle is innervated and split into slips, as illustrated, to restore segmental motion. The long thoracic nerve segment is kept short and is anastomosed to a previously placed cross-facial nerve graft.

SUMMARY

The serratus anterior muscle flap can be transferred as a free flap. It is particularly applicable for facial reanimation, as three or more slips can be used separately.

References

1. Buncke HJ, Alpert BS, Gordon L, Evans HB, eds. *Atlas of clinical reconstructive microsurgery.* Philadelphia: Lea and Febiger, 1986.
2. Buncke HJ, Alpert BS, Gordon L, et al. The serratus anterior muscle for unilateral facial paralysis. In: Buncke HJ, Gordon L, Alpert BS, eds. *Atlas of clinical reconstructive microsurgery.* Philadelphia: Lea and Febiger, 1986.
3. Takayanagi S, Tsukie T. Free serratus anterior muscle and myocutaneous flaps. *Ann Plast Surg* 1982;8:277.
4. Gordon L, Rosen J, Alpert BS, Buncke HJ. Free microvascular transfer of second toe ray and serratus anterior muscle for management of thumb loss at the carpometacarpal joint level. *J Hand Surg* 1984;9:642.

 Online Chapter

CHAPTER 152. Microneurovascular Free Transfer of Extensor Digitorum Brevis Muscle for Facial Reanimation *V. K. Rao and J. A. Butler*

www.encyclopediaofflaps.com

CHAPTER 153 ■ MICRONEUROVASCULAR FREE TRANSFER OF PECTORALIS MINOR MUSCLE FOR FACIAL REANIMATION

J. K. TERZIS

The pectoralis minor muscle seems to have the best qualities of both the gracilis and extensor digitorum brevis muscles, previous choices for facial reanimation, but without their disadvantages. The pectoralis minor is an ideal shape, has adequate bulk, and possesses a dual nerve supply that allows for independent movements of its upper and lower portions. These characteristics make the muscle a more intelligent choice than either the gracilis or extensor digitorum brevis for substitution of atrophied facial musculature (1–7).

INDICATIONS

The best indication for use of the pectoralis minor muscle flap is in developmental facial paralysis in young children. For use in a 4- or 5-year-old child, the muscle dimensions are ideal (i.e., 6 to 10 cm long and 0.4 to 0.6 cm wide). In these patients, the muscle can be used totally, without thinning or shortening. The muscle also can be an excellent choice for adults, especially patients who are not athletic and have not built up muscles of the upper torso through sports or exercise. Its use is not recommended in well-developed patients, especially weightlifters or swimmers, because of excessive bulk, unless substantial debulking is undertaken.

Donor-site morbidity is minimal, limited to a small incision over the anterior axillary fold, an imperceptible loss of pectoralis major bulk that is not appreciated by the patient but only by careful inspection of the upper thoracic area, and no reportable functional loss.

The muscle is flat and is composed of several slips that can be separated in a distoproximal fashion for a substantial length without fear of vascular and neural compromise. It has sufficient bulk to substitute for the lower face and can yield adequate excursion in the needed directions of pull. If the hilus of the muscle is placed over the zygomatic arch, its slips of origin can be separated and fashioned to substitute not only for the zygomatic major muscle, but also for the elevators of the upper lip and for the retractors of the commissure. A multidirectional pull can be obtained that is ideal if the patient has a "canine" type of smile in the contralateral normal face.

Possibly, the most important advantage of the pectoralis minor is its dual innervation, a proof of its segmental origin during development. The upper third of the muscle is innervated by a branch of the lateral pectoral nerve, while the lower two thirds receive nerve supply from the medial pectoral nerve, an offshoot from the medial cord of the brachial plexus. This dual innervation allows for independent movements of the upper part quite separately from the lower part of the muscle. These separately moving muscle subunits can be used to address the separate needs of animation of the eye and mouth, a quality not present in previously described muscle units.

ANATOMY

The pectoralis minor is a flat, thin, triangular muscle situated beneath the pectoralis major. The muscle arises from the outer surfaces of the third, fourth, and fifth ribs near their costochondral junctions and from the fasciae covering the intercostal muscles. The fibers ascend upward and laterally and converge to form a flat tendon that inserts in the upper surface of the coracoid process of the scapula. Frequently, there is an additional slip that originates from the second rib.

The normal action of the muscle is pulling the scapula forward and downward, assisting simultaneously in adduction of the arm by rotating the scapula. If the scapula is maintained in a fixed position by the levator scapulae, the pectoralis minor raises the corresponding ribs in forced inspiration.

Blood Supply

There is great variability in the arterial supply of the pectoralis minor, with contributions received from three main sources: the lateral thoracic artery, the thoracoacromial artery, or directly from a branch of the axillary artery. Infrequently, the latter arterial source is present when contributions to the muscle from the other two arterial trunks are minimal. I call this direct artery the "lateral thoracic artery" because, in the few clinical encounters in which a direct artery from the axillary to the pectoralis minor occurred, there was no visible contribution to the muscle from other arterial sources more inferiorly. In the original ten dissections, a separate branch from the axillary artery was never encountered.

By far the predominant vascular pattern is from branches of the lateral thoracic or thoracoacromial arteries. The former passes around the lateral margin of the muscle after it has supplied it with a branch, while the latter passes around the medial margin of the muscle after it has issued an arterial branch, usually to the superior part of the muscle. One or the other branch is dominant, but in a clinical series, the dominant branch came more frequently from the lateral thoracic artery. When the two branches share the blood supply to the pectoralis minor, harvesting the muscle on the lateral thoracic contribution has been the choice, but in these patients, the superior portion of the muscle was not as well perfused and appeared duskier.

There is also extensive variability in the venous drainage of this muscle. More often than not, there is a separate vein that will drain the muscle adequately; however, in many cases, one of the venae comitantes must be used because the direct vein is absent. If there is some doubt about dominant venous drainage, it is best to harvest all the available veins and to observe under magnification which one best drains the muscle unit after microvascular transfer.

Nerve Supply

The nerve supply to the muscle has minimal variations. The majority of the pectoralis minor (four fifths) receives innervation from the medial pectoral nerve, while the most superior part of the muscle receives a tiny branch from the lateral pectoral nerve. Another substantial branch of the lateral pectoral nerve destined to innervate the pectoralis major uses the pectoralis minor only as a passway; thus harvesting the pectoralis minor necessitates taking of that nerve. However, these axons need not be lost, and if time is taken to redirect these fibers back to the pectoralis minor, additional innervation can be obtained through a process of direct neurotization.

The nerve supply to the pectoralis minor is multisegmental, receiving contributions from all five spinal nerves contributing to the brachial plexus, namely, C5, C6, C7, C8, and T1. Motor fibers from these spinal nerves reach the pectoralis minor through branches of two nerves, the lateral and medial pectoral nerves. The dominant innervation to the pectoralis minor is through the medial pectoral nerve, with contributions from C8 and T1. A major branch from this nerve is responsible in all cases for three fourths or two thirds of the muscle, depending on whether the muscle has three or four slips. Also constant is the innervation of the superior part of the pectoralis minor, which, in all cases, comes through a tiny branch from the lateral pectoral nerve. A larger lateral pectoral branch also penetrates the muscle, but it usually does not supply the muscle; instead, it courses through it on its way to the pectoralis major.

Contrary to reported variability in the nerve supply of the pectoralis major, the innervation of the pectoralis minor is relatively constant. Variations are limited to the presence or absence of the communicating loop, with fiber exchange between the medial and lateral pectoral nerves. It is worth mentioning that in two clinical cases of severe brachial plexopathy, with documented neuroradiologic and electrical findings of C8 and T1 avulsion, the inferior segment of the pectoralis minor responded to intraoperative electrical stimulation, raising the possibility that some motor fibers from T2 may contribute to the innervation of this muscle.

The dual innervation of the pectoralis minor makes it a unique muscle for facial reanimation procedures because the upper leaves can be motored separately from the lower portion of the muscle. This characteristic opens possibilities for independent eye and mouth movements, one of the greatest advantages of using this muscle for facial-muscle substitution (Figs. 1–4).

FLAP DESIGN AND DIMENSIONS

In the adult, the individual slips of the muscle measure 10 to 14 cm long. The upper leaves are shorter, and the lower leaves are longer. In a child or baby, pectoralis minor leaflets are only 6 to 10 cm long, making it ideal for facial reanimation procedures, since the muscle can be used in toto without any trimming. The width of the muscle is less than 0.5 cm in very young patients, but it can be up to 2 or 3 cm in athletic adults, a situation that would require extensive debulking.

Flap design is carried out by precise preoperative measurements of the patient's face in repose and during extremes of facial movement. A mold is made of the exact shape needed for a particular reanimation procedure.

Before harvesting, the tension of the muscle is measured, and 6–0 silk sutures are placed over its inferior margin 1 to 2 cm apart. Once the muscle is harvested from the anterior thorax, it is placed on a wet sponge.

There is a 30% to 50% shrinkage of the muscle following harvesting because of the elastic recoil of its fibers. By placing holding sutures along its origins and insertion, an attempt is made to reexpand the muscle to its previous dimensions. Then the mold is placed on the stretched muscle, and appropriate trimming and debulking are carried out.

It is important to allow for more muscle length than merely the length-width measurements of the facial mold. Supported by experience in facial reanimation procedures and contrasting to extremity free-muscle transplantation, it proved to be a poor idea to reproduce in situ length in the face. In a few patients in whom the muscle was placed under too much tension, the muscle force generated was too great for the requirements of the recipient site. Subsequently, the muscle had to be weakened. Thus, during a revisional stage, the transplanted muscle was loosened by advancing it medially; this invariably corrected the deformity.

In children between 4 and 5 years of age, no trimming or debulking is necessary, since the muscle usually fits the facial dimensions of children perfectly.

OPERATIVE TECHNIQUE

The patient is placed on his or her back, and the face and neck areas, as well as the contralateral upper extremity and upper thorax, are prepped and draped. One surgical team prepares the recipient site. The following tasks need to be addressed: (a) face-lift incision, (b) undermining a cheek flap extending from the preauricular area to the upper and lower lip up to the philtrum—the superior margin of the cheek flap is the infraorbital rim and the inferior margin is the submandibular area, (c) identification of the facial artery and vein and microsurgical isolation of this vascular pedicle from 2 cm below the mandible to the level of the alar base, and (d) identification and microsurgical isolation of the distal ends of the cross-facial nerve grafts up to the region of the upper lip.

A separate team harvests the pectoralis minor muscle simultaneously by working on the opposite side of the operating table; this shortens operating time appreciably. The following procedures are followed:

1. Placement of the incision over the posterior border of the anterior axillary fold, so that it is not easily visualized
2. Identification of the inferior margin of the pectoralis major muscle
3. Identification and isolation of the lateral thoracic vascular pedicle as it enters the inferior margin of the pectoralis major
4. Microsurgical pursuit of the lateral thoracic pedicle to the undersurface of the pectoralis minor muscle and isolation of the dominant arterial trunk that supplies the pectoralis minor
5. Identification of the inferior margin of the pectoralis minor and demarcation of the outer surface over the thorax by blunt dissection
6. Distal dissection freeing the undersurface of the pectoralis minor muscle from the intercostals, investing fasciae, and outer costal surface
7. Proximal exploration clearly defining the outer and inner surfaces of the origin of the muscle up to the coracoid process

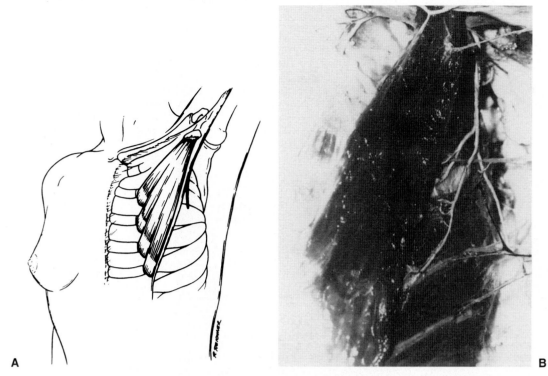

FIG. 1. A: The location of the pectoralis minor on the anterior thorax showing the four slips of origin near the costal cartilages and the coracoid tendinous insertion. Note the *heavy line* over the anterior axillary fold, which signifies the incision for microsurgical harvesting of this muscle. **B:** Corresponding fresh dissection specimen showing the pectoralis minor exposed after removal of the pectoralis major muscle. (From Terzis, ref. 7, with permission.)

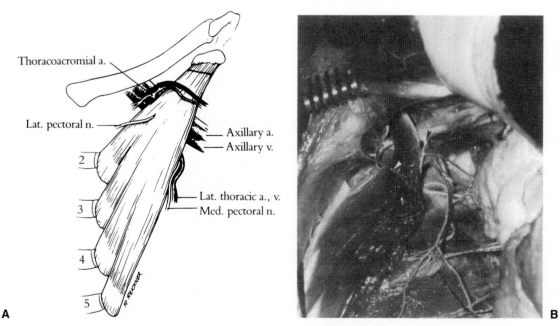

FIG. 2. A: The left pectoralis minor in situ showing the two vascular pedicles, namely, the thoracoacromial and the lateral thoracic, as they emerge around the muscle medially and laterally after they have contributed their branches. Note the *lateral pectoral branch* that uses the pectoralis minor as a passageway in its journey to the undersurface of the pectoralis major. **B:** Fresh specimen showing the left pectoralis minor in situ. The pectoralis major is elevated with the retractor. Note the two arterial branches (*black arrows*), one emerging medially and one laterally, that contribute to the blood supply of this muscle. The superior branch from the thoracoacromial trunk is a small arterial twig, and in this case, as in most cases, one has to transfer the muscle on the branch from the lateral thoracic artery. Note also the branch from the lateral pectoral nerve (*white arrow*) as it pierces through the pectoralis minor to reach the undersurface of the pectoralis major. (From Terzis, ref. 7, with permission).

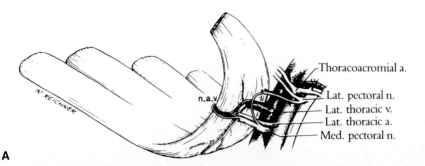

A

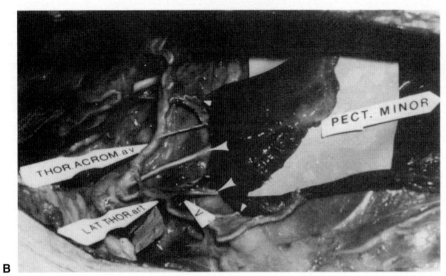

B

FIG. 3. A: The exemplary vascular and neural pattern that supplies the pectoralis minor muscle. Note that the arterial branch from the lateral thoracic artery is larger and enters the muscle more centrally. This artery is closely accompanied by the medial pectoral nerve, which is in all cases the predominant nerve supply to this muscle. The superior portion of the muscle, however, more frequently than not, receives its innervation from contributions of the lateral pectoral nerve. Note the communicating loop between medial and lateral pectoral nerves, which is a common occurrence. B: The right pectoralis minor is reflected toward its origin showing the hilar structures. Note the extensive vascular variability. In this specimen, the thoracoacromial and lateral thoracic arteries contribute two branches each to the pectoralis minor, a small and larger branch, for a total of four. Two are tiny twigs and enter the muscle at its margins (*small white arrows*). The other two branches are of larger caliber (*large white arrows*). Clinically, this muscle would have been transferred on the dominant artery (*upper large arrow*), which in this case is a branch of the thoracoacromial trunk. (From Terzis, ref. 7, with permission.)

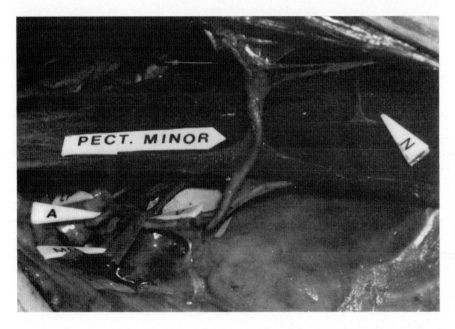

FIG. 4. The inferior margin of the pectoralis major is visualized superiorly. Note the lateral thoracic artery as it ascends from the axillary artery and after supplying the pectoralis minor passes over the lateral margin of the pectoralis minor to enter the inferior margin of the pectoralis major. This is an important surgical landmark because identification of the lateral thoracic vessels at the lower border of the pectoralis major allows easy isolation by following these vessels in a distoproximal fashion. This invariably leads to isolation of the branch of the lateral thoracic to the pectoralis minor muscle. (From Terzis, ref. 7, with permission.)

8. Placement of two holding sutures over the inferior margin of the muscle and averting the muscle so that the hilar structures become apparent
9. Identification of the medial and lateral pectoral nerves and communicating loop, tracing the pectoral nerves to gain as much length as possible, and marking with 8–0 microsutures and subsequent severance of the nerves
10. Identification and clarification of the dominant arterial supply and dominant venous drainage
11. Marking of muscle tension in situ by placing black 6–0 sutures every 1 cm along its inferior margin
12. Separating the origin of the muscle from the thoracic wall and freeing it completely (An attempt is made to incorporate as much fascia as possible in the terminal portion of the individual slips.)
13. Severance of the coracoid insertion
14. Keeping the muscle warm until the recipient site in the face is completely prepared to receive the transfer

Before microsurgical transfer, the previously prepared facial mold is placed on the face and measurements are rechecked. Then, with a preoperative videotape on a TV terminal in the operating room that shows the patient talking or smiling, 4–0 and 5–0 Mersilene sutures are placed to the alar base, upper lip, nasolabial fold, oral commissure, and lower lip. Each suture is tested to see if pulling on the suture reproduces the exact pull needed to match the animation of the contralateral normal face. Then the vascular pedicle of the muscle is severed, and the muscle is photographed as a free unit. It is brought to the face after appropriate trimming and/or debulking.

Both surgical teams are working together at this critical point in a methodical fashion with minimal ischemia time to inset the muscle in the cheek using the previously placed sutures. This usually takes from 20 to 40 minutes.

The diameter of the branch of the lateral thoracic artery that supplies the pectoralis minor ranges from 0.5 to 0.9 mm, depending on the age and vascular variability of the patient. Such a caliber is not too dissimilar to the distal end of the facial artery. If there is a question about the condition of venous drainage, the arterial clamps are released and the hilar structure is carefully observed. The vein that bleeds most profusely is the one chosen for microvascular reconnection with the facial vein.

Once the vascular anastomoses are completed, the insetting of the muscle is checked and the final tension is adjusted. If additional sutures are needed, they are provided at this point. Depending on the preoperative videotapes and the facial mold measurements, facial tension is adjusted, not to exceed the tension in situ. In most cases, 60% to 70% of in situ tension is recommended, depending on the strength of desired pull.

At completion of muscle placement, the operating microscope is brought back to the field and microneural coaptations are carried out. Usually, two cross-facial nerve grafts are placed for smile substitution. The upper graft is coapted with the lateral pectoral nerve, and the lower graft is sutured to the medial pectoral nerve.

At completion of the microneural repairs, the medial and lateral pectoral nerves are stimulated, and intraoperative videotapes of the resulting facial movements are obtained. Finally, the cheek flap is closed, and a tiny stitch is placed as a marker over the cheek to facilitate postoperative Doppler monitoring of the arterial pulse. Usually, no dressing or drains are necessary. The face lift incision is covered with antibiotic ointment, and the face is left open for direct inspection. Extubation of the patient is carried out carefully to ensure that no structures are disrupted (Figs. 5 and 6).

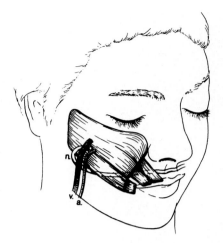

FIG. 5. The pectoralis minor after it has been transferred to the face. The placement of the muscle is such that the coracoid insertion is anchored at the zygomatic arch and preauricular area. The lower slip of the muscle is directed to the commissure or lower lip depending on the preoperative measurements. The central slips are dedicated for the upper lip and nasolabial folds. The upper slip usually ends at the alar base and is also anchored in the medial region of the infraorbital rim about 1 cm below the medial canthus. This slip is placed for nasalis substitution if the patient has a strong nasalis function in the contralateral normal face. The microneurovascular repairs are always done on the external surface of the muscle to facilitate their execution. (From Terzis, ref. 7, with permission.)

CLINICAL RESULTS

One disadvantage of the pectoralis minor flap is that because of its deep position underneath the pectoralis major, debulking cannot be done easily in situ. Thus the muscle must be debulked after harvesting and before reestablishment of its blood supply through microvascular anastomoses with recipient vessels. This increases ischemic time substantially and can have functional repercussions. A further disadvantage is the short and complex neurovascular pedicle, which makes familiarity with the vascular and inaccessible neural networks of the infraclavicular region mandatory if this flap is to be safely used.

Another disadvantage is that the vascular supply of the muscle can vary, and the surgeon should be prepared to make judgments intraoperatively about whether the lateral thoracic artery is of sufficient caliber to carry the whole muscle. If the contributing branch from the thoracoacromial trunk is of large caliber, its severance may lead to duskiness of the upper portion of the pectoralis minor (Figs. 7–10).

SUMMARY

The pectoralis minor is a highly versatile muscle that should be included in the armamentarium of surgeons who treat patients with developmental or late acquired facial paralysis. It is not a substitute for the highly specialized and densely innervated normal facial musculature, but its dual innervation, multileaf origin, and flat, thin shape make it a second-best choice for use in restoration of facial symmetry and coordinated function in cases of chronic or developmental facial paralysis.

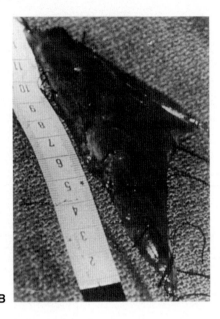 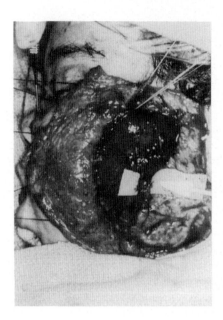

A,B

FIG. 6. **A:** The right pectoralis minor muscle was harvested using the technique described in the text. The outer surface of the muscle is shown. Note the sutures placed every 2 cm to mark the tension of the muscle in situ. **B:** The right pectoralis minor muscle has been transferred to the left cheek. The microvascular anastomoses have been completed (note *white arrow*). The final tension of the muscle will be adjusted prior to the execution of the microneural coaptations. (From Terzis, ref. 7, with permission.)

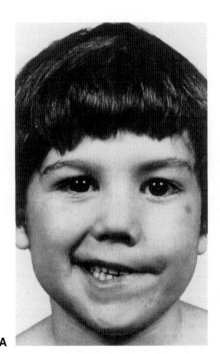 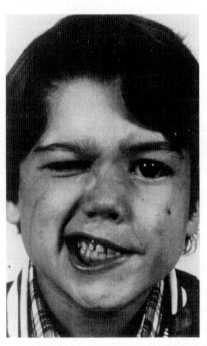

A   **B**

FIG. 7. **A:** A 6-year-old boy with developmental left facial paralysis. Note the absence of left nasolabial fold, lowering of left alar base, lack of left lower lip depressor, and weak buccinator. He also was unable to close the left eye completely and presented with 4-mm scleral show. Note small degree of "puckering" around left commissure, implying a partial paralysis. **B:** Patient is shown here 1 year after three cross-facial (sural) nerve grafts were placed in his face and just prior to the free pectoralis minor transfer to the left face. Direct neurotization through the cross-facial nerves accounts for the increased animation present in the left face. However, this is never enough to restore symmetry. (In 1982, I used to make a nasolabial fold incision to facilitate placement of the cross-facial nerve graft. I have stopped using this incision because the resulting nasolabial scar was not acceptable to me. This has made preparation of the recipient site somewhat more difficult and lengthy, but I think it has paid off now, because there are no visible scars on the anterior face.) (From Terzis, ref. 7, with permission.)

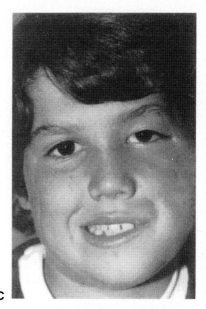
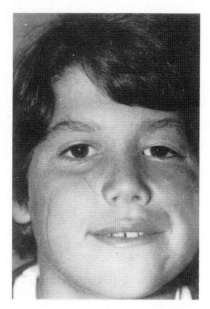
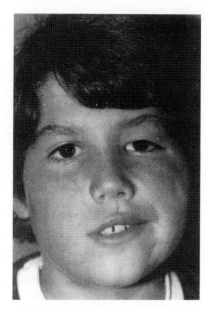

A–C

FIG. 8. A–C: Patient is seen here at 10 years of age and 3 years after microneurovascular transfer of the right pectoralis minor to the left cheek. As is the case with most developmental facial paralysis patients, he has completely synchronous and coordinated animation of the left paralyzed face with the right normal face (B). In addition, the patient is demonstrating a phenomenon that depicts an intriguing degree of plasticity, since he is able to voluntarily move the right (A) or the left side of his face independently (C) despite the fact that both sides of his face are controlled by his right cerebral cortex (i.e., peripheral fibers of the right facial nucleus innervate the right facial musculature as well as cross through the cross-facial nerve grafts to supply innervation to the free pectoralis minor transplanted to the left face). (From Terzis, ref. 7, with permission.)

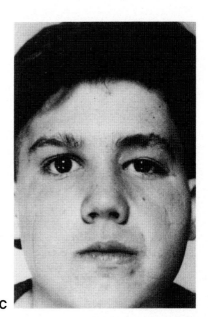
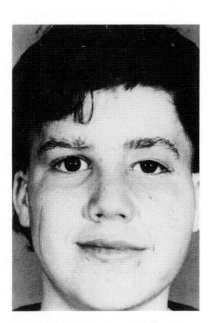
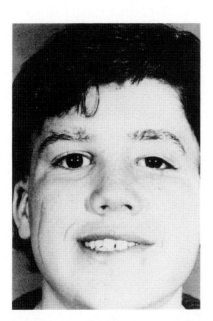

A–C

FIG. 9. Patient is shown here in 1988 at age 13 (i.e., 5 years following microneurovascular transfer of the right pectoralis minor to the left face). A: In repose, (B) showing a small grin, and (C) a broader smile. (From Terzis, ref. 7, with permission.)

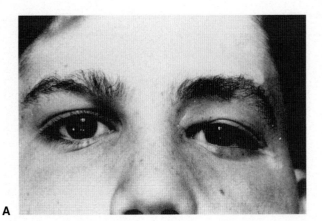
A

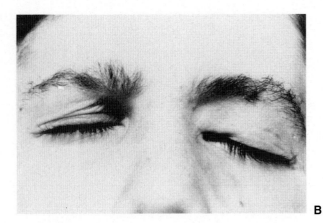
B

FIG. 10. **A,B:** The upper slip of the pectoralis minor, elongated with the incorporation of fascia from its costal origin, was split and placed in a preseptal position to substitute for the paralyzed left eye sphincter. This segment of the muscle was innervated by a separate cross-facial nerve graft to the lateral pectoral nerve. The patient has independent eye movements that are synchronized only with his contralateral eye as well as complete restoration of his blink reflex in the left eye, which was previously delayed and incomplete. There is no evidence of synkinesis with the left lower face. Patient is shown here in close-up with the eyes open (**A**) and closed (**B**). Minimal revisions are planned to correct the excess skin that is shown in the medial aspect of the left upper eyelid. (From Terzis, ref. 7, with permission.)

References

1. Harii K, Ohmori K, Torii S. Free gracilis muscle transplantation with microneurovascular anastomoses for the treatment of facial paralysis. *Plast Reconstr Surg* 1976;57:133.
2. Terzis JK, Sweet RC, Dykes RW, Williams HB. Recovery of function in free muscle transplants using microneurovascular anastomoses. *J Hand Surg* 1978;3:37.
3. O'Brien BMcC, Franklin JD, Morrison WA. Cross-facial nerve grafts and microneurovascular free muscle transfer for long-established facial palsy. *Br J Plast Surg* 1980;33:202.
4. Manktelow RT, McKee NH, Vettese T. An anatomic study of the pectoralis major muscle as related to functioning free muscle transplantation. *Plast Reconstr Surg* 1980;6:610.
5. Mayou BJ, Watson JSD, Harrison DH. Free microvascular and microneurovascular transfer of the extensor digitorum brevis muscle for the treatment of unilateral facial paralysis. *Br J Plast Surg* 1981;34:362.
6. Terzis JK, Manktelow RT. Pectoralis minor: A new concept in facial reanimation. *Plast Surg Forum* 1982;5:106.
7. Teris JK. Pectoralis minor: A unique muscle for correction of facial palsy. *Plast Reconstr Surg* 1989;83:767.

CHAPTER 154 ■ LIP-SWITCH ABBÉ FLAP FOR PHILTRUM

D. R. MILLARD, JR.

The lip-switch flap is popularly known as the Abbé flap (1). The technique involves a composite flap of lip tissue, including skin, muscle, and mucosa, based on one coronary vessel. It has been found to live on a narrow mucosal pedicle (2).

INDICATIONS

In unilateral cleft lip, when the initial surgery has destroyed natural landmarks and the discarding of tissue has tightened the upper lip, not only is there a lack of soft tissue, but the constricting effect on growth of underlying structures compounds the defect. It will be noted that the unrestrained lower lip will show a relatively severe protrusion. The lip-switch flap will, of course, reduce the lower lip slack as it releases the upper lip tightness.

FLAP DESIGN AND DIMENSIONS

The flap can be taken from either lip, but it is most commonly switched from the lower to the upper lip (3–5). Its shape has been varied in form from triangular to rectangular to square to even more odd and irregular configurations. The shape and size of the flap depend, of course, on the defect to which the flap is to be transposed, bearing in mind that it need not necessarily be the exact size of the apparent defect. When the flap is taken out of one lip to be inserted into the other, the donor lip is reduced. This may lessen the amount needed for the opposite lip if normal lip proportions are to be maintained.

It was the previous routine of reconstructive surgeons to insert the lip-switch flap into the upper lip scar. This improved the tissue deficit, but it did not take aesthetic landmarks into consideration, and it resulted in a patchwork effect that seemed to fall short of possibilities.

In postoperative unilateral cleft lip patients in whom the philtrum and cupid's bow had been violated or destroyed, it seemed more logical to ignore the unilateral scar and to use the lip-switch flap to create a new philtrum. Accomplishing this means using a midline releasing incision in the upper lip and transposing a philtrum-shaped flap from the lower lip (Fig. 1A). To be truly philtrum-shaped, the flap should be

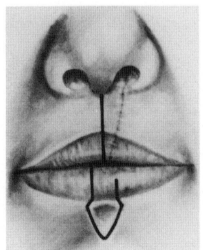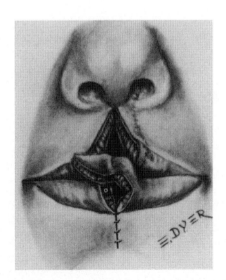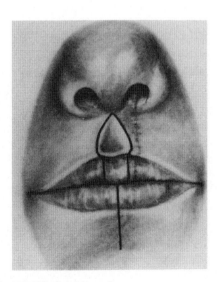

A–C

FIG. 1. **A:** When no philtrum or cupid's bow is present in a postoperative unilateral cleft, then ignore the unilateral scar and divide the upper lip in the midline. Take a shield-shaped lower lip flap from the midline to carry whatever dimple is present to the upper philtrum. **B:** Composite flap based on coronary vessel and small amount of mucosa is being transposed 180 degrees. **C:** Construction of a midline philtrum camouflages the unilateral deformity and scar.

formed somewhat like a shield, and if it is fashioned slightly narrower at the mucocutaneous ridge before it swells into a shield, it also will help to effect a cupid's bow. It should be taken from the middle of the lower lip, where often a dimple is present. This can be spared in the lower lip, but it is most desirable as a philtrum dimple in the upper lip. The flap is transposed 180 degrees (Fig. 1B).

The same aesthetic shape of flap is applicable in secondary bilateral clefts when the scarred prolabium must be shifted into the columella to release the depressed nasal tip. Obviously, a midline shield-shaped lower lip flap is an ideal replacement for the upper lip philtrum.

OPERATIVE TECHNIQUE

Both the donor area and the flap insertion in the upper lip are closed in three layers: mucosa, muscle, and skin. After 7 to 10 days, the pedicle is divided and the upper and lower lip are revised at the division area (Fig. 1C).

CLINICAL RESULTS

Of course, three new scars have been added, but remarkably enough, they are not noticeable because they form the boundaries of the philtrum of the upper lip and only a midline seam of the lower lip. The reconstruction of the philtrum reduces the dominance of the old unilateral cleft scar, rendering it less noticeable. Because it has been relaxed, it can be better revised or even excised totally up to one side of the philtrum flap.

SUMMARY

A midline shield-shaped lower lip flap is an ideal replacement for the upper lip philtrum.

References

1. Abbé R. A new plastic operation for the relief of deformity due to double harelip. *Med Rec* 1898;53:477.
2. Millard DR Jr., McLaughlin, CA. Abbé flap on mucosal pedicle. *Ann Plast Surg* 1979;3:544.
3. Blair VP, Letterman GS. The role of the switched lower lip flap in upper lip reconstruction. *Plast Reconstr Surg* 1950;5:1.
4. Millard DR Jr., Composite lip flaps and grafts in secondary cleft deformities. *Br J Plast Surg* 1964;17:1.
5. Millard DR Jr. *Cleft craft: the evolution of its surgery,* Vol. 2. Boston: Little, Brown, 1977;636–653, 684–710.

CHAPTER 155 ■ LOWER-LIP SANDWICH ABBÉ SKIN FLAP TO UPPER LIP

I. T. JACKSON

EDITORIAL COMMENT

The results that the author shows are outstanding. We wonder whether contraction of the upper lip also occurs when a small Abbé flap is transferred to the upper lip and the orbicularis is sutured to the Abbé flap on either side.

The aim of the cross-lip operation is to improve the appearance of the lip by releasing the tightness, establishing lip balance, and restoring the cupid's bow. In addition, the function of the upper lip should not be compromised; ideally, it should be improved.

INDICATIONS

If there has been a poor primary lip repair with sacrifice of much tissue, the upper lip is tight. This condition can vary from being slight and acceptable to severe, with gross lip imbalance and an unacceptable deformity. There may be central shortness with a whistling deformity and incisor show. The lip imbalance is accentuated by redundancy of the lower lip and, in some cases, maxillary retrusion. This condition is due entirely to skin sacrifice and not to muscle deficiency.

To achieve good upper lip function, orbicularis continuity is essential. A lip may be aesthetically acceptable at rest but not when functioning if that continuity is not established. From personal experience, and according to the literature, it has been noted that the prolabium has no muscle fibers in the complete bilateral cleft. Similarly, in the unilateral cleft, the orbicularis is abnormally inserted (1,2). If the muscle is not correctly dissected out and reconstructed, the coordinated upper lip function is poor.

In severely mutilated lips requiring a cross-lip flap, one can be sure that the level of sophistication in the original repair was low, and it is unlikely that any muscle reconstruction was performed. That being so, the orbicularis is probably intact and can be used to reconstruct muscular continuity in the

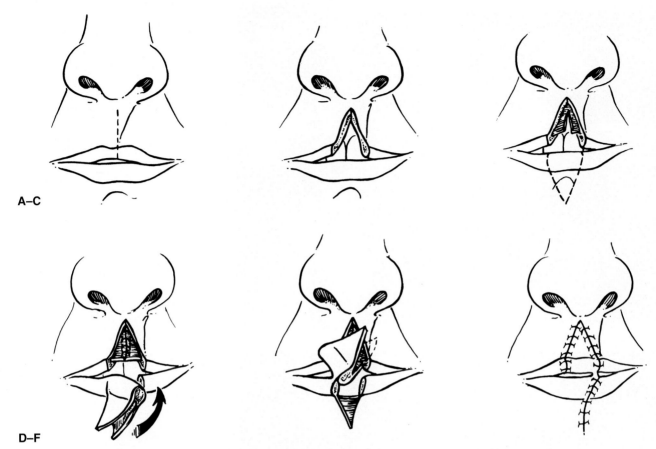

A–C

D–F

FIG. 1. **A:** The midline incision in the upper lip is shown. The junction of skin and vermilion is tattooed with Bonney's blue. **B:** The upper lip is divided completely. **C:** The orbicularis muscles have been widely dissected and can now be comfortably approximated in the midline. The design of the Abbé flap is shown in the lower lip. **D:** The sandwich flap is elevated from the lower lip, leaving the orbicularis of the lower lip intact. **E:** The flap is swung round in such a way that the mucosa is positioned behind the orbicularis and the skin in front of the reconstructed orbicularis. **F:** The flap is sutured in position, and the lower lip defect is closed in layers.

upper lip. The requirements for cover of the reconstructed muscle are skin, vermilion, and mucosa; this is the sandwich cross-lip flap (3).

In the past, cross-lip flaps were lifeless curtains that moved in a secondary fashion when the lateral segments moved. The sandwich cross-lip flap is a functional flap, allowing one to sidestep the question of function in cross-lip flaps, which has its proponents (4,5) and its antagonists (6,7). Other advantages of this procedure are early pedicle division, a clinical impression of an improved lower lip scar, and the flexibility of having the mucosa and the skin separated, allowing for variation in design in the two layers.

FLAP DESIGN AND DIMENSIONS

The three main faults seen in Abbé flap designs are that they are too large, too long, and too square. The flap should be triangular like the philtrum, and it should be as wide and as long as a normal philtrum. It should end in the lip and not be introduced into the nasal floor or columella, as has been suggested (8), except in very exceptional circumstances. The flap always must be inserted into the midline of the upper lip, even if it means disregarding old scars. In some cases, where bulk is required in the lower half of the lip and a cupid's bow is to be established, one should not hesitate to insert a flap of half the lip height.

OPERATIVE TECHNIQUE

Preoperatively, the discontinuity of the orbicularis is demonstrated by asking the patient to purse his or her lips. In the unilateral case, the upper lip is divided completely in the midline. In the bilateral case, the old scars are excised and the prolabium and underlying subcutaneous tissue are used to effect columellar lengthening (Figs. 1 and 2).

The orbicularis muscle bellies are dissected out from the skin and from their periosteal attachments at the alar base and columellar areas. These now can be rotated downward and advanced. It should be noted that there is often brisk bleeding just lateral to the alar base, and attention must be paid to this. The muscles are then sutured together with nonabsorbable suture material. The complex anatomy of the orbicularis (9) cannot be duplicated, but a secure anastomosis is desirable. The muscular sphincter has now been reconstituted, and the skin and mucosal deficiency can be measured.

The dimensions are transferred onto the lower lip. It is helpful to tattoo the mucocutaneous junction on both sides of every incision; this makes for easier approximation later in the procedure. The skin and mucosa are incised down to the orbicularis; on the nonpedicle side, the labial vessels are cut through. This indicates their position, and thus on the side of the pedicle these vessels are virtually skeletonized. The skin and mucosa are now elevated from the orbicularis, the vermilion is divided from it transversely, and the flap is now free on its pedicle. Rotation is

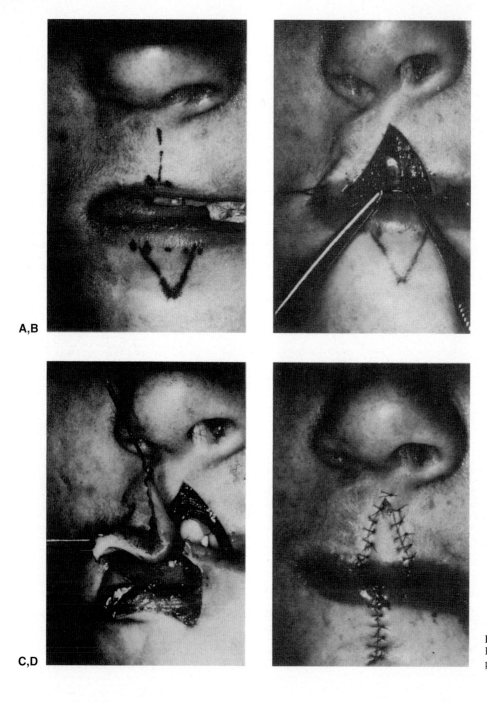

A,B

C,D

FIG. 2. A–D: The operative steps as shown in Fig. 1. (From Jackson and Soutar, ref. 3, with permission.)

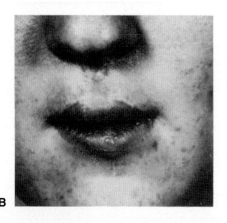

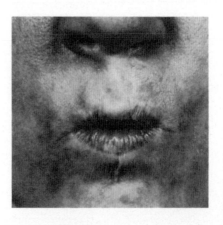

A,B

FIG. 3. A: The lip, having been augmented with a sandwich Abbé switch flap. B: The functional integrity of the upper lip is illustrated. (From Jackson and Soutar, ref. 3, with permission.)

accomplished with facility, and the skin and mucosa are sutured in position. The lower lip is closed in layers.

Division of the flap can safely be performed at 3 to 5 days under local anesthesia.

CLINICAL RESULTS

Since using this technique in most patients requiring a cross-lip flap, the results have been satisfactory from an aesthetic and functional point of view (Fig. 3).

SUMMARY

The cross-lip-sandwich flap can be effectively used to improve both the cosmetic and functional aspects of an upper lip deformity.

References

1. Estlander JA. En ny operationsmetod att atersrall en forstord lapp ellekkind. *Finsak Lak-Sall SK Handl* 1872;14:1.
2. Fara MD, Smahel J. Postoperative follow-up of restitution procedures in the orbicularis oris muscle after operation for complete bilateral cleft of the lip. *Plast Reconstr Surg* 1967;40:13.
3. Jackson IT, Soutar DS. The sandwich Abbé flap in secondary cleft lip deformity. *Plast Reconstr Surg* 1980;66:38.
4. Smith JW. The anatomical and physiological acclimation of tissue transplanted by the lip switch technique. *Plast Reconstr Surg* 1960;26:40.
5. Thompson N, Pollard AC. Motor function in Abbé flaps. *Br J Plast Surg* 1961;14:66.
6. Isaksson I, Johanson B, Peterson I, Sellden U. Electromyographic study of the Abbé and fan flaps. *Acta Chir Scand* 1962;123:343.
7. Schuh FD, Crikelair GF, Cosman B. A critical appraisal of the Abbé flap in secondary cleft lip deformity. *Br J Plast Surg* 1970;23:142.
8. McGregor IA. The Abbé flap: its use in single and double lip clefts. *Br J Plast Surg* 1963;16:46.
9. Briedis J, Jackson IT. The anatomy of the philtrum: observations made on dissection in the normal lip. *Br J Plast Surg* 1980;34:128.

CHAPTER 156 ■ LIP FLEUR-DE-LIS FLAP

D. R. MILLARD, JR.

EDITORIAL COMMENT

This is a classic technique that attempted to replace the lost central portion of the lip. Such substantial deformities were created when the premaxilla or the columella was sacrificed as part of a cleft-lip repair, a sacrifice that fortunately is no longer made.

Through cancer ablation, radiation, or secondary congenital cleft lip deformities, a relative side-to-side tightness of a lip often occurs. There also may be deficiency in the free border vermilion. One lip may be tight and thin, with only a minimum of vermilion visible. The opposite lip may be loose, with voluminous vermilion in view (Fig. 1). In such circumstances, the lip fleur-de-lis flap has been found to be effective in two planes (1).

INDICATIONS

By extending the standard lip-switch flap with lateral mucosal flaps, it is possible to double its dimension of effectiveness. The standard lip-switch portion of the flap will reduce the relative slack of the donor lip while it releases the tightness of the opposite lip.

Simultaneously, the mucosal extensions on the lip-switch flap, taken out of the voluminous vermilion of one lip, are transported and inserted behind the thin free-border vermilion

of the other lip. This has a balancing effect because the excessive vermilion is reduced while simultaneously bolstering the deficient vermilion of the opposite lip.

FLAP DESIGN AND DIMENSIONS

The design of this double-dimension flap depends on the coronary vessels. The composite vertical lip-switch flap is marked, with its horizontal mucosal extensions placed along the coronary vessel just posterior to the free border of the lip. This places the horizontal scar just out of sight (Fig. 2A).

OPERATIVE TECHNIQUE

The order of progression in the cutting of this flap is vital. The mucosal extension away from the future coronary vessel pedicle can pick up the coronary vessel in its body. Then the standard lip-switch flap is cut through and through on that side. The through-and-through incision on the other side of the lip-switch flap is carried up near the coronary vessel, crossing the mucocutaneous junction in front, but preserving the coronary vessel and cutting the other mucosal extension superficial to the coronary vessel (Fig. 2B). This completes the development of the fleur-de-lis, which, with its mucosal limbs, will pivot 180 degrees on the coronary vessel to be transposed into two axes of the opposite lip.

The opposite lip is prepared for the fleur-de-lis by releasing it vertically at the chosen position and by incising the

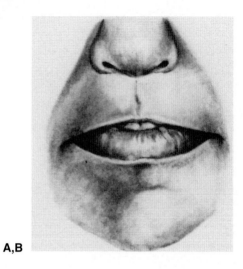

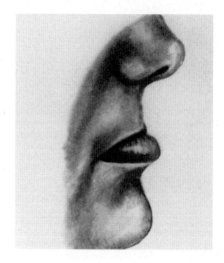

A,B

FIG. 1. **A:** Tight, thin upper lip. **B:** Loose, full lower lip.

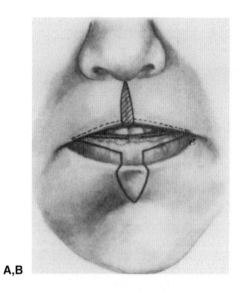

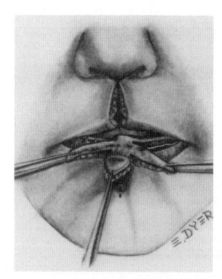

A,B

FIG. 2. **A:** Fleur-de-lis flap marked on the lower lip along the coronary vessel. Upper lip marked for scar excision and posterior mucosal release along the free border. **B:** Fleur-de-lis flap cut, based on coronary vessel on the left.

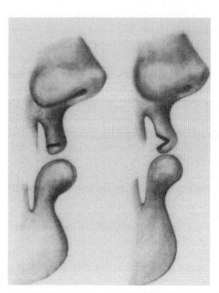

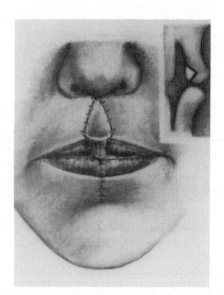

A,B

FIG. 3. **A:** Thin vermilion of the upper lip released by a posterior mucosal incision. **B:** Fleur-de-lis flap transposed into the upper lip with mucosal wings fitting into posterior releasing incisions in the mucosa.

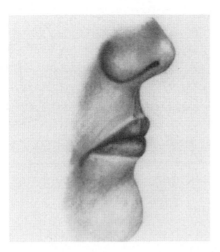

FIG. 4. After division of the pedicle, the upper and lower lip relationship has been improved in two planes.

vermilion horizontally, just posterior to its free border, to allow turndown of mucosa (Fig. 3A). Into this double release, the fleur-de-lis is transposed with a rather flamboyant fit. The lip-switch flap fills the vertical defect, as the mucosal limbs slide in behind the mucosal turndown flaps (Fig. 3B).

SUMMARY

The lip fleur-de-lis flap can release and thicken a thin, tight lip while tightening and thinning the opposite loose, thick lip to the mutual benefit of both (Fig. 4).

Reference

1. Millard DR Jr. A lip fleur-de-lis flap. *Plast Reconstr Surg* 1964;34:34.

CHAPTER 157 ■ ONE-STAGE LIP-SWITCH

H. OHTSUKA

By modifying the Abbé lip-switch procedure for repair of full-thickness defects or deformities of the upper lip (1), a one-stage lip-switch technique was developed (2). This modification obviates the 1- to 2-week waiting period required for separation of the vascular pedicle.

INDICATIONS

The one-stage procedure shortens the time required, thus ameliorating communication problems and discomfort in patients with significant disproportion between the upper and lower lip, especially in unilateral or bilateral cleft-lip deformities. An arterialized one-stage lip-switch operation can be rather risky compared to the traditional Abbé flap. Indications should be limited to properly selected patients. Various degrees of venous congestion or even necrosis in the traditional flap are not rare (3). Therefore, a sufficient quantity of submucosal

tissue must be preserved for the long pedicle of a one-stage lip-switch flap.

ANATOMY

Asymmetries or variations in lower-vermilion vascularization have been described (3,4), including cases with an equal distribution of the bilateral inferior labial arteries; predominant inferior artery of one side; the inferior labial artery present only on one side; or the inferior labial artery present as the terminal branch of the sublabial artery. The inferior labial artery may arise from a common trunk at the level of the labial commissure or directly from the superior labial artery (4,5). In any case, numerous branches and terminals of the inferior labial, sublabial, mental, and submental arteries constitute an abundant labial network.

The facial artery and inferior and superior labial arteries run close to the oral mucous membrane. The main routes of these arteries can be palpated manually between the fingers. A Doppler evaluation is also of value for the precise determination of vessel location both preoperatively and intraoperatively. The venae comitantes do not always parallel the arterial routes and are sometimes absent despite the rich venous network in the submucosa concentrating near the arteries (2,3). In addition, the proper arteries and veins may meander, especially in older people.

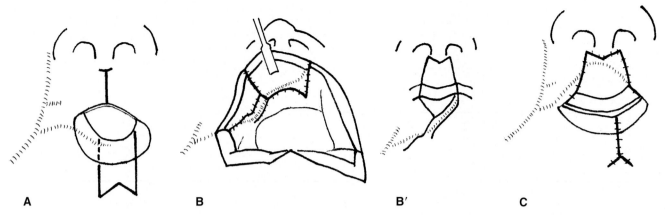

FIG. 1. Diagram of operative procedure. **A:** Preoperative design. Facial and lower labial arteries are illustrated. **B:** Mucosal closure of the transferred flap and pedicle. Modification of closure is shown in **B'**. **C:** Completion of the procedure.

FLAP DESIGN AND DIMENSIONS

The most significant point in the success of this procedure lies in the route of venous drainage. If the inferior labial vein runs exactly along the labial artery as a vena comitans, the procedure is not risky; however, the vein does not always parallel the artery (3), and it is difficult to identify and isolate without damage in some instances. A 7- to 10-mm-wide (or more) mucous pedicle flap, including the inferior labial artery, is recommended as the vascular pedicle for flap survival.

About a quarter to a half of the lower lip is used, depending on assessment of the defect volume in the upper lip. To obtain a good quantity of submucosal tissue and to avoid shortness of the pedicle from the lower lip, the flap must be designed to the side, with the requirements of the upper-lip defect in mind, instead of merely opposing the defect (3).

OPERATIVE TECHNIQUE

An inverted M-shaped lower-lip flap is raised as usual, except for the long pedicle side (Fig. 1); a V-shaped mucosal incision is sometimes recommended (Fig. 1B'). The flap pedicle is extended to the commissure along the inferior labial artery,

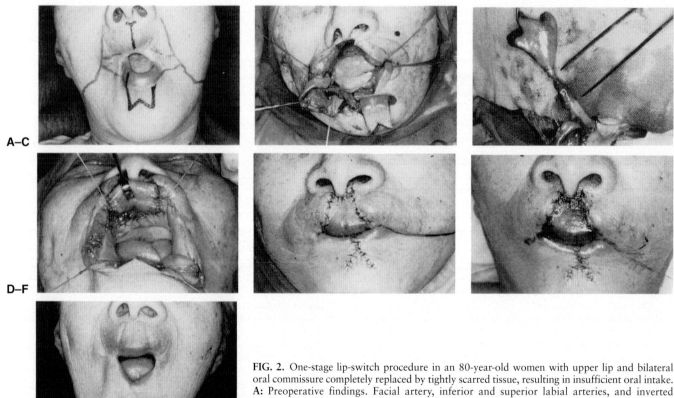

FIG. 2. One-stage lip-switch procedure in an 80-year-old women with upper lip and bilateral oral commissure completely replaced by tightly scarred tissue, resulting in insufficient oral intake. **A:** Preoperative findings. Facial artery, inferior and superior labial arteries, and inverted M-shaped lip flap are depicted. **B:** Raised flap with long, narrow pedicle, including inferior labial artery. **C:** Deepithelialized vascular pedicle shown between forceps. **D:** Completion of mucosal closure of the transferred lower-lip flap and pedicle. **E:** Completion of the procedure. **F:** Twenty-four hours postoperatively. **G:** One month later. (From Ohtsuka, ref. 2, with permission.)

including a thin layer of orbicularis oris muscle about 6 to 8 mm wide. A small amount of tissue in the upper lip, especially near the commissure, may be excised to accommodate the pedicle. Deepithelialization of mucosal tissue may be performed in half of the vascular pedicle on the lip flap side. In this situation, the distal portion of the flap is incised a little closer to the mucous membrane to pass the deepithelialized vascular pedicle through it.

Three-layer fine sutures in the upper lip and loose fixation of the flap pedicle are carried out, followed by primary closure of the flap donor site and the incised site of the vascular pedicle (Fig. 1C). Most cases of venous stasis are reversible with drainage if a nourishing labial artery (or labial coronary arterial arch) is not injured (3). Several dressing changes per day with wet gauze are used (2). Thermographic evaluation may help in postoperative assessment of flap circulation.

CLINICAL RESULTS

Postoperative results were excellent in the case illustrated (Fig. 2). The elderly patient presented with many accompanying cardiovascular and mental problems. During the first 9 postoperative days, mild pulmonary congestion, slight anemia, hypokalemia, arrhythmia, and an unsettled mental state were present. Postoperative venous congestion was treated by

removal of several sutures and insertion of drains. Marginal bleeding was controlled by frequent dressing changes with wet gauze.

SUMMARY

The arterialized one-stage lip-switch procedure can be useful in repairing upper-lip defects and disproportions between upper and lower lips, despite some additional risks compared with the traditional Abbé flap. Careful selection of patients for the procedure is suggested.

References

1. Abbé R. A new plastic operation for the relief of deformity due to double harelip. *Med Rec* 1898;53:477.
2. Ohtsuka H. One-stage lip-switch operation. *Plast Reconstr Surg* 1985;76:613.
3. Hu H, Song R, Sun G. One-stage inferior labial flap and its pertinent anatomic study. *Plast Reconstr Surg* 1993;91:618.
4. Midy D, Mauruc B, Vergnes P, et al. A contribution to the study of the facial artery, its branches and anastomoses: application to the anatomic vascular bases of facial flaps. *Surg Radiol Anat* 1986;8:99.
5. Kamijyo Y. Arterial and venous systems in the head and neck. In: *Oral Anatomy (angiology)*. Vol. 3: Tokyo: Anatomu Co., 1966;462–463, 551 (in Japanese).

CHAPTER 158 ■ SUBCUTANEOUS PEDICLE FLAPS TO THE LIP

J. N. BARRON* AND M. N. SAAD

The use of subcutaneous pedicle flaps in lip reconstruction is limited, partly because of the multitude of excellent standard flaps available and partly because of the difficulty in achieving a mobile lip unless functioning orbicularis muscle is incorporated in the flap when repairing full-thickness defects (1). For these reasons, subcutaneous pedicle flaps usually are limited only to skin defects (2–4). Platysma musculocutaneous flaps from the neck are excellent for reconstructing the lower lip (see Chap. 170).

FLAP DESIGN AND DIMENSIONS

In men, it is important to repair lip defects with a hair-bearing flap, and whenever possible, bulky mushroomed flaps should be avoided, especially when replacing a concave surface, such as the mentolabial groove. The main sources of subcutaneous

pedicle flaps for the repair of lip defects are the nasolabial fold, the chin, and the lip itself.

Flaps from the Nasolabial Fold

The nasolabial fold provides an ample supply of tissue with a good color and texture match. It has a robust blood supply based on the facial artery, and it leaves a linear scar at the donor site. In reconstruction of the upper lip, subcutaneous pedicle flaps should be based inferiorly, and in suitable patients, bilateral flaps can be used to resurface most of the upper lip. Fig. 1 illustrates a defect of the upper lip repaired with an inferiorly based nasolabial subcutaneous pedicle flap.

Flaps from the Chin

Lining defects of the lower lip can be repaired by flaps raised on the chin in hairless patients and based on the subcutaneous

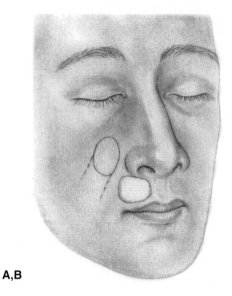
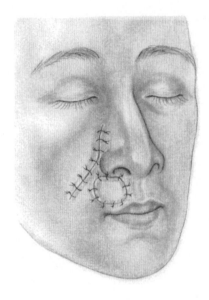

A,B

FIG. 1. **A:** Upper lip defect. Planned repair with an inferiorly based nasolabial flap. **B:** Flap inset and donor site sutured.

tissue at the edge of the defect. The flap then is turned in and sutured to the mucosal defect. The skin defect is repaired with a standard flap.

Flaps from the Lip

Small defects of the lip can be corrected by subcutaneous pedicle flaps from the lip itself. This is particularly well illustrated in the correction of the "whistle tip" deformity seen in cases of

bilateral cleft lips (Fig. 2). Two horizontal V-Y flaps based on subcutaneous pedicles are advanced medially and sutured to each other to provide the required fullness in the midline.

OPERATIVE TECHNIQUE

The general principles, design, and operative technique illustrating the use of subcutaneous pedicle flaps are described in Chapter 44.

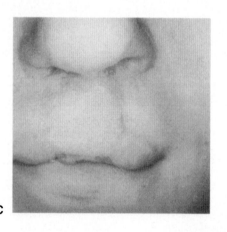
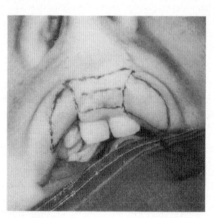
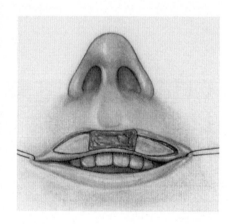

A–C

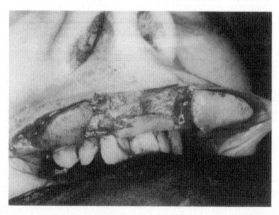
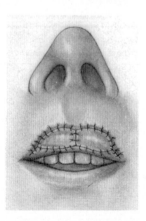
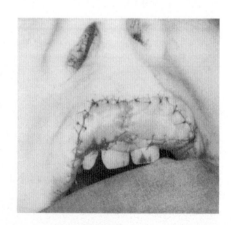

D–F

FIG. 2. **A:** "Whistle tip" deformity in a repaired bilateral cleft lip. **B:** The median segment is deepithelialized. The two flaps, based on anterior or posterior subcutaneous pedicles, are raised. **C–F:** The V–Y flaps are sutured in position, providing the required fullness in the midline.

SUMMARY

Subcutaneous pedicle skin flaps are indicated for lip defects that involve skin or mucosal lining only. Muscle loss should be replaced by other techniques.

References

1. Karapandžić M. Reconstruction of lip defects by local arterial flaps. *Br J Plast Surg* 1974;27:93.
2. Barron JN, Emmett AJJ. The subcutaneous pedicle flaps. *Br J Plast Surg* 1965;18:51.
3. Spira M, Gerow FJ, Hardy SB. Subcutaneous pedicle flaps on the face. *Br J Plast Surg* 1974;27:258.
4. Chongchet V. Subcutaneous pedicle flaps for reconstruction of the lining of the lip and cheek. *Br J Plast Surg* 1977;30:38.

CHAPTER 159 ■ ADVANCEMENT MUSCULOCUTANEOUS AND SKIN FLAPS FOR UPPER LIP REPAIR

E. J. VAN DORPE

Tissue replacement in the central part of the upper lip, the area defined laterally by a vertical line from the alar base to the free margin of the lip, is described. The flaps used are based on the principle of lip advancement by perialar crescentic excision (1–3).

INDICATIONS

Even small skin lesions in the central upper lip region may be difficult to treat by simple elliptical excision without disturbing the anatomic relationship between lip margin, alar base, and philtral ridge. Vertical ellipse excision cannot be done if the lesion is adjacent to the alar base. If the lesion lies between the alar base and the lip margin, an elliptical excision will produce vertical lengthening of the lip when it is sutured. The lengthening is caused by the approximation of the curved edges, making a straight line that is longer than the axis of the ellipse.

Repair of defects larger than half the central upper lip with this method using bilateral flaps is not recommended because it results in a significant discrepancy in length between upper and lower lips. The perialar flap can be used to cover any larger defect in the columella, the nostril floor, or both.

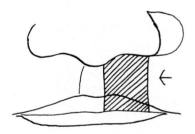

FIG. 2. The size of the perialar crescent is determined by the extent of the advancement to be achieved.

OPERATIVE TECHNIQUE

For smaller defects, lengthening of the lip may be avoided by using a small advancement flap with perialar crescentic excision (Fig. 1). It may be considered an elliptical excision, with its upper part shifted laterally to avoid the nostril.

When the defect is larger (up to half the central upper lip), with involvement of muscle, a vertical segment of the lip is excised down to vermilion (Fig. 2). If possible, the mucosa is

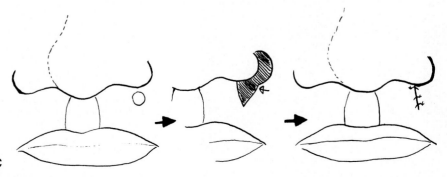

FIG. 1. A–C: Skin lesion of the upper lip adjacent to the nostril. V excision and perialar crescent. Closure after undermining of the lateral flap.

A–C

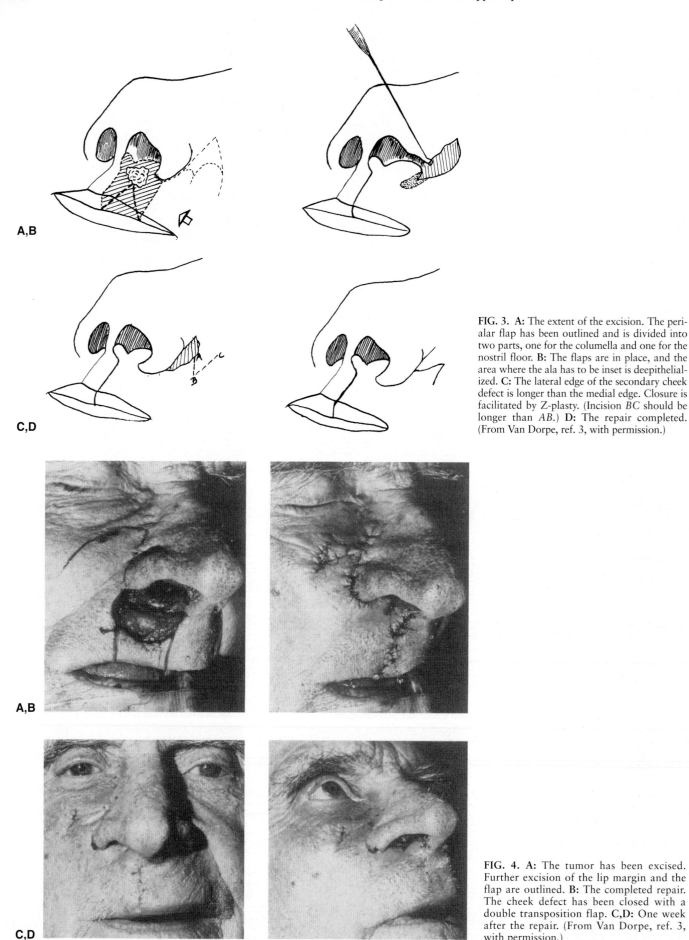

FIG. 3. A: The extent of the excision. The perialar flap has been outlined and is divided into two parts, one for the columella and one for the nostril floor. **B:** The flaps are in place, and the area where the ala has to be inset is deepithelialized. **C:** The lateral edge of the secondary cheek defect is longer than the medial edge. Closure is facilitated by Z-plasty. (Incision *BC* should be longer than *AB*.) **D:** The repair completed. (From Van Dorpe, ref. 3, with permission.)

FIG. 4. A: The tumor has been excised. Further excision of the lip margin and the flap are outlined. **B:** The completed repair. The cheek defect has been closed with a double transposition flap. **C,D:** One week after the repair. (From Van Dorpe, ref. 3, with permission.)

excised as an inverted V. Lateral lip advancement is obtained by perialar crescentic excision. If the defect extends into the nostril floor and columella, the perialar skin is preserved to reconstruct these areas (Fig. 3). It is raised as a caudally based flap, with its width at the base equal to the width of the lip defect.

The alar base then is detached from the lip and cheek, the lateral segment of lip is moved medially to close the defect, and suturing is done in three layers. Care should be taken to set in the alar base at the correct position, which is determined by measuring up from the columella laterally and from the lip margin inferiorly. Often the ala will have to be partly inset across the base of the perialar flap. In this case, the area where ala must be inset is deepithelialized to preserve the blood supply to the flap.

The lateral edge of the secondary cheek defect is often longer than the medial edge. Closure is facilitated by a double transposition flap (Figs. 3C, D and 4).

SUMMARY

Defects of the upper lip can be closed with a good cosmetic result by using various modifications of lip advancement and perialar crescentic excision.

References

1. Dieffenbach JF. *Die Operatieve Chirurgie.* Leipzig: Brockhaus, 1845;423.
2. Webster JP. Crescentic perialar cheek excision for upper lip flap advancement, with a short history of upper lip repair. *Plast Reconstr Surg* 1955;16:434.
3. Van Dorpe EJ. Simultaneous repair of the upper lip and nostril floor after tumour excisions. *Plast Reconstr Surg* 1977;60:381.

CHAPTER 160 ■ SUBMENTAL HAIR-BEARING SKIN FLAP TO UPPER LIP

H. SCHAUPP

EDITORIAL COMMENT

The finesse of this procedure is that it produces a hair-bearing upper lip that has normal-looking hair in the proper direction, as opposed to an island temporal hair-bearing scalp flap that more closely resembles a Groucho Marx moustache. This procedure could be applied to female patients in a similar manner if a hairless resurfacing of the upper lip is required, but it should be limited to severe cases.

Donor sites for hair-bearing skin flaps used in the reconstruction of the upper lip are the scalp (bitemporal flaps), the cheeks (advancement flaps), and the cervical and submental regions (unilateral or bilateral pedicle flaps) (1). The submental flap is preferable for defects of the upper lip and adjacent cheeks in which at least part of the labial mucosa is preserved.

INDICATIONS

In reconstructing the upper lip, the aims are (a) to provide the upper lip with sufficient skin and subcutaneous tissue to cover defects after incision or elevation of scarred and retracted lip tissue; (b) to replace hairless, ugly scars with hair-bearing skin in males; and (c) to lengthen the columella if necessary.

In patients with a cleft lip/nose deformity, the submental hair-bearing skin flap can correct the nasal malformation and improve respiratory function as well as allow active movement of the upper lip. Other indications are large scars and deformities after injuries of the lip and adjoining cheek and defects after tumor resection.

The skin of the submental region is quite similar to that of the lip. As a substitute, it is aesthetically well accepted, even in women. In men, the new moustache is an additional excellent camouflage. Most of our male patients, unable to hide the deformity preoperatively, proudly presented with a moustache postoperatively.

An important advantage of the flap is the hidden donor site, which normally contains a surplus of skin, and a fine scar that lies within relaxed skin tension lines. In most cases, the linear submental scar is scarcely noticeable. The shape of the untubed flap preserves skin and, in addition, makes a skin graft unnecessary (2).

OPERATIVE TECHNIQUE

Between mastoid and submental regions on both sides, 2-cm-wide handle-like flaps containing skin, subcutaneous tissue, and fat are excised and elevated (Fig. 1B). The resulting wounds under the flaps are closed after mobilizing the adjacent skin, and the untubed strips are covered with nonadhering dressing.

The midline "pillar" (which should be wider than the upper lip to cope with shrinkage) is incised, delayed, and finely transected about the tenth day in two to three sessions until the flap can be swung up to the upper lip to cover the

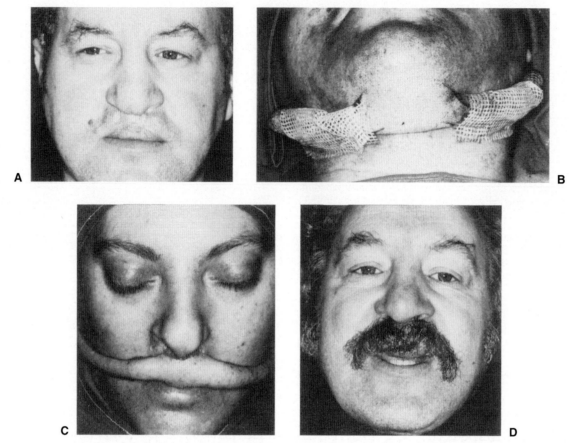

FIG. 1. A: A 36-year-old patient after multiple corrective operations for bilateral cleft lip and palate deformity in childhood. **B:** Elevation of the handle-like pedicles. **C:** Flap inset on the upper lip. **D:** Postoperative view. The columella was lengthened by using the hairless skin on the upper lip.

defect. Five days later, depending on the viability of the medial part of the flap, the pedicles can be transected, first on one side and, 1 to 2 days later, on the other side.

CLINICAL RESULTS

Nasal respiration was improved in every case of bilateral cleft lip in which the tip of the nose was previously dropped and the nostrils were in a horizontal position. In patients in whom the mobility of the upper lip was restricted by scars, induration, or narrowing, the reconstructed lip showed an almost free mobility. In men, the aesthetic results were quite good. In women, without the camouflage possibilities of a moustache, the results were satisfactory, but I suggest that the procedure be limited to severe cases.

Further disadvantages arise from the necessity of at least four operative procedures and the consequent length of time necessary until the pedicles can be removed (at least 16 days)

because the flap has no anatomically defined vessels. Keeping the surgical wound open may be unpleasant for the patient compared with the use of a tubed flap, but this disadvantage is outweighed by the avoidance of split-thickness skin grafts.

SUMMARY

A submental hair-bearing skin flap can be used in several stages to cover a scarred upper lip. The columella can be lengthened at the same time.

References

1. Denecke HJ, Meyer R. *Plastische Operationen an Kopf and Hals,* Vol. 1: *Nasenplastik*. Berlin: Springer-Verlag, 1964.
2. Schaupp H. Spatkorrektur der Oberlippen-Columella-Region bei operierten beidseitigen Lippen-Kiefer-Gaumenspalten unter Verwendung des Submentallapens. *Laryngol Rhinol Otol (Stuttg.)* 1977;56:244.

CHAPTER 161 ■ HAIR-BEARING SKIN FLAPS

J. S. P. WILSON AND M. D. BROUGH

Hair-bearing skin flaps of the scalp can be used for reconstruction of hair-bearing areas of the scalp itself and also of sideburns and the moustache and beard areas in men. Bald areas of the scalp may be used to reconstruct non-hair-bearing areas of the face or oral cavity. Immediate skin cover to large defects of the cranium may be provided by large, narrow-based flaps or single or multiple, broad-based flaps.

Scalp flaps used to reconstruct defects of the scalp may be axial pattern or random pattern, but those used in reconstructing other areas are almost invariably axial-pattern flaps and most commonly are based on the posterior branch of the superficial temporal artery and its associated veins. Much of this chapter is devoted to flaps based on this vessel, as they are the most versatile and most useful flaps of the hair-bearing scalp.

RECONSTRUCTION OF HAIR-BEARING AREAS OF THE FACE (1–5)

Hair-bearing Margin of the Forehead

Defects of this margin, other than the receding hairline of male pattern baldness, are not common but, when present, cause a significant deformity. They usually can be reconstructed with transposition flaps based on the posterior branch of the superficial temporal artery. A secondary defect may leave an obvious bald patch at the back of the scalp. If the flap is large and the galea is cross-hatched with multiple

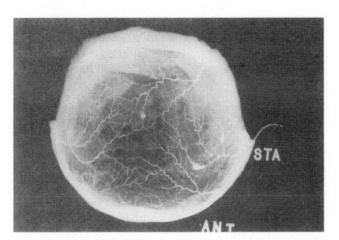

FIG. 1. Radiograph of cadaveric scalp after injection of Micropaque showing the vascular anastomoses. *STA,* superficial temporal artery; *ANT,* anterior branch.

incisions, it will expand and a secondary defect may be avoided. Fig. 5 shows how three flaps were expanded in a girl aged 8 years to reconstruct the anterior hairline, which had been destroyed by a burn injury in infancy.

Eyebrows

Eyebrows help frame the forehead and divide the upper third from the middle third of the face. When thick, as commonly found in men, they can be reconstructed readily on narrow-pedicled flaps based on the posterior branch of the superficial temporal artery. The reconstruction of a hairy eyebrow, because it is the narrowest area of hair-bearing skin, provides an excellent model to explore the potential of the narrow-pedicled hair-bearing flaps; however, it is not always possible to give adequate cover to the vascular pedicle in the grafted forehead of the burned patient.

A narrow-pedicled, hair-bearing flap may be used as an alternative. As long as the pedicle includes the posterior superficial temporal vessels, the hair-bearing flap can be angled to improve the direction of the hair. Bilateral hair-bearing flaps were used in a patient with burn scarring of the forehead (Fig. 6).

It may well be, however, that one of the posterior superficial temporal vessels has been divided or used previously for the construction of a forehead. It is then necessary to raise a flap with an even longer pedicle to allow bilateral reconstruction of the eyebrow. Such a case is illustrated in Fig. 7A. The contralateral eyebrow could be shaped primarily, however. The ipsilateral eyebrow was too large and had to be revised subsequently (Fig. 7B). Still, this exercise does indicate the potential of narrow-pedicled flaps.

Frontal Temporal Hairlines and Sideburn

Two cosmetic units can be reconstructed by a superiorly based transposition flap of postauricular scalp. The position of the normal hairline and sideburn is delineated (Fig. 8A), and the scar tissue is excised. A bipolar flap is raised (Fig. 8B). The anterior flap completes the frontal hairline. The large posterior flap provides hair-bearing skin to create the lateral temporal hairline and sideburn (Fig. 8C).

Sideburns

Sideburns, particularly in men, are important in framing the face. They may be reconstructed by a flap based on the posterior branch of the superficial temporal artery, but this flap needs to be rotated through almost 180 degrees at its base. Sometimes the pathology causing loss of the sideburn or its treatment also has caused loss of the posterior branch of

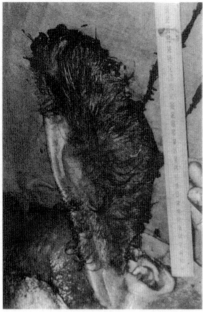
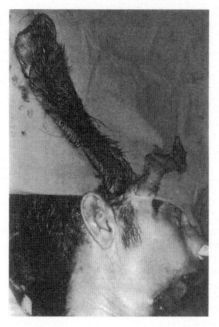
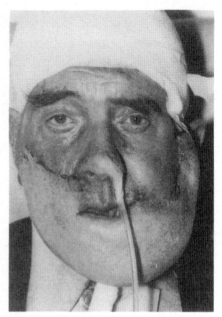

A–C

FIG. 2. Varying applications of hair-bearing scalp flaps. They show the potential diversity in design that is provided by the superficial temporal artery, its posterior branches, and anastomoses. A: Thirty-centimeter scalp flap based on a narrow pedicle containing the superficial temporal artery. B: Combined scalp and forehead flap. C: Inset of narrow-based scalp flap to two thirds of the lower face.

the superficial temporal artery. This may occur, for example, following radical parotid surgery. If this has occurred, a transverse local transposition flap from the scalp based anteriorly, as illustrated in Fig. 9, may be used for reconstruction.

Moustache

Large areas of full-thickness skin losses in the upper lips of men are readily reconstructed with a scalp flap based on the posterior branch of the superficial temporal artery. Many

FIG. 3. Large scalp flap based on a narrow pedicle.

different shapes of moustache can be fashioned (6), but the standard reconstruction is shown in Fig. 4. The reconstruction should be symmetrical, so the defect may have to be enlarged to the size of the cosmetic unit. The scars introduced by the flap are well concealed by the hair of the flap. The reconstruction of a philtrum by introduction of an Abbé flap from the lower lip will improve the appearance.

Full-thickness reconstruction of the upper lip can be achieved using a bipolar flap with a hair-bearing flap based on the posterior branch of the superficial temporal artery providing skin cover; a hairless forehead flap based on the anterior branch of the superficial temporal artery provides buccal cavity lining. When this reconstruction is executed, it is usually necessary to add a tongue flap to reconstruct the vermilion border. This not only prevents hairs turning into the oral cavity, causing irritation, but also improves the contour of the lip.

Beard

Reconstruction of areas of skin loss in the bearded patient should be repaired with hair-bearing skin. This is well illustrated in a patient with severe acne keloid (Fig. 10A). Free skin grafts had been unsatisfactory. The creation of a hemi-beard restored the cosmetic appearance with no recurrence of the keloid (Fig. 10B to D).

A total beard area may be required, and it is important to note the position of the crown on the scalp and to take scalp tissue in front of this for the reconstruction whenever possible. Transfer of the scalp from the crown is safe, but it can produce a bizarre appearance owing to the centrifugal direction of hair growth at this point.

The lower lip, following full-thickness loss, can be reconstructed like the upper lip. Again, a tongue flap should be introduced to provide a vermilion border. It is also possible to reconstruct both the moustache and beard areas with one flap (Fig. 11). When this is done, a central incision is made in the flap, taking care to avoid dividing any major

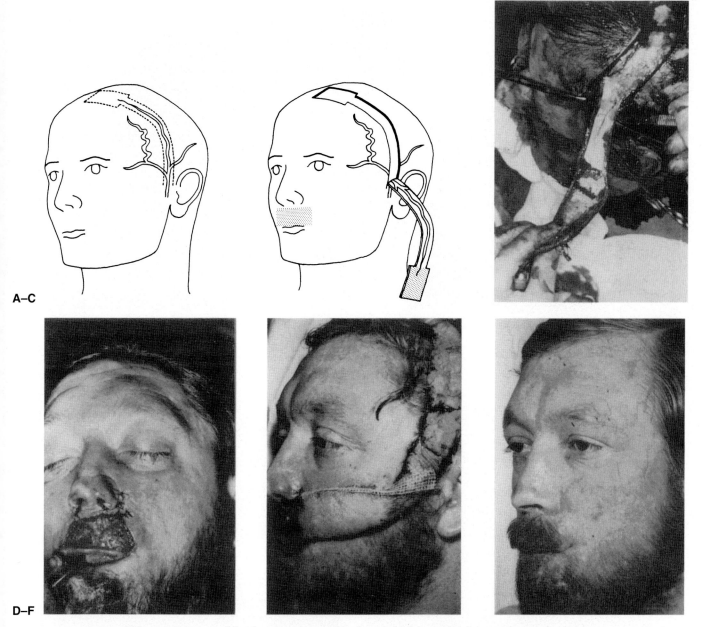

A–C

D–F

FIG. 4. A: Diagram of flap based on the posterior branch of the superficial temporal artery for moustache reconstruction. **B:** Diagram of flap after being raised. **C:** A narrow-based scalp flap raised for reconstruction of moustache. **D:** Upper lip defect created by excising extensive scar tissue from trauma. **E:** Moustache reconstruction. **F:** Final result.

vessels, to provide an oral stoma. A tongue flap is introduced to provide a vermilion border to the lower lip and to the upper lip, if necessary. Local transposition flaps may have to be introduced into the commissures to increase mobility between the lips.

extensive intraoral reconstruction. Smaller areas of bald scalp may be found in a receding anterior hairline, and these also can be used for reconstructing non-hair-bearing areas with benefit.

RECONSTRUCTION OF NON-HAIR-BEARING AREAS OF THE FACE AND ORAL CAVITY

Areas of baldness in men can be used to reconstruct non-hair-bearing areas of the face and lining of the oral cavity. A large central area of baldness on the vertex can be used for

RECONSTRUCTION OF HAIR-BEARING AREAS OF SCALP

Many small defects of the scalp can be reconstructed by expanding local flaps. This is achieved by reflecting the flaps back to their base at the edge of the scalp and dividing the galea with multiple incisions, allowing advancement or expansion of the flap into the defect (7). Flaps may be raised on

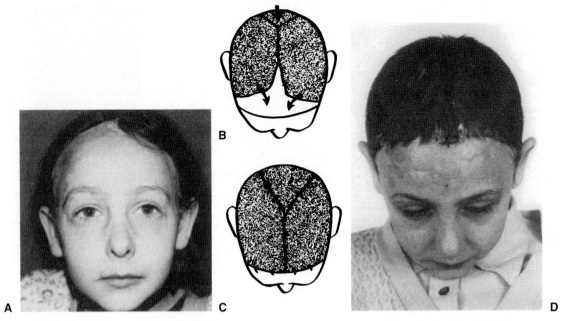

FIG. 5. **A:** Anterior hairline defect following burn injury in infancy. **B:** Plan of flap movement. **C,D:** Early postoperative view of anterior hairline reconstruction.

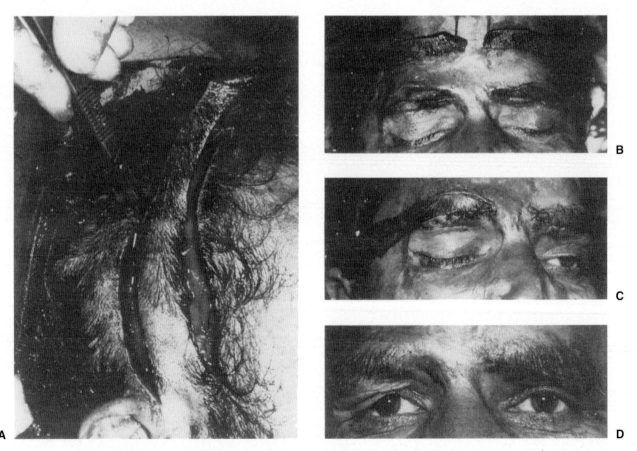

FIG. 6. **A:** Narrow-pedicle flap being raised to reconstruct the right eyebrow. **B–D:** Composite picture of bilateral reconstruction of eyebrows as narrow-pedicle flaps.

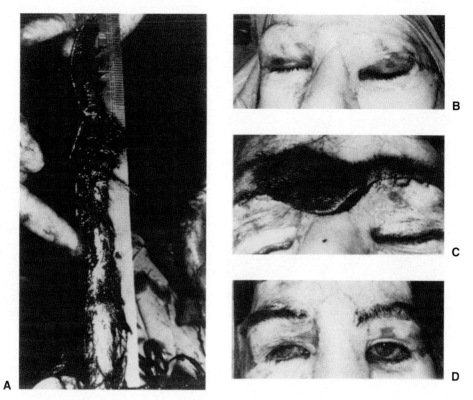

FIG. 7. A: Extended narrow-pedicle flap for the bilateral reconstruction of the eyebrows. **B–D:** Composite photograph showing bilateral reconstruction of the eyebrows with a single pedicle.

either side of the defect to achieve closure. Each flap should be broad based, but it can be narrow if one of the named vessels lies within its base.

Larger scalp defects are reconstructed with transposition flaps. The ideal donor site is in the occipital region, where the resultant defect is repaired with a split-thickness skin graft. This is subsequently covered by hair growing down from the vertex above. Flaps from this region can be based anteriorly on the supraorbital vessels or posteriorly on the occipital vessels. Greater versatility is achieved when the

flaps are based on the contralateral posterior branch of the superficial temporal artery.

REPAIR OF DEFECTS OF THE FACE AND SKULL

Occasionally, scalp flaps based on the posterior branch of the superficial temporal artery can be used to provide immediate

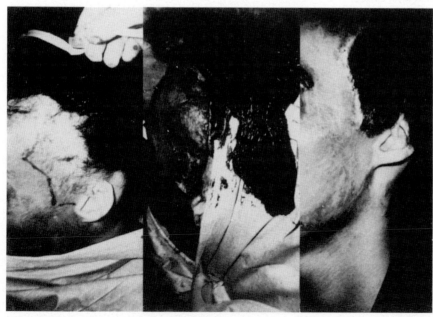

FIG. 8. A–C: Composite photograph showing reconstruction of frontal temporal hairline and sideburns by a superiorly based bipolar flap.

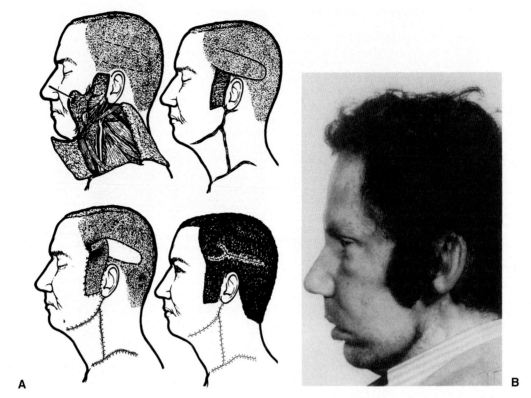

FIG. 9. A: Diagram illustrating reconstruction of preauricular defect following radical resection of the parotid by transposed flap. **B:** Postoperative result.

cover to large defects of the face and skull and may be useful in extensive trauma or following failure of other flaps. They are perhaps more often applicable following extensive craniofacial resections (Fig. 13A). A large posteriorly based combined scalp and forehead flap (Fig. 13B) can be used to line the orbital cavity, adjacent areas, and the craniotomy suture line of the osteoperiosteal flap (7) (Fig. 13C). When the wounds have healed, the hair-bearing part may be excised or partly returned, leaving the galea to be covered with split-thickness skin grafts or other flaps (6).

A single broad, posteriorly based flap may be used to cover the defect following radical resection of the temporal bone (7).

ANATOMY

The scalp consists of soft tissue lying external to the calvaria. It is bounded by the eyebrows overlying the supraorbital ridges and laterally and posteriorly by the margins of the hair-bearing skin. Some hair-bearing skin usually extends onto the nape of the neck below the superior nuchal line of the occipital bone. The scalp contains a large non-hair-bearing area, the forehead. The anatomy of the latter is described in Chapter 105. The scalp has five tissue layers: skin, subcutaneous tissue, the galea aponeurotica and its muscle bellies of frontalis and occipitalis, a layer of loose areolar tissue, and pericranium. The principal blood vessels lie in the subcutaneous layer of the galea.

The blood supply of the scalp is rich and is derived from the terminal branches of both the internal and external carotid arteries. There is a rich network of vessels throughout the scalp, fed by six principal arteries (Fig. 1). The supraorbital and supratrochlear arteries are derived from the internal carotid artery and emerge from the roof of the orbit to pass

vertically upward, supplying the forehead and anterior part of the hair-bearing area of the scalp. The superficial temporal artery (see Fig. 1) is a terminal branch of the external carotid artery. It emerges from the parotid gland to pass over the zygomatic process of the temporal bone, against which it can be palpated 1 cm in front of the tragus. It passes vertically upward for approximately 4 cm before dividing into anterior and posterior branches. The anterior branch follows a convoluted path forward to supply the non-hair-bearing skin of the forehead. The posterior branch passes vertically upward in a straighter course toward the vertex of the scalp. Variations of the normal distribution have been reported (8).

The posterior auricular artery is a small branch of the external carotid artery given off above the digastric muscle. It passes under the parotid gland toward a groove between the cartilage of the auricle and the mastoid process, where it divides to supply branches to the area of scalp behind the pinna.

The occipital artery is another branch of the external carotid artery. It is given off below the origin of the posterior auricular artery. It arises from the posterior aspect of the external carotid artery and passes along the deep surface of the posterior belly of the digastric muscle. It ascends toward the mastoid process, where it divides into several branches supplying the surrounding muscles. The terminal branch supplies the posterior aspect of the scalp and the occipitalis muscle.

Within the scalp, the venous drainage is similar to the arterial supply, although it differs beyond its limits. The lymphatic drainage follows the venous drainage, but there are no lymph nodes on the scalp.

Although the anatomy of the scalp has been known and well documented for centuries, it was recognized only recently that the blood flow pattern within the scalp does not necessarily follow the basic anatomic vascular arrangements. Because

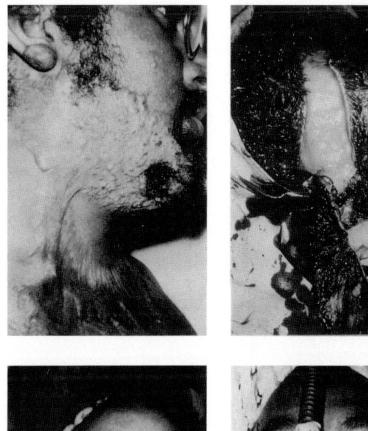

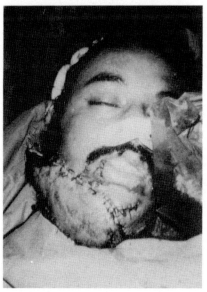
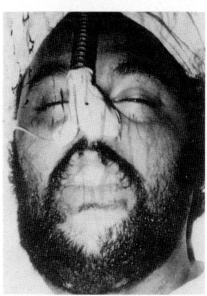

A,B

C,D

FIG. 10. **A:** Massive acne keloid of right bearded area. **B:** Raising of narrow-pedicle scalp flap. **C:** Scalp flap inset. **D:** Final result showing reconstruction of the beard and absence of keloid.

of the rich network of vessels, changes can occur in the flow pattern without any significant change in the viability of tissue that these vessels supply.

Investigations on cadaver scalps and on clinical cases (1,2) revealed that an area of hair-bearing skin could be safely carried on a long narrow pedicle containing the posterior branch of the superficial temporal artery, and as long as the vessel was contained in the pedicle of the flap, anastomoses with adjacent angiotomes or vascular territories were adequate to maintain viability of the flap. Clinical cases of scalp replantation have demonstrated that the entire scalp can survive on one set of vessels (9).

The posterior branch of the superficial temporal artery is the longest vessel in the scalp, and it supplies directly the largest territory of the scalp. This, together with its position, makes it the most versatile vessel for transferring scalp flaps

outside the region of the scalp. It can be used to transfer small delineated areas of the scalp or, indeed, the entire scalp by forming a two- or three-angiotome system similar to the multiangiotome system in the forehead (3).

FLAP DESIGN AND DIMENSIONS

Scalp Flaps Based on the Posterior Branch of the Superficial Temporal Artery

Investigation of the vascular anatomy of the scalp and clinical practice have confirmed that it is possible to raise a narrow-pedicled hair-bearing flap of sufficient length to reconstruct any defect on the face. The flap with the best blood supply extends transversely across the vault of the scalp from ear to ear, including the ipsilateral and contralateral posterior branches of the superficial temporal vessels. The flap may be 30 cm long and only a few centimeters wide, provided these vessels are included in the flap. Fig. 2A and B illustrates a combined forehead and scalp flap. Fig. 2C illustrates the level to which it can be taken on the contralateral side. The total hair-bearing area of the scalp can be transposed on a narrow pedicle if it contains the posterior branches of the superficial temporal vessels. We have not had to raise such a flap, but we had one patient in whom two thirds of the hair-bearing area of the scalp was raised and successfully transposed (Fig. 3). The entire scalp, including the forehead, could be raised if based on the superficial temporal vessels at a point just anterior to the tragus of the ear. This would provide a flap of adequate length and size to cover any defect on the face or upper neck, but a clinical situation requiring this procedure must be rare.

Most scalp flaps used in clinical practice vary in size between the long, narrow pedicle flap and the total hair-

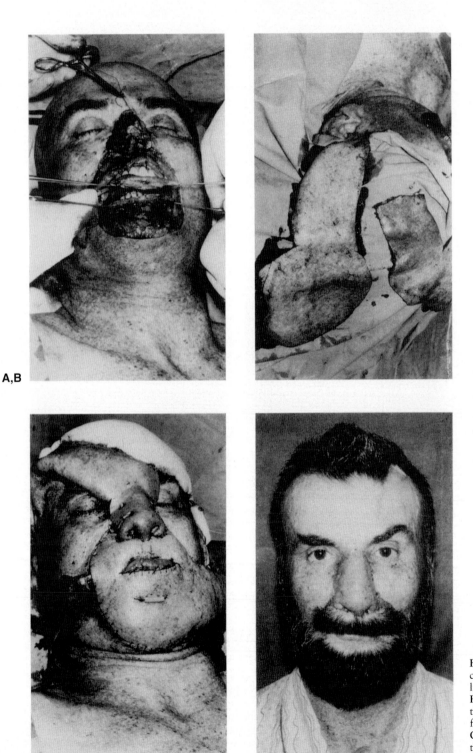

A,B

C,D

FIG. 11. A: Excision of multiple squamous carcinomas of the upper lip, nose, and lower lip in a patient with xeroderma pigmentosa. B: A single flap raised for reconstruction of the upper and lower lip and simultaneous forehead flap for reconstruction of the nose. C: Flaps inset. Central flap incised to create the mouth and tongue flap introduced. D: Postoperative result.

bearing area of the scalp. Provided the posterior branch of the superficial temporal artery remains patent entering the base and within the pedicle, the flap will remain safe and can be cut to produce any reasonable shape required. Fig. 4 illustrates the use of a flap to reconstruct an upper lip defect with a moustache.

At operation, the defect to be reconstructed should be enlarged to the shape of an appropriate cosmetic unit. It is preferable that beards and moustaches be made symmetrical where possible. A template of the appropriate defect is made. The template is swung onto the vertex of the scalp, with a pivot point based 1 cm above the zygomatic arch of the temporal bone, over a point where the superficial temporal artery can be palpated. If a longer pedicle is required to avoid tension, it can be extended to a pivot point just anterior to the tragus of the ear. The template is placed on the scalp in front of the crown in order that hair growth will be in the correct direction, particularly for reconstructing the moustache and beard areas of the face. The flap is marked out with a 2-cm pedicle down to the zygomatic arch.

Other Scalp Flaps

Scalp flaps based on the other named vessels of the scalp can be used to transfer large areas of hair-bearing scalp. Very long flaps across the scalp can be raised, but their base should be 12 cm wide to ensure inclusion of the named vessels, as these are smaller than the posterior branches of the superficial temporal vessels and are less easily identified preoperatively or perioperatively until the flap is almost fully raised.

Combined scalp and forehead flaps are used to provide immediate cover following craniofacial resections (10).

OPERATIVE TECHNIQUE

Careful preoperative preparation of the scalp is essential when using scalp flaps. The superficial temporal artery and its branches are palpated, and their course in the scalp is marked. The Doppler probe is not normally necessary for tracing the vessels. The hair in the area to be used should be cut short enough to identify any previously unrecognized scars. With dense hair, the scalp should be shaved, but with sparse hair, this step may not be necessary; preservation of hairs 0.5 cm long allows identification of direction of hair growth. It is always desirable to shave the planned margins of the flap completely. After the hair has been cut, the whole scalp should be shampooed and thoroughly washed to remove all cut hairs.

The flap is raised from the contralateral side first. It is raised in the plane beneath the galea aponeurotica. Care must be taken to avoid raising the pericranium, which must be preserved for subsequent application of a split-thickness skin graft.

As the flap is raised across the midline, the posterior branch of the superficial temporal artery and its accompanying veins come into view on the undersurface. The pedicle then is fashioned to include these vessels in the center of the pedicle as it is raised down to the zygomatic arch (Fig. 4). The anterior branch of the superficial temporal artery is divided as this is done. The pedicle then can be turned safely at its base to allow the flap to be inset into the defect.

In most cases, 90% of the flap can be inset, which allows safe division of the flap at 2 weeks. Occasionally, it may be desirable to leave the flap longer before dividing the pedicle. There is no necessity to cover the posterior aspect of the pedicle with grafts; indeed, to do so would make return of

the pedicle more difficult. Normally, the posterior aspect of the pedicle can be covered with paraffin gauze. The donor defect of the scalp usually is covered with a split-thickness skin graft. If the defect is small, it may be closed primarily, and this can be made easier by reflecting back the local scalp flaps and incising the galea before advancing them into the defect (1).

If the posterior branches of the superficial temporal vessels are not available, it may be possible to use the contralateral posterior branches of the superficial temporal vessels. If these vessels are not available, a broad-based 12-cm flap may be required; however, a broad-pedicled flap is less mobile and therefore should be 1½ times longer than the appropriate pedicled flap. The flap is raised in the same manner.

Modifications in Technique

Split Flap

Where two adjacent hair-bearing areas require reconstruction, the flap may be axially split into two parts. This is well illustrated in Fig. 12A, in a patient with an unsatisfactory repair of a gunshot wound of the lower third of the face. The pedicle skin of the previous repair was used to provide adequate lining, and the resultant defect in the upper lip and chin was repaired by providing hair-bearing flaps shaped as a beard and moustache carried on a single pedicle containing the posterior superficial temporal artery (Fig. 12).

Multiple Flaps

Bilateral scalp flaps can be synchronously combined with a modified Converse forehead flap to create an eyebrow and moustache and to reconstruct the nose. Additional hair-bearing skin can be gained by using the hair-bearing pedicle of the moustache flap following a delay procedure at 14 days to fill in the defect in the bearded area of the chin (Fig. 11).

Two-flap Repair

Very large craniofacial defects require the introduction of two flaps (Fig. 13). Immediate skin cover to the face and left lateral skull is provided by a combined forehead and scalp flap based on the posterior superficial temporal vessels. This supplies support to the frontal lobe of the brain. A broad-based contralateral flap is transposed forward to overlie the part of the craniotomy suture line not covered by the first flap. The hair-bearing scalp in the forehead region subsequently may be excised, and a nonhairy split-thickness skin graft is applied to the forehead.

CLINICAL RESULTS

We have used long, vascularly based flaps in more than 180 patients. Most were used in reconstructions of defects in the moustache and beard area, and in these patients, the cosmetic results have been excellent, primarily because the hair growth conceals the quality of the underlying skin and camouflages surrounding scars.

Owing to their vascularity, these flaps are not only easy to raise but relatively free of complications. We have had only six patients in whom there has been a small area of flap necrosis. The area of loss was small, and the defect was reconstructed by further advancement of the scalp flap. We have not encountered a case of total loss.

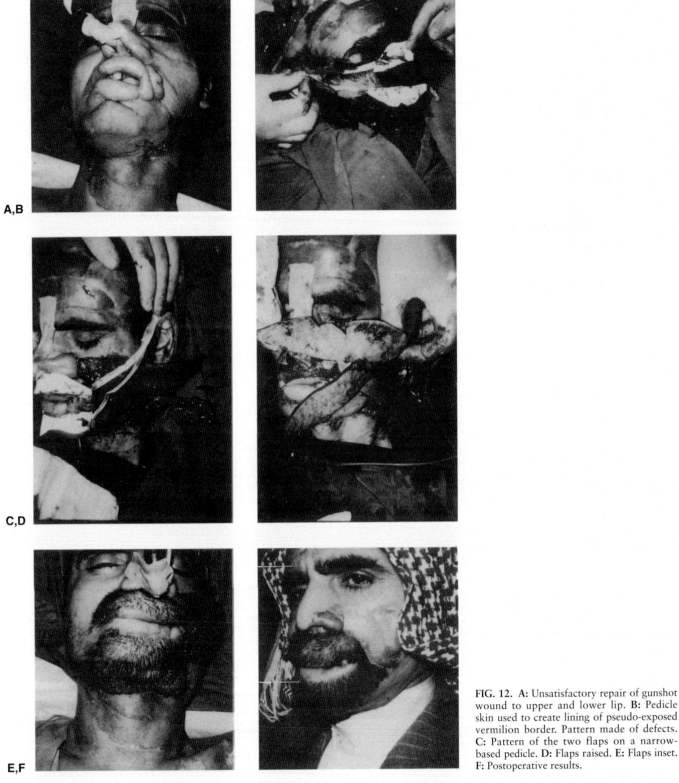

A,B

C,D

E,F

FIG. 12. A: Unsatisfactory repair of gunshot wound to upper and lower lip. B: Pedicle skin used to create lining of pseudo-exposed vermilion border. Pattern made of defects. C: Pattern of the two flaps on a narrow-based pedicle. D: Flaps raised. E: Flaps inset. F: Postoperative results.

In only two patients was any significant infection detected. There was no problem with hematoma formation in any flap, undoubtedly owing to the fact that there is no overt bleeding from the galea. The only significant bleeding from the flap is from the edges. This is controlled, of course, as the flap is inset.

On several occasions we noted some hair loss from the flap, but it was temporary and there was subsequently normal growth of hair in the flap. In one patient, the pericranium was inadvertently raised from the skull, and the defect had to be covered with a local transposition flap.

Asymmetry of reconstructed hair-bearing cosmetic units can be corrected by electrolysis or the subcutaneous excision of hair follicles. Major irregularities of hair growth in comparison with the normal side can be adjusted by the excision of

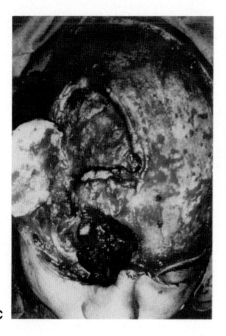
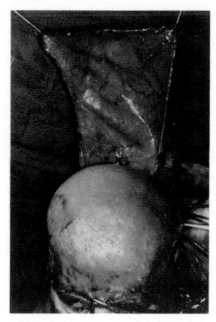
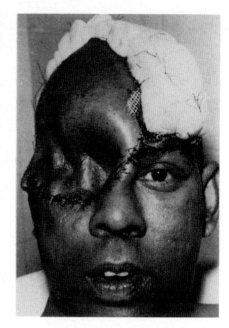

A–C

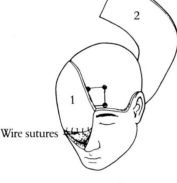
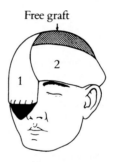

D

Planning of flaps

Flap 1 transposed
to cover excisional defect

Wire sutures

Free graft

Flap 2 transposed
to cover site of
osteoperiosteal flap

FIG. 13. **A:** Defect following craniofacial resection of tumor of the orbit and middle cranial fossa. **B:** Entire remaining scalp raised on a broad pedicle flap. **C:** Flap transposed and sutured into position to cover the defect. **D:** Two-flap repair to reconstruct the right upper half of face and to cover the craniotomy.

the hair-bearing skin and its replacement by a full-thickness skin graft or local flap.

The donor area of the flap has not proved to be a significant problem, as many elderly patients readily accept a small grafted area on the scalp. When small flaps are used, the donor defect sometimes can be closed primarily, although this is often difficult in elderly patients. Expansion flaps can be used to assist this primary closure, particularly in the younger patient. Transposition flaps can be used to cover obvious bald areas at the expense of less obvious areas. Alternatively, serial excision of the bald area successfully repairs the bald area. Large defects are most readily concealed by a toupee or wig. Wigs have been acceptable to a few female patients on whom we have used this flap. There is always an area of loss of sensation of the scalp following the use of these flaps, but only one of our patients has complained of this.

SUMMARY

Various modifications of hair-bearing scalp flaps can be used to reconstruct multiple defects about the face.

References

1. Wilson JSP, Galvao MSL, Brough MD. The application of hair-bearing flaps in head and neck surgery. *Head Neck Surg* 1980;2:386.
2. Wilson JSP, Galvao MSL. Some observations on facial reconstruction by the use of hair-bearing flaps. In: *Proceedings of the VIIth International Congress of Plastic and Reconstructive Surgery, Rio de Janeiro, May 1979*. São Paulo: Sociedade Brasileira de Cirurgia Plastica, 1980.
3. Wilson JSP. Major flaps in the reconstruction of defects of the head and neck. In: Chambers RG, ed. *Cancer of head and neck: proceedings of an international symposium*. Amsterdam: Excerpta Medica, 1975;256–279.
4. Brent B. Reconstruction of ear, eyebrow, and sideburn in the burned patient. *Plast Reconstr Surg* 1975;55:312.
5. Wilson JSP. 478 Major flaps in head and neck reconstruction: some observations on scalp, narrow pedicle forehead and deltopectoral flaps. In: *Transactions of the Sixth International Congress of Plastic and Reconstructive Surgery*. Paris: Masson, 1975.
6. Edgerton MT, Snyder GB. A combined intracranial-extracranial approach and the use of the two-stage split-flap technique for reconstruction with craniofacial malignancies. *Am J Surg* 1965;110:595.
7. Westbury G, Wilson JSP, Richardson A. Combined craniofacial resection for malignant disease. *Am J Surg* 1975;130:463.
8. Stock AL, Collins HP, and Davidson TM. Anatomy of the superficial temporal artery. *Head Neck Surg* 1980;2:466.
9. Miller GDH, Anstee EJ, Snell JA. Successful replantation of an avulsed scalp by microvascular anastomosis. *Plast Reconstr Surg* 1976;59:133.
10. Wilson JSP, Westbury G. Combined craniofacial resection for tumours involving the orbital walls. *Br J Plast Surg* 1973;26:44.

CHAPTER 162 ■ STEPLADDER SKIN-MUSCLE-MUCOSAL FLAP FOR LOWER LIP RECONSTRUCTION

A. D. PELLY AND E.-P. TAN

It is generally accepted that the orbicularis oris should be reconstructed following major resections of the lower lip. Many methods involving full-thickness flaps from the upper lip are likely to produce further functional disruptions of the circumoral sphincter. Dissatisfaction with these methods of repair led surgeons to develop alternative techniques (1–3).

INDICATIONS

We present a technique of lower lip repair that allows adequate excision of the primary lesion, respects the functional integrity of the upper lip, and permits reconstruction of the circumoral sphincter in the same operation (4). This technique has been used without complication in reconstruction of defects of half the lower lip extending to the commissure (Figs. 1 and 2). The technique has been extended to restore the oral sphincter following damage to the ramus mandibularis of the facial nerve.

OPERATIVE TECHNIQUE

The extent of a full-thickness excision of the lip is outlined along with a stepladder incision over the right side of the lower lip (Fig. 1A). The lesion is excised, and the right lower lip is advanced by the stepladder technique (Fig. 1B). A pro-phylactic vermilionectomy is carried out on the remainder of the right lower lip.

A mucosal flap then is fashioned in the left lower buccal sulcus. This incision extends backward to the molar region, and with the help of a generous back cut in the cheek mucosa, the mucosal flap then can be rotated and advanced to meet the mucosa over the right side of the lower lip. A flap of skin only is designed over the left cheek (Fig. 1B). This is advanced medially and rotated superiorly to provide skin cover. No muscle is included in this flap.

The cheek mucosal flap then is sutured to the lip exci-sional defect to provide complete mucosal lining. The stepladder incision is advanced and sutured. The covering skin flap is raised and advanced into position (Fig. 1C). The skin is sutured, and the only residual raw area is over the free border of the lower lip close to the commissure, where the mucosal lining flap and the external skin flap are apposed (Fig. 1D)

A mucomuscular flap then is fashioned on the buccal aspect of the left upper lip. It is based at the modiolus, is 3 cm long and 1 cm wide, and contains the full thickness of the middle third of the orbicularis muscle. The flap is in the general horizontal line of the circumoral sphincter (Fig. 1E).

The flap is transposed and sutured into the defect at the free border of the left lower lip. The muscular component is sutured to the orbicularis of the right side of the lip to restore the continuity of the circumoral sphincter. The mucosal com-ponent completes the lip border (Fig. 1F).

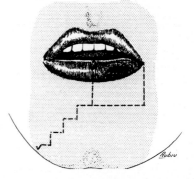

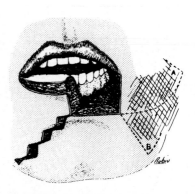

FIG. 1. A: Extent of the excision and the stepladder flap outlined. B: Flap (*B*) (including all of cross-hatched area) consists of skin only. A prophylactic vermilionectomy is carried out over the remainder of the lower lip.

(Continued)

A,B

476

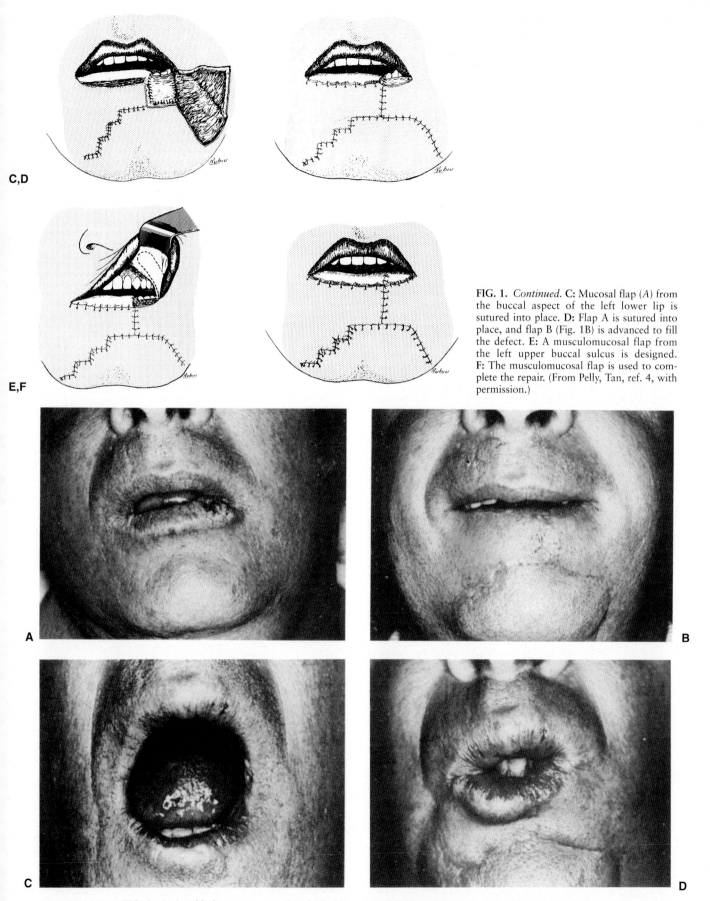

C,D

E,F

FIG. 1. *Continued.* **C:** Mucosal flap (*A*) from the buccal aspect of the left lower lip is sutured into place. **D:** Flap A is sutured into place, and flap B (Fig. 1B) is advanced to fill the defect. **E:** A musculomucosal flap from the left upper buccal sulcus is designed. **F:** The musculomucosal flap is used to complete the repair. (From Pelly, Tan, ref. 4, with permission.)

A

B

C

D

FIG. 2. A: An elderly man presented with a malignant lesion that required surgical excision of the left half of the lower lip. The lesion was excised and repaired as described. **B:** Result 6 weeks postoperatively. **C,D:** Three months later, electromyography showed normal electrical activity in the transposed muscle flap. The appearance and function of the mouth, both at rest and in action, were satisfactory. (From Pelly, Tan, ref. 4, with permission.)

SUMMARY

The stepladder skin-muscle-mucosal flap combination can be used to provide a functional lower lip reconstruction without unnecessarily violating the upper lip.

References

1. Fries I. Advantages of a basic concept in lip reconstruction after tumour resection. *J Maxillofac Surg* 1973;1:73.
2. Johanson B, Aspelund E, Breine U, Holmstom H. Surgical treatment of non-traumatic lower lip lesions with special reference to the step technique. *Scand J Plast Reconstr Surg* 1974;8:232.
3. Puckett CL, Neale HW, Pickrell KL. Dynamic correction of unilateral paralysis of the lower lip. *Plast Reconstr Surg* 1975;55:397.
4. Pelly AD, Tan E-P. Lower lip reconstruction. *Br J Plast Surg* 1981;34:83.

CHAPTER 163 ■ "BANDONEON" TECHNIQUE: MUCOMYOCUTANEOUS STRETCHED FLAPS IN LIP RECONSTRUCTION

I. J. PELED AND Y. ULLMANN

EDITORIAL COMMENT

The innovative nomenclature of this flap is appropriate in that the musical instrument called a bandoneon is like an accordion that stretches and contracts as required. The authors have used this principle in stretching the tissue for lip reconstruction.

Up to two thirds of the lip can be repaired by using a mucomyocutaneous flap in the remaining lip, which is stretched as a "bandoneon," following a zigzag release incision (Fig. 1). Results are quite satisfactory, with no alteration of the commissure, no significant decrease of mouth opening, and well-located scars.

INDICATIONS

Tumors of the lip are quite frequent, especially squamous cell carcinomas. The best treatment is adequate surgical excision, with immediate repair of the defect. Depending on the remaining defect after tumor excision, the choice can be as simple as direct suture, or more sophisticated techniques may be required. The flap described here is suitable for the repair of rather large defects in partial reconstruction of the lip using one or two mucomyocutaneous flaps of the remaining lip in a single-stage procedure. Following wide excision of the tumor and frozen sections of the borders, the remaining defect, from one third to two thirds of the lip, is reconstructed by the bandoneon technique.

Other reports have described use of this procedure for the vermilion only (1,2) or for lip reconstruction without incising the mucosa (3). Some techniques leave unacceptable scarring and may alter the angle of the mouth (4,5).

ANATOMY

This is an arterial flap supplied by the inferior coronary (orbicularis) artery.

FLAP DESIGN AND DIMENSIONS

The commissure is not sacrificed, and the scar is strategically placed in the labiomental junction or nasolabial groove. Continuity of the remaining orbicularis oris muscle is preserved, and by suturing the cut edges the sphincter mechanism can be reconstructed.

OPERATIVE TECHNIQUE

With the patient under local or general anesthesia, the tumor is excised with reasonable margins, and adequacy is established by intraoperative frozen sections. For defects in the lower lip, the horizontal line of the excision at the junction of the lip with the mental area is laterally prolonged in a zigzag or running double W up to or passing the level of the contralateral corner of the mouth (Fig. 1A). This is a full-thickness incision including skin, muscle, and mucosa of the lip.

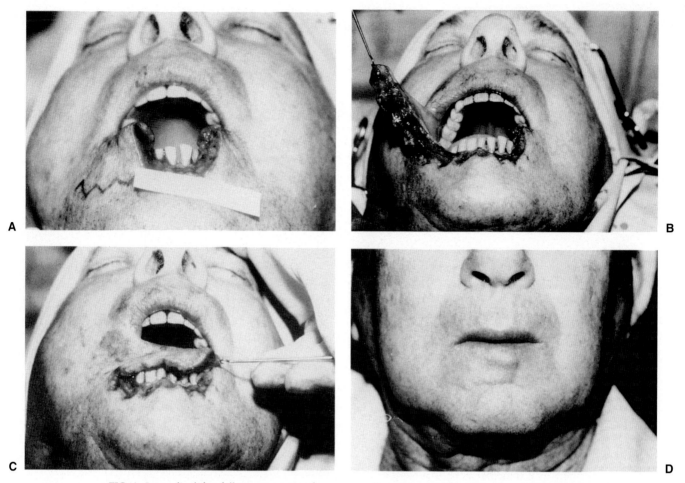

FIG. 1. Lower-lip defect following excision of squamous cell carcinoma. **A:** Zigzag drawn at labiomental horizontal junction delimits the flap. **B:** Following incision and complete release of the flap from buccal mucosa. **C:** The "bandoneon" stretched flap is advanced to bridge the gap. **D:** Early postoperative result showing scar and satisfactory cosmetic result.

The remaining lip is raised as a flap and completely freed from the soft-tissue mandibular attachment (Fig. 1B). The flap is stretched toward the lateral border of the lip defect (Fig. 1C) and sutured in three planes (i.e., mucosa, muscle, and skin) without tension. The running double W facilitates horizontal advancement, and the small triangles are further positioned and indented. The broken scar line makes it less visible, and there is less scar contracture (Fig. 1D).

In medial defects of the lower lip, the same principles can be followed. Two lateral lip flaps in the remaining tissue, adjacent to the angle of the mouth, can be horizontally advanced to bridge the gap. This allows reconstruction of a defect of two thirds of the lower lip. The same procedure can be performed in defects of the upper lip. In these cases, the running W horizontal incision is placed at the nasolabial groove, resulting in an inconspicuous scar.

CLINICAL RESULTS

Using well-vascularized mucomyocutaneous flaps, all cases healed primarily without any complication. Minimal scarring and good placement of scars, as well as the unaltered angle of the mouth, are significant contributors to a good aesthetic and functional result. The strategic location of the scars is in the natural labiomental junction or nasolabial groove, and dog-ears are avoided. Continuity of the remaining orbicularis oris muscle is preserved. By suturing the cut edges, the sphincter mechanism can be reconstructed.

SUMMARY

This simple procedure offers reconstruction of a defect of up to two thirds of the lip, with no alteration of the angle of the mouth, with well-located scars, and with good aesthetic and functional results in suitable cases.

References

1. Goldstein MH. A tissue-expanding vermilion myocutaneous flap for lip repair. *Plast Reconstr Surg* 1984;73:786.
2. Mutaf M, Sensoz O, Tuncay E. The split-lip advancement technique (SLAT) for the treatment of congenital sinuses of the lower lip. *Plast Reconstr Surg* 1993;92:615.
3. Galli JJ. Reconstrucion del labio inferior. *Rev Cir Plast Argent* 1985;8:3.
4. Webster RC, Coffey RJ, Kelleher RE. Total and partial reconstruction of the lower lip with innervated muscle bearing flaps. *Plast Reconstr Surg* 1960;25:360.
5. Karapandžić M. Reconstruction of lip defects by local arterial flaps. *Br J Plast Surg* 1974;27:93.

CHAPTER 164 ■ NASOLABIAL (GATE) SKIN-MUSCLE-MUCOSAL FLAP TO LOWER LIP

R. FUJIMORI

EDITORIAL COMMENT

This procedure certainly accomplishes what it sets out to do; however, the editors are concerned with the innervation to the upper lip unless care is taken not to damage the muscle while making the nasolabial incisions.

There are only a few reports in the literature on total lower lip reconstruction using innervated muscle-bearing flaps (1,2). However, when planning a complete reconstruction of the lower lip, the following points should be considered: First, the flaps used should be local flaps, including innervated muscle. Second, all the suture lines should be in natural facial creases or follow the function lines of the various facial aesthetic units. Finally, the flaps should be large enough to replace tissue loss.

INDICATIONS

Some previous techniques (3–5), although producing excellent functional and aesthetic results, created a tight lower lip with obvious protrusion of the upper lip. Other procedures also produced a large dog-ear on either side of the mentolabial groove, requiring that large amounts of skin be discarded postoperatively for correction.

The gate flap (6), which uses a flap from each nasolabial fold, is an improvement over previous procedures. The main advantages of this design are (a) the flap can be made 3 cm larger than nasolabial rotation flaps, (b) rotation of the flap is possible without the formation of a dog-ear, (c) the flap contains innervated muscle, and (d) the procedure can be carried out in one stage.

OPERATIVE TECHNIQUE

The whole of the affected lower lip is excised as a rectangle (Fig. 1A, $BB'DD'$). The inferior margin of resection (DD') follows the mentolabial groove. Whenever possible, a 3- to 4-mm-wide strip of labial mucous membrane is left attached near the labioalveolar sulcus. The lateral margin of resection (BD and $B'D'$) is usually placed 0.5 to 1.0 cm laterally to perpendiculars dropped from the labial commis-

sures (OO'), but it may extend 2 cm laterally in older patients with wrinkled faces. The width of the nasolabial skin-muscle-mucosal flaps ($BC = DE$, $B'C' = D'E'$) is usually 3 cm, and the suture lines of the flap donor sites (AED, $A'E'D'$) should follow the natural nasolabial fold. The dotted lines (AlB, AmC, $A'l'B'$, $A'm'C'$) represent incisions made through the mucous membrane, which should be about 1 cm wider than the flap itself, so excess mucous membrane can be available for reconstruction of the new red lip.

When making flap incisions CED and $C'E'D'$ below the line CC' that connects both labial commissures, only skin and subcutaneous tissue should be cut, keeping the muscle, and mucous membrane intact in the flap pedicle. Further undermining of the flap pedicle skin is required to allow flap rotation. Flaps prepared in this fashion contain innervated muscles: orbicularis oris, caninus, zygomaticus major or minor, risorius, triangularis, and buccinator.

As soon as the flaps have been mobilized, incisions should be closed in the four layers of mucous membrane, muscle layer, subcutaneous tissue, and skin. The excess mucous membrane above the upper border of the transposed flap is used to replace vermilion. This new red lip will be thinner than the normal lip. Because of cicatricial contraction, the newly reconstructed lower lip tends to become puffy and rounded. This distortion can be effectively corrected by keeping continuous pressure on the lower lip by the sponge fixation method for 3 months postoperatively.

A final procedure involving Z-plasties or scar revision is often required 3 months postoperatively, after the tissues have become supple (Figs. 2 and 3).

CLINICAL RESULTS

Because these flaps contain innervated muscle, the newly reconstructed lower lip has good motor function. These flaps have a good blood supply and can be moved into the excisional defect in one stage without any delay procedure.

SUMMARY

The gate skin-muscle-mucosal flap can be used to provide a functional reconstruction of the entire lower lip.

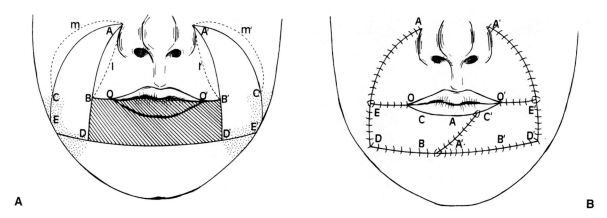

FIG. 1. Gate flap. **A:** Distance $OB = O'B' = 0.5$ to 1.0 cm in normal patients, but it can be extended to 2 cm in the case of older patients with wrinkled faces. Distance $BC = B'C' = 3$ cm. Skin incision along AB and AC should be made through-and-through into the mouth. Skin incision along CE and ED should be made only through subcutaneous tissue. Incision in the mucous membrane is performed along the dotted lines (AlB, AmC, $A'l'B'$, $A'm'C'$) that run laterally to the skin incision lines (AB, AC). Dotted area is undermined subcutaneously. **B:** Suture lines run along the nasolabial fold and mentolabial groove centrally. (From Fujimori, ref. 6, with permission.)

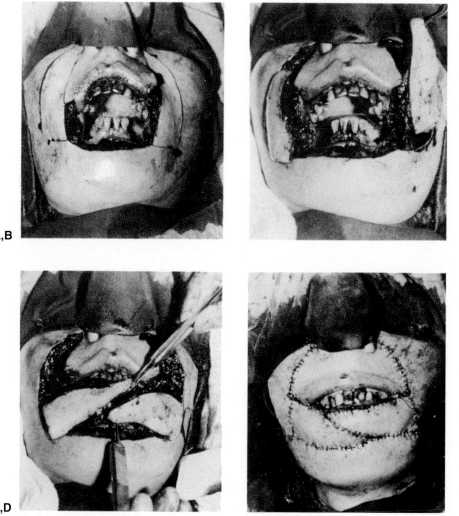

FIG. 2. **A:** The carcinoma was excised and skin incisions for the flap were made in the nasolabial folds. **B:** The flaps raised. **C,D:** Flaps rotated and sutured. (From Fujimori, ref. 6, with permission.)

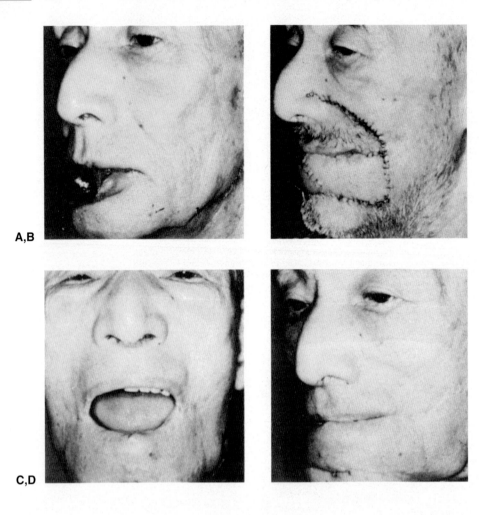

A,B

C,D

FIG. 3. **A:** Squamous cell carcinoma of the lower lip. **B:** Gate flap rotated. **C,D:** Six months postoperatively.

References

1. Webster RC, Coffey RJ, Kellecher RE. Total and partial reconstruction of the lower lip with innervated muscle-bearing flaps. *Plast Reconstr Surg* 1960;25:360.
2. Karapandžić M. Reconstruction of lip defects by local arterial flaps. *Br J Plast Surg* 1974;27:93.
3. Wang MKH, Converse JM, Macomber WB, Wood-Smith D. Deformities of the Lips and Cheeks. In: Converse JM, ed. *Reconstructive plastic surgery.* Philadelphia: WB Saunders, 1967;851.
4. Lentrodt J, Luhr HG. Reconstruction of the lower lip after tumor resection combined with radical neck dissection. *Plast Reconstr Surg* 1971;48:579.
5. Bretteville-Jensen G. Reconstruction of the lower lip after central excisions. *Br J Plast Surg* 1973;26:247.
6. Fujimori R. "Gate flap" for the total reconstruction of the lower lip. *Br J Plast Surg* 1980;33:340.

CHAPTER 165 ■ STEEPLE SKIN-MUSCLE-MUCOSAL FLAP FOR LOWER LIP RECONSTRUCTION

M. F. STRANC AND G. A. ROBERTSON

The repair of extensive lower lip defects has challenged the ingenuity of reconstructive surgeons for many years (1–7). The methods that have evolved can be broadly classified into three categories: those using lip tissues, those that rely on head and neck tissues, and those in which reconstructive material is brought in from a distance.

INDICATIONS

Satisfactory reconstruction of the lower lip must provide a lip curtain of adequate dimensions with sufficient muscular activity and sensory appreciation to allow normal speaking, drinking, and eating. It also must provide adequate access to all parts of the oral cavity and present an acceptable appearance.

Only locally available tissues are likely to meet these criteria. The problems become particularly acute when more than half the lip is missing. The steeple flap was designed to help this group of patients (8).

FLAP DESIGN AND DIMENSIONS

Following marking of the extent of the incision, the defect is converted into a rectangle, with the short side indicating the height of the lip resection and the long border marking the length of the excised lip. The island flap is marked out by extending the lower line of excision laterally for a distance equal to the height of the resected lip. Vertical sides of the island equal to the length of the resected lip are marked. A skin triangle is marked at the top to allow straight-line wound closure (Fig. 1A). The facial artery and its labial branches are located and marked. A Doppler device is of considerable assistance at this stage.

OPERATIVE TECHNIQUE

The lesion is excised as planned. The skin and subcutaneous tissues are incised around the flap. The incision is deepened to full thickness superiorly, inferiorly, and medially. The facial artery is identified on the superomedial aspect of the flap and tied. Tension on the tied vessel helps precise and safe location of the artery on the lateral side (Fig. 1B). Once the vessel is located, incisions above and below it are deepened to full thickness to within 5 mm of the vessel. Mucosa deep to the artery is divided, allowing transposition of the cheek tissues into their new site.

The planning of mucosal incisions for reconstruction of the vermilion relates directly to the site of entry of the facial artery into the flap. When the artery enters the flap low, cheek tissues are "tumbled" into the lip defect, with mucosa along the lateral border cut to excess to provide material for vermilion reconstruction (Fig. 1C). When the artery enters the flap high, the cheek tissues are slid into the lip defect; mucosa along the medial border of the island is used for vermilion reconstruction (Figs. 1D and 2).

CLINICAL RESULTS

This method was used in ten patients. In two patients, total lip reconstruction with bilateral steeple flaps was undertaken. A satisfactory lip curtain was produced in all instances. It is interesting that significant microstomia was avoided in all patients. The average intercommissural distance for the group was 4.9 cm. The lowest recorded distance was 3.8 cm in a patient who had a total lower lip reconstruction. The recovery of cutaneous sensation varied, depending on the interval between surgery and assessment. All patients showed evidence of motor activity, both clinically (Fig. 3) and electromyographically. The length of follow-up varied from 6 to 27 months. Occasional dribbling of fluids, caused by an incomplete motor and sensory recovery, was noted in three patients.

The appearance of the reconstructed lip pleased all patients but one. From our point of view, the appearance of the lips was satisfactory, but an unpleasant fullness of lip was noticeable during lip closure, almost certainly the result of slow resolution of edema, scar contraction, and an incorrect orientation of the underlying muscle fibers.

There were no instances of flap loss. In one patient, excessive swelling postoperatively necessitated the removal of mucocutaneous sutures. No tissue loss occurred, but healing was delayed.

A patient with total lower lip reconstruction using bilateral steeple flaps, an 80-year-old man, suffered minor dehiscence of the suture line between the two flaps (Fig. 4). Spontaneous healing occurred without significant scarring.

SUMMARY

The steeple skin-muscle-mucosal flap has been designed for functional lower lip reconstruction. Bilateral flaps can be used to reconstruct the entire lower lip.

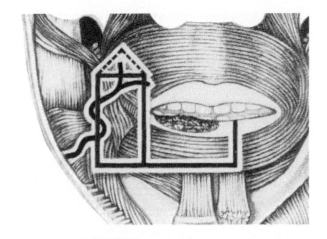

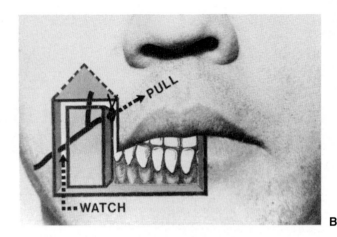

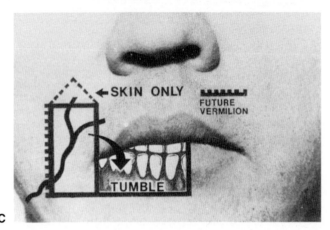

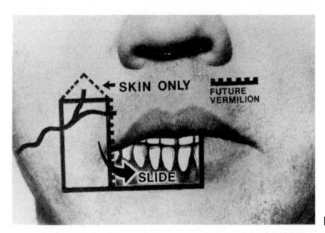

FIG. 1. **A:** Plan of surgery. **B:** Maneuver for safe identification of the facial artery. **C:** Island flap "tumbled" into position. **D:** Island flap slid into position. (From Stranc, Robertson, ref. 8, with permission.)

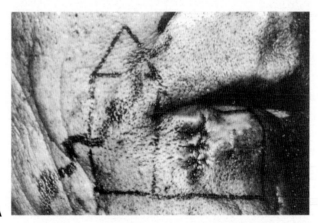

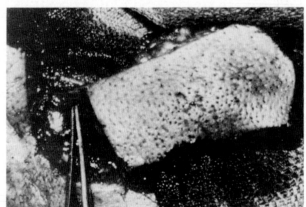

FIG. 2. **A:** Planning of surgery following positive biopsy for squamous cell carcinoma in a 50-year-old man. **B:** Island flap fully mobilized. *(Continued)*

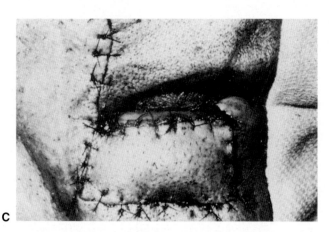

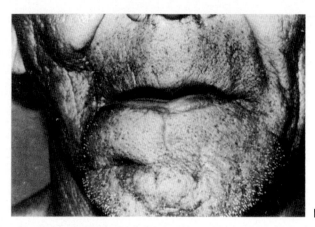

FIG. 2. *Continued.* C: Formation of new lip. D: Appearance 18 months after reconstruction.

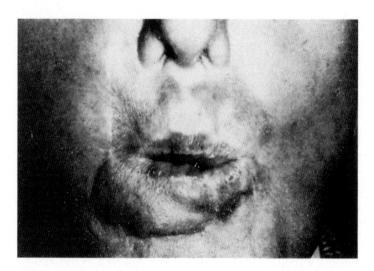

FIG. 3. A 55-year-old man showing clinical evidence of motor function of reconstructed lip 27 months after surgery.

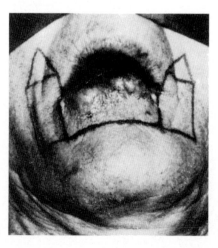

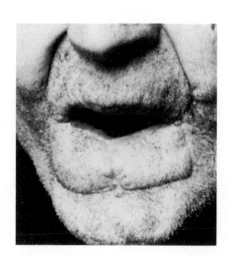

FIG. 4. An 80-year-old man with squamous cell carcinoma. A: Bilateral steeple flaps for total lower lip reconstruction. B: Final result. (From Stranc, Robertson, ref. 8, with permission.)

References

1. Owens N. Simplified method of rotating skin and mucous membrane flaps for complete reconstruction of the lower lip. *Surgery* 1994;15:19.
2. May H. The modified Dieffenbach operation for closure of large defects of the lower lip and chin. *Plast Reconstr Surg* 1946;1:194.
3. Gillies H, Millard DR, eds. *The principles and art of plastic surgery,* Vol. 2. Boston: Little, Brown, 1957;507.
4. Freeman BS. Myoplastic modification of the Bernard cheiloplasty. *Plast Reconstr Surg* 1958;21:453.
5. O'Brien BM. A muscle-skin pedicle for total reconstruction of the lower lip. *Plast Reconstr Surg* 1970;45:395.
6. Olivari N. One-stage reconstruction of the whole lower lip. *Br J Plast Surg* 1973;26:66.
7. Karapandžić M. Reconstruction of lip defects by local arterial flaps. *Br J Plast Surg* 1974;27:93.
8. Stranc MF, Robertson GA. Steeple flap reconstruction of the lower lip. *Ann Plast Surg* 1983;10:4.

CHAPTER 166 ■ UPPER LIP ANGULAR SKIN-MUSCLE-MUCOSAL FLAP TO LOWER LIP

C. R. BALCH

A cross-lip flap from the upper lip provides the best repair for many defects of the lower lip (1). The angular musculocutaneous flap minimizes the resulting deformity in the donor (upper) lip that is frequently associated with other flap designs (2,3).

rectangular, or trapezoidal defects of the lower lip. After creation of the flap, its shape may be modified to fit the defect. The scar of the upper lip is partly concealed in the nasolabial fold (see Fig. 2).

INDICATIONS

The elasticity of the lips and the design of the angular flap allow this flap to be used for reconstruction of large wedge,

FLAP DESIGN AND DIMENSIONS

An angular flap is designed on the upper lip (Fig. 1A). Line *a* is in the nasolabial fold. Line *c* is perpendicular to the vermilion border and is placed as far laterally as possible with-

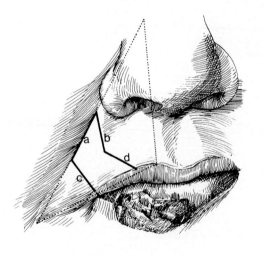

A

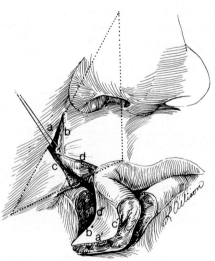

B

FIG. 1. A: Design of the angular cross-lip flap. **B:** Rotation of the flap and closure of the donor site. (From Balch, ref. 1, with permission.)

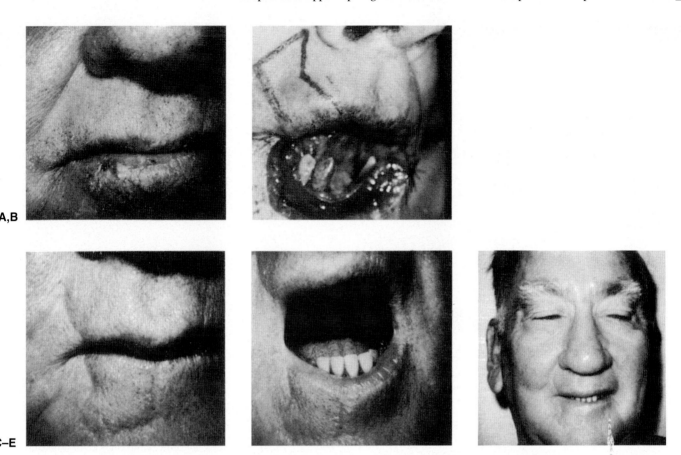

FIG. 2. A: Cancer of the lower lip. **B:** Defect of the lower lip with the design of the angular flap. Note that the commissure is preserved. **C,D:** Four months postoperatively. **E:** The final result. (From Balch, ref. 1, with permission.)

out sacrificing the commissure. The position of line *d* is determined by the width of the lower lip defect. The width of the flap should be approximately half the width of the lower lip defect. Line *b* then is placed so an angle is created at the intersection of lines *b* and *d*. The combined length of lines *a* and *c* needs only to approximate the combined length of lines *b* and *d*.

OPERATIVE TECHNIQUE

The lower lip lesion is excised, and the ipsilateral commissure is preserved, if possible. The angular flap designed on the upper lip may be based medially (Fig. 2) or laterally on the coronary vessels. A standard three-layer closure of both the donor and recipient sites is done. Ten to 14 days later, the pedicle is divided and inset.

CLINICAL RESULTS

The triangular relationship of the ipsilateral pillar of the philtrum, the nasolabial fold, and the line through the commissure and peak of the cupid's bow is maintained (Figs. 1B

and 2). An S- or C-shaped deformity of the nasolabial fold is avoided, and the commissure is preserved. The final scar is within the lines of expression, and notching of the border of the lips is avoided.

SUMMARY

The upper lip angular musculocutaneous flap provides not only a functional reconstruction of the lower lip, but also an excellent cosmetic result.

References

1. Balch CR. Modification of cross lip flap. *Plast Reconstr Surg* 1978;61:457.
2. Kazanjian VH. Supporting flaps used in reconstruction of the lower lip. In: Kazanjian VH, Converse JM, eds. *The surgical treatment of facial injuries.* Baltimore: Williams & Wilkins, 1949.
3. Estlander JA. Classic reprint. Eine Methode aus der einen Lippe Substanzverluste der Anderen zu Erstetzen (A method of reconstructing loss of substance in one lip from the other lip. Translated from the German by B. Sundell). *Arch Klin Chir* 1872;14:622. (*Plast Reconstr Surg* 1968; 42:360.)

CHAPTER 167 ■ FUNCTIONAL LOWER LIP AND ORAL SPHINCTER RECONSTRUCTION WITH INNERVATED DEPRESSOR ANGULI ORIS FLAPS

G. R. TOBIN

EDITORIAL COMMENT

The objective of the procedure, which is to restore the oral sphincter with innervated muscle, is correct. In practice, the technique is cumbersome, because in most cases simple reapproximation of the remnants of the orbicularis muscle may suffice. Further experience with this flap, particularly applicable to postcancer patients, demonstrates that the flap can be extended down along the so-called jowls below the horizontal ramus of the mandible. This is most helpful in reconstructing the upper portion of the lower lip, providing sufficient height with good sphincter restoration.

The innervated depressor anguli oris (DAO) musculocutaneous-mucosal flap is a compound flap that provides functional lower lip and oral sphincter reconstruction with all the necessary components: skin cover, mucosal lining, vermilion, oral sphincter, and sensation.

INDICATIONS

Depressor anguli oris flaps reconstruct sensate lips and functional oral sphincters of normal dimensions in one operation without invading or denervating the upper lip. All previously described methods of lower lip reconstruction suffer from one or more of the following disadvantages:

1. Partial sacrifice or denervation of the upper lip and its orbicularis oris sphincter
2. Transection of the orbicularis oris sphincter lateral to the oral commissure
3. Obliteration of the oral commissure
4. Microstomia

Lip-switch flaps (1,2) sacrifice upper lip and transect its orbicularis oris sphincter, denervate the orbicularis oris medial to the donor site, fail to restore oral circumference, and produce denervated reconstructions (although partial reinnervation subsequently occurs (3)). Inferiorly based nasolabial flaps (4) denervate the upper lip and produce partially or totally denervated reconstructions. They also destroy functional orbicularis oris around the commissure. Inferior pedicle cheek transposition flaps (5) transect the orbicularis oris at the commissure and fail to reconstruct

the lower lip sphincter or provide sensation. Lateral advancement cheek flaps (6–9) denervate the upper lip, transect the orbicularis oris muscle at the commissure, and fail to reconstruct the lower lip sphincter. The myoplastic modification of the Bernard method (10) overcomes some of these disadvantages by preserving upper lip innervation and by avoiding transection of orbicularis oris at the commissure when short advancements are done for small defects. Microstomia and obliteration of the oral commissure occur with Estlander, "fan" (11,12), and Karapandžić (13) flaps; however, the Karapandžić method is the only technique that reconstructs the oral sphincter and preserves motor and sensory innervation to the extent of depressor anguli oris reconstructions.

One depressor anguli oris flap reconstructs over half of a lower lip (Figs. 1 and 2), and bilateral depressor anguli oris flaps reconstruct an entire lower lip of normal length (Fig. 3). The principal advantages of this technique are (a) reconstructed lips with normal sensation and functional oral sphincters, (b) avoidance of microstomia in reconstruction of large defects, (c) preservation of upper lip structure and function, and (d) provision of all lip elements by one flap in one operation. The principle of innervated facial musculocutaneous flap lip reconstruction can be extended to innervated depressor labii inferioris and facial platysma flaps, which also restore sensation and sphincter function in specific anatomic circumstances.

Depressor anguli oris flaps are my first choice for lateral defects involving between one third and two thirds of the lower lip. Based on the preceding discussion, my total approach to lower lip reconstruction is as follows:

1. Defects involving less than a third of the lip are closed directly with V or W excisional preparation.
2. Lateral defects involving between one third and two thirds of the lip are reconstructed with an innervated depressor anguli oris flap.
3. Central lower lip defects involving between one third and two thirds of the lip are closed with either the Karapandžić (13) or myoplastic techniques (10).
4. Total lower lip loss is reconstructed with bilateral depressor anguli oris flaps.
5. Innervated depressor labii inferioris flaps are used for central lower lip defects with preserved vermilion and mucosa (Figs. 4 and 5).
6. Innervated facial platysma flaps are used for defects that destroy the depressor anguli oris musculocutaneous unit along with the lower lip (Fig. 5).

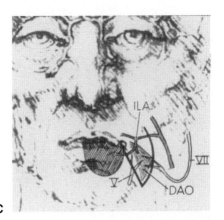
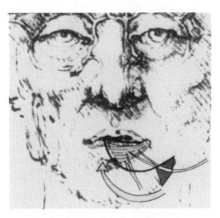
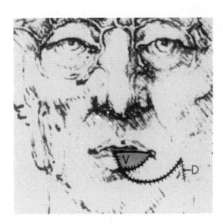

A–C

FIG. 1. Depressor anguli oris flap anatomy and transfer technique. **A:** Flap outline and components shown. These include skin, depressor anguli oris muscle (*DAO*), inferior labial artery (*ILA*), mental nerve (*V*), marginal mandibular nerve (*VII*), and mucosa. **B:** Flap transposition into lip defect reorients the muscle to restore the oral sphincter. **C:** Mucosal advancement restores vermilion (*V*). Donor defect (*D*) is closed directly.

ANATOMY

The depressor anguli oris, or triangularis, is the muscle of facial expression that joins the oral commissure to the lower mandibular border in the line of the nasolabial fold. It functions to depress the oral commissure in facial expression. The depressor anguli oris lies lateral to the depressor labii inferioris and medial to platysmal extensions crossing the mandible into the lower cheeks. The vascular pedicle of the flap is the lower labial branch of the facial vessels, which enter the flap base at the oral commissure (see Fig. 1A).

Flap sensory innervation is the trigeminal nerve mental branch, which also supplies the vermilion and lip that this flap replaces. Depressor anguli oris motor innervation is the facial nerve mandibular branch, which also supplies the orbicularis oris sphincter that this flap reconstitutes. These two nerves are dissected and preserved in the creation of the flap (see Figs. 1 and 2).

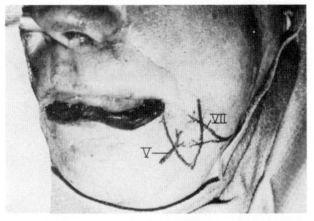
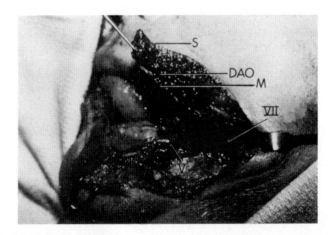

A,B

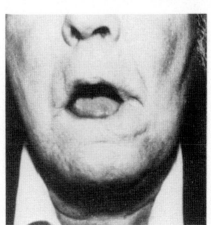
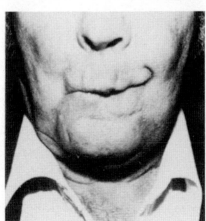

C,D

FIG. 2. Transfer technique illustrated in reconstruction of half the lower lip resected for squamous cell carcinoma. **A:** Flap outlined and nerve positions marked (*V, VII*) after tumor resection and contralateral vermilionectomy. **B:** Flap transposition. The motor nerve (*VII*) and sensory nerve (*V*) to the flap have been dissected. The same incision is used for submental and supraomohyoid lymphadenectomy. *S,* skin; *DAO,* muscle; *M,* mucosa. **C:** The result is a lower lip and oral sphincter of normal dimensions. **D:** Normal lip sensation and oral sphincter function result.

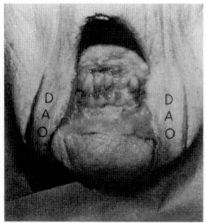
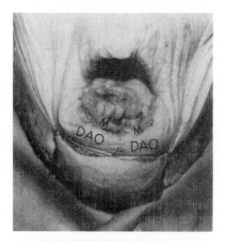
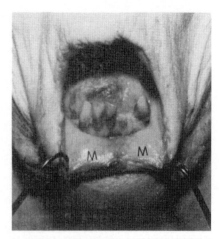

A–C

FIG. 3. Total lower lip reconstruction with bilateral innervated depressor anguli oris flaps demonstrated in a cadaver. **A:** Lower lip totally resected and bilateral depressor anguli oris flaps (*DAO*) with squared distal ends incised. **B:** Flap transposition and mucosal advancement (*M*) restore total lip and sphincter of normal length. **C:** Mucosal components (*M*) restore labial sulcus and vermilion.

FLAP DESIGN AND DIMENSIONS

To restore lips with normal dimensions, flap dimensions are matched to the defect size. The depressor anguli oris muscle is approximately 4 cm long and 2 cm wide. These dimensions allow reconstruction of up to two thirds of a lower lip. The skin component can be safely extended longer than 4 cm by inclusion of submental skin, but the distal flap then has no motor component for sphincter reconstruction. The length of the mucosal component is limited by the depth of the labial-gingival sulcus to approximately 3 cm. Reconstruction of longer mucosal defects requires enlarging the mucosal component with a lateral extension from the labial-gingival sulcus or advancing mucosa from the margins of the recipient defect.

The flap is marked on the skin overlying the depressor anguli oris muscle, which is located preoperatively by palpation during scowling. The flap is superiorly based at the level of the oral commissure, and its axis is the nasolabial fold extended distally to the jaw line (see Figs. 1A and 2A). The medial border originates at the oral commissure.

Bilateral innervated depressor anguli oris flaps reconstruct a total lower lip and are designed with squared distal ends.

Muscle, mucosa, and skin are joined in the midline. The flaps are each made one half of the lower lip length, approximately 2.5 cm long each (see Fig. 3).

OPERATIVE TECHNIQUE

After the skin is incised, the motor and sensory nerves are dissected. First, the facial nerve mandibular branch is approached by a horizontal incision in the shadow area beneath the body of the mandible (see Fig. 2B). This incision also can serve to approach a submental and cervical lymphadenectomy, if indicated. The motor nerve is located by careful dissection of the plane deep to the platysma. If the nerve is difficult to locate, techniques exploiting the anatomic relationship of the nerve to the cervical vessels are useful (1,2). Once the nerve trunk is identified, it is dissected distally to the flap.

Next, the mental nerve is approached by incising the tip of the flap through the muscle to enter the submuscular space above the periosteum. This loose areolar plane is easily dissected to locate the mental foramen. Lateral branches of the mental nerve are then dissected to the flap (see Fig. 2B). Once the nerves are dissected, the remaining deep tissues and

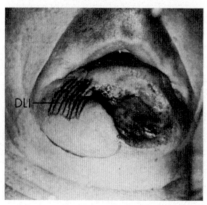
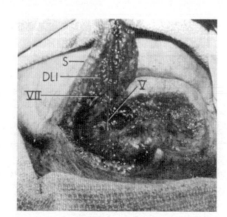
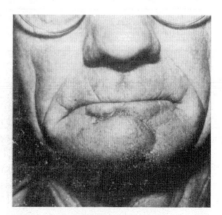

A–C

FIG. 4. Innervated depressor labii inferioris flap reconstruction of lower lip, sphincter, and mental prominence. Lip vermilion and mucosa were preserved. **A:** Flap outlined and muscle position marked (*DLI*). **B:** Flap elevated. *S*, skin; *DLI*, muscle; *V*, mental nerve; *VII*, mandibular nerve. **C:** A functional oral sphincter and a sensate lip and chin are the result.

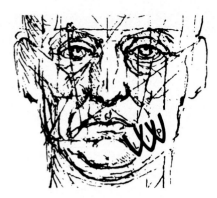

FIG. 5. Depressor labii inferioris (*L*), depressor anguli oris (*I*), and fascial platysma (*P*) innervated musculocutaneous flaps are marked directly over the respective muscles.

mucosal components of the flap are incised. The depressor anguli oris musculocutaneous unit without mucosa is used if mucosa is preserved in the recipient defect.

Flap transposition into the lip defect reorients the muscle to restore the oral sphincter and reroutes the motor and sensory nerves (see Fig. 1B).

Vermilion is provided by advancement of flap mucosa (which is made approximately 1 cm wider than the skin and muscle medially) over the medial flap border in similar fashion to a vermilionectomy procedure (see Fig. 1C). Mucosal, muscle, and skin layers are closed individually, and the donor defect is closed directly.

If clinical circumstances dictate use of an innervated depressor labii inferioris or fascial platysma flap, the sequence of dissection is the same, except that medial branches of the mental nerve supply sensation to the innervated depressor labii inferioris flap and the sensory supply of the innervated fascial platysma flap is division II of the fascial nerve, not the mental nerve.

CLINICAL RESULTS

The depressor anguli oris flap is highly reliable. Complete flap survival and restoration of lip structure and function have followed all uses to date.

A small but definable functional donor defect is seen in the early postoperative period. In a balanced smile, the ipsilateral oral commissure rises more than the contralateral one, and in scowling, the ipsilateral oral commissure depresses less than the contralateral one. In repose and in a full smile, this defect is not evident. With training before a mirror, this minor defect can be eliminated. The skin donor-defect scar is inconspicuous because it falls in the extended nasolabial fold between the cheek and chin aesthetic units.

SUMMARY

Innervated depressor anguli oris musculocutaneous-mucosal flaps reconstruct total or subtotal sensate lower lips and functional oral sphincters with normal dimensions and function as a consequence of preserved innervation.

References

1. Kazanjian VH, Roopenian A. The treatment of lip deformities resulting from electric burns. *Am J Surg* 1954;88:884.
2. Estlander JA. Eine Methode aus der einen Lippe Substanzverluste der Anderen zu Erstetzen (A method of reconstructing loss of substance in one lip from the other lip. Translated from the German by B. Sundell). *Arch Klin Chir* 1872;14:622. *Plast Reconstr Surg* 1968;42:360.
3. Smith JW. The anatomic and physiologic acclimatization of tissue transplanted by the lip-switch technique. *Plast Reconstr Surg* 1960;26:40.
4. Fujimori R. "Gate flap" for the total reconstruction of the lower lip. *Br J Plast Surg* 1980;33:340.
5. Diffenbach JF. *Chirurgische Erfahrungen, besonders ueber die Wiederherstellung Zerstoerter Theile des menchlichen Koerpers nach neuen Methoden.* Berlin: Enslin, 1829–1834.
6. Bernard C. Cancer de la lèvre inférieure. restauration à l'aide de lambeaux quadrilataires-latereaus. In: *Guérison.* Vol. 5. Liege: Scapel, 1852–1853; 162–164.
7. Fries R. The merits of Bernard's operation as a universal procedure for lower lip reconstruction after resection of carcinoma. *Chir Plast* 1971;1:45.
8. Webster RC, Coffey RJ, Kelleher RE. Total and partial reconstruction of the lower lip with innervated muscle-bearing flaps. *Plast Reconstr Surg* 1960; 25:360.
9. Meyer R, Farlot ASA. New concepts in lower lip reconstruction. *Head Neck Surg* 1982;4:240.
10. Freeman BS. Myoplastic modification of the Bernard cheiloplasty. *Plast Reconstr Surg* 1958;21:453.
11. Gillies HD. *Plastic surgery of the face.* London: Henry Frowde, Oxford University Press, 1920.
12. Gillies HD, Millard DR Jr., eds. *Principles and art of plastic surgery.* Boston: Little, Brown, 1957.
13. Karapandžić M. Reconstruction of lip defects by local arterial flaps. *Br J Plast Surg* 1974;27:93.

CHAPTER 168 ■ ORBICULARIS ORIS MUSCLE FLAPS

C. L. PUCKETT, K. L. PICKRELL,* AND J. F. REINISCH

Mobilization of the orbicularis oris muscle flap has been useful in reconstruction for paralysis or discontinuity of the orbicularis muscle.

INDICATIONS

The two clinical circumstances in which we have used this technique most successfully have been (a) dense paralysis of the lip associated with injury to the marginal mandibular branch of the facial nerve (1), and (b) sphincteric discontinuity of the orbicularis oris muscle in the bilateral cleft lip patient (2).

ANATOMY

The orbicularis oris muscle is a sphincter that has no clearly defined origin and insertion; however, its lateral attachments at the modiolus can be considered the origin, with the insertion being into its contralateral half in the center of the upper and lower lips. The muscle is flattened, somewhat ribbon-like, with a thickness of approximately 0.5 cm, and it varies from 1 to 2 cm in width. It is innervated in quadrants (although there is significant overlap) by the zygomatic

*Deceased

branches of the facial nerve for the upper half and the marginal mandibular branch of the facial nerve for the lower half (3). There is variable input by the buccal branch. Three or more filaments of these nerves may enter the muscle quadrant. Blood supply is from the facial artery by means of the labial branches.

FLAP DESIGN AND DIMENSIONS

Because of a rich blood supply, the muscle can be used as a flap based either medially or laterally. When based laterally, flap innervation can be maintained, but if based medially, the flap is effectively denervated.

Unilateral Lower Lip Paralysis

Following marginal mandibular branch injury in which nerve repair is not feasible, a medially based flap of the atrophic orbicularis oris muscle can be combined with a wedge resection of the lip to improve the appearance of the defect. This is particularly helpful when the paralysis is dense and associated with atrophy of the orbicularis oris muscle and droop of the lateral lower lip. A V-shaped wedge of lower lip is marked, with the width of the V matching the amount of orbicularis atrophy (Fig. 1A). The lateral limb of the V is 1 or 2 mm medial to the commissure of the lip.

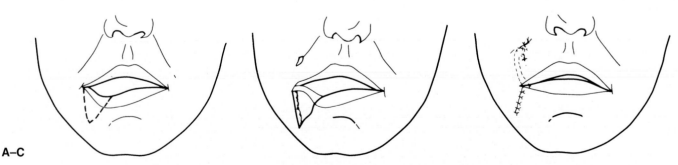

A–C

FIG. 1. A: The wedge resection outlined. The lateral limb of the V is a few millimeters medial to the commissure. The approximate width of the atrophic segment indicates the width of the V. B: The wedge has been resected through and through, preserving only the atrophic strand of orbicularis oris. Note the incision in the nasolabial fold above the commissure. C: The wedge has been approximated, and the orbicularis oris muscle flap has been brought through the subcutaneous tunnel and sutured to the region of the insertion of the zygomaticus major. (From Puckett et al., ref. 1, with permission.)

Bilateral Cleft Lip

In the bilateral complete cleft lip deformity, there is no orbicularis oris muscle in the prolabium. Because many bilateral lip repairs do not incorporate orbicularis oris reconstruction, there is frequently an absent segment of muscle in the central portion of the lip. The resultant incomplete sphincter can add to the aesthetic deformity in these patients. On contraction of the orbicularis oris muscle with animation, two bulges appear in the upper lateral segments. These have been colloquially referred to as the "double-bump deformity." Additionally, there is flattening of the prolabial central segment that may contribute to a rather bizarre appearance. With time, these bulges become apparent even at rest. By creating two laterally based orbicularis oris muscle flaps and bringing them together in the midline, the sphincteric continuity of the muscle can be restored and the double-bump deformity eliminated or minimized.

OPERATIVE TECHNIQUE

Unilateral Lower Lip Paralysis

The previously marked V-shaped wedge on the lower lip is incised, and all tissue is resected, except for the orbicularis oris muscle (Fig. 1B). The muscle is freed circumferentially and detached at the commissure, but it is left attached medially as a flap. A tunnel then is made by both sharp and blunt dissection traversing lateral to the commissure and passing superficially in the region of the modiolus. A 5-mm incision is made in the nasolabial fold 1.5 to 2.0 cm above the commissure. A hemostat is passed from the nasolabial incision through the tunnel to grasp the end of the muscle flap. Advancement of the flap laterally through the tunnel will bring the wedge together, and the lip is closed in three layers with accurate approximation of the vermilion border. The muscle flap then is sutured to the underlying insertion of the zygomaticus major (Fig. 1C).

Use in Bilateral Cleft Lip Patients

The procedure may be incorporated into lip scar revisions or other procedures being done simultaneously in bilateral cleft lip patients. Access to the muscle usually is gained by excising the vertical scars at the edges of the prolabium. We have usually included a Z-plasty at the apex of the scar excisions to lengthen and change the orientation slightly.

Infiltration with epinephrine aids in identifying the muscle. The muscle flap is dissected circumferentially, leaving some of the scar of the previous lip repair attached to the muscle medially. This serves as a handle and as reinforced tissue for suture placement. Dissection is carried laterally almost to a point above the commissure. Intermittent traction on the muscle may reveal skin dimpling, indicating that additional release is necessary. When the two muscle flaps can be approximated in the midline without dimpling the skin, the dissection has been adequate. A tunnel is developed in the prolabial segment. Usually, some tissue resection is necessary to accept the bulk of the muscle and simultaneously create a philtral dimple. The muscle repair is an imbricating one using horizontal mattress sutures of nonabsorbable material. We have found that a tiny suction drain is helpful in decreasing postoperative swelling.

CLINICAL RESULTS

Unilateral Lower Lip Paralysis

The procedure used in unilateral lower lip paralysis has proven helpful in minimizing the deformity resulting from unilateral marginal mandibular branch injury (Fig. 2). We emphasize that its most precise indication is dense paralysis associated with some degree of orbicularis oris atrophy and lip ptosis. Although repair of the injured nerve is the foremost consideration when feasible, a number of occasions exist in which this is either not appropriate or not possible. Because this operation does not provide depressor reanimation, it may be of little value in patients in whom the only defect is absence of depressor function.

Bilateral Cleft Lip

This procedure also has been useful in eliminating or minimizing one of the many aspects of the bilateral cleft lip deformity. Disruption has been evident in only one patient in 20, and a distinct improvement in the double-bump deformity has been observed in approximately 90% of patients. The procedure often exaggerates the lateral vermilion pout, which is corrected easily by a horizontal wedge resection of the vermilion, but we have been reluctant to do this at the same time as the initial procedure for fear that we would misjudge the amount needed.

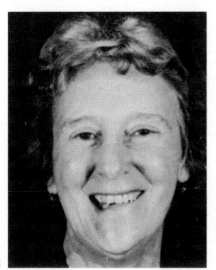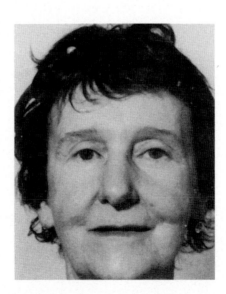

A,B

FIG. 2. **A:** A patient with dense marginal mandibular branch paralysis. Note atrophy in the right lateral lip segment and ptosis of the vermilion. **B:** Two years after wedge resection and orbicularis oris muscle flap. (From Puckett et al., ref. 1, with permission.)

SUMMARY

Orbicularis oris muscle flaps can be used for either the upper or lower lip to restore a more natural functional appearance. This has been especially useful both in patients with unilateral lower lip paralysis and in patients with bilateral cleft lip deformities.

References

1. Puckett CL, Neale HW, Pickrell, KL. Dynamic correction of unilateral paralysis of the lower lip. *Plast Reconstr Surg* 1975;55:397.
2. Puckett CL, Reinisch JF, Werner RS. Late correction of orbicularis discontinuity in bilateral cleft lip deformity. *Cleft Palate J* 1980;17:34.
3. Dingman RO, Grabb WC. Surgical anatomy of the mandibular ramus of the facial nerve based on the dissection of 100 facial halves. *Plast Reconstr Surg* 1962;29:266.

Online Chapter CHAPTER 169. Paired Deltopectoral Skin Flap to the Lip *M. Soussaline*
www.encyclopediaofflaps.com

CHAPTER 170 ■ PLATYSMA MUSCULOCUTANEOUS FLAP TO THE LOWER LIP

J. N. BARRON* AND M. N. SAAD

EDITORIAL COMMENT

The anatomic description and blood supply for the standard platysmal flap apply here. The illustrative case provided by Drs. Barron and Saad shows an innovative way of using the platysmal flap.

* Deceased.

For anatomy, flap design, and operative technique see Chapter 122.

CLINICAL RESULTS

If the nerve supply to the platysma is preserved, the tone of the transplanted muscle is sufficient to prevent the development of a labial ectropion. Careful fixation to the cheek musculature at each lateral margin of the defect is, of course, necessary.

If neck skin is used to reconstruct the vermilion, a subtle color change takes place so that a natural, smooth pink appearance can be expected.

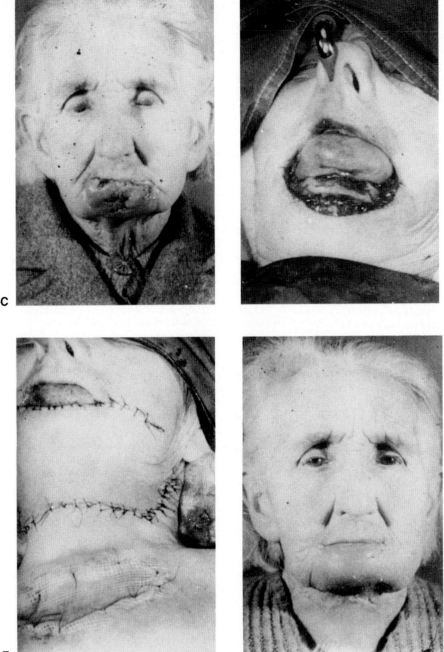

A–C

D,E

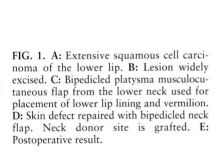

FIG. 1. A: Extensive squamous cell carcinoma of the lower lip. B: Lesion widely excised. C: Bipedicled platysma musculocutaneous flap from the lower neck used for placement of lower lip lining and vermilion. D: Skin defect repaired with bipedicled neck flap. Neck donor site is grafted. E: Postoperative result.

CHAPTER 171 ■ FAN FLAPS

W. R. MULLIN AND D. R. MILLARD, JR.

These flaps were given the name "fan flaps" because of their resemblance to the rotational opening of an oriental folding fan.

INDICATIONS

The fan flap procedure is used today to correct larger full-thickness defects of both upper and lower lips. Attributes of the fan flap are as follows. Two basic principles (1) are observed using this flap: (a) losses should be replaced with similar types of tissue, and (b) tissue from an area of relative excess to supply an area of need should be used. Few conventional axial flaps allow such freedom of movement of such large amounts of tissue based on such a small pedicle. Also, most donor-area scars may be located close to the natural junction lines of facial units.

The fan flap has found its best use for reconstruction of large central full-thickness defects of both upper and lower lips. In such defects, the use of bilateral symmetrical flaps rotated medially usually affords the most satisfactory final result.

FLAP DESIGN AND DIMENSIONS

Owing to the marked elasticity of the lips, evaluation of defects must be determined in the absence of induration and edema. The exact amount of lip loss usually can be judged quite accurately, especially in primary surgical losses resulting from resections for carcinoma if there has not been a large inflammatory response to the tumor. Defects secondary to burns or infection should be allowed to heal to stability and softness before planning reconstruction.

It is most important to recognize that the amount of tissue required to reconstruct an attractive lip is always less than the size of the original defect. It must be stressed that the edges of the defects actually must be grasped and approximated to the desired location so that the true defect to be reconstructed can be visualized and measured. One may see exact percentages quoted, stating X percent of a lip defect can be closed primarily; however, this is a general rule and only a rough guide. More important are the actual examination and the final relationship of the lip to the opposite lip once the defect is closed. For example, one may be able to close an upper lip tightly without the use of a flap; however, the lower lip may have an unsightly protruding appearance relative to the upper lip.

The units of the lips always must be honored. In large central upper lip defects, a midline shield-shaped Abbé flap from the lower lip to reconstruct a philtrum may be in order (2,3); however, this should be done as a secondary procedure so as not to compromise any blood supply traversing the circumoral labial vessel.

Large full-thickness defects of the lateral lip may be repaired using the unilateral fan flap. One also should consider the use of an off-center Abbé flap (4) or an Estlander flap (5), which may be a less elaborate solution to the problem.

Once the true defect that requires reconstruction has been determined, considering laxity and opposite lip relationship, one may proceed to the outline of the flap. A dot is placed at the desired location of the new mouth corner. The length of the defect to be filled is transferred along the adjacent vermilion, and from the point marked, a line is dropped perpendicular from the white roll. The length of this line establishes the bulk and size of the flap, and usually it is at least 1 to 1.5 cm long.

An angle of approximately 60 degrees is turned toward the nasolabial fold. Once the nasolabial fold area is transected, the line follows this area to a point that will provide adequate height and bulk to the flap. In general, approximately no more than one half the upper lip (Fig. 1) and two thirds of the lower lip (Fig. 3) should be attempted using a unilateral fan flap (1).

OPERATIVE TECHNIQUE

The rules of oncologic surgery must be honored if one is dealing with carcinoma as the primary lesion; that is, one must have every assurance that the patient is free of his or her original tumor, and one must not include precancerous tissue in the flap.

Defects of the Upper Lip

Cutting the flap is accomplished nicely using a no. 11 blade pushed through the lip beginning at the dot so that the back of the blade protects the vascular pedicle. The only other landmarks that should be noted are the surface area of the internal lining and, in larger flaps, the exit of Stensen's duct. As the fan flap is rotated into position, the trailing 60-degree triangular segment of tissue finds its own new location, and the most appropriate cut is made so that this point may be inset, thus forming a Z-plasty. Once this point is positioned satisfactorily, a three-layer closure is accomplished, closing mucous membrane, muscle, and then skin. Of course, natural landmarks are carefully approximated, namely, the white roll and vermilion border (Figs. 1 and 2).

Defects of the Lower Lip

Basic steps of design are the same as for the upper lip. Because the lower lip is responsible for oral competence and prevention of drooling, the amount of tissue to be brought in must not be underestimated. Careful attention to closure of the vertical axis to maintain height is paramount to prevent notching in this area and thus incompetence and drooling. A Z-plasty of the labial sulcus mucous membrane closure is often useful (Figs. 3 and 4).

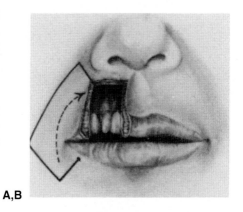
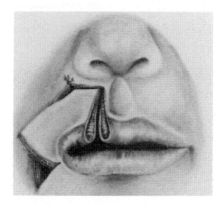

A,B

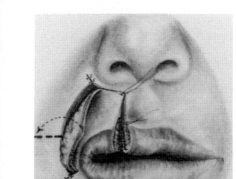
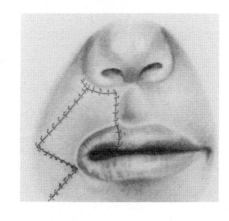

C,D

FIG. 1. A–D: Unilateral fan flap for the upper lip.

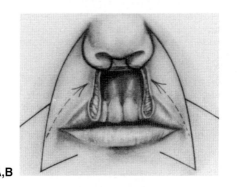
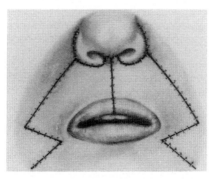

A,B

FIG. 2. A, B: Diagrams of bilateral fan flaps for upper lip defect.

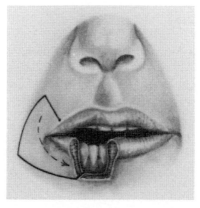
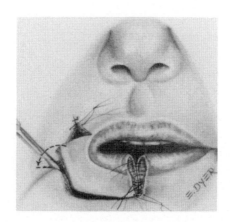
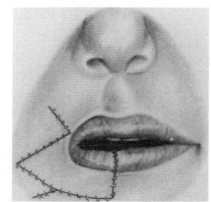

A–C

FIG. 3. A–C: Unilateral fan flap for the lower lip.

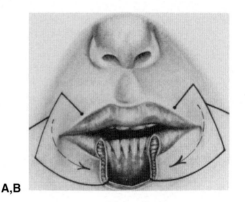 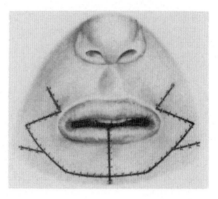

A,B

FIG. 4. A, B: Diagrams of bilateral fan flaps for lower lip defects.

Secondary Procedures

The microstomia and rounded lip corners resulting from the use of fan flaps must now be corrected as a secondary procedure. Time should be allowed for the flaps and scars to soften, and this usually takes a minimum of 2 to 3 months. During this time, the patient who has dentures may have difficulty, and this problem must be taken into consideration.

The commissuroplasty is performed as follows (Fig. 5). The new apex of the commissure is located by noting the normal location on the opposite side, or if this is absent, a perpendicular line is dropped from an area below the pupil of the eye. This gives an approximate lateral extent of where a normal commissure should lie. A triangle of skin is excised, leaving the vermilion rim intact. A point is located along the lower aspect of the vermilion that would reach the new commissure point when lifted and outfolded into that area.

Next, the vermilion is lifted with a few fibers of orbicularis oris muscle. Once this component is freed, full division through the orbicularis is accomplished; in some cases, thinning is required. The vermilion flap then is rolled laterally into the new position. The raw surface along the lateral aspect of the lower lip must be covered using a flap of mucous membrane dissected from within and rolled out onto this area. The mucous membrane substitution for vermilion may be satisfactory; however, in some cases, it is markedly redder than normal vermilion. Also, in some cases, an entropion of this area is caused by contracture of the flap. If this is a problem, one may consider a full-thickness graft of true vermilion from an area that can afford to donate to this area.

Modifications in Operative Technique

A modification of the traditional fan flap is described by other authors (6,7) in which a rectangular segment of tissue is rotated into position and the raw surface must be covered by advancing mucosa or an inferior surface tongue flap. Because the location of the commissure is unchanged, the secondary revision and microstomia are avoided; however, donor-area scars do not seem to follow the natural lines of facial units as well as those of traditional fan flaps, and the area of vermilion to be covered with the advanced mucosa or tongue flap is larger.

CLINICAL RESULTS

Criticism that may be directed toward the use of fan flaps is as follows: Two stages are required to correct the relative microstomia and to reconstruct a new commissure following rotation of a fan flap. Motor nerves innervating the orbicularis oris muscle are divided.

Addressing this problem, Karapandžić (8) (see Chapter 172) describes a similar flap based on mucosal lining. He carefully describes microdissecting the neural filaments in this area to prevent division. In certain circumstances, leaving these nerves intact may hinder the mobility of this flap compared with a completely dissected fan flap.

Branches of the facial motor units divided medial to the lateral canthus of the eye regenerate, or new attachments are formed so that reanimation is possible (1,6,9). Such may be the case when fan flaps are used, for after some time has been

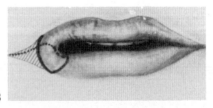 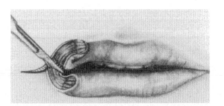

A,B

FIG. 5. A–E: Commissuroplasty done as a secondary procedure.

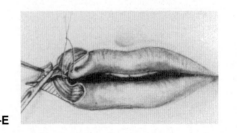 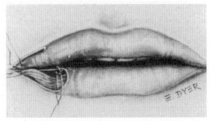 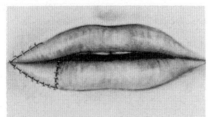

C–E

allowed for the area to soften and settle, voluntary circumferential contracture in the rotated flap may be observed. This may represent real muscle contracture as a result of ingrowth of new motor nerves, new anastomotic connections, or simply transmitted vectors from the animation of the opposite lip. Neurologic return in transplanted flaps (6) has shown that pain returns first, followed by tactile sensation, temperature sensation, and sympathetic function, in that order, with total return at 2 years.

SUMMARY

The fan flap is a versatile and satisfactory flap to use in the reconstruction of certain large full-thickness defects of the lips.

References

1. Gillies HD, Millard DR, Jr., eds. *Principles and art of plastic surgery.* Boston: Little, Brown, 1957.
2. Grabb W, Smith JW, eds. *Plastic surgery,* 3d ed. Boston: Little, Brown, 1979.
3. Millard DR Jr. Composite lip flaps and grafts in secondary cleft deformities. *Br J Plast Surg* 1974;17:40.
4. Abbé RA. A new plastic operation for the relief of deformity due to double harelip (Classic Reprint). *Plast Reconstr Surg* 1968;42:481.
5. Estlander JA. A method of reconstructing loss of substance in one lip from the other lip (Classic Reprint). *Plast Reconstr Surg* 1968;42:360.
6. Smith JW. The anatomical and physiologic acclimatization of tissue transplanted by the lip-switch technique. *Plast Reconstr Surg* 1960;26:40.
7. Stranc MF. Steeple flap reconstruction of the lower lip. *Ann Plast Surg* 1980; 10:4.
8. Karapandžić M. Reconstruction of lip defects by local arterial flaps. *Br J Plast Surg* 1974;27:93.
9. McGregor IA. Reconstruction of the lower lip. *Br J Plast Surg* 1983;36:40.

CHAPTER 172 ■ INNERVATED MUSCULOCUTANEOUS LIP AND CHEEK FLAPS

M. KARAPANDŽIĆ

EDITORIAL COMMENT

This is a classic description of one of the most important procedures currently used to reconstruct defects of the upper and lower lips. This is so particularly because of the attention paid to functional restoration of the oral sphincter.

The aim of reconstruction of lip defects by innervated musculocutaneous lip and cheek flaps is to form new lips that are anatomically and functionally able to satisfy the everyday needs of feeding, phonation, emotional expression, and communication. The reconstructed lip should be able to match the normal one, with parallel appearance, color, texture, hairiness, shape, thickness, elasticity, and dynamics of movement.

The reconstructive method of innervated musculocutaneous arterial flaps is based on the principle of replacing lost tissue with labial or cheek tissue that most closely resembles that of the lips. The flaps should contain skin, muscle, and mucous membrane with discrete blood and nerve supplies. This makes possible immediate mobility and normal sensibility with preservation of vegetative functions in a newly formed vermilion-bordered lip (1–3).

INDICATIONS

The procedure is applied in all patients in whom lip defects cannot be sutured directly without functional consequences. It is most frequently applied in defects caused by radical excision of malignant tumors and traumatic avulsion.

ANATOMY

Flaps are formed from all the anatomic elements of the lip and part of the cheek tissue. Essential elements of the flap are lip muscles covered with skin.

Lip muscles can be classified as either constrictors or dilators. The muscles are arranged in three layers: peripheral, medial, and deep. According to their position and function, these muscles may act as synergists or antagonists in the coordination of lip movement.

The orbicularis oris muscle is the most significant muscle. It is included in the structure of innervated musculocutaneous arterial flaps, together with the buccinator, both forming an orbicularis–buccinator complex that makes a newly formed lip equal in functional quality to the normal lip.

The orbicularis oris muscle is composed of several layers of muscle fibers that surround the lip orifice and stretch in

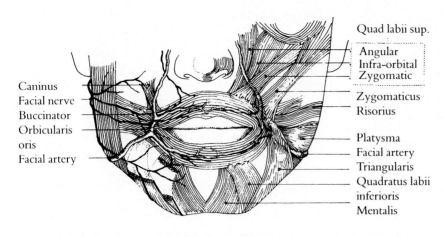

FIG. 1. Anatomy of the lip muscles in layers and their participation in forming the peripheral ring of the orbicularis oris muscle. Position of the facial artery and its branches in relation to the muscles is shown. The branches of the facial nerve enter the orbicularis oris and the other lip muscles.

various directions (Fig. 1). Its muscular structure may be divided into two concentric rings according to the origin of the fibers. The peripheral ring consists of muscle fibers that are radially located and inserted into upper and lower lips. The central ring consists of its own semicircular fibers that stretch obliquely through the thickness of the lip, running from the deep skin surface of one commissure toward the mucous membrane of the opposite commissure. The function of the centrally positioned orbicularis oris muscle is primarily sphincteric; the other lip muscles serve a supporting and dilatating function.

The facial artery with its branches, the inferior and superior labial arteries, supplies the innervated musculocutaneous flaps (Fig. 2). Adequate blood circulation in these flaps is extremely important, especially in elderly and previously irradiated patients. The anterior facial vein with its branches, the upper and lower labial veins, provides venous drainage. Lymphatic drainage is to the regional submental and submandibular glands.

The sensory innervation of the flaps originates from the second and third branches of the trigeminal nerve. Parts of the flap from the upper lip are innervated by the infraorbital nerve, and those formed from the remaining lower lip are innervated by branches of the mental nerve. The commissure area derives sensory innervation from the buccinator nerve.

The motor nerves that are preserved with the flap originate from the buccal and mandibular rami of the facial nerve. The superficial buccal branches pass under the skin and over the superficial facial muscles, which they innervate. Deep fibers supply the zygomatic and quadratus muscles of the upper lip; the deep buccal branches innervate the buccinator and orbicularis oris muscles. The ramus marginalis passes forward under the platysma and the triangularis, supplying innervation to the lower lip muscles and the chin (see Figs. 1 and 2).

FLAP DESIGN AND DIMENSIONS

The dimensions of innervated musculocutaneous arterial lip and cheek flaps depend on the size, position, and cause of the defect. Flaps can be located in the lower and upper lips in the area of lip angles or in both lips simultaneously. Defects are most frequently partial and rarely involve the whole lip. The most frequent defects are those of the lower lip, and they usually are located between the medial line and the commissure, rarely involving the central part.

Dimensions of defects that are suitable for lip reconstruction with this kind of flap are generally from 3 to 9 cm long. Flap width and length vary, depending on the pathologic process that caused the defect. Flaps are formed on both sides of the defect, and their width is equal to the height of the defect. The most suitable width of flaps is from 18 to 25 mm, and the flap should, in principle, have the dimensions of the orbicularis oris muscle.

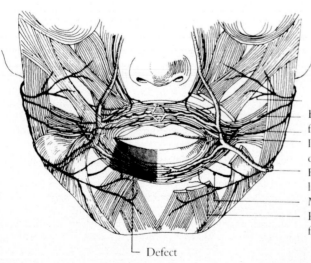

FIG. 2. The separated orbicularis oris muscle with preserved motor and sensory nerves and the facial artery with its branches form the innervated musculocutaneous arterial lip and cheek flaps.

Planning the flap begins with measurement of the lengths of the lower and upper lips and rima oris. The part of the lip to be excised is marked and measured. The defect is planned as a quadrilateral because this form is most convenient for the sliding and rotation of musculocutaneous flaps. From the edge of the planned defect, the width and length flap dimensions are marked on both sides and should follow the course of the orbicularis oris muscle and the natural lines of the face so that scars will not be noticeable.

The planned flaps should be long enough and wide enough that the newly formed lip may be constructed with an adequate rima oris for normal feeding, intelligible speech, and easy approach to the oral cavity for further therapeutic procedures. Adequate flap width allows encircling of the lip and prevents dribbling.

OPERATIVE TECHNIQUE

Defects of the Lower Lip

Full-thickness defects of the lower lip are reconstructed by the formation of two flaps from the remaining healthy lip tissue and tissue from the opposite lip, with the addition, in large defects, of some cheek tissue.

The operative procedure in forming innervated musculocutaneous arterial lip and cheek flaps is a continuous process in which nerve elements and blood vessels are sought simultaneously with selective cutting of some muscle fibers and separation of the orbicularis oris muscle into a special functional unit. From the edge of the defect, the incision advances at an equal distance from the mucocutaneous vermilion line, curving in the direction of the orbicularis oris muscle toward the lip commissure, which it curves around.

Then the incision continues at an equal distance over the nasolabial sulcus to the upper lip, to the area of the vertical projection of the nasal wing. The flap is of equal width along its full length. The incision continues deep to the lip muscles toward the region of the commissure to the site where the surrounding muscles intermingle with the orbicularis oris muscle. To this point, the muscle fibers are gradually cut so that the incision reaches only the mucous membrane in the initial part of the flap. Then, with the preparation of surrounding supporting muscle, some muscle bundles are selectively cut and the orbicularis oris muscle is separated. In the region of the lip commissure, muscle fibers are cut only in the superficial layer, while the deeper fibers of the orbicularis and buccinator muscles are preserved. It is especially important to preserve the medial part of the buccinator muscle because these decussated fibers are contained in the composition of lower and upper lip muscles (see Fig. 2).

If the defect is not large, a smaller part of the triangularis muscle fibers (which continue toward the upper lip) and part of the caninus muscle fibers (which continue to the lower lip) can be preserved in the region of the commisure. Preservation of the triangularis and caninus muscle fibers is necessary so that the mobility of the musculocutaneous flap will not be damaged. In large defects, the orbicularis oris muscle is separated completely from the surrounding muscles; thus, the mobility of the flaps is increased. In all cases, buccinator muscle fibers are saved to maintain functional harmony of the facial muscles with the orbicularis oris muscle. In the upper lip region, only the superficial muscle layer is cut to separate the orbicularis oris muscle and to improve the mobility of the musculocutaneous flaps.

In flap preparation that selectively cuts muscle fibers to separate the orbicularis oris muscle, full attention must be given to preserving the motor and sensory nerves and the facial artery and all its branches. The whole surgical procedure is directed mainly toward finding and preserving the nerve elements and the vascular network. It is usually necessary to use magnifying loupes during preparation of the nerve elements.

While preparing flaps from the remaining lower lip and cutting the superficial muscle fibers at the initial part of the flap, it is necessary to find the fibers of the mental nerve. Usually, one big branch is found, but sometimes there are two. Then the triangularis muscle is cut, preserving the branches of the marginal mandibular nerve that go toward the orbicularis oris muscle. In the region of the commissure, the buccal branches that lie immediately by the facial artery are prepared and preserved. Advancing in the direction of the upper lip, the other motor fibers that innervate the orbicularis oris muscle are gradually revealed. It is usually possible to preserve several buccal branches. Nerve fibers enter the flaps radially; during the preparation and cutting of the muscle fibers, this fact must be kept in mind (Fig. 3D and E).

In the region of the commissure, when cutting the superficial muscles, the facial artery that lies under the triangularis muscle must be preserved. At this site, lower and upper labial arteries can be found. When the facial artery is discovered, it should be carefully prepared in the direction of its central flow so that when the flaps are moved, blood flow will not be strangulated and reduced. Careful attention must be given at the start of cutting muscles in the initial preparation of the flaps because of the variable position of the lower labial artery.

Mucous membrane is cut only enough to ensure sliding of the flaps and to set medial sutures. The rest of the mucous membrane is preserved.

The innervated arterial lip and cheek flaps are now completely mobile and can be raised from the base and brought into the defect by sliding and rotation. First, the flaps are sutured together in the middle, beginning with mucous membrane through the muscles to the skin. In this way, the sphincteric lip ring is formed, completely surrounded by vermilion. To gain a symmetrical lip aperture, flap position is centered, and the medial suture line of the two flaps usually lies in the middle of the previous defect. Mucous membrane and muscle layers then are sutured slowly and carefully to preserve flap innervation and to maintain arterial supply and venous drainage. The muscle suture must be exact, especially in the region of convergence of the dilator muscles in the lip commissure, set symmetrically on the flaps, so that these muscles may retract equally and give a symmetrical lip aperture.

Formation of the new commissure after reconstruction of the reduced lip sphincter is carried out by suturing the cut muscle fibers of the zygomaticus, risorius, and triangularis muscles into their new position. These retract the new commissure by their tonus. In the same way, the volume of the secondary defect is reduced by the sutures, and correct redistribution of the flaps into the defect is undertaken. If there is a marked disproportion between the outer circumference of the flaps and the secondary defect, a triangular excision of skin is performed downward in the direction of the nasolabial furrow or upward in the region of the upper lip. Lip construction is finished by suturing muscles, subcutaneous tissue, and skin.

Defects of the Whole Lower Lip

Defects of the whole lower lip are most generally from 6 to 9 cm long and include all structural muscles. Reconstruction of such large defects should be planned carefully. If the lower lip defect stretches toward both the commissures, innervated

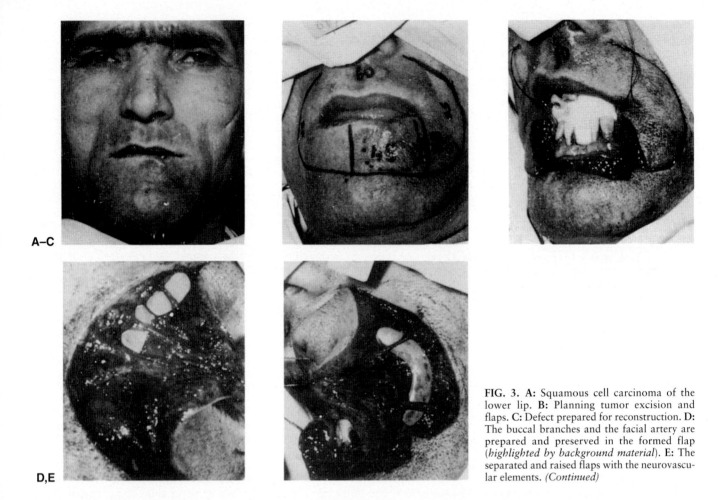

A–C

D,E

FIG. 3. **A:** Squamous cell carcinoma of the lower lip. **B:** Planning tumor excision and flaps. **C:** Defect prepared for reconstruction. **D:** The buccal branches and the facial artery are prepared and preserved in the formed flap (*highlighted by background material*). **E:** The separated and raised flaps with the neurovascular elements. *(Continued)*

musculocutaneous arterial lip and cheek flaps can be formed from the remaining tissue of the commissure and the upper lip according to the principles mentioned earlier (Fig. 4B). This sort of lip reconstruction reduces the circumference of the lip sphincter somewhat and can be accompanied by varying degrees of microstomia. To avoid microstomia, which sometimes entails secondary reconstruction, and to manage defects that include both lip commissures and portions of the upper lip, reconstruction can be performed using a larger part of the cheek tissue.

Innervated musculocutaneous arterial lip and cheek flaps for the reconstruction of the largest lower lip defects begin with an incision parallel to the mucocutaneous line, over the upper lip, toward the nasolabial sulcus. Then, at the same distance, alongside the defect of the commissure curving downward over the cheek tissue, the incision continues toward the projection of the mental foramen. A curved incision is made from the lower edge of the lip defect, parallel to the previous one, and adequate flap width is maintained. The width of the flaps in the region of the upper lip and cheek is equal to the height of the lower lip defect.

In the mental region, the flap is completed by a horizontal incision. The length of the flap from the edge of the defect (exactly from the commissure to the mental region) should be half the length of the lower lip defect. The second half of the length of the lower lip defect is replaced by a flap from the opposite side (Fig. 4C). The full thickness of the

cheek tissue is cut at the beginning of the flap that lies below the lower edge of the lip defect. The other part of the flaps in the region of the commissure and toward the upper lip is prepared according to the principles discussed earlier. Motor nerve fibers are preserved in both the region of the commissure and in the upper lip as well as in other parts of the flaps if possible. The facial artery is preserved during flap preparation.

The mobilized flaps are raised from the donor region and transposed into the defect without any tension. After the flaps are brought into the defect, sutures are placed in the medial surfaces of the flaps, and continuity of the new lip is formed. The mucous membranes of the flaps cover the fresh surface, and so the new lip vermilion is formed. A tongue flap can be used for reconstruction of the vermilion.

Secondary defects in the region of the cheek and mental area are sutured in accordance with anatomic layers, attending to nerve fibers and the facial artery. Flaps are positioned in primary and secondary defects following anatomic layers and paying attention to the depth of the labial sulcus and the height of the newly formed lip. After suturing, the reconstruction is completed, and the newly formed lip has almost the same length and width as the patient's previous lip. This can be ensured by measuring the dimensions of the defect and rima oris preoperatively and the newly formed lip and rima oris postoperatively. The results of reconstruction by such flaps are absolutely satisfactory, because microstomia does not

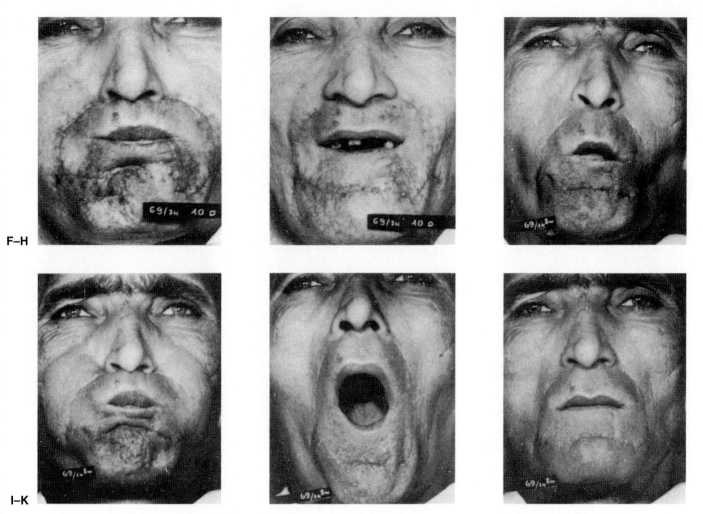

F–H

I–K

FIG. 3. *Continued.* F: The patient 10 days after formation of the new sphincter can keep water under pressure in the mouth. G: Ten days postoperatively, coordinate action of the orbicularis oris and other lip muscles is present. H: Eight months postoperatively, the sphincteric action of the newly formed lip is shown in whistling. I: In the same period, the sphincteric action of the newly formed lip is equal to that of the normal lip. J: The normal aperture of the newly formed lip covered with vermilion. K: Final result with symmetrical lip angles and normal appearance of newly formed lip.

occur and the functional abilities of the newly formed lip are completely adequate.

Defects of the Upper Lip

Innervated musculocutaneous arterial lip and cheek flaps for the reconstruction of upper lip defects are formed from the remaining parts of the resected upper lip and healthy lower lip in dimensions that correspond in width and length to the size of the defect. The same principles that are valid for reconstructing lower lip defects are used (Fig. 5).

Defects of Both Upper and Lower Lips

The simultaneous presence of upper and lower lip defects of larger size considerably reduces the quantity of labial tissue. The process of simultaneous reconstruction of such defects

becomes more complicated. Often the cause of such simultaneous defects on both lips is malignant tumors whose treatment requires radical excisions of the attacked lip parts in the same operative procedure. Defects of both lips also occur after voluminous lip and facial traumas that are accompanied by the avulsion of soft tissues. Reconstruction of full-thickness upper and lower lip defects of large dimensions during the same operative procedure would be impossible without innervated musculocutaneous arterial lip and cheek flaps.

Surgery is planned to remove the tumors of both lips by radical excision. Then, by a curved incision from the base of the lower lip defect at an equal distance, following the orbicularis oris muscle and the necessary width of the flap, the incision is continued over the cheek toward the base of the upper lip defect. A curved incision on the opposite side, symmetrical to the previous one, follows the orbicularis oris muscle to join the base of the upper and lower lip defects (Fig. 6).

In the region of the lip commissure, the muscle fibers of the superficial layer are gradually cut, and the buccal

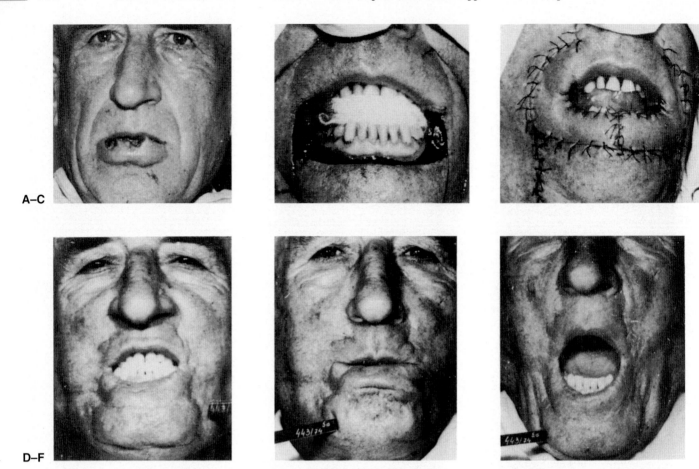

A–C

D–F

FIG. 4. **A:** Squamous cell carcinoma involving the whole lower lip. **B:** Defect of the whole lower lip over the region of both commissures. Lip and cheek flaps are designed. **C:** Innervated musculocutaneous lip and cheek flaps transposed into lip defect. **D:** Newly formed lip is completely mobile, showing the coordinating action of the orbicularis oris muscle. **E:** Result 5 years later, with expressed sphincteric action. **F:** Five years postoperatively, the normal appearance of the reconstructed lip with all functions preserved. (From Karapandžić, ref. 1, with permission.)

branches of the facial nerve and facial artery with its branches are immediately found. The preparation continues with selective cutting of the muscle fibers that are intermingled with the orbicularis oris muscle. Separation of the orbicularis oris muscle in the direction of the bases of the upper and lower lip defects is performed. The buccinator muscle is preserved.

The beginnings of the musculocutaneous lip and cheek flaps are separated from the surrounding muscles right up to the mucous membrane, which is cut only as far from the defects as will make possible the movement of flaps toward each other. The mobilized flaps are raised from their bases and moved simultaneously to the middle of the upper and lower lip defects, and then they are sutured along the medial surfaces in accordance with the anatomic layers.

In this way, the oral sphincter is formed by two semicircular innervated musculocutaneous arterial flaps from the remaining parts of the upper and lower lips and part of the cheek. The bases of these flaps are in the region of both lip angles. After formation of the circular ringlike flap, a symmetrical lip aperture is achieved by redistributing and centralizing the flaps. The flaps are redistributed to the primary and secondary defects by suturing according to the anatomic layers.

Although the defects are large, simultaneous reconstruction of the upper and lower lips by innervated musculocutaneous arterial lip and cheek flaps, surrounded by intact vermilion, is possible. Microstomia is not marked, although it could be expected in view of the dimensions of both lip defects.

Defects in the Region of the Lip Commissure

Innervated musculocutaneous arterial flaps of the upper and lower lips are used. Flap preparation is carried out according to the usual principles. For this location, the flaps are not begun at angles of 90 degrees. Rather, the angles are about 60 degrees on the outer flap circumference, while the angle toward the vermilion border of the flaps is about 120 degrees. This form makes the creation of an adequate lip commissure, which is not always easily achieved, quite possible. The problem is in the exact positioning and symmetry of the commissure with the normal side. Satisfactory shape and symmetry can be obtained by reducing the secondary defect and correctly redistributing the flaps according to the primary defect.

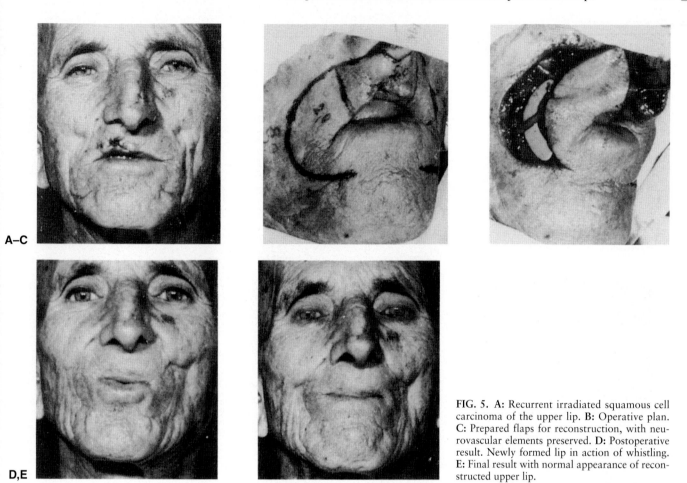

A–C

D,E

FIG. 5. **A:** Recurrent irradiated squamous cell carcinoma of the upper lip. **B:** Operative plan. **C:** Prepared flaps for reconstruction, with neurovascular elements preserved. **D:** Postoperative result. Newly formed lip in action of whistling. **E:** Final result with normal appearance of reconstructed upper lip.

CLINICAL RESULTS

The value of innervated musculocutaneous arterial lip and cheek flaps was tested in 522 patients from 1966 to 1982. Tests included those for arterial and venous blood circulation and lymphatic drainage, both intraoperatively and postoperatively. Sensibility to pain, touch, temperature, modalities of superficial sensibility, and vegetative function also were tested. Special attention was paid to motor functions. Electromyographic results on functional values were checked by clinical methods, studying muscle movement in carrying out basic and complicated lip functions. The results of these tests showed that the reconstructed lip preserved motility, sensibility to all qualities, vegetative functions, and complete circulatory networks (see Figs. 3–6).

The newly formed lip was mobile so that it not only achieved contact with the opposite lip in action but participated in all dynamic movements. It retained liquid in the mouth even under the highest pressure (Fig. 3F). Motility and sensibility in the newly formed lip prevented the uncontrolled dribbling of liquid and saliva, and no patient had drooling. The restored labial sphincter that contained innervated muscles made normal feeding and intelligible speech possible as well as whistling, blowing, smiling, kissing, sucking, pursing, and other everyday lip movements (see Figs. 3–6).

Besides functional ability, characteristics of the newly formed lip were symmetry and the absence of changes in flap volume due either to atrophy or to the presence of edema. The smooth contour of the newly formed lip that was covered with vermilion was flexible and enabled the lip to open sufficiently to fulfill its functions. The adequate height of the newly formed lip had the corresponding depth of the labial sulcus. The position of the lip corners suited facial proportions; the position of the lip did not differ from the opposite one in protrusion. By its position and similarity of tissue to the normal lip and the mobility accompanied by changes in the size of the rima oris, the reconstructed lip gave the impression of a normal one. Therefore, the aesthetic results of this procedure were completely satisfactory (see Figs. 3–6).

The limited quantity of labial and cheek tissues for the formation of innervated musculocutaneous arterial lip and cheek flaps in large lip defects is a shortcoming of this procedure for surgical reconstruction in the lip area. Microstomia, which may occur as a result of applying these flaps, may be avoided by using larger areas of cheek tissue as well as by wider mobilization and correct redistribution of the flaps on the primary and secondary defects. Another drawback might be the appearance of a noticeable scar, in the medial line of the flaps, but a Z-plasty may be used to ameliorate this problem.

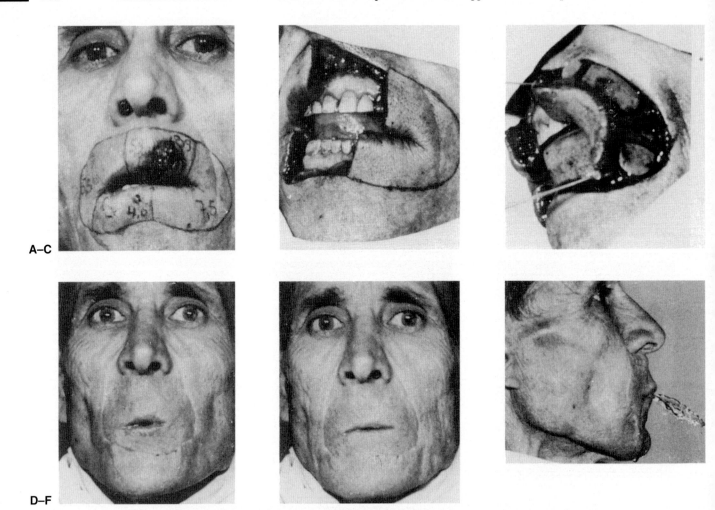

A–C

D–F

FIG. 6. A: Simultaneous presence of lower and upper lip carcinoma and planned flaps. **B:** Excised larger parts of lower and upper lips. Design of flaps for simultaneous reconstruction of both lip defects. **C:** Innervated musculocutaneous arterial lip and cheek flaps prepared, with neurovascular elements preserved. **D:** Sphincteric action after reconstruction of both lips is shown. **E:** Final result with normal appearance of both reconstructed lips with adequate rima oris. **F:** Patient can eject water out of mouth in a thin jet, owing to reconstructed lip sphincter. (From Karapandžić, ref. 1, with permission.)

SUMMARY

Innervated musculocutaneous arterial lip and cheek flaps can be used for all local applications, depending on the defects presented. The number, size, and position of the defects lend themselves to varying specific techniques for flap design and deployment. These flaps also may be applied in combination with other flaps for larger defects in the immediate lip area.

References

1. Karapandžić M. Reconstruction of lip defects by local arterial flaps. *Br J Plast Surg* 1974;27:93.
2. Jabaley ME, Orcutt TW, Clement RL. Applications of the Karapandžić principle of lip reconstruction following excision of lip cancer. *Am J Surg* 1976;132:529.
3. Jabaley ME, Clement RL, Orcutt TW. Musculocutaneous flaps in lip reconstruction: applications of the Karapandžić principle. *Plast Reconstr Surg* 1977;59:680.

CHAPTER 173 ■ TONGUE MUCOSAL AND MUSCULOMUCOSAL FLAP FOR LIP RECONSTRUCTION

J. GUERREROSANTOS

The tongue provides a valuable and versatile mucosal and musculomucosal unit for reconstruction of the vermilion border and lining of the inner aspect of the lip (1–4).

INDICATIONS

The tongue musculomucosal flap can be used in reconstruction of both the upper and lower lips. For carrying out surgical repairs, one can use one or two tongue flaps that can be combined, when necessary, with skin flaps. Most frequent indications for this procedure are defects subsequent to removal of benign or malignant tumors, defects after trauma, and secondary deformities because of clefting.

ANATOMY

The principles of tongue mucosal and musculomucosal flaps are based on the fact that the blood supply to the mucous membranes is derived from the perforating vessels of underlying muscle (5,6). The tongue is a mobile mass of striated muscle covered by mucous membrane. It may be divided into a fixed part, which is the root, and a mobile part, which is formed by the body and apex. The body is divided into two halves by a median raphe that is seen externally as the median sulcus (Fig. 1).

The areas of the tongue covered by the mucous membrane are the apex or tip, the dorsum, the right and left margins, and the inferior surface. The root of the tongue is irrigated by the lingual artery and vein, which have transverse branches; from this part, transverse flaps can be taken. The mobile part of the tongue is irrigated by the ranine arteries and veins. The ranine arteries course next to the deep muscular mass and, forward of this point, have 10 to 12 collaterals.

The terminal branches anastomose in the lingual apex, forming the ranine arch. The median raphe separates both sides perfectly in the lingual body without any vascular anastomosis; this was recently confirmed in arteriographic studies. Longitudinal flaps can be obtained on the lingual body; it is not advisable to design flaps that cross the median raphe. Longitudinal as well as transverse and bipedicle flaps can be created on the apex because of the rich vascularity (see Fig. 1).

FLAP DESIGN AND DIMENSIONS

Three basic factors must be considered in designing a successful tongue flap. First, the exact location, width, and length of the flap depend on the location and size of the defect at the recipient site in the lip. Second, the outlines of the flap should be made following the direction of the blood supply in the root, body, and apex. Third, tension and distortion are the main enemies of successful tongue flap

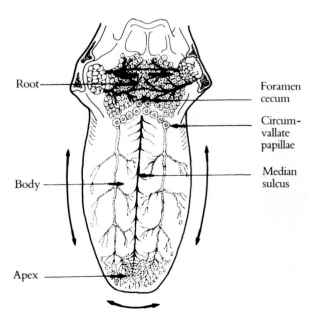

FIG. 1. Anatomy and blood supply of the tongue. Abundant communicating arterial branches and arcades in lingual apex.

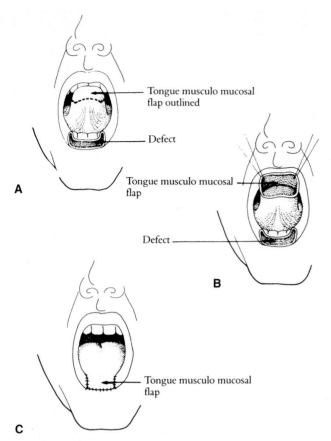

FIG. 2. Direct tongue musculomucosal flap in reconstruction of the lower lip. **A:** The defect and the tongue musculomucosal flap outline are shown. **B:** Tongue musculomucosal flap has been elevated. **C:** Tongue musculomucosal flap sutured in single layer. After 3 weeks, the flap is ready for division.

repair; good arterial and venous blood supply and gentle handling of the tissue are the only allies. A flap site that avoids tension from the mobility of the tongue should be selected (Fig. 2).

Although tongue musculomucosal flaps can be obtained equally well from the dorsum, lateral margins, or inferior

surface, it is recommended that flaps for labial reconstruction be taken from the margins or the undersurface because the mucosa of these areas is smooth and resembles vermilion. It is not wrinkled and does not have papillae like the mucous membrane of the lingual dorsum.

OPERATIVE TECHNIQUE

Reconstruction of the Lower Lip

Direct Tongue Musculomucosal Flap

When total vermilion reconstruction is planned, a single flap is taken from the tip and margin and applied to the lower lip as a single unit. This flap can be used when a lip shave is done in cases of leukoplakia or multiple small epitheliomas. The flap is designed with a single pedicle, including the right amount of muscle for aesthetic reconstruction (Figs. 2 and 3). After careful hemostasis, the flap is sutured in a single layer, with a small raw area left in the pedicle. After 3 weeks, the flap is ready to be divided along a line 1.5 cm behind the posterior margin of the defect. In some cases, a surgical revision is made some months later to correct a residual bulge. Occasionally, the flap has a dark red color because of vascular congestion, and this coloration may last for some months; it later fades.

Direct Marginal Tongue Musculomucosal Flap

The edge of the tongue is a good flap site for lip reconstruction. This flap is useful for primary or secondary reconstruction of half the vermilion border as well as for reconstruction of the labial commissure (Fig. 4). I have used this flap for primary repair in patients who have hemangiomas invading the vermilion border (7), the muscular portion, and mucosa of the lower lip (Fig. 5) and for secondary repair in patients with vermilion border deficits after burns and other trauma. The buccal commissure can be successfully reconstructed after trauma or electrical burn (8,9).

Total Reconstruction of the Lower Lip

By using a combined technique using skin flaps and tongue musculomucosal flaps, it is possible to totally reconstruct the lower lip (10).

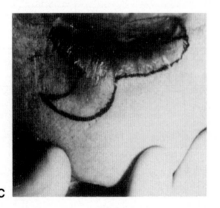
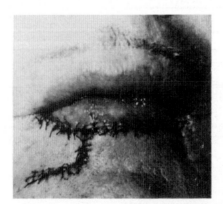
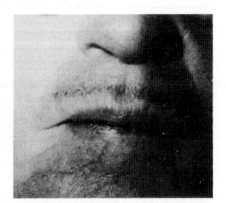

FIG. 3. Patient with squamous cell carcinoma on the right side and cheilitis of the lower lip vermilion. Note the vertical scar on the left side of the lip from a previous squamous cell carcinoma removed 1 year before. **A:** Excision of the vermilion and part of the lower lip is outlined. **B:** Lower lip has been sutured and tongue musculomucosal flap from the apex used to repair vermilion wound. **C:** Patient 8 months postoperatively.

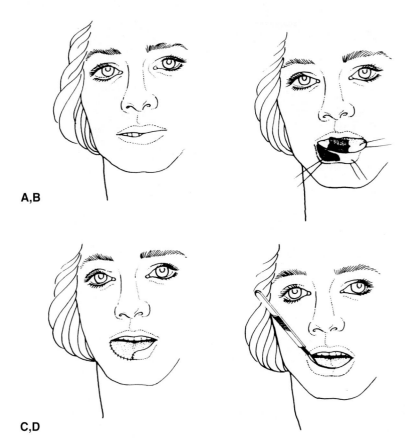

FIG. 4. Direct marginal tongue musculomucosal flap. **A:** Lower lip defect. **B:** Tongue flap obtained from marginal edge of the tongue; loss of lip substance is exposed. **C:** Tongue flap is sutured in a single layer. **D:** Three weeks later, the pedicle is sectioned.

Reconstruction of the Upper Lip

Direct Tongue Flap (11,12)

The tip of the tongue and anterior margins are good donor sites for direct flaps in upper lip reconstruction. The thickness of the vermilion, which may be very thin after trauma, tumor removal, or cleft lip repair, can be increased. When the integument of remaining vermilion is altered by scar tissue or pigmentation, it can be aesthetically improved if the flap is obtained from the margins or inferior aspect of the tongue. The surgical procedure is simple and consists of making a correctly sized flap and suturing it onto the raw surface of the lip, leaving it in that position for 3 weeks (Fig. 6) and then sectioning the pedicle. When sectioning the pedicle, the surgeon

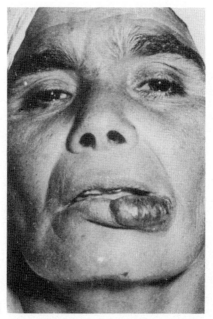
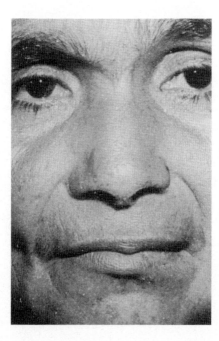

FIG. 5. A: A 52-year-old patient with angioma involving the entire half of the lower lip vermilion. **B:** Postoperative view 1½ years later. (From Guerrerosantos et al., ref. 7, with permission.)

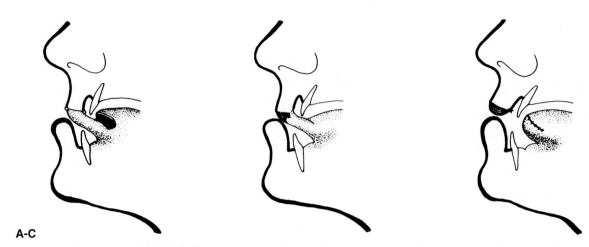

A-C

FIG. 6. Reconstruction of the upper lip using direct tongue musculomucosal flap. **A:** Tongue flap has been transferred into and sutured to the lower border of the defect. **B:** At a later stage, the pedicle of the flap is severed. Dotted area shows new vermilion. **C:** Operation is completed.

should be careful to create a rounded vermilion border that is aesthetically acceptable (Fig. 7).

Buried Denuded Tubular Tongue Flap

This flap provides filling for a labial defect in which the vermilion border has an epithelial covering without scars or color abnormalities. After primary reconstruction of the upper lip in some patients with cleft lip, some sequelae may be observed: notching, extremely narrow vermilion border, unilateral lack of tissue, and a short, tense vermilion border. The filling provided by this flap makes the fissures disappear and the narrow vermilion fill out, and it corrects asymmetries caused by a lack of tissue.

The mucosa is removed, and the tip of the flap is introduced into a pocket made in the lip through an incision in the posterior surface of the lip (Figs. 8 and 9). The flap that is introduced is left in position for a period of 3 weeks, after which the pedicles are sectioned. The quantity of mucosa that is denuded depends on the size of the defect and the volume required. The minimum amount to be denuded and introduced into the pocket should be 1.5 cm. The tubular

tongue-tip flap heals well because of its excellent blood circulation.

CLINICAL RESULTS

In a series of 198 tongue musculomucosal flaps used in lip repair at the Jalisco Reconstructive Plastic Surgery Institute, only two patients had problems with healing. Severe infection in these patients resulted in complete flap separation.

When the flap is obtained from the lingual dorsum, the mucosa is roughened by lingual papillae and looks different from the integument of the vermilion border. In long-term observations in a series of 36 patients, I noted that only two patients had rough mucosa in the flap after more than 2 years. In 20 to 90 days in most patients, the rough papillary appearance of the lingual mucosa gradually changes into the smooth appearance of the vermilion border after passing through a period of hyperkeratinization. I have not seen any lingual dysfunction after tissue donation for lip repair.

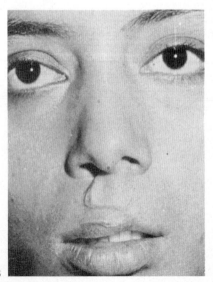
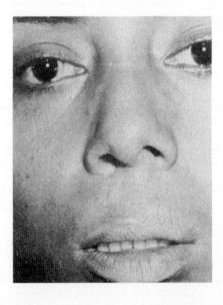

A,B

FIG. 7. **A:** A 22-year-old patient with a cutaneous scar and asymmetry resulting from a deficiency of vermilion on the left. **B:** Result 2 years after revision and direct tongue flap to the lip. (From Guerrerosantos et al., ref. 11, with permission.)

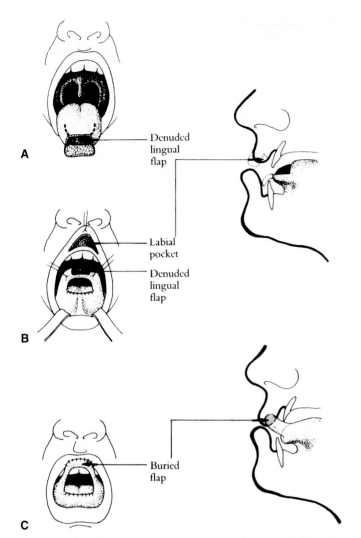

SUMMARY

The tongue can be used to reconstruct the upper and lower lip vermilion as either a mucosal or a musculomucosal flap. This flap can be used in conjunction with other flaps to reconstruct the entire lip, or it can be used alone to build bulk in an otherwise acceptable lip.

References

1. Bakamjian V. Use of tongue flap in lower lip reconstruction. *Br J Plast Surg* 1964;17:76.
2. Guerrerosantos J, Vasquez-Pallares R, Vera-Strathmann A, et al. Tongue flap in reconstruction of the lip. In: *Transactions of the Third International Congress of Plastic Surgeons*. Amsterdam: Excerpta Medica, 1964;1055.
3. Grosserez M, Stricker M. La langue, materiaux de choix dans la réparation des pertes de substance labiale. In: *Transactions of the Third International Congress of Plastic Surgeons*. Amsterdam: Excerpta Medica, 1964;551.
4. McGregor IA. Tongue flap surgery. *Br J Plast Surg* 1966;19:253.
5. Cadenat H, Combelles R, Fabie M. Lambeaux de langue: Vascularisation, morphologie et utilization. *Ann Chin Plast Esthet* 1973;18:223.
6. Bracka A. The blood supply of dorsal tongue flaps. *Br J Plast Surg* 1981;34:379.
7. Guerrerosantos J, Castaneda A, Barba A. Surgery for labial angioma. *Arch Surg* 1967;94:728.
8. Zarem HA, Greer DM Jr. Tongue flap for reconstruction of lips in electrical burns. *Plast Reconstr Surg* 1974;53:310
9. Ortiz-Monasterio F, Factor R. Early definitive treatment of electric burns of the mouth. *Plast Reconstr Surg* 1980;65:169.
10. Fujino I. Reconstruction of an extensive defect of the lower lip with Bernard's muscle-bearing flap and a tongue flap after radical surgery of a lower lip tumor. *Jpn J Plast Reconstr Surg* 1969;12:24.
11. Guerrerosantos J. Use of a tongue flap in secondary correction of cleft lips. *Plast Reconstr Surg* 1969;44:368.
12. Jackson IT. Use of a tongue flap to resurface lip defects and close palatal fistulas in children. *Plast Reconstr Surg* 1972;49:537.

FIG. 8. Buried denuded tubular musculomucosal tongue flap. **A:** The tubular flap is outlined on the tongue tip, and the mucosa of the upper surface is removed. **B:** A pocket is formed in the upper lip. **C:** The tongue flap is inserted into the pocket, and 3 weeks later, the pedicle is sectioned.

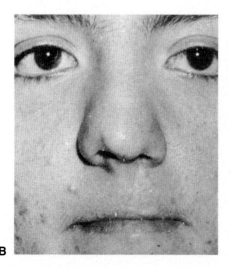
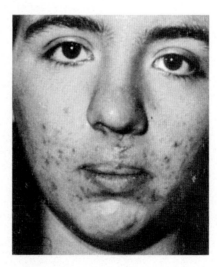

FIG. 9. A,B: A 21-year-old woman with cleft lip sequelae shown before and after reconstruction with a buried denuded tubular tongue flap. The discrete contours of the entire vermilion border are an advantage of this procedure.

CHAPTER 174 ■ BILATERAL LATERAL VERMILION BORDER TRANSPOSITION FLAPS

K. MATSUO

Bilateral lateral vermilion border transposition flaps can be used to correct the "whistling lip" deformity after cleft-lip repair. The procedure is a modification of a V-Y advancement of lateral vermilion flaps transposed 90 degrees (1,2).

INDICATIONS

When patients with the whistle deformity have relatively ample lateral vermilion, these flaps can be used to reconstruct the absent median tubercle. The flaps can easily reconstruct a natural-appearing peaked and everted tubercle, decrease upper-lip tension, and deepen the labiogingival sulcus. They reduce the need for additional surgery, as in the creation of a cross-lip Abbé flap. The flaps can be used to repair a symmetric whistle deformity after bilateral cleft-lip repair and also to repair an asymmetric whistle deformity after unilateral cleft-lip repair.

FLAP DESIGN AND DIMENSIONS

The lateral vermilion flaps are marked inside the vermilion-mucosal junction (Fig. 1). These flaps tend to be wider than planned because the central-lip deficiency usually requires more tissue than expected. Lambdoidal markings in the midposterior prolabium should be located so as to decrease horizontal lip tension and to deepen the labiogingival sulcus after flap transposition. When used to correct an asymmetrical deformity, the width of the flaps and the location of the markings should be considered even more carefully.

OPERATIVE TECHNIQUE

The flaps, which involve mucosa, submucosa, and orbicularis oris muscle, are elevated laterally to medially. They are based on the prolabium and should be raised without leaving a cicatricial connection between the flaps and the surrounding tissue to avoid distortion. The flaps are transposed into a lamboidal incision in the midposterior prolabium. The donor sites in the lateral lip are closed primarily. A dog-ear at the end of the closure between the lateral vermilion flaps is necessary to construct a natural-appearing peaked tubercle; when the result is too peaked, careful trimming should be done (see Figs. 1 and 2D–G).

CLINICAL RESULTS

When used for patients with the whistle deformity, these flaps have produced satisfactory results from both static and dynamic viewpoints. Although the lateral lip donates a compound flap to the tubercle, its thickness appears undiminished. Some patients require secondary reduction of the reconstructed tubercle because the width of the flaps was larger than necessary (Fig. 2A–C, H–J).

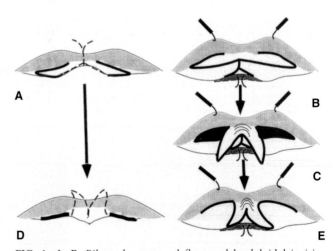

FIG. 1. **A, B:** Bilateral compound flaps and lambdoidal incision markings are drawn inside the vermilion–mucosal junction. **C:** Compound flaps are transposed into the midposterior area of the prolabium. **D,E:** Flaps are sutured into position and donor sites are closed primarily.

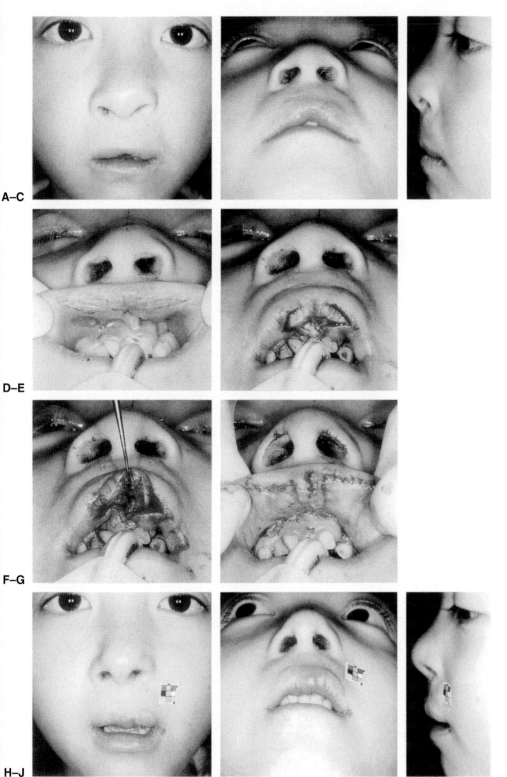

A–C

D–E

F–G

H–J

FIG. 2. Bilateral cleft lip. A–C: Preoperative views. D–G: Operative steps as shown in Fig. 1. H–J: Postoperative views.

SUMMARY

Bilateral lateral vermilion border transposition flaps to correct the whistle deformity can be effectively used to reconstruct a natural-appearing peaked and everted tubercle, decrease upper-lip tension, and deepen the labiogingival sulcus.

References

1. Matsuo K, Fujiwara T, Hayashi R, et al. Bilateral lateral vermilion border transposition flaps to correct the "whistling lip" deformity. *Plast Reconstr Surg* 1993;91:930.
2. Kapetansky KI. Double pendulum flaps for whistling deformities in bilateral cleft lips. *Plast Reconstr Surg* 1971;47:321.

CHAPTER 175 ■ BILATERAL VERMILION FLAPS FOR LOWER LIP REPAIR

H. OHTSUKA

Bilateral vermilion flaps, a modification of a single arterialized vermilion flap used for small defects (1), can be used for median or central and rather lateral, larger defects of the lower lip (2).

INDICATIONS

These flaps are indicated for vermilion defects spanning two fifths to three fifths of the lower lip. Smaller defects also can be repaired, with better postoperative symmetrical balance than can be achieved by the unilateral flap (3). Advantages over other standard techniques include simplicity and safety, the requirement for little or no sacrifice of healthy tissue, and the promotion of rapid wound healing because the flaps are very well vascularized (2).

Bilateral vermilion flaps have been used for squamous cell carcinomas, malignant melanoma, and blue nevus. Where vermilion-only defects were present, the flaps were raised as myocutaneous tissue-expanding vermilion flaps, according to Goldstein (1). Where the defects extended to the white lip, a subcutaneous V–Y advancement flap of the lower lip was added to the bilateral vermilion flaps.

ANATOMY

The inferior labial artery runs close to the mucous membrane. There may be asymmetries or variations of lower-lip vermilion vascularization, including the equal distribution of the bilateral inferior labial arteries, the predominance of the artery on one side, the presence of the artery on only one side, or the artery presenting as the terminal branch of the sublabial artery (4,5). In any case, an abundant vascular network is constantly recognized in the vermilion.

FLAP DESIGN AND DIMENSIONS

The mucocutaneous junction of the vermilion with lip skin is outlined with a marking pen preoperatively. Each vermilion

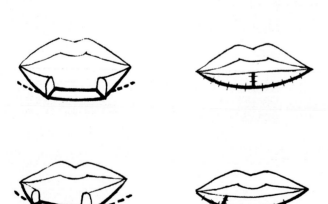

FIG. 1. Diagram of operative procedure for median and lateral vermilion-only defects using bilateral vermilion flaps (*dotted line* shows the mucosal incision).

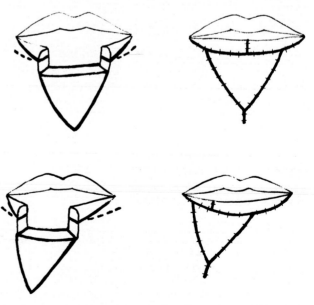

FIG. 2. Diagram of operative procedure for median and lateral vermilion defects extending to the white lip using bilateral vermilion flaps and a subcutaneous V–Y advancement flap.

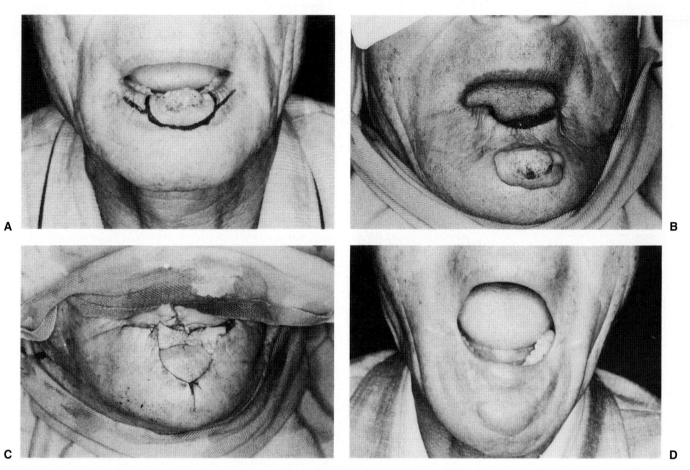

FIG. 3. A 71-year-old man with squamous cell carcinoma of the lower lip. **A:** Preoperative findings: depiction of incision line and vermilion border. **B:** Resected tumor and horizontal defect of the lower lip. **C:** First stage of wound closure. **D:** Eleven months postoperatively.

flap extension to the commissure depends on the location and size of the defect.

OPERATIVE TECHNIQUE

At tumor resection, the labial artery is recognized as an important landmark on each side. Cutting through the mucocutaneous junction of the vermilion will expose the orbicularis oris muscle. A wider mucosal incision is recommended near the labial commissure (3). After mucosal incision, the entire thickness of the vermilion is excised, including the labial artery. If the vermilion defects extend to the white lip, a subcutaneous V–Y advancement flap of the lower lip is added (Fig. 1). A long and narrow horizontal lip defect (perhaps within 1.5 cm downward from the vermilion border) may be effectively repaired by a combination of unilateral or bilateral vermilion flaps and a V–Y advancement flap without sacrificing any additional healthy tissue (Figs. 2 and 3).

CLINICAL RESULTS

The procedure was used in eight patients with both vermilion-only defects and defects extending into the white lip; follow-ups ranged from 4 months to 6 years. In all patients, cosmetically and functionally satisfactory results

were obtained. Complete sensory recovery was observed about 6 months postoperatively. Electromyographic evaluations in two patients revealed that the motility of the orbicularis oris muscle was almost normal within 11 and 12 months, respectively.

SUMMARY

Bilateral vermilion flaps are of value in the repair of larger vermilion defects because of their inherent elasticity and the use of a common anatomic unit. Long and narrow horizontal lip defects may be effectively treated by a combination of vermilion flap(s) and a V–Y advancement flap of the lower lip.

References

1. Goldstein MH. A tissue-expanding vermilion myocutaneous flap for lip repair. *Plast Reconstr Surg* 1984;73:768.
2. Ohtsuka H, Nakaoka H. Bilateral vermilion flaps for lower lip repair. *Plast Reconstr Surg* 1990;85:453.
3. Mutaf M, Sensoz O, Tuncay E. The split-lip advancement technique (SLAT) for the treatment of congenital sinuses of the lower lip. *Plast Reconstr Surg* 1993;92:615.
4. Hu H, Song R, Sun G. One-stage inferior labial flap and its pertinent anatomic study. *Plast Reconstr Surg* 1993;91:618.
5. Midy D, Mauruc B, Vergnes P, et al. A contribution to the study of the facial artery, its branches and anastomoses: Application to the anatomic vascular bases of facial flaps. *Surg Radiol Anat* 1986;8:99.

CHAPTER 176 ■ COMMISSURE RECONSTRUCTION: OVERVIEW

H. G. THOMSON

Bakamjian (1) in 1964 stated that molding the lip commissure with functional fidelity is an almost impossible task. The aim of surgical reconstruction is to give symmetry to the commissure in repose and to permit full opening without webbing. The former goal is much easier to attain than the latter. The subtle flow line of the red lip to its termination at the angle of the commissure and its ability to move up, down, and laterally, as well as vertical mucosal stretching, were well described by Stricker in 1981 (2). The Z distribution of the skin and the accordion effect of the mucosa were emphasized. To achieve this is the goal of reconstructive surgery, but the most common shortfall is the apparent fullness in the commissure owing to a lack of contouring.

INDICATIONS

Defects of the commissure apex are rare; most problems are pericommissural in nature and involve the apex. The most common indication is trauma, especially electrical oral burns.

ANATOMY

To apply the tenets of reconstruction properly, we must first appreciate the topographic location of the commissure on the face. Broadbent and Matthews (3) described the normal location of the oral commissure. With the normal in mind, various landmarks can be chosen and methods for locating the apex of the proposed commissure can be applied (Fig. 1). There should be a special awareness of the tapering effect of the commissure, and this begins at a vertical line through the medial canthus.

FLAP DESIGN AND DIMENSIONS

Tongue Flaps

Bakamjian (1) described several types of tongue flap designs, in particular a ventrolateral, anterior-based flap, which he

included in commissure reconstruction as part of partial or total red lip reconstruction after cancer ablation. Guerrerosantos et al. (4) in 1963 were really the first authors to describe the use of a tongue flap that could give not only mucosal functional and aesthetic advantages but also a degree of much needed bulk in the area. They also described the microscopic papillary appearance of tongue mucosa, which, after 20 to 90 days, takes on a smooth red lip appearance. They usually used the tongue tip.

McGregor (5) also described a tongue flap. Jackson (6) reported the use of tongue flaps in oral electrical burns and the need for awareness of the fact that the tongue flap can be separated by young patients' sharp teeth. To prevent this, he fabricated a prophylactic bite block. He reported an anterior-based sublingual flap that required lanolin three times a day for a few months to prevent desiccation. Jackson makes a point that the tongue papillae do not always disappear, and therefore, his sublabial flap, which is smooth and less red, provides better cosmetic coverage.

In 1974 Zarem and Greer (7) described a sublabial or ventral flap that is anteriorly based and applied to only one surface of the commissure; the other surface is closed with simple mucosal advancement. They did this in an attempt to reduce ultimate bulk excess. They emphasized the shortfall of the color match provided by the vivid pink of the tongue mucosa. They prefer this reconstruction to be initiated 3 weeks after injury and have found that the pedicle can be separated at 2 weeks. A similar technique was reported by Converse in 1977 (8) (Fig. 2). In 1980 Ortiz-Monasterio and Factor (9) described an anterior-based, split, lateral sublabial tongue flap for commissure reconstruction that provides significant tissue

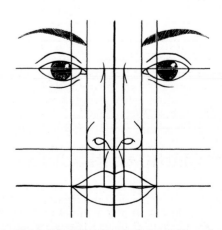

FIG. 1. Wright's facial landmarks for commissure location.

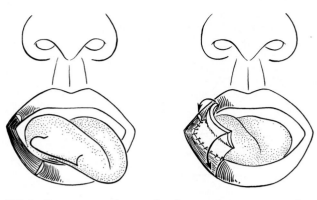

FIG. 2. Converse type of tongue flap for commissure reconstruction.

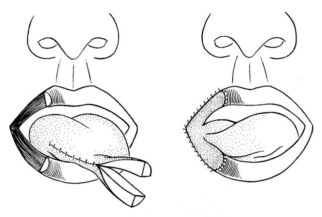

FIG. 3. Ortiz-Monasterio and Factor split pedicle tongue flap.

to the commissure area and, indeed, may create difficult problems with debulking (Fig. 3).

Cheek Flaps

Reconstructions of the lips with cheek flaps are legend. Those related to the commissure only are somewhat limited in number and relate to primary tumor resection and reconstruction.

Tumors of the commissure constitute fewer than 6% of those involving the lip area. Zisser (10) in 1975 reported a technique for cheek advancement and mucosal flap reconstruction of the commissure. The deepithelialized flaps are rotated up into the defect to give both bulk and alignment (Fig. 4). Brusati (11) in 1976 described a similar technique for commissure reconstruction (Fig. 5) that is also based on a Burow's triangle principle. Attempts are made to keep the major scar lines in the axis of the smile crease. This flap is more suitable for horizontal defects compared with the Zisser flap, which is more applicable to vertical problems.

Red Lip Flaps

In 1931 Joseph (12) described a "back-flip" mucosal flap with direct closure of the donor site in the buccal gingival sulcus area. Kazanjian and Roopenian (13) in 1954 described simple advancement flaps of existing red lip for defects less than 1 to 1.5 cm long (Fig. 6). Gillies and Millard (14) in 1957 reported a partial leading edge "back-flip" flap. These flaps can function adequately if the donor site is not deficient and additional bulk is not necessary (Fig. 7).

Buccal Mucosal Advancement Flaps

In 1959 Converse (15) described his technique for elongation of the oral fissure and restoration of the angle of the mouth. This consisted of a triangular scar excision with advancement of three mucosal flaps (Fig. 8). Pons in 1968 (16) described an additional attempt to establish continuity of the orbicularis oris by repositioning the muscle and fibrous tissue remnants. In 1971 Wustrack (17) emphasized his method of dermomuscle stocks to ensure competence of the oral commissure. This concept was further elaborated by Villoria (18) in 1972, who used two muscle and fibrous tissue flaps, coupled with Converse's principle (Fig. 9). Argamaso et al. (19) in 1974 reemphasized the translocation of orbicularis oris remnants.

A slightly different mucosal rotation advancement using a portion of the reepithelialized commissure as a flap for the upper lip and a rotation advancement of the endoral mucosa for the lower lip (Fig. 10) was described by Gillies and Millard in 1957 (14). Muhlbauer in 1970 (20) used an "out of series" double Z-plasty, interposing red and white lip flaps, with possible secondary color match problems (20) (Fig. 11).

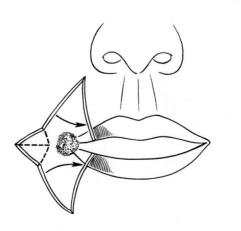
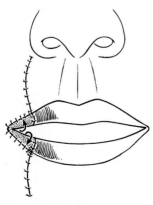

FIG. 4. Zisser method of advancement commissure reconstruction for vertical defects.

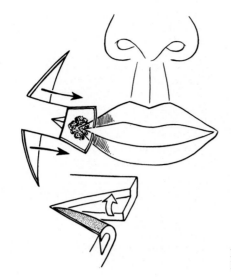

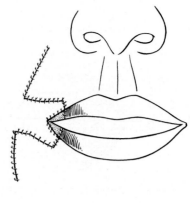

FIG. 5. Brusati technique for more horizontal commissure defect.

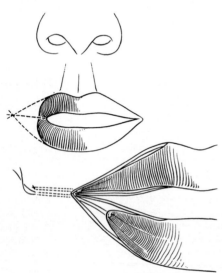

FIG. 6. Kazanjian and Roopenian advancement flaps.

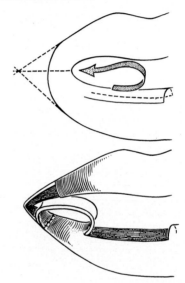

FIG. 7. Gillies and Millard back-flip flap.

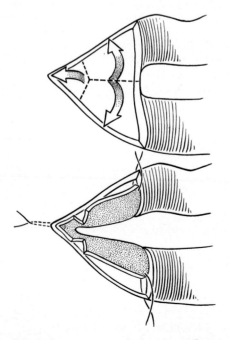

FIG. 8. Converse mucosal advancement flaps.

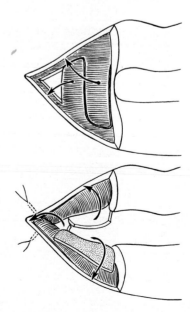

FIG. 9. Villoria muscle-fibrous tissue flaps with Converse commissure reconstruction.

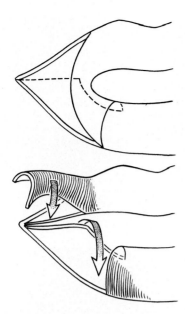

FIG. 10. Gillies and Millard single flap with additional mucosal advancement.

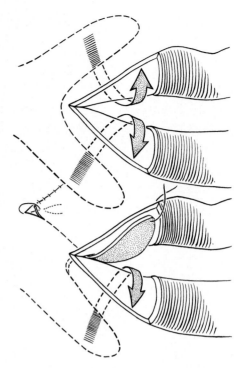

FIG. 12. Kazanjian and Roopenian double mucosal pedicle.

Buccal Mucosal Rotation Flaps

Kazanjian and Roopenian in 1954 (13) described a laterally based double mucosal pedicle to reconstruct the commissure (Fig. 12). This is the basis of my methods of reconstruction (21,22). The biggest hurdle created by this technique is the inappropriate color match and a pouting commissure due to an overabundance of mucosa and poor tailoring of the flap. I have outlined the difficulties of this type of reconstruction in previous publications (21–24).

The most critical aspect of the operation is to establish the location of the commissure apex with some degree of accuracy. This is done by using basic landmarks (medial canthus, philtrum, normal commissure, alar base, and so forth). The measurements are achieved by using suture material rather than a ruler or compass (Fig. 13A and B).

A single-pedicle flap similar to that described by Limberg is simple to design and will provide good opening, but excess mucosal bulk in the commissure is common (Fig. 13C-E). A more satisfactory technique is to use two marginally based rotation flaps that meet in the commissure apex, with primary closure of the donor site (Fig. 14). If two isolated Limberg-like flaps are used, with the apex of the commissure as the juncture point, good tailoring and aesthetics also can be achieved (Fig. 15).

CLINICAL RESULTS

There is no "best" technique for commissure reconstruction with a simple or composite flap. It is impossible to reconstruct a commissure that has a normal, unoperated appearance, particularly when additional white lip scarring is present. Various interpositional and tunnel flaps can be used to eliminate this latter problem, but there is a risk of additional secondary scarring being created in attempts to eliminate the original. In view of these difficulties, it is important to program the patient for additional revisionary surgery after a delay of 1 year.

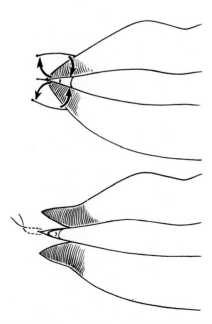

SUMMARY

This chapter outlines the many various methods designed to reconstruct the lip commissure.

FIG. 11. Muhlbauer double white and red Z-plasties.

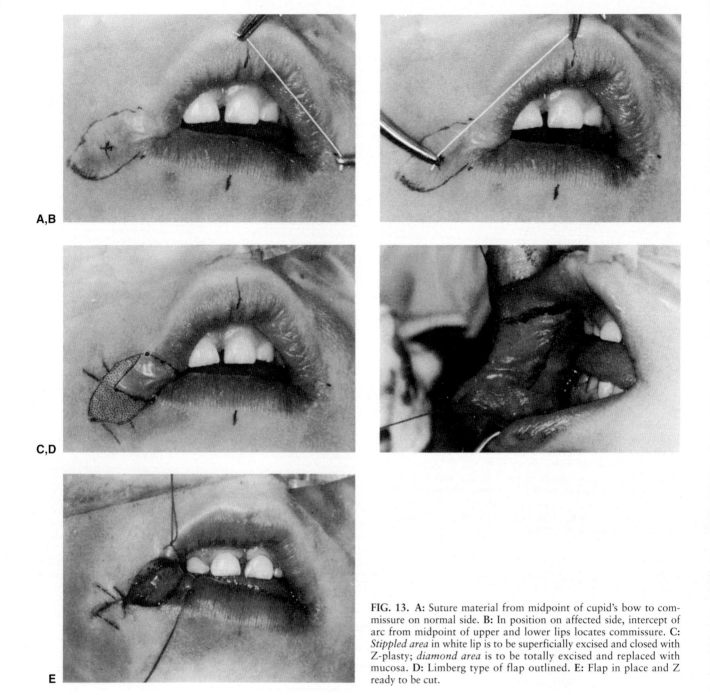

FIG. 13. A: Suture material from midpoint of cupid's bow to commissure on normal side. **B:** In position on affected side, intercept of arc from midpoint of upper and lower lips locates commissure. **C:** *Stippled area* in white lip is to be superficially excised and closed with Z-plasty; *diamond area* is to be totally excised and replaced with mucosa. **D:** Limberg type of flap outlined. **E:** Flap in place and Z ready to be cut.

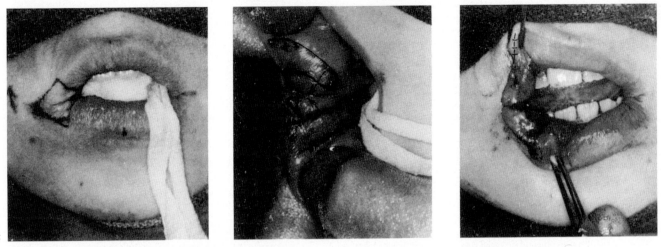

A–C

FIG. 14. A: *Diamond area* to be excised. B: Two marginally based sickle flaps outlined; *dotted area* to be removed. C: Flaps in position with juncture point in commissure apex.

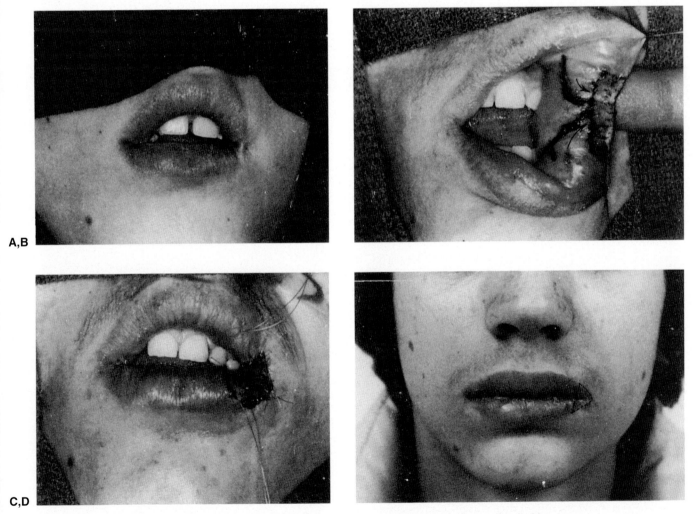

A,B

C,D

FIG. 15. A: Left oral commissure stenosed. B: Two rotation-advancement flaps outlined; oblong area to be excised. C: Flaps in place. D: Late result outlined by *stippled area*.

References

1. Bakamjian V. Use of tongue flaps in lower lip reconstruction. *Br J Plast Surg* 1964;17:76.
2. Stricker M. La commissure buccale. *Ann Chir Plast* 1981;26:131.
3. Broadbent TR, Matthews NL. Artistic relationships in surface anatomy of the face: Application to reconstructive surgery. *Plast Reconstr Surg* 1957;20:1.
4. Guerrerosantos J, Vasquez-Pallaves R, Vera-Strathman A, et al. The tongue flap in reconstruction of the lip. In: *Transactions of the Third International Congress of Plastic Surgery.* Amsterdam: Excerpta Medica, 1963.
5. McGregor IA. The tongue flap in lip surgery. *Br J Plast Surg* 1966;19:253.
6. Jackson IT. Use of tongue flaps to resurface lip defects and close palatal fistulas in children. *Plast Reconstr Surg* 1972;49:537.
7. Zarem HA, Greer DM. Tongue flap for reconstruction of the lips after electrical burns. *Plast Reconstr Surg* 1974;53:310.
8. Converse JM, ed. *Reconstructive plastic surgery.* Philadelphia: WB Saunders, 1977.
9. Ortiz-Monasterio F, Factor R. Definitive treatment of electric burns of the mouth. *Plast Reconstr Surg* 1980;65:169.
10. Zisser G. A contribution to the primary reconstruction of the upper lip and labial commissure following tumor excision. *J Maxillofac Surg* 1975;3:211.
11. Brusati R. Reconstruction of the labial commissure by a sliding U-shaped cheek flap. *J Maxillofac Surg* 1979;7:11.
12. Joseph J. *Nasenplastik and sonstige Gesichtsplastik nebst einen Anhang über Mammaplastik und einige weitere Operationen aus dean Gebiete der ausseren korperplastik.* Leipzig: Kabitsch, 1931.
13. Kazanjian VH, Roopenian A. The treatment of lip deformities resulting from electric burns. *Am J Surg* 1954;88:884.
14. Gillies HD, Millard DR, eds.: *Principles and art of plastic surgery.* Boston: Little, Brown, 1957.
15. Converse JM. *Surgical treatment of facial injuries.* Baltimore: Williams & Wilkins, 1959;795.
16. Pons J. À propos du temps musculaire clans les commissurotomies labiales. *Ann Chir Plast* 1968;13:4.
17. Wustrack KO. Reconstruction of incompetent oral commissures with dermal muscle flaps from the lips. *Plast Reconstr Surg* 1971;62:118.
18. Vittoria JM. A new method of elongation of the corner of the mouth. *Plast Reconstr Surg* 1972;49:52.
19. Argamaso RV, Strauch B, Lewin ML, et al. Lip-commissuroplasty after electrical burns. *Chir Plast* 1975;3:27.
20. Muhlbauer WD. Elongation of mouth in postburn microstomia by a double Z-plasty. *Plast Reconstr Surg* 1970;45:400.
21. Thomson HG, Juckes AW, Farmer AW. Electric burns to the mouth in children. *Plast Reconstr Surg* 1965;35:466.
22. Thomson HG. Electric burns to the mouth. In: Feller I, and Grabb WC eds. *Reconstruction and rehabilitation of the burned patient,* Ann Arbor, Mich.: National Institute for Burn Medicine, 1979. Chap. 62;216.
23. Al-Qattan M, Gillett D, Thomson HG. Long-term objective lip assessment following electrical burns to the oral commissure in infancy and childhood. *Can J Plast Surg* 1996;4:2.
24. Al-Qattan MM, Gillett D, Thomson HG. Electrical burns to the oral commissure: does splinting obviate the need for commissuroplasty? *Burns* 1996;22:555.

CHAPTER 177 ■ COMMISSURE RECONSTRUCTION

R. V. ARGAMASO

EDITORIAL COMMENT

The technique demonstrated here is a functional restoration of the commissure, which should be kept in mind for relatively large defects, particularly following cancer resection. On the other hand, for children who occasionally suffer from electrical burns of the commissure, the simple technique of an angle prosthesis to stretch the area and to soften the scar tissue should also be considered.

The lips form an aesthetic unit of the face and are multifunctional. When an electrical burn occurs at the commissure of the mouth (an injury more likely to be acquired by inquisitive infants and young children), some functional impairment and structural asymmetry may result. Deep burns disrupting the orbicularis oris muscle are a challenge to adequate reconstruction (1).

INDICATIONS

The vermilion tapers and disappears at the corners of the mouth. A full-thickness destruction of tissue at the commissure invariably includes muscle fibers. As a consequence, the normally closed interval between the lips at the corner when the mouth is at rest is transformed into a gap. During the acute stage of the injury, this corner of the mouth becomes incompetent and allows continuous drooling of saliva, which is both untidy and unsightly.

An acute injury is treated conservatively to allow healing with the least sacrifice of viable tissue. As a result of scar deposition and contracture, the oral circumference is reduced. The resulting postburn microstomia is disfiguring and, in severe cases, causes feeding difficulties.

ANATOMY

The orbicularis oris muscle, unlike the orbicularis oculi, is formed by complex strata of muscle fibers surrounding the

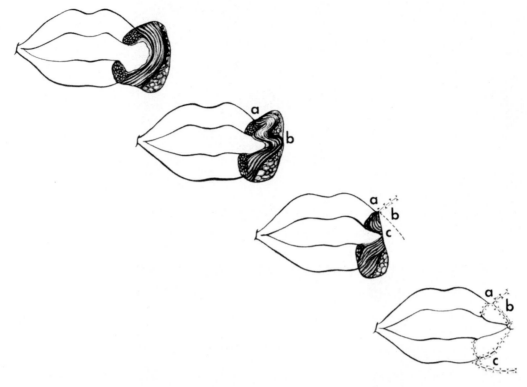

FIG. 1. Stages in reconstruction of the commissure (see text).

mouth. These fibers originate from other muscles of the face and therefore come from several directions.

At the commissure, the buccinator sends upper and lower fibers to the upper and lower lips, respectively. Its middle fibers decussate with those of the levator anguli oris to pass to the lower lip and with those of the depressor anguli oris to pass to the upper lip. The zygomaticus inserts obliquely into the angle of the mouth and blends with the levator and depressor anguli oris. The risorius runs horizontally and inserts into the constituted orbicularis muscle and the skin at the corner of the mouth. These muscles are innervated by the buccal branches of the seventh nerve.

FLAP DESIGN AND DIMENSIONS

When there has been only minor tissue loss, skin and mucosal flaps may be shifted to the area involved. With significant damage to the orbicularis muscle, however, a restoration of muscle continuity within the area of the vermilion is an important aspect of the procedure described (Fig. 1).

OPERATIVE TECHNIQUE

Once the scar has been excised, the original area of the defect is recreated. Assessment of the orbicularis remnant is undertaken by a careful skin dissection. The stumps of the destroyed segment are identified, and the ends are cut squarely. The intact component fibers of the muscle are mobilized gently toward these stumps. Continuity of the orbicularis ring at the vermilion then is reestablished by an end-to-side suture of the discontinuous stumps to the continuous, contiguous muscle fibers.

The new position of the translocated muscle segments now will form the substance or framework of the new commissure.

The skin defect toward the upper lip is repaired by approximating the skin margins, marked *a* and *b* in Fig. 1, in a lateral to medial direction. A straight-line closure is directed vertically to the lip or slightly obliquely. The skin sutures stop at the vermilion, the final suture catching some fibers directly underneath, to maintain the transposed muscle in the medial position.

The apex of the new commissure then is determined by plotting the distance between the corner of the lip and the peak of the cupid's bow on the uninvolved side and then transposing this measurement from the corresponding peak of the cupid's bow to that point on the involved side. A slight overcorrection is advisable because healing generally involves some shortening of this distance.

The skin now is incised in line with the vermilion ridge of the upper lip to the point indicated as the apex of the reconstructed commissure. A triangular flap (*c*) is thus created. This is transposed for coverage of the skin defect of the lower lip.

Finally, buccal mucosal flaps are fashioned and tailored into the corner of the mouth to line the new vermilion. Dogears that develop are trimmed accordingly (Figs. 2 and 3).

CLINICAL RESULTS

The suture lines are usually subjected to some degree of tension. Inflammation is common, but it is easily controlled with local hygiene and topical antibiotics. The functional results generally are gratifying, but the prominence of postoperative scars almost always requires their future revision.

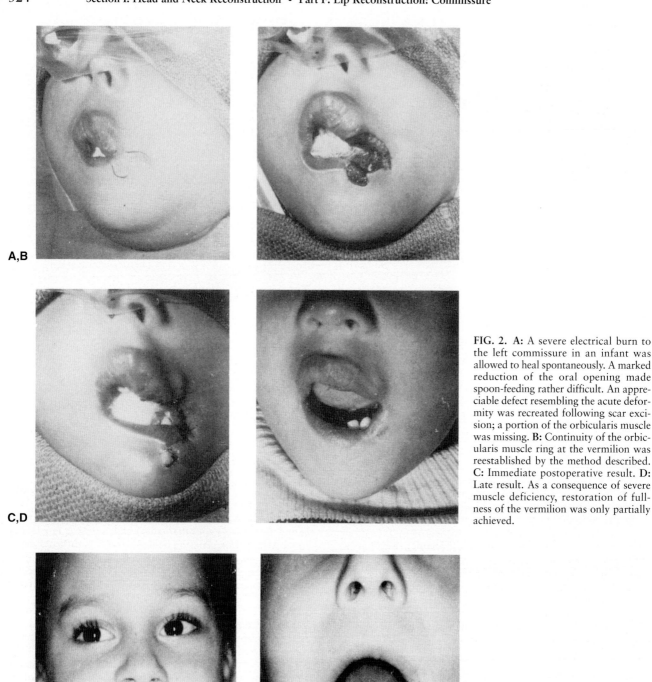

FIG. 2. A: A severe electrical burn to the left commissure in an infant was allowed to heal spontaneously. A marked reduction of the oral opening made spoon-feeding rather difficult. An appreciable defect resembling the acute deformity was recreated following scar excision; a portion of the orbicularis muscle was missing. **B:** Continuity of the orbicularis muscle ring at the vermilion was reestablished by the method described. **C:** Immediate postoperative result. **D:** Late result. As a consequence of severe muscle deficiency, restoration of fullness of the vermilion was only partially achieved.

FIG. 3. A: A 1-year-old burn to the mouth was characterized by obliteration of the left commissure and a marked asymmetry of the lip form during animation. **B:** Reconstruction of the commissure with the same technique was performed to restore some symmetry to the mouth during repose and active motion.

Readvancement of healthy mucosal flaps to replace scarred areas also contributes to the patient's acceptance of the final outcome of repair.

cal burn, is described. A successful reconstruction helps to restore lip competency at the angle of the mouth and also improves the contour and symmetry of the vermilion.

SUMMARY

A method of reestablishing continuity of the orbicularis oris muscle at the commissure, commonly disrupted by an electri-

Reference

1. Argamaso RV, Strauch B, Lewin ML, et al. Lip-commissuroplasty after electrical burns. *Chir Plast* 1975;3:27.

CHAPTER 178 ■ NASOLABIAL FLAPS TO ANTERIOR FLOOR OF MOUTH

I. A. MCGREGOR AND D. SOUTAR

The functional integrity of the anterior floor of the mouth is probably more important in maintaining tongue mobility and consequent normality of articulation and deglutition and control and disposal of saliva than any other part of the oral cavity. Even minor loss of tongue mobility results in a serious disturbance of function. As a result, small defects of this area that elsewhere in the mouth might be suitably managed by direct suture require a formal reconstruction.

For the small defect, a suitably matching small flap reconstruction is required, and it is in this situation that the nasolabial flap provides a simple, safe, and effective method of reconstruction. The reconstruction involves the raising of an inferiorly based nasolabial flap on one side (1) or, much more frequently, both sides (2), depending on the site and size of the intraoral defect. The flap or flaps are tunneled through the cheek and brought into the mouth. There the single flap is sutured to the defect or, in the case of bilateral flaps, interdigitated and sutured to the defect. Division of the pedicle and insetting are carried out 3 weeks later.

INDICATIONS

Defects of the anterior floor of the mouth that are most suitable for a bilateral nasolabial flap reconstruction often involve the floor itself and part of the ventral aspect of the tongue. Frequently, it is found that one flap covers the defect of the floor while the other covers the defect of the tongue, the combined flaps forming a rectangle. The method works best in the edentulous mouth where the loss of the teeth and the alveolar resorption that follows leave a shallow floor of the mouth.

Certain virtues of the technique are obvious: the good cosmetic result on the face because of the scar line in the nasolabial fold and the fact that most adults can spare tissue in the nasolabial site. Less obvious, but possibly more important, is the direction of any pull of the bridge segment. This is upward and laterally and has the effect of holding the tongue up and preventing it from sinking down into the mouth during healing. This plays a significant role in maintaining tongue mobility.

Nearly all the defects in the anterior floor that are potential candidates for the method require bilateral flaps, and it is this technique that will be described.

FLAP DESIGN AND DIMENSIONS

Inferiorly based nasolabial flaps are outlined on each cheek and raised with sufficient subcutaneous tissue to ensure a good blood supply, although remaining superficial to the facial muscles. The base of the flap should be maintained at just above the level of the angle of the mouth (Fig. 1). It is desirable to place the base of the flap at this point because just below this level several branches from the facial artery and inferior labial artery pass into the nasolabial skin and subcutaneous tissue (3). The flap relies on the subcutaneous and dermal vascular system, augmented by these vessels in the base of the flap. Placing the base of the flap at this level also ensures that the flaps enter the oral cavity from well above the "sump" area and so minimize any tendency to fistula formation.

OPERATIVE TECHNIQUE

The tunnel is made through the soft tissue of the cheek near the base of the flap, gaining entrance to the mouth through previously intact buccal mucosa, and sited to take the most direct route to the defect. The passage must be made wide enough to accommodate the flap easily. There is no tendency to strangulation of the flap unless the tunnel is made unduly narrow or the secondary defect on the cheek is closed too tightly in the vicinity of the tunnel. Each flap is led into the oral cavity and interdigitated with its fellow. It is surprising how often the two flaps, adapting to a natural position, lie with one flap anterior to the other (Fig. 2).

The secondary defect is closed, taking care (as previously stressed) to leave a small triangular area inferiorly unsutured to avoid constricting the base of the flap. The flaps are sutured to the margins of the intraoral defect and finally to each other. The flaps are divided, and insetting is completed at the end of 3 weeks, with the bridge segment usually discarded. The flaps at this stage look bulky, and the appearance before division is made worse by the presence of the bridge segment of each flap passing laterally and the natural tendency of each flap to tube itself. The bulky appearance should be ignored because the appearance of pin-cushioning settles quite quickly to complete flatness (Fig. 3).

The technique described is two-stage; although there is no doubt that it could be made into a single-stage procedure by raising the flaps as skin islands relying on a pedicle of subcutaneous tissue, this is unwise. In the area of the base of the flap, the pilosebaceous follicles extend deeply in the subcutis, and the pedicle of an island would be a somewhat tenuous structure with a dubious blood supply. We consider that to jeopardize the blood supply of the flap in this way is not justified. A further reason for using a two-stage technique concerns the presence in males of hair-bearing skin in the flap, particularly at its base. The 3-week interval between the two stages allows hair to grow on the flap in its intraoral site. When the bridge segment is divided, it is a simple matter to ensure that no hairs remain on the part of the flap that is to be left in the mouth permanently.

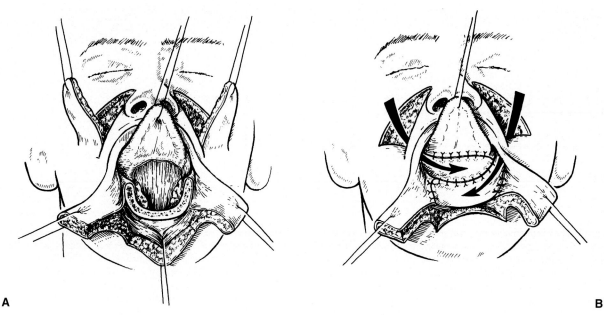

A   B

FIG. 1. A,B: The principle of bilateral inferiorly based nasolabial flaps brought into the mouth through a cheek tunnel, interdigitated, and sutured to the defect of the anterior floor of the mouth.

CLINICAL RESULTS

The presence of teeth in the symphyseal region makes the flap technically much more difficult. The distance required to reach the defect is considerably increased, and the area of inset tends to be smaller. The possibility of biting through the flap pedicle is also a deterrent to using the flap, and the use of bite blocks to prevent this makes the transfer, if anything, technically even more difficult. All in all, it is best restricted to the edentulous patient.

Dental state aside, the main restriction to use of the flap concerns the lateral extent of the defect. The length of each flap raised on the face is strictly limited above by the presence of the eye and the need to avoid ectropion when the secondary defect is closed. It is equally limited below in males by the commencement of beard area skin at approximately the level of the angle of the mouth. This limitation of length means that the defects these flaps can fill in the mouth are correspondingly limited in width.

The nasolabial flap has proved reliable in intraoral reconstruction. Necrosis is not common and, in our experience, has

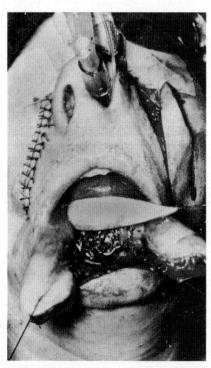
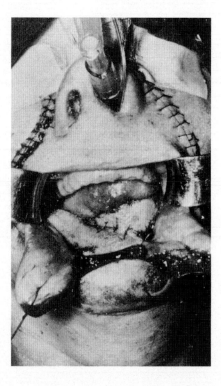

A,B

FIG. 2. The steps in transfer of bilateral nasolabial flaps in a patient following resection of a small squamous cell carcinoma of the anterior floor of the mouth. A: The left nasolabial flap raised, and the right flap tunneled through into the mouth, with the secondary defect sutured. B: The flaps interdigitated and sutured in position.

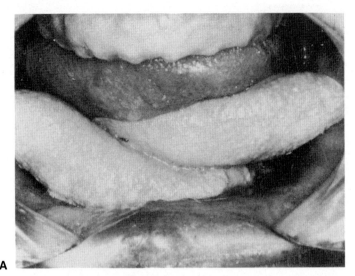
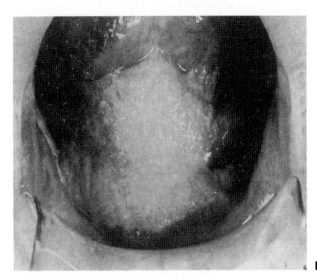

A

B

FIG. 3. Subsequent stages of the transfer. **A:** The flap just prior to division of the pedicles with obvious pin-cushioning. **B:** Late result showing how the pin-cushioning corrects as the flaps flatten out.

been the result of technical error. Although the flaps may appear bulky at the time of division (Fig. 3A), the temptation to thin at this stage should be resisted because the flaps flatten out rapidly (Fig. 3B); this is particularly evident when excision of tumor also has involved resection of the alveolar rim of mandible.

SUMMARY

Only by reconstruction with flaps such as bilateral nasolabial flaps can the anterior free segment of the tongue, where so

much of the function of that organ resides, be kept in its normal position and state, untethered, freely mobile, and separate from the anterior floor of the mouth.

References

1. Zarem HA. Current concepts in reconstructive surgery in patients with cancer of the head and neck. *Surg Clin North Am* 1971;51:149.
2. Cohen IK, Edgerton MT. Transbuccal flaps for reconstruction of the floor of the mouth. *Plast Reconstr Surg* 1971;48:8.
3. Herbert DC, Harrison RG. Naso-labial subcutaneous pedicle flaps. *Br J Plast Surg* 1975;28:85.

CHAPTER 179 ■ ONE-STAGE NASOLABIAL SKIN FLAPS FOR ORAL AND OROPHARYNGEAL DEFECTS

R. A. ELLIOTT

The nasolabial region is a well-known donor site for a variety of flaps. In most older patients, this area can yield a sizeable flap without significant distortion. When the flap is based inferiorly, the beard usually can be avoided, and when the flap is carried on a subcutaneous pedicle, one-stage repair of many oral and oropharyngeal defects is feasible.

INDICATIONS

The nasolabial skin flap is quite versatile. Numerous authors have extolled its virtues for repair of ipsilateral surgical defects of the palate and a variety of other intraoral defects. Until the 1970s, most employed two-stage procedures and protected the flap with a bite block (1–4). Development of a safe one-stage technique enhanced its value significantly, particularly in the edentulous patient. The repair of antral fistulae, prompt rehabilitation of elderly and poor-risk patients, and combination with radical neck dissection became more routine, and bilateral flaps were interdigitated to repair defects of the anterior floor of the mouth and liberate the tongue (5).

ANATOMY

The facial artery enters the face lateral to the mandible at the anterior border of the masseter and passes upward and forward on a tortuous course to the corner of the mouth, giving off the inferior labial artery branches, which supply the base of the flap and adjacent muscles. Although not dissected in this operation, the facial artery can be mobilized readily until it becomes fixed beneath the risorious and zygomaticus major muscles near the mouth. After giving off the superior labial artery deep to the latter muscle, a smaller main trunk passes on and through facial muscles to reach the inner canthus. No vessels enter the deep surface of the distal portion of the flap superiorly.

All named arteries are accompanied by one or more veins; most drain into the facial vein. The terminal branches of the facial nerve lie deep in the facial muscles and are not endangered by flap elevation superficial to the muscle, as recommended [see Operative Technique section]. Rich anastomoses between the facial vessels and the deep perforators of the infraorbital and transverse facial vessels further assure an abundant blood supply to and from the flap. Division of the facial artery at the level of the mandible, for example, during radical neck surgery, is not a limiting factor, primarily because of similar rich anastomoses between the facial, masseteric, and buccal vessels (6).

FLAP DESIGN AND DIMENSIONS

The skin and subcutaneous flap is based inferiorly near the angle of the mouth and may extend to the inner canthus. The medial border lies in the paranasal sulcus above and in the nasolabial fold below (Fig. 1A). The flap width and length are judged to fill the defect without tension and permit safe closure of the donor site. The full width is maintained for most of the length. Flap width has varied from 1.5 to 3.0 cm, and narrower flaps have never been used.

The design proximal to the skin-bearing triangle is held at full width for at least 1.5 cm to define a subcutaneous pedicle to tunnel through the cheek. The remainder of the inferior pattern then tapers sharply to facilitate donor site closure without a dog-ear (Fig. 1B).

A liberal arc of rotation similar to that of the arterialized flap (7) delivers this flap to most points in the oral cavity and lateral pharynx with ease. The point of entry into the mouth can be varied slightly to bring the skin-bearing tissue directly to the defect (Fig. 1C) but should remain above the angle of the mouth to assure the best flap circulation (6).

OPERATIVE TECHNIQUE

The entire design pattern is outlined sharply through the dermis. Then the flap is elevated superficial to the facial muscles, from superior to inferior, until the selected point for passage of the subcutaneous pedicle through the cheek is reached.

A liberal tunnel is created through the cheek to avoid constriction of the pedicle. Blunt dissection minimizes the threat of damage to the facial nerves and vessels as the flap is delivered into the defect beneath its nearest border. After testing briefly for position and adequacy, the flap is marked to define the near border of the defect and withdrawn.

The pattern is deepithelialized inferior to the mark, any hair follicles are removed conservatively, and the flap is returned to the defect and inset with a single layer of nonabsorbable sutures. Tension must be avoided, especially along the long axis of the flap. The donor site is closed superiorly by advancement or direct suture and inferiorly by undermining and advancing the lateral cheek over the base of the pedicle to avoid distortion or compression of the pedicle.

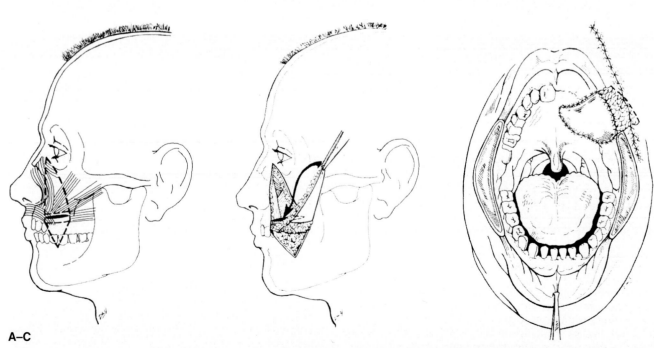

A–C

FIG. 1. A–C: Flap design and technique. (From Elliott, ref. 5, with permission.)

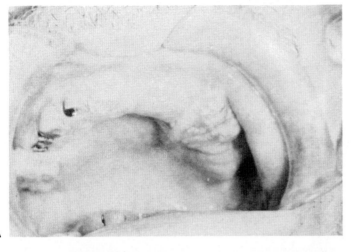
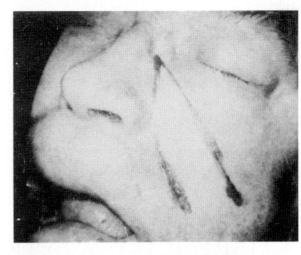
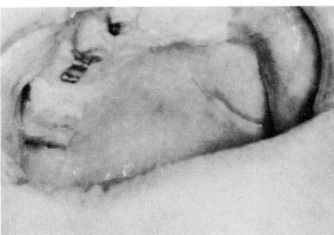
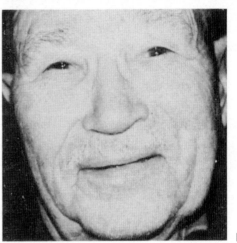

FIG. 2. Squamous cell carcinoma excision of alveolus and palate in 85-year-old man. A: Lesion for full-thickness excision through lining of maxillary antrum. B: Design of usable flap. C: Inset flap after 5 months. D: Donor site at 33 months. (From Elliott, ref. 5, with permission.)

CLINICAL RESULTS

Over the past 20 years, I have used this flap for the one-stage repair of significant surgical defects of anterior and posterior palate, including the uvula; tonsil and base of tongue; lateral tongue; oropharyngeal wall; and floor of mouth, both lateral and anterior. It provided one-stage repair of alveolar and palatal defects involving the maxillary sinus for three elderly, edentulous patients, one of whom is illustrated in Fig. 2.

My first candidate, a hearty 85-year-old man, was spared an antral fistula, had full rehabilitation after radical neck surgery for metastatic disease, and remained free of clinical disease to his death at age 92. Other operated patients had emphysema, heart failure, renal disease, obesity, diabetes, and alcoholism. Three had a radical neck dissection as part of the procedure.

There have been no complications with this flap. Hair delivered into the oral cavity on one flap remained a curiosity without clinical significance. No cysts have been seen; except for some flattening of facial contour and a permanent scar, there is little evidence of surgery. Most facial scars become barely noticeable in elderly patients, especially those following normal skin lines.

This flap design obviates the need for more complicated and risky techniques in the repair of a variety of significant intraoral defects. It is my closure technique of choice whenever an ade-quate nasolabial donor site can be matched with a significant intraoral defect, especially in the edentulous patient.

SUMMARY

An inferiorly based nasolabial skin flap, transposed on a subcutaneous pedicle buried in an ipsilateral cheek tunnel, is proposed for the safe, one-stage repair of a variety of significant intraoral defects. This technique has many advantages for elderly and high-risk patients and can be combined with radical neck dissection.

References

1. Rosenthal W. Verschluss traumatischer Gaumendefekte durch Weichteile des Gesichts. *Zentralbl Chir* 1868;43:596.
2. Esser JFS. Deckung von Gaumendefekten mittels Geslielter Naso-labial Haclappon. *Dtsch Z Chir* 1918;147:128.
3. Wallace AF. Esser's skin flap for closing large palatal fistulae. *Br J Plast Surg* 1966;19:322.
4. Georgiade N, Mladick R, Thome F. The nasolabial tunnel flap. *Plast Reconstr Surg* 1969;43:463.
5. Elliott RA. Use of nasolabial skin to cover intraoral defects. *Plast Reconstr Surg* 1976;58:201.
6. Herbert D, Harrison R. Nasolabial subcutaneous pedicle flaps. *Br J Plast Surg* 1975;28:85.
7. Rose EH. One-stage arterialized nasolabial island flap for floor of mouth reconstruction. *Ann Plast Surg* 1981;6:71.

CHAPTER 180. Buccal Fat Pad Flap Plus Skin Graft to Oroantral and Oronasal Defects *P. Egyedi and H. Müller*
www.encyclopediaofflaps.com

CHAPTER 181 ■ INTRAORAL RECONSTRUCTION WITH TONGUE MUSCULOMUCOSAL FLAPS

J. GUERREROSANTOS

EDITORIAL COMMENT

A good study of the vascular anatomy of the tongue and its relevance in the design of tongue flaps can be found in Bracka, A. The blood supply of dorsal tongue flaps. *Br J Plast Surg* 34;379, 1981.

The tongue musculomucosal flap provides the most dependable means of reconstructing the lining of the oral cavity. The tongue flap is especially useful in the surgical correction of palatal perforations that are large or surrounded by thickened fibrous tissue. Using tongue flaps, a surgeon can be more aggressive in removing tumors and still give the patient the opportunity for successful rehabilitation through immediate reconstruction.

INDICATIONS

Palatal Reconstruction

The tongue flap is particularly useful in heavily irradiated patients by providing additional muscle coverage of the bones. It plays an important role in the treatment of large fistulas (1–9). The closure of perforations in the soft palate is preferably done with the use of the palatal tissues themselves, and in extensive perforations, we can use a combined reconstructive method that uses a tongue flap and a pharyngeal flap.

Buccal Reconstruction

In the buccal area, tissue losses that include the mucosa alone or some or all of the anatomic layers can be reconstructed with a tongue flap (10,11). The flap can be designed to vary the amount of muscle that is considered necessary for reconstructing the defect (see Fig. 5). For full-thickness cheek losses,

the tongue musculomucosal flap can be used for the inner lining, and the outer covering can be provided by either a forehead flap or a large pectoralis major musculocutaneous flap.

Floor of the Mouth and Tonsillar Area Reconstruction

The tongue flap can be used for reconstructing either a primary or a secondary defect in both the floor of the mouth (12–15) and the tonsillar area (16,17).

ANATOMY

A thorough appreciation of the anatomy of tongue flaps and their clinical applications is given in Chapter 173.

FLAP DESIGN AND DIMENSIONS

Palate

Proper planning of a tongue flap is essential to the success of the operation to ensure that the orientation of the flap will be correct at each stage and that it will fit the defect without tension, kinking, or torsion. All possible sites and orientations for the flap should be considered to ensure that the most suitable one is selected. Planning of the tongue flap in reverse is probably the most important phase of the operation. Using a pattern of the defect, the steps in the operative procedure are carried out in reverse order until the donor site is reached. The final pattern should be larger than needed, particularly in length.

For reconstructing the palatal lining, it is advisable to use an anteriorly based tongue musculomucosal flap (Fig. 1). On the basis of my experience and that of some other authors, incisions should be made following the longitudinal direction of the blood circulation of the tongue, always avoiding crossing the midlingual raphe. The following dimensions should be

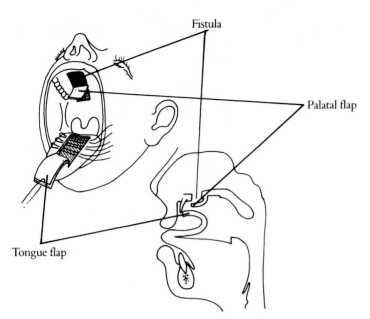

Fistula

Palatal flap

Tongue flap

FIG. 1. Anteriorly based tongue musculomucous flap used for the closure of perforation in the hard palate. The flap should be 5 cm long, 3.5 cm wide, and quite thick. It is sutured into the fistula, and the pedicle is sectioned 2 or 3 weeks later. (From Guerrerosantos, ref. 5, with permission.)

used: 5 cm long, 3.5 cm wide, and two thirds of the thickness of the lingual dorsum.

Buccal Area

To succeed in cheek reconstruction using a tongue flap, the following rules should be observed. Flaps should be planned with a minimum width of 2 cm and a minimum thickness of 5 mm. I prefer dorsal or marginal flaps whose pedicles are near the lingual apex. The pedicle should be long enough to permit mobility of the tongue without allowing traction on the tip of the flap. If the loss of cheek mucosa is very extensive a large direct flap may be used, taking care that the pedicle does not cross the median lingual raphe.

OPERATIVE TECHNIQUE

Palatal Reconstruction

The margins of the palatal fistula are first pared. About a 2-cm layer of tongue muscle is raised with the flap to ensure that a full quota of blood vessels remains. Elevation of the flap is done in the direction of the pedicle as far as necessary,

checking at intervals to see at which point the flap is capable of reaching its destination without tension.

The donor site is easily closed in two or three layers, leaving a small area open next to the flap pedicle to avoid tension at the base of the pedicle and disturbance of the blood supply. The tip of the flap is sutured to the margins of the fistula. The palatal closure of these wounds is critical to prevent added morbidity from small fistula formation. Simple running sutures or simple interrupted palatal sutures often fail to evert the mucosa. I have used a separate horizontal mattress suture to ensure the close approximation of tissues with minimal chance of inversion of the epithelium (Fig. 2).

After 3 weeks, the flap can be divided and sutured along the line 1.5 cm behind the posterior margin of the defect. The bridge segment of the flap is turned upward to its original site, and insetting of the distal transferred segment is completed. The bridge segment often tends to entube, and this must be undone by scoring and, if necessary, by excising contracted scar tissue (Figs. 3 and 4).

Floor of the Mouth and Tonsillar Area Reconstruction, Buccal Area

The technique used in palatal reconstruction can be adapted to reconstruction of other intraoral areas (Figs. 3–5)

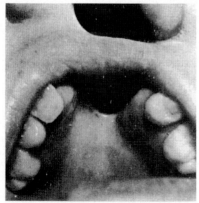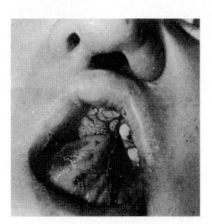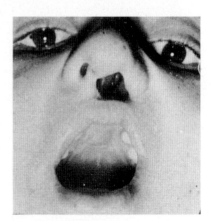

A–C

FIG. 2. A: Palatal-alveolar fistula after noma. B: Closure of the fistula with tongue flap. C: Result is shown 18 months after repair. (From Guerrerosantos and Altamirano, ref. 17, with permission.)

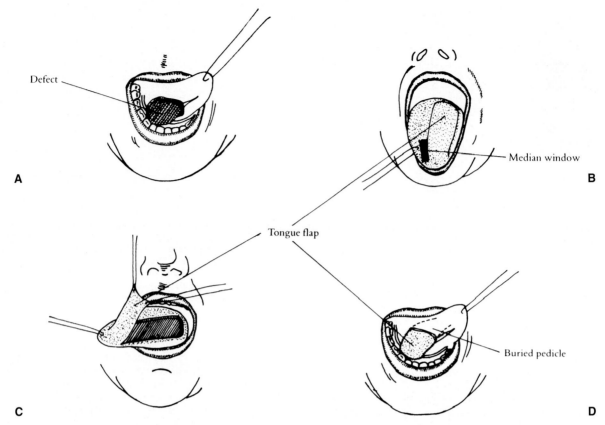

FIG. 3. Tongue and floor of the mouth reconstruction. **A:** Defect on the lower aspect of the tongue and floor of the mouth. **B:** An anteriorly based tongue flap is outlined, and a median window is made on the midlingual line near the tip. **C:** Raising of the tongue flap. **D:** Suture of the flap into the defect. The flap passes through a median window, its pedicle being buried. (From Guerrerosantos, ref. 5, with permission.)

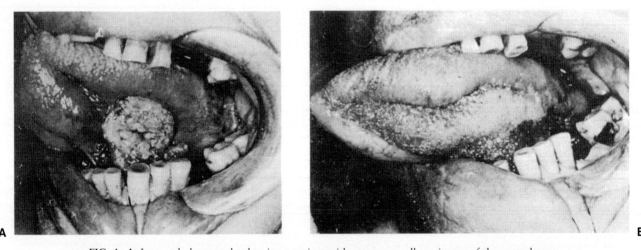

FIG. 4. **A:** Intraoral photographs showing a patient with squamous cell carcinoma of the ventral surface of the tongue and floor of the mouth. **B:** This patient was treated surgically using the technique shown in Fig. 3.

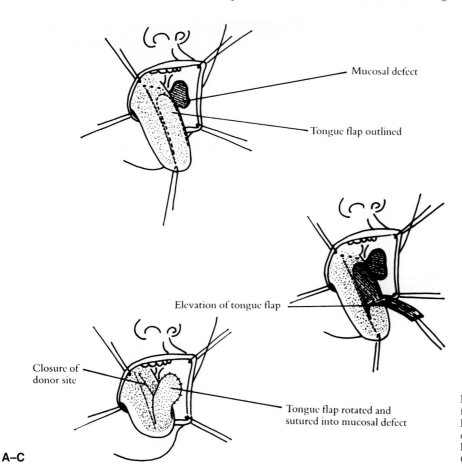

Mucosal defect

Tongue flap outlined

Elevation of tongue flap

Closure of donor site

Tongue flap rotated and sutured into mucosal defect

A–C

FIG. 5. Cheek area reconstruction. **A:** A flap is planned on the lingual apex. **B:** Elevation of the tongue flap. **C:** Suture of the flap into the defect. Three weeks later, the pedicle is sectioned. (From Guerrerosantos, ref. 5, with permission.)

CLINICAL RESULTS

Like any other flap, the tongue musculomucosal flap is subject to complications if it is not used with judicious care. All general flap principles should be observed faithfully. Complications have been generally associated with local wound problems, such as localized infections and limited wound dehiscence. Tension and distortion are the main enemies of successful tongue musculomucosal flap repair. Good arterial and venous blood supply and gentle handling of tissue are its only allies.

Using the technique correctly, I have achieved success in 90% of my tongue flap patients, as far as flap integration and healing are concerned. I caution that the surgeon should never design a transverse flap across the lingual raphe because the distal portion of the flap will necrose. Also, the tongue flap can fail in oral reconstruction if a short, thin flap is designed, if the flap is sutured under tension, if the circulation is deficient, and if there is danger of the tongue separating the flap from the palate.

SUMMARY

The tongue musculomucosal flap can be used to close various intraoral defects.

References

1. Conley JJ, De Amesti F, Pierce MK. Use of tongue flaps in head and neck surgery *Surgery* 1957;41:745.
2. Conley JJ. The use of lingual flaps in repair of fistulas of the hard palate. *Plast Reconstr Surg* 1966;38:123.
3. Guerrerosantos J, Garay J, Tones A, Altamirano JT. Tongue flap with triple fixation in secondary cleft palate surgery. In: *Transactions of the Fourth International Congress of Plastic Surgeons.* Amsterdam: Excerpta Medica, 1969;369.
4. Guerrerosantos J, Fernandez JM. Further experience with the tongue flap in cleft palate repair. *Cleft Palate J* 1973;10:192.
5. Guerrerosantos J. Tongue flaps. In: Grabb WC, Myers MB, eds. *Skin flaps.* Boston: Little, Brown, 1975;216.
6. Jackson IT. Use of tongue flaps to resurface lip defects and close palatal fistulas in children. *Plast Reconstr Surg* 1972;49:537.
7. Jackson IT. Closure of secondary palatal fistulas with intraoral tissue and bone grafting. *Br J Plast Surg* 1972;25:73.
8. Klopp CT, Schurter M. Reconstruction of palate with tongue flap and repair of tongue. *Cancer* 1956;9:1.
9. Quetglas J. Perforaciones del paladar. *Rev Esp Cir Plast* 1973;6:131.
10. Kleinschmidt O. Operaciones en las partes blandas y esqueleto de la cara. In: Kirschner M., ed. *Tratado de tecnica operatoria general y especial.* Barcelona: Editorial Labor, 1948;378.
11. Schultz RC. Regional considerations in repairing soft tissue. In: Schultz RC ed., *Facial injuries.* Chicago: Year Book Medical Publishers, 1970;118.
12. Oneal RN. Oronasal fistulas. In: Grabb WC, Rosenstein SW, Bzoch KR, eds. *Cleft lip and palate.* Boston: Little, Brown, 1971;490.
13. Papaioannou A, Farr H. Reconstruction of the floor of the mouth by a pedicle tongue flap. *Surg Gynecol Obstet* 1966;122:807.
14. Pilhew FR. Tongue flap in oral surgery. *Boll Soc Cirug (Buenos Aires)* 1964;48:442.
15. Som ML. Marginal resection of the mandible with reconstruction by tongue flap, for carcinoma of the floor of the mouth. *Am J Surg* 1971;121:679.
16. Fernandez-Villoria JM. Tonsillar area reconstruction. *Plast Reconstr Surg* 1967;40:220.
17. Guerrerosantos J, Altamirano JT. The use of lingual flaps in repair of fistulas of the hard palate. *Plast Reconstr Surg* 1966;38:123.

CHAPTER 182 ■ BUCKET-HANDLE VESTIBULAR MUCOSAL FLAP TO ANTERIOR PALATE

P. EGYEDI AND H. MÜLLER*

The problem of minor residual fistulas and clefts adjacent to the premaxilla or in the palate has received little attention in the literature compared with other aspects of clefting. The reason may be that these fistulas are often symptomless, and surgical correction may be difficult and disappointing. Also, prosthetic covering of these fistulas is sometimes successful, although the long-term effect of any partial prosthetic appliance on the remaining dentition must be taken into account.

INDICATIONS

Some indications for closure of palatal fistulas are (a) escape of liquids through the nose, (b) escape of air through the nose during speech, (c) impaction of solid food particles in the fistula, and (d) the need to immobilize the premaxilla with a bone graft for prosthetic purposes.

ANATOMY

As Fig. 1 demonstrates, the pedicle of the flap is situated laterally, and the base is well vascularized (1), unlike the base of the vestibular flap, which can be used most successfully in unilateral clefts and is situated medially in the region of the cleft. The vessels involved are branches of the labial and infraorbital arteries. The midpart of the flap, however, is composed partly of scar tissue, a condition that must be noted.

FLAP DESIGN AND DIMENSIONS

In unilateral clefts, the average fistula can be closed with a vestibular flap (2). In major openings, the tongue flap (see Chapter 181) can be used advantageously (3). In bilateral cleft patients in whom a Y-shaped opening around the premaxilla exists, bilateral vestibular flaps can be used, but the failure rate seems fairly high. Because the base of the vestibular pedicle is usually scarred by previous operations, the blood supply must be assumed to be marginal, and where the two flaps meet, tip necrosis occurs frequently.

OPERATIVE TECHNIQUE

Two parallel incisions are made in the vestibulum (Fig. 1A). The width of the flap is between 0.4 and 1 cm, depending largely on the local anatomy and the depth of the vestibular sulcus. Exact measurements cannot be given, because irregularities in the scarred area are considerable. If the vestibulum is quite shallow, the surgeon should be careful not to remove too much tissue from the inner aspect of the lip unless correction with an Abbé flap is planned.

The inner of the two incisions is carried to the alveolar bone. The periosteum can be raised over a small distance (e.g., 0.2 cm), but then the flap leaves the bone to enter the vestibular tissue to meet the outer incision just labial to the vestibular "crest." At this stage, after the bucket-handle flap has been raised, an attempt is made to obtain a nasal layer of epithelial tissue on both sides of the premaxilla.

A "circumcision" of the Y-shaped area is done, the periosteum of the premaxilla and the lateral alveolar segments are raised, and the nasal layer is closed with inverted sutures. Access may be extremely difficult in these patients, and if a reliable closure is not possible, one sometimes must resort to deepithelialization of the fistula and to closing it with a single layer of tissue on the oral surface. In this latter case, however, introduction of a bone graft into the cleft cannot be done in the same operation. As a rule, the bulk of the bucket-handle flap is such that the alveolar gap can be plugged over a considerable area. Whenever a more or less reliable nasal layer closure can be obtained, introduction of autogenous bone is usually indicated, since the success rate of closure is greatly increased (4). Suturing should be done with fine atraumatic sutures (Fig. 2).

After treatment, a petrolatum-impregnated iodoform gauze is lightly applied over the whole area and kept in place with sutures fixed to adjacent teeth, forming a network over the area. Sutures and pack are covered by cold-cure acrylic. Additionally, 600,000 units of penicillin G are administered for 2 days.

CLINICAL RESULTS

Eighteen patients have been treated with this flap. In one patient, necrosis of the area of the flap behind the premaxilla resulted, and this should be considered a failure. In all other patients, flap survival was satisfactory, although in a few

* Deceased.

534

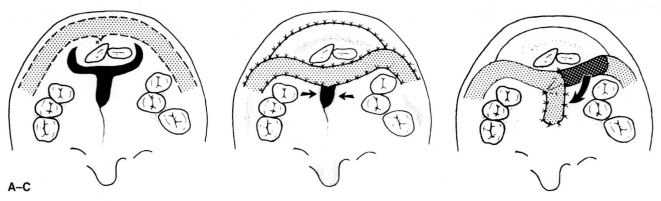

A–C

FIG. 1. **A:** Schematic drawing of the bucket-handle vestibular mucosal flap. At *X,* the extension mentioned in the text could be made to cover the dorsal part of a Y-shaped fistula. In the situation depicted here, this would be useless. **B:** The flap was sutured into the anterior part of the fistula. The defect dorsal to the flap sometimes can be closed by mobilizing the palatal mucoperiostea (*arrows*) and suturing them together. **C.** Alternative method of closure of the dorsal part of the defect using one end of the bucket-handle flap at a second operation (see text). (From Egyedi, ref. 1, with permission.)

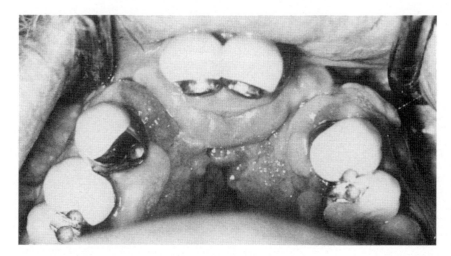

FIG. 2. Typical end result after stabilization of the premaxilla and closure of the residual cleft with the bucket-handle vestibular mucosal flap. The pedicles and the slight bulging immediately dorsal to the incisors can be seen clearly.

patients, superficial necrosis with loss of epithelium was seen; however, these patients had reepithelialization within a few weeks, and the desired closure in the alveolar area was invariably obtained. In three patients, the most distal part of the fistula of the anterior palate remained patent. In two patients, persistent fistulas were closed at a second operation because of subjective complaints. Significant bone loss in this area was observed in two of seven patients in whom bone was inserted. Total loss of the bone graft occurred in the patient in whom there was necrosis of the flap.

A significant disadvantage is the unavoidable reduction of the vestibulum oris, especially anterior to the premaxilla. Correction with a vestibuloplasty in a second operation is possible, or if indicated, an Abbé flap can be done.

Sometimes it is necessary to displace the premaxilla to get a satisfactory occlusion. In such instances, the bucket-handle flap, unlike two vestibular flaps, cannot be used in the same operation. In vestibular flaps, the soft-tissue pedicle to the premaxilla serves also as the blood supply; however, the difficulty of getting a proper nasal layer makes this combined operation rather risky anyway.

The pedicle of the bucket-handle flap sometimes presents an obstacle for construction of an anterior bridge; also, the pedicles may produce a sensation of restricted movement of the lip for the patient. In such instances, the pedicles should be divided at the height of the alveolar process and replaced in their original position.

In Y-shaped fistulas, the dorsal leg of the Y cannot, as a rule, be covered properly by the bucket-handle flap unless the leg is very short. In this instance, the bucket-handle flap can be provided with an extension to cover this part of the fistula also (Fig. 1A). If the latter procedure is not possible, one can secondarily dissect half the palatal part of the bucket-handle flap and swing it over to the dorsal leg of the Y (Fig. 1C), with the blood supply provided by the opposite part of the flap. Alternatively, one can try to obtain closure of this part of the gap by approximating two palatal flaps (Fig. 1B), but the results are often disappointing.

SUMMARY

The bucket-handle vestibular mucosal flap can be used to close small anterior palatal fistulas.

References

1. Egyedi P. The bucket-handle flap for closing fistulas around the premaxilla. *J Maxillofac Surg* 1976;4:212.
2. Burian F. *Chirurgie der Lippen- and Gaumenspalten.* Berlin: Verlag, 1963.
3. Guerrerosantos J, Altamirano JT. The use of lingual flaps in repair of fistulas of the hard palate. *Plast Reconstr Surg* 1966;38:123.
4. Perko M. Gleichzeitige Osteotomie des Zwischenkiefers, Restspaltenverschluss und Zwischenkieferversteifung durch sekundare Osteoplastik bei Spatfallen von beidseitigen Lippen-, Kiefer, and Gaumenspalten. *Dtsch Zahn Mund Kieferheilk* 1966;47:1.

CHAPTER 183 ■ PALATAL MUCOPERIOSTEAL ISLAND FLAP

P. J. GULLANE AND S. ARENA

EDITORIAL COMMENT

This procedure appears to provide adequate coverage in the adult after tumor resection or trauma. The editors believe it should not be used in the growing child because of possibly severe secondary effects on the dentition and palatal growth.

The palatal mucoperiosteal island flap serves to resurface defects of the soft palate, retromolar trigone, buccal region, tonsillar fossa, and posterior third of the floor of the mouth. Palatal flaps have been used for some time in palate-lengthening procedures, in closure of oroantral fistulas, and in resurfacing intraoral defects (1–7). The success of this flap depends on the external carotid system and an intact palate.

INDICATIONS

Soft Palate Reconstruction

This flap provides adequate local tissue to reconstruct the soft palate after tumor ablation. The periosteal surface that faces cephalically does not require coverage (see Fig. 2). Alternatively, two separate mucoperiosteal island flaps can be used and tailored to fit the defect (see Fig. 3).

Tonsil and Retromolar Trigone Defects

Ablation of cancer in the tonsillar and retromolar trigone areas frequently leaves a defect that is too small for a regional flap but is suitable for local flap reconstruction. Various reconstructive techniques include skin grafts and local tongue flaps. The palatal mucoperiosteal island flap provides adequate tissue, good reliability, and excellent healing, even when used over exposed bone.

Buccogingival Sulcus Relining

Many benign tumors and occasionally low-grade cancers (verrucous carcinoma) occur in the region of the buccogingival sulcus. Wide surgical extirpation leaves a defect that, if it is lined with a skin graft, leads to cheek contracture. The palatal flap with a "free up" procedure in the greater palatine foramen will provide adequate tissue coverage in a one-stage operation without the disadvantages inherent in the use of skin grafts.

The many advantages of the palatal mucoperiosteal island flap include a local source of tissue, a strong flap with good blood supply, excellent mobility (it can be positioned anywhere through an arc of 180 degrees), adequate bulk and length, a limited impairment of speech, and a success rate of 96%. These many advantages compensate for the relatively prolonged 2 to 3 months required for epithelialization of the donor site over the hard palate.

ANATOMY

The hard palate is composed of the premaxilla, maxilla, and palatine bones. The main mass of the hard palate is made up of the palatal processes of the maxilla, and posteriorly, the horizontal plate of the palatine bones completes the bony shelf. The greater palatine foramen lies between the palatine bone and the maxilla. The lesser palatine foramina perforate the palatine bone itself.

The mucous membrane of the anterior hard palate is strongly united with the periosteum, forming the mucoperiosteum, which can be readily stripped from the bone. The attachment of the periosteum to the bone is secured by multiple fibrous tissue pegs (Sharpey's fibers).

The blood supply to the hard palate is provided by the greater palatine artery, which emerges from the greater palatine foramen and courses anteriorly along the lateral margin of the palate to enter the incisive foramen. Venous drainage accompanies the artery back to the pterygoid plexus.

OPERATIVE TECHNIQUE

Approximately 85% of the soft tissue over the hard palate may be elevated on one greater palatine artery and rotated through 180 degrees to resurface an intraoral defect. The incisions are carried through the periosteum, and the opposite greater palatine artery is ligated. At the junction of the soft and hard palates, 0.5 to 1.0 cm of overlap should be provided to prevent a nasopalatine fistula (Fig. 1).

The vascular bundle then is carefully identified, and if further length to the pedicle is necessary, a greater palatine foramen "free up" procedure can be accomplished with a fine burr and a fracture of the hook of the hamulus. In freeing up the neurovascular bundle from its foramen by this maneuver, a further 1.0 cm of length can be provided to the flap. This flap now will provide 8 cm^2 of tissue. The palatal defect is left to epithelialize spontaneously. By 3 months, there is complete healing of the denuded donor site (Figs. 2 and 3).

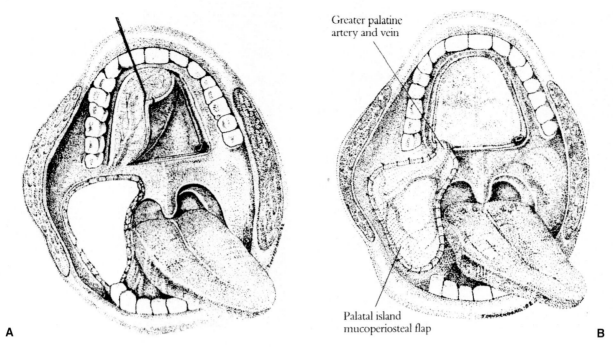

Greater palatine
artery and vein

Palatal island
mucoperiosteal flap

A

B

FIG. 1. A: Outline and elevation of mucoperiosteal island flap. B: Flap elevated and rotated through 180 degrees into the operative defect.

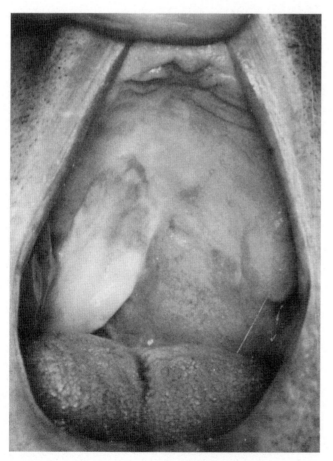

FIG. 2. Palatal flap reconstructs half the soft palate. Note the good epithelialization of the donor site.

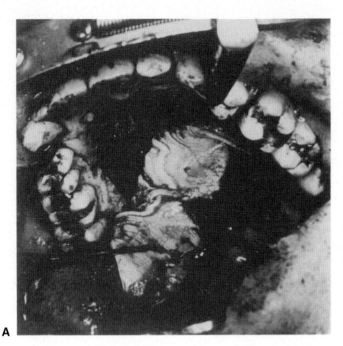

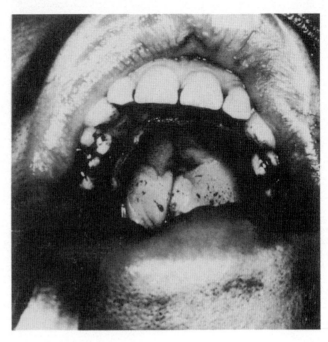

A   B

FIG. 3. **A:** Two separate mucoperiosteal island flaps used to reconstruct the total soft palate. **B:** Flaps sutured in position.

CLINICAL RESULTS

This flap has been used in 52 patients over an 8-year period. No fistulas of the palate have occurred; however, flap necrosis developed on two occasions. The high success rate is attributable to excellent blood supply and careful identification and preservation of the vascular pedicle. The greater palatine foramen "free-up" provides an extra 1.0 cm of length to the flap, but extreme caution should be exercised to prevent damage to the neurovascular bundle.

SUMMARY

The palatal mucoperiosteal island flap can be used to cover defects in the soft palate, the tonsil area, and the retromolar trigone regions as well as to provide lining for the buccogingival sulcus.

References

1. Millard DR. The island flap in cleft palate surgery. *Surg Gynecol Obstet* 1963;116:197.
2. Wilson JSP. The application of the two-centimeter pedicle flap in plastic surgery. *Br J Plast Surg* 1967;20:278.
3. Henderson D. Palatal island flap in closure of oroantral fistula. *Br J Oral Surg* 1974;12:141.
4. Herbert DC. Closure of a palatal fistula using mucoperiosteal island flap. *Br J Plast Surg* 1974;37:332.
5. Millard DR, Seider HA. The versatile palatal island flap: its use in soft palate reconstruction and nasopharyngeal and choanal atresia. *Br J Plast Surg* 1977;30:300.
6. Gullane PJ, Arena S. Palatal island flap for reconstruction of oral defects. *Arch Otolaryngol* 1977;103:598.
7. Montandon D, Lehmann W. An island palatal flap for velum reconstruction. *Chir Plast* 1980;5:257.

CHAPTER 184 ■ CERVICAL SKIN FLAP FOR INTRAORAL LINING

V. Y. BAKAMJIAN

Before the post-World War II era of advances in reconstructive surgery, most repairs after cancer surgery of the head and neck involved direct suturing of oral wound edges. Reconstruction was often postponed for an arbitrary 6 or 12 months to rule out recurring cancer before embarking on a protracted plan of reconstruction with flaps migrated from distant sites.

The next reconstructive advance—choosing cervical skin to replace losses of oral lining—seemed a natural choice (1–4). A skin flap could be outlined on the neck in either a transverse,

oblique, or vertically downward direction from a superolateral base below the mastoid process and angle of the mandible (Fig. 1A). This location was chosen for its proximity to oral sites as well as for the blood supply from branches of the external carotid artery.

In view of the limitations imposed on the use of cervical skin following radical neck dissection, however, it is not at all surprising that cervical neck flaps have been almost completely abandoned for intraoral lining in favor of later more versatile

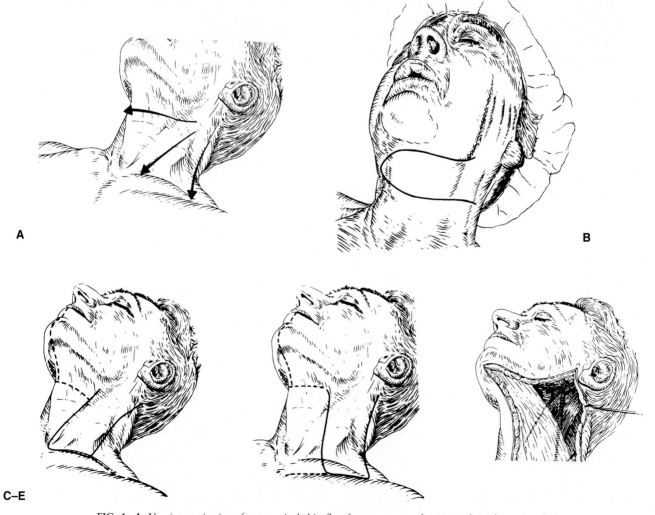

FIG. 1. A: Varying projections for a cervical skin flap from a more or less superolateral common base under the mastoid process and angle of the mandible. **B–E:** Varying incisional patterns that may provide good exposure for neck dissection simultaneously with the formation of a flap for intraoral lining. Absence of the layer of platysma muscle from the base area that is common for cervical flaps.

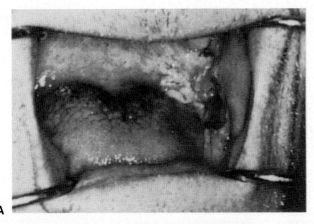
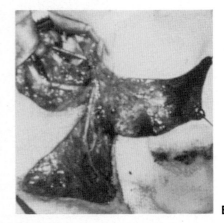

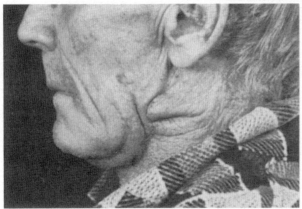
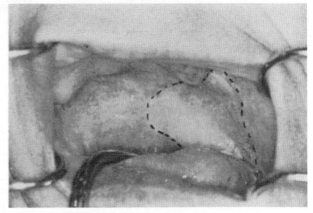

FIG. 2. An obsolete example of the oblique variant of cervical flap that could be used in male patients to obtain hairless supraclavicular skin, if it were available, for the intraoral defect. **A:** A faucial and soft palatine lesion. **B:** The raised flap and the defect viewed from below. **C:** The fistula of flap entry. **D:** Oral view of the reconstruction.

techniques that followed the introduction of deltopectoral (5,6), musculocutaneous (7,8), and free flaps (9,10).

INDICATIONS

Advantages of the cervical skin flap are (a) proximity for direct transfer to intraoral common defects, (b) thinness and pliability of the flap, (c) better than average random-pattern vascularity than in skin on the torso or extremities, and (d) the laxity of aging cervical skin from which it is convenient to borrow flap material. In the form described herein, it is capable of lining moderate-sized oral defects fairly well, leaving only an inconspicuous linear scar on the neck.

If a cervical flap is to be used, it is important that this option not be destroyed by the routine incisions habitually employed for radical neck dissection (5). Instead, by accurately anticipating reconstructive requirements before the recipient defect is created by resection, the surgeon should tailor neck incisions for each patient to meet the requirements for the formation of an appropriate flap for reconstruction.

FLAP DESIGN AND DIMENSIONS

Generally, only the transverse variant of the flap for use in elderly female patients remains a practical option (Fig. 1B).

This is only possible with no more than a supraomohyoid neck dissection. In this form, the flap is outlined so that its maximal width permits direct closure of the donor wound. The safe length of the flap may be to the anterior border of the contralateral sternocleidomastoid muscle.

OPERATIVE TECHNIQUE

Raising the flap may or may not include the thin platysma layer of muscle with the skin, as the surgeon chooses. Either choice cannot significantly influence the success or failure of the flap because the platysma does not extend to the base area of the flap over the upper third of the sternocleidomastoid muscle (Fig. 1D).

Depending on the location of the recipient defect, the flap will pass to its destination either buccally or lingually in relation to the mandible through a portal generally in the vicinity of its angle (Figs. 2 and 3). The passage is treated with the caution that is usual for avoiding injury to the marginal mandibular branch of the facial nerve. After the flap is sutured distally into the defect, its basilar segment within the short tunnel is entubed, skin side inward, forming a skin-lined fistula, and the donor neck wound is closed by direct suturing of its edges. A minor second-stage procedure some 2 to 3 weeks later will divide the pedicle and close the fistula.

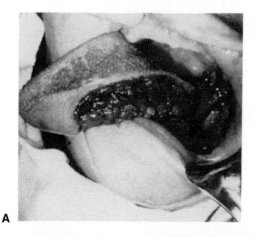
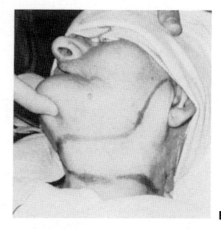

A

B

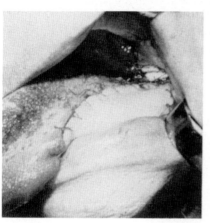
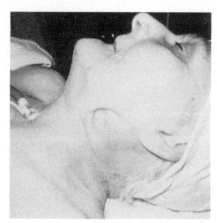
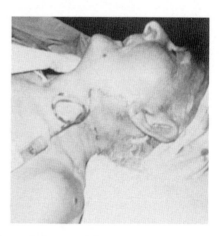

C–E

FIG. 3. A bilobed version of the transverse cervical flap to a glossal and glossopalatine area defect. A: The defect. B: Outline of the flap. C: Intraoral view of the repair. D: The fistula. E: Division of the pedicle and closure of the fistula.

CLINICAL RESULTS

In an early series of 20 patients in whom a cervical skin flap was used for intraoral lining, 18 had had radical neck dissection and two had had supraomohyoid neck dissection. Four of the 20 flaps failed, all the failures occurring in patients with radical neck dissection and with flaps of an oblique or vertically downward orientation.

SUMMARY

Cervical skin flaps once were used extensively for intraoral lining. They recently were supplanted by the more versatile and reliable techniques introduced by deltopectoral, musculocutaneous, and free flaps. The transverse cervical flap still has some value for the elderly female patient in whom node dissection is limited to the supraomohyoid area.

References

1. Edgerton MT. Replacement of lining to oral cavity following surgery. *Cancer* 1951;4:110.
2. Edgerton MT, DesPrez JD. Reconstruction of the oral cavity in the treatment of cancer. *Plast Reconstr Surg* 1957;19:89.
3. DesPrez JD, Kiehn CL. Methods of reconstruction of anterior oral cavity and mandible malignancy. *Plast Reconstr Surg* 1959;24:238.
4. Bakamjian VY, Littlewood M. Cervical skin flaps for intraoral and pharyngeal repair following cancer surgery. *Br J Plast Surg* 1964;17:191.
5. Bakamjian VY, Marshall D. Plastic and reconstructive considerations in selecting incisions used for radical neck dissection. *Aust N Z J Surg* 1967;36:184.
6. Bakamjian VY. The reconstructive use of flaps in cancer surgery of the head and neck. In: Saad MN, Lichtveld P, eds. *Reviews in plastic surgery: general plastic and reconstructive surgery.* Amsterdam: Excerpta Medica, 1974.
7. Brown RG, Fleming WH, Jurkiewicz MJ. An island flap of the pectoralis major muscle. *Br J Plast Surg* 1977;30:161.
8. Ariyan S. The pectoralis major myocutaneous flap: a versatile flap for reconstruction in the head and neck. *Plast Reconstr Surg* 1979;63:73.
9. Daniel RK, Taylor GI. Distant transfer of an island flap by microvascular anastomosis. *Plast Reconstr Surg* 1973;52:111.
10. Harii K, Ohmori K, Ohmori S. Hair transplantation with free scalp flaps. *Plast Reconstr Surg* 1974;53:410.

CHAPTER 185 ■ SUBMENTAL SKIN FLAP FOR INTRAORAL LINING

M. SOUSSALINE

A submental skin flap for the reconstruction of mucosal cheek defects after cancer resection is described (1–3). Mucosal cheek defects up to 6 × 6 cm with overlying intact cheek skin can be closed with this flap.

small T1–T2 cheek cancers, where the cheek skin is in good condition, are most satisfactory. Radiation therapy to the submental skin is a contraindication to the use of this flap.

INDICATIONS

Women with an excess of skin in the submental area yield the best results. The quality and flexibility of the skin are quite close to those of the mucosa. Male bearded skin is less desirable. Reconstructions following the primary resection of

ANATOMY

The flap includes the underlying muscular fascia. Blood supply is from the anterior and inferior branches of the facial artery, and venous drainage is provided by the anterior jugular vein, which must be preserved. The dissection is started at the distal end of the flap to preserve venous drainage.

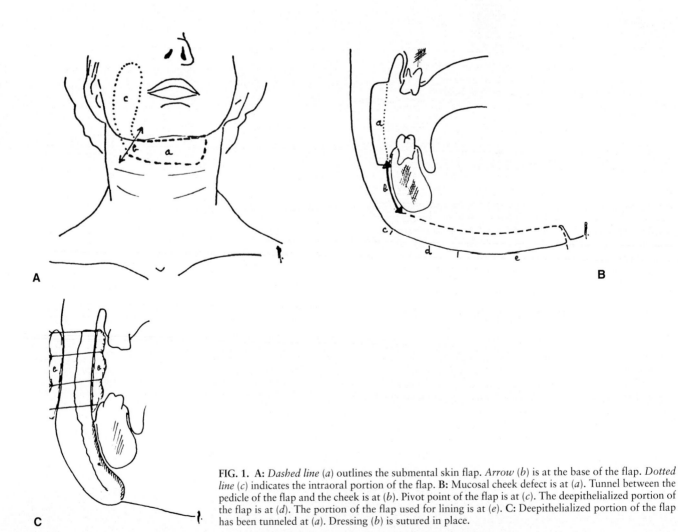

FIG. 1. **A:** *Dashed line* (a) outlines the submental skin flap. *Arrow* (b) is at the base of the flap. *Dotted line* (c) indicates the intraoral portion of the flap. **B:** Mucosal cheek defect is at (a). Tunnel between the pedicle of the flap and the cheek is at (b). Pivot point of the flap is at (c). The deepithelialized portion of the flap is at (d). The portion of the flap used for lining is at (e). **C:** Deepithelialized portion of the flap has been tunneled at (a). Dressing (b) is sutured in place.

FLAP DESIGN AND DIMENSIONS

This flap is based on a 6- to 7-cm-wide pedicle in the submental region. The flap is 10 to 12 cm long, and its long axis is horizontal. The posterior side of the flap lies in the fold between the submental anterior cervical areas (Fig. 1A).

OPERATIVE TECHNIQUE

After the flap is raised, a tunnel is made along the buccal surface of the lateral anterior mandible to reach the buccal sulcus and the inferior margin of the cheek resection. The flap then is turned into the mouth (Fig. 1B). The tunneled portion of the flap is deepithelialized, and the flap is then sutured to the mucosal defect with 3–0 nylon.

The flap donor area is closed by approximation of the wound edges. A dressing to provide soft compression on the flap is sutured in place (Fig. 1C). The dressing is removed after 5 days. A feeding tube is used until healing has taken place.

CLINICAL RESULTS

I have used this technique in three patients with good results. There has been no flap necrosis, and healing was complete in 3 weeks. The cosmetic result at the flap donor site was acceptable.

SUMMARY

The submental skin flap can be used in one stage for intraoral lining of cheek defects.

References

1. Hadjistamoff B. Restoration of cheek by using the skin of the jaw-neck region. *Plast Reconstr Surg* 1947;2:127.
2. De Cholnoky T. Cheek repair of extensive soft-tissue losses. *Plant Reconstr Surg* 1955;16:288.
3. Soussaline M, Senechal G, Cachin M, et al. *La chirurgie reparatrice en carcinologie cervico-faciale.* Paris: Ste. Franc ORL et path cervico-faciale, 1977.

CHAPTER 186 ■ ANTERIOR CERVICAL AND LATERAL CERVICAL APRON SKIN FLAPS

B. W. EDGERTON

EDITORIAL COMMENT

This clever way of obtaining thin skin to resurface the floor of the mouth has the disadvantage that it cannot be used in postradiation neck dissections, particularly if the carotid vessels are exposed. The temporary fistula would be a serious disadvantage if radiation were contemplated postoperatively. The fistula can be avoided (see text). The author continues to believe that the safest and simplest techniques should be used when the results are comparable; regional flaps do sometimes get neglected.

Following World War II, the need for a method of immediate reconstruction of the lining of the oral cavity following surgical resection of large malignant tumors stimulated the design of a variety of new pedicle skin flaps about the head and neck (1–3). One of the most useful of these new regional flaps proved to be the cervical apron flap. Even in the 1990s this method offers certain advantages over the use of free flaps in cancer reconstruction.

INDICATIONS

The reconstruction of large lining defects in the oral cavity continues to be one of the (if not the most) important features in satisfactory functional rehabilitation of speech, eating, and appearance after the removal of large cancers of the head and neck. Resected lining of the oropharynx may be satisfactorily replaced by free skin grafts, but if good functional results are to be expected following resections of the anterior cavity, with or without removal of the symphysis of the mandible, a pedicle flap must be used. Bilateral nasolabial fold flaps will provide lining for the oral cavity in modest amounts (up to 2 inches), but usually the defects following adequate cancer resections are too large. The surgeon should consider the use of an apron cervical pedicle flap.

There are several advantages to the use of this particular flap in the treatment of oral cavity malignancy. The flap allows transfer of non-hair-bearing skin from the anterior or lateral neck region into the oral cavity by means of a transverse superior pedicle that is based along the lower border of the mandible. This apron of skin is used to provide needed lining for the floor of the mouth or the alveolar and buccal

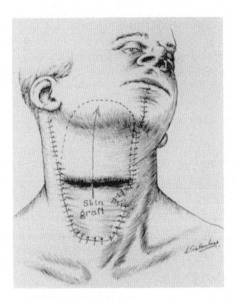

FIG. 1. In the first stage, a primary cancer of the right floor of the mouth was removed in continuity with a right radical neck dissection. The contents of the deep neck were exposed by the design and shape of the apron flap. The lower part of this flap, or the "apron," must be raised from a part of the neck below the hairline in men. In most instances, the chin and lower lip-splitting incision used here for exposure is unnecessary. I currently extend this medial incision at the hyoid level toward the mastoid process on the contralateral side. A deliberate dart is created along the anterior border of the skin graft to avoid any later linear contracture.

regions. It also will serve to replace resected tongue or to line the lower lip.

Elevation of the flap exposes the underlying deep contents of the neck, thus facilitating neck dissection and the removal of cervical lymph nodes that so often accompany the surgical excision of squamous cancer of the oral cavity. The apron cervical flap may be elevated, folded, and transferred at the time of tumor resection without prior delay procedures. It may be transferred, along with closure of the orocutaneous fistula, as a one-step procedure if desired (4).

I have continued to find the apron flap to be the most reliable and dependable "workhorse" for anterior oral cavity lining reconstruction. This flap also has proved to be of significant value in the repair of certain congenital defects, such as aglossia-adactylia, and in the repair of gunshot wounds with major losses of the floor of the mouth and mandible.

ANATOMY

The circulation to the flap is highly reliable in the absence of preoperative intensive radiation therapy to that portion of the neck. The blood supply of this flap is so vigorous that it has proved to be one of the few regional flaps in the head and neck region that will support an immediate free bone graft to a defect in the mandible—providing a high probability of bone graft osteosynthesis. Pedicle flaps of less vigor, such as those from the chest or shoulders, often are associated with slow bone graft absorption when used to cover an immediate bone graft. Although this is treated as a random pedicle flap, it does in fact receive descending branches from the labial vessels and from vessels reaching the flap from each lower cheek region.

In most instances, the flap is elevated so that it includes the platysma muscle underlying the entire apron flap. This muscle

provides a vigorous layer of blood vessels to nourish the flap, analogous to the additional circulation provided through the deep fascia in modern fasciocutaneous flaps.

FLAP DESIGN AND DIMENSIONS

This flap must be planned from the outset of treatment because it is not possible to use it once a neck dissection has been performed through the usual neck incisions. It is a flap that should be used with caution even in a nonoperated neck if that patient's neck has been exposed to a heavy dose of preoperative radiation.

Certain anatomic points need to be considered in the design and planning of an apron cervical flap. In female patients, the absence of hair-bearing skin in the neck gives one the latitude to design the flap so that the apron lies at a somewhat higher level on the neck than in male patients. With men, that portion of the flap destined for permanent intraoral replacement should be marked carefully to lie inferior to the normal beard line in the lower neck (Figs. 1 and 2). The width of the expected lining defect within the oral cavity should be estimated carefully. The width of the apron part of the flap need not exceed that measurement.

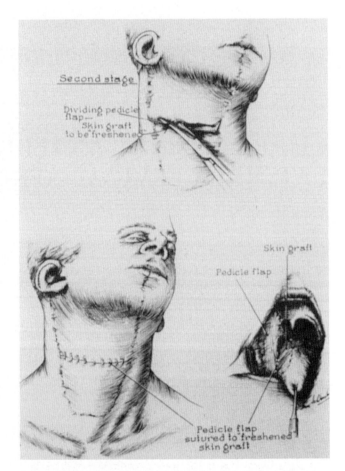

FIG. 2. The second stage is carried out 3 to 4 weeks later. The upper margin of the previous skin graft is slightly elevated and sutured to the divided margin of the skin flap just above. The non-hair-bearing portion of the apron flap then is drawn into the oral cavity and fitted to the remaining defect, with the excess being trimmed. When desired, a portion of this flap can be carried across the floor of the mouth and used to replace tongue that may have been resected with the primary tumor.

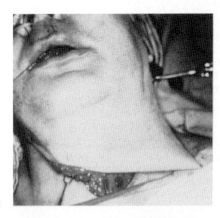
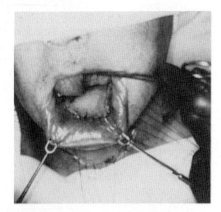
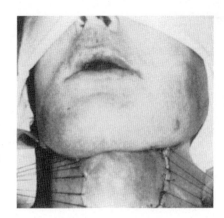

A–C

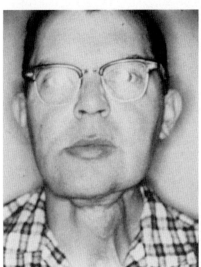
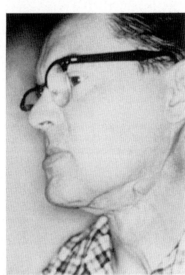

D,E

FIG. 3. A: This patient had a large cancer of the floor of the mouth penetrating the lingual cortex of the mandible. A single 1.5-cm-diameter lymph node in the left carotid triangle was positive for squamous cell carcinoma. At the outset of stage 1, the incision shown was used to elevate a large apron flap from the lower left neck region with a wide pedicle extending from one mastoid tip to the other. (The incision for this flap must be planned before the neck dissection is undertaken.) The platysma muscle is lifted with the skin flap. The tumor then was removed in continuity with a complete left neck dissection and a supraomohyoid neck dissection on the right side. The involved mandible was resected with the specimen over a 12-cm-wide central area. The floor of the mouth and a small portion of the anterior tongue were included for good tumor margin. B: The mandible has been replaced with an iliac bone graft and small transosseous steel bar. The apron flap has been folded about the bone graft and may be seen with its margin sutured to the remaining mucosa on the deep surface of the lower lip. The tongue thus remains free for the important functions of talking and eating. C: At the end of the first stage, the patient's mandible has been satisfactorily reconstructed. A narrow fistula extends from the neck up into the oral cavity along the pedicle of the flap and is left for several weeks until stage 2 is performed. D,E: The postoperative appearance of the patient following the second stage of the apron flap procedure. At that operation, the pedicle of the flap was divided and its intraoral portion was attached to the underside of the tongue tip. The neck fistula then was closed by suturing the skin in the left submaxillary region to the upper margin of the previously applied skin graft. At 11 years after surgery, there was no recurrence of the squamous cell carcinoma. (A, B, and C from Edgerton, DesPrez, ref. 4, pp. 100–101, with permission.)

There is essentially no limit to the width of this flap. The pedicle will easily carry sufficient non-hair-bearing skin from the lower neck to replace the entire width of the anterior oral cavity. I have moved flaps with aprons up to 14 cm wide and 10 cm long. It is unusual to require this much flap tissue for oral cavity repair.

OPERATIVE TECHNIQUE

After designing the flap to meet width requirements for the lining defect within the oral cavity, the incisions in the neck above the apron are allowed to widen out toward the tip of the mastoid process on the ipsilateral side and laterally toward the angle of the mandible on the contralateral side of the neck. This gives an extremely wide pedicle that receives circulation from both sides of the skin of the upper neck (Fig. 3A). The platysma muscle is usually left on the deep surface of the apron flap and elevated with the skin and subcutaneous tissue.

The facial artery and vein may be sacrificed on both sides of the neck at the lower border of the mandible along with the removal of the tumor without serious jeopardy to the blood supply of this flap. When one reaches the level of the cervical branch of each facial nerve to the lower lip, that nerve is identified and lifted upward with the pedicle, thus preserving good lower lip function bilaterally.

The elevated flap then is reflected upward onto the patient's face. The neck dissection is carried out on one or both sides of the neck along with the indicated removal of mandible, floor of mouth, and a margin of normal oral cavity mucosa around the tumor. When a segment of the mandible has been resected, a bone graft from the iliac crest is fashioned and fit to the defect. A small steel bar below the bone graft provides additional fixation by wiring to the mandibular fragments (bone and bar technique).

The apron then is folded inward and around the lower border of the bone graft and bar so that the skin from the lowest margin of the apron flap is brought up into the oral cavity (Fig. 3B). This edge is sutured to the remaining mucosa on the deep surface of the lower lip at the anterior border of the mucosal defect created by resection of the cancer. The lap thus surrounds the bone graft, covering its anterior, inferior, and posterior surfaces. The lower neck is closed with a split-thickness skin graft so that a deliberate fistula is left leading from the oral cavity outward along the pedicle of the apron flap to the surface of the neck (Fig. 3C). The orocutaneous fistula is closed at a second operation 3 to 4 weeks later (Fig. 3D). It is of interest that very few mechanical problems are experienced by the patient during the 4-week interval, and minimal salivary discharge occurs through the fistula. This is important because many patients also will have a tracheostomy during that period.

Variations in Operative Techniques

The cervical apron flap may be transferred along with closure of the orocutaneous fistula as a one-step procedure, if desired, by removing the epidermis over that portion of the pedicle that transverses the submaxillary and submental spaces of the neck (4). This method will leave a permanent blood-bearing pedicle supplying the apron portion of the flap that constitutes the new lining of the oral cavity. The donor site in the lower neck causes minimal deformity and may be closed either by a simple split-thickness skin graft or by rotation of an adjacent regional flap.

I have used the cervical apron flap as a one-stage island flap technique by removing the epidermis of the folded pedicle and closing the cervical skin and fistula at the primary operation. There are two disadvantages to this one-stage method: (a) unless the tongue remnant is mobile, the approximation of the lining portion of the flap to the posterior part of the oral cavity defect (usually along the residual resected body of the tongue) is more difficult and less ideal; and (b) the closure of the neck incision is likely to be dimpled or puckered at the point of the pedicle. For these reasons, I usually carry out the apron flap as a two-stage technique.

At times, the skin of the lower lip or chin may be involved in a malignant process that also extends into the oral cavity. When this is the case, the apron flap technique still may be used, but it is designed as a double-pedicle flap. The involved skin of the chin and lip is resected, but a pedicle base is left on either side of the chin defect. Each lateral pedicle may extend to the lobe of the ear. These two lateral pedicles appear to be quite adequate to allow an apron of skin from the lower neck to be brought upward and folded in a similar fashion to the standard cervical apron flap. The central upper border of the flap is advanced up into the chin and lip area to close the defect in that region. The apron then is turned under the reconstructed mandible to line the cavity in the fashion described above.

In a few instances, I have included a segment of the clavicle in the soft tissue beneath the apron of the flap, using this as a bone graft for the mandible. Because free bone grafts do well when placed within the standard apron flap, it is difficult to know whether inclusion of the clavicle adds significantly to the technique (5). The blood supply that this segment of clavicle receives from the undersurface of the apron flap must be relatively small, but the bone ends do bleed modestly at the time of transfer.

CLINICAL RESULTS

The vigorous blood supply to the cervical apron flap has made flap necrosis an uncommon occurrence. In approximately 3%

of the elevated flaps, some degree of full-thickness necrosis occurs postoperatively along the lining portion of the apron flap. In most instances, these are small areas of demarcation along the sutured edges of the flap only a few millimeters in width. In no instance have I experienced a major loss of a flap requiring an additional flap from another source.

Vilray Blair et al. (6) pointed out years ago that the blood supply about the head and neck of males, even those of advanced age, was so satisfactory that age was little or no contraindication to the design and transfer of flaps in that region. I have found this to be the case. The exception occurs in elderly men who also are severely malnourished or dehydrated. Appropriate preoperative nutrition and hydration are, of course, essential for consistent flap success. Women have more delicate circulation to the skin of the head and neck. This must be taken into consideration in planning their cervical apron flaps. In a few instances, the vertical straight-line portions of residual scar in the apron donor site of the lower neck required later Z-plasty. This problem can be avoided by appropriate design of the skin graft (including triangular darts) used to replace the apron of skin (see Fig. 1).

In one instance, the apron flap separated completely from its line of attachment to the inner surface of the lower lip 8 days following surgery. The underlying large bone graft to the mandible was exposed. To my surprise, conservative management over a period of 8 weeks produced spontaneous healing within the oral cavity and a successful take of the bone graft. The skin pedicle to the apron flap was not divided until this healing was complete.

SUMMARY

The anterior and lateral cervical apron flap technique is a reliable method of immediate reconstruction of large defects of the anterior oral cavity. The proximity of this tissue to the oral cavity and the vigorous blood supply of the tissue make it the most reliable of all of the regional flaps for reconstruction of this part of the body. It may be combined with immediate bone grafting of the mandible (bone and bar technique). Although today the use of a free flap may be considered an alternative reconstructive technique for these defects, the added operative time and greater risk of circulatory failure make this a somewhat dubious choice. The apron flap should be considered whenever there has been no prior major neck surgery or irradiation.

References

1. Brown JB. Rehabilitation of patients with head and neck tumors. In: *Symposium on cancer of the head and neck.* Chicago: American Cancer Society, 1957;263.
2. Edgerton MT, McKee DM. Reconstruction with loss of the hyomandibular complex in excision of large cancer. *Arch Surg* 1959;78:425.
3. Ward G, Edgerton MT. Recent improvements in resection of the maxilla. *Am J Surg* 1950.
4. Edgerton MT, DesPrez JD. Reconstruction of the oral cavity in the treatment of cancer. *Plast Reconstr Surg* 1957;19:89.
5. Davis JS. *Plastic surgery.* Philadelphia: Blakiston, 1919;504.
6. Blair VP, Moore S, Byars LT. *Cancer of the face and mouth.* St. Louis: Mosby, 1941.

CHAPTER 187 ■ OMENTAL FLAP FOR CHEEK, NECK, AND INTRAORAL RECONSTRUCTION

S. K. DAS AND M. A. LESAVOY

The good vascularity, unique arrangement of blood vessels, and ability to accept skin grafts with ease allow the omentum, which is dispensable, to be an excellent salvage flap.

INDICATIONS

Typical indications for use of the omentum are (a) to protect the exposed, irradiated carotid vessels following block dissection of the neck as well as to prevent carotid blowout (1) (see Chapter 137); (b) to reconstruct the pharyngostome; (c) to reconstruct full-thickness cheek defects (2); (d) to contour the face, and (e) to use as cover for the face with the addition of split-thickness skin grafting following massive tissue loss (3,4).

ANATOMY

See Chapter 137.

FLAP DESIGN AND DIMENSIONS

For pedicle transfer of the omentum from within the abdominal cavity to distal targets, such as the neck or face, various lengthening procedures are mandatory (5–8). Following omentocololysis (6), there is a gain in omental length of 2 to 12 cm. For the omentum to reach the neck, however, omentogastrolysis (freeing of the omentum from the greater curvature of the stomach, based on a right or left gastroepiploic pedicle) is necessary. Usually, the right gastroepiploic vessels are larger than the left, and at least one other major artery should be preserved and left attached to the stomach. The gastroepiploic arch is maintained with the omentum (Fig. 1).

It is now possible to mobilize the omentum superiorly to the root of the neck in 88% of patients and to the ear in 79% of patients. If the omentum does not reach the target area of the neck or face after this stage, it is almost certain that a definitive omental lengthening is needed.

Planning the incisions (5,6) for elongation of the omentum and preserving the continuity of the vascular arcades will allow the omentum to reach to the vault of the skull. The only deficiency in lengthening the omentum for distal target areas is the reduction in the quantity of omentum available for use. Thus, when the quantity of the omentum limits the lengthening procedure, transfer of the omentum by microvascular anastomoses is appropriate, provided healthy recipient vessels are available. This will allow a large piece of the omentum to be transferred to distal areas without losing bulk.

OPERATIVE TECHNIQUE

For pedicle transfer of the omentum from the abdomen to the face or neck, the best route is subcutaneous. After the omentum is harvested and lengthened, it is brought out of the abdomen through the upper end of the laparotomy wound and tunneled subcutaneously along the presternal area to the target area over the neck or face. Care should be taken to make the tunnel big enough that the pedicle of the omentum is not strangulated (Fig. 2).

CLINICAL RESULTS

The success rate with omental flaps, both on a pedicle and with microvascular free transfer, in reconstructing difficult defects over face, neck and head, is extremely high. An interesting reported finding is that overall increase in body weight is reflected in the transplanted omentum. Because of the size of the donor and recipient vessels in vascularized omental transfer (1.5 mm and greater), the procedure is not difficult. Any complications related to this procedure are due mostly to omental harvesting.

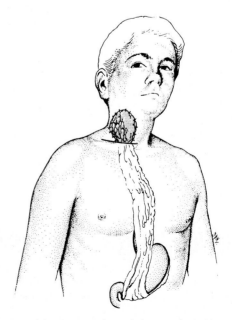

FIG. 1. Route of the omentum for pedicle transplantation to the neck through a subcutaneous tunnel. (From Das, ref. 6, with permission.)

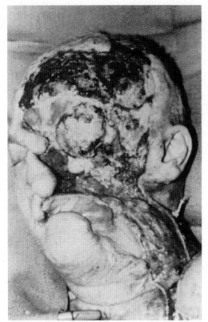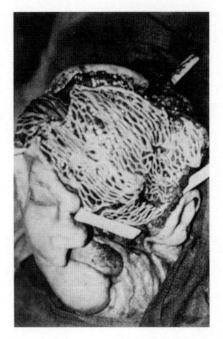

A,B

FIG. 2. A: Craniofacial area before reconstruction with omentum. Massive craniofacial resection of left frontal bone, orbit, globe, maxilla, left half of the mandible, and left radical neck dissection. Pectoralis major, latissimus dorsi, multiple random, scalp, and other flaps had failed. The patient originally had a carcinoma of the maxillary antrum and had refused surgery. B: Omentum in place over the scalp and face. The right gastroepiploic vessels were anastomosed to the contralateral right facial vessels, so that the omentum could span the skull to arrive at left side of the face. Ipsilateral recipient vessels were nonexistent. The omentum was covered with a meshed split-thickness skin graft. The omentum and graft did well, and later the unit was elevated without compromise to drain a brain abscess.

SUMMARY

The omentum, either pedicled or as a free-tissue transfer, is an excellent salvage flap for defects of the head and neck.

References

1. Goldsmith HS, Beattie EJ. Carotid artery protection by pedicled omental wrapping. *Surg Gynecol Obstet* 1970;130:57.
2. Harashina T, Imai T, Wada M. The omental sandwich reconstruction for full-thickness cheek defect. *Plast Reconstr Surg* 1979;64:411.
3. Arnold PG, Irons GB. One stage reconstruction of massive craniofacial defect with gastroomental free flap. *Ann Plast Surg* 1981;6:26.
4. Brown RG, Nahai F, Silverton JA. The omentum in facial reconstruction. *Br J Plast Surg* 1978;31:58.
5. Alday ES, Goldsmith HS. Surgical technique for omental lengthening based on arterial anatomy. *Surg Gynecol Obstet* 1972;135:103.
6. Das SK. The size of the human omentum and methods of lengthening it for transplantation. *Br J Plast Surg* 1976;29:170.
7. Das SK. Use of the omentum in reconstructive surgery. In: Barron J, Saad MN, eds. *Operative manual of plastic and reconstructive surgery.* Edinburgh: Churchill-Livingstone, 1980; Chap. 5.
8. Das SK. Assessment of the size of the human omentum. *Acta Anat (Basel)* 1981;110:108.

CHAPTER 188 ■ CERVICAL MUSCULOCUTANEOUS FLAP FOR INTRAORAL LINING

H. SAITO

EDITORIAL COMMENT

In effect, this is a variation of the platysmal myocutaneous flap. Because the blood supply to the platysma usually comes from branches along the facial artery, the flap must be designed in order not to jeopardize the blood supply.

The lateral and median cervical skin flap (1), a modified version of previously reported methods (2,3), is suitable for a reconstruction of intraoral defects smaller than 6 × 6 cm.

INDICATIONS

The lateral cervical musculocutaneous flap is used for reconstruction of lateral defects in the mouth and pharynx (Fig. 1).

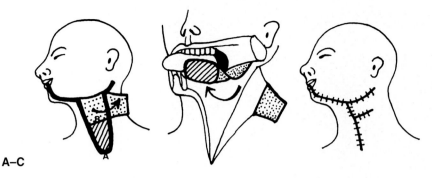

A–C

FIG. 1. Schematic drawing of the lateral cervical musculocutaneous flap. **A:** To make the subcutaneous tissue–platysma muscle pedicle of this flap, a laterally based epidermal–dermal flap was raised and turned back on itself (*arrow*). The thick line indicates the incision line of the vertical lateral cervical flap. **B:** The flap is rotated as the arrow indicates and sutured to the mucosal defect. **C:** Final external appearance. (From Saito et al., ref. 1, with permission.)

The median cervical musculocutaneous flap is used for reconstruction of the anterior median floor of the mouth (Fig. 2).

FLAP DESIGN AND DIMENSIONS

For the lateral cervical musculocutaneous flap, a vertical rectangular flap, usually 6 × 5 cm, is outlined on the lateral neck and is designed to be large enough to cover the defect. The tip can extend to just above the clavicle. The location of the base is usually 2 cm below the posterior half of the mandible and is 8 cm wide.

The procedure for the median cervical musculocutaneous flap is essentially the same as for the lateral flap, except the pedicle is based on the median submental region and is about 7 cm wide.

OPERATIVE TECHNIQUE

The subcutaneous tissue–platysma muscle pedicle of both the lateral and median cervical musculocutaneous flaps is developed on the bearded portion of the flap, adjacent to its base. This is done by first raising a laterally based epidermal–dermal rectangular skin flap, which is temporarily turned back on itself, until it can be used at the end of the operation to close the upper neck wound (see Figs. 1 and 2). Then the lateral or median cervical flap can be raised to include the platysma muscle. Intravenous fluorescein is used to assess the viability of the flap.

The lateral flap is used to cover the intraoral defect and can be turned upward to the tonsillar region or half rotated and extended horizontally to the region of the tongue and oral floor. The flap is sutured in place and usually fixed with a tie-over

dressing. The neck is easily closed by using all or part of the laterally based epidermal–dermal skin flap and by advancing the anterior and posterior neck skin.

The median flap is sutured into the anteromedian floor of the mouth after the appropriate neck dissection. Excision of the lower lip should be avoided, and suspension of the hyoid bone is unnecessary (Fig. 3).

CLINICAL RESULTS

Lateral cervical musculocutaneous flaps were used in 37 patients and the median flap was used in three. The primary tumors involved the floor of the mouth, tongue, tonsil, gingiva, buccal mucosa, root of the tongue, and mandible. All but three of the tumors were squamous cell carcinomas. Either conservative or radical neck dissections were performed on one or both sides in 36 of 40 patients. Mandibular resection, marginal or sectional, was used in 16 patients. Combination therapy with radiation was carried out in 28 patients.

The flap survived without complications in 38 of 40 patients (95%). One patient who received a preoperative full dose of radiation for gingival cancer had an oral fistula that was, however, easily repaired by fistulectomy. Another patient with carcinoma of the oral floor developed a fistula that healed spontaneously. Preoperative radiation of less than 3,000 rads and postoperative full-dose radiation did not interfere with wound healing. The intraoral tissue looked like skin (histologically, dermis) in 112 patients and like mucous membrane (histologically, connective tissue or scar) in 28 patients.

The epidermal–dermal flap used to close the donor site became necrotic in a few patients; however, enough connective tissue to protect the carotid artery survived. When the neck wound could be closed easily by advancing the skin, the epidermal–dermal flap was excised.

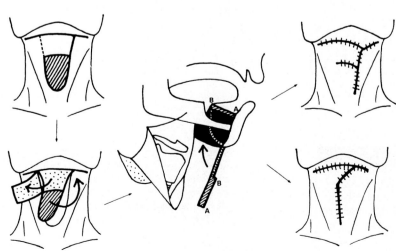

A–C

FIG. 2. Schematic drawing of the median cervical musculocutaneous flap. **A:** Incision lines. **B:** The flap and laterally based epidermal–dermal flap. **C:** The flap (*AB*) is rotated into the floor of the mouth as the arrow indicates and sutured into the defect. **D:** Final external appearance. (From Saito et al., ref. 1, with permission.)

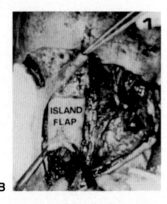
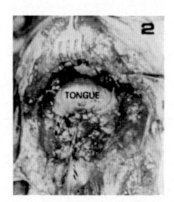
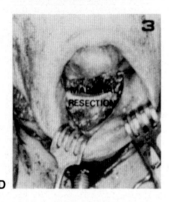
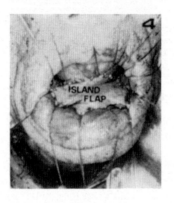

A,B

C,D

FIG. 3. **A:** The median cervical musculocutaneous flap prepared. The forceps hold the end of the epidermal–dermal flap. **B:** The tongue is seen through the defect left after resection of the floor of the mouth. **C:** Marginal resection of the mandible. **D:** Reconstructed floor of the mouth. A tie-over dressing is usually employed.

SUMMARY

A median or lateral cervical musculocutaneous flap can be used to cover many of the smaller (up to 6 × 6 cm) intraoral defects.

References

1. Saito H, Nishimura H, Matsui T, et al. Primary reconstruction by modified cervical island skin flap following resection of oral and pharyngeal cancer. *Arch Otorhinolaryngol* 1978;221:203.
2. DesPrez JD, Kiehn CD. Methods of reconstruction following resection of anterior oral cavity and mandible for malignancy. *Plast Reconstr Surg* 1959;24:238.
3. Farr HW, Jean-Gillies B, Die A. Cervical island skin flap repair of oral and pharyngeal defects in the composite operation for cancer. *Am J Surg* 1969;118:759.

CHAPTER 189 ■ BUCCINATOR MYOMUCOSAL ISLAND PEDICLE FLAP

D. J. HURWITZ

Complex anatomy and confined space make closure of large intraoral wounds and oronasal fistulae a formidable undertaking. To solve the problems of distant donor sites, multistaged procedures, and the sequelae of failed cleft-palate repairs, a well-vascularized, single-staged, buccal mucosal flap was developed (1–6).

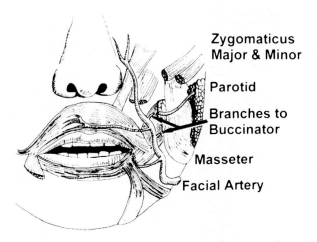

FIG. 1. Diagrammatic frontal composite view of anatomy relevant to the buccinator muscle and facial artery.

INDICATIONS

The anteriorly based buccinator mucosal island flap (BMIF) yields up to a 5 × 7-cm patch of oral mucosa and muscle that can reach most regions of the oral cavity with minimal donor-site morbidity. Bilateral flaps can reconstruct both nasal and oral surfaces.

ANATOMY[1]

The buccinator muscle joins the orbicularis oris sphincteric complex. The deepest muscle of facial expression, it forms a quadralateral canopy from maxillary to mandibular alveoli, and from oral commissure to pterygomandibular raphe. The buccinator forces food against the teeth during chewing and permits forceful blowing of air through the lips.

The muscle is innervated by the buccal branch of the facial nerve, which crosses the masseter along the parotid duct, branches to the superficial surface of the muscle, and continues through the buccal fat pad to innervated medial upper lip musculature, The buccal branch of the mandibular division of the trigeminal nerve provides sensation to mucosa via a deeper traverse across the medial pterygoid muscle.

The buccal fat pad separates the buccinator from the masseter. Beyond the anterior border of the masseter, the buccomasseteric fascia covers the fat pad. The parotid duct crosses the masseter, enters the buccal fat pad, and then perforates the superior midportion of the buccinator to empty into the oral cavity. The deep surface of the buccinator is adherent to mucosa. If approached through a nasolabial incision, the buccinator lies immediately lateral to the orbicularis oris muscle. It is deep to the orbicular, the zygomaticus major, and levator anguli oris muscles (Fig. 1). The surgeon also encounters the masseter muscle, buccal fat pad, and buccomasseteric fascia. Between the buccomasseteric fascia and the buccinator are an areolar connective tissue plane and fat pad that facilitate blunt separation of the muscle.

The facial artery forms the blood supply of the BMIF (4,7). It originates from the external carotid and ascends the neck, sprouting submandibular gland, platysma, and submental branches. After the artery crosses the antegonial notch of the mandible, it gives off twigs to the masseter and depressor anguli oris muscles (Figs. 1 and 2). Under cover of the lip depressors, the facial artery branches into the inferior labial artery that encircles the lower lip. Between the mandible and maxilla, the artery obliquely crosses and supplies two or three branches to the anterior portion of the buccinator (5). After it courses between and supplies twigs to the zygomaticus and levator anguli oris, the facial artery branches into the superior labial artery which runs across the upper lip. After sprouting the lateral nasal artery, the facial artery usually terminates through the levator labii superioris alaeque nasi as the angular artery.

Generous anastomoses to the infraorbital (from the internal maxillary), to the transverse fascial (from the superficial temporal), and to the dorsal branch of the ophthalmic (from the internal carotid) allow the option of a distally based flap. The marked tortuousity of the facial artery in the face can be unraveled for additional centimeters of pedicle length. The anterior racial vein takes a more direct and posterior course to drain into the jugular vein. Small venae comitantes travel with the artery.

There is an independent and anastomotic deep posterior blood supply to the buccinator throughout the buccal branch of the internal maxillary artery and venous drainage through the pterygoid plexus. This system forms the basis of posteriorly based buccinator mucosal flaps (5,6).

FLAP DESIGN AND DIMENSIONS

Flaps for fistulas of the hard palate that do not involve the alveolus are pedicled on the proximal facial artery for a direct intermaxillary course and greater vascular length. The flap crosses the dental arch through an edentulous segment or may have to be divided later. Both proximally and distally based facial artery pedicles can repair fistulas that include the aveolus

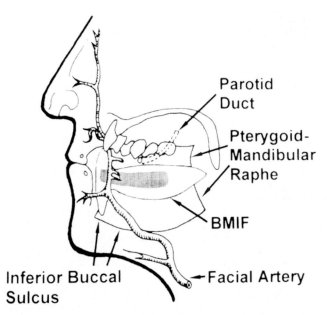

FIG. 2. Sagittal composite intraoral view, schematically illustrating T-shaped flap (in *gray*). Note its relationship to the buccal mucosa and facial artery.

---

[1]*Superficial* and *lateral* denote toward the external surface or skin. *Deep* or *medial* is toward the oral cavity or mucosa. *Anterior* is in the direction of the oral commissure. *Posterior* is the pharynx. *Inferior* is the mandible; *superior* is the maxilla.

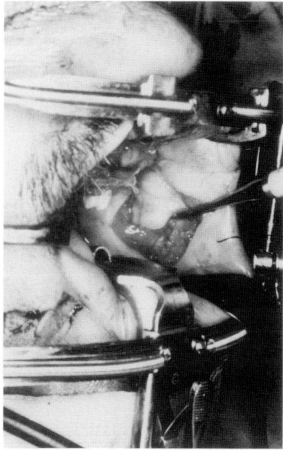

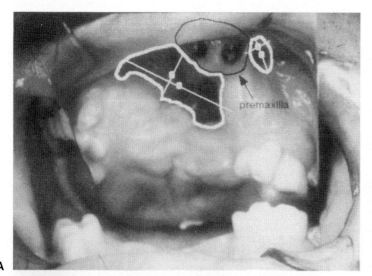

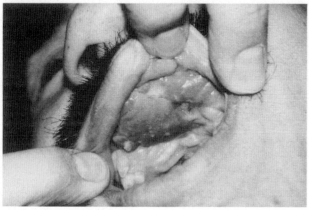

FIG. 3. A 43-year-old man with previously repaired bilateral complete cleft lip and palate who suffered from large anterior oronasal fistulas on either side of the premaxilla. After uneventful healing of bilateral T-shaped buccinator mucosal island flaps (BMIFs), an alveolar iliac crest bone graft was performed 4 months postoperatively, to create a continuous alveolus for functional dental reconstruction. **A:** In this mirror view of the anterior palate, the isolated premaxilla is demonstrated by the *arrow* and is surrounded by fistula. **B:** After the fistula margins were opened, bilateral T-shaped BMIFs were harvested. On the left side, a turnover, distally based flap resurfaced the nasal side. Elevation of the left flap, with forceps holding the facial artery. **C:** On the right side, a proximally based advancement flap repaired the oral surface of the anterior hard palate.

as well as the palate or when the approach to the palatal fistula is through an opening in the maxillary sinus. Up to a third of the vertical buccal sulcus span can be harvested, with only temporary oral opening restriction. Wider flaps require skin grafting of the donor site.

In moderate-sized, cleft-related fistulas (Fig. 3A), turnover marginal oral flaps are developed to close the nasal side, leaving a larger but exclusively oral wound to close. If the enormity of the fistula prevents this approach or this is a fresh cancer resection, then bilateral buccal flaps repair both the oral and nasal sides.

A myomucosal island flap is most often designed as a transverse ellipse originating near the oral commissure (Fig. 3B). The upper margin of the flap is inferior to the parotid duct, and the lower margin approaches the mandibular buccal sulcus. In addition to the midsulcus transversely oriented

ellipse, a vertically oriented flap anterior to the parotid duct or a combined T-shaped flap is designed (see Fig. 2).

OPERATIVE TECHNIQUE

The recipient site is created; the buccal flap is drawn with methylene blue as the labial commissure is pulled medially. Bimanual cheek palpation locates the oblique course of the facial artery across the cheek. Good retraction, magnification, and lighting are essential. The Dingman cleft-palate gag is useful if the upper tongs are positioned in the buccal sulcus instead of under the incisors. Several 2–0 silk sutures pull the labial commissure toward the mouth gag. The parotid duct orifice may be cannulated for extra safety. Because the facial artery is superficial to the buccinator and takes a sinuous pathway through the cheek, a nasolabial counterincision aids the dissection (see Flap Design and Dimensions section).

Intraoral Start

With marked stretch on the buccal mucosa, the outline of the flap is incised with a scalpel through to the buccinator muscle (Fig. 3B). The transversely oriented fibers are seen easily, and the minimal bleeding is stopped by electrocautery. Excessive penetration threatens injury to the facial artery anteriorly and premature entry into the buccal fat pad posteriorly. If extraoral accessory exposure is elected, a gauze sponge can be placed in the buccal sulcus and the cutaneous incision done.

Extraoral Exposure

The nasolabial fold is incised through subdermal fat and the superficial fascia and fat dissected to identify the facial artery just inferior to the labial commissure, where it is most superficial. The vessel is followed up to the alar base and inferiorly toward the mandible by teasing away overlying facial muscles. The artery is intertwined with terminal twigs from the buccal and zygomatic branches of the facial nerve as well as the infraorbital nerve. Dissection should be done superficial and anterior to the vessel, leaving the branches to the buccinator undisturbed. Using microhemoclips, the inferior labial, superior labial, and lateral nasal branches are ligated, leaving most of the blood flow through the facial artery to the buccinator muscle. The artery defines the anterior margin of the buccinator muscle. When a proximally vascularized flap is chosen, the distal end is ligated near the nasal branches.

Next, dissection is done medial to the buccal fat pad, and the muscle is freed from the buccomasseteric fascia. Once into the fat pad, dissection is easier as one hugs the muscle. It is important to stay deep to the buccal motor branches and end posteriorly at the anterior border of the masseter muscle. With distally based flaps, the facial artery is ligated inferior to the labial commissure. After the superficial surface of the muscle is exposed, the mouth is reentered.

Intraoral Return

To conserve the buccinator muscle, the posterior 40% of the mucosa in dissected off the muscle. The mucosa also may be raised from the portion of the flap that lies anterior to the facial artery. After hemostasis is obtained, an incision is made through the small segment of buccinator muscle to the buccal fat pad, preserving the facial vein with the flap, if possible. The anterior mucosal dissection places the facial artery at risk; so the nasolabial exposure is referred to as often as necessary. The remaining attachments are cut and the flap is delivered to the fistula without twisting the pedicle.

An extraoral counterincision maintains the recognizable orientation of the pertinent anatomy, allows direct visualization of the facial arterial system, and is the safest way to avoid inadvertent vascular injury to the small branches to the buccinator. The choice of proximally or distally based flaps depends on the proximity of the defect.

Exclusive Intraoral Approach

Such an approach, which avoids a facial scar, suffers from poor exposure and disorientation; the facial artery descends deep within the wound (see Fig. 2). With experience, however, the intraoral approach is possible. After the perimeter mucosal flap incision is made, the buccinator muscle is perforated, conserving as much muscle as possible, as noted above. A thin membrane contains the buccal fat pad, and preserving it avoids spewing fat into the field. The proximal artery is easier to identify and therefore should be found first; its inferior labial branch is isolated and divided. The anterior buccinator that intertwines with other facial muscles at the labial modiolus is separated. Vital branches to the buccinator are anticipated and preserved. Ligation of the superior labial branches signal the end of the critical segment of blood supply to the flap. There are multiple layers of facial muscles that must be teased and cut away until the facial artery and its venae comitantes remain as the only restraint to transferring the flap to the palate. For a proximally based flap, the distal vessel is ligated.

The myomucosal flap is now hanging on a vascular cord. It is essential not to twist or overly pull on the pedicle as the flap is sewn into the defect. When there are two flaps, the nasal flap is flipped over (usually on a distal pedicle) and sewn to the nasal edge of the fistula with 4–0 chromic catgut. The oral-side flap (usually on a proximal pedicle) is advanced across the disrupted alveolus to be sutured (Fig. 3C). Even with a relatively small segment of buccinator muscle, the two flaps are rather thick and go on to swell generously. For these reasons, and because the facial artery pedicle tethers across the cheek to the palate, if alveolar discontinuity demands an iliac crest bone graft, it is best delayed (Fig. 3).

CLINICAL RESULTS

Division of the pedicle is safe after 6 weeks. Two of nine patients have reported asymptomatic numbness in the lateral upper lip. Facial nerve dysfunction has not been noted, although subtle changes in the smile have been observed. Mouth-opening exercises are encouraged and, in this group of patients, the extreme intraoral pressures associated with playing wind instruments have not been an issue.

SUMMARY

For large intraoral wounds and oronasal fistulas, the anteriorly based buccinator mucosal island flap provides a generous amount of oral mucosa and muscle to reach most regions of the oral cavity with minimal donor-site morbidity.

References

1. Jackson IT. Closure of secondary palatal fistulas with intra-oral tissue and bone grafting. *Br J Plast Surg* 1972;25:93.
2. Bozola AR, Gasques JA, Carriquiry CE, de Oliveria MC. The buccinator myomucosal flap: anatomical study and clinical application. *Plast Reconstr Surg* 1989;84:250.
3. Killey H, Kay L. An analysis of 250 cases of orantral fistulas treated by buccal flap operation. *J Oral Surg* 1967;24:726.
4. Sasaki T, Baker HW, McConnell DB, et al. Cheek island flap for replacement of critical limited defects of the upper aerodigestive tract. *Am J Surg* 1986;152:43.
5. Carstens MH, Stofman GM, Hurwitz DJ, et al. A new approach for repair of oro-antral-nasal fistulae: the anteriorly based buccinator myomucosal island flap. *J Craniomaxillofac Surg* 1991;19:64.
6. Carstens MH, Stofman GM, Hurwitz DJ, et al. The buccinator myomucosal island pedicle flap: anatomic study and case report. *Plast Reconstr Surg* 1991;88:39.
7. Niranjan NS. An anatomical study of the facial artery. *Ann Plast Surg* 1988;21:14.

CHAPTER 190 ■ STERNOCLEIDOMASTOID MUSCLE AND MUSCULOCUTANEOUS FLAP

S. ARIYAN

The sternocleidomastoid muscle and musculocutaneous flap can be used for reconstruction of the tongue, floor of the mouth, tonsillar fossa, and cheek (1–7). It also can be used for pharyngoesophageal defects (see Chapter 216). There are several advantages to the sternocleidomastoid flap. It uses local tissue for one-stage reconstruction of oropharyngeal defects of moderate size, with donor sites that may be closed primarily without the necessity of skin grafts. The flap can be used successfully in patients who have had previous radiation to the neck if the skin is soft and supple over the muscle and there is no clinical evidence of radiation fibrosis or induration.

ANATOMY

The sternocleidomastoid muscle is a round muscle that arises by two tendinous fascicles from the sternum and the medial third of the clavicle, passes obliquely across the side of the neck, and inserts on the lateral surface of the mastoid process. Fresh and preserved cadaver dissections have demonstrated that the sternocleidomastoid has three blood supplies (7,8) (Fig. 1). These vessels enter the muscle at various sites as nutrient vessels to circulate within the muscle and provide musculocutaneous branches to the overlying skin. Although sonic small branches may travel for a centimeter or two along the undersurface of the muscle, there is no axial distribution of vessels along the length of the undersurface of the muscle.

The blood supply to the superior portion of the sternocleidomastoid is a branch from the occipital artery that enters the muscle just below the mastoid region (Fig. 1). The blood supply to the inferior portion is from a branch of the thyrocervical trunk. Midway between its origin and insertion, the sternocleidomastoid is supplied by a branch of the superior thyroid artery as well as by smaller vessels from the adjacent strap muscles.

FLAP DESIGN AND DIMENSIONS

Flaps can be designed with only a "paddle" of skin attached over one end of a pedicle of the sternocleidomastoid muscle, which then is used to transport this skin (7,9). The muscle pedicle may be based on either the superior or inferior blood supply (Fig. 2), the choice being made according to the ease with which the flap may be transported to the defect. In each case, the donor site can be closed either by local advancement of the neck skin or by local transposition flaps.

Surgical defects from resections in the oral cavity may be reconstructed with a 6 × 8-cm paddle of skin transported on a pedicle of sternocleidomastoid muscle based on its superior blood supply (Fig. 3). The skin paddle should be kept overlying the muscle above the level of the clavicle. Although large paddles of skin may have sufficient circulation to the portion that is extended over the clavicle or below, the blood supply to this extended portion is tenuous and unreliable.

Tongue and Floor of Mouth

Resection of lesions in the anterior or lateral floor of the mouth resulting in wounds of moderate size may be recon-

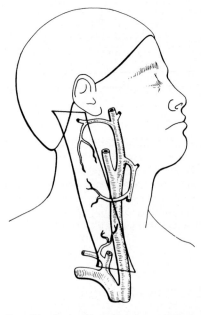

FIG. 1. The three blood supplies to the sternocleidomastoid are the occipital artery superiorly, superior thyroid artery midway, and thyrocervical trunk inferiorly. (From Ariyan, ref. 7, with permission.)

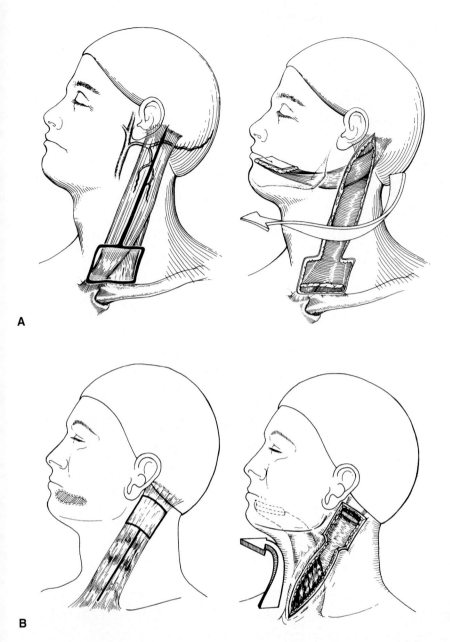

A

B

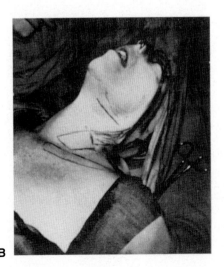

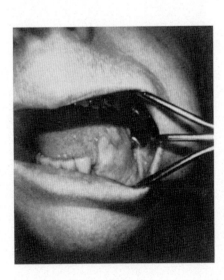

A,B

FIG. 2. A: A paddle of skin outlined on the inferior portion of the sternocleidomastoid above the clavicle may be elevated on its superior blood supply and transported under the mandible to the oral cavity. B: A paddle of skin outlined on the superior portion of the sternocleidomastoid may be elevated on its inferior blood supply and transported under the mandible.

FIG. 3. A: The skin paddle is outlined over the lower portion of the sternocleidomastoid but kept above the level of the clavicle. B: The sternocleidomastoid muscle is dissected as high as necessary to allow this muscle pedicle to be rotated under the mandible to reach the area of the surgical defect.

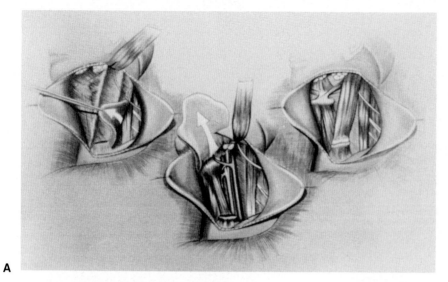

A

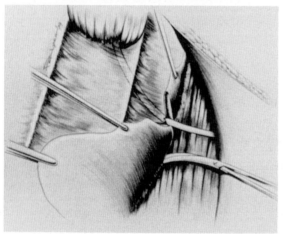

B,C

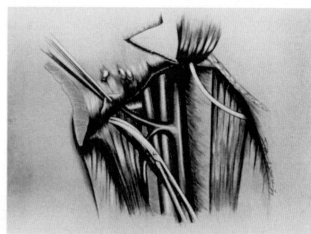

FIG. 4. **A:** A prophylactic neck dissection may be performed by preservation of the spinal accessory nerve and jugular vein. **B:** The fascia of the posterior triangle is incised at the border of the trapezius muscle to dissect and preserve the spinal accessory nerve. **C:** Once the spinal accessory nerve is freed to the sternocleidomastoid, the remainder of the neck contents may be dissected as one specimen from the vessels and nerves in the carotid sheath. (From Ariyan, ref. 10, with permission.)

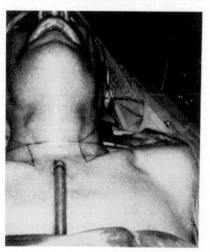

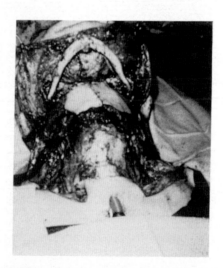

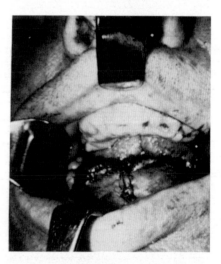

A–C

FIG. 5. **A:** A large tumor of the floor of mouth may require two sternocleidomastoid flaps based on the superior blood supplies. **B,C:** Following resection of the tumor and a rim mandibulectomy, the two sternocleidomastoid flaps may be sutured to each other in the midline, to the tongue posteriorly, and to the labial sulcus anteriorly.

structed with a single paddle of skin based over the inferior portion of the sternocleidomastoid transported on its superior blood supply. This allows for coverage of the wound and preserves the free motion of the tongue.

Larger resections of the floor of the mouth that may require resection of a portion of the tongue, with or without a rim mandibulectomy, may require two sternocleidomastoid flaps (Fig. 5). The required resection may result in a defect too large for these flaps, however, and it may be necessary to reconstruct the area with a large flap, such as the pectoralis major musculocutaneous flap.

Tonsillar Fossa and Posterior Floor of Mouth

Surgical defects of moderate size may be covered with a 6 × 8-cm paddle of skin transported on a pedicle of sternocleidomastoid muscle. This area is particularly suited for an inferiorly based sternocleidomastoid flap because the flap can be pivoted on its longitudinal axis and passed under the mandible for a more direct approach to the area (Fig. 6). A superiorly based sternocleidomastoid flap may be used, but it often results in a bulky mass under the mandible as a result of the muscle folding on itself to reach the tonsillar area.

Cheek

Large through-and-through defects of the cheek need inner lining as well as outer covering. These may be reconstructed with a large superiorly based sternocleidomastoid muscle flap for inner lining that is closed in two layers to provide a watertight seal. The outer covering can be provided with a skin graft, a cervical skin flap, or a musculocutaneous flap, such as the trapezius or pectoralis major muscle. Another alternative is to reconstruct with two skin paddles on an axial (flat muscle) musculocutaneous flap such as the pectoralis major or latissimus dorsi muscle.

OPERATIVE TECHNIQUE

The skin paddle is incised down to the muscle fascia, and it is "tacked down" to the muscle with several interrupted sutures from the dermis to the muscle fascia. Traction must not be placed on the skin paddle because the attachments to the underlying muscle are loose and areolar and the musculocutaneous vessels within this tissue will be damaged. One or two traction sutures are placed through the muscle fascia at the

distal end of the muscle pedicle to help elevate the sternocleidomastoid during its dissection.

The muscle may be dissected and elevated by incising the fascia along the anterior and posterior borders of the sternocleidomastoid muscle belly. This separates the muscle from the cervical fascia of the anterior and posterior triangles as they split to cover the two surfaces of the sternocleidomastoid muscle. The dissection then is continued by scissors to free and elevate the muscle pedicle from the deeper half of the split cervical fascia. Only the amount of dissection necessary to transport the skin paddle under the body of the mandible to reach the oral cavity is needed. The middle blood supply from the superior thyroid can often be preserved, but it may be cut and tied if necessary to provide the mobility to reach the defect. Care must be taken to avoid damaging the spinal accessory nerve passing through or under the sternocleidomastoid.

If a prophylactic neck dissection is to be performed concurrently, the dissection is carried further cephalad (Fig. 4). The spinal accessory nerve will need to be cut to elevate the sternocleidomastoid sufficiently to reach the inframastoid area. Occasionally, this nerve passes under the sternocleidomastoid rather than through the muscle and gives a motor branch to the muscle. In such a case, the branch to the sternocleidomastoid may be cut and the main trunk of the spinal accessory nerve may be preserved if the patient is a proper candidate for a "functional" radical neck dissection (10); however, if it is necessary to carry the dissection to the inframastoid area, care must be taken to avoid damage to the occipital artery supplying this muscle.

Once the flap is dissected sufficiently to allow it to pass under the mandible and reach the surgical defect, the tension on the flap is placed on the muscle by suturing from the deeper portion of the wound margins to the muscle pedicle. This not only permits the skin paddle to be sutured to the mucosal margin without tension but also provides a second layer of closure to protect the deeper wound from the salivary products and bacteria.

CLINICAL RESULTS

Despite its many advantages, the sternocleidomastoid flap has significant limitations. The musculocutaneous blood supply from the muscle to the overlying skin is delicate and can be damaged easily through the loose areolar tissue attaching the skin to the underlying muscle. This makes the sternocleidomastoid musculocutaneous flap technically one of the most delicate and tenuous for survival of the skin paddle.

In flaps with compromised circulation, ischemia was manifested by early venous congestion, ecchymosis, and blistering

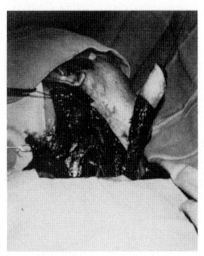
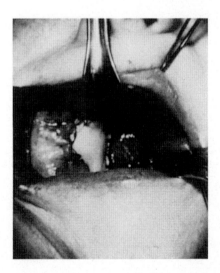

A,B

FIG. 6. **A,B:** A paddle of skin over the superior portion of the sternocleidomastoid muscle may be pivoted 180 degrees on its longitudinal axis to reach a defect in the tonsillar fossa.

of the skin paddle within 48 hours. These paddles resulted in loss of the epithelium in 10 of the 24 flaps. Nevertheless, each of these flaps healed with intact wound margins and survival of the dermis of the skin paddle. In each case, the dermis resurfaced with epithelium without requiring surgery. Histologic examination of these flaps demonstrated squamous epithelium of the surface and survival of the deeper dermis, even though there was absence of the keratin layer and absence of the glandular elements, indicating loss of the upper dermis.

In two patients, a small pharyngocutaneous fistula was noted in the first few postoperative days. These fistulas closed by contraction of the wound within 2 weeks despite oral intake of a liquid diet by each patient.

One potential objection to the use of a sternocleidomastoid musculocutaneous flap might be that it violates the general principles of cancer surgery. For many years, this muscle has been removed as part of the specimen in the classic radical neck dissection, even if it did not contain invasive tumor; however, the safety of preserving the sternocleidomastoid muscle in patients treated with prophylactic neck dissections and in selected patients with clinically positive necks has been demonstrated (11,12). As mentioned earlier in this chapter, the investing layer of the cervical fascia over the anterior cervical triangle splits into anterior and posterior sheets to envelop the sternocleidomastoid and converges again to cover the posterior triangle. Therefore, if the muscle is dissected out of this enveloping sheet, the posterior layer of this split cervical fascia may be left intact, leaving the underlying neck contents undisturbed and permitting the resection of the entire remaining neck contents (10).

SUMMARY

Sternocleidomastoid muscle and musculocutaneous flaps can be used successfully either alone or with other flaps to reconstruct various cheek, neck, and intraoral defects.

References

1. Owens NA. A compound neck pedicle designed for the repair of massive facial defects: formation, development and application. *Plast Reconstr Surg* 1955;15:369.
2. Bakamjian VY. A technique for primary reconstruction of the palate after radical maxillectomy for cancer. *Plast Reconstr Surg* 1963;31:103.
3. Littlewood AHM. Compound skin and sternomastoid flaps for repair in extensive carcinoma of the head and neck. *Br J Plast Surg* 1967;20:403.
4. Jabaley ME. Reconstruction of patients with oral and pharyngeal cancer. *Curr Probl Surg* 1977;14:1.
5. McCraw JB, Magee WP, Kalwaic H. Uses of the trapezius and sternomastoid myocutaneous flaps in head and neck reconstruction. *Plast Reconstr Surg* 1979;63:49.
6. O'Brien BM. A muscle-skin pedicle for the total reconstruction of the lower lip. *Plast Reconstr Surg* 1970;45:395.
7. Ariyan S. One-stage reconstruction for defects of the mouth using a sternocleidomastoid myocutaneous flap. *Plast Reconstr Surg* 1979;63:618.
8. Jabaley ME, Hedder FR, Wallace WH, et al. Sternocleidomastoid regional flaps: a new look at an old concept. *Br J Plast Surg* 1979;32:106.
9. Ariyan S. The sternocleidomastoid myocutaneous flap. *Laryngoscope* 1980;90:676.
10. Ariyan S. Functional radical neck dissection. *Plast Reconstr Surg* 1980;65:768.
11. Bocca E, Pignataro O. A conservative technique in radical neck dissection. *Ann Otol Rhinol Laryngol* 1967;76:975.
12. Bocca E. Conservative neck dissection. *Laryngoscope* 1975;85:1511.

CHAPTER 191 ■ TRAPEZIUS OSTEOMUSCULOCUTANEOUS ISLAND FLAP FOR RECONSTRUCTION OF THE ANTERIOR FLOOR OF THE MOUTH AND MANDIBLE

W. R. PANJE

The trapezius osteomusculocutaneous island flap can be successfully used in the reconstruction of the anterior floor of the mouth and the mandibular arch (1,2).

INDICATIONS

Indications for use of the trapezius osteomusculocutaneous island flap are (a) anterior mandibular defects, (b) compound defects (i.e., floor of mouth, tongue, or buccal area) in addition to bone (mandibular defect), (c) osteoradionecrosis, and (d) facial contouring in which bone is necessary.

This flap offers the following advantages over previous approaches: (a) it has the potential of a one-stage immediate reconstruction; (b) it offers the alternative of available skin, muscle, or bone for reconstruction of defects of the lower two thirds of the face and oral cavity; and (c) it eliminates the need for microsurgical transplantation of tissue. In addition, in

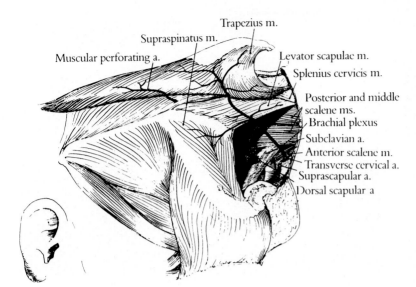

FIG. 1. Major branches of the transverse cervical artery and associated structures, with patient lying prone.

patients in whom oncologic surgery has resulted in denervation of the trapezius muscle, the trapezius osteomusculocutaneos island flap has the advantage of using the already paralyzed trapezius muscle without the need for damaging additional muscles (such as the chest muscle in the pectoralis bone flap).

ANATOMY

Multiple arteries supply the trapezius muscle, but the major blood supply is provided by the transverse cervical artery arising from the thyrocervical trunk (3). The transverse cervical artery begins deep to the sternal head of the sternocleidomastoid muscle, crosses the posterior triangle, and enters the trapezius muscle on its deep surface about 4 cm medial to the acromion. The artery is identified easily as it passes deep to the posterior belly of the omohyoid muscle (Fig. 1).

The transverse cervical vein usually travels in the same fascial plane as the artery; however, the vein can travel superficial to the omohyoid muscle. If it is seen in this area, it should be preserved. It usually empties into the subclavian vein 2 to 3 cm lateral to where the thyrocervical trunk originates from the subclavian artery. The vein is usually the limiting factor in extending the arc of rotation of this flap.

The accessory nerve generally enters the trapezius muscle in the area of the vascular pedicle. Because of its multiple innervations of the muscle, the nerve usually can be preserved if properly dissected.

To use the scapular spine as part of this compound flap, the trapezius muscle attachment to the scapular spine must be preserved. Accessory nutrient arteries penetrate the scapular spine at the fascial attachment of the trapezius muscle to the spine (4).

OPERATIVE TECHNIQUE

The first step in the formation of the trapezius osteomusculocutaneous island flap is the harvesting of a composite flap of the trapezius muscle based on the transverse cervical artery and vein, overlying skin, and all or a portion of the scapular spine. The flap can be developed once the transverse cervical artery and vein supply has been identified entering the deep surface of the trapezius muscle (Fig. 1).

To preserve the attachment of the trapezius muscle to the bone, an incision should be made inferior to the scapular spine. This incision will detach the infraspinatus muscle from

the bone. The inferior side of the spine should be bluntly dissected free of any muscle attachments. By bringing the dissection laterally along the spine, the fossa will be identified just deep to the acromial part of the spine. This part of the scapular bone should be palpated, and the arch covering the fossa must be maintained.

The scapular spine that is to be used to reconstruct the anterior mandibular defect is removed from the body of the scapula by a sharp chisel or osteotome, proceeding from a lateral to a medial direction (Fig. 2). The acromial attachment to the clavicle should be maintained to preserve normal shoulder joint function. By this method, approximately 12 × 2 cm of spine can be obtained without compromising shoulder girdle stability. Once the scapular spine has been delivered, the surgeon will proceed in a manner similar to the procedure used in the development of the trapezius musculocutaneous island flap.

In reconstructing the mandible, the scapular spine can be fractured in a green-stick manner at its midpoint to conform to the mentum of the mandible. The scapula is attached to the remaining mandibular segments by wire. External fixation is also needed (Morris biphase). The mentum area of the newly reconstructed mandible also needs anterior support. This can be accomplished by attaching wire between the biphase and the mandible or by neck bandage support, in which a bulky dressing is applied beneath the chin and maintained in place for at least 2 weeks. A 4- to 6-week period of stabilization is needed for bony union to occur (Fig. 3).

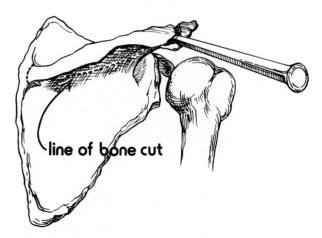

FIG. 2. Line of chisel cut when removing scapular spine for mandible reconstruction is indicated.

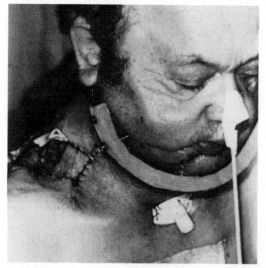
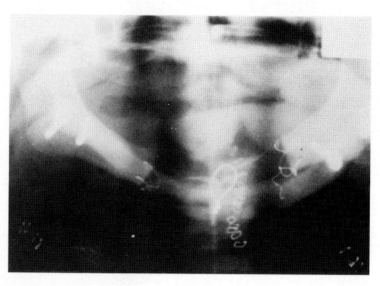

A,B

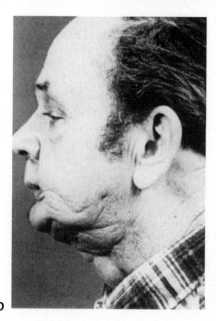

C,D

FIG. 3. **A:** Five days after trapezius osteomusculocutaneous island flap primary restoration of an anterior mandibular and floor of mouth defect. **B:** Orthopantomogram radiograph demonstrating scapular spine replacement of an anterior mandibular defect. **C:** Two months after restoration of the anterior mandible and floor of the mouth. **D:** Three years after restoration of the anterior mandible and floor of the mouth. Note that dentures have been fitted to the reconstructed mandible.

The scapular spine also can be used simply based on the trapezius muscle by means of occipital artery vascular nutrition only (5), that is, if the transverse cervical artery and vein have been interrupted, as with a previous radical neck dissection, the occipital artery perforators usually will take over the blood supply to the trapezius muscle. By maintaining the integrity of the muscle attachments to the scapular spine as well as by carrying the muscle back to the region of the occipital artery, a pedicled flap based on the occipital artery and paraspinous artery perforators attached to the scapular spine then can be used to reconstruct the anterior mandibular defect. Skin also can be used in a nondelayed manner in reconstructing the anterior floor of the mouth at the same time as when the mandible is reconstructed, as long as it is not extended caudal to the scapular spine. The skin of the superior-based unipedicle compound trapezius osteomusculocutaneous flap does not survive as well as that of the island flap.

CLINICAL RESULTS

When using the trapezius osteomusculocutaneous island flap for reconstruction of the anterior floor of the mouth and the mandible, a 90% success rate may be expected, even when used in irradiated fields. There is a 70% success rate in restoring osteoradionecrotic bone loss and in preventing the spread of osteoradionecrosis.

SUMMARY

The trapezius osteomusculocutaneous flap can be used to reconstruct the anterior floor of the mouth and the mandible.

References

1. Panje WR, Cutting C. Trapezius osteomyocutaneous island flap for the reconstruction of the anterior floor of the mouth and the mandible. *Head Neck Surg* 1980;3:66.
2. Panje WR. Mandible reconstruction with the trapezius osteomusculocutaneous flap. *Arch Otolaryngol* 1985;111:223.
3. Huelke D. A study of the transverse cervical and dorsal scapular arteries. *Anat Rec* 1958;132:233.
4. Lexer E, Kuliga B, Turk W. *Untersuchungen über Knochenarterien.* Berlin: Hirschwald, 1904;15–16.
5. McCraw JB, Magee WR, Kalwaic H. Uses of the trapezius and sternomastoid myocutaneous flaps in head and neck reconstruction. *Plast Reconstr Surg* 1979;63:49.

CHAPTER 192 ■ RIB–PECTORALIS MAJOR OSTEOMUSCULOCUTANEOUS FLAP

M. S. G. BELL

The rib–pectoralis major osteomusculocutaneous flap has been used to provide replacement for mandibular defects and lining tissue in the oral cavity, especially for reconstruction of the soft palate, floor of the mouth, and lateral pharyngeal wall (1). It may be used as a pedicle flap or as a free flap.

ANATOMY

Both the fifth and sixth ribs have been used, and each seems to obtain sufficient blood supply from the overlying pectoralis major muscle to allow flap transfer and survival to provide a reasonably reliable composite flap for complicated reconstructions (2,3). (For details of the muscle anatomy, see Chapter 132.)

FLAP DESIGN AND DIMENSIONS

I have taken a portion of skin up to 15 cm² for reconstruction of the soft palate, floor of the mouth, and lateral pharyngeal wall. The inferior margin of the cutaneous portion of the pectoralis major flap may be extended below the costal margin by at least 5 cm.

The skin flap should be cut larger than necessary because the bulk of muscle and fat beneath the skin must be accommodated in closure of the mouth defect, and underestimating this area is easy. Because the rib does provide some degree of rigidity, swelling in the area may increase skin tension on the suture line, and a rather redundant flap will minimize this degree of tension. (I believe that development of fistulas in my series of patients may have been, in part, a result of this problem.)

The cutaneous portion of the flap always should be planned so that the superior margin begins as high as possible to include the perforating musculocutaneous arteries along the lower margin of the pectoralis major muscle. In female patients in whom the inframammary fold must be taken as the upper margin of the skin flap, dissection may be beveled upward, just beneath the breast tissue, preserving cutaneous perforating vessels that may be seen running obliquely downward. This factor may be critical in preserving the cutaneous blood supply.

Either the fifth or sixth rib can be used. In 21 of my 22 patients, the sixth rib was taken. In the reconstruction in which the fifth rib was used, the muscle pedicle was under a little greater tension than with sixth-rib flaps. The fifth-rib flap is useful when an external skin and lip defect also must be covered because a longer skin component can be used.

Access to the base of the pectoralis major flap may be achieved in several ways. A vertical incision is used by many surgeons, with the incision running downward from the mid-portion of the clavicle to the point at which the cutaneous portion of the pectoralis major flap is raised. Access to the flap also may be gained by raising a standard deltopectoral flap. This procedure displays the entire clavicular origin of the muscle and the musculotendinous junction in the axilla, which is subsequently divided.

Access to the sternal origin of the pectoralis major flap is gained by raising a laterally based flap about 10 cm wide at the level of the anterior axillary line that extends medially to the sternum. This flap usually contains the nipple and is designated so that its inferior limb runs right along the proposed skin flap to be carried into the mouth (Fig. 1A, B). The amount of skin undermining with this technique is greater than in the vertical incision technique; however, the standard Bakamjian flap is preserved and may be used for help in closure of the chest defect when a large flap is taken. It also may be used for closure of the neck skin should a defect be present there or should a subsequent complication require use of a local flap.

OPERATIVE TECHNIQUE

The pectoralis major muscle is raised from the chest wall along its lateral margin. There is a discrete fascial plane allowing blunt dissection. The sternal and clavicular origins of the pectoralis major muscle are separated, and the vessels entering the deep surface of the muscle are easily seen and preserved. The sternal portion of the muscle that will carry the skin and bone is defined laterally to its musculotendinous junction in the axilla.

The muscle is divided at this point (Fig. 1). The sternal origin of the muscle then is divided with the cutting cautery. At this point, the rib with the largest muscular attachment can be chosen The skin flap overlying the rib is incised, and the intercostal muscles above and below the rib that are to be taken are divided with the cutting cautery. Periosteum of the rib is preserved to ensure maximum blood supply. The costal cartilage is disarticulated at the sternum, and the rib is divided laterally

561

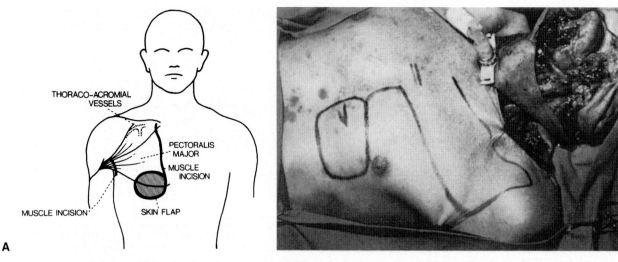

FIG. 1. A: The pectoralis major osteomusculocutaneous flap using a vertical incision for access (see text for details). **B:** Variation in design to preserve a deltopectoral flap for either immediate or later use. (From Bell, Barron, ref. 1, with permission.)

according to the bone length required. The angle of the costochondral junction, especially in the sixth rib, corresponds well to the angle between the body and vertical ramus of the mandible. The intercostal artery is ligated where it leaves the internal mammary artery, anterior to the thoracis internus muscle.

Because the perichondrium is taken with the rib, entry into the pleural space may occur as dissection proceeds laterally. If care is taken, using the wide end of the Howarth elevator, the rib usually can be elevated without damaging the pleura.

The rib–pectoralis major osteomyocutaneous flap then is raised on its neurovascular bundle and tunneled beneath the skin in the supraclavicular area into the neck and mouth (Fig. 2). The bone is tailored to the appropriate length and may be bent by kerfing to conform to the desired contour of the new mandible. Fixation with intramedullary Compere wires and wire loops has been satisfactory. The rib and the costal cartilage are soft, and I have found that plates and screws are less secure than intramedullary fixation (see Fig. 3).

The vascularity of the bone and cartilage appears to be adequate for healing. Bleeding will be observed from the perichondrium and periosteum of the rib after the flap has been elevated. I considered performing a microvascular anastomo-

sis of the intercostal artery and vein to suitable vessels in the neck, but this effort was judged unnecessary because there was visible bleeding.

If the pleural space has been entered, the defect is narrowed by using a rib approximator and wiring the adjacent ribs with 25-gauge wire loops. The chest wall skin defect is closed with a combination of the lateral chest wall flap and the deltopectoral flap as required. Figure 1B shows the lateral chest flap bearing the nipple used to close the chest defect. A free skin graft to the donor bed of one of these flaps may be required.

In one patient, I used this flap as a free composite flap to repair a large soft-tissue defect in the face. The patient had had mucormycosis and required removal of two thirds of his hard and soft palate, his left maxilla, his ethmoid sinus and left eye, and the cribriform plate and floor of his left anterior cranial fossa (Fig. 4). The pectoralis major flap was easily revascularized by means of the facial vessels.

CLINICAL RESULTS

I have used this osteomyocutaneous flap on 22 occasions to reconstruct mandibular defects. One free flap for reconstruc-

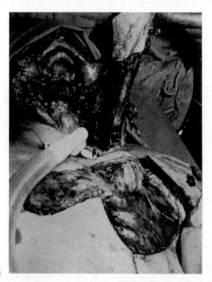
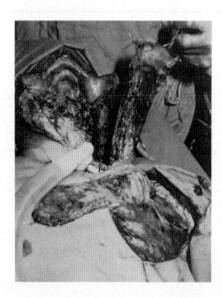

FIG. 2. A,B: The flap elevated and passed beneath the skin bridge over the clavicle. Note the large muscle attachment to the rib. (From Bell, Barron, ref. 1, with permission.)

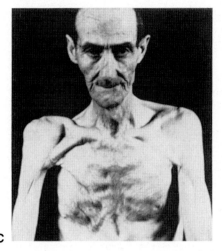
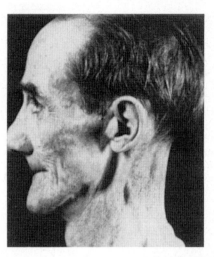
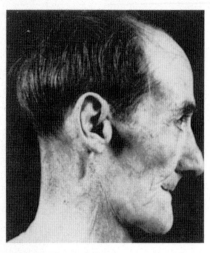

A–C

FIG. 3. A–C: Postoperative views of a patient who had a postradiation recurrent squamous cell carcinoma on his right tonsil extending onto his soft palate and pharyngeal wall and anteriorly onto the floor of his mouth. He required an en bloc resection of his entire soft palate, the right third of his oral pharynx and hypopharynx, and the entire vertical and horizontal half of his right mandible. A right radical neck dissection was performed in continuity with this. Reconstruction was done with a sixth-rib composite pectoralis major musculocutaneous flap. The nasal lining of the soft palate was created by a mucosal flap from the hard palate; the oral right half of the soft palate was reconstructed from the musculocutaneous flap. The flap also lined the oral and hypopharyngeal defects and replaced the floor of the mouth and mandible. Healing of both the donor and recipient areas was uneventful. The threaded Kirschner wires were removed from the mandible at 3 months, and the patient has clinical union of the mandible. His speech is hypernasal but clear. He eats without difficulty, although he did have problems initially with swallowing. The cosmetic result is excellent. (From Bell, Barron, ref. 1, with permission.)

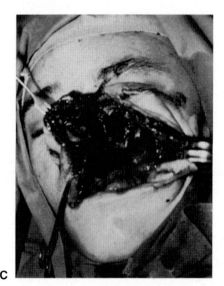
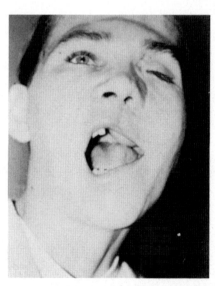
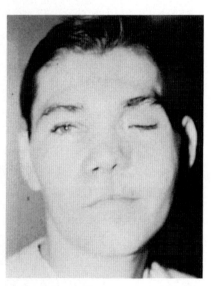

A–C

FIG. 4. A: This 22-year-old man had an extensive composite resection for mucormycosis. Two thirds of his hard and soft palate were removed, along with his left maxilla, eye, floor of orbit, nasal septum, cribriform plate, and floor of his anterior cranial fossa. After a 6-week course of amphotericin B and dressing changes, a delayed composite free-flap reconstruction was performed using the pectoralis major rib flap. B,C: This free flap was anastomosed to the facial vessels in the neck, and it healed without difficulty. Portions of this flap were deepithelialized where the bulk of the flap was in contact with the inner surface of the cheek and along the lining of the nose. A nasopharyngeal tube was left in place to stent this area for a period of 3 weeks. The patient now has excellent air entry through both nostrils. The skin was left on the flap to line the eye socket, and the patient wears a plastic prosthesis to give some bulk to his eyelid. The nipple is located in the center of his palate. It is now 2 years since surgery, and the patient has had no problems with this flap, aside from a small abscess that developed after it was perforated with a lamb bone. The abscess was drained and healed without difficulty. The cosmetic result is excellent, and the patient's speech is mildly hypernasal.

tion of the hard and soft palate and left maxillary defect has been done. The skin portion of the flaps replaced the floor of the mouth and the pharyngeal wall in four patients and the soft palate as well in two others (see Fig. 3). All patients, with the exception of the free-flap patient, have had a full course of radiation therapy preoperatively.

The pectoralis major muscle pedicle appears to allow excellent protection for the great vessels in the neck, and its bulk gives a cosmetically satisfying contour to the neck. I have lost two flaps because of compression of the vascular pedicle within the arch of the rib. This was a technical error, and the encircling rib evidently constricted the pedicle. Seven ribs became exposed with delayed healing, requiring total removal of the bone in five. I have thus had major complications in seven of 22 patients.

The chest wall defects have healed without complication. Persistent pleural effusions in two patients necessitated maintenance of the chest tube for 10 days. I have noted no appreciable loss of shoulder function as a result of using this muscle flap.

Hospitalization varied from 2 to 4 weeks in the patients who did not develop complications with local wound healing. Two patients with extensive pharyngeal wall reconstructions had prolonged deglutition problems. With time, they have managed to take oral nourishment. Cosmetically, the results are equal to currently described reconstructive techniques (4–7). Bony union was firm in all my patients at pin removal 3 months postoperatively. A bone biopsy taken from two patients at 4 and 12 weeks after surgery showed viable, architecturally normal bone. The rib appears to have been adequately vascularized in my group of 15 patients, and it has evidently not resorbed. Bony union has been painless and clinically firm (fibrous union). Despite the advantages of the rib in providing a more total replacement of tissue loss, there was a significant rate of complications detracting from its advantages.

In contrast, a musculocutaneous flap has a much lower incidence of complications (8,9), with no flaps lost in my ongoing series. While the stability of the mandible is not restored and the cosmetic appearance may be less pleasing, the reliability is evidently much higher. Therefore, the osteomusculocutaneous flap should be restricted in use because of its high complication rate. The proportion of breakdowns was higher in midline reconstructions, with only one of four flaps healing uneventfully. The success rate of this procedure would likely be greater in nonirradiated patients, but there were none in my series of mandible reconstructions.

SUMMARY

The osteomusculocutaneous flap should be restricted in use probably to fairly large defects of the lateral mandible where there is concern about instability and rotation of the opposite hemimandible.

References

1. Bell MSG, Barron PT. The rib-pectoralis major osteomyocutaneous flap. *Ann Plast Surg* 1980;6:347.
2. Ariyan S, Finseth FJ. The anterior chest approach for obtaining free osteocutaneous rib. *Plast Reconstr Surg* 1978;62:676.
3. Hendel PM, Huttner RS, Rodrigo J, Buncke HJ. The functional vascular anatomy of the rib. *Plast Reconstr Surg* 1982;70:578.
4. Cuono CB, Ariyan S. Immediate reconstruction of a composite mandibular defect with a regional osteomusculocutaneous flap. *Plast Reconstr Surg* 1980;65:477.
5. Daniel RK. Mandibular reconstruction with free tissue transfers. *Ann Plast Surg* 1978;1:346.
6. McKee DM. Microvascular bone transplantation. *Clin Plast Surg* 1978;5:283.
7. Rosen IB, Bell MSG, Barron PT, et al. Use of microvascular flaps including free osteocutaneous flaps in reconstruction after composite resection for radiation and recurrent oral cancer. *Am J Surg* 1979;138:544.
8. Ariyan S. The pectoralis major myocutaneous flap: a versatile flap for reconstruction in the head and neck. *Plast Reconstr Surg* 1979;63:73.
9. Ariyan S. Further experiences with the pectoralis major myocutaneous flap for the immediate repair of defects from excisions of head and neck cancers. *Plast Reconstr Surg* 1979;64:605.

CHAPTER 193 ■ LATERAL PECTORAL OSTEOMUSCULOCUTANEOUS FLAP

J. W. LITTLE III AND J. R. LYONS

An obvious further extension of the pectoralis musculocutaneous flap is the inclusion of skeletal tissue deep to the muscle as a composite flap to allow one-stage immediate reconstruction of the mandible (1).

Others have included rib (2–6), but because the costal origins of the pectoralis major muscle arise only from the cartilaginous portions of the second through sixth ribs (7), we contend that these flaps represent essentially chondromusculocutaneous flaps with bony rib extensions. Certainly, exclusion or resection

of the cartilage component would render the bony parts little more than free grafts. While cartilaginous rib serves, perhaps, as an effective mandibular spacer, it surely cannot allow the solid reconstruction through bony interposition and union that is preferred in mandibular repair.

A component of the pectoral muscle system does have its origin from the true bony rib cage: the pectoralis minor muscle arising from the third through fifth bony ribs lateral to the costochondral junction. We recommend, therefore, a composite system that incorporates a key portion of this muscle in a lateral pectoral flap—formally, a pectoralis major–pectoralis minor osteomusculocutaneous flap.

INDICATIONS

Such a composite transfer is indicated whenever mandibulectomy is performed, whether or not accompanied by neck dissection. Although conventional secondary bone grafting remains a satisfactory alternative for mandibular restoration in the nonirradiated patient without undue scarring, we consider vascularized bony transfer mandatory in unfavorable situations.

Osteomusculocutaneous flaps based on the sternocleidomastoid system are negated by surgical and radiation therapy to the neck (8). Sternal transfer on the pectoralis system is useful (9), but we prefer our bony component and donor site. Although dissection of the lateral pectoral composite flap is demanding and practiced elevation requires 2 hours, it offers obvious advantages compared with free bony transfer by microvascular techniques.

ANATOMY

The blood supply of the pectoral muscles by way of the thoracoacromial artery is well described (10–14). The pectoral branch sends a significant vessel to the pectoralis minor muscle before continuing on the deep surface of the pectoralis major as its dominant vascular supply. The descending portion of the vessel, while closely applied to the undersurface of the pectoralis major muscle, remains free from the muscle in a distinct fibroareolar layer that is further protected on its deep surface by a significant fascial sheet.

A secondary supply to the pectoralis comes by way of the lateral thoracic artery. After a highly variable origin from the second part of the axillary artery, the subscapular trunk, or the thoracoacromial artery, the vessel follows the lateral border of the pectoralis minor, supplying this muscle and the serratus anterior before reaching the undersurface of the pectoralis major. It anastomoses freely with the pectoral branch of the thoracoacromial artery, the thoracodorsal artery of the subscapular trunk, and the intercostal arteries of the lateral thoracic wall.

It is the arborized bed of the lateral thoracic artery that we consider the collateral bridge between the thoracoacromial supply of the pectoralis major free border and, through pectoralis minor and serratus anterior attachments, the lateral bony fifth rib. It is perhaps surprising that the lower half of the pectoralis minor muscle alone can serve this function without the need to include the entire unit with its proximal blood supply, but such has consistently been the case.

The lateral pectoral osteomusculocutaneous flap includes a lateral segment of vascularized fifth rib that is carried within a soft-tissue bloc that contains the entire musculature of the chest wall from the superior border of the fourth rib to the inferior border of the sixth between the costochondral and anterior axillary lines. This muscle bloc includes a segment of free-border pectoralis major, the lower half of pectoralis minor, and portions of serratus anterior, external oblique, and external and internal intercostal muscles.

FLAP DESIGN AND DIMENSIONS

The major part of the pectoralis major muscle can be spared, minimizing both functional and aesthetic deformities to the chest wall. The resulting narrow, flat pedicle is far more appropriate for passage through most necks. If muscle bulk is truly required throughout the neck, we suggest including the entire pectoralis minor muscle with its proximal blood supply, detaching the muscle from the coracoid while continuing to preserve the pectoralis major span intact. Incidentally, we have found the thin pedicle as effective as the bulky muscular one in protecting an irradiated carotid where overlying neck flaps have failed.

The pectoralis major–pectoralis minor osteomusculocutaneous flap differs from previous flaps in three respects: (a) the attached rib is lateral and therefore bony, (b) the accompanying skin paddle is lateral and therefore hairless even in relatively hirsute patients, and (c) the pedicle is muscle free and therefore thin.

We prefer a lateral inframammary location for the skin island, even in cases not involving rib transfer. Not only is the subcutaneous tissue of this region frequently scant, but so also is the hair production. Although others advocating fascial-cutaneous extensions beyond the muscle have selected more medial sites for their paddles, recent in vivo injection studies suggest that a lateral distribution of the thoracoacromial axis may predominate, at least under the influence of competing hemodynamic territories.

Inframammary skin islands have measured up to 12×12 cm. The pivot point of this island flap occurs immediately below the midclavicle. The arc of rotation allows the skin island to reach the posterior pharynx and the rib to reach the contralateral mandibular angle.

Following extirpation or preparation of the defect, the course of the pectoral branch of the thoracoacromial artery is outlined on the chest wall (see Chapter 132). If neck dissection has been performed, the lower limb of the preferred parallel incisions of McFee will have been adjusted downward to the level of the clavicle. The skin island is marked according to the requirements of the defect. If both lining and cover are missing, a sizable paddle is required to replace both and to include an intervening deepithelialized zone for passage from extraoral to intraoral sites.

The island is routinely ovoid in configuration, with specific tailoring to await the stage of "fitting in." It extends from just below the nipple-areola in men (just above the inframammary fold in women) to as far inferior as necessary (approaching the costal margin), and from the costochondral line medially (slightly medial to the nipple line in men) to as far lateral as necessary (approaching the anterior axillary line). The fifth rib is palpated precisely and indicated beneath the upper third of the skin island. If there has been no incision at the level of the clavicle, one is marked (Fig. 1).

OPERATIVE TECHNIQUE

The skin island is incised on all margins down to underlying muscle. Beginning at the superior margin, where the pectoralis major muscle is now exposed some brief distance above its free border, the skin and subcutaneous tissues of the upper pectoral region are rapidly elevated from the muscle as a broad bipedicle flap to the level of the clavicular incision.

Dissection of the flap proper then is begun, starting at the inferior margin, raising skin, subcutaneous tissue, and investing muscle fascia from the underlying muscle slips of external oblique and serratus anterior, until the lower border of the sixth rib is reached. If this dissection is not "bloody," sufficient muscle fascia is not being retained with the flap and portions of the distal skin island may be jeopardized (15).

Over the sixth rib, dissection is deepened onto periosteum, exposing this layer until the superior border of that rib is reached. Dissection is now further deepened through the intercostal musculature of the fifth intercostal space onto pleura.

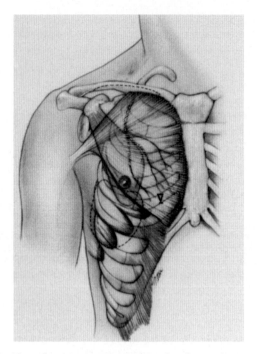

FIG. 1. Planned incisions. (From Little et al., ref. 1, with permission.)

Here a few protective fibers of internal intercostal muscle may be retained on the endothoracic fascia overlying the pleural surface as the dissection approaches the inferior margin of the key fifth rib.

The medial flap margin is deepened through remaining soft tissues onto the fifth rib at the costochondral junction. The rib is freed circumferentially over a short subperiosteal zone and divided just lateral to the junction so that no cartilage will be included in the future osteosynthesis. The cut end of the rib then is lifted with a prying motion, and superior and lateral dissection is resumed between the periosteum and pleura. With practice, a somewhat forceful yet blunt technique allows rapid performance of an otherwise tedious step, sparing an intact pleura. This is continued from medial to lateral, progressively lifting the rib away from pleura, until the necessary length has been freed.

If the resected portion of mandible has been measured with a curved wire at the time of extirpation, precise determination of required rib length is possible. Of course, an additional 2 to 3 cm is included to allow mortised unions. When the deter-

mined length is freed, the rib is divided laterally, along with its intercostal bundle.

This same level of dissection, immediately above the pleura, is continued superiorly another centimeter, clearing the fourth intercostal space up to the inferior border of the fourth rib, which can be palpated from beneath as the flap is folded upward. Because this rib will be left with the chest wall, its inferior edge is sharply incised through the soft tissue and periosteum of the flap superficial to its intercostal bundle.

The dissection now proceeds, lifting periosteum from denuded fourth rib, until its superior border is reached. Until this point, dissection has proceeded en bloc with easily defined peripheral and deep margins to the bloc (Fig. 2). No attention to specific anatomic particulars has been required.

Now a finger is insinuated around and behind the free border of the pectoralis major muscle just above the hinged attachment of the flap at the superior border of the fourth rib, entering the space between the pectoralis major and the remaining upper portion of pectoralis minor muscle. A sweep of the finger superiorly clears this space to the clavicle, leaving the upper portion of the pectoralis minor muscle against the chest wall.

It would be possible to include within the flap the entire pectoralis minor muscle with its major vascular supply from above, but this has not been necessary to ensure rib survival and would otherwise increase the bulk of the pedicle beyond the aesthetic requirements of most patients.

The remaining narrow attachment of the flap to the bony wall—consisting of fourth-rib periosteum, intercostal fascia, and a few pectoralis minor fibers—is now divided flush with the superior border of the fourth rib, leaving the entire composite bloc attached only along the free lateral border of the pectoralis major muscle. Now that the composite paddle has been raised, attention must be directed to dissection of the vascular paddle.

The bipedicle skin flap is retracted superiorly to expose the pectoralis major muscle. A site is selected some 2 to 3 cm above the superior margin of the skin island (three to four fingerbreadths above the free-muscle border) for complete division of the muscle down to the submuscular fatty layer with its pectoral vessels. This division of muscle is performed with care over a semilunar arc that, when completed, will leave a defect in the free border of the pectoralis major muscle that has a serrated edge (Fig. 3).

This step is aided by lifting the pectoralis major and attached composite bloc to determine the course of the pectoral branch underneath the muscle, thereby predicting the precise zone of the arc under which they will be encountered. Once the vessels themselves are found, dissection proceeds

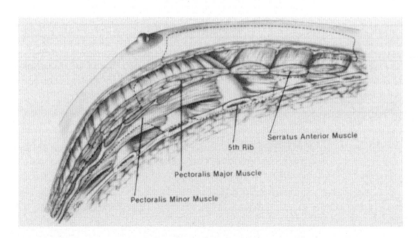

Serratus Anterior Muscle

5th Rib

Pectoralis Major Muscle

Pectoralis Minor Muscle

FIG. 2. Staggered cross section of composite bloc. (From Little et al., ref. 1, with permission.)

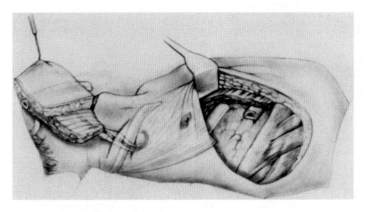

FIG. 3. The lateral pectoral composite flap and secondary defect. (From Little et al., ref. 1, with permission.)

rapidly as the vessels are freed within their fatty compartment from the deep muscular surface.

Perforating branches into the overlying muscle are divided between microclips, and the submuscular fascia is progressively divided on either side of the vessels until the clavicle is reached. Here the vessels can be freed totally from the muscle and allowed to drop away, rendering a true vascular island of the composite bloc. The clavicular origin of the muscle then is sharply divided along the clavicle, creating a bipedicle flap of muscle paralleling the overlying bipedicle flap of skin and fat. The muscle rent need be only large enough to allow passage of the entire compound paddle up through the muscle and skin onto the chest.

If neck dissection has not been done, the skin and platysma of the neck also are elevated as a broad bipedicle flap to the level of the defect, and the flap again is passed through. A half-twist of the ribbon-like pedicle is necessary to bring the curve of the rib into accord with that of the mandible, or the rib can be rolled down one-half turn to accomplish the same alignment.

If, on bringing the rib and skin island to their respective defects, there is tension on the pedicle as it crosses the clavicle, a broad half-thickness notch in that structure will bring relief (as we have added on two occasions). Assuming proper elevation and handling of the flap, bleeding can be elicited from the muscle cuff about the rib and from the rib ends.

If symphysis replacement is required, burred grooves through the concave cortical rib surface will cause free flow of blood and allow appropriate bending for chin contour, which is maintained by wires. For such symphysis replacement, the rib ends are freed of soft tissue, burred of outermost cortex, and inserted within the cleared cancellous portions of the cut mandibular ends, where they are transfixed. For horizontal and ascending ramus replacement, overlapping mortised joints are fashioned and wired. In all cases, prolonged external biphasic splinting is added, allowing full jaw motion throughout the postoperative period.

Skin islands have replaced lining from the levels of the hypopharynx and contralateral posterior pharyngeal wall to the anterior floor of the mouth, tongue, and cheek. When concomitant cover is required, an intervening buried deepithelialized strip is necessary between intraoral and extraoral portions of the flap.

Small defects of the pleura are closed directly, while larger ones require a chest tube. When direct closure of the skin defect is possible without tension, such as when the skin island is needed for lining alone, an anterior border strap flap of latissimus dorsi muscle is transposed to cover the pleura and fill out the muscle defect of the chest wall. When defects are closed in the wake of skin islands needed to replace both lin-

ing and cover, a latissimus dorsi musculocutaneous flap allows secure closure without displacement of chest wall landmarks (Fig. 4).

CLINICAL RESULTS

The bony fifth rib within a composite bloc based on a nonmuscular pedicle has been transferred to the mandible of six patients. All had massive (T_3 or T_4) or recurrent cancers, and all had received prior irradiation to the jaw and neck (two with added interstitial dosage). Half required replacement of cover, as well as lining, during their jaw reconstructions. All flaps survived and healed under these unfavorable conditions.

One patient suffered a minor partial-thickness marginal loss to a portion of the chest paddle extended beyond the anterior axillary line. This healed spontaneously without treatment. Three patients died within 4 months of surgery (two from tumor and one of postoperative stroke), all with satisfactory reconstructions essentially intact. The remaining three patients demonstrate a solid mandible with good range of motion and residual occlusion. Speech and oral function have been good.

One patient developed a minor anterior separation of lining and required a chest tube for 1 week because of a pleural tear that was otherwise without consequence. No chest tube was required in the remaining five patients.

In a prior patient in whom a full-thickness muscular pedicle was used, total flap loss followed efforts to reduce the muscular element to allow passage through an undissected neck. We consider the recommended nonmuscular technique safer in achieving a truly narrower pedicle.

In using the skeletonized, nonmuscular pedicle, functional pectoral loss is minimized. We do not suggest that total function is preserved by this maneuver, however, because the remaining muscle must be denervated to a greater or lesser degree when the nutrient pathways with their inevitable neural components are freed from the muscle. Some muscle wasting results, producing a deformity, but the deformity is mild and subtle compared with the alternative of complete muscle division with retraction of medial and lateral parts.

SUMMARY

One-stage reconstruction of the mandible, including both cover and lining, with the lateral pectoral (pectoralis major-pectoralis minor) osteomusculocutaneous flap is well worth the extra surgical effort involved.

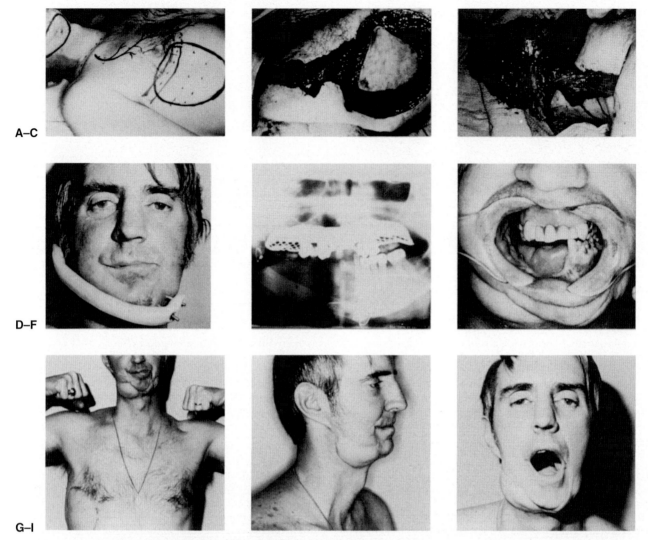

FIG. 4. A: A 44-year-old man with osteoradionecrosis of the mandible and recurrent mucoepidermoid carcinoma treated by composite excision, including lining, mandibular body, and skin. Extirpation and reconstruction marked. **B:** Flap elevated and laid over chest, showing thin pedicle, pectoralis muscle, and skin paddle. **C:** Flap elevated and laid over neck showing bleeding fifth rib. **D:** Early postoperative view with mandibular splint in place. **E:** Postoperative Panorex of jaw at 14 months. **F:** Postoperative occlusion. **G:** Postoperative donor site; note latissimus dorsi musculocutaneous patch. **H,I:** Postoperative views at 14 months. (From Little et al., ref. 1, with permission.)

References

1. Little JW III, McCulloch DT, Lyons JR. The lateral pectoral composite flap in one-stage reconstruction of the irradiated mandible. *Plast Reconstr Surg* 1983;71:326.
2. Ariyan S. Pectoralis major, sternomastoid, and other musculocutaneous flaps for head and neck reconstruction. *Clin Plast Surg* 1980;7:89.
3. Ariyan S, Cuono CB. Myocutaneous flaps for head and neck reconstruction. *Head Neck Surg* 1980;2:321.
4. Cuono CB, Ariyan S. Immediate reconstruction of a composite mandibular defect with a regional osteomusculocutaneous flap. *Plast Reconstr Surg* 1980;65:477.
5. Landra AP. One-stage reconstruction of a massive gunshot wound of the lower face with a local compound osteomusculocutaneous flap. *Br J Plast Surg* 1981;34:395.
6. Biller HF, Baek S, Lawson W, et al. Pectoralis major myocutaneous island flap in head and neck surgery: analysis of complications in 42 cases. *Arch Otolaryngol* 1981;107:23.
7. Williams PL, Warwick R, eds. *Gray's anatomy,* 36th Ed. Philadelphia: Saunders, 1980.
8. Siemssen SO, Kirkby B, O'Connor TPF. Immediate reconstruction of a resected segment of the lower jaw using a compound flap of clavicle and sternomastoid muscle. *Plast Reconstr Surg* 1978;61:724.
9. Green MF, Gibson JR, Bryson JR, Thomson E. A one-stage correction of mandibular defects using a split sternum pectoralis major osteomusculocutaneous transfer. *Br J Plast Surg* 1981;34:11.
10. Ariyan S, Finseth FJ. The anterior chest approach for obtaining free osteocutaneous rib grafts. *Plast Reconstr Surg* 1978;62:67.
11. Ariyan S. The viability of rib grafts transplanted with periosteal blood supply. *Plast Reconstr Surg* 1980;65:140.
12. Manktelow RT, McKee NH, Vettese T. An anatomical study of the pectoralis major muscle as related to functioning free muscle transplantation. *Plast Reconstr Surg* 1980;65:610.
13. Freeman JL, Walker EP, Wilson JSP, Shaw HJ. The vascular anatomy of the pectoralis major myocutaneous flap. *Br J Plast Surg* 1981;34:3.
14. Nakajima H, Maruyama Y, Kocla E. The definition of vascular skin territories with prostaglandin E1: the anterior chest, abdomen and thigh-inguinal region. *Br J Plast Surg* 1981;34:258.
15. Magee WP, Gilbert DA, McInnis WD. Extended muscle and musculocutaneous flaps. *Clin Plast Surg* 1980;7:57.

CHAPTER 194 ■ VASCULARIZED OUTER TABLE CALVARIAL BONE FLAP

J. M. PSILLAKIS

The outer table of the calvarium has become an increasingly important donor site for bone grafts in craniofacial surgery (1–5). It is close to the operative field, it has a membranous origin similar to that of the facial skeleton, there is an inconspicuous donor-site scar, and there is relatively little postoperative pain.

The vascularized outer table calvarial bone flap can be taken from any part of the skull, but in most cases I use the parietal region as the donor area, and the blood supply is carried by the periosteum in continuity with the deep fascial layer of the temporal aponeurosis.

INDICATIONS

This flap is useful for bone loss in the frontal area, supraorbital region, zygomatic region up to the level of the nose, maxillary area in the middle third of the face, and the mandibular area up to the level of the chin.

ANATOMY

The superficial temporal artery continues cranially anterior to the ear at the level of the superficial fascia of the head, more commonly known as the SMAS, and gives off large branches to the parietal and frontal areas. Relatively large perforators of the superficial temporal artery are given off that penetrate into the calvarium primarily at suture lines. There are multiple anastomoses between the superficial temporal system and the middle meningeal arterial arcade within the diploic space.

The periosteum over the frontal parietal region continues with a thin layer over the deep temporal fascia. At the level of the zygomatic arch, proximal branches from the superficial temporal vessels anastomose within the deep temporal muscle. This system irrigates the periosteum even in the absence of large perforating branches from the distal superficial temporal artery. The outer table of the calvarial bone in the frontal parietal region receives numerous small perforators from the vascular network within the periosteum. These perforators do not significantly contribute to the blood supply of the inner table. The inner table is more vascularized by the meningeal vessels. Because of the existence of this random system of anastomosing vessels from the superficial and deep arteries through the temporalis fascia and periosteum, a periosteal flap can be designed using this layer as a pedicle carrying a segment of the outer table of the calvarium (Fig. 1). If only the outer table is to be used, it is unnecessary to include the galea and the superficial temporal artery to maintain the blood supply to the bone. If the full thickness of the bone is to be used, it is important to include the galea and the superficial temporal vessels in the flap. The thickness of the calvarium is variable from one region to the other, but a special study performed in 100 cadavers showed that the thickness of the parietal area is 5 mm, with a range of 4 to 6 mm.

FLAP DESIGN AND DIMENSIONS

With a pivot point in the zygomatic arch, the vascularized outer table calvarial bone flap can reach the forehead, the zygomatic region, and the mandible up to the level of the chin. The bone can be as long as needed to go from one temporal region to the other. The width can be variable, but it is easier to take bone flaps from a maximum width of 5 cm. If larger areas are necessary, a more careful cut of the bone is necessary to avoid damage to the inner table. I was able to take up to 10 cm in width without creating a lesion in the inner table. The pedicle must include the deep temporal fascia and the loose tissue that is found over it. If a long pedicle is needed, the temporal fascia must be cut in a curved shape with the pivot point more posteriorly on the zygomatic arch. The width of the fascia at the level of the zygomatic arch may range from 5 to 8 cm.

OPERATIVE TECHNIQUE

The skull is exposed through a coronal incision and subgaleal dissection. Care is taken to avoid injury to the proximal branches of the superficial temporal artery within 2 cm of the zygomatic arch. The size and shape of the bone graft are determined, and an appropriate pattern of the graft is marked in the periosteum of the parietal or frontal bone behind the hairline. This pattern is at least 2 to 3 mm larger than the actual graft needed.

The periosteum along the perimeter of the pattern is cut, except inferiorly, where the bone is to be pedicled. With a pneumatic saw, the bone then is cut through the outer cortex into the diploic space. The groove created by the pneumatic saw then is used to insert the pediatric Gigli saw into the distal extremity of the flap to cut through the diploic space. As the saw approaches the pedicle proximally, gentle upward pressure will cut the inferior bony margin without disrupting the

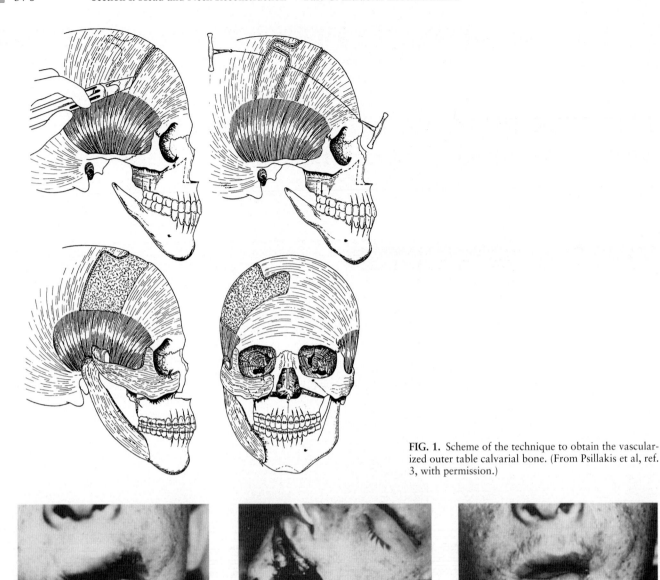

FIG. 1. Scheme of the technique to obtain the vascularized outer table calvarial bone. (From Psillakis et al, ref. 3, with permission.)

A–C

FIG. 2. A: Partial loss of the mandible from a gunshot wound. **B:** Intraoperative view of the technique described. **C:** Postoperative appearance.

delicate fascial pedicle. This method can be used to elevate bone flaps up to 5 cm in width. If a larger bone flap is necessary, long, flexible, thin saw blades can be used. For segments of bone up to 3 cm, the thin and flexible pneumatic saw can be used for cutting through the diploe. The chisel also can be used for narrow segments, and specific designs of chisels have been published, but I think the chisel is much more risky to take bone from the skull than the method just described.

CLINICAL RESULTS

The results of this operation have been very satisfactory (Fig. 2). The outer table calvarial bone has almost no resorption, and it retains volume well. It is also quite hard, and its curvature is ideal for modeling the bone and creating projection where necessary.

SUMMARY

The outer table of the skull can be brought down as a vascularized bone flap for various facial defects.

References

1. McCarthy JG. Zide BM. The spectrum of calvarial bone grafting: introduction of the vascularized calvarial bone flap. *Plast Reconstr Surg* 1984;74:10.
2. Pensler J, McCarthy JG. The calvarial donor site: an anatomic study in cadavers. *Plast Reconstr Surg* 1985;75:648.
3. Psillakis JM, Grotting JC, Casanova R, et al. Vascularized outer table calvarial bone flaps. *Plast Reconstr Surg* 1986;78:309.
4. Casanova R, Cavalcante D, Grotting JC, et al. Anatomic basis for vascularized outer-table calvarial bone flaps. *Plast Reconstr Surg* 1986;78:300.
5. McCarthy JG. Vascularized outer-table calvarial bone flaps (Discussion). *Plast Reconstr Surg* 1986;78:318.

CHAPTER 195 ■ MICROVASCULAR FREE TRANSFER OF A DORSALIS PEDIS FLAP FOR INTRAORAL LINING

L. A. SHARZER

The oral cavity, it was thought, had certain characteristics that rendered it unsuitable as a free-flap recipient site (1,2). Subsequent reports (3–7) indicated that it is possible to transfer free flaps safely to the oral cavity, and although this mode of reconstruction has not become the first-line treatment of choice, it is nevertheless an essential part of the reconstructive surgeon's armamentarium.

INDICATIONS

Of the available free-flap donor sites for intraoral reconstruction, the dorsum of the foot has several distinct advantages. Its thinness and pliability make it especially suitable to replace oral lining. The free dorsalis pedis flap is of suitable size, and it has a long vascular pedicle. It is also possible to transfer it as an osteocutaneous flap by including the second metatarsus (see Chapter 203). Finally, the distance between the foot and the mouth makes a two-team approach very practical, without increased operating time.

ANATOMY

The vascular anatomy and technique of elevation of the dorsalis pedis flap are described in Chapter 518.

FLAP DESIGN AND DIMENSIONS

Arteriography of the dorsum of the foot is routine prior to dorsalis pedis flap elevation. It is necessary to assess the patency, location, and source of the dorsalis pedis artery as well as the adequacy of the posterior tibial circulation. Two views are necessary, particularly the lateral view, if an augmented flap is required, and a decision must be made regarding the need for delay.

A reasonable approximation of size and shape, however, can be made from preoperative evaluation of the lesion. The flap then should be designed slightly larger than the anticipated need. The vascular pedicle should be taken long enough to allow for sufficient leeway in choice of recipient vessel. This is particularly important in the irradiated patient, because it is best to choose a recipient artery outside the area of irradiation. Venous drainage of the flap is by means of the greater saphenous vein and the venae comitantes of the dorsalis pedis artery; therefore, both should be taken long enough to allow freedom in choosing a recipient vein. Either one will provide adequate venous drainage.

It is important to remember that because free-flap reconstruction is planned, possible recipient vessels should not be sacrificed unnecessarily. It is, of course, axiomatic that the choice of this method of reconstruction must not compromise the adequacy of the resection for cure of the cancer. Unlike free-flap transfer to other sites, where a specific recipient artery is planned, the surgeon must be well versed in the vascular anatomy of the head and neck area and have in mind a variety of possible recipient vessels. Frequent choices are the facial artery and vein (retrograde from the face), lingual or superior thyroid artery (if end-to-end arterial anastomosis is desired), or the external carotid artery (if end-to-side anastomosis is preferred).

OPERATIVE TECHNIQUE

Delay is rarely necessary before intraoral transfer of a dorsalis pedis flap. The only indication for delay is the requirement for a large flap that includes the "random" portion of the dorsal foot skin. This is the portion of skin distal to the perforating branch of the dorsalis pedis artery in those patients in whom the first dorsal metatarsal artery is of a type II configuration. In these patients, my method of delay is to elevate the distal portion of the flap as far proximally as the perforating branch and to ligate this branch. The flap then is replaced in situ and reelevated 7 to 10 days later. Most oral cancers, even large ones, have a small enough mucosal presentation that an undelayed flap will suffice.

For details of flap elevation see Chapter 518. If marginal circulation is in question, it can be tested with fluorescein. The flap is transferred to the oral cavity and held in place with a few sutures, and the vascular anastomoses are carried out (Fig. 1). It is my preference to perform the arterial anastomosis first; however, the order of vascular connections is probably not important. Once circulation is established, a watertight intraoral closure is performed, followed by routine wound closure. Monitoring of the flap in the postoperative period is by hourly observation of color and capillary refill as well as by palpation or Doppler examination of the dorsalis pedis artery.

CLINICAL RESULTS

There are two disadvantages to this type of intraoral reconstruction. Free flaps are generally an all-or-nothing procedure. Early vascular thrombosis leads to complete flap necrosis, in contrast to pedicle flap reconstruction, where partial necrosis or fistula formation is the most common complication, but

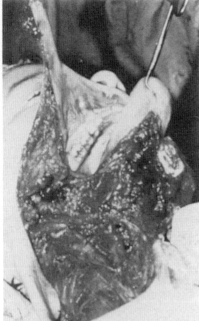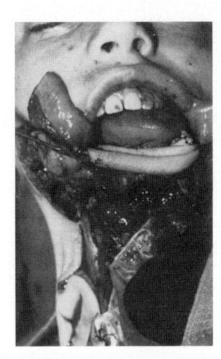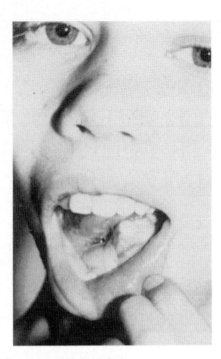

A–C

FIG. 1. A: Large intraoral wound following composite resection for mandibular sarcoma. B: Dorsalis pedis flap being inset. Flap has been sutured to base of tongue; anterior border is free. C: Postoperative appearance of flap.

complete flap loss is rare. Specific disadvantages of the dorsalis pedis flap relate to donor-site morbidity; however, because these flaps are relatively small, donor-site complications are unusual.

SUMMARY

Free dorsalis pedis flap transfer for intraoral lining is not the usual first-line treatment. Nevertheless, it is a reliable, safe alternative and a valuable addition to our choice of reconstructive procedures.

References

1. Kaplan EN, Buncke HJ, Murray DE. Distal transfer of cutaneous island flaps in humans by microvascular anastomoses. *Plast Reconstr Surg* 1973;52:301.
2. Finseth F, Kavarana N, Antia N. Complications of free-flap transfers to the mouth region. *Plast Reconstr Surg* 1975;56:562.
3. Leek D, Ben-Hur N, Mazzarella L. Reconstruction of the floor of the mouth with a free dorsalis pedis flap. *Plast Reconstr Surg* 1977;59:379.
4. Sharzer LA, Horton CE, Adamson JE, et al. Intraoral reconstruction in head and neck cancer surgery. *Clin Plast Surg* 1976;3:495.
5. Panje WR, Bardach J, Krause CJ. Reconstruction of the oral cavity with a free flap. *Plast Reconstr Surg* 1976;58:415.
6. Franklin JD, Withers EH, Madden JJ, Lynch JB. Use of the free dorsalis pedis flap in head and neck repairs. *Plast Reconstr Surg* 1979;63:195.
7. Schlenker JD, Robson MC, Parsons RW. Methods and results of reconstruction with free flaps following resection of squamous cell carcinoma of the head and neck. *Ann Plast Surg* 1981;6:362.

CHAPTER 196 ■ INNERVATED GRACILIS MUSCULOCUTANEOUS FLAP FOR TOTAL TONGUE RECONSTRUCTION

N. J. YOUSIF AND W. W. DZWIERZYNSKI

EDITORIAL COMMENT

A number of flaps for reconstruction of the total tongue have been described, and they include—besides the innervated gracilis—the radial forearm, the lateral arm flap, as well as the rectus abdominis. One should not forget that possibly the most important factors for deglutition are the remaining muscles in the undersurface of the resected tongue. Restoration of sensibility should also be an important objective and can be achieved by performing an anastomosis either end-to-end or end-to-side to the lingual nerve.

Reconstruction after total glossectomy is a difficult problem in head and neck reconstructive surgery. The tongue is essential in swallowing, speech, and airway protection (1). Tongue function is achieved by the complex interactions of the intrinsic and extrinsic musculature and their nerve innervation (2,3). To obtain active muscle function for a neo-tongue, we utilize an innervated transverse gracilis myocutaneous flap. Recreating all the complex motions of the tongue is currently impossible, but the innervated gracilis flap is used in an attempt to recreate one of these functions—elevation (4). Elevation of the neo-tongue can potentially help the glossectomy patient achieve airway protection and improved propulsion of the food bolus.

INDICATIONS

Innervated tongue reconstruction is indicated for total glossectomy defects after cancer extirpation surgery (5,6). Most conventional tongue reconstructions provide only bulk (7,8). For partial glossectomy defects, in which some muscle innervation remains, addition of bulk may be sufficient (9). For patients undergoing total glossectomy, innervated gracilis reconstruction offers the cancer patient hope of restoration of some aspects of tongue function.

ANATOMY

The dominant vascular pedicle from the profunda femoris artery to the gracilis enters the muscle 10 cm below the pubic tubercle. The artery at its origin is 1.5 to 2 mm in diameter. It is accompanied by two venae comitantes. The main arterial pedicle divides into three to six vessels, ranging in length between 1 and 2 cm, before entering the muscle. In the upper third of the gracilis muscle, three to six musculocutaneous perforators supply the overlying skin. A septocutaneous perforator can sometimes be found running between the gracilis and the adductor longus muscle. The middle and distal thirds of the skin overlying the gracilis muscle are supplied by vessels from the superficial femoral and saphenous arteries. The unreliability of this distal skin component of the traditional longitudinally designed gracilis myocutaneous free flap has limited its usefulness in the treatment of larger defects (10). Vertical orientation of the skin paddle allows a more robust and reliable blood supply to the cutaneous paddle (11).

The motor-nerve supply to the gracilis muscle is the anterior branch of the obturator nerve, which is located between the abductor magnus and the abductor longus muscles. The nerve enters the muscle immediately superior to the dominant vascular pedicle, on its deep medial surface.

FLAP DESIGN AND DIMENSIONS

The skin paddle is designed to reconstruct the bulk of the resected tongue and pharynx. Skin paddles as large as 10 × 20 cm can be harvested for tongue reconstruction. With the patient in the supine position, the knee and hip are flexed, and the lower extremity is abducted. A line is drawn 10 cm inferior to the pubic tubercle, perpendicular to the axis of the gracilis muscle. This line marks the center of the cutaneous paddle of the transverse gracilis flap. A crescent-shaped skin paddle is designed; the width of the cutaneous segment is determined by the amount of skin in the upper medial thigh that can be removed, while allowing direct closure (Fig. 1). An incision is made along the anterior margin of the flap down to, and including, the fascia lata. Flap dissection continues from anterior-to-posterior in a subfascial plane until the intermuscular septum.

The septofasciocutaneous and myofasciocutaneous perforators from the dominant pedicle are identified, protected, and included in the flap. The adductor longus muscle is retracted anteriorly, to gain better exposure of the flap pedicle. Dissection of the pedicle continues to the profunda femoris artery and vein. A pedicle length of 6 to 8 cm can be achieved. The nerve to the gracilis lies immediately superior to the vessels; it is dissected to its branching point. A posterior incision is made along the flap margin, including the deep fascia of the thigh, and dissection proceeds anteriorly to the posterior border of the gracilis. The gracilis muscle is then separated from the adductor longus and adductor magnus muscles. The entire gracilis muscle is included with the flap for fabrication of a dynamic sling. The donor site is reliable and well known to most microsurgeons.

OPERATIVE TECHNIQUE

The initial flap dissection can be started simultaneously with the cancer extirpative surgery. The width of the gracilis skin

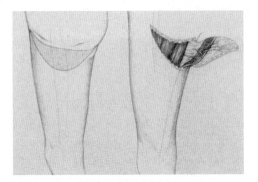

FIG. 1. Drawing of donor site (**left**) and shin paddle (**right**).

paddle is chosen to allow direct closure of the donor site; this is usually 6 to 10 cm. After cancer extirpation, the recipient vessels are identified in the neck. For the recipient vessel, the external carotid artery can be used in an end-to-side fashion; or one of its branches, the lingual or superior thyroid artery, can be used with an end-to-end anastomosis. The external jugular vein or one of its branches is usually chosen for the venous outflow. The hypoglossal nerve stump is preserved for neurotization of the neo-tongue (4).

The orientation of the gracilis muscle is critical. The muscle is oriented transversely to form a sling, achieving elevation of the neo-tongue with active muscle contraction. The ends of the muscle are fastened laterally to the mandibular arch. This is achieved with a Mitek suture anchor (DePuy Mitek, Raynham, MA) inserted into the mandible body or its remnant (Fig. 2). If a mandible reconstruction is required, the gracilis muscle is suspended to the periosteum of the remaining mandible or by using direct suture fixation to the reconstruction plate on the fibula flap. The muscle is centrally secured to the hyoid bones. The skin pedicle, which is oriented perpendicularly to the muscle, is used to close the intraoral defect and is folded to produce a neo-tongue (12). Sufficient bulk must be available to allow palatoglossal contact. After the gracilis is suspended, the vascular anastomoses are performed. The motor nerve to the gracilis is coapted to the hypoglossal nerve on one side.

CLINICAL RESULTS

Surgical difficulties encountered in creating a neo-tongue with the transverse gracilis technique are minimal. Because of the abundant subcutaneous tissue on the flap, attachment of the gracilis to the mandible is the greatest challenge. In all patients, bulk was maintained during postoperative follow-up; however, decreased bulk in the flap may occur following radiation therapy. Excessive bulk may also pose a problem: in one patient, a suction lipectomy was required to achieve tracheostomy decannulation. Prognosis in patients requiring a total glossectomy is generally poor. The innervated gracilis musculocutaneous flap offers palliation and, in the occasional survivor, long-term improved reconstruction (13).

SUMMARY

The innervated gracilis musculocutaneous flap is currently our preferred method of reconstruction of large total glossec-

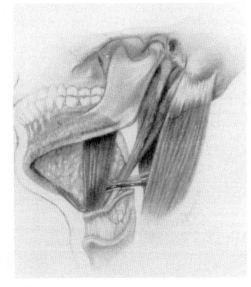

FIG. 2. Attachment of gracilis muscle to mandible transversely as seen from below.

tomy defects. The bulk of the cutaneous pedicle and muscle is superior to other methods of static reconstruction. The donor site is reliable and well known to most microsurgeons. With the addition of a single-nerve anastomosis, the innervated gracilis flap offers a reconstructive option that can replace bulk and can offer the potential for improved physiologic motion.

References

1. Yu P, Robb GL. Reconstruction for total and near-total glossectomy defects. *Clin Plast Surg* 2005;32:411.
2. McConnell FMS. Analysis of pressure generation and bolus transit during pharyngeal swallowing. *Laryngoscope* 1988;98:71.
3. Urken ML, Moscoso J, Lawson W, Biller HF. A systematic approach to functional reconstruction of the oral cavity following partial and total glossectomy. *Arch Otolaryngol Head Neck Surg* 1994;120:589.
4. Yousif NJ, Dzwierzynski WW, Sanger JR, et al. The innervated gracilis musculocutaneous flap for total tongue reconstruction. *Plast Reconstr Surg* 1999;104:916.
5. Urken ML, Turk JB, Weinberg H, et al. The rectus abdominis free flap in head and neck reconstruction. *Arch Otolaryngol Head Neck Surg* 1991;117:857.
6. Sultan MR, Coleman JJ III. Oncologic and functional considerations of total glossectomy. *Am J Surg* 1989;158:297.
7. Matloub H, Larson D, Kuhn J, et al. Lateral arm free flap in oral cavity reconstruction: a functional evaluation. *Head Neck* 1989;11:205.
8. Sanger JR, Campbell BH, Ye Z, et al. Tongue reconstruction with a combined brachioradialis-radial forearm flap. *J Reconstr Microsurg* 2000;16:7.
9. Cheng N, Shou B, Zheng M, Huang A. Microneurovascular transfer of the tensor fasciae latae musculocutaneous flap for reconstruction of the tongue. *Ann Plast Surg* 1994;33:136.
10. Whetzel TP, Lechtman AN. The gracilis myofasciocutaneous flap: vascular anatomy and clinical application. *Plast Reconstr Surg* 1997;99:1642.
11. Yousif NJ, Matloub HS, Kolachalam R, et al. The transverse gracilis musculocutaneous flap. *Ann Plast Surg* 1992;29:482.
12. Yoleri L. Total tongue reconstruction with free functional gracilis muscle transplantation: a technical note and review of the literature. *Ann Plast Surg* 2000;45:181.
13. Wechselberger G, Schoeller T, Bauer T, et al. Surgical technique and clinical application of the transverse gracilis myocutaneous free flap. *Br J Plast Surg* 2001;54:423.

CHAPTER 197 ■ SCAPULAR OSTEOCUTANEOUS FLAP

W. M. SWARTZ

Scapular and parascapular cutaneous flaps of the back (1–6) may be combined with the osseous territory of the lateral border of the scapula to provide versatile osteocutaneous free flaps based on the circumflex scapular artery. A wide variety of tissue combinations have been used extensively for head and neck reconstruction of both the mandible and maxilla (7) and also for reconstruction of tibial osseous defects (8).

INDICATIONS

The principal indication for the scapular osteocutaneous flap in head and neck surgery has been mandibular reconstruction.

Osseous defects of the mandible of up to 14 cm, in conjunction with large cutaneous or intraoral mucosal defects, are well suited for this application. Great freedom in spatial orientation of skin and bone is allowed. Through-and-through defects of the cheek, combined with sagittal mandibular defects, also can be reconstructed with this flap, as can anterior mandible defects (9). The length of the vascular pedicle easily reaches the external carotid system under most conditions. In addition, the scapular bone can be used for the maxilla and the infraorbital rim in maxillectomy defects. A great amount and variety of soft tissues are available for restoring cheek skin, palatal tissue, or obliteration of the maxillary sinuses.

ANATOMY

The blood supply to the lateral border of the scapula is derived from a descending branch of the circumflex scapular artery just before its emergence through the triangular space, where it then arborizes to supply the cutaneous circulation. The distal third of the scapula is supplied additionally by the terminal branches of the thoracodorsal artery (Fig. 1). This anatomic relationship

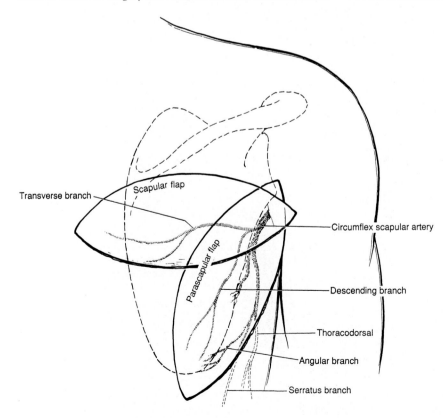

FIG. 1. Diagrammatic rendition of blood supply to the lateral border of the scapula.

is important when planning osteotomies of the distal third of the scapula: If the thoracodorsal circulatory system is not included in the flap, osteotomies in the distal third risk necrosis of the bone. The entire border of the scapula, including the tip, may be well served by the proximal blood supply, provided that osteotomies in the distal third are not performed.

After giving off branches to the muscles surrounding the lateral border of the scapula, the circumflex scapular artery emerges through the triangular space, bound by the long head of the triceps and the teres major and teres minor muscles. The skin circulation then arborizes into a transverse branch and a descending branch, which provide the directional basis for the parascapular flap and transverse scapular flap. The skin flap also can be oriented toward the margin of the breast into the axilla.

The vascular pedicle is derived from the subscapular artery and, as such, derives a length about 4 to 5 cm to the lateral border of the scapula. Should a skin-only flap be used, a longer pedicle of 6 to 9 cm is possible. The diameter of the subscapular artery is 2.0 to 2.5 mm. Paired venae comitantes accompany the circumflex artery; they join into a single large vein near the axillary vein.

FLAP DESIGN AND DIMENSIONS

The osseous portion of the flap extends from just below the glenoid fossa to the tip of the scapula and may include the entire tip should reconstructive needs require. Up to 14 cm of bone length are available in the adult male. The cutaneous flap can be designed either transversely or obliquely, depending on soft-tissue requirements. Additionally, multiple skin paddles can be developed with separation of the skin, leaving connections in the subdermal plexus. This kind of arrange-

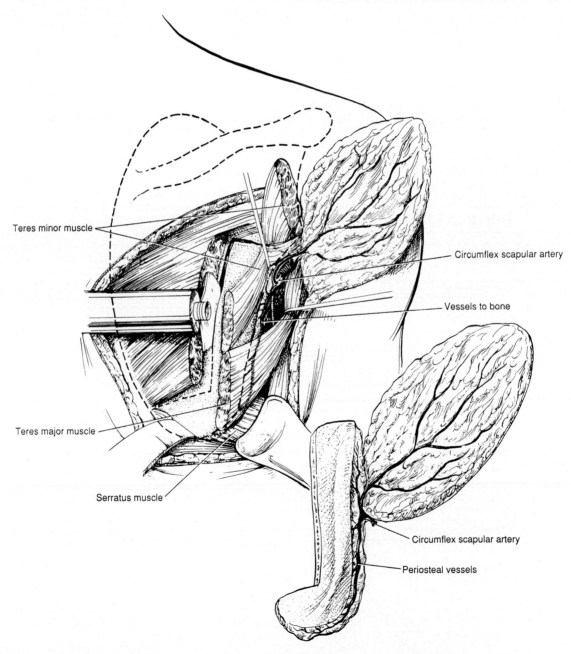

FIG. 2. Diagram illustrating anatomic landmarks involved in sharp division of teres major along with the branches of the serratus muscle. The bone is then cut through.

ment is helpful for providing intraoral and extraoral skin requirements.

OPERATIVE TECHNIQUE

The surgical procedure is carried out in either the prone or lateral positions, depending on recipient-site requirements. The proximal portion of the skin paddle is centered over the triangular space, which, in turn, lies along the upper border of the scapula. Preoperatively, the cutaneous distribution of the lateral and descending branches of the circumflex scapular artery is identified using transcutaneous ultrasonic Doppler evaluation. The arm is draped with a stockinette, allowing freedom of arm motion during the dissection. The skin then is incised down to the loose areolar plane directly above the infraspinatus muscle.

I prefer to elevate the skin island from medial to lateral, identifying the vessels in the subcutaneous plane on the underside of thy, flap. The subscapular artery then is followed into the triangular space at the lateral border of the scapula. It is important not to separate the circumflex scapular artery from the lateral border of the scapula in this dissection. The dissection is carried on the lateral border of the circumflex scapular artery through the triangular space. Several branches to the teres major and subscapular muscles are ligated to accomplish the vascular preparation.

If the latissimus dorsi muscle or the angular branch of the thoracodorsal vessels is required for a complex, multitissue reconstruction, an additional incision is made in the axilla and the thoracodorsal system is dissected. This maneuver is not necessary unless the latissimus or the terminal branch of the thoracodorsal vessel is required.

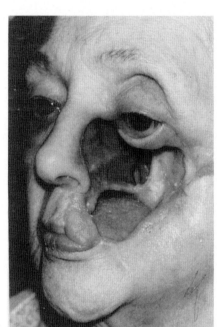
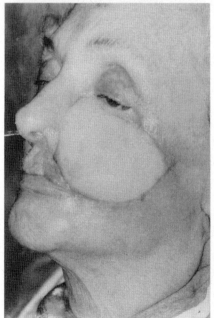

A,B

C

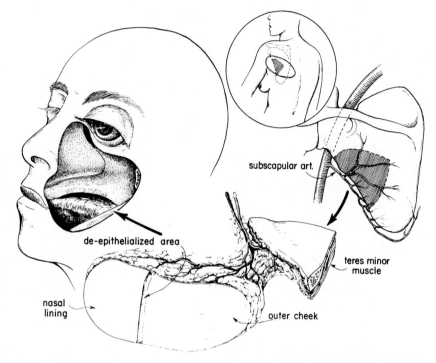

FIG. 3. An 86-year-old woman, following radical maxillectomy for squamous-cell carcinoma. **A:** Preoperative condition showing missing septum of nose, left nasal side wall, orbital floor, hard palate, and external cheek skin. **B:** Proposed surgical plan. Lateral border of scapula was designed to become new alveolar bone, stretching from the midline of the maxilla to the zygomatic arch. The thickest portion of the scapula was suitable for osteointegrated implants for later dental restoration; the thinner scapular blade formed the hard palate. A skin graft was used on the palatal surface over periosteum and muscle that accompanied the scapular bone. A large double-paddle scapular skin flap then formed the basis of the soft-tissue restoration, which included the nasal lining and external cheek skin. **C:** Early postoperative result.

At this time, the lateral border of the scapular bone is palpated as it joins the thinner central portion, and this is the site of the longitudinal osteotomy. Using a periosteal elevator, the teres major muscle is divided sharply along with the branches of the serratus muscle toward the tip of the scapula. Then, using an oscillating saw, the bone is cut through, either angulating toward the tip, if desired, or straight along the border (Fig. 2). A second cut is made transversely across the lateral border of the scapula about one finger breadth below the glenoid fossa. This portion of the dissection is somewhat bloody, and periosteal bleeders will require coagulation. An osteotome is used to complete the saw cuts, if necessary. Muscular attachments of the scapular border to the serratus muscle and teres muscle are sharply divided, and the bone then is elevated completely on its vascular pedicle. Vessels that contribute to the blood supply of the scapula will be identified at the time of cutting through these muscles.

When large flaps that need both the circumflex scapular artery and the thoracodorsal systems are required with an osteotomy in the central portion of the scapula, both the thoracodorsal and circumflex scapular systems are dissected. The teres major muscle straddles these two blood supplies. Either the teres major can be divided from its origin and resutured, or a portion of the flap can be passed through the triangular space to complete the dissection. With adequate retraction and a bit of a stretch, all but the largest flaps can be delivered into the axilla to join with the latissimus dissection and the thoracodorsal pedicle, thus avoiding division of the teres major muscle.

The scapular osteocutaneous donor site requires reattachment of the serratus and the teres muscle to the border of the scapula. These muscles are reapproximated with 2-0 Vicryl or Dexon sutures, without needing to drill holes in the border of the scapula. A drain is placed in the axilla, and the skin is closed primarily. Postoperatively, the shoulder is kept immobilized for 1 week, and gradual stretching exercises are begun. An example of the scapular osteocutaneous flap used for complex three-dimensional reconstruction requiring bone and soft tissue is presented (Fig. 3).

CLINICAL RESULTS

Our experience using this flap for a wide variety of mandibular and maxillary defects has encouraged us to recommend the flap without reservation. Donor-site morbidity is low, and shoulder motion is regained in most patients through a course of physical therapy commencing 1 week postoperatively.

SUMMARY

This flap provides a segment of corticocancellous bone up to 14 cm long that is well perfused on a vascular pedicle separate from the overlying skin island. Because of the rich subdermal plexus of the scapular and parascapular systems, extremely large multilobulated flaps can be fabricated for a wide variety of bone and soft-tissue defects. The rich blood supply to the scapular bone contributes to early bone union.

References

1. Dos Santos LF. The scapular flap: a new microsurgical free flap. *Rev Bras Cir* 1980;70:133.
2. Dos Santos LF. The vascular anatomy and dissection of the free scapular flap. *Plast Reconstr Surg* 1984;73:599.
3. Nassif TM, Vidal L, Bovet JL, Baudet J. The parascapular flap: a new cutaneous microsurgical free flap. *Plast Reconstr Surg* 1982;69:591.
4. Rowsell AR, Davis DM, Eisenberg N, et al. The anatomy of the subscapular-thoracodorsal arterial system: a study of 100 cadaver dissections. *Br J Plast Surg* 1984;37:574.
5. Gilbert A, Teot L. The free scapular flap. *Plast Reconstr Surg* 1982;69:6011.
6. Teot L, Bosse JP, Monfarrege R, et al. The scapular crest pedicled bone grafts. *Br J Microsurg* 1981;3:257.
7. Swartz WM, Banis JC, Newton ED, et al. The osteocutaneous scapular flap for mandibular and maxillary reconstruction. *Plast Reconstr Surg* 1986;77:530.
8. Sekeguchi J, Kobaygashi S, Ohmori K. Use of the osteocutaneous free scapular flap on the lower extremities. *Plast Reconstr Surg* 1993;91:1103.
9. Coleman JJ, Sultan MR. The bipedicled osteocutaneous scapular flap: a new subscapular system free flap. *Plast Reconstr Surg* 1991;87:682.

CHAPTER 198 ■ RADIAL FOREARM FREE FLAP IN INTRAORAL RECONSTRUCTION

D. S. SOUTAR AND I. A. MCGREGOR

EDITORIAL COMMENT

Postoperatively, the radius must be protected from undue stress because the incidence of fracture can be significant when a segment of the radius has been removed with the flap. The ulnar artery version of the forearm flap has not been included in the Encyclopedia because the safety of this flap is still being debated.

The radial forearm flap is a fasciocutaneous flap based on the radial artery and venae comitantes, together with the subcutaneous forearm veins. Several reports (1–5) already have demonstrated the versatility, usefulness, and reliability of this flap both as a pedicled flap in reconstructive surgery of the hand and as a free flap in the expanding field of free tissue transfer. This flap can be used as either a fasciocutaneous flap or as an osteofasciocutaneous flap (6,7) for reconstructing defects resulting from excision of intraoral malignancies.

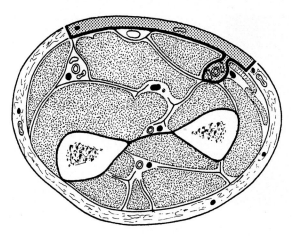

FIG. 1. Fasciocutaneous flap. Cross section through the forearm distal to pronator teres showing the position of the radial artery and the plane of dissection for elevation of the fasciocutaneous flap. (From Soutar et al., ref. 7, with permission.)

INDICATIONS

Resection techniques that preserve all or part of the mandible and reconstructive techniques that aim to restore mandibular continuity result in smaller intraoral defects. Such defects do not readily accommodate large bulky flaps without distorting the oral cavity and disturbing oral function and competence.

The radial forearm flap offers thin, pliable predominantly hairless skin that is well suited to replace oral mucosa following tumor excision. The flap readily conforms to the varying contours within the oral cavity and subsequently settles remarkably quickly, showing little or no evidence of contracture or "pincushioning" (Fig. 8). This may be related to the presence of the deep fascia on the undersurface of the flap that, perhaps, does not contract to the same degree as subcutaneous fat.

Bone may be included as an osteocutaneous flap to reconstruct the mandible and oral mucosa in a single stage (see Fig. 9). The fascial attachment of skin to bone allows a mobility of the skin that simplifies closure of the oral mucosa.

The donor defect is relatively painless, even in patients from whom bone has been removed. This causes the patient minimal discomfort in the early postoperative period, thus facilitating recovery and early mobilization. In the longer term, skin grafts on the forearm appear to give a satisfactory cosmetic result, particularly in elderly patients.

ANATOMY

Much of the skin of the forearm is supplied by the radial artery, which is covered proximally by the fleshy belly of the brachioradialis. It soon emerges distally between the brachioradialis and the flexor carpi radialis to lie superficially, covered only by skin, subcutaneous tissue, and the deep fascia.

The artery, together with its two venae comitantes, is invested in a condensation of the deep fascia known as the lateral intermuscular septum (Fig. 1). This septum separates the flexor and extensor compartments of the forearm and is attached to the periosteum of the radius distal to the insertion of pronator teres.

The artery gives off branches that pass through the deep fascia to supply the underlying flexor muscles and branches that spread out on the deep fascia to form a fascial plexus and supply the overlying skin. By means of this vascular network, the radial artery can supply the skin of the palmar and radial aspects of the forearm and provide a periosteal blood supply to the distal radius.

Venous drainage of the forearm flap is provided by two venae comitantes that accompany the artery and a variable pattern of subcutaneous forearm veins that drain into the cephalic, basilic, and median cubital veins. Routinely, both venous systems communicate by means of a constant branch from the venae comitantes, which drains into the median cubital vein.

The forearm flap is ideally suited for free-tissue transfer because the artery can be readily palpated for much of its length and the superficial subcutaneous veins of the forearm are easily identified. The diameter of the artery, usually in excess of 3 mm, remains relatively constant from its origin to the wrist joint, making anastomosis of either proximal or distal ends equally straightforward. Furthermore, the absence of significant arterial disease, particularly atheroma in elderly patients, has been most remarkable.

FLAP DESIGN AND DIMENSIONS

Using a template, a radial forearm flap can be designed to replace the amount of resected tissue accurately, thereby minimizing distortion and functional disturbance within the oral cavity. The radial artery, which is subcutaneous for much of its length in the forearm, can be palpated and its course marked on the skin surface. The superficial subcutaneous forearm veins are similarly marked, and the appropriately designed flap is outlined.

The arteriovenous system on which the forearm flap is based is capable of supplying all the skin of the forearm from above the elbow to the wrist, except for a narrow strip overlying the ulna posteriorly. In practice, such large flaps are not required in intraoral reconstruction.

The quality of the skin and the length of the vascular pedicle required for easy anastomosis most often influence the choice of donor site. The presence and distribution of hair on the forearm may influence site selection (Fig. 2), although

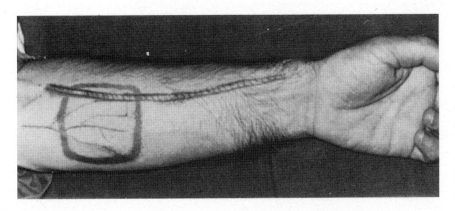

FIG. 2. Proximal fasciocutaneous flap. The radial artery and superficial veins were marked on the skin surface and a flap was designed on the non-hair-bearing skin. A distal arterial pedicle was raised and subsequently anastomosed to provide a retrograde arterial flow. (From Soutar et al., ref. 7, with permission.)

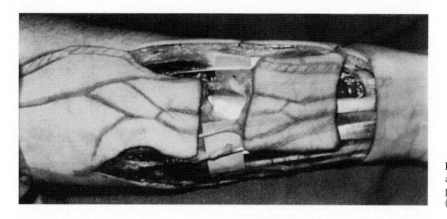

FIG. 3. Distal fasciocutaneous flap. The radial artery and subcutaneous veins are dissected out proximally. Note the exposed tendons distally. (From Soutar et al., ref. 7, with permission.)

such hairs tend to be short and fine and cause little following flap transfer.

Distally designed flaps are thinner than proximal flaps, and this is most evident in woman and obese patients. In addition, the distal design is chosen when bone is to be included (as an osteocutaneous flap) or when a long vessel pedicle is required. The advantages of the distal flap have to be balanced against the donor defect. In practice, the mid-forearm flap has proved to be most useful. It combines the advantages of ease of elevation and donor defect found in proximal flaps with the skin quality of distal flaps.

An added bonus of the midforearm flap lies in the possibility of raising both a proximal and distal vascular pedicle, allowing a certain freedom with regard to subsequent anastomosis because either end of the artery can be anastomosed in an antegrade or retrograde fashion and the free end ligated. Alternatively, the artery can be used as an interpositional graft. In this situation, the arterial flow appears to be more physiologic, matching more closely the preexisting conditions in the forearm.

OPERATIVE TECHNIQUE

Elevation of the forearm flap is straightforward and can be performed simultaneously with the intraoral resection without altering the patient's position on the operating table. Also, the vessels that supply this flap can be assessed accurately preoperatively and are fairly large and constant. This greatly simpli-

fies the technical aspects of this free-tissue transfer and may explain, in part, the reliability of the technique.

It can be difficult to determine which vein to use for anastomosis in free-tissue transfer, and on occasions, it has seemed prudent to anastomose both a superficial vein and a deep vena comitans. In other cases, useful information can be gained by selective clamping of the veins prior to transferring the flap. Where doubt exists, it is safer to perform the arterial anastomosis first, and following release of the arterial clamps, the pattern of venous outflow can be accurately determined and the appropriate vein then chosen for anastomosis.

The length of venous pedicle should never be a problem, since this can be extended well above the elbow, and in this

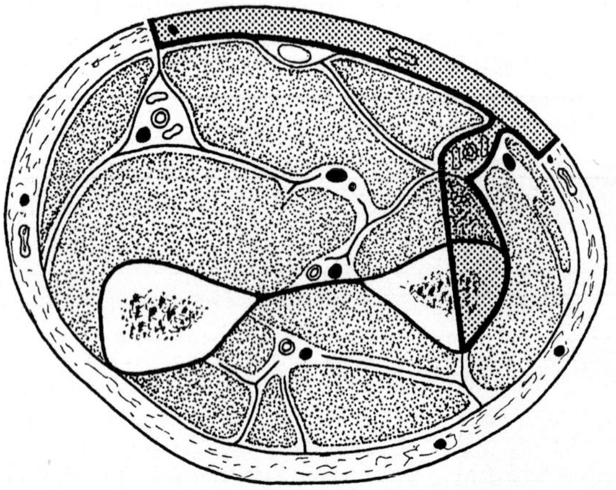

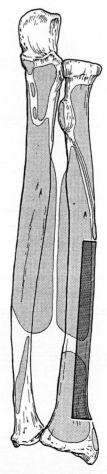

FIG. 4. Osteofasciocutaneous flap. Cross section through the forearm distal to pronator teres showing the plane of dissection for elevation of the osteocutaneous flap. (From Soutar et al., ref. 7, with permission.)

FIG. 5. The muscle attachments to the radius limit the length of bone available for transfer. (From Soutar et al., ref. 7, with permission.)

situation, a single venous anastomosis obviously will provide drainage for both superficial and accompanying venous systems.

Donor Site

After outlining an appropriately designed flap, dissection proceeds under tourniquet control following elevation exsanguination. This technique is preferred to more complete exsanguination methods, since it permits easier identification of vessels that still contain some blood. This aids the dissection and preservation of superficial veins and, in addition, facilitates the identification of the numerous vessels on the undersurface of the fascia that require ligation and division.

The margins of the flap are incised down to the deep fascia, preserving subcutaneous veins as required. It is easier to incise the fascia overlying muscle rather than that which overlies tendon, and for this reason, elevation of the flap commences proximally, most often at the posterior ulnar border, where the fascia is thickest and most readily identified.

The flap is raised in a subfascial plane, exposing muscle bellies proximally and tendons distally (Fig. 3). Intermuscular septa passing deeply are divided, as are the vessels that pass through the deep fascia to supply the underlying flexor mus-

cles. More distally, care must be taken to preserve the paratenon covering the flexor tendons to retain a defect suitable for skin grafting. The plane of dissection on the undersurface of the deep fascia ensures that the radial artery, lying in the lateral intermuscular septum, is included in the flap (see Fig. 1).

When raising a fasciocutaneous flap, the attachment of the lateral intermuscular septum to the periosteum of the radius must be divided to allow elevation of the radial artery and venae comitantes. With the vascular pedicle thus secured in the flap, the radial margin incision can be completed, again dissecting in a subfascial plane.

Retraction of the brachioradialis allows identification of the radial nerve, which may be isolated and preserved. The fasciocutaneous flap is now separated from the underlying musculature, but it remains attached by the radial artery and venae comitantes proximally and distally and by the previously isolated subcutaneous veins proximally. Longitudinal incisions can be made, as required, in a proximal or distal direction to dissect out sufficient length of vascular pedicle.

When bone is to be included as an osteocutaneous flap, the attachment of the lateral intermuscular septum to the periosteum of the radius must be preserved intact (Fig. 4). To reach the medial border of the radius, the plane of dissection passes deeply through the muscle bellies of the flexor pollicis longus and pronator quadratus. The lateral border of the radius has

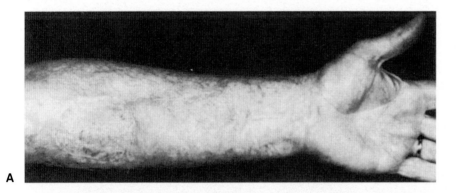

A

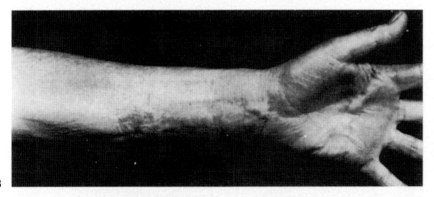

B

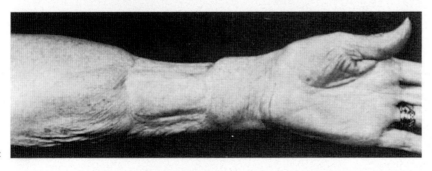

C

FIG. 6. Donor defect. A: Proximal defect at 6 months. B: Distal defect at 6 months. C: Distal defect extending over radial border at 9 months. (From Soutar et al., ref. 7, with permission.)

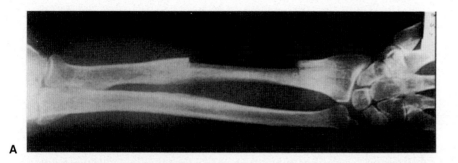

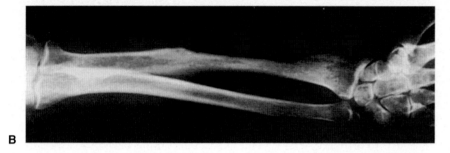

FIG. 7. Defect in radius at 3 weeks (**A**) and at 9 months (**B**) following removal of a 7-cm length of bone in a 72-year-old patient. (From Soutar et al., ref. 7, with permission.)

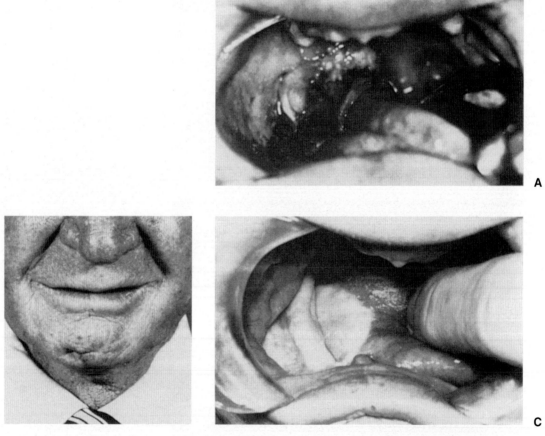

FIG. 8. The forearm flap as a fasciocutaneous flap. **A:** Squamous carcinoma involving the right lower alveolus, floor of mouth, and retromolar trigone in a 64-year-old patient. **B:** Postoperative appearance at 8 months following excision that included a rim resection of mandible. **C:** Intraoral appearance 8 months after operation. (From Soutar et al., ref. 7, with permission.)

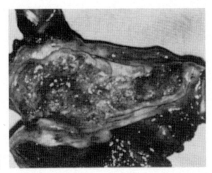
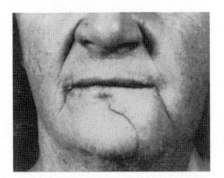

A,B

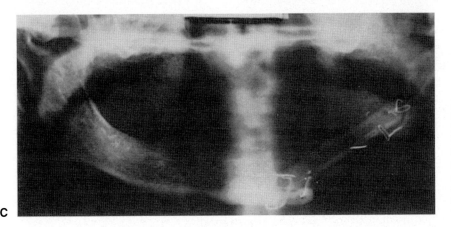

C

FIG. 9. The forearm flap as an osteocutaneous flap. **A:** Squamous cell carcinoma involving the left lower alveolus in a 63-year-old patient. Resection included 6.5 cm of underlying mandible. **B:** Appearance 5 weeks after operation. **C:** Postoperative radiograph at 3 weeks shows the position of a 6.5-cm segment of radius that was used to reconstruct the mandibular defect. (From Soutar et al., ref. 7, with permission.)

no such muscle attachments, but here the attachment of the lateral intermuscular septum, as it passes into the lateral periosteum of the radius, can be identified and preserved intact.

The length of bone that can be removed is limited by the muscle attachments to the radius and is restricted to that part which is attached to the lateral intermuscular septum (Fig. 5). This extends distally from the insertion of the pronator teres, and a length of up to 10 cm of bone extending to the insertion of brachioradialis can be obtained. The thickness of radius that can be removed safely is often difficult to determine in practice.

It is advisable to obtain preoperative radiographs of the forearm to exclude disease or deformity and to assess the thickness of the radius and cortices. Certainly, no more than half the cross section of the radius should be removed, and it is safer to err on the side of conservatism rather than to weaken the radius and risk subsequent fracture.

Occasionally, small defects in the forearm can be closed directly, but by far the majority require a split-thickness skin graft. Both graft survival and the late cosmetic result are often better in the proximal defect overlying muscle than on the paratenon of the distal defect. Confining the donor area to the palmar aspect of the forearm and avoiding the radial border also result in a more favorable cosmetic result (Fig. 6).

When bone is removed, immobilization in protective plaster is mandatory to limit use of the limb in the immediate postoperative period. Fracture of the radius has been reported in patients in whom such protective measures have not been carried out. Postoperative radiographs of the forearm can be used to monitor progress and to determine the degree and extent of immobilization required (Fig. 7).

An Allen test is performed routinely preoperatively to ensure viability of the hand devoid of a radial arterial input, and repair of the radial artery is therefore not essential. In practice, repair of the radial artery is performed when it is technically straightforward, and a segment of the cephalic vein that lies adjacent to the defect and has a caliber similar to the radial artery is a convenient donor for a reverse vein graft (Figs. 8 and 9).

CLINICAL RESULTS

The radial forearm flap has already proved to be safe and reliable in free-tissue transfer, and the use of this technique in intraoral reconstruction is similarly rewarding, with over 90% success reported in the authors' own series. Although the donor site is quite painless, there can be a problem with healing of the skin graft on the donor defect; however, delayed wound healing does not significantly alter the patient's progress or discharge from hospital. The risk of fracture following removal of bone from the radius has been mentioned, and in the authors' only such patient, the fracture healed uneventfully following immobilization in plaster for 6 weeks.

SUMMARY

The radial forearm flap offers thin, pliable, hairless skin that can conform well to the contours of the oral cavity. This technique has proved to be a safe, reliable, versatile, and convenient method of intraoral reconstruction.

References

1. Yang G, et al. Forearm free skin flap transplantation. *Natl Med J China* 1981;61:139.
2. Song R, Gao Y, Song Y, et al. The forearm flap. *Clin Plast Surg* 1982;9:21.
3. Muehlbauer W, Olbrisch RR, Herndl E, Stock W. Die Behandlung der Halskontraktur nach Verbrennung mit dem freien Unterarmlappen. *Der Chir* 1981;52:635.
4. Muehlbauer W, Hemdl E, Stock W. The forearm flap. *Plast Reconstr Surg* 1982;70:336.
5. Stock W, Muehlbauer W, Biemer E. Der neurovaskulaere Unterarm-Insel-Lappen. *Z Plast Chir* 1981;5:158.
6. Biemer E, Stock W. Total thumb reconstruction: A one-stage reconstruction using an osteocutaneous forearm flap. *Br J Plast Surg* 1983;35:52.
7. Soutar DS, Scheker LR, Tanner NSB, McGregor IA. The radial forearm flap: A versatile method for intraoral reconstruction. *Br Plast Surg* 1983; 36:1.

CHAPTER 199 ■ FACIAL ARTERY MUSCULOMUCOSAL (FAMM) FLAP

H. O. B. TAYLOR AND J. J. PRIBAZ

EDITORIAL COMMENT

This is an excellent arterialized flap for reconstructions of the lower lip, particularly those including the vermilion. The donor site is usually quite acceptable, and there is no functional deficit. One should remember that *wet* mucosa transferred to the outside tends to dry and needs constant lubrication.

Refinements of previously used buccal mucosal flaps have led to the facial artery musculomucosal (FAMM) flap, which, through its axial pattern blood supply, oblique orientation, and high length-to-width ratio, provides a robust donor for the reconstruction of mucosal defects throughout the mouth and nose, with minimal donor-site morbidity With attention to detail, and inclusion of the facial artery along the full length of the flap, a long and narrow flap may be harvested in either a superiorly or inferiorly based manner, with few donor-site or flap complications.

INDICATIONS

Oral and perioral reconstruction requires the transfer of surrogate specialized tissues to reconstruct form and function. In the past, the buccal mucosa was utilized as a random musculomucosal flap (1,2). The subsequent FAMM flap has been used in the reconstruction of a broad array of nasal and oral defects, including those in the palate, alveolus, nasal lining, maxillary antrum, tonsillar fossa, and floor of the mouth (3). It is particularly useful for reconstructing lip defects that may be too large to reconstruct with transfer of adjacent vermilion (4). The color, texture, and moisture of the mucosa carried by the FAMM flap combine to make it an excellent option for wet vermilion reconstruction. Although a number of other options exist for lip reconstruction, including mucosal grafts, labia minora grafts, two-stage flaps such as the tongue flap, cross-lip flap, bilateral island vermilion flaps, and free-tissue transfer (5), the FAMM flap provides a hardy source of axially perfused musculomucosal tissue in a single-stage procedure.

ANATOMY

The FAMM flap is an axial buccal flap based on the facial artery, a branch of the external carotid system, which curves beneath the lower border of the mandible, at the anterior aspect of the masseter muscle. Passing in a serpentine fashion, upward toward the commissure, the facial artery lies deep to the risorius and zygomaticus major muscles, but superficial to the deepest perioral muscles, the buccinator, levator anguli

oris, and the deep lamina of the orbicularis (Fig. 1A and B). Here it gives rise to multiple perforators of the cheek and continues superiorly toward the medial canthus of the ipsilateral eye as the angular artery. Anastomoses exist along its course with the buccal and infraorbital arteries. There is no named vein that drains this region, but a rich network to the anterior facial vein and posterior pterygoid plexus and internal maxillary vein provides a robust outflow. The position of the facial artery superficial to the buccinator requires that the FAMM flap include layers of mucosa, submucosa, and buccinator muscle in order to capture the vessel.

FLAP DESIGN AND DIMENSIONS

If one is careful to include the facial artery along the full length of the flap, it is possible to design a long (7 to 8 cm) and narrow axially perfused flap. It may be based superiorly (Fig. 2A), or inferiorly (Fig. 2B). The flap includes layers of mucosa, submucosa, a strip of buccinator muscle, and the facial artery above it. Inclusion of the required layers deep to the facial artery makes the flap approximately 8 to 10 mm in thickness. Using a Doppler ultrasound, the surgeon marks the course of the facial artery intraorally. No effort is made to include identifiable venous drainage, particularly in the superiorly based flaps, but despite this, it is rare for these flaps to become congested.

OPERATIVE TECHNIQUE

For the superiorly based flap, after Doppler ultrasound is used for the facial artery, the first incision is made anteroinferiorly through the mucosa, submucosa, and buccinator, to identify the axial vessel. Before proceeding, the facial artery is ligated and divided. The edges of the rest of the flap are incised and elevated from inferior to superior, including the three soft-tissue layers (mucosa, submucosa, buccinator) and the axial facial artery along the full length of the flap. For inferiorly based flaps, a mirror-image procedure is performed. The first incision is made anterosuperiorly, to identify and divide the facial artery in the upper lip. The flap is then elevated toward its inferior base. In this circumstance, the facial vein may be seen in the lateral inferior dissection.

CLINICAL RESULTS

We have used the FAMM flap to reconstruct a broad array of defects, including those secondary to inherited anomalies (e.g., lip vermilion in hemifacial microsomia, cleft palate), oncologic resections, vascular anomalies, and trauma. The tissue and color match provide a good substitute for native tissue,

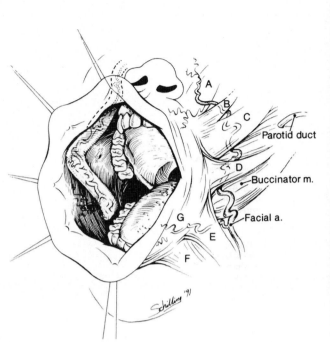

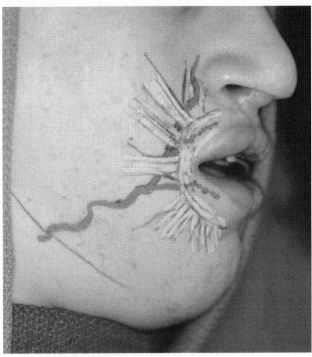

A,B

FIG. 1. **A,B:** The anatomy of the facial artery. A branch of the external carotid system, the facial artery hooks around the mandible just anterior to the border of the masseter. It courses toward the commissure and then toward the medial canthus, as the angular artery. With respect to the perioral muscles, it lies deep to the zygomaticus minor (*B*), zygomaticus major (*C*), risorius (*D*), depressor anguli oris (*E*), and depressor labia inferiors (*F*), and the superficial lamina of the orbicularis oris (*G*). It lies superficial to the buccinator, the deep lamina of the orbicularis oris (*G*), and the levator anguli oris (*A*).

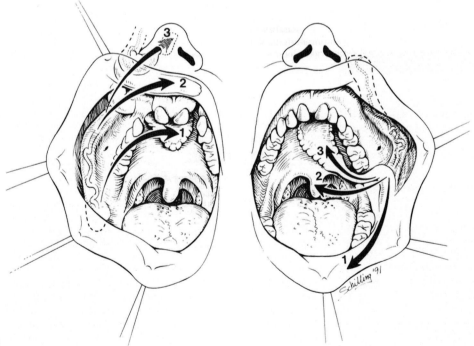

A,B

FIG. 2. **A:** The superiorly based FAMM flap can reach the hard plate (*1*), the upper lip and alveolus (*2*), the maxillary antrum, nose, and even the inferior orbit (*3*). **B:** The inferiorly based FAMM flap can reach the lower lip and floor of mouth (*1*), the soft palate and tonsillar fossa (*2*), and the hard palate and alveolus (*3*).

and the fullness of the flap is useful for reconstructing the appropriate lip contour, particularly for central and full-thickness defects. We have used this flap for vermilion reconstruction, in conjunction with free-tissue transfer reconstructions of larger perioral composite defects. Donor-site morbidity is low, with few complications in wound healing and minimal interference in facial animation.

SUMMARY

The FAMM flap is a flexible and safe flap that provides excellent tissue match for lip and vermilion reconstruction, as well as for multiple other defects around the mouth and nose.

References

1. Rayner CR, Arscott GD. A new method of resurfacing the lip. *Br J Plast Surg* 1987;40:454.
2. Bozola AR, Gasques JA, Carriquiry CE, et al. The buccinator musculomucosal flap: anatomic study and clinical application. *Plast Reconstr Surg* 1989;84:250.
3. Pribaz J, Stephens W, Crespo L, et al. A new intra-oral flap: facial artery musculomucosal (FAMM) flap. *Plast Reconstr Surg* 1992;90:421.
4. Pribaz JJ, Meara JG, Wright S, et al. Lip and vermilion reconstruction with the facial artery musculomucosal flap. *Plast Reconstr Surg* 2000;105:864.
5. Langstein HN, Robb GL. Lip and peri-oral reconstruction. *Clin Plast Surg* 2005;32:431.

CHAPTER 200 ■ RADIAL FOREARM FREE OSTEOCUTANEOUS FLAPS FOR INTRAORAL RECONSTRUCTION

J. B. BOYD

EDITORIAL COMMENT

This is an excellent description of the harvesting of bone with the radial forearm flap. The bone is quite useful for short defects of up to 10 cm in a straight line. The procedure is not intended for use around the mentum, where a curving bone is needed. Postoperatively, the forearm requires splinting for at least 6weeks to decrease the incidence of radial bone fractures.

The radial forearm osteocutaneous flap, basically a fasciocutaneous flap based on the radial artery, is thin, supple, and easy to elevate. It has large vessels, a long pedicle, and a capacity to be sensate or to carry a bone supply (1–5). It also has the advantage of allowing simultaneous dissection in two-team head and neck surgery. This flap is especially useful for low-volume, short (2–10 cm) mandibular defects.

INDICATIONS

The capacity of the forearm flap to carry two separate skin paddles allows it to reconstruct full-thickness defects (6) with an ease not matched by the fibula or iliac crest (7). It also provides mucosal replacement second to none. The skin flap is thin, supple, and, with reinnervation, capable of sensation approaching that in the normal mouth, which enhances oral continence and may improve speech, mastication, and swallowing (4).

The segmental supply of the radial bone by the artery allows it to be osteotomized once or twice for accurate contouring in the symphysial and parasymphysial regions. A lateral segment of mandible may be handled as a "straight shot," using the radial bone as a biocompatible reconstruction plate.

ANATOMY

The bone carried by this flap is approximately one third of the cross-sectional area of the distal anterolateral radius (Fig. 1). Although small, the bone is quite strong and will accept osseointegrated implants for dental rehabilitation (8).

The skin of the anterior forearm receives a significant blood supply from the radial artery via septocutaneous vessels passing along the septum between the brachioradialis and the flexor carpi radialis muscles (the lateral intermuscular septum). These perforators are plentiful in the distal third of the forearm, but proximally, where tendons give way to muscle bellies, they become rather sparse. Nevertheless, it is probably safe to raise a septum-based skin flap anywhere along the course of the radial artery. In this way, two skin islands may be raised, one proximal and one distal, to facilitate reconstruction of the through-and-through defect.

After emerging from the septum, the vessels branch laterally and medially, piercing the deep fascia and quickly passing to the subdermal plexus to supply the skin. Contrary to previ-

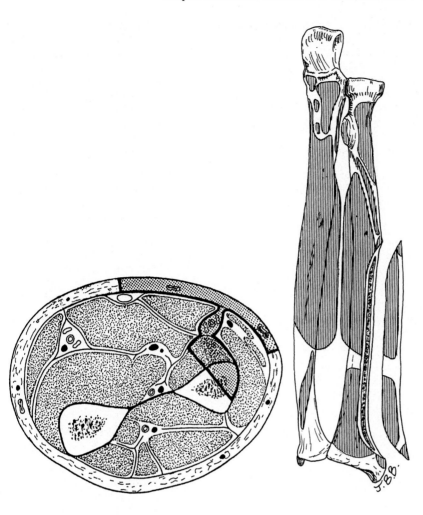

A,B

FIG. 1. **A:** Section of distal forearm showing disposition of radial artery with respect to vascular septum, flexor pollicis longus, and the osteotomy. One third of the radial cross section is taken with an osteotomy, which passes posteriorly and laterally from the midline of its anterior surface. The skin paddle is situated over the dorsoradial aspect of the wrist to include the cephalic vein. This improves vessel access in the neck but is admittedly detrimental to the postoperative cosmetic appearance at the wrist. **B:** Muscular attachments to the left anterior radius and ulna with respect to the radial bone graft. The graft extends between the insertions of the pronator teres and brachioradialis (some of which are included for extra length). Note that the osteotomy is "boat-shaped" to avoid cross cutting at the corners and excessive weakening.

ous teachings, these vessels do not travel on the surface of the deep fascia for any significant distance; as a result, little of the deep fascia needs to be harvested with the flap.

The brachial artery bifurcates into radial and ulnar arteries a few centimeters distal to the antecubital fossa. The radial artery and its venae comitantes are invested by the fascia of the lateral intermuscular septum. The artery passes distally along the radial side of the pronator teres, initially lying between the biceps tendon and the bicipital aponeurosis. It then crosses anterior to the pronator teres, just proximal to that muscle's insertion into its tubercle on the lateral surface of the radius. On entering the distal third of the forearm, it first overlies the flexor pollicis longus and finally the pronator quadratus. These two muscles intimately clothe the flat anterior surface of the distal radius (Fig. 1). Muscular branches from the radial artery give periosteal twigs to the underlying bone and are the basis for the osseous portion of the flap.

Classically, there are three major subcutaneous veins in the anterior forearm: the cephalic, the median, and the basilic. There are significant variations on this basic pattern. Perforating veins connect the superficial veins to the deep system at various points. Of most interest here is the communication at the level of the brachial artery bifurcation, which may be single or multiple and may be from any of the superficial veins (commonly the median).

Either the venae comitantes or the large subcutaneous veins of the forearm are capable of draining the osteocutaneous forearm flap. The superficial veins are often preferred because of their greater diameter and their independence from the arterial pedicle. Care should be taken, however, to ensure that

the superficial veins have not been canalized previously and undergone partial or complete thrombosis.

The medial antebrachial cutaneous nerve (C8, T1) enters the forearm in the company of the basilic vein. It soon gives off a number of large anterior branches that pass down the radial side of the basilic vein and supply the ulnar half of the anterior forearm as far as the wrist. An ulnar branch supplies the ulnar border of the forearm. The lateral antebrachial cutaneous nerve (C5, C6) is the forearm continuation of the musculocutaneous nerve. It enters the forearm on the ulnar side of the cephalic vein and, via multiple branches, supplies the radial half of the forearm as far as the wrist as well as the dorsoradial aspect of the forearm.

FLAP DESIGN AND DIMENSIONS

It is useful to mark the radial artery and the larger subcutaneous veins on the skin surface. The skin flap is usually positioned over the anterior or anterolateral aspect of the distal wrist. Here the subcutaneous tissue is thinnest, the skin is reasonably hairless, and the pedicle length is maximized. The relationship of the skin flap to the bone graft should be assessed carefully in view of the expected recipient defect. The bone graft will extend proximally for up to 12 cm from a point 2 cm proximal to the tip of the styloid process (see Fig. 1). Usually, the recipient defect requires the skin paddle to lie over the midpoint of the bone, but this is not always the case. It is advantageous to position the flap anterolaterally in such a way that part of it overlies the cephalic vein. This vessel can be used for venous drainage. In hirsute patients, the flap may be positioned purely on the anterior aspect of the distal wrist where the skin is less hairy for a superior cosmetic result. Unfortunately, the median vein is often quite small in the distal wrist. If an innervated flap is required, it should be noted that the watershed between the neurosomes of the lateral and medial antebrachial cutaneous nerves lies down the midline of the anterior forearm. Those positioned centrally, and straddling two neurosomes, require both superficial nerves (4).

The flap may be of almost any dimensions as long as a significant portion of it overlies the vascular septum. Practically, the whole anterior forearm skin may be taken safely, but this is rarely required. Limits extend from the antecubital fossa to the transverse wrist crease and from the ulnar border of the forearm to the posterolateral aspect of the radial border. Raising a flap of such dimensions would require the entire vascular septum to be preserved. The "base" of any radial forearm skin flap is that portion in direct contact with the vascular septum. Like any flap, if the base is small, the surviving length is accordingly reduced.

When small skin islands are required (less than 6 × 4 cm), it is sometimes possible to perform primary closure at the donor site (9). Such a flap is positioned transversely with one edge overlying the radial artery. Closure is effected by means of a long, ulnar-based rotation-advancement of the entire proximal forearm skin. The proximal defect is closed as a V to Y. Wrist flexion facilitates closure.

OPERATIVE TECHNIQUE

A preoperative Allen's test should always be done, but its meaning is open to question. Only in a severe arteriopathy would grafting of the radial artery be necessary. Many cases have been performed in the presence of an unfavorable Allen's test, with no adverse sequelae. One possible cause for an ischemic hand following this surgery is the inadvertent ligation or division of a *superficial* ulnar artery, which can lie in the superficial tissues along the medial border of the flap. With the tourniquet up, this may take the appearance of a large vein. Such a vessel is at most risk with skin paddles that intrude onto the ulnar border of the wrist.

A tourniquet is placed around the upper arm. The arm is *incompletely* exsanguinated using an Esmarch or an Ace bandage before dissection commences.

The skin flap is incised around its periphery, and dissection is carried down to the underlying muscle fascia. Care is taken at the proximal margin of the flap to identify and preserve the cephalic vein or any other superficial veins. An incision is made from the proximal edge of the flap incision straight up the forearm toward the antecubital fossa. Dissection is carried through the subcutaneous tissue, and the selected venous system is traced proximally. If an innervated flap is desired, all the subcutaneous nerves entering the flap should be preserved in a sheath of fascia; they tend to lie just superficial to the deep fascia. Precise identification of the nerves is best made in the proximal forearm, where they are large and located next to the cephalic and basilic veins. These nerves and their relevant branches then can be traced distally into the proximal margin of the flap.

The ulnar side of the flap then is elevated at a level just superior to the deep fascia, working toward the intermuscular septum between the brachioradialis and the flexor carpi radialis. Approximately 1 cm on the ulnar side of this septum, the deep fascia is incised, and dissection then passes under it. Preservation of the deep fascia in this way facilitates skin grafting of the donor site. Dissection proceeds over the surface of the flexor carpi radialis tendon, leaving paratenon behind. It then extends around the radial edge of the tendon into the space beneath. Usually, the superficial fibers of the flexor digi-

torum superficialis muscle are now visible. Dissection around the radial side of this muscle allows it to be retracted in an ulnar direction. When this is done, the fibers of the flexor pollicis longus are seen arising from the flat anterior surface of the distal radius and the adjacent interosseous membrane. This completes dissection on the ulnar side.

The radial dissection is similar to that on the ulnar side. It passes immediately superficial to the deep fascia until a point is reached 1 cm lateral to the intermuscular septum, where the deep fascia is divided and dissection then proceeds at this deeper level. The brachioradialis tendon is seen, and the dissection hugs this tendon in the same way as the ulnar dissection hugged that of the flexor carpi radialis. Paratenon is preserved. Once around the ulnar border of the brachioradialis tendon, the plane of dissection remains close to its undersurface. A space filled with loose adventitial tissue is soon entered. Blunt dissection in this space exposes the dorsoradial *bare area* of the radius.

Distally, the radial artery and its venae comitantes are easily identified; these are ligated and divided. The brachioradialis tendon is elevated somewhat from its attachment to the distal radius; however, care is taken to preserve its distal attachment. This maneuver allows a little more radius to be included in the osteocutaneous flap because the attachment of the brachioradialis defines the distal limit of the bone graft. The cephalic vein is ligated and divided distally, as are other small veins in the region.

It should be noted that the superficial branch of the radial nerve passes through the deep portion of the flap and is visible during the radial dissection. This nerve is *not* to be used for innervation purposes. The nerve can be easily dissected from the undersurface of the flap, and *it is virtually never necessary to sacrifice it.*

The proximal portion of the intermuscular septum between the brachioradialis and the flexor carpi radialis is entered and communicated with the more distal dissection. The radial artery and its venae comitantes are immediately visible between these muscles. Proximal to the skin island, it is not necessary to maintain any skin perforators, septal or otherwise.

The vascular leash is dissected free of surrounding tissues. It can be taken all the way up to the origin of the radial artery from the brachial artery, just distal to the antecubital fossa. The superficial venous system communicates with the deep system of veins just distal to this point. This communication may be preserved as part of a combined venous pedicle (10). Both cephalic vein and superficial nerves may be dissected into the upper arm to obtain greater length.

Now attention is focused on perhaps the trickiest part of the operation: the osteotomy (Fig. 2). At this point, the radius is totally obscured from view: its anterior surface is clothed by the muscle fibers of the flexor pollicis longus. The lateral border of the radius is palpated easily, but the medial border is not, due to the tightness of the interosseous membrane. Passing a fine hemostat through the flexor pollicis longus muscle is a way of establishing where the bone ends and where the interosseous membrane begins. In this way, it is possible to visualize mentally the radius as it lies underneath the flexor pollicis longus muscle. A line is drawn longitudinally down the anterior surface of the flexor pollicis longus muscle at a point corresponding to the exact midline of the flat anterior face of the radius. The osteotomy will pass from here, dorsally and laterally, toward the bare area (Fig. 1). If the osteotomy were to pass perpendicularly through the radius, then half the cortex would be harvested. By angling the osteotomy laterally toward the bare area, however, it is ensured that only one third of the circumference of the radius is taken as a graft (Fig. 2).

The muscle fibers of the flexor pollicis longus muscle then are divided. The incision passes all the way down to bone. It extends from the distal radius proximally for about 12 to

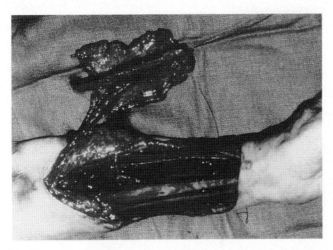

FIG. 2. A square-shaped osteotomy has been completed and the flap isolated on its pedicle. This radius went on to undergo fracture! Boat-shaped osteotomies are probably safer.

14 cm. The periosteum is elevated for a short distance on either side of the incision so that the radius can be visualized along the line of the proposed osteotomy. The proximal extension of the osteotomy eventually will exit the radius laterally. This point will be situated either at or near the pronator tubercle. Insertion of the pronator teres has been widely accepted as defining the most proximal permissible extent of the osteotomy, just as the insertion of the brachioradialis tendon has been said to set the limit for the distal extent.

By now, the bone has been prepared for osteotomy medially, laterally, and proximally. It remains only to communicate the flexor pollicis longus splitting incision distally with the bare area of the radius immediately proximal to the remaining insertion of the brachioradialis muscle. There is nothing of vital importance that can be divided in this area, but some large branches of the radial artery may need to be tied off.

It is hoped that the dissection will take less than 2 hours of tourniquet time. The tourniquet is released, and hemostasis is established by the usual means. The osteotomy is best performed using a fairly powerful reciprocating saw with a narrow blade not exceeding 1.5 cm in width; this is essential if the saw is to be guided in its course through the bone. With assistants retracting the vital structures and providing irrigation, the reciprocating saw enters the distal radius under the tendon of the brachioradialis muscle at approximately 45 degrees to the bone surface and angled proximally. The osteotomy passes proximally until it is in the vicinity of the pronator teres insertion, and then it is angled out through the lateral cortex. Again, it follows the predetermined cut that has already been made in the soft tissues. Because one continuous osteotomy has been made (Fig. 1), the graft is boat- or keel-shaped and there is no cross cutting (11,12) (Fig. 2).

The bone is observed to bleed from its cut surface, and the flap is observed to have a good capillary return. After 15 min of perfusion, the pedicle is divided and the flap removed to the recipient site.

Perfusion of the hand by the ulnar artery should be assessed at this stage. With proper preoperative assessment, there should be no surprises. Nevertheless, the surgeon should be prepared to graft the radial artery if faced with obvious arterial insufficiency; in practice, this is extremely rare.

To facilitate wound closure, the palmaris longus tendon usually is removed and discarded. The proximal portion of the wound is closed directly. Although the paratenons of the flexor carpi radialis and the brachioradialis have been preserved and probably would accept a skin graft, it is often better to bury the tendons among the fibers of the flexor digitorum superfi-

cialis muscle. By whatever means, a flat, well-vascularized bed is produced to receive an unmeshed skin graft held in place by a meticulous tie-over dressing. The graft remains unmeshed to maximize the *bridging phenomenon*, which may help to avoid tendon exposure. The immediate result of harvesting a radial bone graft is a diminution in the breaking strength of the radius by 76% (11). The risk of fracture following relatively minor trauma mandates cautious rehabilitation.

The wrist, including the thumb, then is immobilized in a palmar splint, which is generally not removed for 7 days. When it is removed, the patient is fitted with an above-elbow cast (preferably fiberglass) or splint with a window, if necessary, to continue dressings at the skin-graft recipient site. The cast should hold the elbow at right angles and the wrist in moderate extension. The thumb can be free at this stage. The patient wears the above-elbow cast for a period of 2 months, and then the upper portion is removed, converting it to a below-elbow cast for a further month.

At the recipient site, the bone is osteotomized (if necessary), trimmed, and fitted into the defect. Closing wedge osteotomies are performed after elevating periosteum and guarding the radial artery with a Freer elevator. Fixation of the osteotomy is best achieved by a five-hole miniplate applied to the cut surface of the bone. Fixation of the graft to the recipient mandible may be performed in a number of ways. Miniplates can be used with end-to-end abutment of a graft to residual mandibular fragments. Alternatively, the mandibular fragments may have their outer cortices removed and the graft overlapped and lag-screwed to them (Fig. 3). The cut surface of the bone graft is thus brought into contact with decorticated mandibular bone. The final option is to fix the mandibular fragments with a large reconstruction plate and then trim the graft to fit the interosseous defect. Then it may be simply wired or screwed to the plate. Any of these methods gives excellent fusion rates (13).

The skin flap is sutured to the intraoral defect using mattress sutures of 3-0 Dexon or Vicryl. Microvascular anastomoses are performed to the ipsilateral facial artery and external jugular vein, if available. Otherwise, alternative vessels may be selected (14). The radial forearm flap is one of the few flaps where the arterial and venous pedicles may simultaneously access opposite sides of the neck.

The lateral antebrachial cutaneous nerve is trimmed and anastomosed to the stump of the ipsilateral lingual nerve. If this is intact or absent, the inferior alveolar nerve is equally effective. Exposure may require drilling out the mandibular fragments. Alternatively, an end-to-side anastomosis between the lateral antebrachial cutaneous nerve and an intact lingual nerve may be attempted, with some expectation of success (15).

CLINICAL RESULTS

The donor defect is cosmetic rather than functional (16) but, when bone is taken, 2–3 months of splinting are required to lessen the risk of radial fracture. Fear of fracture and limited bone stock explain why this radial forearm osteocutaneous flap does not enjoy universal acclaim; however, donor defects may be minimized by meticulous surgical technique, limiting the bone graft to one third of the distal radial circumference, direct wound closure when possible, and appropriate postoperative splinting.

In low-volume resections, the cosmetic results are excellent and the lap is extremely suitable for a full-thickness defect. The cosmetic outcome is less satisfactory when the requirement is for bulkier tissue. Bony defects exceeding 10 cm are probably unsuitable for reconstruction with this flap. Poor results occur when the indications are exceeded and the patient ends up with a soft-tissue or bony deficiency, particularly disastrous at the

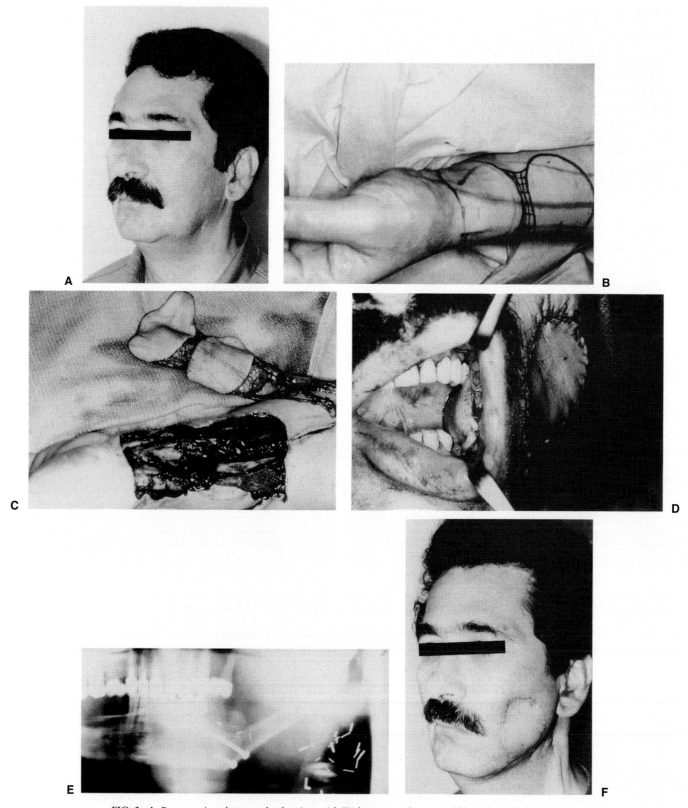

FIG. 3. A: Preoperative photograph of patient with T4 lesion invading mandible and cheek skin, requiring through-and-through excision. B: Resection including oral mucosa, cheek skin, mandibular body, and angle. Radial artery and cephalic vein marked on the skin. Two skin paddles are designed to straddle these structures; their size is estimated using a template of the defect. One paddle will be used for oral lining and the other for cheek cover. C: Noninnervated osteocutaneous flap isolated on its pedicle. There is sufficient mobility within the tissues to allow some independent movement of the skin paddles with respect to the bone. D: At termination of the procedure, both skin paddles are visualized and found to be perfusing well. E: Postoperative radiograph showing the lag-screw fixation technique. F: Postoperative result. (From Soutar et al., ref. 5, with permission.)

mentum. As with most osteocutaneous free flaps, the external skin paddle is a poor match for facial skin.

Even though functional impairment has been minimal at the donor site, the radius is significantly weakened (11), which could be troublesome in manual workers and elderly patients with osteoporosis; however, radial fracture is uncommon in centers where the flap is routinely used (12) and where appropriate steps are taken to minimize the risk. Cold sensitivity does not seem to be a problem (16); however, the skin graft is in a very prominent position, is often subject to delayed healing, and represents a significant cosmetic deformity. In young members of both sexes, this may be of vital concern.

SUMMARY

The radial forearm osteocutaneous flap is arguably the best flap for the restoration of intraoral function following oromandibular reconstruction. Extensive amounts of thin, supple skin are available, with excellent potential for reinnervation.

References

1. Song R, Gao Y, Yu Y, et al. The forearm flap. *Clin Plast Surg* 1982;9:21.
2. Urken ML, Weinberg H, Vickery C, et al. The neurofasciocutaneous radial forearm flap in head and neck reconstruction: a preliminary report. *Laryngoscope* 1990;100:61.
3. Dubner S, Heller KS. Reinnervated radial forearm free flaps in head and neck reconstruction. *J Reconstr Microsurg* 1992;8:467.
4. Boyd B, Mulholland S, Gullane P, et al. Lateral antebrachial cutaneous neurosome flaps in oral reconstruction: are we making sense? *Plast Reconstr Surg* 1994;93:1350.
5. Soutar DS, Scheker LR, Tanner NSB, McGregor IA. The radial forearm flap: a versatile method for intraoral reconstruction. *Br J Plast Surg* 1983;36:1.
6. Boyd JB, Morris SF, Rosen IB, et al. The "through and through" oromandibular defect. *Plast Reconstr Surg* 1994;93:44.
7. Boyd JB, Rosen IB, Freeman J, et al. The iliac crest and the radial forearm flap in vascularized oromandibular reconstruction. *Am J Surg* 1990;159:301.
8. Mounsey RA, Boyd JB. Mandibular reconstruction with osseointegrated implants into the free vascularized radius. *Plast Reconstr Surg* 1994;94:457.
9. Elliot D, Bardsley AF, Batchelor AG, et al. Direct closure of the radial forearm flap donor defect. *Br J Plast Surg* 1988;41:358.
10. Gottlieb LJ, Tachmes L, Pielet RW. Improved venous drainage of the radial artery forearm flap: use of the profundus cubitalis vein. *Ann Plast Surg* 1993;9:281.
11. Swanson E, Boyd JB, Mulholland RS. The radial forearm flap: a biomechanical study of the osteotomized radius. *Plast Reconstr Surg* 1990;85:267.
12. Weinzweig N, Jones NF, Shestak KC, et al. Oromandibular reconstruction using a keel-shaped modification of the radial forearm flap. *Ann Plast Surg* 1994;33:359.
13. Boyd JB, Mulholland RS. Fixation of the vascularized bone graft in mandibular reconstruction. *Plast Reconstr Surg* 1993;91:1.
14. Mulholland S, Boyd JB, McCabe S, et al. Recipient vessels in head and neck microsurgery: radiation effect and vessel access. *Plast Reconstr Surg* 1993;92:628.
15. Viterbo F, Trindade JC, Hoshino K, Neto AM. End to side neurorrhaphy with removal of the epineural sheath: an experimental study in rats. *Plast Reconstr Surg* 1994;94:1038.
16. Smith A, Bowen VA, Rabczak T, Boyd JB. Donor site deficit of the osteocutaneous radial forearm flap. *Ann Plast Surg* 1994;32:372.

CHAPTER 201 ■ VASCULARIZED RIB–PERIOSTEAL TRANSPLANTATION FOR RECONSTRUCTION OF THE MANDIBLE AND MAXILLA

D. SERAFIN AND V. E. VOCI

EDITORIAL COMMENT

This technique has now been supplanted by free fibular/scapular osteocutaneous flaps and iliac-crest flaps.

Nonvascularized bone grafts have had reasonable success in small, well-vascularized defects. The major problem arises when larger defects require large segments of contoured bone and soft-tissue coverage. The rib is one source of vascularized bone that can be transplanted with or without overlying skin (1,2).

INDICATIONS

Vascularized rib–periosteal transplantation is indicated to reconstruct a moderate deficiency of the maxilla or mandible in a relatively avascular bed. The recipient skin envelope must be adequate to accommodate the relative bulk of the osseous segment and associated bulky musculature.

If the skin envelope is healthy with adequate blood supply and the mandibular or maxillary defect is small to moderate in size, then a nonvascularized bone graft will provide satisfactory results. If the mandibular or maxillary segment to be replaced is large with an associated large cutaneous defect,

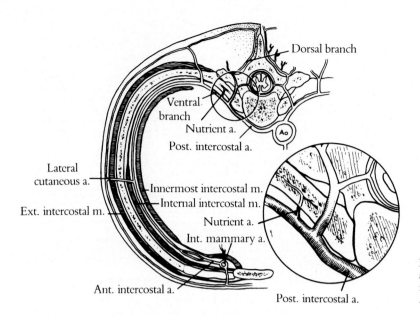

FIG. 1. The vascular anatomy of the intercostal artery. Note that the artery of Adamkiewicz arises from one of the dorsal branches between T7 and L2. Also note the location of the nutrient artery to the rib.

then a vascularized iliac osteocutaneous flap based on the deep circumflex iliac vessel is the donor tissue of choice (3).

The major advantage of the vascularized rib–periosteal transplant is the ability to provide vascularized osseous tissue in a relatively avascular bed. Osteocyte survival has been confirmed by subsequent biopsies, arteriography, and serial radiographs (4–6). lone union occurs with callus formation similar to that noted at a fracture site.

ANATOMY

There are nine paired posterior intercostal arteries. They arise from the dorsal aspect of the aorta. At their origin, they lie midway in the intercostal space and course obliquely upward as they proceed laterally. The arteries on the right are longer because the aorta lies to the left of the vertebral column. Opposite the heads of the ribs, the posterior intercostal artery divides into a ventral and dorsal branch (Fig. 1). The dorsal branch supplies the spinal cord, its meninges, and the vertebrae. It then continues dorsally to supply muscular branches to the paraspinous muscles and cutaneous branches to the skin. The artery of Adamkiewicz arises from one of these dorsal branches between T7 and L2. This is an extremely important vessel because it provides the major blood supply to the thoracolumbar spinal cord. Injury to this vessel may result in paraplegia.

Proximally, the ventral branch of the posterior intercostal artery lies between the posterior intercostal membrane and pleura. By the time it has reached the angle of the rib, however, it has penetrated the posterior intercostal membrane and internal intercostal muscle and continues anteriorly between the external and internal intercostal muscles. It courses upward in the interspace obliquely to lie inferior to the corresponding rib and continues anteriorly in the costal groove between the pleura and the posterior intercostal membrane. It eventually anastomoses with the anterior intercostal artery, a branch of the internal thoracic artery, at about the midclavicular line. Each intercostal artery is accompanied by a vein and an intercostal nerve. The vein is superior and the nerve is inferior to the artery (Fig. 2).

The ventral branch gives off multiple branches. The first branch is the nutrient artery to the rib above. This nutrient branch is given off near the tubercle of the rib and enters the bone through a nutrient foramen (see Fig. 1). It quickly

divides into proximal and distal medullary arteries in the medullary cavity of the rib. Collateral intercostal branches are given off at regular intervals, beginning at the angle of the rib. They course down to the superior border of the rib below, supplying the surrounding soft tissue. Musculocutaneous perforators are also given off at regular intervals, supplying the pectoralis, serratus, and intercostal muscles as well as the overlying skin. The overlying skin is also supplied by a lateral cutaneous arterial branch that arises at the midaxillary line and courses with the lateral cutaneous nerve. The direct and musculocutaneous perforators supply the skin portion of an osteocutaneous flap. Mammary branches are given off by the third, fourth, and fifth intercostal arteries.

The veins on the right side empty into the azygos vein. On the left side, the upper veins empty into the accessory hemiazygous vein, and the lower veins empty into the hemiazygous vein.

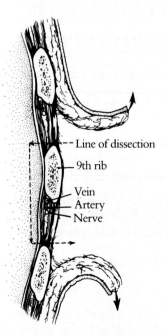

FIG. 2. A cross section of the rib and the corresponding interspaces. Note the location of the intercostal vein, artery, and nerve.

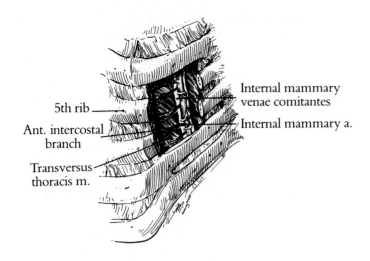

5th rib

Ant. intercostal branch

Transversus thoracis m.

Internal mammary venae comitantes

Internal mammary a.

FIG. 3. The vascular anatomy of the internal thoracic artery and venae comitantes.

OPERATIVE TECHNIQUE

Three operative approaches have been described for rib–periosteal and osteocutaneous rib grafts: anterior, posterolateral, and posterior. Each method has advantages and disadvantages.

Anterior Approach (7,8)

The donor vessels can be either the anterior intercostal artery and vein (which are often small with multiple branches) or the internal thoracic artery and vein (both of which have large diameters and lengthy pedicles). The major advantages are the reliability of a cutaneous portion and accessibility to the head and neck in the supine position. The main disadvantages include the bulk of the pectoralis major muscle, which must be included, and the dissection, which is somewhat difficult.

A rib below the fourth is usually selected, so that the dissection of the internal thoracic vessel is facilitated by the transverse thoracic muscle, which is present below this level. This muscle separates the vessels from the pleura and therefore makes the dissection somewhat less difficult. If the fifth rib is chosen (1), a small transverse incision is made over the costochondral cartilage, which is removed subperichondrally, exposing the internal thoracic vessels and fifth anterior intercostal vessels (Fig. 3). The overlying skin island is dissected down to the rib, preserving the lateral cutaneous nerve, which theoretically can be used to innervate the skin. The bone then is transected laterally and bluntly dissected off the parietal pleura. Although previous authors indicate that the dissection is extrapleural, this has not been our experience.

Posterolateral Approach (9,10)

The flap is based on the posterior intercostal vessels, lateral to the paraspinous muscles. These are usually 1 to 2 mm in diameter. The chief advantages are that the dissection is relatively less difficult than with the other approaches and the pedicle is quite lengthy. The major disadvantages include the need for an open thoracotomy incision, the bulk of the muscle cuff, the lack of a reliable cutaneous portion, and the position of the patient, which limits access to the head and neck region. The ninth or tenth rib is usually selected (2).

With the patient in a lateral thoracotomy position, the incision is made over the chosen rib and extended down through the anterior portion of the latissimus dorsi muscle for exposure. The appropriate length of rib segment is delineated. The pleural cavity is entered anteriorly, and the rib is transected. The dissection of the rib and muscle is then continued posteriorly. Care must be taken to preserve a sufficient muscular cuff around the rib, especially inferiorly along the vascular pedicle. When sufficient length of bone is obtained, the rib is transected posteriorly. The pedicle is dissected out as far posteriorly as is necessary to obtain adequate pedicle length. Fifteen centimeters of pedicle length can be obtained lateral to the paraspinous muscles, depending on the length of the rib segment (Fig. 4). There is no danger of injury to the artery of Adamkiewicz when the dissection is this far lateral.

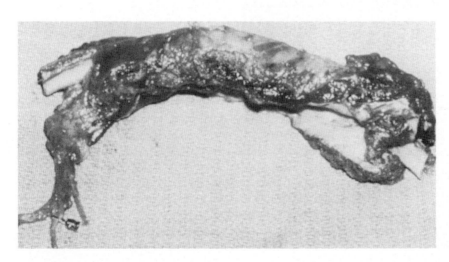

FIG. 4. Intraoperative photograph demonstrating rib–periosteal segment. Note the lengthy neurovascular pedicle (*lower left*). (From Serafin, Riefkohl, ref. 12, with permission.)

If a cutaneous skin island is required, a previous delay should be performed or multiple cutaneous veins anastomosed, in addition to the posterior intercostal vein, at the time of transplantation. In a review of transplanted intercostal osteocutaneous flaps, over half had problems with the skin island.

To provide reliable cutaneous cover, an island latissimus dorsi musculocutaneous flap has been successfully employed with an attached segment of rib (Fig. 5). The osseous segment, however, must be revascularized, because earlier attempts without revascularization resulted in partial loss of the bone.

Recently, posterolateral rib segments have been successfully transplanted based on blood supply from the attached serratus muscle. The thoracodorsal artery and vein with branches to the serratus muscle are selected as the donor vasculature (Fig. 6). "Winging" of the scapula does not occur, provided that the superior slips of origin of the serratus muscle are not violated and the long thoracic nerve of Bell is not injured. A skin island may be included in the dissection.

Posterior Approach (5,11)

The only theoretical advantage to this approach is that the nutrient vessel supplying medullary blood flow is included. Recent evidence, however, shows that this is not necessary for osteoblast survival and bone healing. The disadvantages are many, including a very difficult dissection, possible injury to the artery of Adamkiewicz, the need for a major thoracotomy, and an unreliable cutaneous portion.

The incision is made over the rib (usually the sixth, to avoid injury to the artery of Adamkiewicz), beginning near the midline of the back and extending laterally. The incision is extended down through the latissimus dorsi and lateral aspect

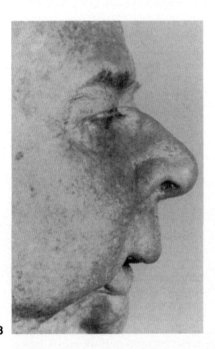
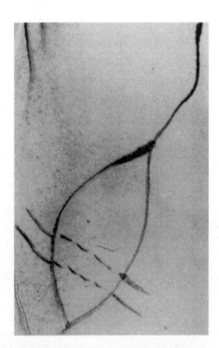

A,B

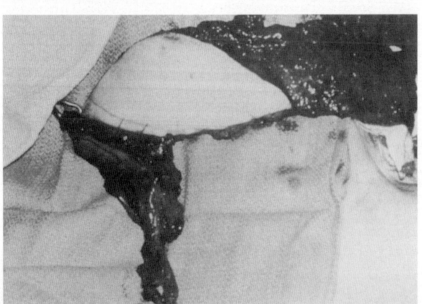

C

FIG. 5. A: Preoperative photograph of a patient with an orocutaneous fistula subsequent to a composite resection and postoperative radiation. B: Intraoperative outline of an island latissimus dorsi musculocutaneous flap with the attached rib periosteal segment. C: Intraoperative photograph demonstrating vascularized rib–periosteal segment attached to the island latissimus dorsi musculocutaneous flap by loose areolar connective tissue. The rib–periosteal segment will be revascularized to branches of the external carotid artery and the facial vein. *(Continued)*

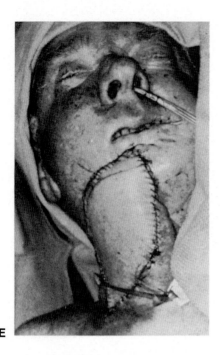
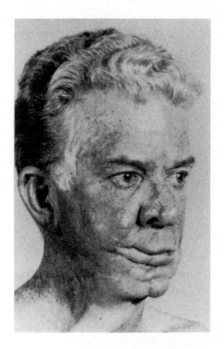

D,E

FIG. 5. *Continued.* **D:** Intraoperative photograph following successful transfer of the island latissimus dorsi musculocutaneous flap. **E:** Late postoperative result. (From Serafin, Riefkohl, ref. 12, with permission.)

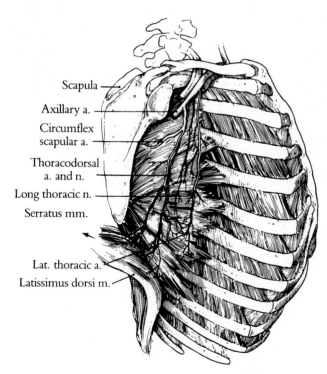

FIG. 6. The vascular anatomy to the serratus muscle. This muscle, with the associated rib–periosteal segment, will be transplanted and revascularized at the recipient site. Note that the vascular basis for the composite tissue is the thoracodorsal artery and vein, with communication to the lateral thoracic artery and vein by means of a branch to the serratus musculature. Also note the long thoracic nerve that must be carefully preserved.

Labels on figure:
Scapula
Axillary a.
Circumflex scapular a.
Thoracodorsal a. and n.
Long thoracic n.
Serratus mm.
Lat. thoracic a.
Latissimus dorsi m.

of the erector spinae muscles. The intercostal muscles in the interspace above are divided, and the pleural cavity is opened. A similar incision is made in the interspace below, staying close to the rib inferiorly to ensure safety of the vascular pedicle in the muscular cuff. The length of rib needed is determined, and the rib is transected laterally. The rib is mobilized enough at this point to visualize the origin of the posterior intercostal vessels through the pleura. The vessels are isolated through the pleura, ligated, and divided. The dorsal spinal branch then is ligated and divided near its origin on the posterior intercostal artery. The vascular pedicle is dissected retrograde, passing it under the sympathetic trunk. The rib can be disarticulated and the thoracotomy incision closed with a chest tube (Figs. 7 and 8).

CLINICAL RESULTS

Twelve patients (86%) underwent the successful transplantation of a vascularized rib–periosteal segment. In this series there were two failures (14%). One transplant failed because of inadequate preoperative planning. The rib selected for transplantation was previously fractured, resulting in an unrecognized associated injury to the posterior intercostal artery and vein. The other failure occurred postoperatively. This patient developed severe hematemesis. During the course of frequent vomiting, both anastomoses were disrupted. This was confirmed by reexploration later in the postoperative period.

A major disadvantage is the lengthy operative procedure, often with attendant thoracic morbidity. Other disadvantages include the structural weakness of the transplanted rib segment, a deficient quantity of bone, and an obligatory large, bulky muscular cuff that must be included with the rib–periosteal segment to ensure adequate cortical circulation. The associated cutaneous segment using the posterolateral approach is unreliable.

SUMMARY

Vascularized osseous transplantation has a definite but limited role in reconstruction of the head and neck subsequent to tumor ablation and trauma.

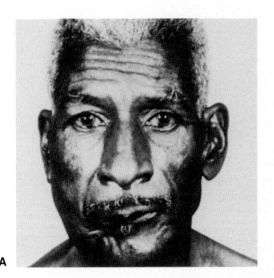

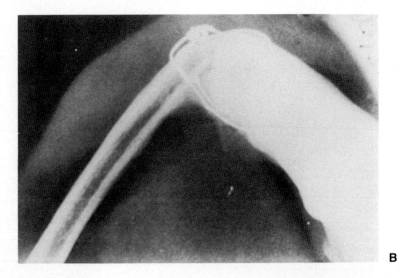

A

B

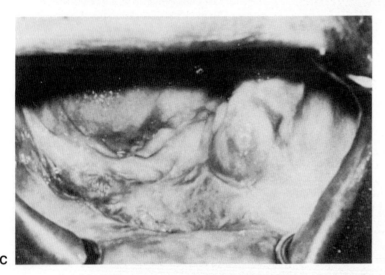

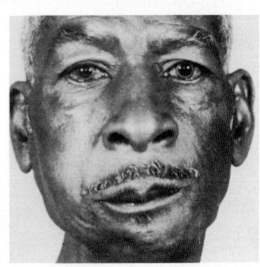

C

D

FIG. 7. **A:** Preoperative photograph of a patient following composite resection and postoperative radiation. **B:** Radiograph at 4 months demonstrating solid bone union between the remaining segment of mandible and the rib–periosteal transplant. Note callus formation. **C:** Intraoral photograph demonstrating results following vestibuloplasty. Note that vestibuloplasty is possible because of the addition of well-vascularized tissue to this relatively avascular area. **D:** Late postoperative result. (From Serafin, Riefkohl, ref. 12, with permission.)

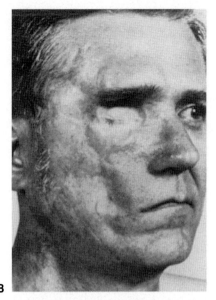
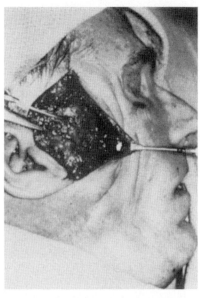

A,B

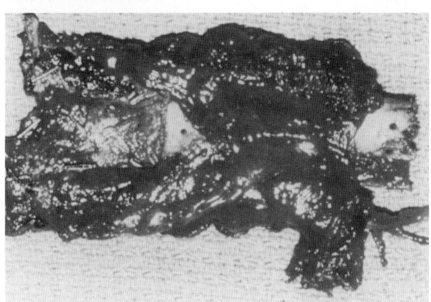
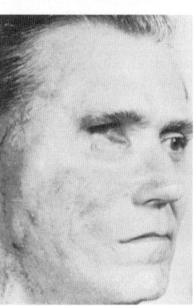

C,D

FIG. 8. **A:** Preoperative photograph demonstrating extensive scarring and relative avascularity secondary to previous trauma. Note depression of the maxilla. **B:** Intraoperative dissection of recipient vasculature through a preauricular incision. **C:** Intraoperative photograph demonstrating rib–periosteal segment. Note the vascular clips on the periosteum for subsequent radiographic follow-up. **D:** Late postoperative result. (From Serafin et al., ref. 2, with permission.)

References

1. Buncke, HJ, Furnas DW, Gordon L, Achauer BM. Free osteocutaneous flap from a rib to the tibia. *Plast Reconstr Surg* 1977;59:799.
2. Serafin D, Riefkohl R, Thomas I, Georgiade NG. Vascularized rib-periosteal and osteocutaneous reconstruction of the maxilla and mandible: an assessment. *Plast Reconstr Surg* 1980;66:718.
3. Taylor GI, Townsend P, Corlett R. Superiority of the deep circumflex iliac vessels as the supply for free groin flaps. *Plast Reconstr Surg* 1979;61:745.
4. Berggren A, Weiland AJ, Dorfman H. Free vascularized bone grafts: factors affecting their survival and ability to heal to recipient bone defects. *Plast Reconstr Surg* 1982;69:19.
5. Östrup LT, Fredrickson JM. Reconstruction of mandibular defects after radiation, using a free, living bone graft transferred by microvascular anastomoses: an experimental study. *Plast Reconstr Surg* 1975;55:563.
6. Ostrup LT. Rib transplantation. In: Serafin D, Buncke HJ Jr, eds. *Microsurgical composite tissue transplantation.* St. Louis: Mosby, 1979.
7. Ariyan S, Finseth FJ. The anterior chest approach for obtaining free osteocutaneous rib grafts. *Plast Reconstr Surg* 1978;62:767.
8. McKee DM. Microvascular rib transplantation in reconstruction of the mandible. Presented at the Annual Meeting of the American Society of Plastic and Reconstructive Surgeons, Montreal, Canada, 1971.
9. Harashina T, Nakajima H, Imai T. Reconstruction of mandibular defects with revascularized free rib grafts. *Plast Reconstr Surg* 1978;62:514.
10. Serafin D, Villareal-Rios A, Georgiade NG. A rib-containing free flap to reconstruct mandibular defects. *Br J Plast Surg* 1977;30:263.
11. Daniel RK. Mandibular reconstruction with free tissue transfers. *Ann Plast Surg* 1978;1:346.
12. Serafin D, Riefkohl R. In: Serafin D, Buncke HJ, Jr, eds. *Microsurgical composite tissue transplantation.* St. Louis: Mosby, 1979.

CHAPTER 202 ■ MICROVASCULAR FREE TRANSFER OF SERRATUS ANTERIOR AND RIB COMPOSITE FLAP

W. C. LINEWEAVER, F. ZHANG, AND A. KELLS

The serratus anterior–rib composite flap is a versatile flap with use in reconstruction of both bone and soft-tissue defects. Clinical applications have shown that the serratus anterior–rib composite flap offers a long thoracodorsal vascular pedicle, large pedicle vessels for anastomoses, relatively simple dissection, soft-tissue coverage without large muscle bulk, and a favorable donor site.

INDICATIONS

By using the serratus as the source of rib blood supply and the thoracodorsal vessels as the pedicle, the serratus anterior–rib composite flap avoids the disadvantages of the short internal mammary or the posterior intercostal pedicles of microvascular rib osseous or osteocutaneous flaps (1,2). Based on its cross-sectional area and curved shape, the rib is an excellent source of vascularized bone to reconstruct defects of the facial bones, particularly the mandible. The serratus anterior–rib composite flap is suitable for repair of mandibular defects with soft-tissue loss, either of the floor of the mouth or of the chin or neck (3). The circumferential thickness of rib and its general shape are also similar to what is found in metacarpal and metatarsal bones. The serratus–rib composite flap can provide an excellent resource for reconstruction of metacarpal and metatarsal defects with associated soft-tissue defects (4,5).

In reconstruction of segmental long-bone defects of the lower extremity, vascularized fibular osteoseptocutaneous flaps are generally recommended as the first choice, because the fibular flap has several advantages (6–8). However, when the fibular flap is not available and the bone defects are greater than 10 cm, serratus anterior–rib flaps become useful alternative flaps. Because the rib flap is curved, rather than straight, and has a limited cross-sectional area to withstand body weight-load, indications in lower-extremity reconstruction at this point are (a) bilateral tibial fibular defects greater than 10 to 12 cm; (b) extensive composite defects of bone and soft tissue; and (c) contralateral fibula damage, making the vascular anatomy and dissection unreliable and difficult. The flap may need to be extended to include two or three ribs, to provide more strength and to support axial weight-bearing (9,10).

ANATOMY

The serratus anterior muscle is located on the lateral thoracic wall. Its fibers arise from the outer surfaces of the upper 9 to 10 ribs anterolaterally and insert into the medial border of the scapula. The serratus anterior muscle receives a dual blood supply. The lateral thoracic artery, located anterior to the subscapular-thoracodorsal artery, enters the lateral surface of the muscle and then courses anteriorly with multiple branches into the muscle. The second blood supply is via the thoracodorsal artery, which has branches to the serratus anterior. Studies of dissections of the thoracodorsal artery showed that in 99% of cases, the thoracodorsal artery gave off one or more branches to the serratus anterior muscle (11). Rarely, this serratus pedicle can branch off directly from the axillary vessels (12).

The rib has a dual blood supply that includes nutrient vessels from the posterior intercostal artery, as well as a periosteal blood supply through the serratus anterior muscle from the serratus anterior branch of the thoracodorsal artery (13). Dye-injection studies of the thoracodorsal system demonstrate continuity between the serratus branch and the intercostal arteries through the periosteal vessels. Arteriograms through the distal thoracodorsal arteries also show consistent filling of the lower sixth to ninth intercostal vessels from the serratus muscle perforators. These findings further demonstrate consistent communication between the serratus branch and the intercostal arteries through the periosteal vessels (5).

FLAP DESIGN AND DIMENSIONS

With the patient placed in the lateral position, the flap is planned anterior to the anterior axillary line and is centered over the sixth rib, with extensions above and below the fifth and seventh ribs. The lower the rib is taken, the longer the pedicle obtained. If necessary, a skin paddle of approximately 6 × 12 cm overlying the ribs can be elevated. For lower-extremity reconstruction, one rib graft is too weak to support body weight. Two or three sections of ribs may be used, to provide more strength and to support axial weight-bearing.

OPERATIVE TECHNIQUE

Initial elevation of the flap is via a midaxial anterior skin flap incision. The anterior border of the latissimus dorsi muscle is identified and retracted posteriorly. The thoracodorsal vessels are exposed between the posterior surface of this muscle and the serratus anterior. The serratus branch of the thoracodorsal

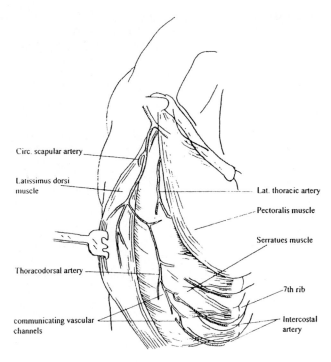

FIG. 1. Operative exposure for flap harvest.

is traced to the desired muscle segment. The serratus muscle is then dissected from the scapula. Generally, the cephalad four slips of the serratus muscle are left intact to anchor the scapula, and the flap is composed of the distal slips.

At the designed rib-muscle segment, the intercostal neurovascular bundle can be easily identified (Fig. 1). Adequate intercostal muscles are left with the periosteum of the chosen rib, particularly at the lower border, to preserve the neurovascular bundle. The rib is then transected immediately lateral to the costochondral junction.

The extrapleural dissection may be difficult because the parietal pleura is densely adherent to the posterior rib periosteum. It may be necessary to sacrifice a portion of the pleura in order to preserve the periosteum. In this situation, the pleura has to be closed by approximating the adjacent ribs, and temporary chest-tube placement is necessary. If two ribs are to be used, harvesting alternative ribs is better than harvesting consecutive rib segments. If three ribs are harvested, the continuous two-rib defect should be protected with a sheet of synthetic Marlex mesh or lyophilized dura, to reinforce the chest wall.

The serratus anterior–rib composite flap is now isolated on the serratus branch of the thoracodorsal pedicle, which is dissected proximally toward the axilla and can be divided at an appropriate level.

CLINICAL RESULTS

In 1984, Richards et al. (3) reported seven cases of microvascular free and pedicled transfer of rib composite flaps, with overlying muscle for reconstructions of mandibular defects caused by injury, tumor resection, and hemifacial microsomia (Fig. 2). In mandibular reconstruction, the vascularized rib was eminently suitable, as lengths of bone between 12 and 16 cm are required. Long segments of rib can be bent by greenstick fracturing, after making cuts on the inner cortex. The reconstructions were proved solid and looked satisfactory on radiographs. Loss of soft tissue of the flap was reported in two of seven cases. Buncke's group (2,14) also reported successful

mandibular reconstruction with microvascular serratus–rib composite free-flap transfer. In a typical case, 18 cm of the sixth rib was contoured into place, by subperiosteal scoring and screw fixation, to the remnant left side of the mandible, after resection of a malignant histiocytoma of the right side of the mandible. Postoperative follow-up showed bony restoration.

In 1999, Hui et al. (5) reported two cases of microvascular serratus–rib composite free-flap transfers for reconstruction of the first metacarpal bone. In these cases, the ribs were placed in the metacarpal defect and secured with Kirschner wires. The first metacarpophalangeal joint was fused. Subsequent healing was uneventful. The results showed that the vascularized rib graft offers ideal structural support, and the circumferential thickness is similar to that of the metacarpal. This flap offers a long vascular pedicle with less muscle bulk in reconstruction of hands with metacarpal and soft-tissue defects. Moscona et al. (4) and Bruck et al. (13) also reported similar results of microvascular serratus–rib composite free-flap transfers for metatarsal reconstruction. In these cases, the ribs were also fixed in placed by axial Kirschner wires. Postoperative technetium-99 bone scan showed good perfusion, and radiographs confirmed union of the metatarsal bones.

Lin et al. (9,10) reported serratus anterior rib flaps that were used for composite tibial bone and soft-tissue reconstruction in 22 patients. Two of these patients underwent bilateral serratus anterior rib flaps for bilateral tibia-fibular open grade IIIB fractures. The number of ribs harvested varied between one and three, depending on the bone defect. The limbs were protected with a brace and with crutch ambulation for up to 1 year, until adequate hypertrophy of the ribs occurred. The results showed that 21 of 24 flaps survived completely. Fifteen of 21 flaps had primary bone union and hypertrophy of the bone. The unhealed tibias were treated with secondary conventional bone grafting or Ilizarov bone transportation.

In addition to recipient complications such as flap loss, nonunion, osteomyelitis, and stress fracture, donor-site

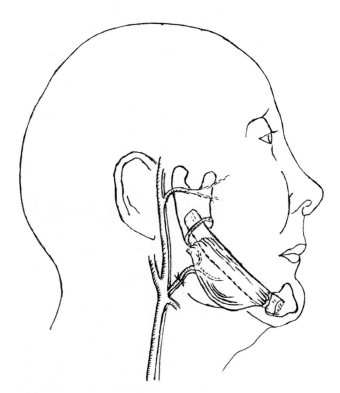

FIG. 2. Flap inset for mandibular reconstruction (pedicle vessels are anastomosed to the facial vessels).

morbidities, including pneumothorax, pleural fibrosis, chest-wall deformities, and chronic chest pain, are rarely reported. Generally, the donor site is inconspicuous and asymptomatic.

SUMMARY

The serratus anterior–rib composite flap, with the advantages of a long thoracodorsal vascular pedicle, simple dissection, soft-tissue coverage without large muscle bulk, and low donor-site complications, can provide excellent bone and soft tissue for reconstruction of mandible, metacarpal, and metatarsal defects combined with soft-tissue loss. When the fibular flap is not available and bone defects are greater than 10 cm, serratus anterior–rib flaps become a useful alternative for repair of tibial bone and soft-tissue defects.

References

1. Buncke HJ, Furnas DW, Gordon L, et al. Free osteocutaneous flap from a rib to the tibia. *Plast Reconstr Surg* 1977;59:799.
2. Buncke HJ. Rib microvascular transplantation. In: Buncke HJ, Ed., *Microsurgery: transplantation-replantation.* Philadelphia: Lea & Febiger, 1991;350–367.
3. Richards MA, Poole MD, Godfrey AM. The serratus anterior/rib composite flap for mandibular reconstruction. *Br J Plast Surg* 1985;38:466.
4. Moscona RA, Ulhmann Y, Hirshowitz B. Free composite serratus anterior muscle-rib flap for reconstruction of the severely damaged foot. *Ann Plast Surg* 1988;20:167.
5. Hui KC, Zhang F, Lineaweaver WC, et al. Serratus anterior-rib composite flap: anatomic studies and clinical application to hand reconstruction. *Ann Plast Surg* 1999;42:132.
6. Malizos KN, Nunley JA, Goldner RD, et al. Free vascularized fibula in traumatic long bone defects and in limb salvaging following tumor resection: comparative study. *Microsurgery* 1993;14:368.
7. Yazar S, Lin CH, Wei FC. One-stage reconstruction of composite bone and soft tissue defects in traumatic lower extremities. *Plast Reconstr Surg* 2004;114:1457.
8. Pollock R, Stalley P, Lee K, Pennington D. Free vascularized fibula grafts in limb salvage surgery. *J Reconstr Microsurg* 2005;21:79.
9. Lin CH, Wei PC, Levin S, et al. Free composite serratus anterior and rib flaps for tibial composite bone and soft-tissue defect. *Plast Reconstr Surg* 1997;99:1656.
10. Lin CH, Yazar S. Revisiting the serratus anterior rib flap for composite tibial defects. *Plast Reconstr Surg* 2004;114:1871.
11. Rowsell AR, Davies DM, Eisenberg N, Taylor GI. The anatomy of the subscapular thoracodorsal arterial system: study of 100 cadaver dissections. *Br J Plast Surg* 1984;37:574.
12. Goldberg JA, Lineaweaver WC, Buncke HJ. An aberrant independent origin of the serratus anterior pedicle. *Ann Plast Surg* 1990;25:487.
13. Bruck JC, Bier J, Kistler D. The serratus anterior osteocutaneous free flap. *J Reconstr Microsurg* 1990;6:209.
14. Whitney TM, Buncke HJ, Alpert BS, et al. The serratus anterior free-muscle flap: experience with 100 consecutive cases. *Plast Reconstr Surg* 1990;86:481.

CHAPTER 203 ■ MICROVASCULAR TRANSFER OF THE COMPOUND DORSALIS PEDIS SKIN FLAP WITH SECOND METATARSAL FOR MANDIBLE AND FLOOR OF MOUTH RECONSTRUCTION

R. M. ZUKER AND R. T. MANKTELOW

EDITORIAL COMMENT

Care must be taken in closure of the donor site to prevent late donor-site problems. By releasing the tendons laterally and medially and shifting them toward the midline, the bony defect can be covered. A skin graft then can be placed over this vascularized surface.

Perhaps one of the most significant contributions to head and neck reconstruction is the use of the free composite osteocutaneous flap (1–8). The dorsalis pedis flap (9,10), when used with the second metatarsal, can reconstruct not only the floor of the mouth but also up to 8 cm of the mandible itself with vascularized tissue.

INDICATIONS

Reconstruction of head and neck defects is most difficult following composite resections. There are occasions when no bony reconstruction of any kind is mandatory, such as hemimandibular resections. We believe reconstruction with vascularized bone provides the patient with the best reconstructive alternative. Thus, a hemimandibular resection would be a relative indication.

Anterior segment defects, on the other hand, leave the patient with a significant functional and aesthetic deformity that requires reconstruction. Conventional techniques often fall short of providing adequate, lasting bone for both contour restoration and function. Problems may ensue with mastication, the production of intelligible speech, and drooling. The dorsalis pedis flap with the metatarsal, when osteotomized, provides an excellent reconstructive tool for the anterior segment defect, one that cannot be provided by any other available means of reconstruction. The anterior segment composite resection, then, does provide an absolute indication for the compound dorsalis pedis skin and metatarsal flap, provided that the bony defect can be reconstructed with the 7 to 8 cm of metatarsal available.

Among advantages of the flap are that it provides vascularized bone for difficult reconstructive problems such as anterior segment defects. It also provides thin, pliable tissue for mucosal resurfacing, a long vascular pedicle, and a donor site that is remote from the recipient site, which may have been radiated.

FLAP DESIGN AND DIMENSIONS

With postoperative lingual swelling, the pedicle could be compromised seriously if its position were between the tongue and mandible. Thus, it is better to have the vascular pedicle external to the mandible. The most likely site of recipient vasculature is identified. Because the position of the vessels should be external to the mandible, it is best to use the contralateral foot. Routine angiography is not necessary if adequate independent dorsalis pedis and posterior tibial pulses are present.

The boundaries of the skin flap include the extensor retinaculum proximally, the interdigital web spaces distally, and 1 cm on either side of the extensor hallucis longus (medially) and extensor digiti quinti (laterally). The second metatarsal then lies beneath the central segment of the skin flap (see Fig. 2B).

OPERATIVE TECHNIQUE

The operation is carried out in three parts. The tumor (Fig. 1A) is resected along with the anterior segment of mandible. Usually, a lip-splitting approach is used (Fig. 1B). A radical neck dissection is often necessary, and the recipient vasculature is prepared on this side. We have used virtually all the branches of the external carotid artery to revascularize this flap. Usually, however, the superior thyroid or facial vessels, if available, are used. To assist in the mandibular reconstruction, the mandible that has been resected is measured on either side of the midline and its angle at the anterior segment is esti-

mated. A template of this resected segment may be useful in planning the osteotomy of the second metatarsal.

Donor Site

The dissection begins distally between the first and second toes, where the first dorsal metatarsal artery is identified (11). This usually lies in the interosseous musculature on a superficial plane. This vessel, then, will be visualized throughout the dissection, and it and any musculature that lies between it and the second metatarsal should be included in the flap.

The extensor tendons to the second toe are divided at the metatarsophalangeal level, and this joint is entered. The second metatarsal is included with the skin flap with transection of the intermetatarsal ligaments and the interosseous musculature along the adjacent borders of the first and third metatarsi.

The skin flap is elevated just superficial to the paratenon overlying the extensor tendons. The fine attachments between the second metatarsal and the skin flap are maintained. The extensor tendons to the second toe remain on the foot to aid in closure. With elevation from distal to proximal, the extensor hallucis brevis tendon is encountered. Because this tendon lies between the skin flap and the first dorsal metatarsal artery, it must be maintained in the flap.

At the medial border of the dissection, care is taken to maintain continuity between the flap and the long saphenous vein. The decision regarding venous drainage will be made at the termination of the dissection, but during elevation, both the long saphenous vein and the venae comitantes of the anterior tibial–dorsalis pedis–first dorsal metatarsal vascular system must be maintained.

The dissection then proceeds proximally to the base of the second metatarsal. Extreme care must be taken at this point not to damage the perforating branch of the dorsalis pedis artery and to preserve the takeoff of the first dorsal metatarsal artery within the flap. The first dorsal metatarsal artery originates from the dorsalis pedis artery as it passes over the second cuneiform bone and plunges down to the plantar arch (see Anatomy, Chapter 278). The perforator must be visualized and transected deep to the takeoff of the first dorsal metatarsal artery. This latter vessel, along with the interosseous musculature adjacent to the second metatarsal, must be maintained in the flap.

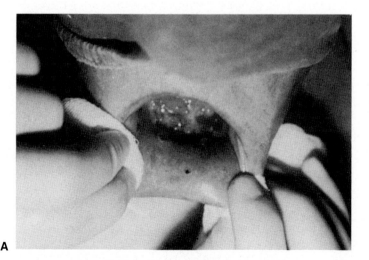
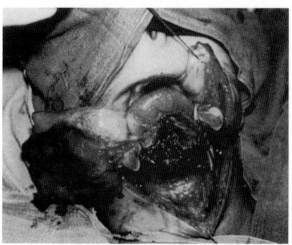

A   B

FIG. 1. A: Squamous cell cancer of sulcus with mandibular involvement. B: Defect after resection of tumor.

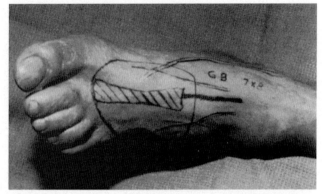
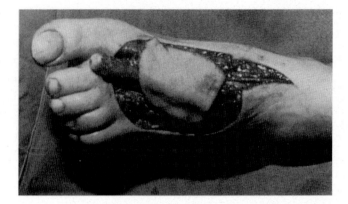

A,B

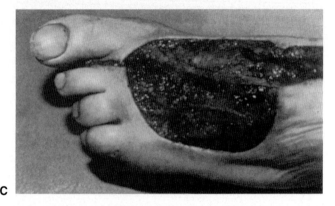

C

FIG. 2. A: The compound dorsalis pedis skin flap with second metatarsal. B: Flap elevated on vascular pedicle. C: Donor site prepared for split-thickness skin grafting.

Before complete separation of the bone, it is helpful to isolate the dorsalis pedis artery and its venae comitantes. The proximal skin incision is made, and the superficial peroneal nerves are sacrificed. This flap has the potential for innervation should this be desirable. The proximal bony attachments at this point are divided. The capsular attachments to the cuneiforms and adjacent metatarsi are transected using a no. 11 blade. Extreme care is taken to protect the dorsalis pedis vessels, the perforating branch, and the first dorsal metatarsal vessels.

Patience is necessary at this point to free the bone from its dense fibrous capsular attachments. Once the bone is freed, the flap attachments consist of only the long saphenous vein and the dorsalis pedis artery and its venae comitantes. Through a more proximal curvilinear incision, the extensor retinaculum is incised, facilitating dissection of the dorsalis pedis vessels and, more proximally, the anterior tibial vessels. The vascular pedicles are dissected to the length required (Fig. 2B). The circulation within the flap is allowed to stabilize before definitive flap separation. The flap is completely separated from the foot and transferred to the recipient site.

Donor-site closure of the foot must not be undertaken lightly. Much of the criticism directed toward this flap has been in regard to difficult donor-site problems, which can be avoided by using proper closure technique. After complete hemostasis has been obtained, the first and third metatarsi are approximated distally using heavy wire or Mersilene sutures. The second toe is amputated with approximation of the first and second web spaces. To obtain a healthy, vascularized bed for skin grafting, the tendon and paratendinous tissue must be approximated. Two bipedicled tendon flaps are elevated. The medial one consists of only the extensor hallucis longus with its paratenon. The lateral flap consists of the extensor tendons to the second, third, fourth, and fifth toes as well as the surrounding paratenon. Bipedicle flaps are elevated directly above the periosteum. These flaps then are mobilized and

directed toward each other to form a continuous vascularized surface. They are approximated with heavy absorbable sutures. All rents in the paratenon must be closed with fine absorbable sutures.

An even vascularized bed then is prepared for grafting (Fig. 2). We prefer a medium-thickness split-thickness skin graft, which is held in place with a tieover bolus dressing. The ankle is maintained in the neutral position with a posterior slab. Elevation and bed rest are maintained for 10 days.

Recipient Site

The flap is transferred to the head and neck area. All bony work must be done before revascularization. In a hemimandibular reconstruction, osteotomy is rarely necessary. The length of the resected mandible then is reconstructed using a similar length of metatarsal. The cartilaginous surface at either end of the metatarsal is removed, so that a direct end-to-end apposition of bone can be achieved. It is best to use as much cancellous segment of the metatarsal as possible for the osteosynthesis. We prefer two interosseous wire loops at either end for bony fixation.

For anterior segment defects, an osteotomy is almost always necessary. The osteotomy need not be symmetrical, as the endosteal blood supply to the metatarsal enters at either end. The periosteal blood supply is also maintained. Accurate lengths of the resected segment then are planned for the reconstruction. The site and angle of the osteotomy are outlined. We prefer a closing-wedge osteotomy (Fig. 3A) that is maintained by two interosseous wire loops. Final tightening and adjustment of these wire loops are left until the bone has been wired in place.

The cartilage from either end of the metatarsal is removed, so that direct apposition between the metatarsal and the resid-

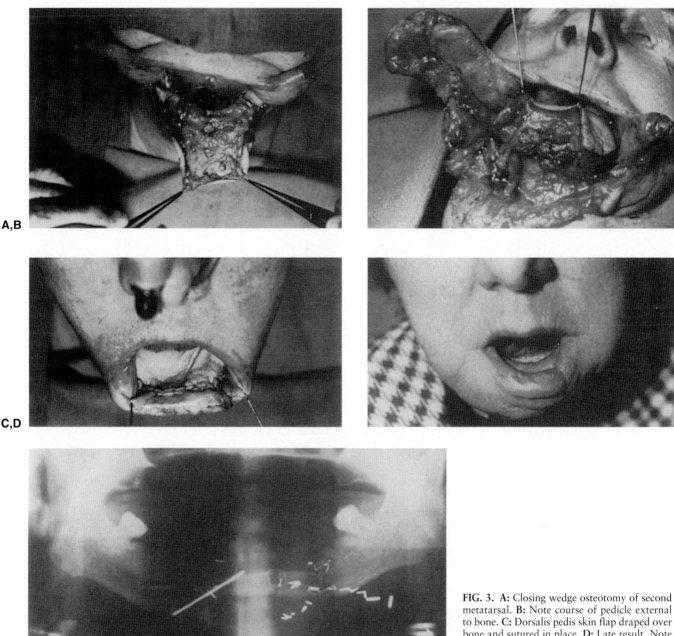

A,B

C,D

E

FIG. 3. **A:** Closing wedge osteotomy of second metatarsal. **B:** Note course of pedicle external to bone. **C:** Dorsalis pedis skin flap draped over bone and sutured in place. **D:** Late result. Note intraoral flap and adequate chin projection. **E:** Radiograph of reconstructed mandible.

ual mandible can be achieved. Again, maximal cancellous contact is preferable. Two accurately placed interosseous wire loops provide for bony fixation at either end (Fig. 3B). The residual mandibular segments should be placed in as near preoperative occlusion as possible. In this way, optimal chin projection can be achieved.

Once the final adjustments and tightening of the wires are done, the flap is revascularized. Generally, the long saphenous vein is used as the venous drainage system; however, if it is small and the vena comitans of the anterior tibial artery is of sufficient size, the vena comitans is used. One artery and one vein are all that are required for anastomosis. With release of the clamps, revascularization is evident not only in the skin but also from the prepared bone ends and the muscle cuff around the second metatarsal.

The skin flap is then definitively sutured in place with watertight interrupted mattress sutures (Fig. 3C). The neck flaps are repositioned with appropriate suction drainage. Great care in oral hygiene is maintained for 2 weeks until oral intake is permitted. A nasogastric tube is sufficient to provide adequate nutritional intake. The skin flap is thin and pliable and thus contours well over the metatarsa. The late reconstructive results are excellent in terms of soft-tissue cover and chin projection (Fig. 3D and E).

CLINICAL RESULTS

Donor-site healing problems may occur if care is not taken in donor-site closure. Also, this is a difficult flap to elevate.

SUMMARY

The dorsalis pedis skin flap with second metatarsal may be useful for composite floor of the mouth and mandibular defects. It is particularly helpful where conventional bone grafting is unlikely to succeed (anterior segment in radiated bed) and the aesthetic and functional consequences of inadequate reconstruction would be disastrous.

References

1. Gilbert A. Composite tissue transfers from the foot: anatomic basis and surgical technique. In: Daniller A, Strauch B, eds. *Symposium on microsurgery.* St. Louis: Mosby, 1976;230.
2. May JW Jr, Chait LA, Cohen BE, O'Brien BM. Free neurovascular flap from the first web of the foot in hand reconstruction. *J Hand Surg* 1977; 2:387.
3. Morrison WA, O'Brien BM, MacLeod AM. The foot as a donor site in reconstructive microsurgery. *World J Surg* 1979;3:43.
4. O'Brien BM, Morrison WA, MacLeod AM, Dooly BJ. Microvascular osteocutaneous transfer using the groin flap and iliac crest and the dorsalis pedis flap and second metatarsal. *Br J Plast Surg* 1979;32:188.
5. Zuker RM, Manktelow RT, Palmer JA, Rosen IB. Head and neck reconstruction following resection of carcinoma using microvascular free flaps. *Surgery* 1980;88:461.
6. Zuker RM, Rosen IB, Palmer JA, et al. Microvascular free flaps in head and neck reconstruction. *Can J Surg* 1980;23:157.
7. Bell MSG. New method of oral reconstruction using a free composite foot flap. *Ann Plast Surg* 1980;5:281.
8. MacLeod AM, Robinson DW. Reconstruction of defects involving the mandible and floor of mouth by free osteocutaneous flaps derived from the foot. *Br J Plast Surg* 1982;35:239.
9. McCraw JB, Furlow LT. The dorsalis pedis arterialized flap. *Plast Reconstr Surg* 1975;1:177.
10. Duncan MJ, Manktelow RT, Zuker RM, Rosen IB. Mandibular reconstruction in the radiated patient: the role of osteocutaneous free tissue transfers. *Plast Reconstr Surg* 1985;76:829.
11. Ohtsuka H. Angiographic analysis of the first metatarsal artery. *Ann Plast Surg* 1981;7:2.

CHAPTER 204 ■ MICROVASCULAR FREE TRANSFER OF A COMPOUND DEEP CIRCUMFLEX GROIN AND ILIAC CREST FLAP TO THE MANDIBLE

G. I. TAYLOR AND R. J. CORLETT

The vascular territory of the deep circumflex iliac artery encompasses a large amount of skin and bone that can be used for one-stage transfer with reliability. The bone graft is well vascularized and provides excellent contour for the mandible, and the donor site has minimal morbidity (1,2). In addition to skin, other soft-tissue elements can be harvested with a common blood supply to provide a functional as well as an aesthetic result. This composite graft is best suited for the difficult problems encountered in head and neck reconstruction (3–5).

INDICATIONS

There have been many significant advances in the past 20 years in reconstruction of major defects of the mandible and the associated soft tissues (6–9). Initially, the forehead and deltopectoral flaps improved soft-tissue repair. They provided better coverage for nonvascularized bone grafts, taken usually from the iliac crest or the rib. Their reliability fell dramatically, however, if the area was heavily irradiated. The musculocutaneous flap provides additional bulk, as well as vascularized muscle, to cover the carotid vessels; however, the supply to associated bone segments has not proved to be reliable.

Although a number of donor sites have been used for this purpose, we believe that the iliac crest flap, designed initially on the superficial circumflex iliac artery and, more recently, on the deep circumflex iliac artery, has a number of advantages, especially when the bone gap is considerable. Large amounts of both iliac bone and groin skin are available from an area that has minimal donor-site morbidity, both cosmetic and functional.

The vessels for anastomosis are large, ranging from 1.5 to 3.0 mm in diameter, permitting reliable anastomoses. The

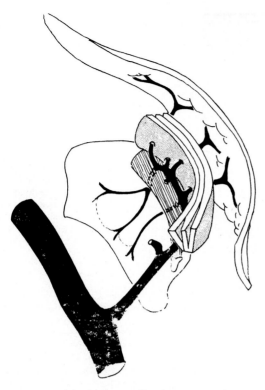

FIG. 1. Diagram of the deep circumflex iliac artery with its periosteal supply to the inner cortex of the ilium and the musculocutaneous perforators that pierce the three muscles of the abdominal wall at intervals to nourish the overlying skin. The iliacus muscle is *cross-hatched*. (From Taylor et al., ref. 2, with permission.)

may lie in a more superficial plane, and when this occurs, the variation usually is associated with an abnormal obturator artery.

The musculocutaneous perforators to the skin arise from the parent artery as it lies adjacent to the inner aspect of the ilium. They penetrate the muscles beyond the anterior superior iliac spine and emerge from the external oblique in a row approximately 1 cm above the iliac crest. The terminal part of the deep circumflex iliac artery usually emerges as the largest perforator 8 to 10 cm from the anterior superior iliac spine.

The deep circumflex iliac artery is 1.0 to 1.5 mm in diameter and is usually suitable for anastomosis. It can be used to provide a distal runoff from the graft or to connect to another vessel (e.g., the superficial circumflex iliac artery) to augment cutaneous circulation. After division of the three layers of the abdominal wall, the deep circumflex iliac artery will be found situated in the fold between the overhanging transversus muscle and the iliacus.

FLAP DESIGN AND DIMENSIONS

We perform angiography on most patients, which provides valuable information on both the donor and recipient vessels (Fig. 2). It outlines the effects of previous surgery, radiation, or tumor expansion on the vascular anatomy. The finding of an abnormal obturator artery in the groin is a preoperative warning that the course of the deep circumflex iliac artery may be more superficial than normal, although we have yet to encounter this in a clinical case.

The presence or absence of suitable recipient vessels on one side of the neck is noted after neck dissection or radiation

pedicle is long, from 5.0 to 9.0 cm. The anatomy is familiar to most surgeons. Not only is the iliac crest the ideal shape for mandibular reconstruction, but sufficient bone is available in an adult to reconstruct an entire mandible with a vascularized graft from one hip.

The bone can be contoured or split, or appropriate osteotomies can be performed to obtain an exact replica of the jaw. Also, soft tissue other than skin may be included in the graft design to reconstruct muscle and ligamentous attachments to the lower jaw.

ANATOMY

The deep circumflex iliac artery arises from its posterolateral side at the level of the inguinal ligament. The artery, together with its paired venae comitantes, courses upward and laterally in its own fascial sheath behind the inguinal ligament toward the anterior superior iliac spine (Fig. 1). The paired venae comitantes join to form a single vein 2 to 3 cm lateral to the external iliac artery. This vein then characteristically diverges upward from its artery to reach the external iliac vein. In so doing, it crosses either in front of or behind the external iliac artery. At this point of divergence, there is usually a communication with one of the venae comitantes of the superficial circumflex iliac artery.

Approximately 1 cm medial to the anterior superior iliac spine, a large ascending muscular branch is given off. This vessel pierces the transversus muscle and the internal oblique. It may be found reliably 1 cm above and lateral to the anterior superior iliac spine. Rarely, the deep circumflex iliac vessels

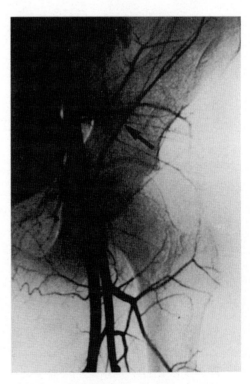

FIG. 2. Angiogram showing the characteristic "paintbrush stroke" of the deep circumflex iliac artery passing upward and laterally at 45 degrees from the region of the hip joint. (From Taylor, Daniel, ref. 11, with permission.)

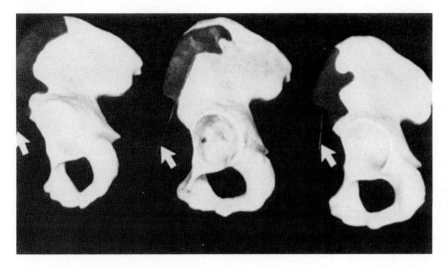

FIG. 3. The three methods of designing the ramus and body of the mandible from the ilium. The first and third technique place the vascular pedicle (*arrow*) at the angle of the jaw. The second method sites the graft pedicle at the jaw midline, where it will reach recipient vessels on either side of the neck. (From Taylor, ref. 12, with permission.)

therapy, and this predicts the need for vein grafts or a modification of graft design.

An acrylic pelvis with detachable iliac crests is a useful aid when selecting the donor hip for planning the correct orientation of the graft. A methyl methacrylate replica of the bone defect is made preoperatively and used both in the planning and as a preoperative check of the size and shape of the graft both at the donor and recipient sites (Fig. 4). The mandible may be designed from the iliac crest in one of three ways, depending on the length of graft required and the position of the vascular pedicle (see Fig. 1).

1. The usual method uses the ipsilateral hip. The lower jaw is designed in such a way that the anterior superior iliac spine becomes the angle of the mandible, the anterior inferior iliac spine becomes the head, and the iliac

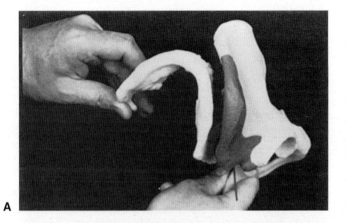

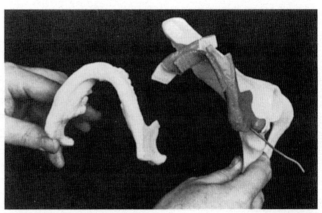

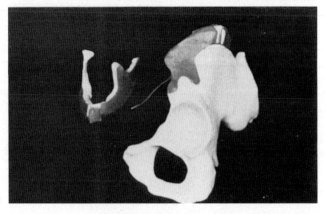

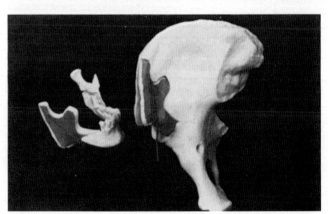

FIG. 4. Bone models used in planning. **A:** The curve of the iliac crest matches the lower border of the body of the mandible to the chin and then veers away. **B:** Osteotomy performed from the outer cortex to recreate the chin contour. This may be done as a step or a wedge osteotomy. **C:** The graft model used to plan case 1. Note the keystone of bone at the chin point. **D:** The graft model used for case 2. The graft was split from the inner aspect of the ilium to leave the outer cortex and hemiapophysis for normal hip contour and growth. (From Taylor, ref. 10, with permission.)

crest becomes the body of the mandible. The vascular pedicle will be situated behind the new angle of the jaw. Here it is readily accessible for anastomosis to one of the branches of the external carotid system (e.g., the facial artery). This design allows the greatest length of graft to be obtained for mandibular construction. A wedge or step osteotomy is performed in the midline to adjust the curvature of the bone when the graft extends beyond the chin (Fig. 5, *left*).

2. For reconstruction of short mandibular segments, the bone graft may be designed so that the anterior iliac crest becomes the ramus of the jaw and the bone between the anterior superior iliac spine and the anterior inferior iliac spine becomes the body (Fig. 5, *center*).

3. Alternatively, the first pattern can be reversed so that the ramus is contoured from the posterior ilium and the body from the anterior part of the crest. This places the pedicle near the midline, and it will reach vessels on the opposite side of the neck. Because of the curvature of the crest, the graft must be designed from the opposite hip (Fig. 5, *right*).

Despite all preoperative planning outlined, it may be difficult to anticipate some of the three-dimensional problems encountered during actual surgery. Rehearsal of the operation on a fresh cadaver has been invaluable in solving these problems before entering the operating room.

A plastic foam replica of the skin defect is shaped, and this pattern is transferred to the hip, taking care to center it over the skin perforators. The skin flap is marked two thirds above and one third below the line of the anterior iliac crest. The flap will survive as far medially as the femoral vessels, but it must incorporate the perforators that emerge above the iliac crest between 2 and 8 cm from the anterior superior iliac spine. The acrylic model is used to outline the bone graft. Doppler studies can be used to locate the recipient vessels in the neck.

OPERATIVE TECHNIQUE

The dissection of the graft is conveniently divided into four steps: (a) a medial isolation of the pedicle, (b) an upper lateral division of the muscles of the anterior abdominal wall, (c) a lower lateral separation of the upper thigh muscles, and (d) a deep section of the ilium (Figs. 5–14).

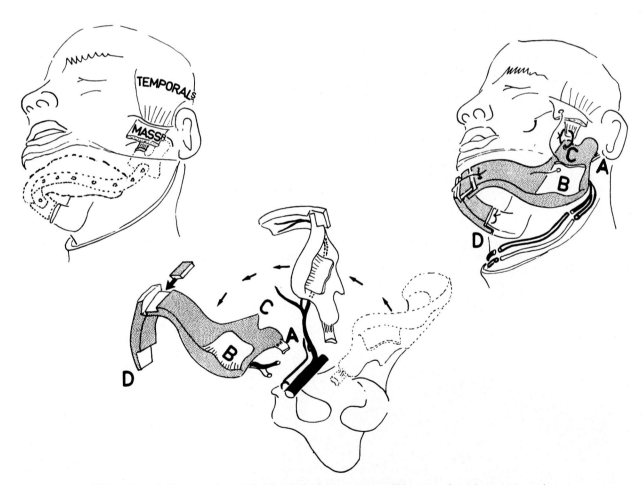

FIG. 5. Case 1. The procedure. *Left:* Resection of the entire mandible except the right ramus, together with the tumor, the metal prosthesis, and the soft tissues from the lower lip to the level of the hyoid bone. *Center:* The graft designed from the ipsilateral hip. A segment of the rectus femoris tendon, *A*, provides capsular ligaments for the temporomandibular joint. A flap of fascia lata, *B*, allows reattachment of the masseter muscle. A coronoid process, *C*, is shaped from the blade of the ilium to secure the temporalis tendon. An osteotomy is made in the midline to recreate the chin and is secured with a free bone keystone. The bone is step-cut at point *D* for fixation to the right ramus. *Right:* The graft in position with vein grafts needed to reach normal recipient vessels on the opposite side of the neck.

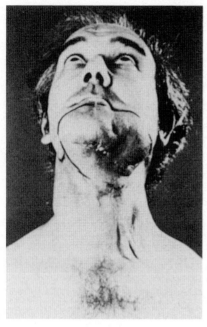

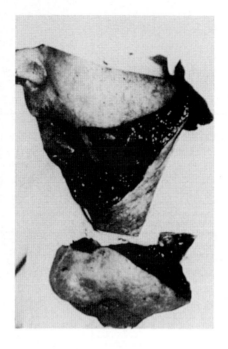

A,B

FIG. 6. Case 1. **A:** A recurrent squamous cell carcinoma with fistula onto the neck. Note the margins of the soft-tissue excision. **B:** Resection of the tumor. (From Taylor, ref. 12, with permission.)

Medial Dissection

In the medial dissection, the skin is incised directly over the inguinal canal, and the external ring is located. The external oblique aponeurosis is split parallel to and 1 cm above the free edge of the inguinal ligament. The external iliac artery is palpated through the posterior wall of the inguinal canal.

The pedicle is dissected laterally, dividing the arching fibers of the internal oblique and the transversus muscles from the inguinal ligament. It is often useful to look for the large ascending muscular branch of the deep circumflex iliac artery (reliably found 1 cm above and lateral to the anterior superior iliac spine) early in the dissection and trace it down to the main pedicle.

Upper Lateral Dissection

In the upper lateral dissection, to retain the musculocutaneous perforators to the skin, a 1.5- to 2.0-cm-wide strip of the three abdominal wall muscles is left attached to the bone, extending posteriorly for 8 to 10 cm. During the course of

this dissection, the ascending branch of the deep circumflex iliac artery is encountered. After division of the three layers of the abdominal wall, this artery will be found situated in the fold between the overhanging transversus muscle and the iliacus. The iliacus muscle is divided 1 cm below and medial to this line, and the remaining muscle is swept from the surface of the iliac bone by blunt finger dissection to preserve the periosteal supply.

Lower Lateral Dissection

Because the deep circumflex iliac artery supplies the ilium from its medial side, in the lower lateral dissection, the muscles attached to its lateral aspect can be safely separated from the bone. It is useful to retain some of the attachments to this side of the bone for use in mandibular reconstruction. A segment of tensor fasciae latae can be left on the outer lip of the iliac crest to reattach the masseter muscle. Similarly, the tendon of the rectus femoris is preserved at the anterior inferior iliac spine for reconstruction of the capsule of the temporomandibular joint.

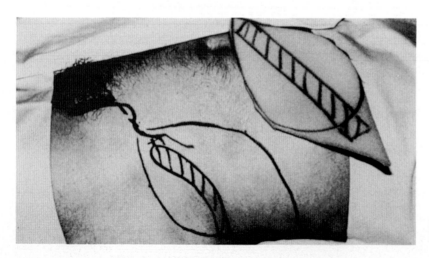

FIG. 7. Case 1. Pattern of the soft-tissue and bone requirements transferred to the ipsilateral hip. The skin flap measured 28 × 15 cm, and the bone graft, which measured 21 × 7 cm, included the entire iliac crest.

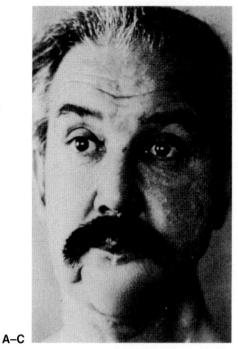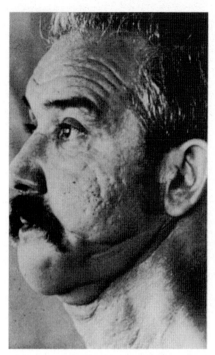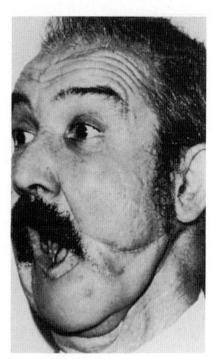

A–C

FIG. 8. A–C: Case 1. The result at 3 years. A bone scan and bone biopsies taken on either side of the osteotomy at day 5 confirmed viability of the entire graft. At 6 weeks, the external fixation was removed, at which stage there was clinical union of the bone. The skin flap was thinned on two occasions, at 3 and 5 months.

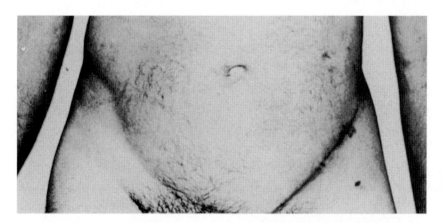

FIG. 9. Case 1. The donor site. Note the hip contour after removing the entire iliac crest and a large skin flap. (From Taylor, ref. 10, with permission.)

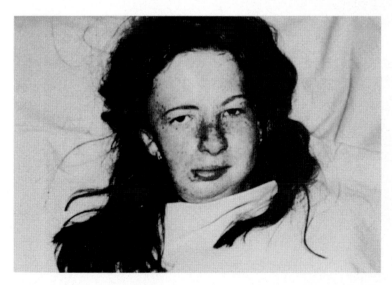

FIG. 10. Case 2. Right hemifacial microsomia in a 13-year-old with deformity of the right ear and partial right facial palsy. The right ramus and a portion of the body of the mandible were absent, the ear and right maxilla were underdeveloped, and the soft tissues of the right side of the face were deficient. Two previous attempts at reconstruction—a silicone block spacer at 2 years of age and a conventional costochondral graft at 11 years of age—had been extruded owing to infection. Electrical studies showed that the right facial nerve was absent and what function the patient had was innervated from the left side. (From Taylor, ref. 10, with permission.)

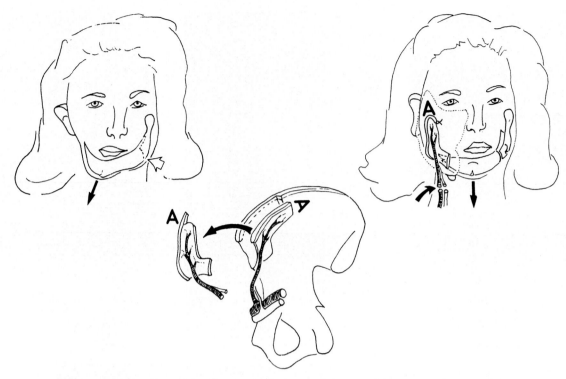

FIG. 11. Case 2. Diagram of the procedure. *Left:* Sagittal osteotomy of the left side of the mandible to centralize the chin. *Center:* Graft split from the hip with an additional flap of hemiapophysis to cap the new head of the mandible, *A.* This was done to retain normal hip development and to provide a possible growth center for the jaw. *Right:* The graft in position with anastomosis of the deep circumflex iliac vessels to the facial artery and common facial vein. The skin flap (*dotted lines*), shaved of epithelium, reconstitutes soft-tissue contour. (From Taylor, Daniel, ref. 11, with permission.)

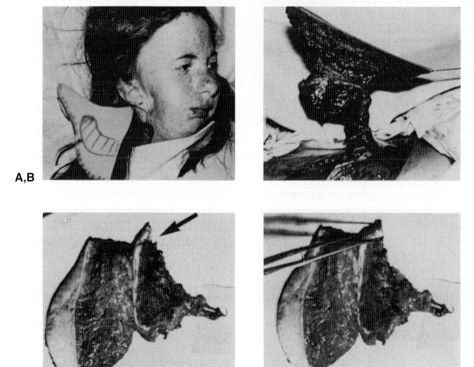

FIG. 12. Case 2. A: Pattern of the soft-tissue and bone requirements. B: The composite graft isolated on the deep circumflex iliac pedicle. A portion of the skin flap has been shaved of epithelium. A small portion of the skin flap was left intact to monitor the vascularity postoperatively. C,D: Flap of apophysial cartilage turned to cap the new head of the mandible. (From Taylor, Daniel, ref. 11, with permission.)

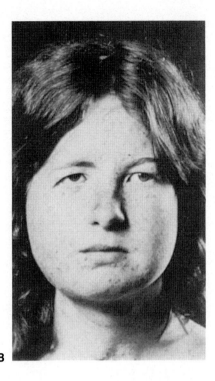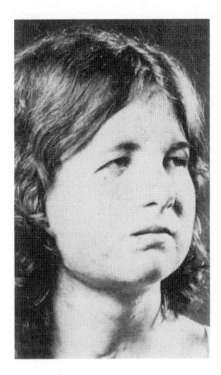

FIG. 13. A,B: Case 2. At 2 years, there is good correction of facial symmetry. No attempt has been made to correct the facial palsy. (From Taylor, Daniel, ref. 11, with permission.)

A,B

The upper and lower lateral parts of this dissection are then joined beyond the tuberosity of the crest. The remaining muscle attachments are separated from the bone as far posteriorly as the posterior superior iliac spine if this length of bone graft is required. The terminal branch of the deep circumflex iliac artery is thereby preserved in this part of the dissection. Finally, the inguinal ligament is detached from the anterior superior iliac spine, and the iliacus muscle is divided as it passes under the vascular pedicle. In so doing, the lateral cutaneous nerve of the thigh will be encountered. In some cases, its continuity can be retained; in others, it may have to be divided and repaired.

Bone Section

Careful preoperative planning and the use of bone models provide an accurate assessment of the required length and shape of the bone graft. The ilium is sectioned with an oscil-

lating or reciprocating saw. The bone is eased medially to prevent tension on the vascular pedicle. Further contouring and any osteotomies are performed while the graft is in situ. This shortens the ischemia time and permits circulatory readjustment in the flap before transfer.

Because the blood supply to the bone enters the medial cortex, it is possible to remove excess bone or, indeed, the entire outer cortex if desired. Osteotomies may be performed to adjust the curvature of the bone. The integrity of the medial periosteum is preserved for distal graft perfusion, together with the attachments of the transversus and iliacus muscle to the inner lip of the iliac crest.

Removal of the wing of the ilium creates a breach in the lateral abdominal wall that requires careful closure. It is essential to repair the transversus muscle to the iliacus or the remaining iliac bone. Because the iliacus muscle is tenuous posteriorly, we have found it useful to drill a number of holes in the cut edge of the ilium to reattach the transversus muscle. The remaining part of the closure involves suture of the glutei and the tensor fasciae latae to the internal and external oblique muscles. A Tanner slide procedure may be useful if there is insufficient laxity in the external oblique.

CLINICAL RESULTS

The main disadvantage of this graft is its bulk, especially in obese or muscular patients; however, the skin and subcutaneous tissues can be omitted and the attached muscle sealed with a split-thickness skin graft. Alternatively, the skin flap may be thinned at a later stage.

SUMMARY

The deep circumflex groin skin and iliac crest flap provides both skin cover and lining, as well as vascularized bone, for mandibular reconstruction.

FIG. 14. Case 2. The hip contour and function are normal. (From Taylor, ref. 10, with permission.)

References

1. Taylor GI, Townsend P, Corlett RJ. Superiority of the deep circumflex iliac vessels as the supply for free groin flaps: experimental work. *Plast Reconstr Surg* 1979;64:595.
2. Taylor GI, Townsend P, Corlett RJ. Superiority of the deep circumflex iliac vessels as the supply for free groin flaps: clinical work. *Plast Reconstr Surg* 1979;64:745.
3. Manchester WM. Some technical improvements in the reconstruction of the mandible and temporomandibular joint. *Plast Reconstr Surg* 1972;50:249.
4. Merritt WH, Acharya G, Johnson ML. Complications in 45 island pectoralis major myocutaneous flaps for head and neck cancer reconstruction: a 13-month follow-up. Presented at the Annual Meeting of the American Society of Plastic and Reconstructive Surgeons, New York, October 23, 1981.
5. Baek S, Lawson W, Biller HF. An analysis of 133 pectoralis major myocutaneous flaps. *Plast Reconstr Surg* 1982;69:460.
6. Mehrhof A, Rosenstock A, Neifeld JP, et al. The pectoralis major myocutaneous flap in head and neck reconstruction: an analysis of complications. *Am J Surg* 1983;146:478.
7. Reid C, Taylor GI. The vascular territory of the acromiothoracic axis. *Br J Plast Surg* 1984;37:194.
8. Serafin D, Buncke HJ. Vascularized rib periosteal transplantation. In: Serafin D, Buncke HJ, eds. *Microsurgical composite tissue transplantation.* St. Louis: Mosby, 1979. Chap. 31.
9. Soutar DS, Scheker LR, Tanner NSB, McGregor IA. The radial forearm flap: a versatile method for intraoral reconstruction. *Br J Plast Surg* 1983;36:1.
10. Taylor GI. The current status of free vascularized bone grafts. *Clin Plast Surg* 1983;10:185.
11. Taylor GI, Daniel RK. Aesthetic aspects of microsurgery. *Clin Plast Surg* 1981;8:333.
12. Taylor GI. Reconstruction of the mandible with free composite iliac bone grafts. *Ann Plast Surg* 1982;9:361.

CHAPTER 205 ■ MICROVASCULAR FREE TRANSFER OF THE MEDIAL WALL OF THE ILIAC CREST ON THE DEEP CIRCUMFLEX ILIAC ARTERY FOR MANDIBULAR RECONSTRUCTION

H. R. STERMAN AND B. STRAUCH

EDITORIAL COMMENT

Use of the medial wall eliminates much of the postoperative discomfort of the patient. Although the osteotomized free fibular flap is more frequently used for mandibular reconstruction, especially when additional lining or skin is needed, the iliac-crest free flap remains an excellent technique when only bone is required.

The deep circumflex iliac artery (DCIA) osteous or osteocutaneous free flap is a technique for oromandibular reconstruction that maximizes function as well as form and maintains the quality of life for patients who may be cured or may only have a few months to live (1–10). A modification of the original flap that uses only the medial wall of the iliac crest has contributed a major advance, now allowing the bone flap to fill the defect precisely, thus refining its bony component and reducing morbidity.

INDICATIONS

The original DCIA flap was used when any defect of the mandible existed, from the condyle to the parasymphysis. Even defects that crossed the mentum could be reconstructed, and grafts up to 16 cm could be harvested along the crest. For extended defects that cross the mentum, a free osteotomized fibula is a better choice.

The DCIA osseous/osteocutaneous flap is better suited for reconstruction of the ramus, angle, and body of the mandible because of its natural curvature. When an osteocutaneous flap is involved, defects of the mucosa and extraoral skin can be replaced by using a large skin paddle. If the soft-tissue defect is relatively large, an accessory flap for mucosal or skin coverage may be required. The medial-wall DCIA free flap can be taken with bone alone or as a myoosseous or even osteocutaneous flap, thus providing for oral lining and bone for the reconstruction, or even provision of external skin. The medial-wall flap has become the flap of choice for segmental mandibular defects.

Advantages of using the medial wall include significantly less donor-site morbidity, such as pain, hernia, deformity, and gait disturbance. The medial cortex is thinner and provides a flap that is less bulky, provides good contour, and is more cosmetically acceptable. Variations include the use of the internal iliac muscle for soft-tissue coverage (10), allowing the muscle to be rotated through any arc, for coverage of any defect, and provision of thin, pliable tissue. This flap allows soft-tissue coverage with reconstruction of almost any mandibular defect except defects that cross the mentum. The thickness of the iliac-crest flap allows placement of osseointegrated implants into the free vascularized bone graft.

CHAPTER 206 ■ INTERNAL OBLIQUE–ILIAC CREST OSTEOMYOCUTANEOUS FREE FLAP IN OROMANDIBULAR RECONSTRUCTION

M. L. URKEN

EDITORIAL COMMENT

This is a good flap when a substantial amount of tissue is needed for internal lining. The internal oblique can be used with the ascending branch at the same time the iliac crest is used.

The iliac crest osteocutaneous flap, based on the deep circumflex iliac artery and vein (DCIA and DCIV), was a major innovation in oromandibular reconstruction and helped to revolutionize the approach to the management of oral cancers (1). The problem with this composite flap was related to the soft-tissue component, which was often too bulky and unreliable, especially when positioning the skin paddle in ways that threatened its normal anatomic relationship to the bone. Such demands on the skin paddle are frequent when reconstructing the three-dimensional geometry of the oral cavity and oropharynx. The internal oblique muscle, supplied by the ascending branch of the DCIA and DCIV, provides a broad sheet of thin, pliable, and well-vascularized soft tissue that enhances the versatility of the iliac donor site.

INDICATIONS

The advantage of the iliac donor site is that it provides the best source of vascularized bone for stable and retentive implant placement among the three donor sites (i.e., ilium, scapula, and fibula) that are most commonly used for oromandibular reconstruction (2). The choice of the best donor site is based on a variety of factors unique to the patient and the disease process. Choice of the correct flap depends on the dimensions, location, components of the defect and, most important, soft-tissue requirements; the patient's body habitus; location and quality of teeth in both jaws; irradiation status of the patient; prognosis for survival of the disease process that led to the segmental mandibulectomy defect; whether the reconstruction is done in a primary or secondary setting; and patient motivation. There is no single flap that solves all the reconstructive needs of all patients. The iliac, scapular, and fibular donor sites must be considered and a choice made for all patients undergoing this type of reconstruction. The ilium continues to have definite indications, despite the increasing popularity of the fibula in these reconstructions, especially for patients in whom preoperative angiography demonstrates that the fibular blood supply is not favorable.

Current indications for iliac-crest osteocutaneous or osteomyocutaneous flaps include (a) primary reconstruction of a lateral oromandibular defect with a minimal to moderate defect of the tongue; (b) reconstruction of the symphyseal region in a patient with a dentate residual mandible to achieve parity of bone height of the native tooth-bearing mandibular segment and the neomandible; (c) reconstruction of the symphysis in conjunction with a total or near-total glossectomy (3); (d) reconstruction of the symphysis in a patient who is not a candidate for dental rehabilitation so that the height of the neomandible that can be achieved with the ilium is sufficient to maintain the position of the lower lip and help insure oral competence; (e) reconstruction of the lateral mandible in conjunction with a portion of the infrastructure of the maxilla, where the internal oblique muscle is used to resurface both the oral and sinus aspects of the defect; and (f) reconstruction of composite defects of the oral cavity involving mucosa, bone, and skin.

ANATOMY

The DCIA and DCIV arise from the external iliac artery and vein within 1 to 2 cm above the inguinal ligament. Although the DCIV may run either deep or superficial to the external iliac artery, it always takes a cephalad turn, to enter the external iliac vein up to 3 cm above the junction of the DCIA and the external iliac artery. The DCIA and DCIV travel in a linear course toward the anterior superior iliac spine (ASIS), where they then assume a more curvilinear course along the inner table of the ilium. The pedicle is easily identified at the junction of the transversus abdominis and iliacus muscles, lying from 0.5 to 2.5 cm beneath the lip of the iliac crest (4). During its course, the deep circumflex pedicle gives rise to the ascending branch, perforators to the ilium and the inner periosteum, and an array of cutaneous perforators that traverse the three muscles of the abdominal wall. These latter perforators exit the external oblique muscle in a zone that extends from the ASIS to a point about 9 cm lateral, where the DCIA terminates as a large cutaneous perforator. The key to ensuring the blood supply to the skin is to be certain to design the skin paddle over this zone of perforators and to harvest a cuff of the three muscle layers to maintain the integrity of these delicate vessels.

The ascending branch(es) of the DCIA and DCIV, which supply the internal oblique muscle, arise at any point from the external iliac vessels to the ASIS. Through cadaver dissections, it has been shown that the ascending branch arises within 1 cm medial to the ASIS in 65% of cases but has a more medial takeoff, from 2 to 4 cm medial to the ASIS, in 15% of cases. In the remaining cases, there is no single dominant ascending branch but rather an array of branches that supply the internal oblique muscle. Therefore, in roughly 80% of cases, the internal oblique muscle has an axial-pattern blood supply with a single dominant ascending branch (1,5–7). Because of this axial pattern, the muscle can be maneuvered safely in virtually any direction relative to the bone to restore the anatomy of this region (6,7).

FLAP DESIGN AND DIMENSIONS

The bone of the ilium can be harvested with an excellent vascular supply for up to 14 cm lateral to the ASIS. The ilium can be harvested either as a unicortical or, more commonly, as a bicortical vascularized bone flap. In the former case, the inner table is harvested while maintaining the muscle attachments to the outer table. Preservation of the muscle insertions of the upper thigh muscles leads to an easier postoperative course of rehabilitation. The disadvantage of harvesting a unicortical segment of bone is that it often leads to insufficient bone width for placement of dental implants.

The skin paddle is designed along an axis that can be drawn from the ASIS to the inferior border of the scapula. As long as the skin paddle is centered over this axis, the zone of perforators is almost certainly incorporated. The maximum dimensions of the skin flap have not been determined; the limiting factor is more often the ability to achieve primary closure

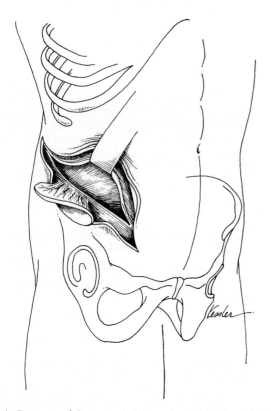

FIG. 1. Exposure of the internal oblique muscle is achieved by incising the skin paddle as well as the external oblique muscle and aponeurosis. The external oblique is incised while preserving a cuff attached to the inner table of the iliac crest. The internal oblique muscle is exposed by blunt dissection to the level of the costal margin, where it is then incised along its medial, lateral, and cephalad margins to reflect it caudally off the transversus abdominis muscle. (From Urken et al., ref. 6, with permission.)

of the abdominal wall rather than pushing the limits of the vascular supply.

The internal oblique muscle arises from the thoracolumbar fascia, the iliac crest, and the inguinal ligament. It inserts into the linea semilunaris of the rectus sheath and the lower three ribs. This muscle usually is harvested in its entirety to ensure adequate tissue for achieving the reconstruction and because harvesting only the lower extent of the muscle does little to maintain the integrity of the abdominal wall (Fig. 1). The patient's body habitus determines the thickness and dimensions of the internal oblique muscle. In all cases, the muscle shrinks in size once its attachments are cut, and it must be stretched during insetting to take advantage of the full extent of tissue harvested. Although any one of the three major components of this tripartite flap can be harvested independently, based on the DCIA and DCIV, the three components are usually harvested together when reconstructing oromandibular defects.

OPERATIVE TECHNIQUE

The skin incision provides exposure of the external oblique muscle and aponeurosis, which, in turn, is incised in the direction of its fibers, leaving a 3-cm cuff of muscle attached to the inner table of the ilium (Fig. 1). The plane between the internal and external oblique muscles is defined, and exposure of the entire span of the internal oblique muscle is obtained, from the ilium to the costal margin, by blunt dissection. Although the internal oblique muscle can be cut at any point to begin dissection of the muscle off the transversus abdominis, it is started most easily in the region just caudal to the twelfth rib.

The internal oblique muscle then is carefully elevated in a cephalad to caudad direction, stopping within 2 cm of the inner table of the ilium. On the deep surface of the muscle, the ascending branch is identified and preserved. This vascular arcade is followed as it courses through the transversus abdominis muscle to its junction with the DCIA and DCIV. With the exposure afforded by transecting the transversus abdominis muscle, leaving a cuff attached to the inner table of the ilium, the DCIA and DCIV can be traced to their takeoff from the external iliac vessels. The DCIA and DCIV must be isolated from the surrounding fascial envelope composed of the condensation of the transversalis and iliacus fasciae while leaving the course of these vessels undisturbed lateral to the ASIS. Complete exposure of the inner table of the ilium is achieved by transecting the iliacus muscle approximately 2 cm deep to the palpable pulse of the DCIA. The lateral aspect of the ilium is exposed by sharp dissection throughout the full extent of the bone to be harvested. The bone flap then is cut from the lateral aspect of the ilium while carefully retracting the abdominal contents. In the region medial to the ASIS, the lateral femoral cutaneous nerve can be identified and preserved in most cases. This nerve may run a course either superficial or deep to the DCIA and DCIV.

Closure of the iliac donor site must be done in a meticulous fashion to prevent weakness or frank herniation of the abdominal contents (Fig. 2). This is accomplished by approximating the transversus abdominis muscle to the iliacus muscle. It is often helpful to drill holes in the cut margin of the ilium to allow greater purchase of these sutures and to ensure a secure inner closure. In select cases, where the strength of the transversus abdominis muscle is questionable, a synthetic mesh can be placed. The second layer of the closure is achieved by suturing the external oblique muscle to the upper thigh muscles and tendons. Flexion of the ipsilateral knee is helpful to relieve tension on the closure. During the postoperative period,

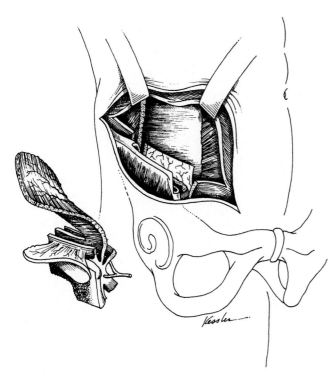

FIG. 2. Internal oblique iliac-crest osteomyocutaneous flap has been harvested from the abdominal wall. The defect must be closed in three layers. The first involves approximation of the transverse abdominis to the iliacus muscle. The external oblique muscle then is sutured to the upper thigh muscles. The skin and subcutaneous tissues are closed to complete the donor-site repair. The flap shown here is unicortical, preserving the external table of the ilium with the attachments of the upper-thigh muscles. (From Urken et al., ref. 6, with permission.)

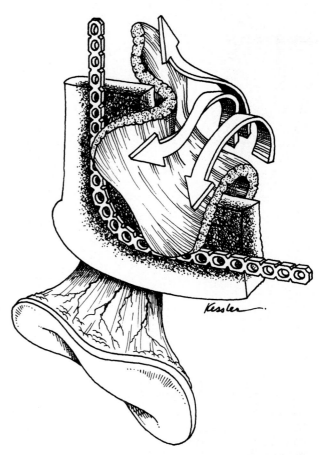

FIG. 4. The iliac crest is usually fixed to the native mandible, using a three-dimensional reconstruction plate. The internal oblique muscle may be transposed over the neomandible and used for coverage of defects of the oropharynx, hypopharynx, as well as the infrastructure of the maxilla. Greater freedom can be obtained in the mobility of the internal oblique muscle relative to the bone by performing a backcut to narrow the soft-tissue attachments surrounding the ascending branch of the DCIA. (From Urken et al., ref. 6, with permission.)

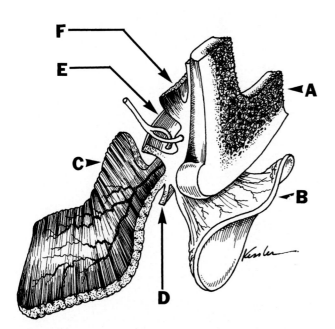

FIG. 3. Various components of the tripartite iliac-crest osteomyocutaneous flap have been labeled: ilium, which may be unicortical or bicortical, A; skin paddle, B; internal oblique muscle, C; cuff of external oblique muscle, D; transversus abdominis muscle, E; iliacus muscle, F. (From Urken et al., ref. 6, with permission.)

assisted ambulation, beginning with a walker and then progressing to a cane, is instituted starting on day 5 or 6 after surgery.

The iliac crest-internal oblique composite flap, consisting of the iliac bone, the broad sheet of the internal oblique muscle, and the skin overlying the iliac crest (Fig. 3), is inset into the oral cavity. The internal oblique muscle is used to resurface the ilium, achieving a thin cover over the neomandible that is ideally suited for dental rehabilitation (Fig. 4). The muscle can achieve maximum mobility relative to the bone by performing a backcut along the muscle to isolate a narrow soft-tissue pedicle surrounding the vascular supply. Although the initial description of the use of this flap in the oral cavity included a primary vestibuloplasty using a split-thickness skin graft, this technique is rarely used currently, except in select situations (6,8) (Fig. 5). These latter cases include patients with a significant loss of either the floor of the mouth or the buccal/labial mucosa. In these cases, mucosalization of the bare muscle may lead to obliteration of the buccal or lingual sulci, which otherwise could be preserved with the application of a skin graft. The internal oblique muscle undergoes significant atrophy as a result of denervation, producing a desirable lining of the oral cavity.

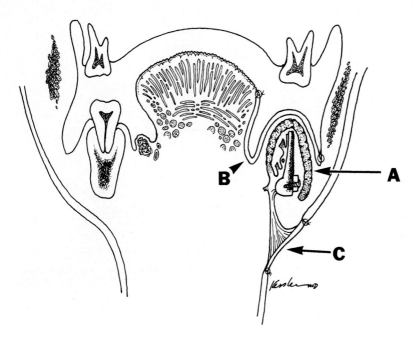

FIG. 5. Coronal section through the reconstructed oral cavity reveals the internal oblique muscle, *A*, transposed over the iliac bone, which is rigidly fixed to the native mandible. A split-thickness skin graft is shown sutured over the muscle to achieve restoration of sulcular anatomy, *B*. The skin paddle of the tripartite flap is sutured into the neck to serve either as a monitor or for closure of an associated cutaneous defect, *C*. (From Urken et al., ref. 6, with permission.)

CLINICAL RESULTS

In a series of 180 vascularized bone-containing free flaps used exclusively in oromandibular reconstruction (including ilium, scapula, and fibula donor sites), the soft-tissue flaps transferred with the ilium (n = 123) included 66 internal oblique flaps and 57 osteocutaneous flaps. The tripartite flap, consisting of bone, skin, and muscle, is ideally suited for reconstructing composite defects that include mandible, mucosa, and overlying skin (8). It is critical to respect the relationship of the skin paddle to the bone so as not to compromise the vascular supply to the skin. In most cases where the skin is used for external cover, it is usually limited in its cephalad extent to defects that do not extend above the level of the oral commissure. Careful attention to this important parameter will result in a high success rate, with a minimum of complications related to skin ischemia.

SUMMARY

The iliac donor site is a valuable source of vascularized bone that can be transferred with two separate soft-tissue flaps. The internal oblique muscle flap provides greater versatility to this donor site, thus expanding its use in oromandibular reconstruction.

References

1. Taylor GI, Townsend P, Corlett R. Superiority of the deep circumflex iliac vessels as the supply for free groin flaps. *Plast Reconstr Surg* 1979;64:595.
2. Moscoso J, Keller J, Genden E, et al. Vascularized bone flaps in oromandibular reconstruction: a comparative anatomic study of bone stock from various donor sites to assess suitability for enosseous dental implants. *Arch Otolaryngol Head Neck Surg* 1984;120:36.
3. Salibian A, Rappaport I, Allison G. Functional oromandibular reconstruction with the microvascular composite groin flap. *Plast Reconstr Surg* 1985;76:819.
4. Frederickson JM, Man SC, Hayden RE. Revascularized iliac bone graft for mandibular reconstruction. *Acta Otolaryngol (Stockh)* 1985;99:214.
5. Ramasastry SS, Tucker JB, Swartz WM, Hurwitz DJ. The internal oblique muscle flap: an anatomic and clinical study. *Plast Reconstr Surg* 1984;73:721.
6. Urken ML, Vickery C, Weinberg H, et al. The internal oblique-iliac crest osseomyocutaneous microvascular free flap in head and neck reconstruction. *J Reconstr Microsurg* 1989;5:203.
7. Urken ML, Vickery C, Weinberg H, et at. The internal oblique-iliac crest osseomyocutaneous free flap in oromandibular reconstruction: report of 20 cases. *Arch Otolaryngol Head Neck Surg* 1984;120:36.
8. Urken ML, Weinberg H, Vickery C, et al. The internal oblique-iliac crest free flap in composite defects of the oral cavity involving bone, skin and mucosa. *Laryngoscope* 1991;101:257.

CHAPTER 207 ■ THORACODORSAL (SERRATUS ANTERIOR) COMPOUND FLAP

A. M. GODFREY AND B. N. BAILEY

Musculocutaneous cover and rib can be prepared as two separately oriented components vascularized by a single long pedicle with large vessels. This double flap may be used as an island or free flap.

INDICATIONS

The component parts of the flap may be used in different combinations and can be used as a free flap wherever skin, bone, and muscle may be required. This includes defects of the limb bones as well as defects of the mandible and maxilla. This flap also can be used as an island flap to reach some head and neck defects as well as the arm and chest wall.

ANATOMY

Muscle

The serratus anterior muscle arises as eight digitations from the upper eight ribs. The first digitation is the largest, and it inserts into the upper costal surface of the vertebral border of the scapula. The next three digitations insert into the whole of the vertebral border, and the lower four digitations insert into the scapular angle. Denervation or removal of the lower four digitations does not produce winging of the scapula if the upper four digitations are intact.

Nerve Supply (Long Thoracic Nerve)

The long thoracic nerve is not at risk during surgery because the supply to the upper four digitations of the serratus anterior lie slightly deeper on the chest wall, separated from the vascular pedicle of the flap by a definite fascial layer.

Vascular Supply (Lateral Thoracic and Thoracodorsal Arteries)

The upper four digitations are supplied mainly by branches of the lateral thoracic artery. The lower four digitations are supplied by a single branch (72%), two branches (24%), and multiple branches (4%) of the thoracodorsal pedicle as well as the lateral thoracic and intercostal vessels (1). The branch(es) pierces the fascia over the serratus anterior superficial to the nerve supply (approximately in the midaxillary line) and runs with it to the lower four digitations. The vascular and nerve supplies to the latissimus dorsi muscle have been described in detail elsewhere (2–4).

There is a rich communication between the intercostal vessels and the thoracodorsal branches supplying the serratus anterior. This has been confirmed by the authors using standard cadaver injection techniques.

The presence of endosteal as well as periosteal blood supply is shown at operation by the bleeding from the rib marrow. This provides a block of serratus anterior muscle, rib(s), and intercostal muscles and vessels for reconstruction, supplied only by the thoracodorsal pedicle. This block may be used alone or with a latissimus dorsi muscle or musculocutaneous flap, all supplied by the thoracodorsal pedicle (Fig. 1).

OPERATIVE TECHNIQUE

The patient is placed in the lateral position with the upper arms supported and abducted to allow access to the axilla. The skin incision is made along the lateral border of the latissimus dorsi muscle from the axilla to approximately the eighth rib. It is made convex anteriorly if skin is to be taken with the latissimus dorsi. The lateral margin of the latissimus dorsi muscle is elevated in the lower half of the wound, and its vascular bundle is traced proximally to the bifurcation of the thoracodorsal trunk, about 10 cm from the origin of the subscapular artery. The branch(es) to the serratus anterior runs from the thoracodorsal pedicle downward and a little anteriorly before piercing the fascia over the serratus anterior and supplying its distal half.

Delineation of the Serratus Anterior-Rib Tissue Block

For single-rib reconstructions (e.g., jaw), the fifth rib is used. When two ribs are required, the fifth and sixth ribs are used (Fig. 2).

Muscle is incised along the inferior margins of the fourth and sixth interspaces to preserve two intercostal bundles. The incision is deepened to the pleura, which is freed from the deep surface of the ribs by digital and scissor dissection.

It is important to include the maximum costal insertion of the serratus anterior, and so the anterior rib division is made just lateral to the costochondral junction. The scapular insertion of the serratus anterior is divided, and the muscle is sutured to the ribs posteriorly to prevent separation during manipulation.

The required length of rib(s) is measured from anteriorly, and the rib is divided posteriorly so that the serratus anterior tissue block is now attached only by its vascular pedicle. The rib curvature may be altered by careful sawcuts through the inner cortex. To straighten the rib(s), greenstick outfractures

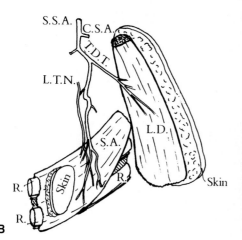

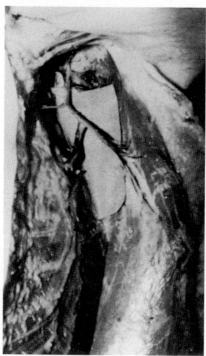

FIG. 1. A: The thoracodorsal trunk (*T.D.T.*) is shown branching to the serratus anterior (*S.A.*) muscle and the latissimus dorsi (*L.D.*) muscle. *R.*, rib; *S.S.A.*, subscapular artery; *C.S.A.*, circumflex scapular artery; *L.T.N.*, long thoracic nerve. B: Cadaver dissection.

are made. To increase rib curvature, inner cortical wedges are excised and greenstick infractures are made.

The intercostal bundles and muscle insertions must be protected. When the curvature of two ribs is altered, the sawcuts should be staggered to retain more stability of the bone unit.

The latissimus dorsi muscle or musculocutaneous flap is raised in the usual way, and its vascular pedicle is traced proximally to obtain the required length. The entire bifid composite flap is left attached to the subscapular vessels during closure of the defect to allow recovery and to maintain perfusion until transfer.

Closure of the Secondary Defect

Pleural tears are closed with fine catgut sutures. A chest tube drain is inserted through a distal intact intercostal space and is brought out through the anterior skin.

The rib defect is covered posteriorly by the scapula. Laterally, the serratus anterior is sutured together from above and below the wound. Direct closure of the skin is possible when latissimus dorsi muscle or musculocutaneous flaps of up to 12 to 14 cm have been raised. Wider defects may be covered with split-thickness skin grafts. Mesh reinforcement of the interspace could be carried out, but so far we have not found it necessary. A single-rib defect is closed by pulling together the adjacent ribs with heavy sutures, and, if possible, the skin defect is closed directly. The scar is concealed mostly by the resting arm.

CLINICAL RESULTS

The following variations have been used in 21 patients: ten patients with lower leg defects of skin and bone, ranging from 8 to 28 cm; one patient with an upper humeral defect of 14 cm; and ten patients with mandibular/facial reconstruction

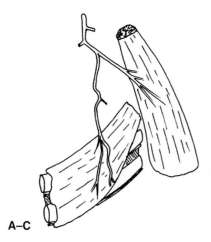

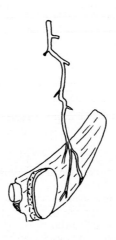

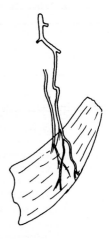

FIG. 2. Possible variations of the thoracodorsal compound flap. A: Two ribs plus muscle cover for major limb reconstruction. B: One rib plus serratus anterior muscle and skin for jaw reconstruction. C: Innervated muscle.

for congenital abnormalities, defects following tumor resection, traumatic defects, and facial palsy.

SUMMARY

The thoracodorsal compound flap can be used either as a free flap or as an island flap. It can be tailored easily to fit many defects, as the amount of bone, muscle, and skin to be included in the flap can be varied in a number of ways.

References

1. Rowsell AR. Personal communication concerning 100 cadaver axillary dissections, Oxford, 1980.
2. Olivari N. The latissimus flap. *Br J Plast Surg* 1976;29:126.
3. Bostwick J, Nahai F, Wallace JG, Vasconez LO. Sixty latissimus dorsi flaps. *Plast Reconstr Surg* 1979;63:31.
4. Bailey BN. Latissimus dorsi flaps: a practical approach. *Ann Acad Med (Singapore)* 1979;8:445.

CHAPTER 208 ■ MICROVASCULAR FREE TRANSFER OF A PARTIAL FIBULA FOR MANDIBULAR RECONSTRUCTION

M. A. SCHUSTERMAN

EDITORIAL COMMENT

This is an excellent chapter describing the procedure that is most commonly known for restoration of continuity of the mandible.

Reconstruction of the mandible, particularly when the defect involves the anterior mandible, is a formidable challenge to the reconstructive surgeon. Most defects consist not only of bone, but also of soft tissue, thus necessitating use of a composite reconstructive modality. Vascularized bone has been well accepted for use in reconstruction of the mandible. Of all the flaps currently available, the fibula has become the flap of choice at many centers.

INDICATIONS

Benign and malignant neoplasms account for about 80% of mandibular resections. Most of these tumors are squamous cell carcinomas that require composite reconstructions wherein both the mandible and the affected extraoral and intraoral soft tissues are replaced. This type of restoration also may be indicated for severe trauma to the lower face.

The advantages of the fibula free flap include (a) ease of flap harvest; (b) excellent quality and quantity of bone, suitable for placement of dental implants; (c) a segmental periosteal blood supply that provides good flow to multiple osteotomy sections, allowing shaping of the bone to match the original mandible; (d) a reliable skin paddle that can be derived from the lateral leg skin; (e) a remote location in relation to the tumor site, which permits a two-team approach that reduces operating time; and (f) less donor-site morbidity (1–3).

If no skin paddle is required, the fibula is harvested from the ipsilateral leg. If skin tissue is needed in the reconstruction, the contralateral leg is selected, allowing for placement of the skin paddle intraorally (Fig. 1).

ANATOMY

The fibula bone lies in the deep posterior compartment, just lateral to the tibia (Fig. 2). The upper end of the fibula does not comprise any part of the knee joint but articulates with the undersurface of the tibial plateau. The lower end of the fibula is the lateral malleous and is involved in ankle-joint articulation. There are four muscles surrounding the fibula: the extensor digitorum longus superiorly, the posterior tibialis medially, the peroneal muscles laterally, and the flexor hallucis longus inferiorly. The blood supply to the fibula comes from the peroneal vessels, which are one of three terminal branches of the popliteal artery; the others are the anterior tibial vessel and the posterior tibial, which branches with the peroneal vessels.

The peroneal vessels lie between the tibialis posterior muscle and the flexor hallucis longus. The posterolateral intermuscular septum is the terminal end of the transverse crural septum; it is through this septum that the cutaneous perforators run. It is therefore important to harvest as much of this septum as possible when harvesting the skin paddle (see Fig. 2).

FLAP DESIGN AND DIMENSIONS

The fibular head at the knee, the peroneal nerve just below the fibular head, and the lateral malleolus at the ankle are marked (Fig. 3). Hash marks are drawn at 10, 15, 20, and 25 cm from the fibular head. The skin paddle is centered between the hash

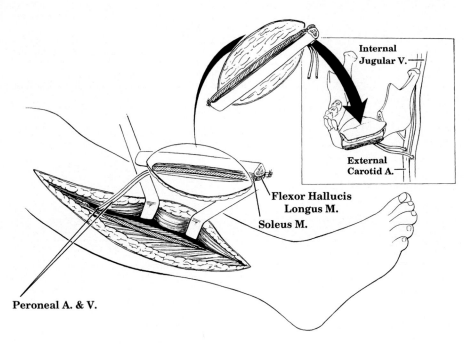

Peroneal A. & V.

Flexor Hallucis Longus M.

Soleus M.

Internal Jugular V.

External Carotid A.

FIG. 1. Use of the contralateral osteocutaneous fibula facilitates intraoral placement of the skin paddle.

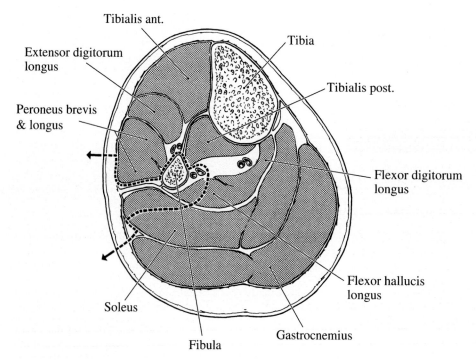

Tibialis ant.

Extensor digitorum longus

Peroneus brevis & longus

Tibia

Tibialis post.

Flexor digitorum longus

Flexor hallucis longus

Soleus

Gastrocnemius

Fibula

FIG. 2. Cross-sectional anatomy of the leg; *dotted line* denotes tissue harvest for osteocutaneous fibula.

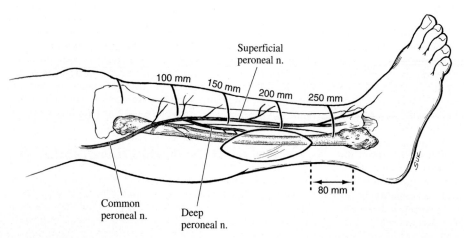

Superficial peroneal n.

100 mm   150 mm   200 mm   250 mm

80 mm

Common peroneal n.

Deep peroneal n.

FIG. 3. Design of flap on the leg; note position of peroneal nerve. Distances are millimeters from fibular head.

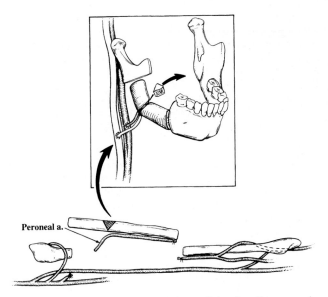

FIG. 4. Posterior reconstruction requires pedicle take off at neoangle, and thus a proximal bone harvest.

marks, taking into account the mandibular area being resected: this determines whether the proximal or distal part of the fibula is used.

In the anteroposterior plane, the paddle is centered along the posterior border of the fibula. A posterior mandibular reconstruction entails the creation (by osteotomy) of a ramus and neoangle; use of the proximal fibula allows pedicle placement at the neoangle, and thus adjacent to the recipient vessels in the neck (Fig. 4). For an anterior mandibular reconstruction, the distal fibula is used to provide long donor vessels from the end of the flap (Fig. 5).

OPERATIVE TECHNIQUE

The designated leg is elevated and a tourniquet inflated. Because the peroneal artery and vein course along the medial side of the fibula, a lateral approach is used in beginning the dissection. An anterior incision down through the deep muscle fascia is made; inclusion of this fascia is crucial. As the dissection continues posteriorly to the posterolateral intermuscular septum, the peroneal muscles are exposed. The anterior surface of the septum then is followed down the fibula, and the peroneal muscles are elevated from the lateral and anterior surfaces of the bone. The anterolateral intermuscular septum is divided close to the fibula to prevent injury to the anterior tibial neurovascular bundle, and the dissection continues down through the interosseous membrane.

Next a posterior incision is made down through the deep muscle fascia, and the skin paddle is elevated to the edge of the soleus muscle. An incision about 1 cm deep is made in the soleus muscle 1 cm from its lateral border. The bone is now cut to the required length with an oscillating saw. The bone should not be cut within 8 cm of the lateral malleolus because the tibiofibular ligaments may be injured, causing ankle-joint instability. The proximal cut in the fibula should be made as high as possible without damaging the peroneal nerve. Even if the proximal fibula will not be used, it should be harvested to expose the trifurcation of the leg vessels, facilitating the pedicle dissection.

Once the fibula is cut, it is retracted laterally, and the dissection proceeds from distal to proximal and from medial to lateral. Medially, the peroneal vessels are located, followed down to their distal aspect, ligated, and divided. With knowl-

edge of their location, flap dissection continues (medially to laterally), with less risk of harming the perforating vessels to the skin paddle.

After elevating the flap, the tourniquet is released and any residual bleeding controlled. By this time, the ablative team should have the mandible exposed and ready for resection. Before osteotomies are undertaken, the reconstruction team bends a reconstruction plate over the native mandible, stabilizes the plate with screws posterior to the planned mandibulectomy cuts, and then removes the plate and screws. Thus, the original shape of the mandible will be reestablished and the condyles correctly positioned relative to the neomandible.

The ablative team now completes the resection while the reconstruction team uses the shaped reconstruction plate (as a template) to cut the fibula with closing wedge osteotomies; during this sequence, the fibula is perfused in situ. Bone fragments are fixed before transfer to limit ischemia time. As soon as the resection is finished and tumor-free margins have been confirmed by frozen sections, the pedicle is divided and the flap is transferred to the recipient site.

First, the skin paddle is inset along the tongue because this is technically easier to do before the bone is in place. Next the bony ends of the fibula/reconstruction-plate complex are trimmed (while being moderately compressed) to make a good fit, and then the plate is fastened to the native mandible with the screws and holes used previously. Microsurgical anastomoses are performed last. The external carotid artery and internal jugular vein used in an end-to-side configuration are the recipient vessels of choice. After the anastomoses are completed, the flap is checked for adequate revascularization, flap insetting is completed, and the wound is closed over suction drains. The leg incision is also closed over suction drains, and a bulky dressing and posterior leg splint are applied.

Postoperatively, the patient is managed and monitored in the surgical intensive care unit. If the patient is stable after 24 to 48 hours and transferred to a regular nursing floor, activity is slowly increased, as tolerated. A feeding tube is used in all patients who have a mandibular, floor-of-the-mouth, or oropharyngeal reconstruction. During the first postoperative week, most patients are seen for physical therapy to initiate walking and range-of-motion exercises, particularly in the donor area.

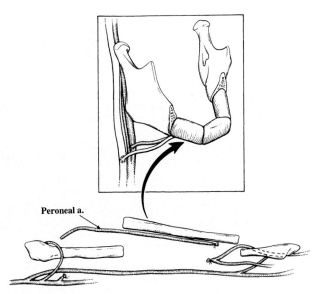

FIG. 5. Anterior reconstruction requires a long pedicle and thus a distal bone harvest.

Following a fibular harvest, the posterior leg splint is removed on the third or fourth day, and the patient begins cautious ambulation in physical therapy. If there is a skin graft to the donor site, walking is postponed for 7 days, and the leg is wrapped with an elastic bandage when it is dependent. In uncomplicated cases without a skin graft, the patient is discharged 10 to 14 days after surgery.

CLINICAL RESULTS

Excellent results have been achieved with this flap (Fig. 6) for immediate and delayed reconstruction defects due to trauma, osteoradionecrosis, and salvage cases after previous flap failure. Flap losses have resulted from the difficult nature of the cases, not from any inherent flaws of the fibula flap. Two main areas of concern involve the vascular supply of the flap.

The first vascular condition of concern is atherosclerosis. Many patients requiring free fibulas are elderly and have a significant history of tobacco use; they are therefore also strong candidates for development of arterial occlusive disease of the lower-extremity vessels. Each candidate for this flap needs to have a detailed history and examination of the cardiovascular system. If there are clinical indications of arterial insufficiency, angiograms are indicated before the procedure to assess the integrity of the peroneal artery and the vascular supply to the leg.

A second issue of concern is the peroneal magnus artery, especially a situation in which the entire lower extremity is fed by a dominant or solitary peroneal artery, so that vessel sacrifice would devascularize the lower extremity. Although this condition has an estimated incidence of 10% in the normal population, we have not seen its occurrence in more than 120 free fibula flaps. We do not perform routine angiography in all patients to rule out the occurrence of this condition; again, the

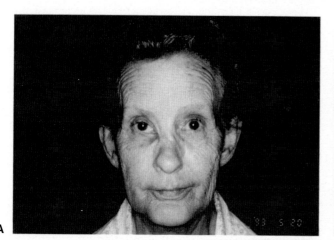

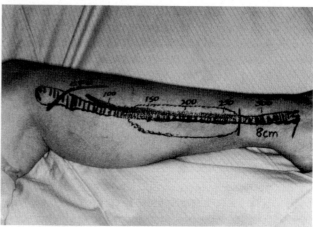

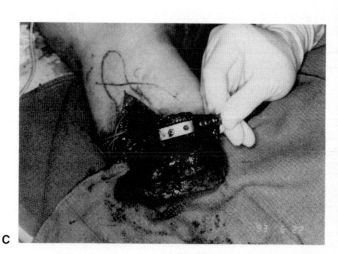

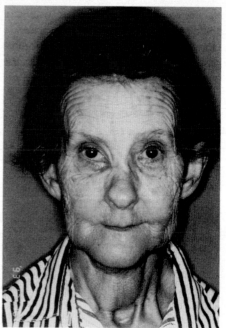

FIG. 6. **A:** Preoperative appearance of patient with recurrent squamous-cell carcinoma. **B:** Preoperative marking of leg; note the position of the peroneal nerve, which should be avoided, and the location of skin in relation to hash marks, measured in millimeters from fibular head. **C:** Prebent plate is taken to the leg, where harvested fibula is osteotomized and fixed to the plate in situ to limit ischemia time. **D:** Postoperative appearance, frontal view.

main indications for angiography are clinical symptoms and signs of vascular insufficiency.

The gravest complication is total flap loss because of thrombosis, which usually occurs during the first 24 hours after surgery. In addition to frequent clinical assessments by experienced personnel, monitoring devices are used for direct imaging of the blood vessels or for measuring tissue perfusion. When a flap is judged to have questionable blood inflow or outflow, the *only* acceptable action is immediate surgical exploration. Early thrombectomy may salvage a flap if the ischemic interval has been less than 2 or 3 hours. Donor-site complications with the free fibular flap have tended to be minor and brief; usually, edema and pain are not significant.

SUMMARY

In the past few years, advances in free-flap composite reconstructions have resulted in reliable methods for quality restoration of the mandible. The fibula is a choice donor, with major advantages and few deterrents.

References

1. Schusterman MD, Reece GP, Miller MJ, Harris S. The osteocutaneous free fibula flap: is the skin paddle reliable? *Plast Reconstr Surg* 1992;90:787.
2. Hidalgo DA. Free fibula flap: a new method of mandible reconstruction. *Plast Reconstr Surg* 1989;84:71.
3. Wei FC, Chen HC, Chuang CC, Noordhoff MS. Fibular osteoseptocutaneous flap: anatomic study and clinical application. *Plast Reconstr Surg* 1986;78:191.

CHAPTER 209 ■ ENDOCULTIVATION: COMPUTER-AIDED TISSUE ENGINEERING OF CUSTOMIZED, VASCULARIZED BONE GRAFTS FOR MANDIBULAR RECONSTRUCTION

P. H. WARNKE

EDITORIAL COMMENT

At present, the standard for mandibular reconstruction, either segmental or, at times, complete, is the use of vascularized fibula, scapula, or iliac crest. The failures are often due to poor lining, particularly in cases of prior irradiation.

The method here described, as the author indicates, is still experimental, but it brings together two principles that are fairly well established. One is the use of the prefabricated flap introduced by Shintomi, from Japan, and the second is the use of computerized technology for preoperative planning. It is still unclear what type of bone regeneration occurs with bone morphogenetic protein-7 in a scaffold made of titanium.

through growing it anew by means of tissue engineering, may offer new solutions for reconstructive surgeons. "Regeneration" means that one repairs the damaged tissue by growing it anew with methods of tissue engineering, thus circumventing the issue of immunologic rejection, as the patient's own cells are used to cultivate the required tissue. I describe a technique of endocultivation, which involves the growing of customized, computer-designed, vascularized replacements for subsequent transfer, to reconstruct previously resected bone. It should be emphasized that endocultivation techniques are still at a basic stage of development and are currently more suited to homogenous tissue like bone. However, they may offer the potential to grow more complex organ replacements in the future.

INDICATIONS

The repair of bony defects from congenital malformations, trauma, infection, or tumor resection remains a challenge in modern orthopaedic and maxillofacial surgical practice (1). The reconstruction of the long bones, the spine, and the skull must meet high mechanical and aesthetic demands. However,

Currently, major bone discontinuity defects of more than 6 cm are repaired with an autologous vascularized fibula, scapula, iliac crest, or rib transplant. Recent advances in the emerging field of regenerative medicine, that is, repairing damaged tissue

a major disadvantage of autologous vascularized bone is that harvesting the required bone graft creates another skeletal defect, which is associated with significant morbidity (2). In vitro tissue engineering has been a focus of many research groups; however, in vivo endocultivation techniques currently offer greater potential (3,4). Patients serve as their own bioreactors, and the required tissue is cultivated inside the patient's own body on an individualized matrix. In vitro bioreactors are not required (4–6).

In 2004, we began using endocultivation techniques to grow customized, computer-designed, vascularized, jaw replacements in the latissimus dorsi muscle of patients, for subsequent transplantation to reconstruct their previously resected jaws (4,5). The latissimus dorsi flap has accrued a broad spectrum of applications in the field of reconstructive surgery. This is due to the large area of tissue available, thereby allowing flexibility in flap design, as well as its long and high-capacity vascular pedicle that permits relatively technically easy microvascular anastomoses (7,8).

The anatomic proximity of the latissimus dorsi to the thoracodorsal artery is fortuitous, as it allows for significant spontaneous neovascularization (9). This subsequently permits free-flap transfer into the desired recipient region. This independent vascular supply makes it possible to grow constructs of the size of a mandible or, in the future (4,5), possibly even a complex organ. For example, the latissimus dorsi is a more suitable incubation site to grow a bone replacement, such as a neomandible, than the site to which it will subsequently be transplanted, as the area containing the bone defect is often compromised by prior radiation therapy. Irradiated tissue demonstrates poor regenerative properties and even soft-tissue injury heals poorly. The choice of a prepared muscle pouch inside the latissimus dorsi has proven to be a highly successful site as a bioreactor in early clinical studies, with substantial evidence of heterotopic bone growth and remodeling within the graft (5).

The special feature of the endocultivation procedure is that the flap can be prefabricated with an individualized bone replacement. Computer-aided design (CAD) provides a practical and exacting method of customizing replacement scaffolds, to produce a perfect fit for each individual defect. Two major advantages of this technique are the production of an optimal three-dimensional aesthetic outcome and the prevention of creating a secondary skeletal defect. It should be emphasized that the endocultivation technique is still very new, and such prefabricated flaps are currently indicated only for patients who have poor potential skeletal donor sites.

ANATOMY

The latissimus dorsi is a flat, fanlike muscle that arises directly from the spinal processes of the lower six thoracic vertebrae, the lumbar and sacral vertebrae, and the dorsal iliac crest via the thoracolumbar fascia. The muscle inserts between the teres and pectoralis muscles at the humerus, and together with the teres major, it forms the posterior axillary fold (7). The main nutrient vessel is the thoracodorsal artery, which regularly gives off a strong branch to the serratus anterior muscle. The length of the extramuscular part of the vessel course varies from 6 to 16 cm and is about 9 cm, on average (8). The extramuscular part gives off several minor branches (7). At the point of origin from the subscapularis vessels, the thoracodorsal vessels have diameters of 1.5 to 4 mm (artery) and 3 to 5 mm (vein after unification of the two concomitant veins) (7,8). Whereas the thoracodorsal artery provides blood mainly to the proximal and lateral two-thirds of the muscle, the distal parts of the muscle are reached by perforating branches of the intercostal arteries (7,8).

FLAP DESIGN AND DIMENSIONS

The flap design is similar to a regular latissimus dorsi flap. The flap can be combined with a skin paddle. Because of its good vascular supply and the size of the latissimus dorsi, the muscle can be surgically divided to form a pouch to insert the replacement scaffold. The pouch is the site of cultivation, and acts as an in vivo bioreactor. The dimensions of the replacement determine the size of the pouch. As the thoracodorsal vessel pedicle is intended to provide the vascular supply of the transplant, the pouch should be located near the lateral rim of the muscle. Therefore, the cultivated-bone replacement will have sufficient blood supply after both transplantation and microsurgical anastomosis of the vessel pedicle.

OPERATIVE TECHNIQUE

The endocultivation procedure has one presurgical step for custom scaffold design and two different surgical steps. These are described for the cultivation of a mandible replacement.

Step 1

Preoperative Planning

The aim is to grow a subtotal replacement mandible inside the latissimus dorsi muscle, with an adequate vascular pedicle to allow for subsequent transplantation of a viable graft into the defect. Furthermore, the replacement should be individually shaped to fit the defect perfectly, thus improving the chances of adequate postoperative function and a satisfactory aesthetic result.

Initially, a three-dimensional computed tomography (CT) scan of the head must be performed, to identify the mandibular defect and to design an ideal virtual replacement of the missing part/s, using CAD-planning techniques (Fig. 1). The data describing the mandible replacement are then directed to a CAD-operated three-axes milling machine, and a Teflon mandible model is created, matching exactly the virtual dimensions of the replacement mandible.

Step 2

Scaffold Loading and Implantation

The Teflon mandible is then used as a mold from which a titanium mesh scaffold is created (Fig. 2). The Teflon mandible is subsequently set aside, and the titanium mesh cage (now serving as an external scaffold) is filled with an internal scaffold—bovine hydroxyapatite matrix. This internal scaffold is then coated with bone morphogenetic protein-7 (BMP-7). Subsequently, 10 to 20 mL of bone marrow is aspirated from the iliac crest and added to the hydroxyapatite matrix, with the intention of providing undifferentiated precursor cells as a target for rhBMP-7.

The loaded titanium mesh cage (Fig. 3) is then implanted into a surgically created pouch of the right or left latissimus dorsi muscle. The pouch serves as an in vivo bioreactor. A 7- to 10-week cultivation phase is required, to allow for both the growth of heterotopic bone and for ingrowth of new vessels from the thoracodorsal artery (Fig. 4).

Computed tomography after implantation and prior to transplantation is helpful to detect heterotopic bone growth or any increase in mineralization (Fig. 5). In addition, bone scintigraphy (600 MBq technetium-99m-oxydronate-tracer)

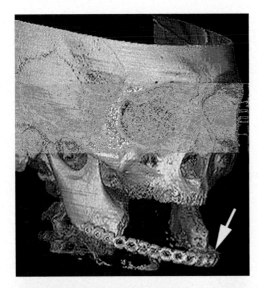

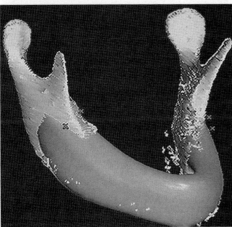

FIG. 1. **Top** : Three-dimensional computed tomography (CT) scan of a 56-year-old patient after ablative surgery for squamous-cell cancer 8 years previously. The mandible was resected from the paramedian left region to the retromolar right region. This critical-sized defect of more than 7 cm was bridged with a titanium reconstruction plate since the initial surgery. **Bottom:** The CT data of the mandible with defect region is separated. Using computer-aided design (CAD)-planning techniques, an ideal virtual mandibular transplant is designed, that would fit exactly into the defect. The data of this virtual transplant are forwarded to a CAD-operated 3-axes milling machine, to form an identical Teflon model (compare with Fig. 2) (4).

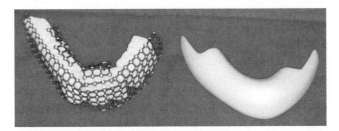

FIG. 2. A Teflon mandible model (*right*) was prepared with a CAD-operated 3-axes milling machine. The model has identical dimensions to the virtually designed transplant (compare with Fig. 1). A titanium mesh scaffold was then formed onto the Teflon model. After removing the Teflon model, the remaining titanium mesh cage (*left*) has dimensions similar to those of the ideal virtual transplant. The cage is loaded with hydroxyapatite blocks serving as internal scaffold. The blocks will be later coated with bone morphogenetic protein–7 and autologous bone marrow (4).

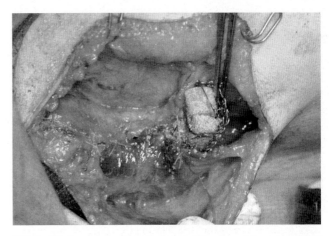

FIG. 3. The loaded titanium mesh cage is implanted into a pouch of the right latissimus dorsi muscle of the patient. The surrounding muscle tissue is fixed on the cage with resorbable sutures, to allow for maximum soft-tissue contact for neovascularization inside the graft (4).

may be used to demonstrate extraskeletal osteoblast activity inside the replacement. This is useful in demonstrating the successful induction of new bone formation.

Step 3

Transplantation

After a cultivation period of a minimum of 7 weeks, the mandible replacement is transplanted to repair a significant mandibular defect. The replacement is harvested with the sur-

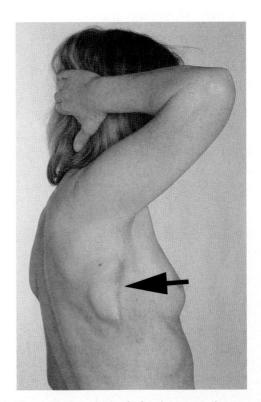

FIG. 4. View on the lateral side of a female patient, where a mandibular replacement (*arrow*) is growing inside her lateral right latissimus dorsi muscle. The shoulder range of motion is not significantly reduced.

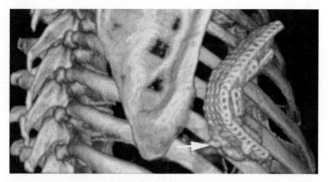

FIG. 5. Three-dimensional (3D) CT scanning of the thorax. The mandible replacement is cultivated without contact to the skeleton laterally anterior to the tip of the scapula. New bone formation is even seen to be occurring through the titanium scaffold around the mandibular replacement (arrow) (4).

rounding muscular tissue and the adjacent vessel pedicle from the thoracodorsal artery and vein (Fig. 6). Transplantation into the defect region is performed via an extraoral approach. Minor bone overgrowth on the ends of the replacement can be curetted, so that the transplant fits easily into the defect. As the replacement has been customized using CAD design, no further correction of the shape or form of the graft should be required. When a titanium mesh cage is being used as the external scaffold, it is helpful to have overlapping edges at the docking points to the original mandible stumps. Thus, the replacement can be easily fixed onto the stumps with miniscrews (Fig. 7). The transplant's vascular pedicle is then anastomosed onto the neck vessels, utilizing standard microsurgical techniques.

CLINICAL RESULTS

Experience in humans with this computer-assisted endocultivation technique is currently very limited (4,10,11). The method is still experimental and, at the time of publication of this chapter, still requires ethics approval, as the use of BMPs at this anatomic site is an off-label use. As such, mandibular reconstructions using vascularized fibula, scapula, or iliac-crest grafts remain the gold standard. Preoperative planning requires experience in CAD planning and rapid prototype development, to allow for the exact fit of the replacement.

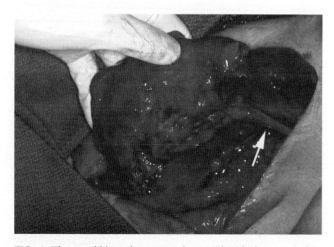

FIG. 6. The mandible replacement is harvested with the surrounding muscle tissue and the adjacent thoracodorsal vessel pedicle (*arrow*) (4).

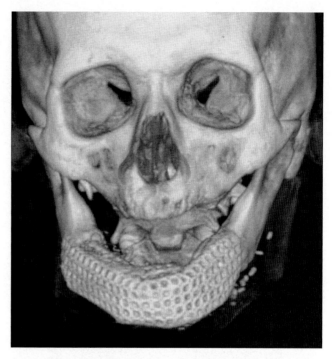

FIG. 7. Three-dimensional CT scan of the patient after transplantation of the endocultivated mandible replacement. The overlapping titanium-mesh wings of the replacement are fixed in the correct position, thus returning the contour of the patient's jaw-line to approximately that present premorbidly (4).

To date, patients undergoing this procedure have not complained of pain or sleep disturbance and have relayed only minor concerns regarding the range of motion of the affected shoulder. Wound closure can be a problem after transplantation of a massive replacement, particularly if the skin is nonelastic in the defect region, with previous irradiation therapy and fibrosis. Although not ideal, a split-thickness skin graft covering the adjacent muscle tissue of the graft may be employed if this proves to be particularly problematic (4). This type of mandible replacement allows for masticatory function, when the external scaffold is properly fixed onto the mandible stumps. Patients are provided with a significantly superior quality of life, given their improved aesthetic appearance and enhanced ability to speak. To date, there has been no experience in the insertion of dental implants into such neomandibles.

The amount of bone that can be induced with BMP is limited. Follow-up CT studies have shown that bone density inside the replacements subsequently enhances, due to masticatory functional loading. It is likely that, with the technique described previously, it may not exceed the density of regular cancellous bone (12). Future studies are focused on improvement of bone induction.

SUMMARY

Endocultivation is a pioneering technique used to grow individually shaped bone replacements within the latissimus dorsi muscle of patients with severe skeletal defects. The goal is to use the patient as the bioreactor, to prevent the common problems of engineering tissue in vitro in the laboratory. The replacement scaffolds are designed prior to surgery, using CAD, to enable a perfect fit. The site of cultivation is a surgically created pouch in the lateral latissimus dorsi, which allows for neovascularization, courtesy of the thoracodorsal artery and vein, thereby allowing subsequent free-flap transfer into the desired recipient region. This independent vascular supply makes it possible to grow constructs of the size of a mandible or, in the future, possibly even a complex organ.

References

1. MacArthur BD, Oreffo ROC. Bridging the gap. *Nature* 2005;433:19.
2. Takushima A, Harii K, Asato H, et al. Mandibular reconstruction using microvascular free flaps: a statistical analysis of 178 cases. *Plast Reconstr Surg* 2001;108:1555.
3. Spector M. *Basic principles of tissue engineering*. Chicago: Quintessence Publishing Co., Inc., 1999:Chap. 1, Tissue engineering.
4. Warnke PH, Springer IN, Wiltfang J, et al. Growth and transplantation of a custom vascularised bone graft in a man. *Lancet* 2004;28:766
5. Warnke PH, Wiltfang J, Springe, IN, et al. Man as living bioreactor: fate of an exogenously-prepared customized tissue-engineered mandible. *Biomaterials* 2006;27:3163.
6. Warnke PH. Repair of a human face by allotransplantation. *Lancet* 2006;15:368:181.
7. Wolff KD, Hölzle F. *Raising of microvascular flaps: a systematic approach.* Berlin, Heidelberg, New York: Springer, 2005.
8. Bartlett SP, May JW Jr, Yaremchuk MJ. The latissimus dorsi muscle: a fresh cadaver study of the primary neurovascular pedicle. *Plast Reconstr Surg* 1981;67:631.
9. Terheyden H, Warnke P, Dunsche A, et al. Mandibular reconstruction with prefabricated vascularized bone grafts using recombinant human osteogenic protein-1: an experimental study in miniature pigs. Part 2: transplantation. *Int J Oral Maxillofac Surg* 2001;30:469.
10. Heliotis M, Lavery KM, Ripamonti U, et al. Transformation of a prefabricated hydroxyapatite/osteogenic protein-1 implant into a vascularised pedicled bone flap in the human chest. *Int J Oral Maxillofac Surg* 2006;35:265.
11. Arnander C, Westermark A, Veltheim R, et al. Three-dimensional technology and bone morphogenetic protein in frontal bone reconstruction. *J Craniofac Surg* 2006;17:275.
12. Warnke PH, Springer IN, Acil Y, et al. The mechanical integrity of in vivo engineered heterotopic bone. *Biomaterials* 2006;27:1081. [Epub 2005 Aug 22]

CHAPTER 210 ■ RECONSTRUCTION OF THE CERVICAL ESOPHAGUS WITH SKIN FLAPS

C. E. SILVER AND R. J. BRAUER

EDITORIAL COMMENT

These adjacent skin flaps are of historical significance only.

Tumors of the hypopharynx and cervical esophagus are often treated by total pharyngolaryngectomy with partial or total esophagectomy. Repair of the surgical defect is a complex task. Reconstructions have been performed using many variations and combinations of local tissues, skin grafts, stents, regional flaps, free flaps, and transpositions or free transplantations of abdominal viscera. The ideal reconstruction would entail a single-stage operation, employ nonirradiated tissues, require no thoracic or abdominal surgery, and have minimal morbidity and mortality. Although marked improvements in reconstructive procedures have occurred, there is still no single procedure that can be applied to all patients with uniformly reliable results. Various methods of pharyngoesophageal reconstruction using skin flaps have the advantage of not requiring abdominal or thoracic operations, but they have other limitations.

INDICATIONS

Many of the standard cervical skin flaps have been replaced by either the deltopectoral flap (see Chapter 211) or the pectoralis major musculocutaneous flap (see Chapter 212) or a combination of these flaps. When these flaps are unavailable or contraindicated for some reason, the cervical skin flap (Wookey) (1,2) or its modifications can be used.

FLAP DESIGN AND DIMENSIONS

The procedure described by Wookey (2) employed a laterally based rectangular cervical skin flap for reconstruction following pharyngolaryngectomy. The upper edge of the flap was sutured to the cut edge of the pharynx and the lower edge to the esophagus. The flap was then folded back onto itself, creating a lateral fissure in the neck. All the pharyngeal and esophageal anastomoses were completed at the first stage. The opposite cervical skin was mobilized to resurface the neck, or if necessary, a skin graft was used. At a second stage, the lateral fissure was closed. In most cases, this could be accomplished by simple incision and direct suture along the edges of the defect (3).

In a modified procedure (4–7), the cephalocaudal length of the flap was increased by including the submental skin. This allowed a greater length of esophagus to be resected. The pharyngeal and esophageal anastomoses were only partially completed at the first stage in order to simplify the procedure. At the second stage, the neoesophagus was completed and the cervical defect was resurfaced by transfer of a thoracoacromial skin flap.

The reconstruction with cervical skin was further modified by others. A U-shaped superiorly based flap with separate incisions for the pharyngostoma and esophagostoma has been described (8). Bilateral skin flaps have been used, where one flap is lined with a skin graft (9). One flap formed the posterior wall, and the skin-lined flap provided the anterior esophageal wall and external surface.

OPERATIVE TECHNIQUE

The modified Wookey reconstruction uses a laterally based skin flap for the initial resection, which can include a radical neck dissection. The superior incision includes the submental skin by following the contour of the mandible (Fig. 1A). The inferior incision parallels the clavicle. The flap extends to the angle of the mandible on both sides. At the conclusion of the resection, the operative site includes the stumps of the trachea, esophagus, and oropharynx (Fig. 1B). The flap is sutured to the posterior edges of the oropharynx and the esophagus, creating two temporary stomata (Fig. 1C). A tracheostoma is constructed through a separate incision in the skin below the flap. The submental area is covered with a split-thickness skin graft. At the second stage, a new gullet is created by tubing the flap (Fig. 1D–F). A previously delayed thoracic skin flap is used to cover the cervical cutaneous defect (Fig. 1G).

CLINICAL RESULTS

The Wookey procedure has several inherent shortcomings. The laterally based flap tends to have marginal circulation at the tip, associated with frequent partial loss. The flap is often in the field of prior radiotherapy. Necrosis may delay completion of reconstruction by several weeks, and several additional procedures often are required to replace the lost tissue. In addition, the wide open pharyngostoma results in constant aspiration of saliva into the dependent tracheostoma, causing the patient to be most uncomfortable until reconstruction is finally completed.

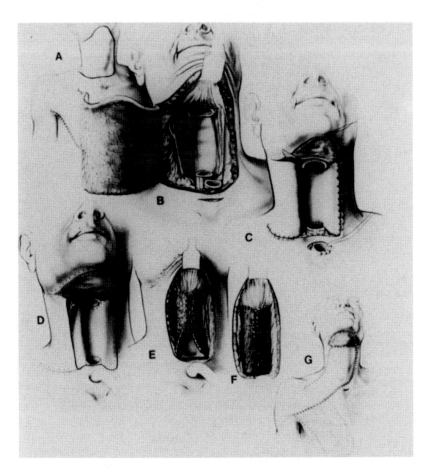

FIG. 1. Modified Wookey operation. **A:** Outline of laterally based flap. **B:** Operative field after resection. Note stumps of oropharynx, esophagus, and trachea. **C:** Completion of first stage. Exteriorization of pharynx and esophagus. Submental skin graft. **D:** Second stage. Incision outlining pharyngoesophageal segment. **E,F:** Closure of skin-lined tube. **G:** Rotation of thoracoacromial flap to resurface neck. (From Silver, ref. 7, with permission.)

In 1960 Mustard (3) reported the results of 44 patients operated on by himself and Wookey. Twenty-four percent of their patients survived 5 years, and six (14%) died before surgery was completed. The average length of hospitalization was not reported, but Mustard recommended 6 to 12 weeks between the primary resection and closure of the lateral sinus.

In eight modified Wookey reconstructions performed by the senior author (4), there was one operative death. All patients developed temporary fistulas after the second stage. Hospitalizations ranged from 6 weeks to 3 months.

In another series of 13 patients (10), an average of three procedures was required to complete reconstruction; hospitalizations ranged from 25 to 210 days. Twelve patients were ultimately able to swallow. One operative death occurred.

SUMMARY

Cervical skin flaps were the standard flaps used to reconstruct the pharyngoesophageal area. They are still useful in some patients, but they have been largely supplanted by the hardier deltopectoral and pectoralis major flaps.

References

1. Mikulicz J. Ein Fall von Resektion des Carcinomatosen Oesophagus mit Plastichen Ersatz des excidirten Stuckes. *Prager Med Wochenschr* 1886; 11:93.
2. Wookey H. The surgical treatment of carcinoma of the pharynx and upper esophagus. *Surg Gynecol Obstet* 1942;75:499.
3. Mustard RA. The use of the Wookey operation for cancer of the hypopharynx and cervical esophagus. *Surg Gynecol Obstet* 1960;111:577.
4. Silver CE, Som ML. Reconstruction of the cervical esophagus after total pharyngolaryngectomy: a modified Wookey operation. *Ann Surg* 1967;165:239.
5. Silver CE. Surgical treatment of hypopharyngeal and cervical esophageal cancer. *World J Surg* 1981;5:499.
6. Silver CE. *Surgery for cancer of the larynx and related structures.* New York: Churchill-Livingstone, 1981.
7. Silver CE. Reconstruction after pharyngolaryngectomy-esophagectomy. *Am J Surg* 1976;132:428.
8. Montgomery WM. *Surgery of the upper respiratory tract,* Vol. 2. Philadelphia: Lea & Febiger, 1973;300–301.
9. Litton WB. Reconstruction of the hypopharynx and cervical esophagus: local flap technique after planned preoperative irradiation. *Trans Am Acad Ophthalmol Otol* 1968;72:85.
10. Demergasso F, Piazza MV. Trapezius myocutaneous flap in reconstructive surgery for head and neck cancer: an original technique. *Am J Surg* 1979; 138:533.

CHAPTER 211 ■ DELTOPECTORAL SKIN FLAP: PHARYNGOESOPHAGEAL RECONSTRUCTION

V. Y. BAKAMJIAN

Reconstruction of the pharynx and cervical esophagus was the initial purpose for which the deltopectoral flap was devised in 1962 to overcome the considerable difficulties and shortcomings of earlier methods, mainly the two-stage technique with a cervical flap (see Chapter 210) and other one-stage techniques with skin grafts (1–7).

ANATOMY

See Chapter 124.

OPERATIVE TECHNIQUE

Radical neck dissection with laryngopharyngectomy that precedes reconstruction with a deltopectoral flap is best served by a transverse pair of parallel neck incisions, modified after MacFee. Contrary to commonly voiced opinions, these incisions amply provide needed exposure for accomplishing the ablative objective adequately (Fig. 1A) while also serving the interest of the reconstruction. The upper incision is placed at hyoid or just below hyoid level in a natural skin crease, and the lower is placed at clavicular level, in common with the upper margin of the deltopectoral flap (Fig. 1B).

The flap is introduced to the midline of the neck, passing beneath the bipedicle flap of cervical skin raised between the incisions of the neck dissection (Fig. 1C). With its raw side facing the prevertebral fascia, suturing begins between the tip of the flap and the excision line in the posterior wall of the oropharynx or epipharynx, as the case may be. The process continues to the sides bilaterally and reflects forward to meet at a point at the base of the tongue, a bit off-center and away from the side of the radical neck dissection. Starting from this point, the longitudinal seam that entubes the flap veers gently backward in its descent to meet the stump of the esophagus behind the transected trachea. Here the lips of the seam part to encircle the esophageal end opening, establishing an end-to-side anastomosis to the skin tube (Fig. 1D). Before this anastomosis is completed, however, a nasally introduced feeding tube is passed down the skin tube and into the esophagus and stomach, after which the seam is continued a short distance more to a fistulous exit over the medial head of the clavicle. The neck wounds are closed, and the donor wound on the chest and shoulder is covered with a skin graft (Fig. 1E).

The saliva-draining fistula, lying to one side and a little below the level of the tracheostoma (Fig. 1F), poses no aspiration problems in the interim of some 3 weeks before the second stage. This procedure consists of reentering the anastomosis site through the scar of the previous clavicular incision, opening the lowermost portion of the skin tube and dividing it, adjusting the disparity in caliber of the tubes, and reconnecting them in more of an end-to-end type of anastomosis (Fig. 1G).

A nearly identical technique is applicable in cases of oropharyngeal high resection without loss of the larynx and cervical portion of the gullet. Here the hollow tube of inverted skin, lying alongside the retained larynx and cervical gullet, serves only as a carrier for the distally used portion of the flap in the recipient defect (Fig. 2A), and it needs to be returned to the chest wall in a later stage. Division of the tube is done by reopening the upper scar of the previous neck incision, through which the oropharyngeal reconstruction is also completed. The remainder of the tube then is dissected downward in the neck and delivered to the outside through the scar of the lower neck incision, where it is untubed and returned to the chest wall (Fig. 2B).

There is also the possibility of rotating the end of the flap into the thoracic inlet instead of upward into the oropharynx (Fig. 3A). This maneuver was found useful in a case of low obstruction of the cervical esophagus with a heavily irradiated recurrent cancer. The resection, including larynx, thyroid gland, and cervical esophagus, extended to approximately 1½ inches below the level of the sternal notch. The mode of entubing and anastomosis is demonstrated by the diagrams in Fig. 3B. A minor complication ensued, with dehiscence and radionecrosis of the damaged cervical skin from around the tracheostoma (Fig. 3C) but was easily corrected at a second stage, when the divided pedicle of the deltopectoral flap was used to replace the unhealthy skin around the tracheostoma (8,9) (Fig. 3D).

SUMMARY

The deltopectoral flap can be adapted to reconstruct either high or low defects of the cervical esophagus.

Text continues on page 636.

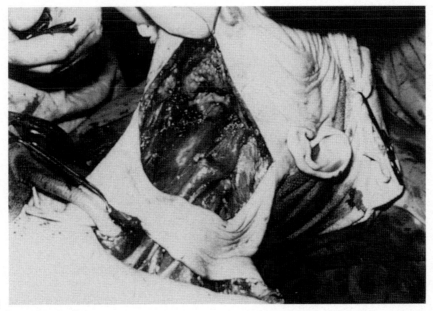

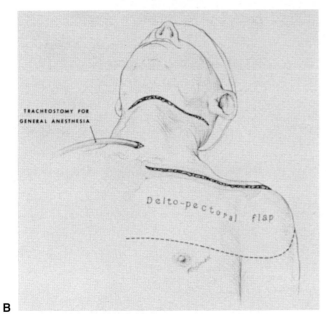

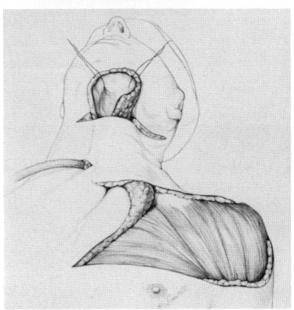

A

B

C

FIG. 1. **A:** Typical exposure obtained through a transverse pair of parallel incisions for laryngopharyngectomy and radical neck dissection. **B:** Outline of the incisions in conjunction with those to be used for raising the deltopectoral flap. **C:** Passage of the deltopectoral flap into the neck, beneath the bipedicle cervical flap of neck dissection. *(Continued)*

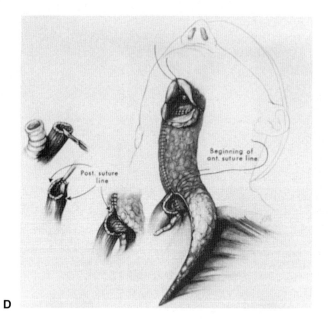

D

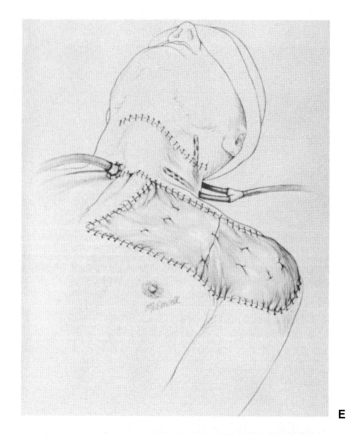

E

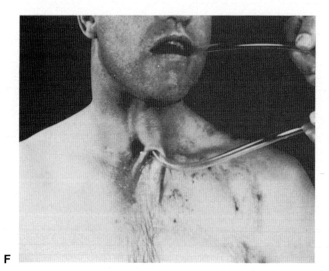

F

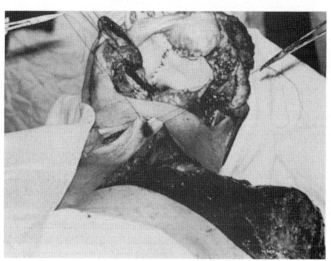

G

FIG. 1. *Continued.* D: Manner of forming the new gullet and its upper and lower anastomoses. E: First stage completed, with closure of neck wounds and skin grafts on donor area. F: Demonstration of the fistulous outlet that remains over the medial head of the clavicle. G: Steps in the second stage for completion of the reconstruction. (From Bakamjian, Calamel, ref. 5, with permission.)

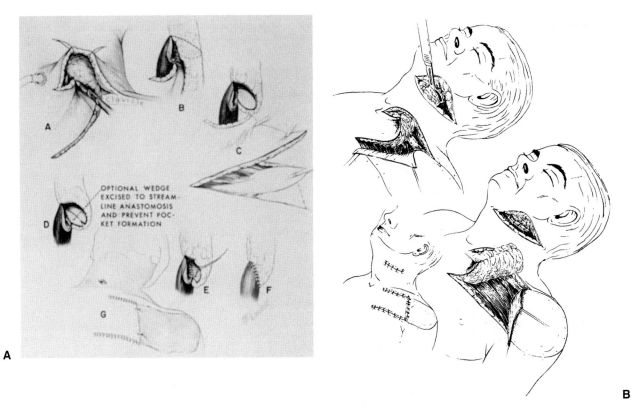

FIG. 2. **A:** The same basic technique employed for an oropharyngeal high defect not involving a loss of the larynx and cervical esophagus. **B:** Steps in the second-stage division of the entubed pedicle and its return to the chest.

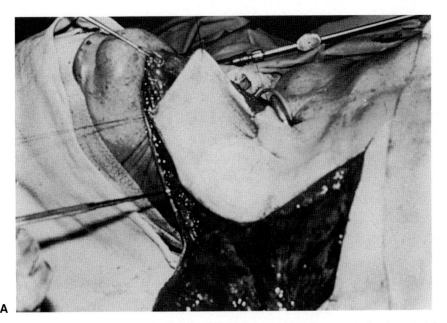

FIG. 3. **A:** Rotation of the tip of the flap to a low-lying esophageal stump in the thoracic inlet. *(Continued)*

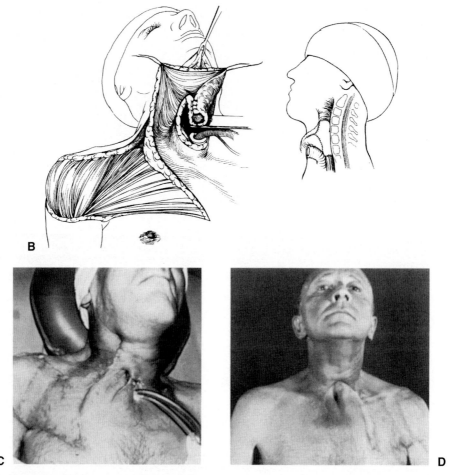

FIG. 3. *(Continued)* **B:** Diagram of the first-stage repair, the width of the flap end forming the length of the new gullet. **C:** The patient ready for the second stage. **D:** Final result. Note that the base of the deltopectoral flap has been used to replace the radiation-damaged skin around the tracheostoma. (From Bakamjian, Calamel, ref. 5, with permission.)

References

1. Bakamjian VY. A two-stage method for pharyngoesophageal reconstruction with a primary pectoral skin flap. *Plast Reconstr Surg* 1965;36:173.
2. Bakamjian VY. Reconstruction of the pharynx and cervical esophagus. In: Gaisford JC, ed. *Symposium on cancer of the head and neck: total treatment and reconstructive rehabilitation.* St. Louis: Mosby, 1969.
3. Bakamjian VY. Surgery for cancers of the hypopharynx and cervical esophagus. In: Cooper P, ed. *The craft of surgery,* 2nd ed. Boston: Little, Brown, 1971.
4. Bakamjian VY. Methods for pharyngoesophageal reconstruction. In: Grabb WC, Smith JW, eds. *Plastic surgery: concise guide to clinical practice,* 2nd ed. Boston: Little, Brown, 1973.
5. Bakamjian VY, Calamel PM. Oropharyngoesophageal surgery. In: Converse JM, ed. *Reconstructive plastic surgery,* 2nd ed. Philadelphia: Saunders, 1977; 2697–2756.
6. Bakamjian VY, Holbrook LA. Prefabrication techniques in cervical pharyngoesophageal reconstruction. *Br J Plast Surg* 1973;26:214.
7. Jackson IT, Lang W. Secondary esophagoplasty after pharyngolaryngectomy, using a modified deltopectoral flap. *Plast Reconstr Surg* 1971;48:155.
8. Selfe RW, Conley JJ. Tracheostoma construction with a deltopectoral flap. *Arch Otolaryngol* 1979;105:290.
9. Virkkula L, Eerola S, Appelqvist P. Repair of stricture and fistula of antethoracic oesophagogastrostoma using reversed pectoralis skin pedicle flap. *Scand J Thorac Cardiovasc Surg* 1977;11:67.

CHAPTER 212 ■ USE OF THE PECTORALIS MAJOR MUSCULOCUTANEOUS FLAP FOR ONE-STAGE CERVICAL, ESOPHAGEAL, AND PHARYNGEAL RECONSTRUCTION

R. F. RYAN

Reconstruction of the cervical esophagus has challenged surgeons for many years (1). Until 15 years ago, it was not unusual for patients needing esophageal replacement to undergo 20 or 30 operations. The two major developments in solving the problem of cervical esophageal replacement were the deltopectoral flap (2) and the development of free microvascular flaps of jejunum (3). The disadvantage of the Bakamjian flap was that it required two or three stages if it required a delay. The jejunal flap required an abdominal procedure and the risk of microvascular failure.

The next step was using a cutaneous flap vascularized by its underlying muscle for partial replacement of the esophagus (4–7). This was a one-stage procedure with the flap buried, and it did not require delay, division of the pedicle, or invasion of the abdominal cavity.

INDICATIONS

The pectoralis major musculocutaneous flap can be used to replace the cervical esophagus and lower pharynx.

OPERATIVE TECHNIQUE

The following is a description of the procedure as performed on the first patient: Preoperative examination of the cervical esophagus in this female patient showed only a small linear lesion about 1 cm wide and 2.5 cm long. The patient had previously undergone extensive radiation over the neck, a left radical neck resection, a right modified neck resection, and a laryngectomy. The oncologic surgeon planned to open the old midline T incision from the laryngectomy radical neck incision and resect the anterior portion of the esophagus. Unfortunately, the tumor extended submucosally and required resection of the entire esophagus from the level of the tracheostomy up to the posterior pharyngeal wall and resection of the gullet after a previous glossectomy and laryngectomy.

I was aware of previous failures in which musculocutaneous flaps had been sutured in a straight line along the borders of the skin to make a skin-lined tube. I also was aware that a hollow tube can be made by a narrow pedicle if it is sutured in a spiral manner, as is done with the cardboard core

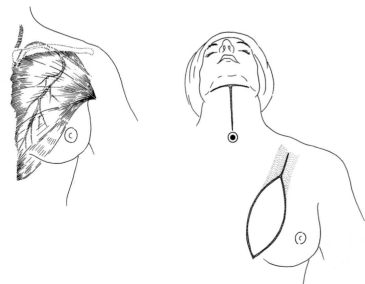

FIG. 1. A: The principal blood supply to the left pectoralis major muscle. B: The pectoralis major musculocutaneous flap, permanent tracheostomy, and old T incision from laryngectomy and right radical neck dissection. (From Ryan et al., ref. 7, with permission.)

A,B

637

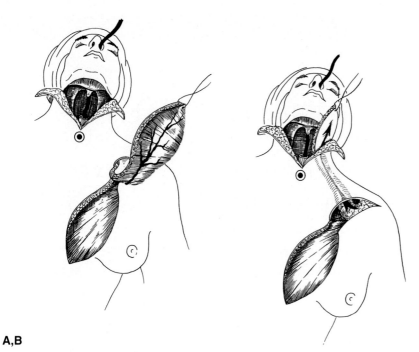

FIG. 2. A: The elevated left pectoralis major musculocutaneous flap. A nasogastric tube is shown entering the distal esophagus and lying on the bare prevertebral fascia after resection of the esophagus. **B:** Drawing shows passage of the musculocutaneous flap up into the neck wound. (From Ryan et al., ref. 7, with permission.)

A,B

for a roll of toilet tissue. Moreover, muscular contractions would tend to seal a spiral tube of skin rather than distract the edges and form fistulas.

A long pectoralis major muscle cutaneous flap was therefore elevated (7), as shown in Figs. 1 through 4. Because this was the first time I had done such a procedure, the pedicle was first tacked to one side. This would not work, so it was sutured to the other side of the oral cavity and then sutured in a spiral fashion. Because the new esophagus was of a much greater diameter than the remaining esophagus, the distal esophagus was split, as when anastomosing vessels of different diameters (Figs. 5 and 6).

CLINICAL RESULTS

The patient did well, but she refused to have the nasogastric tube removed. She did drink and swallow around the tube; however, several weeks postoperatively, the patient accidentally dislodged her nasogastric tube and was unable to swallow. In observing the patient, I noticed that she used her left arm to lift the glass to her mouth and was unable to swallow liquid. I then had the patient use her right hand, and she was able to swallow without difficulty. Thus, I would recommend that the nerve to the flap be divided.

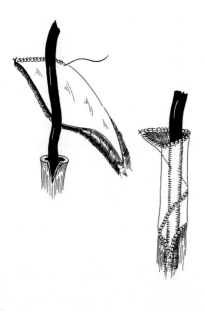

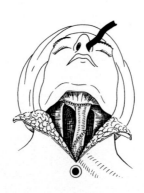

FIG. 3. A: Suturing of the distomedial edge of the left pectoralis major musculocutaneous pedicle flap to the nasal pharynx with the distal tip at the right side. A nasogastric tube enters the distal esophagus, which has been split to give a large anastomotic suture line. **B:** The flap is sutured on its distolateral side to the remaining floor of the mouth. The suturing then was continued in a spiral manner, sewing pedicle edge to pedicle edge to form a new esophagus around the nasogastric tube. Not shown is the bulk of the pectoralis muscle that covered the suture lines. **C:** Drawing shows the completed esophageal tube or gullet from nasopharynx to distal cervical esophagus. The muscle is not shown as it overlaps the tube. (From Ryan et al., ref. 7, with permission.)

A-C

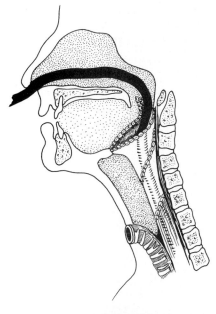

FIG. 4. Lateral drawing to show the total amount of pharynx and esophagus replacing the single-stage reconstruction by a left pectoralis major musculocutaneous flap. (From Ryan et al., ref. 7, with permission.)

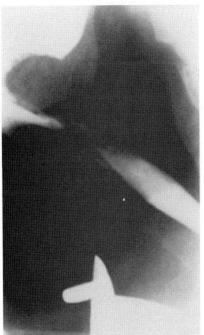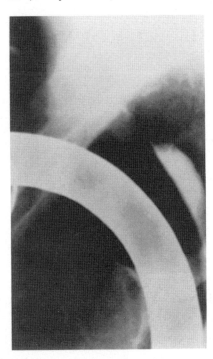

A,B

FIG. 5. Radiographs showing contrast media flowing down around the large nasogastric tube still in place in the reconstructed gullet. (From Ryan et al., ref. 7, with permission.)

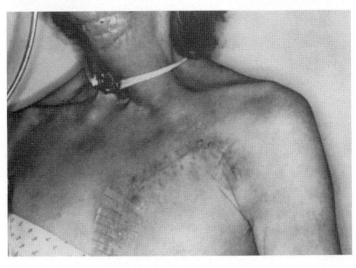

FIG. 6. Photograph showing the skin incisions of the neck and chest wall that healed primarily. (From Ryan et al., ref. 7, with permission.)

This patient is now 2 years postoperative, still has a patent esophagus, and is maintaining her nutrition. She has had a subcutaneous recurrence of the squamous cell carcinoma, however. The patient is still smoking through her tracheostomy.

SUMMARY

The pectoralis major musculocutaneous flap can be used in a spiral fashion to reconstruct the cervical esophagus and lower pharynx.

References

1. Capozzi A, Feierabend TC, Davenport F, Bernard FD. Cervical esophageal reconstruction. *Plast Reconstr Surg* 1966;38:347.
2. Bakamjian VY, Holbrook LA. Prefabrication techniques in cervical pharyngoesophageal reconstruction. *Br J Plast Surg* 1973;26:214.
3. McKee DM, Peters CR. Reconstruction of the hypopharynx and cervical esophagus with microvascular jejunal transplant. *Clin Plast Surg* 1978;5:305.
4. Ariyan S. The pectoralis major myocutaneous flap: a versatile flap for reconstruction in the head and neck. *Plast Reconstr Surg* 1979;63:73.
5. Ariyan S. Further experiences with the pectoralis myocutaneous flap for the immediate repair of defects from excisions of head and neck cancers. *Plast Reconstr Surg* 1979;64:605.
6. Theogaraj SD, Merritt WH, Acharya G, Cohen IK. The pectoralis major musculocutaneous island flap in single-stage reconstruction of the pharyngoesophageal region. *Plast Reconstr Surg* 1980;65:267.
7. Ryan RF, Krementz ET, Cardona O. One-stage cervical esophageal and pharyngeal reconstruction for a fourth primary cancer. *Plast Reconstr Surg* 1981;67:224.

CHAPTER 213 ■ TRAPEZOIDAL PADDLE PECTORALIS MAJOR MYOCUTANEOUS FLAP FOR ESOPHAGEAL REPLACEMENT

B. STRAUCH, C. SILVER, R. FEINGOLD, AND A. SHEKTMAN

EDITORIAL COMMENT

The pectoralis major myocutaneous flap for intraoral reconstruction has a high failure rate caused mainly by inadequate positioning of the skin paddle. The trapezoidal design of the skin paddle, which is placed entirely over the pectoralis major muscle, gives assurance of excellent viability and decreases the complications of intraoral skin necrosis. This alternative is useful in free-flap resurfacing intraorally.

The trapezoidal paddle pectoralis major myocutaneous flap is especially useful for circumferential hypopharyngeal defects and for esophageal reconstruction in elderly patients. It is preferred by the authors to free jejunal autografts.

INDICATIONS

Reconstruction of circumferential defects of the hypopharynx and cervical esophagus remains a challenge. Correction can be accomplished with the use of pedicled myocutaneous flaps or with the use of microvascular free flaps. The trapezoidal pad-dle pectoralis major myocutaneous flap (TPPMMC) is recommended and preferred for its ease of performance over free jejunal flaps, for the rapidity of surgery, and for the absence of an intraperitoneal approach.

Generally, malignant disease in this area carries a poor prognosis; therefore, surgical intervention frequently assumes only a palliative role. For this purpose, a procedure needs to have a low rate of major complications and also should allow the patient to return to a normal or near-normal lifestyle as soon as possible after surgery. Reconstructive efforts should be easily executed, should require little in the way of expensive equipment, and should conserve hospital resources. The trapezoidal paddle pectoralis major myocutaneous flap represents such a procedure.

ANATOMY

The pectoralis major is a type-V muscle, with its dominant vascular supply coming from the pectoral branch of the thoracoacromial artery running on its undersurface. The skin island and muscle are raised together using the origin of the thoracoacromial vessels at the clavicle as the axis of rotation. All the skin attached to the muscle will survive elevation as a myocutaneous flap.

FLAP DESIGN AND DIMENSIONS

The skin island is drawn on the chest wall as a trapezoid, with the shorter parallel side superiorly and the longer parallel side inferiorly. It is situated entirely over muscle with no "random" portion. The height of the trapezoid corresponds to the length of the pharyngoesophageal defect. Once tubed and transposed, the superior narrow base of the trapezoid will become situated in the inferior pole of the defect to be anastomosed to the esophagus. Therefore, the width of this component of the trapezoid must correspond to the diameter of the esophagus. Because this distal suture line represents the narrowest portion of the reconstruction, an 8-cm width is usually required to prevent stricture. After transposition, the inferior wider base of the trapezoid will become situated in the superior pole of the defect, to be anastomosed to the oropharynx. Thus, the width of this component of the trapezoid must correspond to the diameter of the oropharynx.

OPERATIVE TECHNIQUE

After the extirpative part of the procedure is completed, the resultant defect is measured. The vertical height of the defect will become the vertical height of the trapezoidal paddle. The skin paddle is outlined on the chest wall in a trapezoidal shape, with the long edge of the paddle placed inferiorly and the short edge placed superiorly (Fig. 1). The length of these edges should be equal to the circumference of the oropharyngeal and esophageal remnants. The skin paddle should lie entirely over the pectoralis major muscle. No "random" portion should be created.

Once the skin paddle is incised down to the pectoralis fascia, the muscle itself is mobilized, and the entire musculocutaneous flap is rotated into the neck. The flap should be tubed before performing the proximal and distal anastomoses, the long suture line placed laterally (Figs. 2–4), and the muscle placed over the skin tube. The pectoralis major muscle is sutured to the surrounding tissue for support. A split-thickness skin graft is placed on any of the externally exposed muscles, and the chest wound is closed primarily.

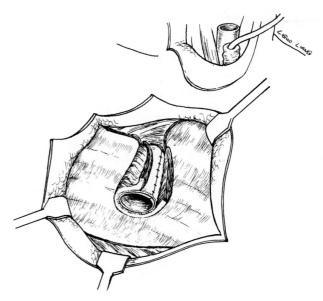

FIG. 2. Flap should be tubed before proximal and distal anastomoses. Long suture line should be lateral and muscle placed over the skin tube.

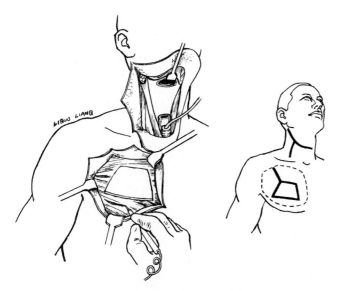

FIG. 1. After extirpation, resultant defect is measured. Vertical defect height will become vertical height of the trapezoidal paddle. Skin paddle is outlined on chest wall in trapezoidal shape, with the long edge of the paddle placed inferiorly, and the short edge is placed superiorly.

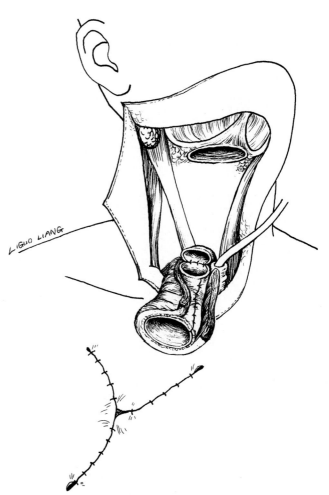

FIG. 3. Muscle and skin paddle are passed subcutaneously into the neck wound. The inferior anastomosis is begun.

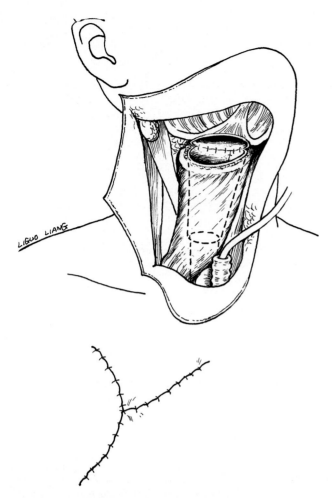

LIGUO LIANG

FIG. 4. Superior repair (the larger circumference) is now closed. Muscle flap is sutured over the neck wound. Any remaining defect not covered with the skin flap is skin grafted.

CLINICAL RESULTS

Among the ten consecutive patients in a series who underwent hypopharyngeal reconstruction with the TPPMMC flap, no flap loss occurred in any of the patients. Normal or near-normal swallowing was attained by all patients. The time to deglutition was 1 to 3 weeks for nonirradiated patients, and 3 to 13 weeks for irradiated patients. Fistulas developed in four

patients, all of whom had been previously irradiated. Two of the four fistulas healed with conservative management. One stenosis developed in this series and was treated successfully by a single dilation.

Compared with results of free jejunal transfers (1–6), the TPPMMC flaps had an appreciable advantage in the rate of flap loss (i.e., 3.0 to 1.5% versus 3.0 to 13.5%), respectively. The TPPMMC flap also has a relative ease of execution, with an average operating time of 2.5 to 3.0 hours, compared with an average of 6.0 to 6.5 hours for the free jejunal graft. Use of the flap also avoids the morbidity associated with opening the peritoneal cavity to harvest the jejunal graft or performing a bowel anastomosis (7). Because many patients in all the series reported are in the advanced-age category, decrease in operating time and the elimination of an intraabdominal procedure weigh heavily in favor of the pedicled procedure.

Because of the anatomy of the TPPMMC flap, the attached muscle serves to cover the suture line closure. This normal muscle cover is lacking in jejunal and free radial forearm flap reconstructions (8).

SUMMARY

The trapezoidal paddle pectoralis major myocutaneous flap has predictably good results and low complication rates, and it requires a relatively short operating time. Compared with free jejunal grafts, it holds a promising position in reconstruction of postextirpative defects of the hypopharynx and cervical esophagus.

References

1. Coleman JJ, III. Reconstruction of the pharynx after resection for cancer. *Ann Surg* 1989;209:554.
2. Coleman JJ, III, Tan K-C, Searles JM, et al. Jejunal free autograft: analysis of complications and their resolution. *Plast Reconstr Surg* 1989;84:589.
3. Reece GP, Schusterman MA, Miller MJ, et al. Morbidity and functional outcome of free jejunal transfer reconstructions for circumferential defects of the pharynx and cervical esophagus. *Plast Reconstr Surg* 1995;96:1307.
4. Cusumano RJ, Silver CE, Brauer RJ, Strauch B. Pectoralis myocutaneous flap for replacement of cervical esophagus. *Head Neck* 1989;11:450.
5. Silver CE, Cusumano RJ, Fell SC, Strauch B. Replacement of upper esophagus: results with myocutaneous flap and with gastric transposition. *Laryngoscope* 1990;99:819.
6. Coleman JJ, III. Jejunal free flap. In: Strauch B, Vasconez L, Hall-Findlay E, eds. *Grabb's encyclopedia of flaps*, 2nd ed. Philadelphia: Lippincott–Raven, 1998; Chap. 204.
7. Shah JP, Haribhakti V, Loree TR, Sutaria P. Complications of the pectoralis major myocutaneous flap in head and neck reconstruction. *Am J Surg* 1990; 160:352.
8. Boyd JB. Radial forearm cutaneous flap for hypopharyngeal reconstruction. In: Strauch B, Vasconez L, Hall-Findlay E, eds. *Grabb's encyclopedia of flaps*, 2nd ed. Philadelphia: Lippincott–Raven, 1998; Chap. 207.

CHAPTER 214 ■ BILOBED CHEST FLAP (DELTOPECTORAL SKIN FLAP AND PECTORALIS MAJOR MUSCULOCUTANEOUS FLAP)

R. M. MEYER

The bilobed chest flap is a double cutaneous and musculocutaneous flap used for head and neck reconstruction. The flap incorporates the pectoralis major musculocutaneous flap and the medially based cutaneous deltopectoral flap in a single bilobed unit. Both flaps come from the ipsilateral chest and provide for both reconstruction of pharyngoesophageal wall defects and external cutaneous coverage in one stage.

INDICATIONS

Solutions to the problem of external coverage at flap donor sites have been numerous, and I have used six alternative methods, according to the type of repair. In my experience with 78 pectoralis major musculocutaneous flaps, I have used the following methods for closure or cover of the external defect (1–3):

1. Skin approximation and suture (21 patients)
2. Using a part of the pectoralis major musculocutaneous flap for two patches (31 patients)
3. Split-thickness skin grafts (18 patients)
4. Advancement shoulder flaps (4 patients)
5. Contralateral deltopectoral flaps (3 patients)
6. Ipsilateral deltopectoral flap (1 patient)

The last method is the subject of this chapter (i.e., the use of the pectoralis major musculocutaneous flaps for pharyngoesophageal reconstruction, combined with the ipsilateral medially based deltopectoral flap for cutaneous coverage). The ipsilateral musculocutaneous and cutaneous flaps, having a common base, thus form a single bilobed flap.

FLAP DESIGN AND DIMENSIONS

The bilobed chest flap is composed of two standard flaps: the pectoralis major musculocutaneous flap and the deltopectoral cutaneous flap. The two flaps share a common base, starting approximately 3 to 4 cm below the medial end of the clavicle and continuing cranially and laterally to the anterior part of the neck. The design of the two flaps resembles an open V (Fig. 1). The outline of the musculocutaneous portion of the bilobed flap should be centered on the thoracoacromial artery.

OPERATIVE TECHNIQUE

First, the musculocutaneous portion of the bilobed flap is raised to repair the deep neck defect in the pharyngoesophageal tract

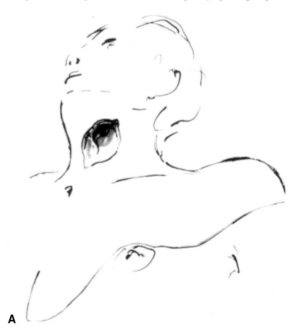

A

FIG. 1. A,B: Outline of the bilobed flap. (From Meyer et al., ref. 2, with permission.) *(Continued)*

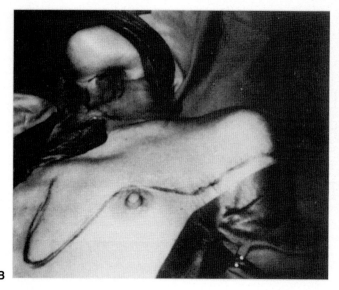

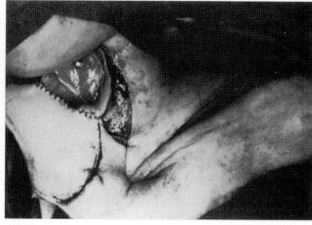

FIG. 2. The lower oblique part of the bilobed flap containing part of the pectoralis major muscle is sutured to the border of the defect.

B

FIG. 1. *(continued)*

after pharyngolaryngectomy. I tailor a new upper digestive tract, making a tube with the pectoralis major musculocutaneous flap (Figs. 2 and 3). The reconstruction begins on the lower side, with the anastomosis to the esophageal remnant. The junction between the mucocutaneous anastomosis and the vertical suture line, which forms the new digestive tract, is placed laterally. At the end of the vertical sutures, the flap has a funnel shape, with the inner layer formed by the cutaneous portion of the pectoralis major flap and the outer one by the muscle portion. The upper anastomosis then is performed in the same manner as the lower, by joining the flap to the remaining

base of the tongue, as well as to the lateral and posterior pharyngeal walls.

After this first part of the cervical reconstruction, the previously outlined deltopectoral cutaneous flap is raised (Fig. 4), starting at its lateral edge. It is then rotated to cover the exposed raw surface of the musculocutaneous flap (Fig. 5).

At this time, care must be taken not to dissect this cutaneous portion of the bilobed flap too medially. A medial base must be preserved in order not to jeopardize the blood supply, which depends on the perforating branches of the internal mammary artery.

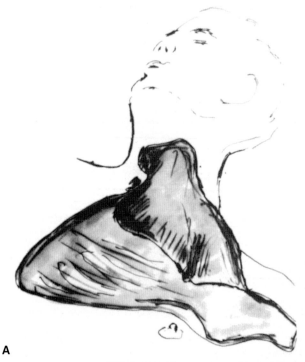

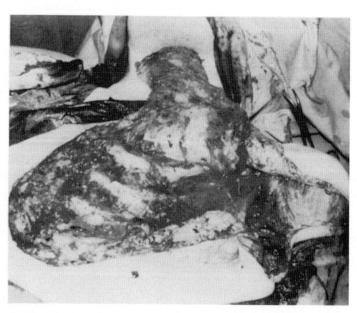

A   **B**

FIG. 3. A,B: The anterior and lateral pharyngeal wall from the esophageal mouth up to the base of the tongue is reconstructed by the pectoralis major musculocutaneous part of the flap. (From Meyer et al., ref. 2, with permission.)

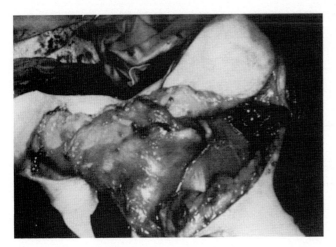

FIG. 4. The donor area of the musculocutaneous part of the flap is closed, and the deltopectoral part of the flap is raised.

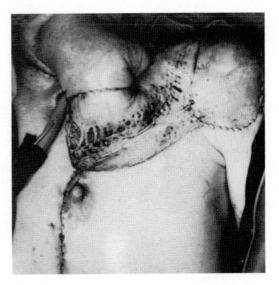

FIG. 6. The donor area of the horizontal deltopectoral part of the composite flap is covered by a split-thickness skin graft. (From Meyer et al., ref. 2, with permission.)

The musculocutaneous lower donor site is closed primarily by joining the edges of the wound. The deltopectoral donor site is covered with a split-thickness skin graft (Figs. 6 and 7).

CLINICAL RESULTS

The use of a combined musculocutaneous and cutaneous flap from the ipsilateral chest permits reconstruction of the cervical pharyngoesophageal tract and simultaneous provision of a pedicled cutaneous cover in head and neck reconstruction. The considerable length, bulk, and excellent blood supply of the pectoralis major musculocutaneous flap render it especially appropriate for pharyngeal reconstruction. Its use has appreciably reduced the incidence of fistula formation. The deltopectoral cutaneous flap has the double advantage of

being a pedicled cutaneous flap and having its base close to the recipient site. This composite flap is a true bilobed flap, having the advantages of one-stage reconstruction without delay and incorporating both musculocutaneous and cutaneous elements from an ipsilateral donor site.

SUMMARY

The advantages discussed render the bilobed chest flap useful for many cases involving inner and outer head and neck reconstruction.

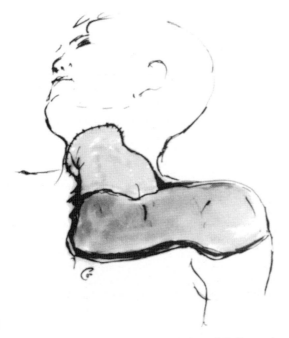

A

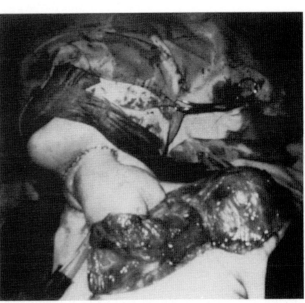

B

FIG. 5. A,B: External coverage by the deltopectoral part of the flap.

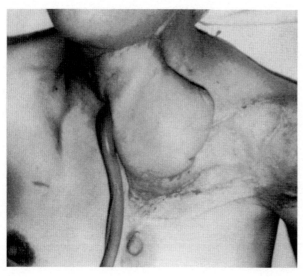

FIG. 7. Result after 4 months (while undergoing endoscopic revaluation).

References

1. Brupbacher JP, Meyer R, Failat ASA, Botta Y. Reconstruction de l'oesophage cervical avec le lambeau musculo-cutané du grand pectoral. *Cah Franc d'Orl* 1981;16:639.
2. Meyer R, Kelly TP, Failat ASA. Single bilobed flap for use in head and neck reconstruction. *Ann Plast Surg* 1981;6:203.
3. Meyer R, Brupbacher JP, Brown WL. Pharyngoesophageal reconstruction by pectoralis major myocutaneous flap. *Chir Plast* 1982;6:249.

CHAPTER 215 ■ LATISSIMUS DORSI MUSCULOCUTANEOUS FLAP FOR PHARYNGOESOPHAGEAL RECONSTRUCTION

F. E. BARTON, JR., J. M. KENKEL, AND W. P. ADAMS, JR.

Despite recent advances in microsurgical techniques, regional pedicled flaps remain the mainstay of reconstructive options for pharyngoesophageal reconstruction. The island pectoralis major musculocutaneous flap continues to be the preferred flap of many reconstructive surgeons; however, the latissimus dorsi musculocutaneous flap is a safe and reliable alternative for reconstruction of partial and circumferential cervical esophageal defects (1–3).

INDICATIONS

The latissimus dorsi musculocutaneous flap may be used for any one-stage pharyngoesophageal reconstruction, but it should be considered the flap of choice in patients with large soft-tissue or cutaneous deficits, infected wounds, or irradiated beds that could not support microvascular transfer. The following are the advantages of the latissimus dorsi musculocutaneous flap for pharyngoesophageal reconstruction:

1. A large area of skin can be transferred while still closing the donor site primarily.
2. The cutaneous paddle is usually hairless, in contrast to flaps from the anterior chest in men.
3. The donor site is on the back, which is more acceptable to women than donor deformities on the anterior chest.
4. There is minimal functional loss from latissimus dorsi harvest.
5. The long vascular pedicle allows for a wide arc of rotation that easily reaches the nasopharynx.
6. The flap can be split into separate musculocutaneous units to be used for lining, soft-tissue fill, and skin cover or to preserve motor function at the flap donor site (4).
7. The vascular pedicle is away from the field of resection or irradiation in head and neck malignancies.

ANATOMY

The latissimus dorsi is a flat muscle extending obliquely across the back. It originates from the lower six thoracic vertebrae, lumbar and sacral vertebrae, iliac crest, and external surface of the lower four ribs, and it inserts on the intertubercular groove of the humerus (5,6). The neurovascular anatomy of the latissimus dorsi flap was expertly described previously (7–11). The thoracodorsal artery originates from the subscapular artery and is the principal blood supply to the latissimus dorsi muscle. One to three arterial branches to the chest wall are given off before the thoracodorsal artery enters the latissimus dorsi muscle (7). The neurovascular pedicle enters the muscle on its undersurface about 8 to 10 cm from its origin (8) and 8 to 12 cm below its humeral insertion. The vessels bifurcate about 2 cm after entering the muscle. The superior branch traverses the muscle parallel to its border approximately 3.5 cm from the upper edge. The lateral branch parallels the posterior border of the muscle some 2 cm from its edge (7). Cutaneous perforators emanate from these branches and appear at regular patterns 3 to 5 cm apart (1,12,13). In cadaveric injection studies of the thoracodorsal artery, the lower third of the muscle and its overlying skin consistently do not fill with contrast medium, which indicates this portion of the muscle and skin are unreliable for use as a musculocutaneous flap (1,12).

FLAP DESIGN AND DIMENSIONS

The vascular status of the musculocutaneous unit is assessed preoperatively. Using a Doppler device, the main thoracodorsal artery is traced through the lower axilla to its entrance into the latissimus dorsi muscle. The large anterior branch that parallels the lateral edge of the muscle is identified, and the specific perforating tributaries from the muscle to the skin are pinpointed. When possible, the cutaneous paddle is placed over the area of maximum density of perforating vessels.

While a large skin island would inevitably include one or more perforators from the muscle, small flaps used in pharyngoesophageal reconstruction are specifically placed over identified perforators to ensure survival. The skin paddle is ideally designed approximately two thirds of the way down the mus-

cle. This location preserves a reliable vascular supply to the skin and yet allows a wide range of motion of the flap on its pedicle. Alternatively, a portion of skin from the lower third of the flap may be carried as a random extension of a more superiorly based island. Skin paddles taken within 8 cm of the posterior iliac crest have been routinely incorporated in large flaps containing abundant muscle (2). On the other hand, a skin island isolated over the lower third of the muscle may not be viable.

Because the flap will be rotated 180 degrees when transposed to the neck, the island is diagrammed upside-down on the back. A trapezoidal paddle is marked obliquely on the muscle so when the flap is transferred to the neck and the cutaneous island is oriented vertically, the muscle pedicle will exit inferiorly and laterally (Fig. 1).

The size of the cutaneous paddle depends on the size of the esophageal defect. For an entire cervicoesophageal segment, the island should be 8 cm wide at its cephalic margin (to match the circumference of the lower esophageal junction) and about 12 cm long caudally. After transfer, an island flap of this size will yield a lumen of 4 to 5 cm at the hypopharynx and 2 to 2.5 cm in the distal esophagus. Smaller defects not involving the full esophageal circumference can be repaired with smaller cutaneous islands of proportional size.

OPERATIVE TECHNIQUE

The patient is placed in a semilateral decubitus position that facilitates simultaneous flap elevation and tumor extirpation. Dissection begins with a transverse axillary incision that is extended down the lateral border of the latissimus dorsi muscle (Fig. 2). The muscle is bluntly dissected from the serratus muscle anteriorly and the thoracolumbar vessels to the latissimus are severed. The thoracodorsal neurovascular pedicle is isolated, and the vessels to the serratus anterior and teres major are ligated and divided. The thoracodorsal artery and vein are skeletonized up to the level of the circumflex scapular vessels, which are left intact to provide collateral flow and to tether the pedicle so that it will not kink. The thoracodorsal nerve is transected to promote atrophy of the muscle postoperatively. Hyperabduction of the upper extremity may injure the brachial plexus and should be avoided (14).

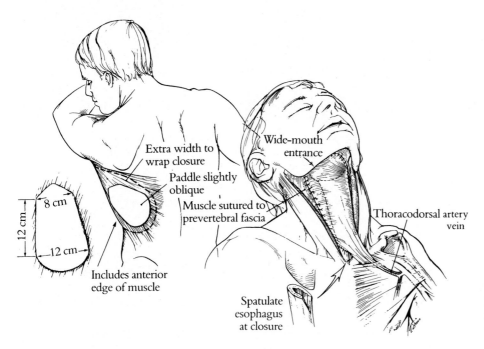

Extra width to wrap closure

Wide-mouth entrance

Paddle slightly oblique

Muscle sutured to prevertebral fascia

8 cm

12 cm

12 cm

Thoracodorsal artery vein

Includes anterior edge of muscle

Spatulate esophagus at closure

FIG. 1. Technique of latissimus dorsi musculocutaneous flap esophageal reconstruction.

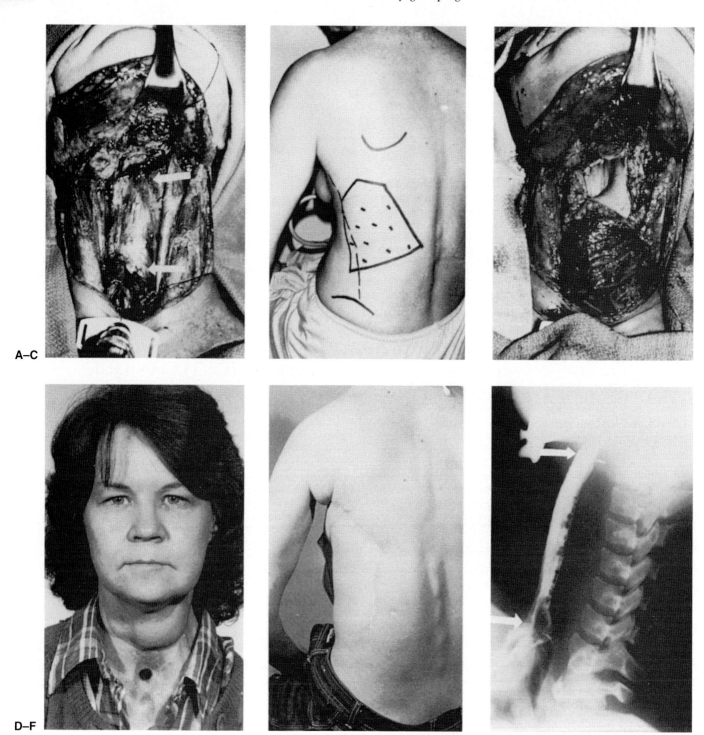

A–C

D–F

FIG. 2. A 40-year-old woman with extensive squamous-cell carcinoma of the piriform sinus and esophagus underwent laryngopharyngectomy and reconstruction of the segmental cervical esophagus with the latissimus dorsi island musculocutaneous flap. **A:** Operative defect. Note the circumferential esophageal loss between *arrows*. **B:** Design of the latissimus cutaneous paddle on the back. Note cutaneous perforators. **C:** Completion of replacement of cervical esophagus with the tubed cutaneous paddle. **D:** Postoperative appearance. **E:** Postoperative donor-site defect. **F:** Lateral cervical esophagogram with *arrows* indicating the reconstructed segment.

The skin island is incised circumferentially down to muscle fascia, and the remaining skin is reflected off the muscle. The muscle, with its attached island, then is freed distally, dissected in a retrograde fashion, and cut at its humeral insertion to increase the arc of rotation. A heavy suture is placed in the lateral muscle and secured to the pectoralis minor muscle or chest wall. This suture prevents stretch injury and torsion of the pedicle and improves control and countertraction during transfer of the flap to the neck (14).

A tunnel is created between the pectoralis major and minor muscles, penetrating the pectoralis major to exit over the clavicle and enter the cervical area. The pectoralis tunnel is made medial to the thoracoacromial pedicle. The tendinous insertion of the pectoralis minor can be transected to prevent compression of the vascular pedicle of the flap as it courses between these two muscles (14). Care is taken to preserve the neurovascular supply of the pectoralis major muscle during preparation of the intermuscular tunnel. The donor site on the back is closed primarily.

Inset of the latissimus dorsi musculocutaneous flap is similar to that of other flaps. If a partial esophageal circumference is needed, the skin island is sutured to the mucosal remnant. In the event of circumferential esophageal loss, the skin island is tubed, the upper end is sutured to the hypopharynx, and the lower end is sutured to the distal esophagus. For combined pharyngeal and cervical or buccal defects, the latissimus dorsi flap can be split based on its consistent medial and lateral arterial branches (4). Postoperative stricture is avoided by rounding the edge of the flap in the hypopharynx to create a wide-mouthed funnel effect and by spatulating the distal anastomosis with a triangular extension of the flap set into an incised esophageal wall (Fig. 1). The latissimus dorsi muscle also can be used as a second-layer closure over the mucosal suture line or to cover one or both carotid vessels by securing the flap to the prevertebral fascia.

CLINICAL RESULTS

The senior author's experience with the latissimus dorsi musculocutaneous flap in pharyngoesophageal reconstruction was reported previously (1). In that series, the latissimus dorsi musculocutaneous flap was found to be most useful for replacement of large amounts of vascularized tissue when previous surgery or irradiation precludes the use of local flaps. The latissimus dorsi musculocutaneous flap was preferred over the pectoralis musculocutaneous flap because the skin of the back is usually hairless and thus better suited for intraoral lining. In addition, the donor defect of the latissimus dorsi musculocutaneous flap was more acceptable to patients than the deficit caused by elevation of other regional flaps from the anterior trunk. The pectoralis major flap, for instance, produces an unsightly infraclavicular hollow and an absent anterior axillary fold that many women find disagreeable.

Disadvantages of the latissimus dorsi musculocutaneous flap for use in head and neck reconstruction include the following:

1. Flap dissection and elevation must be done with the patient in the semilateral position, which may require intraoperative repositioning.
2. Dissection of the neurovascular pedicle must be done through a separate axillary incision and can be somewhat tedious.
3. The flap may be bulky and too thick for small esophageal defects, especially in obese patients.
4. Neuropraxia of the brachial plexus can occur if the shoulder is not carefully supported during flap harvest.

SUMMARY

The latissimus dorsi musculocutaneous flap is an excellent option in pharyngoesophageal reconstruction. It provides generous amounts of hairless skin and muscle while producing an acceptable donor defect.

References

1. Barton FE Jr, Spicer TE, Byrd HS. Head and neck reconstruction with the latissimus dorsi myocutaneous flap: anatomical observations and report of 60 cases. Plast Reconstr Surg 1983;71:199.
2. Watson JS, Lendrum J. One stage pharyngeal reconstruction using a compound latissimus dorsi island flap. Br J Plast Surg 1981;34:87.
3. Yamamoto K, Yokota K, Higaki K. Entire pharyngoesophageal reconstruction with latissimus dorsi myocutaneous island flap. Head Neck Surg 1985;7:461.
4. Tobin GR, Moberg AW, DuBou RH, et al. The split latissimus dorsi myocutaneous flap. Ann Plast Surg 1981;7:637.
5. Hollinshead WH. Textbook of anatomy, 2nd ed. New York: Harper & Row, 1967.
6. Spalteholz W. Hand-Atlas of human anatomy, 7th ed. Philadelphia: Lippincott, 1943; vol 2.
7. Bartlett SP, May JW Jr, Yaremchuk MJ. The latissimus dorsi muscle: a fresh cadaver study of the primary neurovascular pedicle. Plast Reconstr Surg 1981;67:631.
8. Tobin GR, Schusterman M, Peterson GH, et al. The intramuscular neurovascular anatomy of the latissimus dorsi muscle: the basis for splitting the flap. Plast Reconstr Surg 1981;67:637.
9. Cassel JM. Intramuscular anatomy of the latissimus dorsi muscle. Br J Plast Surg 1989;42:607.
10. Rowsell AR, Eisenberg N, Davies DM, et al. The anatomy of the thoracodorsal artery within the latissimus dorsi muscle. Br J Plast Surg 1986;39:206.
11. Rowsell AR, Davies DM, Eisenberg N, et al. The anatomy of the subscapular-thoracodorsal arterial system: study of 100 cadaver dissections. Br J Plast Surg 1984;37:574.
12. Watson JS, Craig RDP, Orton CI. The free latissimus dorsi myocutaneous flap. Plast Reconstr Surg 1979;64:299.
13. Saijo M. The vascular territories of the dorsal trunk: a reappraisal for potential flap donor sites. Br J Plast Surg 1978;31:200.
14. Sabatier RE, Bakamjian VY, Carter WL. Craniofacial and head and neck applications of the transaxillary latissimus dorsi flap. Ear Nose Throat J 1992;71:173.

Online Chapter
www.encyclopediaofflaps.com

CHAPTER 216. Sternocleidomastoid Muscle and Musculocutaneous Flaps *S. Ariyan*

CHAPTER 217 ■ RECONSTRUCTION OF THE CERVICAL ESOPHAGUS BY VISCERAL INTERPOSITION

C. E. SILVER AND R. J. BRAUER

Various segments of abdominal viscera may be transposed or freely transplanted to replace portions of esophagus after resection or stenosis. The main advantage of these procedures, compared to reconstructions using skin (see Chapter 210), is that considerably longer segments of esophagus can be replaced. Visceral interpositions often can be performed in a single stage, thus permitting rapid rehabilitation of the esophagectomized patient; however, the magnitude of surgical trauma is generally greater than with skin reconstructions, and potentially disastrous complications may occur in association with necrosis or anastomotic failure. Thus, a greater degree of risk is assumed with these procedures than with reconstructions using skin to replace esophagus.

INDICATIONS

Reversed Gastric Tube

An antiperistaltic gastric tube (1) has been found to have several advantages over isoperistaltic tubes (2–4), including greater length, simplicity, and versatility, and has been more widely employed (Fig. 1).

Esophagocoloplasty

The colon generally provides a slightly shorter conduit than can be created by a reversed gastric tube and is more difficult to transfer subcutaneously. Thus, we tend to use colon more often in patients in whom substernal transfer is feasible or in whom anastomosis to the lower cervical esophagus is required (5) (Fig. 2).

Despite arguments advanced by advocates of either esophagocoloplasty or gastric tube esophagoplasty, the choice of procedure depends more on the experience and familiarity of the individual surgeon with either method than on any marked inherent advantage of one over the other.

Gastric Transposition (Gastric Pull-Up)

The gastric pull-up operation offers several advantages over other visceral interpositional procedures (6–11). The blood supply of the transposed stomach is superior to that of colon and reversed gastric tube. The procedure is performed in one stage, and the only anastomosis is extraabdominal, which lessens the chance of peritonitis or mediastinitis. The pharyn-gogastric anastomosis is particularly resistant to strictures and dehiscence. Elimination of the thoracotomy markedly lessens the morbidity and mortality of the procedure. When employed in properly selected patients, the gastric transposition operation comes close to being the ideal method for pharyngoesophageal reconstruction (see Chapter 210). There are, however, limitations.

The gastric transposition operation for resection and reconstruction of cervical esophageal carcinoma combines the advantages of two concepts. The scope of resection is increased by including extrathoracic extraction of the entire esophagus with the resection. Reconstruction is then accomplished by pulling the entire stomach through the posterior mediastinal bed of the resected esophagus to the level of the pharynx, to which it is anastomosed. The procedure is performed in a single stage and is technically simpler than other methods of visceral interposition. The well-vascularized stomach is a most reliable esophageal substitute (Fig. 3).

Free Jejunal Transfer

See Chapter 218.

ANATOMY

Reversed Gastric Tube

The reversed gastric tube is pedicled at the fundic end of the stomach and is based on the left gastroepiploic vessels. With splenectomy and mobilization of the tail of the pancreas, a sufficiently long conduit can be developed to easily reach the level of the oropharynx (Fig. 1).

Esophagocoloplasty

Both right and left colon can be used for esophageal replacement. In theory, the right colon has the advantage of assuming an isoperistaltic orientation after interposition; however, a great length of the left colon can be pedicled on the middle colic vessels, and angiographic studies (12) confirmed that the marginal artery of the colon is more consistent on the left side. Although the left colon assumes an antiperistaltic orientation when interposed, this has not proven functionally significant (Fig. 2).

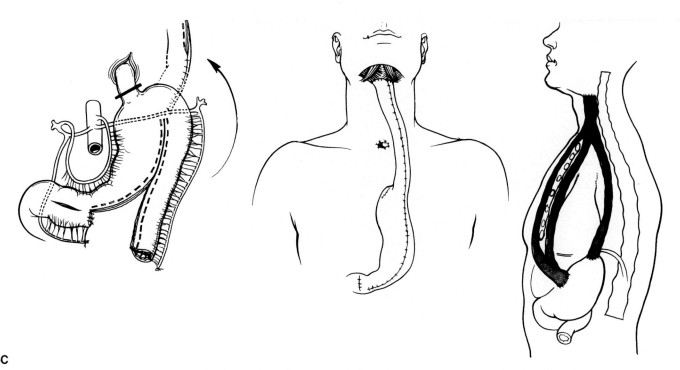

A–C

FIG. 1. Reverse gastric tube esophagoplasty. **A:** Pedicled tube from greater curvature. **B:** Final position of tube with anastomoses to pharynx. **C:** Alternate routes for tubed transfer to neck (subcutaneous, substernal, and posterior mediastinal). (From Silver, ref. 13, with permission.)

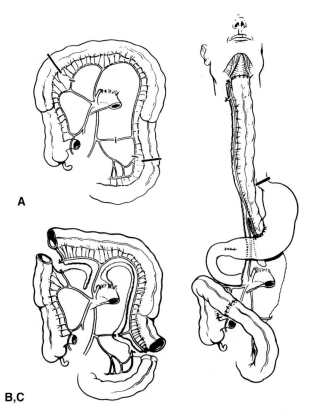

A

B,C

FIG. 2. Esophagocoloplasty (left colon). **A:** Blood supply of colon—outline of transposed segment. **B:** Colon mobilized. **C:** Final position of interposed colon. (From Silver, ref. 13, with permission.)

Gastric Transposition

Blunt digital dissection from abdominal and cervical incisions is used to mobilize the esophagus without a thoracotomy. The stomach is drawn through the posterior mediastinum by traction on the esophagus. The transposed stomach receives its blood supply from the right gastric and gastroepiploic vessels (Fig. 3).

OPERATIVE TECHNIQUE

Reversed Gastric Tube

The procedure (13) may be performed in one stage, with the resection using two surgical teams, or it may be employed as a secondary procedure at an interval following esophagectomy and creation of a temporary pharyngostoma. The abdomen is entered through an upper midline abdominal incision, the gastrocolic and gastrosplenic ligaments are divided, and a splenectomy is performed. A pedicled tube is created along the greater curvature of the stomach using a stapling device (Fig. 1). Care is taken at all times to preserve the gastroepiploic vessels. A pyloroplasty is performed to improve gastric emptying.

The tube may be transferred to the neck by means of a substernal, posterior mediastinal, or subcutaneous route (Fig. 1B and C). Although the posterior mediastinal route (used after total esophagectomy) is shortest, the substernal route has been most often employed. For secondary reconstruction, the subcutaneous route must be used because of obliteration of mediastinal tissue planes. The subcutaneous route, although longer than the others, has the advantage of safety in that the mediastinal

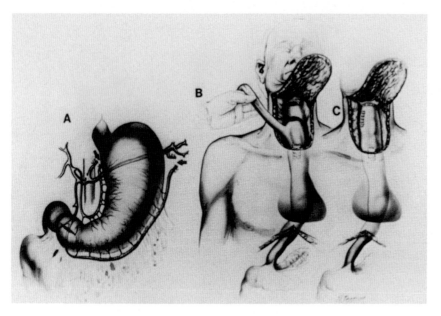

FIG. 3. Gastric transposition or pull-up. **A:** Blood supply of stomach mobilized for transposition. **B:** Stomach transposed through posterior mediastinum. **C:** Pharyngogastric anastomosis. (From Silver, ref. 13, with permission.)

contents are not threatened by massive infection in the event of necrosis or dehiscence.

Left Colon Esophagocoloplasty

An isolated loop of bowel, supplied by the middle colic vessels, is created by dividing the superior left colic artery and the anastomotic connections between the middle colic and right colic and superior and inferior branches of the left colic artery (Fig. 2A) (13). The bowel is mobilized by dissecting the greater omentum from the colon and by dividing the gastrocolic and phrenocolic ligaments and lateral peritoneal reflections (Fig. 2B). Care is taken while mobilizing the bowel to protect its marginal circulation. The bowel is brought posterior to the stomach (to avoid creating an obstructive band) and is transposed to the neck. The same routes are used for transfer to the neck as with the gastric tube, although the substernal route has been the most popular. The distal end of the colon is brought through the tunnel first and is anastomosed to the oropharynx or cervical esophagus. The proximal colon (which has now become distal "esophagus") is anastomosed to the lesser curvature of the stomach as close to the fundus as possible. A pyloroplasty is performed to enhance gastric emptying. A colocolostomy is performed to restore bowel continuity.

Gastric Transposition

After resectability of the lesion has been established by cervical exploration, the abdomen is entered through an upper midline incision by a second surgical team working simultaneously (13,14). The left gastric, short gastric, and left gastroepiploic vessels are divided (Fig. 3A). Mobilization of the stomach continues by dividing the gastrocolic and gastrosplenic ligaments without compromising the arcade of the gastroepiploic vessels on the greater curvature. Preservation of venous drainage is as critical as arterial preservation. Particular care must be exercised to avoid injuring the right gastroepiploic vein. The gastroesophageal junction is mobilized, the vagus nerves are transected, the esophageal hiatus

is enlarged, and a Kocher maneuver is performed to free the duodenum. A pyloroplasty is mandatory, owing to vagal resection.

The thoracic esophagus is mobilized by blunt digital dissection from the cervical and abdominal incisions. The delicate posterior tracheal wall is separated with extreme care to prevent disruption, which can be life threatening. The endotracheal balloon should be deflated before separating the party wall of trachea and esophagus to prevent pressure from the balloon from being transmitted to the tracheal wall, causing or extending a tear. A ring dissector (11) or a vein stripper (13) may be used to facilitate esophageal dissection. When the esophagus has been fully mobilized, the abdominal surgeon feeds the stomach into the posterior mediastinum, while the cervical surgeon gently pulls the esophagus. A no. 28 French tube inserted in the esophagus and secured with sutures may facilitate this maneuver. When the stomach assumes its final position, the pylorus is at the level of the xiphoid and the cardioesophageal junction is at the sternal notch (Fig. 3B). The cardioesophageal junction is transected and closed with staples or continuous suture. A two-layer pharyngogastric anastomosis is created in the dome of the fundus (Fig. 3C).

CLINICAL RESULTS

Reversed Gastric Tube

Anastomotic fistulas and strictures are the most common complications of reversed gastric tube esophagoplasty (3,15). Peptic ulceration has been reported after the procedure (16). The incidence of anastomotic failure possibly may be reduced with a technique that involves separate incision and suture of the seromuscular and mucosal layers (17). A major limitation in the usefulness of this procedure is that the operation is extensive and technically difficult. We found the procedure more useful for secondary reconstruction in patients who had previously undergone resection than as a one-stage procedure (1,13,18). In six patients in whom this technique was used, there was effective palliation in five, with one surgical mortality (13).

Esophagocoloplasty

The problems encountered with esophagocoloplasty are due to the relatively poor blood supply, the difficulty of mobilizing a sufficiently long segment of colon, and the magnitude of the procedure. Necrosis of the colon and anastomotic leakage or dehiscence with resulting infection are the most common complications. A distinct disadvantage of esophagocolostomy, in comparison with other procedures, is the number of anastomoses (esophagocolostomy, gastrocolostomy, colocolostomy, and pyloroplasty) that must be performed, thus increasing operating time, as well as the risk of anastomotic failure at each site. In three colon interpositions for reconstruction after pharyngolaryngectomy (13), there was one surgical mortality. In another series of 14 colon interpositions (19), 10 patients were able to swallow.

Gastric Transposition

The limiting factor for gastric transposition is upward extension of the tumor. While the gastric fundus easily reaches the level of the hyoid bone, anastomosis attempted above this level may result in excessive tension on the suture line with resultant disruption. Creation of a gastric flap can increase the upward reach of the stomach, but such a procedure is technically complex and prone to complications. Thus we do not recommend gastric transposition for esophageal replacement if the level of resection extends above the hyoid bone.

Gastroduodenal ulcers, tumors, and previous gastric surgery may preclude the use of stomach for esophageal replacement. A major disadvantage is that the procedure is suitable only as a one-stage operation (20) and thus may be employed only in patients who are in suitably good condition.

Complications include tears in the posterior tracheal wall, pneumothorax, hemorrhage, pleural effusions, peritonitis, mediastinitis, fistulas, and delayed rupture of the great vessels. The transposed stomach will usually tamponade vessels and raw surfaces within the mediastinum. Because of the absence of a major intraabdominal anastomosis, peritonitis and mediastinitis occur less frequently than with other abdominal organ transpositions.

In the combined results in five series of patients (13) totaling 120 gastric transposition operations, there was an operative mortality of 12% and satisfactory results in 56%. Well-motivated patients can develop esophageal speech after the procedure (21). There are generally few problems with swallowing (11,21).

SUMMARY

The cervical esophagus can be reconstructed with various techniques using visceral interposition. These involve a reversed gastric tube, a left colon esophagocoloplasty, and a gastric pull-up procedure. The free jejunal transfer is discussed in Chapter 218.

References

1. Heimlich B. Reversed gastric tube esophagoplasty for failure of colon, jejunum and prosthetic interpositions. *Ann Surg* 1975;182:154.
2. Ong GB. The Kirschner operation: a forgotten procedure. *Br J Surg* 1973;60:221.
3. Postlethwait RW. Technique for isoperistaltic gastric tube for esophageal bypass. *Ann Surg* 1979;189:673.
4. Yamato T, Hamanaka Y, Hirata S, et al. Esophagoplasty with an autogenous tubed gastric flap. *Am J Surg* 1959;137:597.
5. Goligher JC, Robin IG. Use of left colon for reconstruction of the pharynx and esophagus after pharyngectomy. *Br J Surg* 1954;42:283.
6. Ong GB, Lee TC. Pharyngogastric anastomosis after oesophagopharyngectomy for carcinoma of the hypopharynx and cervical esophagus. *Br J Surg* 1960;48:193.
7. LeQuesne LP, Ranger D. Pharyngolaryngectomy with immediate pharyngogastric anastomosis. *Br J Surg* 1966;53:105.
8. Silver CE. Gastric pull-up operation for replacement of the cervical portion of the esophagus. *Surg Gynecol Obstet* 1976;142:243.
9. Stell PM. Esophageal replacement by transposed stomach. *Arch Otolaryngol* 1970;91:166.
10. Leonard JR, Maran AG. Reconstruction of the cervical esophagus via gastric anastomosis. *Laryngoscope* 1970;80:849.
11. Akiyama H, Hiyama M, Miyazono H. Total esophageal reconstruction after extraction of the esophagus. *Ann Surg* 1975;182:547.
12. Ventemiglia R, Khalil KG, Frazier OH, et al. The role of preoperative mesenteric arteriography in colon interposition. *J Thorac Cardiovasc Surg* 1977;74:98.
13. Silver CE. *Surgery for cancer of the larynx and related structures.* New York: Churchill-Livingstone, 1981.
14. Silver CE. The gastric transposition operation for replacement of cervical esophagus. In: Cohn LH, ed. *Cardiac/thoracic surgery*, Vol. 1, *Modern techniques in surgery.* Mt. Kisco, NY: Futura, 1981.
15. Ein SH, Shandling B, Simpson JS, et al. Fourteen years of gastric tubes. *J Pediatr Surg* 1978;13:638.
16. Gozner A, Stanciu D, Kirilla A, et al. Ulcer on the presternal tube after esophagoplasty of the greater curvature of the stomach. *Rev Chir* 1978;27:213.
17. Sugimachi K, Yaeta A, Ueo H, et al. A safer and more reliable operative technique for esophageal reconstruction using a gastric tube. *Am J Surg* 1980;140:471.
18. Silver CE. Reconstruction after pharyngolaryngectomy—esophagectomy. *Am J Surg* 1976;132:428.
19. DeSanto LW, Carpenter RJ. Reconstruction of the pharynx and upper esophagus after resection for cancer. *Head Neck Surg* 1980;2:369.
20. Silver CE. Surgical management of neoplasms of the larynx, hypopharynx and cervical esophagus. *Curr Probl Surg* 1977;14:1.
21. Harrison KFN. Rehabilitation problems after pharyngogastric anastomosis. *Arch Otolaryngol* 1978;104:244.

CHAPTER 218 ■ MICROVASCULAR FREE TRANSFER OF INTESTINE

R. S. STAHL AND M. J. JURKIEWICZ

The aggressiveness of pharyngoesophageal malignancies and strictures makes unencumbered wide resection and effective palliation essential goals in their treatment. It is applications such as these for which microvascular free transfers of intestine are well suited (1–16).

INDICATIONS

Because of poor survival rates of patients with pharyngoesophageal malignancies, the optimal reconstructive procedure would have one stage, a low complication rate, and a brief hospitalization and would allow an adequate resection of the neoplasm with an acceptable operative mortality. The need for obligate stoma formation should be eliminated. Not only should airway patency be preserved and deglutition be restored early, but these functions would hopefully be retained as long as possible with recurrent disease. Donor tissue should be from beyond the field of preoperative radiotherapy and relatively resistant to harm from postoperative irradiation. Reconstruction would be facilitated by mucosa-bearing tissue and as little violation of body cavities as possible.

Multiple other methods of pharyngoesophageal reconstruction exist, each having its own merits. Disadvantages of these techniques variably include the need for multiple stages and prolonged recuperation, limitations by extent of neck dissection or perioperative radiation, fistula formation, pharyngostomes, stricture formation, multiple gastrointestinal suture lines, violation of multiple body cavities, and the requirement of advanced or highly specialized surgical techniques.

FLAP DESIGN AND DIMENSIONS

While approximation of resection margins is usually possible in the hypopharynx and upper esophagus, excessive tension all too often results in stricture, fistula, or limitation of tongue mobility. Local mucosal flaps are often satisfactory for small or less than circumferential defects. Regional unipedicled cervical flaps (17) provide a logical, regional, albeit multistage, means of reconstruction. The Wookey flap (18) is also limited by the extent of previous neck dissection and radiation and requires the presence of a pharyngostome and an esophagostome.

The medially based deltopectoral flaps (19) employ tissue with a known arterial supply from beyond irradiated or dissected cervical tissue to restore upper aerodigestive continuity. This procedure also requires the interim use of stomata and typically requires two or more stages. Reversed split-thickness skin grafts supported by tantalum or steel mesh (20,21) have

been used, but they frequently result in stricture formation or mesh migration and erosion.

In the fortuitous event that the anterior upper half of the trachea and larynx is spared from tumor, this tissue may be used to reconstitute the anterior esophageal wall (22,23). It has been noted that split-thickness skin grafts may be used for recreation of the posterior pharyngeal wall if necessary. While providing a conservative means of reconstructing the hypopharynx in a single-stage procedure, this technique is limited by the restrictions it places on margins of resection, as well as postoperative stricture formation.

The pectoralis major musculocutaneous flap also has been used to fashion into a pharyngoesophagus (24). While using one procedure to bring healthy tissue into the neck, it may be rather bulky when tubed and it lacks mucosal lining and peristalsis.

The gastrointestinal tract is often employed as a donor for pedicled or free grafts. Gastric, small bowel, or colonic transpositions provide one-stage reconstruction. A long suture line (25) has been applied to a strip of vascularized reversed greater curvature to form a pedicled gastric tube for similar application. These technically challenging procedures develop a segment of bowel on a long pedicle and invade the abdominal or pleural cavity, mediastinum, or chest wall. There are multiple potential gastrointestinal, thoracic, or mediastinal complications that often relate to breakdown of suture lines. Pedicled techniques all too often lead to excessive tension on the superior suture line.

Free transfer of revascularized intestine allows for a standardized approach to difficult problems of upper aerodigestive reconstruction with little regard for size or configuration of the surgical defects. Extirpative procedures may extend from the base of the skull to the mediastinum, and reliable reconstruction is possible with viable mucosa-bearing tissue with relatively few contraindications. Extensive atherosclerosis and radiation injury are only relative contraindications, since extension of the vascular pedicle with vein grafts allows for selection of more suitable recipient vessels. The surgeon's lack of familiarity with microsurgical technique is the prime contraindication to performance of such a free transfer.

OPERATIVE TECHNIQUE

Donor Site

Once the extent of resection and the needs of the recipient site have become apparent, a second team may begin the search for an intestinal segment suitable for transfer. This is usually done through a left upper quadrant transverse incision. After locating the ligament of Treitz, the caliber and the vascular pedicle and arcade are inspected to select an acceptable segment of bowel, typically 10 to 14 cm in length. The requirements of the recipient site are usually met by a segment from the proximal jejunum.

Recipient Site

Once the segment is isolated on its pedicle, the bowel margins are divided and observed for satisfactory bleeding and, hence, viability. While the abdominal team is developing this segment on as long a pedicle as possible, the presumptive recipient vessels may be prepared for anastomosis if their caliber matches the donor vessels appropriately. Branches of the external carotid artery and tributaries of the external jugular vein usually have the most suitable caliber and location. The superior thyroid artery is often selected, since the inferior thyroid, cervical, and intrathoracic vessels often lie too low to receive the free intestinal transfer. Occasionally, contralateral vessels are chosen for anastomosis when preoperative radiotherapy has been administered ipsilaterally. If necessary, any larger vessel, including the carotid itself, may be employed for a side-to-end anastomosis with the donor vessel.

Once the recipient vessel in the neck is prepared and flow is confirmed, the intestine may be harvested. If the bowel needs to be elongated, division of the mesentery at the second level of arcades may help to some extent (26). As the mesenteric donor vessels are being microscopically prepared by one team, the abdomen is simultaneously closed following a bowel anastomosis. Consideration is also given to the performance of a gastrostomy.

The isolated segment is brought to the neck, preferably isoperistaltically, and a proximal anastomosis is performed to the pharyngeal margin. Thus, difficult proximal anastomotic sutures may be placed accurately and the free intestine suspended and secured from motion during the microsurgical portion of the procedure. The veins are anastomosed first. Once both anastomoses are complete, the clamps are released in the same order.

Obvious pulsation of mesenteric vessels, peristalsis, production of secretions, and vigorous bleeding from the non-anastomosed bowel margin should be evident. If discrepancies exist between the caliber of the recipient and donor tissues, antimesenteric incisions in the donor bowel will assist in a proper match.

Before completion of the distal anastomosis, a nasogastric tube may be threaded through the lumen of the neoesophagus. Inclusion of a small silicone window in the neck closure allows for direct observation of flap viability (Fig. 1E). Some forego this direct observation and perform regular postoperative endoscopy instead (27) (Fig. 2).

Although cooling of the isolated bowel prior to transfer has been advocated (28), bowel ischemia time has been reduced to 60 to 90 minutes in the Emory series by awaiting complete preparation of the recipient site and vessels as a prerequisite to transecting the mesenteric pedicle. Similarly, the two-team approach allows for completion of transfer within

1½ to 2 hours following excision. Low-molecular-weight dextran and steroids were administered in the Emory series, while heparinization is used in some centers (27). As a rule, oral liquids may be taken by the patient several days postoperatively. Care must be taken throughout the postoperative course to avoid flap constriction by tracheostomy tube tapes or dressings.

CLINICAL RESULTS

After this single-stage reconstruction, the average patient in the Emory series could swallow at 12 days postoperatively. Twenty-eight of 32 patients were hospitalized less than 21 days following their procedure. Consequently, there was no significant delay in initiating postoperative radiotherapy. Two of 25 patients who underwent this procedure following resection of tumor suffered non-tumor-related stricture formation; four patients developed dysphagia secondary to tumor recurrence. There was no incidence of stenosis following repair of seven preexisting strictures (29).

The intestinal segment used in most cases has been jejunum; however, advantages of colon as an autotransplant should not be overlooked. These include compatibility of the larger lumen with needs of nasopharyngeal construction, smaller amount of bowel secretions and regurgitation, and the larger vascular pedicle.

A gradual return of basal electrical activity has been documented in autotransplanted bowel both experimentally and clinically. Furthermore, the return of good swallowing ability, weight gain, and normal distal esophageal function, correlating with absence of reflux symptoms, have been documented in patients after jejunal transfer (26). Contraction of these grafts in response to either local or gastric antral distension is indicative of retention of intrinsic myoelectric activity, as well as some neurohumoral feedback mechanism (26).

By 1982, more than 100 cases of free intestinal transfer had been reported in the literature, with a cumulative mortality rate of 5.4%. Most of these deaths were from cardiorespiratory causes, as late as 5 weeks postoperatively. Twelve percent of patients suffered major complications, most related to necrosis or infection of the autograft. Half the major complications are now preventable with improvements in venous microanastomosis and vigilant pulmonary care to prevent aspiration pneumonia that arises from graft secretions in the early postoperative period. There was an 11% minor complication rate. These consisted primarily of transient fistulas and three patients who experienced occasional self-limiting dysphagia.

SUMMARY

Free vascularized bowel transfer in the hands of experienced microsurgeons has become a reliable, versatile, and rapid method of restoring pharyngeal or esophageal integrity with functional mucosa-bearing tissue. Although an abdominal procedure is necessary, the dissection is far from extensive, with addition of an intraabdominal anastomosis.

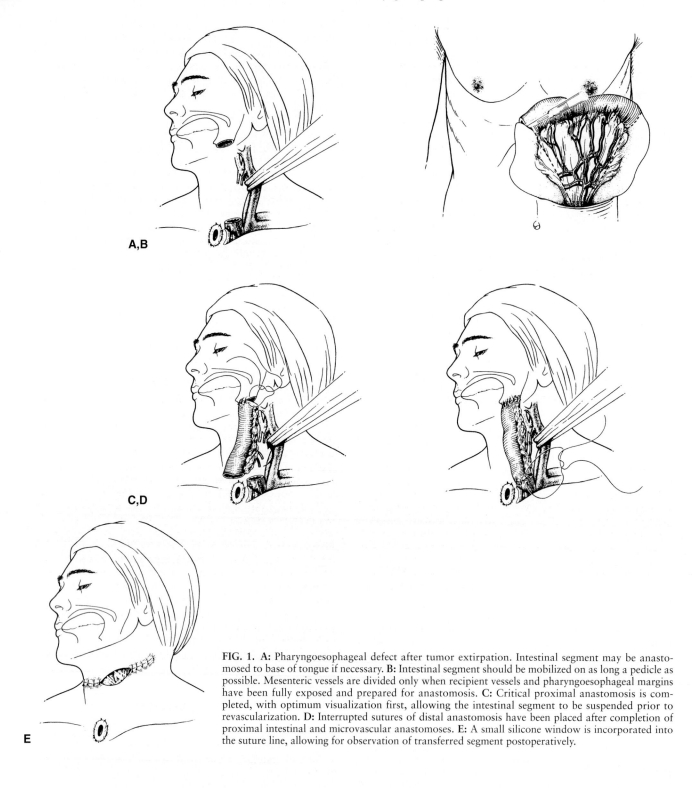

A,B

C,D

E

FIG. 1. A: Pharyngoesophageal defect after tumor extirpation. Intestinal segment may be anasto-mosed to base of tongue if necessary. **B:** Intestinal segment should be mobilized on as long a pedicle as possible. Mesenteric vessels are divided only when recipient vessels and pharyngoesophageal margins have been fully exposed and prepared for anastomosis. **C:** Critical proximal anastomosis is com-pleted, with optimum visualization first, allowing the intestinal segment to be suspended prior to revascularization. **D:** Interrupted sutures of distal anastomosis have been placed after completion of proximal intestinal and microvascular anastomoses. **E:** A small silicone window is incorporated into the suture line, allowing for observation of transferred segment postoperatively.

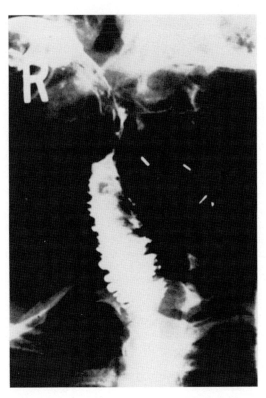

FIG. 2. A barium swallow should be obtained several days postoperatively prior to resumption of oral intake. (From McConnel et al., ref. 15, with permission.)

References

1. Longmire WP Jr. A modification of the Roux technique for antethoracic esophageal reconstruction: anastomosis of the mesenteric and internal mammary blood vessels. *Surgery* 1947;22:44.
2. Seidenberg B, Rosenak SS, Hurwitt ES, Som ML. Immediate reconstruction of the cervical esophagus by a revascularized isolated jejunal segment. *Ann Surg* 1959;149:162.
3. Hiebert AC, Cummings GO. Successful replacement of the cervical esophagus by transplantation and revascularization of a free graft of gastric antrum. *Ann Surg* 1961;154:103.
4. Roberts RE, Douglass FM. Replacement of the cervical esophagus and hypopharynx by a revascularized free jejunal autograft. *N Engl J Med* 1961;264:342.
5. Nakayama K, Yamamoto K, Tamiya T, et al. Experience with free autografts of the bowel with a new venous anastomosis apparatus. *Surgery* 1964;55:796.
6. Jurkiewicz MJ. Vascularized intestinal graft for reconstruction of the cervical esophagus and pharynx. *Plast Reconstr Surg* 1965;36:509.
7. Peters CR, McKee DM, Berry BE. Pharyngoesophageal reconstruction with revascularized jejunal transplants. *Am J Surg* 1971;121:675.
8. Mullens JE, Pezacki ZJ. Reconstruction of the cervical esophagus by revascularized autografts of intestine. *Int Surg* 1971;55:157.
9. Uemichi A, Invi K, Onchi K, et al. Reconstruction of the cervical esophagus by transplantation and revascularization of small intestinal segment: ten year follow-up. *Surgery* 1977;81:343.
10. McKee DM, Peters CR. Reconstruction of the hypopharynx and cervical esophagus with microvascular jejunal transplant. *Clin Plast Surg* 1978;5:305.
11. Chang TS, Hwang OL, Wang-Wei. Reconstruction of esophageal defects with microsurgically revascularized jejunal segments: a report of 13 cases. *J Microsurg* 1980;2:83.
12. Hester TR, McConnel FM, Nahai F, et al. Reconstruction of cervical esophagus, hypopharynx and oral cavity using free jejunal transfer. *Am J Surg* 1980;140:487.
13. Sasaki T, Baker HW, McConnell DB, Vetto RM. Free jejunal graft reconstruction after extensive head and neck surgery. *Am J Surg* 1980;139:650.
14. Oesch I, Helikson MA, Shermeta DW, et al. Esophageal reconstruction with free jejunal grafts: an experimental study. *J Pediatr Surg* 1980;15:433.
15. McConnel FMS, Hester TR, Nahai F, et al. Free jejunal grafts for reconstruction of pharynx and cervical esophagus. *Arch Otolaryngol* 1981;107:476.
16. Harashina T, Kakegawa T, Imai T, Suguro Y. Secondary reconstruction of oesophagus with free revascularized ileal transfer. *Br J Plast Surg* 1981;34:17.
17. Trotter W. Operative treatment of malignant disease of the mouth and pharynx. *Lancet* 1913;1:1075.
18. Wookey H. The surgical treatment of carcinoma of the pharynx and upper esophagus. *Surg Gynecol Obstet* 1942;75:499.
19. Bakamjian VY. A two-stage method for pharyngoesophageal reconstruction of the cervical esophagus and pharynx. *Plast Reconstr Surg* 1965;36:509.
20. Negus VE. Reconstruction of pharynx after pharyngoesophagolaryngectomy. *Br J Plast Surg* 1953;6:99.
21. Edgerton MT. One-stage reconstruction of the cervical esophagus or trachea. *Surgery* 1952;31:23.
22. Asherson N. Pharyngectomy for post-cricoid carcinoma: one-stage operation with reconstruction of the pharynx using the larynx as an autograft. *J Laryngol* 1954;68:550.
23. Som ML. Laryngoesophagectomy: primary closure with laryngotracheal autograft. *Arch Otolaryngol* 1956;63:474.
24. Withers EH, Franklin JD, Madden JJ, Lynch JB. Immediate reconstruction of the pharynx and cervical esophagus with the pectoralis major myocutaneous flap following laryngopharyngectomy. *Plast Reconstr Surg* 1981;68:898.
25. Heimlich HJ. Reconstruction of the esophagus with a reversed gastric tube. *Surg Gynecol Obstet* 1962;114:673.
26. Meyers WC, Seigler HF, Hanks JB, et al. Postoperative function of free jejunal transplants for replacement of the cervical esophagus. *Ann Surg* 1980;192:439.
27. Ancona E. Gastrointestinal microsurgery: colonic and jejunal autotransplants for cervical esophagoplasty. *Int Surg* 1981;66:39.
28. Flynn MB, Acland RD. Free intestinal autografts for reconstruction following pharyngolaryngoesophagectomy. *Surg Gynecol Obstet* 1979;149:858.
29. Hester TR. Personal communication, 1982.

CHAPTER 219 ■ JEJUNAL FREE FLAP

J. J. COLEMAN III

The jejunal free flap or jejunal free autograft is a reliable, frequently used method of transferring a segment of bowel to replace an area lined with mucosa. Because of the length of the small bowel, its constant blood supply, and its more favorable bacterial content, the jejunum has been more popular than segments of the colon or stomach. The size of the jejunal branches of the mesenteric vessels allows revascularization at the site of reconstruction with microscope or loupe magnification.

INDICATIONS

Although usually used to reconstruct circumferential defects of the laryngopharynx, this flap is also useful in reconstruction of partial pharyngeal defects, oral cavity, and vagina. The defect created by extirpation of malignancy in the upper aerodigestive tract is characterized by heavy bacterial contamination, possible previous radiotherapy, and complex functional significance. Because late-stage disease requiring such surgery has a high likelihood of early recurrence, single-stage restoration of function and reasonably normal appearance are crucial.

The predominant functions of the upper aerodigestive tract are alimentation and respiration; more specialized actions include swallowing and speech. Although the precise recreation of speech has been elusive, swallowing is facilitated by providing a patent conduit between the oral cavity and the remaining esophagus. Jejunum is of a similar caliber and structure to the cervical esophagus and pharynx and is thus useful for replacement of total laryngopharyngectomy defects from the nasopharynx at the base of the skull to the thoracic inlet, or occasionally to the aortic arch. It is most useful when the larynx has been removed because its copious secretions may result in aspiration with the larynx in place.

Using the jejunum as a tube-fillet combination, the total or partial glossectomy/laryngectomy defect can be reconstructed with a single segment of bowel (Fig. 1). Partial defects of the hypopharynx, oropharynx, and oral cavity are also amenable to reconstruction using a patch of jejunum, again best suited in the absence of the larynx. The length of the mesentery of the jejunum and the need for midline position of the bowel require recipient vessels in the neck. If previous radical neck dissection or vascular disease result in deficient vessels, a flap with a longer pedicle, such as the gastroepiploic flap or the radial forearm flap, may be necessary to reach branches of the axillary artery. The presence of ascites is a contraindication to this procedure.

Although the jejunum is expendable and useful as both a circumferential and patch repair, other methods are also available (1). When the larynx remains intact, the jejunum should not be used unless the segment is at or below the cricopharyngeus. For patch-type defects or when the larynx is intact, the lateral arm, radial forearm, scapula, and lateral thigh flaps all provide epithelial lining to replace pharyngeal mucosa, with minimal to moderate donor-site morbidity. Circumferential

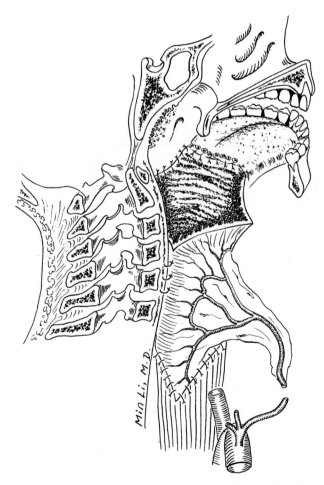

FIG. 1. By splitting the jejunum along its antimesenteric border, a combination tube-fillet configuration can be obtained that will allow reconstruction of defects that have both circumferential and planar components. The pliability of the planar area allows it to conform to the shape of the buccoalveolar mucosa pharyngeal wall or the floor of mouth area.

tion in 2 hours or less. Because the ideal location for the bowel conduit is in the midline (the anatomic site of the pharynx and cervical esophagus), and because there is an obligate length of mesentery necessary before anastomosis can be done, vessels situated in the lateral neck are best for recipients.

OPERATIVE TECHNIQUE

The transverse cervical vessels can be found just lateral to the jugular vein deep to the omohyoid in the medial posterior triangle; these are ideal for anastomosis low in the neck. The facial and occipital branches of the external carotid, which lie just beneath the digastric muscle on the lateral neck and external jugular vein, may be dissected out and placed laterally in the superior neck (Fig. 3). Anastomosis to the main internal jugular or the proximal medial branches of the external carotid requires bowing of the jejunum off the midline or folding of the mesentery. The former impairs subsequent transit of food through the conduit, and the latter increases the risk of venous thrombosis. Whatever vessels are chosen should be completely prepared for micosurgical anastomosis before division of the jejunal vessels.

A supraumbilical midline incision is used to enter the abdomen. After identifying the ligament of Treitz, the jejunum is mobilized to a point that will easily allow the tube jejunostomy to be affixed to the abdominal wall after harvest of the segment of jejunum. Once this general area has been identified, the mesentery is examined (using transillumination, if helpful) to identify a jejunal branch of the mesenteric vessels and follow its arborization distally and to provide a segment of jejunum adequate to cover the defect. Usually, a slightly longer segment is identified and trimmed back later in the

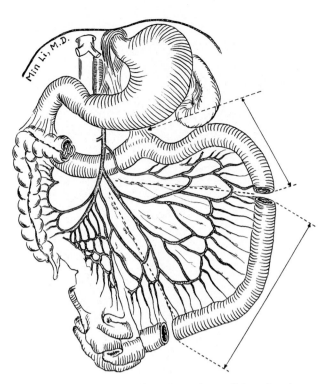

FIG. 2. The pattern of blood supply to the small intestine changes from proximal to distal. In the jejunum, there is usually only one arcade before the vasa recta directly supplying the mesenteric border of the bowel. In the ileum, there are multiple arcades between the main ileal branch and the vasa recta, making determination of the segment of bowel perfused by a single branch more difficult.

defects can be closed with the larger skin flaps of the radial forearm and scapula.

ANATOMY

The jejunum is the second portion of the small intestine, beginning at the ligament of Treitz and extending approximately 8 feet distally. The blood supply includes the jejunal branches of the superior mesenteric artery and vein that pass through the mesentery and arborize to supply the gut. In the proximal mesentery, there is usually only one arcade of vessels distal to the segmental artery and vein, with the vasa recta extending directly off the arcade. This makes the relationship between the branch of the superior mesenteric artery and the segment of gut it supplies more direct than in the ileum, where there are two or three arcades of vessels between the superior mesenteric artery and vein and the vasa recta to the bowel (Fig. 2). When harvested, the diameter of the jejunal vessels from the superior mesenteric artery and vein range from 2 to 4 mm.

FLAP DESIGN AND DIMENSIONS

To some degree, the segment of jejunum available on a single pedicle depends on body habitus and the length of the mesentery. The selection of an appropriate branch and its subsequent blood supply can result in lengths of bowel from 10 to 30 cm. The mesentery of the small bowel varies with body habitus but generally ranges in length from 15 to 20 cm.

Selection of appropriate vessels in the neck before harvesting the jejunal free autograft is of paramount importance. The ischemia tolerance of jejunum is low, requiring revasculariza-

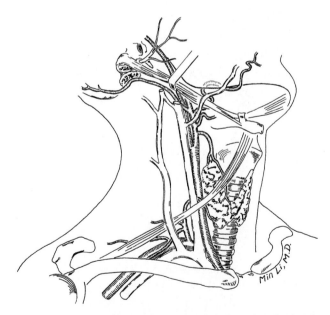

FIG. 3. The omohyoid and digastric muscles are excellent landmarks for vessel selection in the neck. Beneath the omohyoid in the posterior triangle lie the transverse cervical vessels, which usually arise from the thyrocervical trunk of the subclavian artery. These vessels are frequently present even after neck dissection and may even be enlarged as collateral blood supply to the neck. Division of the branches to the scalene muscles and levator scapulae provide an excellent vascular pedicle. Dissection along the posterior belly of the digastric muscle reveals the occipital and facial branches of the external carotid artery, which can be transposed either medially or laterally for vascular anastomosis. The external jugular vein is a satisfactory recipient vessel and should be preserved whenever possible in the initial exposure of the neck.

neck. The proximal and distal ends of this segment are marked to orient the bowel in an isoperistaltic direction.

The mesentery is incised in a triangle, the apex of which is at the origin of the jejunal branch of the superior mesenteric vessels, and the mesentery and vessel branches are divided and ligated, taking care to observe their branching and to avoid injuring vessels that supply the segment. The bowel is divided at its proximal and distal ends with a GIA stapler. At this point, the ends of the divided bowel are observed for several minutes to ensure adequate vascular supply at the sites of future anastomosis. If the bowel is dusky at this point, this indicates injury to its blood supply and requires resection back to viable vascularized tissue (Fig. 4). An end-to-end or end-to-side jejunojejunostomy is performed between the proximal and distal segments and the mesentery repair, leaving the separated segment supplied by its own blood vessels.

Distal to the jejunojejunostomy, a Witzel tube jejunostomy is placed, brought through the abdominal wall, and the serosa around the tube fixed to the peritoneum (Fig. 5). With bowel continuity reestablished, the abdomen is irrigated, and the segment of bowel is left in situ until it is ready to be harvested for the reconstruction. Before removing the segment, careful dissection of the base of the mesentery is important to provide maximal pedicle length and to avoid injury to the pedicle or to the superior mesenteric vessels. Meticulous cleaning of fat and lymphatic tissue and individual ligation of the artery and vein decrease the ischemia time for the segment in the neck and

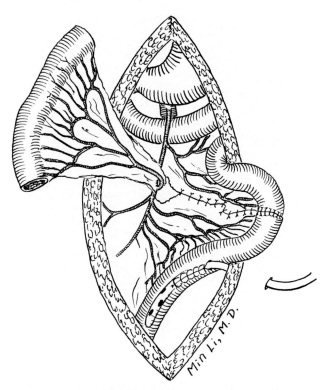

FIG. 5. Reanastomosis of the bowel is performed and the mesentery approximated. A tube jejunostomy is placed distal to the enteric anastomosis, and the bowel is affixed to the parietal peritoneum and abdominal wall. The segment of bowel to be used for reconstruction can be left in situ until the time for revascularization in the neck. Careful dissection of fat and lymphatic tissue off the base of the mesentery will allow the best exposure for ligation and division of the jejunal vessels.

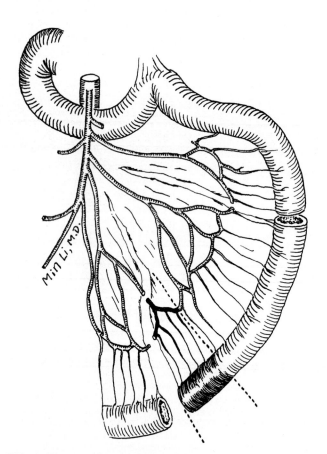

FIG. 4. Transection and ligation of the mesentery may result in ischemia to the bowel to be harvested or to the proximal and distal bowel. Because the intraenteric collateral blood supply is limited to about 2 cm, it is important to observe the ends of the segments carefully before performing reanastomosis or harvest of the segment. Any ischemic-appearing bowel should be resected by ligating directly along the mesenteric border.

minimize the chance of intraabdominal bleeding. As soon as the segment is transferred to the reconstructive team in the neck, the abdominal wall is closed.

Of utmost importance in successful reconstruction and avoidance of fistula, is visualization of the pharyngoenteric anastomosis site, so that precise suturing can be performed. Most often, the proximal anastomosis is more difficult to visualize, particularly when the tumor has extended cephalad into the nasopharynx. Mandibulotomy or other adjunct procedures may be necessary to afford adequate visualization; it should be performed before division of the jejunal vascular branches in the abdomen.

When the jejunum has been situated in a comfortable position in the neck, the most difficult bowel anastomosis is performed using 3–0 absorbable suture in two layers, when possible incorporating seromuscular and musculomucosal sutures. Sometimes single-layer full-thickness sutures are preferable. The most difficult areas to visualize are the lateral aspects of a high circumferential suture line. Placement of several seromuscular sutures from the bowel wall to the prevertebral fascia (Fig. 6) will help suspend the segment and avoid traction on the sutures of the proximal anastomosis.

The mesentery is tacked to the neck to keep it from folding on turning of the neck, and microvascular anastomosis is performed. As previously stated, it is imperative that the recipient vessels lie in a position in which they will not kink, the mesentery will not kink, and the bowel segment can remain in the midline. At this point, if there is some question that the ischemia time may exceed 2 hours, the arterial anastomosis should be performed first. Revascularization of the segment produces vigorous contraction of the bowel and mucorrhea.

Careful reassessment then should be made of the length of bowel necessary to close the defect. The segment should be straight and under slight tension when both visceral anastomoses have been completed, as there is a tendency for elongation of the segment over time, and thus interference with passage of the food bolus. Excess bowel should be removed right along the mesenteric border to avoid damage to the blood supply in the more proximal mesentery. Excess mesentery can be used to reinforce the suture line or to help close a neck wound where skin has been resected. Because stricture may occur at the distal anastomotic line, triangular interdigitation of the jejunum into the esophagus is useful. In cases where the lesion is low and the resection may extend into the thoracic esophagus, the distal enteric anastomosis should be performed first, because it is likely to be the most difficult. The jejunal esophageal anastomosis is performed in two layers, taking care not to narrow the lumen.

Occasionally, there is a size mismatch between the proximal jejunum and the proximal oropharyngeal defect. A wider anastomosis can be obtained by creating an end-to-side anastomosis. The jejunum is opened along its antimesenteric border to the appropriate length and then sutured to the base of the tongue and pharynx (Fig. 7).

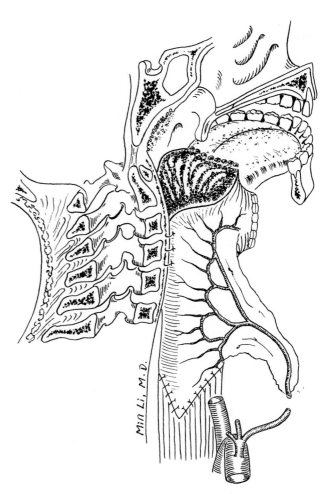

FIG. 7. A wider pharyngojejunal anastomosis is sometimes necessary when the defect includes the base of the tongue. With the proximal bowel oversewn, enterotomy along the antimesenteric border can provide an opening of variable length for end-to-side anastomosis.

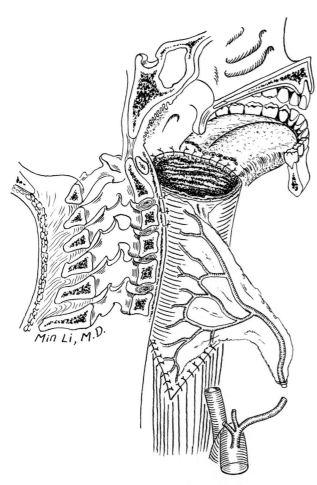

FIG. 6. As much of the pharyngoenteric anastomosis as possible should be done in two layers. Spatulation of the esophagus will help prevent stenosis at the distal suture line. Fixation of the segment to the rigid prevertebral fascia will help relieve tension on the proximal anastomosis and perhaps decrease fistula formation. Any excess length of jejunum should be trimmed so that the conduit is straight between the pharynx and the esophagus.

All positioning of the bowel segment and vessels, both donor and recipient, should be done with recognition that the neck at the time of microvascular anastomosis is frequently hyperextended and turned to its most lateral extent. The vascular anastomosis must be situated well in all positions—neutral, flexion, and contralateral rotation—to avoid vascular compromise.

There are numerous methods of monitoring the vascular integrity of the jejunal free autograft. We prefer the combination of Doppler ultrasound and direct observation. A short segment of the skin suture line is left open over the serosa of the bowel and packed with xeroform gauze; it can be visualized for monitoring and for direct Doppler ultrasound evaluation (Fig. 8). In addition to this, a line is marked on the skin over the site of the anastomosis and along the course of the mesenteric vessels. Hourly Doppler ultrasound checks are performed. After several days, the xeroform gauze is removed, and the defect is closed secondarily or allowed to contract.

CLINICAL RESULTS

Measurement of success in pharyngeal reconstruction evaluates the restoration of ability to provide nourishment adequate to maintain weight perorally. Several large series have shown an 80% to 83% success rate in meeting this goal, using the jejunum as reconstruction for pharyngeal defects

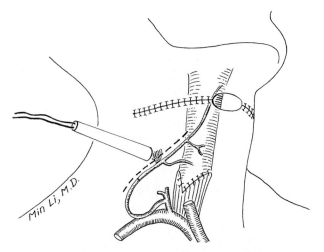

FIG. 8. Monitoring may be performed by a combination of direct observation of the serosa through a small opening in the suture line and Doppler ultrasound. Marking the skin over the jejunal vessel path to the bowel will help localize the vessel itself and avoid confusion with the carotid and its branches.

(2,3). Viability of the jejunal graft was achieved in 95% to 97% of patients (2,3). Several smaller series have corroborated these results. Jejunum transfer thus has been demonstrated to be a reliable method for pharyngeal reconstruction. Complications have been frequent in the neck, but more than 50% of cases resolve without surgical intervention (4). Despite the comorbidities carried by many of the patients, abdominal and pulmonary complications have been low and mortality in the range of 3% to 5% compared with 10% to 25% for gastric pull-up (5).

Voice restoration, another desirable reconstructive goal, can be achieved by immediate or delayed tracheoesophageal puncture through the jejunal segment. The unpredictable contraction of the jejunum may impede the flow of air from the stomach to the mouth, however, and a more flaccid radial forearm free flap may provide superior voice reconstruction (6).

SUMMARY

The jejunal free autograft is an effective, reliable method of reconstructing total or partial pharyngeal defects. Defects of variable length and shape may be addressed with high likelihood of graft viability and functional restoration.

References

1. Coleman JJ. Reconstruction of the pharynx and cervical esophagus. *Surg Rounds* 1991;14:855.
2. Coleman JJ, Searles JM, Hester TR, et al. Ten years experience with the free jejunal autograft. *Am J Surg* 1987;154:394.
3. Reece GP, Schusterman MA, Miller MJ, et al. Morbidity and functional outcome of free jejunal transfer reconstruction for circumferential defects of the pharynx and cervical esophagus. *Plast Reconstr Surg* 1995;96:1307.
4. Coleman JJ, Tan KC, Searles JM, et al. Jejunal free autograft: analysis of complications and their resolution. *Plast Reconstr Surg* 1989;84:589.
5. Surkin ME, Lawson W, Biller H. Analysis of the methods of pharyngoesophageal reconstruction. *Head Neck Surg* 1984;6:953.
6. Anthony JP, Singer MI, Mathes SJ. Pharyngoesophageal reconstruction using the tubed radial forearm flap. *Clin Plast Surg* 1994;21:137.

CHAPTER 220 ■ MICROVASCULAR FREE TRANSFER OF A COMPOUND FLAP OF STOMACH AND OMENTUM

J. BAUDET, B. PANCONI, AND L. VIDAL

Despite the theoretical advantages of musculocutaneous flaps, many complications are still encountered. This is why another technical procedure is often necessary in special cases, namely, the free transfer of greater omentum and stomach (1,2).

INDICATIONS

The merit of this procedure is to allow a one-stage reconstruction that closes large pharyngoesophageal defects with particularly well vascularized tissue. Despite some difficulties, it is a safe and reliable procedure. Anastomoses are located away from the recipient site in the axillary area where vessels run deep, and the donor site has not been irradiated and is usually free of major atherosclerotic processes. Also, the reconstruction is functional. Obviously, the procedure should not replace well-known simpler methods (local skin flaps, distant cutaneous or musculocutaneous flaps) that are recommended whenever possible. Furthermore, free flaps

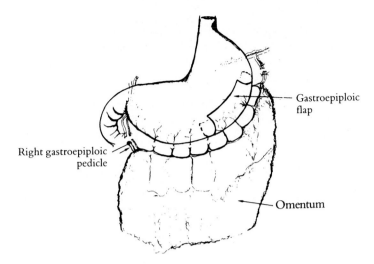

FIG. 1. Schematic diagram of the compound free transfer of omentum and stomach based on the right gastroepiploic pedicle.

to the oral cavity, even with moderately irradiated tissues and vessels (3), have their own indications, as do free transfers of gastrointestinal tissue of other types, such as jejunum (4–7) (see Chapter 218), sigmoid (8–12), and gastric antrum (13).

The compound stomach–omentum flap should be selectively used with the following indications: for closure of inveterate pharyngostoma in heavily irradiated tissue, most likely after several unsuccessful previous attempts at closure by other methods; for closure of long-standing partial or subtotal defects of the cervical esophagus under unfavorable local conditions; and for primary reconstruction of large defects of the pharyngeal wall.

The portion of stomach included in the transfer has an excellent blood supply and provides an especially good solution for reconstruction of any partial and subtotal defect of pharyngeal or esophageal wall. The greater omentum, thanks to its own rich blood supply, also is known for its properties of defense against infection, its ability to participate in biologic debridement, its potential for adapting its shape to any anatomic contour, and its ability to granulate, thus offering an excellent bed for skin grafting. Apart from general contraindications, such as diabetes, severe atherosclerosis, malnutrition, and anemia, this procedure is also not feasible in patients who have had past gastric surgery such as gastrectomy or gastrostomy.

ANATOMY

The greater curvature of the stomach receives its blood supply from short vessels emerging from the right and left gastroepiploic vessels. The right gastroepiploic pedicle is predominant from both anatomic and dynamic viewpoints (14). This pedicle is constant, and the artery and vein have large diameters. The most appropriate part of the greater curvature of the stomach to be included in continuity with the omentum must be located as distally as possible from the origin of the right gastroepiploic pedicle in order to obtain the longest pedicle (Fig. 1). Finally, the whole greater omentum, depending on the vascular territory of the right gastroepiploic pedicle, must be freed and included in the transfer.

FLAP DESIGN AND DIMENSIONS

The considerable length of the pedicle (about 30 cm) allows vascular anastomoses to be located at a suitable distance from the cervical area, where postoperative or postradiotherapeutic sclerosis precludes reasonable chances for another type of transfer (Fig. 2). These anastomoses are located in the axillary area. The dimensions of the largest flap available are about 13 cm long and 8 cm wide.

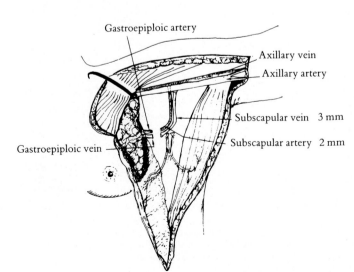

FIG. 2. Schematic diagram of the axillary area showing anastomoses of the right gastroepiploic pedicle with the subscapular pedicle.

OPERATIVE TECHNIQUE

Donor Site

The right gastroepiploic artery and vein are identified and exposed through a median abdominal incision located above the umbilicus. The greater omentum is then progressively freed from the transverse colon and mesocolon and subsequently, from right to left, from the stomach through a complete ligation of the short gastric vessels. The stomach is clamped level with the great curvature, and the gastric flap is excised in continuity with the greater omentum, preserving the short gastric vessels that supply the flap at this level. Bleeding from the gastric wall is then checked, and the right gastroepiploic pedicle is severed. The transfer is immersed in a chilled heparinized serum (15,000 U intravenously per 100 cc) and any remaining blood is squeezed out by gentle finger manipulation.

The stomach is finally closed over a suction nasogastric tube in two layers with deep interrupted extramucosal stitches and running superficial sutures. Removal of this gastric flap produces narrowing of the lumen in the midsection of the stomach that is reduced to 2.5 cm in diameter but without functional consequences (2,15).

Recipient Site

The axillary artery and vein are identified, and further dissection provides adequate exposure of the origin and course of the subscapular artery and vein.

Revascularization of the transfer is carried out by end-to-end anastomoses of the right gastroepiploic artery (2.5 mm) to the subscapular artery and the right gastroepiploic vein to the subscapular vein (3 mm) (see Fig. 2). After release of the arterial clamp, the quality of the revascularization of the gastric wall section is observed, as well as pulsation of the gastroepiploic vessels.

The skin of the left anterior chest wall is then widely undermined from the axilla to the neck. The long transfer then is

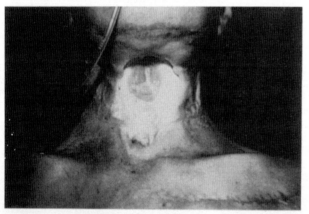
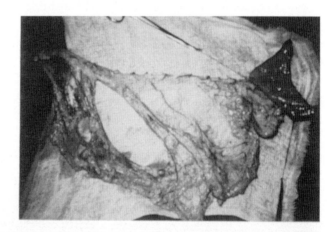

A,B

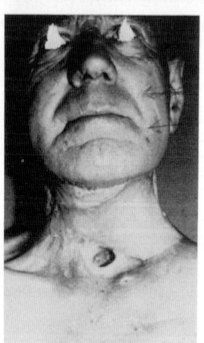
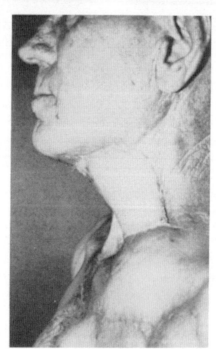
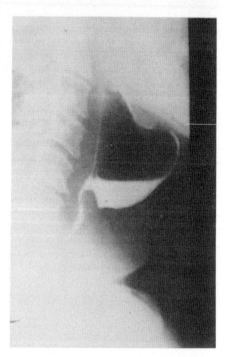

C–E

FIG. 3. **A:** Wide inveterate pharyngostoma after removal of carcinoma of the piriform sinus, bilateral radical neck dissection, and radiation therapy. An attempt at closure by a deltopectoral flap had failed. **B:** Appearance of the compound transfer. **C,D:** Good cosmetic result. Oral feeding resumed at the third postoperative week. **E:** Restoration of a spacious gullet shown at barium swallow.

brought through this spacious tunnel to the recipient site, adequately prepared by a large excision of pharyngeal or esophageal wall and any necrotic, infected, or scarred tissue (Fig. 3). The anterior pharyngeal and/or esophageal wall is then reconstructed by suturing of the gastric flap using one layer of full-thickness 3–0 absorbable interrupted sutures, and this is covered by several layers of folded over omentum extending laterally past the suture line of the gastric flap to obtain a thick padding and efficient packing of any early postoperative fistula.

A pharyngoesophageal tube is inserted for permanent suction of saliva. The omentum is left to granulate for about 10 days and then is skin-grafted. As soon as bowel function is restored, feeding by nasogastric tube is resumed. This tube usually is removed at the end of the second week, and oral alimentation by liquid and semisolid food is started (2,15).

CLINICAL RESULTS

The free transfer of omentum and stomach restores a roomy pharyngeal gullet and functional cervical tract, as proved by barium studies and cineradiography, with evidence of satisfactory contractions and transit time (Fig. 3E). Endoscopy demonstrates almost normal-appearing gastric mucosa but with the presence of some degree of edema and inflammation; this is confirmed by biopsy. Finally, pH measurement using calorimetric methods shows a persistent biochemical property with a pH value of 5. There has been no sign of peptic ulcer in the esophageal mucosa.

SUMMARY

Free transfer of a compound stomach and omentum flap is responsible for significant progress in one of the most challenging areas of reconstructive surgery.

References

1. Baudet J. Reconstruction of the pharyngeal wall by free transfer of the greater omentum and stomach. *Int J Microsurg* 1979;1:53.
2. Baudet J, Guimberteau JC, Laisne D, et al. La révascularisation par microchirurgie d'un transfert mixte gastro-épiploïque: technique et indications. Presented at the Société Chirurgie Bordeaux et SudOuest, April 20, 1978.
3. Ohtsuka H, Kamiishi H, Saito H, et al. Successful free-flap transfers with diseased recipient vessels. *Br J Plast Surg* 1976;29:5.
4. Germain M, Gremillet C, Patricio J. Replacement of the esophagus by a jejunal loop revascularized by vascular microanastomoses. *Int J Microsurg* 1979;1:60.
5. Germain M, Gremillet C, Morales-Chavez, et al. Replacement of the cervical esophagus and pharynx by transplantation and microsurgical revascularization of a free digestive graft. *Int J Microsurg* 1980;2:23.
6. Katsaros J, Tan E. Free bowel transfer for pharyngoesophageal reconstruction: an experimental and clinical study. *Br J Plast Surg* 1982;35:268.
7. Robinson DW, MacLeod A. Microvascular free jejunum transfer. *Br J Plast Surg* 1982;35:358.
8. Nakayama K, Tamiya T, Yamamoto K, Akimoto S. A simple new apparatus for small-vessel anastomosis (free autograft of sigmoid included). *Surgery* 1962;52:918.
9. Maillet P, et al. Cancer de l'oesophage cervical: rétablissement du transit par transplant sigmoïdien révascularisé. *Lyon Chir* 1965;61:420.
10. Ancona E, Cusumano A, Frasson P, et al. Notiva in campo di microchirurgia clinica: la sostituzione dell'esofago cervicale mediante auto trapiante di ans intestinale. *Terapia* 1976;61:203.
11. Baudet J, Traissac JL, Laisne D, et al. Reconstruction de l'oesophage cervical après pharyngo-laryngectomie circulaire par anse sigmoïde transplantée avec micro-suture vasculaire. *Rev Laryngol* 1977;98:481.
12. Baudet J, Guimberteau JC, Traissac JL, et al. La reconstruction du pharynx et de l'oesophage cervical par transfert libre d'intestin et d'estomac. *Chirurgie* 1978;504:873.
13. Hiebert CA, Cummings GO, Jr. Successful replacement of cervical esophagus by transplantation and revascularization of a free graft of gastric antrum. *Ann Surg* 1961;154:103.
14. Bourgeon A, Tran DD, Abbes M, et al. Etude de la revascularisation du grand épiploon: applications chirurgicales. *Bull Assoc Anat (Nancy)* 1973;57:59.
15. Papachristou D, Fortner JC. Experimental use of a gastric flap on an omental pedicle to close defects in the trachea, pharynx, or cervical esophagus. *Plast Reconstr Surg* 1977;59:382.

CHAPTER 221 ■ MICROVASCULAR TRANSFER OF THE DORSALIS PEDIS SKIN FLAP FOR HYPOPHARYNGEAL RECONSTRUCTION

R. M. ZUKER AND R. T. MANKTELOW

The dorsalis pedis skin flap can be used for lining in most areas of the head and neck, but it is particularly useful for areas of difficult access (1–4). The pharyngoesophageal area is often difficult to reconstruct with conventional pedicle flaps, but it poses no problem when a free flap is used (5–7).

INDICATIONS

The dorsalis pedis skin flap is useful in the smaller hypopharyngeal defects, particularly when a tube is not needed because the defect is not circumferential. The flap is especially useful when the more commonly used flaps, such as the pectoralis major or deltopectoral, have already been used. This flap provides ease of access, thin pliable tissue for mucosal resurfacing, a long pedicle, and a remote site (nonradiated tissue).

ANATOMY

See Chapter 518 (8,9).

FLAP DESIGN AND DIMENSIONS

The procedure should be planned in reverse, even though the extent of the defect is not precisely known. One should know,

however, whether a portion of the anterior or posterior wall can be preserved. The more likely side of available recipient vessels is chosen, and then the more appropriate foot is selected. (For example, with a hypopharyngeal defect with a residual posterior wall and vessels likely on the right, select the left foot.)

The flap can extend distally to the interdigital web spaces (10). Its proximal extent is to the distal portion of the extensor retinaculum. Its lateral boundaries are 1 cm medial to the extensor hallucis longis tendon and 1 cm lateral to the extensor digiti quinti tendon (Fig. 1B).

OPERATIVE TECHNIQUE

The procedure is carried out in three stages. The recipient site is prepared following resection of the lesion, and a suitable

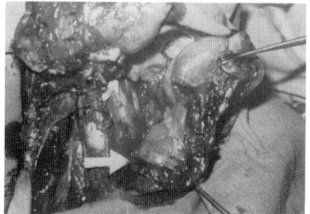
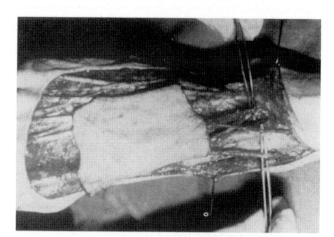

A,B

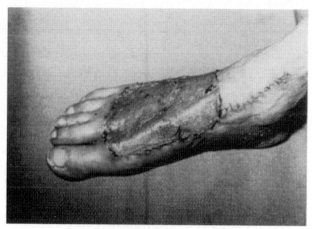
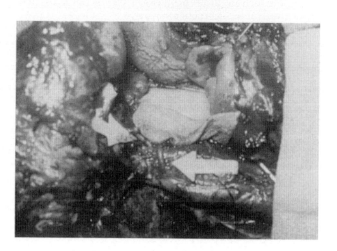

C,D

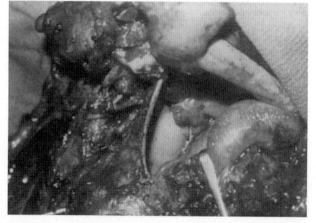

E

FIG. 1. **A:** Recipient-site preparation. *Arrow* denotes extent of hypopharyngeal defect (posterior wall). **B:** Dorsalis pedis flap isolated on vascular pedicle. **C:** Healed donor site. **D:** Flap tacked in place and revascularized. **E:** Flap sutured in position, closing hypopharyngeal defect.

artery and vein are found (Fig. 1A). We have used virtually all vessels in the head and neck and, for the hypopharynx, have found the transverse cervical and inferior thyroid most useful. Meticulous hemostasis is mandatory.

Donor Site

The dissection begins at the web space between the first and second toes. Here the first dorsal metatarsal artery is identified as it lies in the interosseous musculature, usually at a superficial level. The vessel is doubly ligated and divided. The flap then is carefully elevated from distal to proximal below the level of the first dorsal metatarsal artery, including it in the flap. The flap must be elevated above the paratenon of all extensor tendons and must leave a suitable bed for split-thickness skin grafting.

As the dissection proceeds more proximally, the extensor hallucis brevis tendon is encountered. Because this structure passes between the first dorsal metatarsal artery and the skin, it must be maintained in the flap. It is divided, and the dissection proceeds beneath it. Also, on the medial side of the flap, care is taken to maintain the continuity of the long saphenous vein and the flap. Toward the base of the second metatarsal, a critical point in the dissection is reached. Here the first dorsal metatarsal artery originates from the dorsalis pedis artery as it passes over the second cuneiform bone and plunges down to the plantar arch. It is imperative to maintain communication between the dorsalis pedis artery and the first dorsal metatarsal artery.

The perforating vessel is doubly ligated and divided deep to the takeoff of the first dorsal metatarsal artery. Flap elevation then proceeds proximally, maintaining the dorsalis pedis artery in the flap. The venae comitantes of this vessel are preserved, along with the long saphenous vein. At the termination of flap elevation, the decision will be made as to which vein will be used.

Proceeding further proximally, the superficial peroneal nerve is encountered when the proximal skin incision is made. (This flap does have the potential for innervation.) After the proximal skin incision is made, the extensor retinaculum is divided to facilitate the dissection of the dorsalis pedis vessels and, more proximally, the anterior tibial vessels. At this point, the flap is isolated on the long saphenous vein and the anterior tibial artery and its venae comitantes (Fig. 1B). A long pedicle can be dissected out for this flap, but in our experience, this has not been necessary for the hypopharyngeal region. The flap is then completely divided from the foot.

Donor-site closure must be carried out with extreme care. Any rents in the paratenon are carefully closed with absorbable sutures. A vascularized bed must be present for grafting. We prefer to use a medium-thickness split-thickness graft, which is gently held in place with a tie-over bolus dressing. The ankle is maintained in neutral position with a posterior slab. This dressing is not changed for 10 days, and strict bed rest with foot elevation is maintained. If a longer flap is necessary, such that the interdigital web space is transgressed, then hyperkeratosis may ensue. This is a difficult problem,

and it is best to restrict the flap to the area just proximal to the interdigital web spaces (Fig. 1C).

Recipient Site

The site of the recipient vessels will determine in which direction the flap is situated, since the pedicle will go toward the recipient vessels. The flap is loosely tacked in place, and vessel length is adjusted. Usually, the long saphenous vein is used. This has a relatively thick wall compared to the veins of the head and neck. The venous anastomosis is done first, and then the arterial anastomosis is done (Fig. 1D). The flap is then sutured definitively into place with a watertight closure of interrupted mattress sutures (Fig. 1E). The neck flaps that were used for access to the hypopharyngeal region are then returned to their original position.

CLINICAL RESULTS

Donor-site healing problems will occur if vascularized paratenon is not preserved. Also, this flap is difficult to elevate.

SUMMARY

The dorsalis pedis skin flap can be used for smaller noncircumferential mucosal defects in the hypopharynx, particularly when the conventional pedicle flaps about the head and neck have been previously exhausted. Access is not a problem, and thin pliable tissue is provided; however, this is a difficult flap to elevate, and unless care is taken, donor-site healing problems can occur.

References

1. Gilbert A. Composite tissue transfers from the foot: anatomic basis and surgical technique. In: Daniller AI, Strauch B, eds. *Symposium on microsurgery.* St. Louis: Mosby, 1976;230.
2. Morrison WA, O'Brien BM, MacLeod AM. The foot as a donor site in reconstructive microsurgery. *World J Surg* 1979;3:43.
3. Robinson DW. Dorsalis pedis flap. In: Serafin D, Buncke HJ, eds. *Microsurgical composite tissue transplantation,* Part II, Section 1. St. Louis: Mosby, 1979;257–284.
4. Ben-Hur N. Reconstruction of the floor of the mouth by a free dorsalis pedis flap with microvascular anastomosis. *J Maxillofac Surg* 1980;8:73.
5. Zuker RM, Manktelow RT, Palmer JA, Rosen IB. Head and neck reconstruction following resection of carcinoma using microvascular free flaps. *Surgery* 1980;88:461.
6. Zuker RM, Rosen IB, Palmer J, et al. Microvascular free flaps in head and neck reconstruction. *Can J Surg* 1980;23:157.
7. Zuker RM, Manktelow RT. The dorsalis pedis flap: technique of elevation, foot closure, and flap application. *Plast Reconstr Surg* 1986;77:93.
8. McCraw JB, Furlow LT. The dorsalis pedis arterialized flap. *Plast Reconstr Surg* 1975;55:177.
9. Ohtsuka H. Angiographic analysis of the first metatarsal artery. *Ann Plast Surg* 1981;7:2.
10. May JW, Chait LA, Cohen BE, O'Brien BM. Free neurovascular flap from the first web of the foot in hand reconstruction. *J Hand Surg* 1977;2:387.

CHAPTER 222 ■ RADIAL FOREARM CUTANEOUS FLAP FOR HYPOPHARYNGEAL RECONSTRUCTION

J. B. BOYD

The radial forearm flap (1) is extremely versatile because of its thin, supple nature; its ease of elevation; its large vessels and long pedicle; and its capacity to be sensate (2–4). To these advantages must be added the possibility of simultaneous dissection in two-team head and neck surgery and the ease of tubing the flap for pharyngeal reconstruction (5,6). The donor defect is cosmetic rather than functional, but the patient must endure 2 weeks of immobilization to allow the skin graft to take.

INDICATIONS

The radial forearm flap may be used as a patch for noncircumferential defects, or it may be tubed when a complete section of the hypopharynx has been removed. A patch is indicated when at least one third of the circumference remains following resection of the tumor. If less than a third remains, the remanent may just as well be discarded, for its only contribution would be to impose a second longitudinal suture line on the repair (7).

Many would argue that the radial forearm flap is second choice to free jejunum for circumferential pharyngeal and hypopharyngeal defects. The jejunum, being tubular, requires only superior and inferior enteric anastomoses; the radial forearm flap has a longitudinal seam as well. The potential for leakage and fistula development is correspondingly greater. It should be noted that swallowing is often quite slow with a jejunal graft, even though peristalsis is orthodromic (8). The tubed radial flap, although only a passive conduit, seems to offer less delay. Furthermore, there are circumstances in which the radial forearm flap might be preferred over enteric substitutes. For example, multiple previous abdominal surgeries or active Crohn disease would make the necessary laparotomy excessively risky.

When a patch repair is required, however, the jejunum has no advantages over the forearm. In fact, the long pedicle of this flap, its capacity for reinnervation, and its more accessible donor site give it the edge. When the larynx is still present, reinnervation may help prevent aspiration (2). Patch repair is indicated following a pharyngectomy or pharyngolaryngec-

tomy when there is insufficient pharyngeal wall for a tension-free closure. The closure of such defects without a patch may lead to dehiscence and a pharyngocutaneous fistula. Such fistulas, when large, are themselves another indication for patch repair using a radial forearm flap. In this case, there is a requirement for a two-layer closure. The radial forearm flap can bear two skin paddles, but it is probably more effective to use a single paddle for the inner layer and to cover the repair with pectoralis muscle (Fig. 1), which has the ability to overlap, adhere to, and seal the anastomotic suture line (7).

ANATOMY

The skin of the anterior forearm receives a significant blood supply from the radial artery via perforating septocutaneous vessels passing to the skin along the vascular septum between the brachioradialis and the flexor carpi radialis muscles (Fig. 2). These perforators are plentiful in the distal third of the forearm; proximally, where tendons give way to muscle bellies, they become sparser. Nevertheless, it is probably safe to raise a septum-based skin flap anywhere along the course of the radial artery. In this way, two skin islands may be raised, one proximal and one distal, thereby facilitating two-layer closure of a large pharyngeal fistula.

After emerging from the septum, the vessels branch laterally and medially, piercing the deep fascia and quickly passing to the subdermal plexus to supply the skin. Contrary to previous teaching, these vessels do not travel on the surface of the deep fascia for any significant distance. As a result, little of the deep fascia needs to be harvested with the flap.

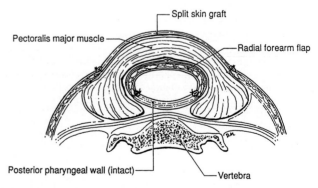

FIG. 1. Diagram showing how pectoralis muscle overlaps the mucosal anastomosis in the radial forearm flap and fills the dead space laterally. This is believed to contribute to the reliability of the repair.

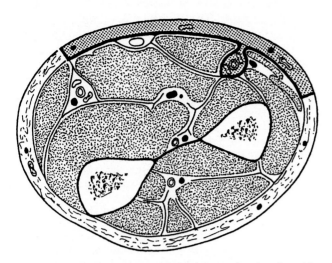

FIG. 2. Diagrammatic section of distal forearm showing disposition of radial artery in respect to vascular septum, brachioradialis, and flexor carpi radialis. The skin paddle extends over the dorsoradial aspect of the wrist to encompass the cephalic vein. This improves vessel access in the neck but is admittedly detrimental to the cosmetic result at the wrist.

Practically the whole anterior forearm skin can be safely taken. Limits extend from the antecubital fossa to the transverse wrist crease, and from the ulnar border of the forearm to the posterolateral aspect of the radial border. Raising a flap of such dimensions would require preservation of the entire vascular septum. The "base" of any radial forearm skin flap is that portion in direct contact with the vascular septum. Like any flap, if the base is small, the surviving length is accordingly reduced. Length-to-width ratios of 2 or more should be avoided.

The brachial artery bifurcates into radial and ulnar arteries a few centimeters distal to the antecubital fossa. The radial artery passes distally along the radial side of the pronator teres, initially lying between the biceps tendon and the bicipital aponeurosis. It crosses anterior to the pronator teres just proximal to that muscle's insertion into its tubercle on the lateral surface of the radius. On entering the distal third of the forearm, it first overlies the flexor pollicis longus and finally the pronator quadratus. Septocutaneous branches from the radial artery pass along the vascular septum between the brachioradialis and flexor carpi radialis muscles to supply the skin (see Fig. 2).

The radial artery is accompanied by two venae comitantes. These vessels are constant but of variable diameter. Often, they are inconveniently small for microvascular anastomosis. In the region of the bifurcation of the brachial artery, there is a confluence of veins. Here, the venae comitantes of both ulnar and radial arteries communicate with each other as well as with one or more of the large subcutaneous veins of the forearm.

Classically, there are three major subcutaneous veins in the anterior forearm: the cephalic, the median, and the basilic. In the distal forearm, the cephalic vein lies on the dorsoradial, and the basilic on the dorsosulnar aspect of the wrist. They pass around their respective borders at the midforearm level and then proceed proximally on the radial and ulnar sides of the anterior forearm. The median vein lies in the midline of the anterior forearm. Just distal to the antecubital fossa, it bifurcates into two: the median cephalic and the median basilic; the former angles radially to join the cephalic, the latter ulnarly to join the basilic. The cephalic and basilic veins then pass up the arm on either side of the biceps muscle, although there are significant variations on this basic pattern. Perforating veins connect the superficial veins to the deep sys-

tem at various points. Of most interest here is the communication at the level of the brachial artery bifurcation. This communication may be single or multiple and from any of the superficial veins (commonly, the median).

Both the venae comitantes and the large subcutaneous veins of the forearm are capable of draining the flap alone. The superficial veins are often preferred because of their greater diameter and their independence from the arterial pedicle. Care should be taken to ensure that the superficial veins have not previously been canalized and not undergone partial or complete thrombosis.

The median antebrachial cutaneous nerve (C8,T1) enters the forearm in the company of the basilic vein. It soon gives off a number of large anterior branches that pass down the radial side of the basilic vein and supply the ulnar half of the anterior forearm as far as the wrist. An ulnar branch supplies the ulnar border of the forearm. The lateral antebrachial cutaneous nerve (C5,C6) is the forearm continuation of the musculocutaneous nerve. It enters the forearm on the ulnar side of the cephalic vein and via multiple branches supplies the radial half of the forearm as far as the wrist as well as the dorsoradial aspect of the forearm.

FLAP DESIGN AND DIMENSIONS

The skin flap usually is positioned over the anterior or anterolateral aspect of the distal wrist. Here the subcutaneous tissue is thinnest and the pedicle length maximized. It is advantageous to position the flap anterolaterally in such a way that part of it overlies the cephalic vein (see Figs. 1 and 3). This vessel then can be used for venous drainage. In hirsute patients, the flap may be positioned purely on the anterior aspect of the distal wrist where the skin is less hairy. Unfortunately, the median vein is often quite small at the distal wrist. Furthermore, it is a favorite target for the frustrated phlebotomist. If an innervated flap is required, it should be noted that the watershed between the neurosomes of the lateral and medial antebrachial cutaneous nerves lies down the midline of the anterior forearm. It follows that flaps positioned over the cephalic vein and extending to the midline need only the lateral antebrachial cutaneous nerve for full reinnervation. Those positioned centrally, and straddling two neurosomes, require both superficial nerves (4).

The flap may be of almost any dimension so long as a significant portion of it overlies the vascular septum. For tubular pharyngeal reconstruction, a quadrangular flap is required (see Fig. 3). To produce a 3-cm tube, the flap must be 9.4 cm long ($\pi \times 3$). Its width is governed by the length of the pharyngeal gap. By making the flap trapezoidal in shape, allowance may be made for the discrepancy in diameter between the narrow esophagus and the wider base of the tongue. On the other hand, making it a perfect rectangle retains flexibility in the final orientation. The dimensions of patch reconstructions are determined by the size and shape of the defect.

OPERATIVE TECHNIQUE

A preoperative Allen's test should always be done, but its meaning is open to question. Only in a severe arteriopathy would grafting of the radial artery be necessary. In many cases, the flap was elevated in the presence of an unfavorable Allen's test, with no adverse sequelae. One possible cause for an ischemic hand after this surgery is the inadvertent ligation or division of a superficial ulnar artery, which can lie in the superficial tissues along the medial border of the flap. With the tourniquet up, this may take the appearance of a large

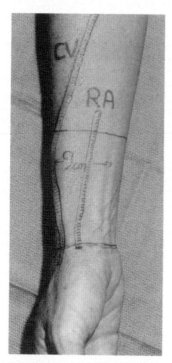

FIG. 3. Preoperative markings for a tubular reconstruction, approximately 3 cm in diameter.

vein. Such a vessel is at most risk with skin paddles that intrude onto the ulnar border of the wrist.

A tourniquet is placed around the upper arm. The arm is incompletely exsanguinated using an Esmarch or an Ace bandage before dissection commences. Totally empty vessels are difficult to identify.

The skin flap is incised around its periphery, and dissection is carried down to the underlying muscle fascia. Care is taken at the proximal margin of the flap to identify and preserve the cephalic vein or any other superficial veins that may be recruited for venous drainage. A whole network of veins may be selected. An incision is made from the proximal edge of the flap incision straight up the forearm toward the antecubital fossa. Dissection is carried through the subcutaneous tissue and the selected venous system traced proximally. If an innervated flap is desired, all the subcutaneous nerves entering the flap should be preserved in a sheath of fascia. They tend to lie just superficial to the deep fascia; however, they are extremely delicate and somewhat difficult to locate at this level. Precise identification of the nerves is best made in the proximal forearm, where they are large and located next to the cephalic and basilic veins. These nerves and their relevant branches then can be traced distally into the proximal margin of the flap.

The ulnar side of the flap then is elevated at a level just superficial to the deep fascia, working toward the intermuscular septum between the brachioradialis and the flexor carpi radialis (see Fig. 1). About 1 cm on the ulnar side of this septum, the deep fascia is incised and dissection then proceeds under it. Preservation of the deep fascia in this way facilitates skin grafting of the donor site. Dissection proceeds over the surface of the flexor carpi radialis tendon, leaving paratenon behind. It then extends around the radial edge of the tendon into the space beneath. Usually, the radial artery and its venae comitantes are now visible. This step completes dissection on the ulnar side.

The radial dissection is similar to that on the ulnar side. It passes immediately superficial to the deep fascia until a point is reached 1 cm lateral to the intermuscular septum, where the deep fascia is divided; dissection then proceeds at this deeper level. The brachioradialis tendon is seen, and the dissection hugs this tendon in the same way as the ulnar dissection hugged that of the flexor carpi radialis. Paratenon is preserved.

The radial artery and its venae comitantes are easily identified at the distal margin of the flap. These are ligated and divided. The cephalic vein is ligated and divided distally, as are other small veins in this region.

It should be noted that the superficial branch of the radial nerve passes through the deep portion of the flap and is visible during the radial dissection. This nerve is not to be used for innervation purposes because it passes right through the flap and out the other side. Furthermore, its loss may give rise to a painful neuroma, as well as sensory loss, on the dorsum of the hand. The nerve can be easily dissected from the undersurface of the flap, and *it is virtually never necessary to sacrifice it.*

The proximal portion of the intermuscular septum between the brachioradialis and the flexor carpi radialis then is entered and communicated with the more distal dissection. The radial artery and its venae comitantes are immediately visible between these muscles. Proximal to the skin island, it is not necessary to maintain any skin perforators, septal or otherwise.

The vascular leash is dissected free of surrounding tissues and, together with its attached skin island, lifted clear of the forearm. This involves bipolar coagulation and the clipping or ligation of numerous small muscular branches. It can be stripped all the way up to the origin of the radial artery from the brachial artery just distal to the antecubital fossa. The superficial venous system communicates with the deep system of veins just distal to this point. This communication may even be preserved as part of a combined venous pedicle (9). Both cephalic vein and superficial nerves may be dissected into the upper arm to obtain greater length.

It is to be hoped that the dissection will take less than 2 hours of tourniquet time. The tourniquet is released and hemostasis is established by the usual means. Perfusion of the hand by the ulnar artery should be assessed at this stage. With proper preoperative assessment, there should be no surprises. Nevertheless, the surgeon should be prepared to graft the radial artery when faced with obvious arterial insufficiency. In practice, this is extremely rare. Perfusion of the flap also is assessed. To save ischemia time, the flap may be tubed in situ with a single mattress layer of 3–0 polyglycolic acid tied internally. When required, the vascular pedicles are divided between ligatures and the preformed neopharynx transferred to the head and neck region.

To facilitate wound closure, the palmaris longus tendon usually is removed and discarded. The proximal portion of the wound closes directly. Although the paratenons of the flexor carpi radialis and the brachioradialis have been preserved and would probably accept a skin graft, it is often better to bury the tendons among the fibers of the flexor digitorum superficialis muscle. Soft tissues are sutured over the exposed tendon using 4–0 chromic catgut. By whatever means, a flat, well-vascularized bed is produced to receive an unmeshed skin graft, held in place by a meticulous tie-over dressing. The graft remains unmeshed to maximize the bridging phenomenon, which may help avoid tendon exposure. The wrist, including the thumb, then is mobilized in a palmar splint that is generally not removed for 7 days. When it is removed, the graft is inspected. If the take is less than 100%, further splinting and dressings are required.

At the recipient site, the flap is anastomosed to the proximal and distal pharynx with a single layer of internally tied mattress sutures (3–0 polyglycolic acid). Patch reconstructions are sutured directly into the defect using a similar technique. Arterial microanastomosis is performed to one of the major branches of the external carotid artery if the defect is high and to the transverse cervical artery if it is low. The external jugular vein, if available, provides the most convenient venous drainage. Otherwise, alternate vessels may be selected (10). The radial forearm flap is one of the few in which the arterial and venous pedicles may access opposite sides of the neck simultaneously. In cases of pharyngeal fistula, where there is a requirement for a two-layer closure, it is advantageous to use a pectoralis major flap for the outer layer (see Figs. 1 and 4). The muscle may be overlapped around the suture line to seal off the anastomosis and minimize the risk of leakage. If the patient is thin, the skin paddle of the flap can be used for skin closure. If there is too much bulk, the muscle can simply be skin grafted. In cases where the larynx is still present, the lateral and medial antebrachial cutaneous nerves may be trimmed and anastomosed to the greater auricular nerve (2).

Postoperative monitoring may be done by transcutaneous Doppler readings taken from the radial artery, which lies on the outside of the neopharynx in the subcutaneous plane. Alternatively, a small "monitor flap," supplied by the radial vessels, may be brought out on the skin surface. Buried laser Doppler probes have also been used. Patients are mobilized after a few days and usually commence a progressive oral diet at 2 weeks (3 weeks, if irradiated).

CLINICAL RESULTS

Similar to most free flaps in the head and neck, the radial forearm flap enjoys a 95% success rate in terms of survival. Specific complications in pharyngeal reconstruction involve fistula and stricture formation. For tubular reconstructions, the fistula rate approaches 50% and is believed to be significantly higher than that associated with jejunal reconstruction (6). These fistulas, like those occurring with free jejunal grafts, tend to close spontaneously with conservative treatment. (Fistulas are thought to be much rarer with patch repairs, particularly when reinforced by vascularized muscle.)

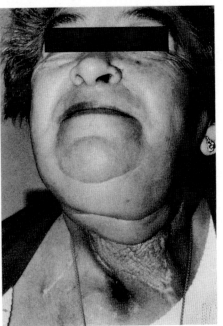

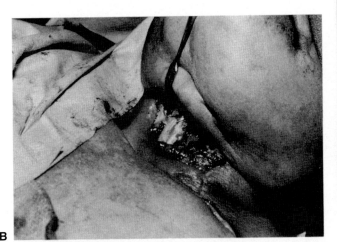

A,B

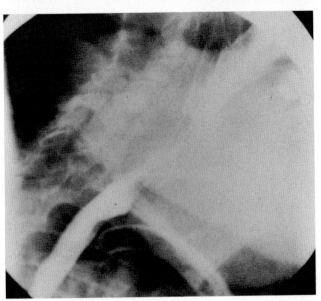

C

FIG. 4. A: Pharyngeal fistula following laryngopharyngectomy, with attempted primary repair of pharyngeal remnant. Two thirds of the circumference has been lost. B: Final results using radial forearm flap used as shown in Fig. 3. C: Barium swallow.

Swallowing may be superior with the radial forearm flap due to the absence of peristalsis; however, comparative trials have not been undertaken. Late strictures have been reported in 5% of tubular radial forearm flap reconstructions (6) and in fewer than 20% of jejunal cases (11). Most respond to endoscopic dilatation.

Tubular reconstructions usually leave a considerable cosmetic defect on the forearm because a large amount of skin is harvested. Functional problems are rare, however, and rehabilitation is more rapid than when abdominal surgery is involved.

Trachoesophageal puncture for the placement of a voice prosthesis may be performed 6 weeks after laryngopharyngeal reconstruction using a tubed radial forearm flap. The puncture is placed within 1 cm of the inferior suture line. Voice rehabilitation is reported to be excellent in those patients in whom there is residual tongue function (6).

SUMMARY

For patients undergoing pharyngolaryngectomy who require reconstruction of part or all of the pharyngeal circumference, the radial forearm flap may be used either as a patch or as a tube. The graft may be tailored to fit the defect, accommodating the discrepancy in diameters between the oropharynx and esophagus. Like the jejunum, the flap tolerates postoperative radiation extremely well, and it is favored in the presence of intraabdominal pathology and general debility.

References

1. Song R, Gao Y, Yu Y, et al. The forearm flap. *Clin Plast Surg* 1982;9:21.
2. Urken ML, Weinberg H, Vickery C, et al. The neurofasciocutaneous radial forearm flap in head and neck reconstruction: a preliminary report. *Laryngoscope* 1990;100:161.
3. Dubner S, Heller KS. Reinnervated radial forearm free flaps in head and neck reconstruction. *J Reconstr Microsurg* 1992;8:467.
4. Boyd B, Mulholland S, Gullane P, et al. Lateral antebrachial cutaneous neurosome flaps in oral reconstruction: Are we making sense? *Plast Reconstr Surg* 1994;93:1350.
5. Harii K, Ebihara S, One I, et al. Pharyngoesophageal reconstruction using a fabricated forearm free flap. *Plast Reconstr Surg* 1985;75:463.
6. Anthony JP, Singer MI, Mathes SJ. Pharyngoesophageal reconstruction using the tubed free radial forearm flap. *Clin Plast Surg* 1994;21:137.
7. Peat BG, Boyd JB, Gullane PJ. Massive pharyngo-cutaneous fistulae: salvage with two-layer flap closure. *Ann Plast Surg* 1992;29:153.
8. Meyers WC, Seigler HF, Hanks JB, et al. Postoperative function of "free" jejunal transplants for replacement of the cervical esophagus. *Ann Surg* 1980;192:439.
9. Gottlieb LJ, Tachmes L, Pielet RW. Improved venous drainage of the radial artery forearm flap: use of the profundus cubitalais vein. *Ann Plast Surg* 1993;9:281.
10. Mulholland S, Boyd JB, McCabe S, et al. Recipient vessels in head and neck microsurgery: radiation effect and vessel access. *Plast Reconstr Surg* 1993;92:628.
11. Reece GP, Bengston BP, Schusterman MA. Reconstruction of the pharynx and cervical esophagus. *Clin Plast Surg* 1994;21:125.

Page numbers followed by *f* indicate illustrations; *t* following a page number indicates tabular material.